Pediatric
ICD-10-CM 2021
A MANUAL FOR PROVIDER-BASED CODING

❖ 6th Edition ❖

American Academy of Pediatrics

Cindy Hughes, CPC, CFPC, Consulting Editor

Becky Dolan, MPH, CPC, CPEDC, Staff Editor

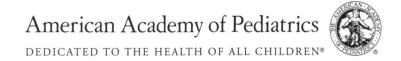

American Academy of Pediatrics

DEDICATED TO THE HEALTH OF ALL CHILDREN®

American Academy of Pediatrics Publishing Staff

Mary Lou White, *Chief Product and Services Officer/SVP, Membership, Marketing, and Publishing*

Mark Grimes, *Vice President, Publishing*

Mary Kelly, *Senior Editor, Professional/Clinical Publishing*

Laura Underhile, *Editor, Professional/Clinical Publishing*

Meghan Corey, *Editorial Assistant*

Jason Crase, *Senior Manager, Production and Editorial Services*

Leesa Levin-Doroba, *Production Manager, Practice Management*

Peg Mulcahy, *Manager, Art Direction and Production*

Mary Jo Reynolds, *Marketing Manager, Practice Publications*

Published by the American Academy of Pediatrics
345 Park Blvd
Itasca, IL 60143
Telephone: 630/626-6000
Facsimile: 847/434-8000
www.aap.org

The American Academy of Pediatrics is an organization of 67,000 primary care pediatricians, pediatric medical subspecialists, and pediatric surgical specialists dedicated to the health, safety, and well-being of all infants, children, adolescents, and young adults.

While every effort has been made to ensure the accuracy of this publication, the American Academy of Pediatrics (AAP) does not guarantee that it is accurate, complete, or without error.

Any websites, brand names, products, or manufacturers are mentioned for informational and identification purposes only and do not imply an endorsement by the American Academy of Pediatrics (AAP). The AAP is not responsible for the content of external resources. Information was current at the time of publication.

This publication has been developed by the American Academy of Pediatrics. The contributors are expert authorities in the field of pediatrics. No commercial involvement of any kind has been solicited or accepted in development of the content of this publication.

Please visit www.aap.org/coding for an up-to-date list of any applicable errata for this publication.

Special discounts are available for bulk purchases of this publication. Email Special Sales at nationalaccounts@aap.org for more information.

Printed in the United States of America.

11-114E

1 2 3 4 5 6 7 8 9 10

MA0989

ISBN: 978-1-61002-448-8
eBook: 978-1-61002-449-5
ISSN: 2475-9708

Disclaimer

Every effort has been made to include all pediatric-relevant *International Classification of Diseases, 10th Revision, Clinical Modification* (*ICD-10-CM*) codes and their respective guidelines. It is the responsibility of the reader to use this manual as a companion to the official *ICD-10-CM* publication. Do not report new or revised *ICD-10-CM* codes until their published implementation date, at time of publication set for October 1, 2020. Further, it is the reader's responsibility to access the American Academy of Pediatrics (AAP) Coding at the AAP website (www.aap.org/coding) routinely to find any corrections due to errata in the published version.

Contents

Tabular List

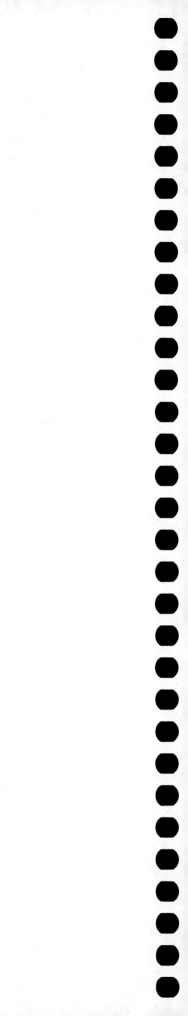

Foreword

The American Academy of Pediatrics (AAP) is pleased to publish this sixth edition of *Pediatric ICD-10-CM: A Manual for Provider-Based Coding,* a pediatric version of the *International Classification of Diseases, 10th Revision, Clinical Modification* (*ICD-10-CM*) manual. The AAP believes it is vital to publish an *ICD-10-CM* manual that is more manageable for pediatric providers. The expansive nature of the code set from *International Classification of Diseases, Ninth Revision, Clinical Modification* to *ICD-10-CM* overwhelmed many physicians, providers, and coders, so we condensed the code set by only providing pediatric-relevant diagnoses and their corresponding codes. However, as we move forward, we want members to have access to more codes and those that are less common in pediatrics but still need to be included. We reduced the guidelines so that only those applicable to the physician or provider are included, while those only relevant to facilities are removed. When needed, those codes can be located in the larger *ICD-10-CM* manual. Lastly, guidelines that exist for topic-specific chapters or specific codes can now be found in their respective tabular chapter or right where the specific code is listed. This will aid the user in identifying any chapter- or code-specific guidelines where they are needed most. This should assist in reducing any coding errors caused by reporting services that go against the guidelines that were once solely kept in the front of the manual, away from applicable codes. In addition, tips are included throughout to aid in your coding. These are unique to this manual.

The AAP is committed to the clinical modification of the *ICD* code set and, for the past several years, has sent an AAP liaison to the *ICD* Coordination and Maintenance Committee Meeting. We are especially grateful to Edward A. Liechty, MD, FAAP, and Jeffrey F. Linzer Sr, MD, FAAP, our appointed liaisons. The *ICD* Coordination and Maintenance Meeting is the semiannual meeting where all new *ICD* codes are presented, as well as revisions to the tabular list, index, and guidelines. Having dedicated expert liaisons aids in presenting pediatric and perinatal issues at the meeting. The AAP is also very pleased to continue its work with the *ICD* Editorial Advisory Board for *Coding Clinic for ICD-10-CM and ICD-10-PCS. Coding Clinic* is responsible for publishing *ICD* coding guidance and clarifications to supplement the *ICD-10-CM* manual. Dr Linzer sits on the Editorial Advisory Board, and Dr Liechty is our alternate. They sit on the board to represent pediatric issues, and both are experts on all *ICD-10-CM* matters.

The AAP will continue to support its members on issues regarding coding, and the AAP Health Care Financing Strategy staff at the AAP headquarters stands ready to assist with problem areas not adequately covered in this manual. The AAP Coding Hotline can be accessed at https://form.jotform.com/Subspecialty/aapcodinghotline.

Acknowledgments

Pediatric ICD-10-CM: A Manual for Provider-Based Coding is the product of the efforts of many dedicated individuals. First and foremost, we must thank Cindy Hughes, CPC, CFPC, consulting editor, for her professional input and particularly for her ongoing work to make this manual more user friendly.

We would also like to thank members of the American Academy of Pediatrics (AAP) Committee on Coding and Nomenclature, past and present, and the AAP Coding Publications Editorial Advisory Board. They support all coding efforts here at the AAP. These members contribute extensive time, reviewing and editing various coding content for the AAP.

We would also like to extend a very special thank-you to members of various subspecialty sections of the AAP who contributed their expertise and knowledge to the development of the original manual.

Lastly, we would like to acknowledge the tireless work of Jeffrey F. Linzer Sr, MD, FAAP, and Edward A. Liechty, MD, FAAP. Both Dr Liechty and Dr Linzer are advocates for pediatrics and neonatology and ensure that our issues are heard. They advocate for all pediatric patients in helping get codes established for conditions that need to be tracked for purposes of research and quality. They both keep the AAP and pediatric issues at the forefront of diagnostic coding, and we are very grateful for their time and expertise!

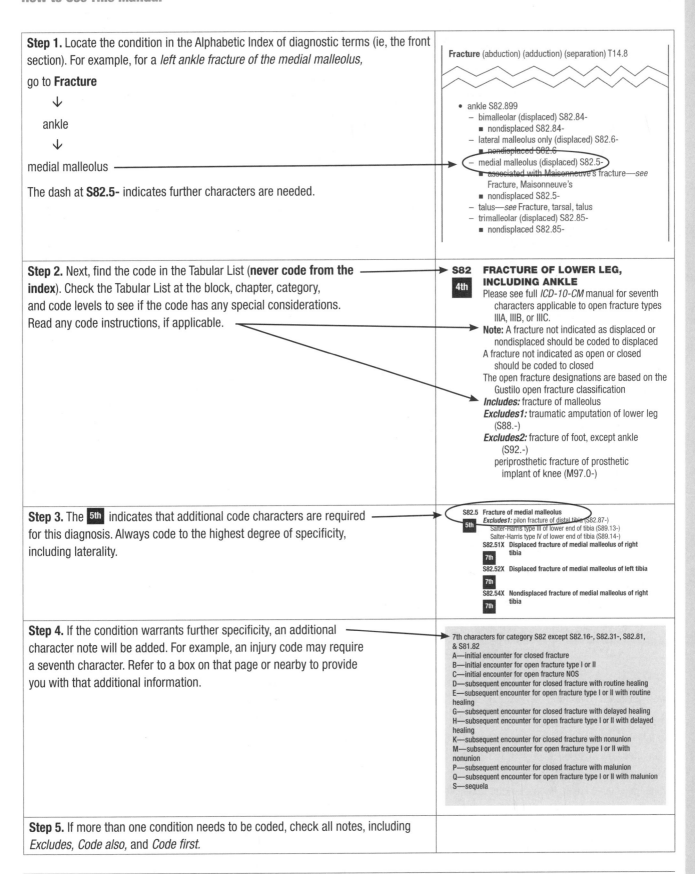

Step 1. Locate the condition in the Alphabetic Index of diagnostic terms (ie, the front section). For example, for a *left ankle fracture of the medial malleolus*,

go to **Fracture**

↓

ankle

↓

medial malleolus ——————————————

The dash at **S82.5-** indicates further characters are needed.

Fracture (abduction) (adduction) (separation) T14.8

- ankle S82.899
  - bimalleolar (displaced) S82.84-
    - nondisplaced S82.84-
  - lateral malleolus only (displaced) S82.6-
    - nondisplaced S82.6
  - medial malleolus (displaced) S82.5-
    - associated with Maisonneuve's fracture—*see* Fracture, Maisonneuve's
    - nondisplaced S82.5-
  - talus—*see* Fracture, tarsal, talus
  - trimalleolar (displaced) S82.85-
    - nondisplaced S82.85-

Step 2. Next, find the code in the Tabular List (**never code from the index**). Check the Tabular List at the block, chapter, category, and code levels to see if the code has any special considerations. Read any code instructions, if applicable.

S82 **FRACTURE OF LOWER LEG, INCLUDING ANKLE**

4th

Please see full *ICD-10-CM* manual for seventh characters applicable to open fracture types IIIA, IIIB, or IIIC.

Note: A fracture not indicated as displaced or nondisplaced should be coded to displaced

A fracture not indicated as open or closed should be coded to closed

The open fracture designations are based on the Gustilo open fracture classification

Includes: fracture of malleolus

Excludes1: traumatic amputation of lower leg (S88.-)

Excludes2: fracture of foot, except ankle (S92.-)

periprosthetic fracture of prosthetic implant of knee (M97.0-)

Step 3. The **5th** indicates that additional code characters are required for this diagnosis. Always code to the highest degree of specificity, including laterality.

S82.5 Fracture of medial malleolus

5th ***Excludes1:*** pilon fracture of distal tibia (S82.87-)

Salter-Harris type III of lower end of tibia (S89.13-)

Salter-Harris type IV of lower end of tibia (S89.14-)

S82.51X Displaced fracture of medial malleolus of right tibia

7th

S82.52X Displaced fracture of medial malleolus of left tibia

7th

S82.54X Nondisplaced fracture of medial malleolus of right tibia

7th

Step 4. If the condition warrants further specificity, an additional character note will be added. For example, an injury code may require a seventh character. Refer to a box on that page or nearby to provide you with that additional information.

7th characters for category S82 except S82.16-, S82.31-, & S82.81, & S81.82

A—initial encounter for closed fracture

B—initial encounter for open fracture type I or II

C—initial encounter for open fracture NOS

D—subsequent encounter for closed fracture with routine healing

E—subsequent encounter for open fracture type I or II with routine healing

G—subsequent encounter for closed fracture with delayed healing

H—subsequent encounter for open fracture type I or II with delayed healing

K—subsequent encounter for closed fracture with nonunion

M—subsequent encounter for open fracture type I or II with nonunion

P—subsequent encounter for closed fracture with malunion

Q—subsequent encounter for open fracture type I or II with malunion

S—sequela

Step 5. If more than one condition needs to be coded, check all notes, including *Excludes, Code also,* and *Code first.*

While attempting to stay true to the complete *International Classification of Diseases, 10th Revision, Clinical Modification* (*ICD-10-CM*) manual, *Pediatric ICD-10-CM: A Manual for Provider-Based Coding* is meant specifically for pediatrics and only includes those conditions more commonly seen in pediatrics. We have attempted to remove all adult-only conditions, as well as those conditions not typically found in the United States. Because *ICD* classification is used worldwide, many conditions listed in the official manual are not found in this part of the world.

Some codes are included under *Excludes* notes in the Tabular List for reference purposes only and to be consistent with the coding guidance. However, not every code included under *Excludes* will be found in the Tabular List if the condition is not specific to US pediatric health care. In addition, some codes that can be found in the Alphabetic Index might not also appear in the Tabular List. Again, these conditions are not commonly found in US pediatric health care, and the codes are included in the Alphabetic Index for reference purposes only. These conditions can be found in the larger Tabular List on the National Center for Health Statistics website (https://www.cdc.gov/nchs/icd/icd10cm.htm).

Guidelines

Guidelines relevant to all pediatric codes are still included. Note that some chapter-specific guidelines will appear at the beginning of the related chapter when they are overarching to most of that chapter. However, chapter-specific guidelines that are relevant only at specific category or code levels will be found at those category or code levels. The beginning of each chapter will reference the category(ies) or code(s) where the guidelines can be found. Guidelines that are **bold** have been revised or added for 2021. Guideline updates for the current year in the front matter and chapter-specific guidelines are printed in **bold.**

Abbreviations

We use our own abbreviations throughout that may not appear in *ICD-10-CM;* however, all abbreviations are defined on the inside front cover for easy access as you navigate through the manual.

Unspecified Laterality

While unspecified codes can still be found throughout and in certain instances will be the most appropriate code, we have removed nearly every code that uses unspecified laterality. We feel it is important that laterality is documented in nearly all conditions. You will see a footnote in those chapters where we have specifically left out laterality in nearly all conditions. If you need to report unspecified laterality for a condition and it is not listed in the chapter, refer to the full *ICD-10-CM* manual. Those codes will typically have a final character of 0 (zero) or 9.

Three-Character Codes

Three-character codes still exist in *ICD-10-CM.* Those will be noted specifically throughout the chapters as well.

E15   NONDIABETIC HYPOGLYCEMIC COMA
Includes: drug-induced insulin coma in nondiabetic
hyperinsulinism with hypoglycemic coma
hypoglycemic coma NOS

Abbreviated Code Descriptors

To help keep the size of the manual manageable, some codes are only written out fully at the category or subcategory level. The category or subcategory will be notated with a semicolon (;) and the code will begin with a lowercase letter. For example,

A37.0   Whooping cough due to Bordetella pertussis;
A37.00   without pneumonia
A37.01   with pneumonia

At the subcategory level (**A37.0**) you see the semicolon (;), and at the code levels (**A37.00** and **A37.01**), the codes begin with a lowercase letter. Therefore, code **A37.00** reads, "Whooping cough due to Bordetella pertussis without pneumonia."

Symbols

The following symbols are used throughout the text:
• Identifies new codes
▲ Identifies revised codes
▫ Identifies codes linked to social determinants of health

Reminder: New guidelines have been bolded.

The Centers for Medicare and Medicaid Services (CMS) and the National Center for Health Statistics (NCHS), two departments within the U.S. federal government's Department of Health and Human Services (DHHS), provide the following guidelines for coding and reporting by using the International Classification of Diseases, 10th Revision, Clinical Modification (*ICD-10-CM*). These guidelines should be used as a companion document to the official version of the *ICD-10-CM* as published on the NCHS website. The *ICD-10-CM* is a morbidity classification published by the United States for classifying diagnoses and reason for visits in all health care settings. The *ICD-10-CM* is based on the ICD-10, the statistical classification of disease published by the World Health Organization (WHO).

These guidelines have been approved by the four organizations that make up the Cooperating Parties for the *ICD-10-CM*: the American Hospital Association (AHA), the American Health Information Management Association (AHIMA), CMS, and NCHS.

These guidelines are a set of rules that have been developed to accompany and complement the official conventions and instructions provided within the *ICD-10-CM* itself. The instructions and conventions of the classification take precedence over guidelines. These guidelines are based on the coding and sequencing instructions in the Tabular List and Alphabetic Index of *ICD-10-CM*, but they provide additional instruction. Adherence to these guidelines when assigning *ICD-10-CM* diagnosis codes is required under the Health Insurance Portability and Accountability Act (HIPAA). The diagnosis codes (Tabular List and Alphabetic Index) have been adopted under HIPAA for all healthcare settings. A joint effort between the healthcare provider and the coder is essential to achieve complete and accurate documentation, code assignment, and reporting of diagnoses and procedures. These guidelines have been developed to assist both the healthcare provider and the coder in identifying those diagnoses that are to be reported. The importance of consistent, complete documentation in the medical record cannot be overemphasized. Without such documentation, accurate coding cannot be achieved. The entire record should be reviewed to determine the specific reason for the encounter and the conditions treated.

The term encounter is used for all settings, including hospital admissions. In the context of these guidelines, the term provider is used throughout the guidelines to mean physician or any qualified health care practitioner who is legally accountable for establishing the patient's diagnosis. Only this set of guidelines, approved by the Cooperating Parties, is official.

The guidelines are organized into sections. Section I includes the structure and conventions of the classification and general guidelines that apply to the entire classification and chapter-specific guidelines that correspond to the chapters as they are arranged in the classification. Section II includes guidelines for selection of principal diagnosis for non-outpatient settings. Section III includes guidelines for reporting additional diagnoses in non-outpatient settings. Section IV is for outpatient coding and reporting. It is necessary to review all sections of the guidelines to fully understand all the rules and instructions needed to code properly.

Note: Updates have been bolded.

Section I. Conventions, general coding guidelines, and chapter-specific guidelines

The conventions, general guidelines, and chapter-specific guidelines are applicable to all health care settings unless otherwise indicated. The conventions and instructions of the classification take precedence over guidelines.

A. Conventions for the *ICD-10-CM*

The conventions for the *ICD-10-CM* are the general rules for use of the classification independent of the guidelines. These conventions are incorporated within the Alphabetic Index and Tabular List of the *ICD-10-CM* as instructional notes.

1. The Alphabetic Index and Tabular List

The *ICD-10-CM* is divided into the Alphabetic Index, an alphabetical list of terms and their corresponding code, and the Tabular List, a structured list of codes divided into chapters based on body system or condition. The Alphabetic Index consists of the following parts: the Index of Diseases and Injury, the Index of External Causes of Injury, the Table of Neoplasms, and the Table of Drugs and Chemicals.

> *See Section I.C2. General guidelines*
> *See Section I.C.19. Adverse effects, poisoning, underdosing and toxic effects*

2. Format and Structure

The *ICD-10-CM* Tabular List contains categories, subcategories, and codes. Characters for categories, subcategories, and codes may be either a letter or a number. All categories are 3 characters. A three-character category that has no further subdivision is equivalent to a code. Subcategories are either 4 or 5 characters. Codes may be 3, 4, 5, 6, or 7 characters. That is, each level of subdivision after a category is a subcategory. The final level of subdivision is a code. Codes that have applicable 7th characters are still referred to as codes, not subcategories. A code that has an applicable 7th character is considered invalid without the 7th character.

The *ICD-10-CM* uses an indented format for ease in reference.

3. Use of codes for reporting purposes

For reporting purposes, only codes are permissible, not categories or subcategories, and any applicable 7th character is required.

4. Placeholder character

The *ICD-10-CM* utilizes a placeholder character "X." The "X" is used as a placeholder at certain codes to allow for future expansion. An example of this is at the poisoning, adverse effect, and underdosing codes, categories T36-T50. Where a placeholder exists, the X must be used in order for the code to be considered a valid code.

5. 7th Characters

Certain *ICD-10-CM* categories have applicable 7th characters. The applicable 7th character is required for all codes within the category, or as the notes in the Tabular List instruct. The 7th character must always be the 7th character in the data field. If a code that requires a 7th character is not 6 characters, a placeholder X must be used to fill in the empty characters.

6. Abbreviations

a. Alphabetic Index abbreviations

NEC "Not elsewhere classifiable"—This abbreviation in the Alphabetic Index represents "other specified." When a specific code is not available for a condition, the Alphabetic Index directs the coder to the "other specified" code in the Tabular List.

NOS "Not otherwise specified"—This abbreviation is the equivalent of unspecified.

b. Tabular List abbreviations

NEC "Not elsewhere classifiable"—This abbreviation in the Tabular List represents "other specified." When a specific code is not available for a condition, the Tabular List includes an NEC entry under a code to identify the code as the "other specified" code.

NOS "Not otherwise specified —This abbreviation is the equivalent of unspecified.

7. **Punctuation**

   [ ] Brackets are used in the Tabular List to enclose synonyms, alternative wording, or explanatory phrases. Brackets are used in the Alphabetic Index to identify manifestation codes.

   ( ) Parentheses are used in both the Alphabetic Index and Tabular List to enclose supplementary words that may be present or absent in the statement of a disease or procedure without affecting the code number to which it is assigned. The terms within the parentheses are referred to as *nonessential modifiers.* The nonessential modifiers in the Alphabetic Index to Diseases apply to subterms following a main term, except when a nonessential modifier and a subentry are mutually exclusive, in which case the subentry takes precedence. For example, in the *ICD-10-CM* Alphabetic Index under the main term *Enteritis,* "acute" is a nonessential modifier and "chronic" is a subentry. In this case, the nonessential modifier "acute" does not apply to the subentry "chronic."

   : Colons are used in the Tabular List after an incomplete term, which needs one or more of the modifiers following the colon to make it assignable to a given category.

8. **Use of "and"**

   Refer to Section I.A.14 (page XV). Use of the term "And"

9. **Other and Unspecified codes**

   a. "Other" codes

   Codes titled "other" or "other specified" are for use when the information in the medical record provides detail for which a specific code does not exist. Alphabetic Index entries with NEC in the line designate "other" codes in the Tabular List. These Alphabetic Index entries represent specific disease entities for which no specific code exists so the term is included within an "other" code.

   b. "Unspecified" codes

   Codes titled "unspecified" are for use when the information in the medical record is insufficient to assign a more specific code. For those categories for which an unspecified code is not provided, the "other specified" code may represent both other and unspecified.

   See Use of Sign/Symptom/Unspecified Codes, page XVIII

10. **Includes Notes**

    This note appears immediately under a three-character code title to further define, or give examples of, the content of the category.

11. **Inclusion terms**

    List of terms is included under some codes. These terms are the conditions for which that code is to be used. The terms may be synonyms of the code title, or, in the case of "other specified" codes, the terms are a list of the various conditions assigned to that code. The inclusion terms are not necessarily exhaustive. Additional terms found only in the Alphabetic Index may also be assigned to a code.

12. **Excludes Notes**

    The *ICD-10-CM* has two types of excludes notes. Each type of note has a different definition for use, but they are all similar in that they indicate that codes excluded from each other are independent of each other.

    a. Excludes1

    A type 1 Excludes note is a pure excludes note. It means "NOT CODED HERE!" An Excludes1 note indicates that the code excluded should never be used at the same time as the code above the Excludes1 note. An Excludes1 is used when two conditions cannot occur together, such as a congenital form versus an acquired form of the same condition.

    b. Excludes2

    A type 2 Excludes note represents "Not included here." An Excludes2 note indicates that the condition excluded is not part of the condition represented by the code, but a patient may have both conditions at the same time. When an Excludes2 note appears under a code, it is acceptable to use both the code and the excluded code together, when appropriate.

13. **Etiology/manifestation convention ("code first," "use additional code," and "in diseases classified elsewhere" notes)**

    Certain conditions have both an underlying etiology and multiple body system manifestations due to the underlying etiology. For such conditions, the *ICD-10-CM* has a coding convention that requires the underlying condition be sequenced first, followed by the manifestation. Wherever such a combination exists, there is a "use additional code" note at the etiology code and a "code first" note at the manifestation code. These instructional notes indicate the proper sequencing order of the codes, etiology followed by manifestation.

In most cases, the manifestation codes will have in the code title, "in diseases classified elsewhere." Codes with this title are a component of the etiology/manifestation convention. The code title indicates that it is a manifestation code. "In diseases classified elsewhere" codes are never permitted to be used as first-listed or principal diagnosis codes. They must be used in conjunction with an underlying condition code, and they must be listed following the underlying condition. See category F02, Dementia in other diseases classified elsewhere, for an example of this convention.

There are manifestation codes that do not have "in diseases classified elsewhere" in the title. For such codes, there is a "use additional code" note at the etiology code and a "code first" note at the manifestation code, and the rules for sequencing apply.

In addition to the notes in the Tabular List, these conditions also have a specific Alphabetic Index entry structure. In the Alphabetic Index, both conditions are listed together with the etiology code first, followed by the manifestation codes in brackets. The code in brackets is always to be sequenced second.

An example of the etiology/manifestation convention is dementia in Parkinson's disease. In the Alphabetic Index, code G20 is listed first, followed by code F02.80 or F02.81 in brackets. Code G20 represents the underlying etiology, Parkinson's disease, and must be sequenced first, whereas codes F02.80 and F02.81 represent the manifestation of dementia in diseases classified elsewhere, with or without behavioral disturbance.

"Code first" and "Use additional code" notes are also used as sequencing rules in the classification for certain codes that are not part of an etiology/manifestation combination.

See Section I.B.7. Multiple coding for a single condition.

14. **"And"**

The word "and" should be interpreted to mean either "and" or "or" when it appears in a title.

For example, cases of "tuberculosis of bones," "tuberculosis of joints," and "tuberculosis of bones and joints" are classified to subcategory A18.0, Tuberculosis of bones and joints.

15. **"With"**

The word "with" or "in" should be interpreted to mean "associated with" or "due to" when it appears in a code title, the Alphabetic Index (either under a main term or subterm), or an instructional note in the Tabular List. The classification presumes a causal relationship between the two conditions linked by these terms in the Alphabetic Index or Tabular List. These conditions should be coded as related even in the absence of provider documentation explicitly linking them, unless the documentation clearly states the conditions are unrelated or when another guideline exists that specifically requires a documented linkage between two conditions (e.g., sepsis guideline for "acute organ dysfunction that is not clearly associated with the sepsis"). For conditions not specifically linked by these relational terms in the classification or when a guideline requires that a linkage between two conditions be explicitly documented, provider documentation must link the conditions in order to code them as related.

The word "with" in the Alphabetic Index is sequenced immediately following the main term or subterm, not in alphabetical order.

16. **"See" and "See Also"**

The "see" instruction following a main term in the Alphabetic Index indicates that another term should be referenced. It is necessary to go to the main term referenced with the "see" note to locate the correct code.

A "see also" instruction following a main term in the Alphabetic Index instructs that there is another main term that may also be referenced that may provide additional Alphabetic Index entries that may be useful. It is not necessary to follow the "see also" note when the original main term provides the necessary code.

17. **"Code also note"**

A "code also" note instructs that two codes may be required to fully describe a condition, but this note does not provide sequencing direction. The sequencing depends on the circumstances of the encounter.

18. **Default codes**

A code listed next to a main term in the *ICD-10-CM* Alphabetic Index is referred to as a default code. The default code represents that condition that is most commonly associated with the main term, or is the unspecified code for the condition. If a condition is documented in a medical record (for example, appendicitis) without any additional information, such as acute or chronic, the default code should be assigned.

B. General Coding Guidelines

1. Locating a code in the *ICD-10-CM*

To select a code in the classification that corresponds to a diagnosis or reason for visit documented in a medical record, first locate the term in the Alphabetic Index, and then verify the code in the Tabular List. Read and be guided by instructional notations that appear in both the Alphabetic Index and the Tabular List.

It is essential to use both the Alphabetic Index and Tabular List when locating and assigning a code. The Alphabetic Index does not always provide the full code. Selection of the full code, including laterality and any applicable 7th character, can only be done in the Tabular List. A dash (-) at the end of an Alphabetic Index entry indicates that additional characters are required. Even if a dash is not included at the Alphabetic Index entry, it is necessary to refer to the Tabular List to verify that no 7th character is required.

2. Level of Detail in Coding

Diagnosis codes are to be used and reported at their highest number of characters available.

ICD-10-CM diagnosis codes are composed of codes with 3, 4, 5, 6, or 7 characters. Codes with three characters are included in *ICD-10-CM* as the heading of a category of codes that may be further subdivided by the use of fourth and/or fifth characters and/or sixth characters, which provide greater detail.

A three-character code is to be used only if it is not further subdivided. A code is invalid if it has not been coded to the full number of characters required for that code, including the 7th character, if applicable.

3. Code or codes from A00.0 through T88.9, Z00–Z99.8

The appropriate code or codes from A00.0 through T88.9, Z00–Z99.8 must be used to identify diagnoses, symptoms, conditions, problems, complaints, or other reason(s) for the encounter/visit.

4. Signs and symptoms

Codes that describe symptoms and signs, as opposed to diagnoses, are acceptable for reporting purposes when a related definitive diagnosis has not been established (confirmed) by the provider. Chapter 18 of *ICD-10-CM*, Symptoms, Signs, and Abnormal Clinical and Laboratory Findings, Not Elsewhere Classified (codes R00.0 – R99), contains many but not all codes for symptoms.

See Use of Sign/Symptom/Unspecified Codes, page XVIII

5. Conditions that are an integral part of a disease process

Signs and symptoms that are associated routinely with a disease process should not be assigned as additional codes, unless otherwise instructed by the classification.

6. Conditions that are not an integral part of a disease process

Additional signs and symptoms that may not be associated routinely with a disease process should be coded when present.

7. Multiple coding for a single condition

In addition to the etiology/manifestation convention that requires two codes to fully describe a single condition that affects multiple body systems, there are other single conditions that also require more than one code. "Use additional code" notes are found in the Tabular List at codes that are not part of an etiology/manifestation pair where a secondary code is useful to fully describe a condition. The sequencing rule is the same as the etiology/manifestation pair; "use additional code" indicates that a secondary code should be added, if known.

For example, for bacterial infections that are not included in Chapter 1, a secondary code from category B95, Streptococcus, Staphylococcus, and Enterococcus, as the cause of diseases classified elsewhere, or B96, Other bacterial agents as the cause of diseases classified elsewhere, may be required to identify the bacterial organism causing the infection. A "use additional code" note will normally be found at the infectious disease code, indicating a need for the organism code to be added as a secondary code.

"Code first" notes are also under certain codes that are not specifically manifestation codes but may be due to an underlying cause. When there is a "code first" note and an underlying condition is present, the underlying condition should be sequenced first, if known.

"Code, if applicable, any causal condition first" notes indicate that this code may be assigned as a principal diagnosis when the causal condition is unknown or not applicable. If a causal condition is known, then the code for that condition should be sequenced as the principal or first-listed diagnosis.

Multiple codes may be needed for sequela, complication codes, and obstetric codes to more fully describe a condition. See the specific guidelines for these conditions for further instruction.

8. **Acute and Chronic Conditions**

If the same condition is described as both acute (subacute) and chronic, and separate subentries exist in the Alphabetic Index at the same indentation level, code both and sequence the acute (subacute) code first.

9. **Combination Code**

A combination code is a single code used to classify:

Two diagnoses, or

A diagnosis with an associated secondary process (manifestation)

A diagnosis with an associated complication

Combination codes are identified by referring to subterm entries in the Alphabetic Index and by reading the inclusion and exclusion notes in the Tabular List.

Assign only the combination code when that code fully identifies the diagnostic conditions involved or when the Alphabetic Index so directs. Multiple coding should not be used when the classification provides a combination code that clearly identifies all of the elements documented in the diagnosis. When the combination code lacks necessary specificity in describing the manifestation or complication, an additional code should be used as a secondary code.

10. **Sequela (Late Effects)**

A sequela is the residual effect (condition produced) after the acute phase of an illness or injury has terminated. There is no time limit on when a sequela code can be used. The residual may be apparent early, such as in cerebral infarction, or it may occur months or years later, such as that due to a previous injury. Examples of sequela include: scar formation resulting from a burn, deviated septum due to a nasal fracture, and infertility due to tubal occlusion from old tuberculosis. Coding of sequela generally requires two codes sequenced in the following order: The condition or nature of the sequela is sequenced first. The sequela code is sequenced second.

An exception to the above guidelines are those instances where the code for the sequela is followed by a manifestation code identified in the Tabular List and title, or the sequela code has been expanded (at the fourth, fifth or sixth character levels) to include the manifestation(s). The code for the acute phase of an illness or injury that led to the sequela is never used with a code for the late effect.

Application of 7th characters refer to Chapter 19

11. **Impending or Threatened Condition**

Code any condition described at the time of discharge as "impending" or "threatened" as follows:

If it did occur, code as confirmed diagnosis. If it did not occur, reference the Alphabetic Index to determine if the condition has a subentry term for "impending" or "threatened" and also reference main term entries for "Impending" and for "Threatened." If the subterms are listed, assign the given code. If the subterms are not listed, code the existing underlying condition(s) and not the condition described as impending or threatened.

12. **Reporting Same Diagnosis Code More Than Once**

Each unique *ICD-10-CM* diagnosis code may be reported only once for an encounter. This applies to bilateral conditions when there are no distinct codes identifying laterality or two different conditions classified to the same *ICD-10-CM* diagnosis code.

13. **Laterality**

Some *ICD-10-CM* codes indicate laterality, specifying whether the condition occurs on the left, right or is bilateral. If no bilateral code is provided and the condition is bilateral, assign separate codes for both the left and right side. If the side is not identified in the medical record, assign the code for the unspecified side.

14. **Documentation by *Clinicians Other Than the Patient's Provider***

Code assignment is based on the documentation by patient's provider (i.e., physician or other qualified healthcare practitioner legally accountable for establishing the patient's diagnosis). There are a few exceptions, such as codes for the Body Mass Index (BMI), depth of non-pressure chronic ulcers and pressure ulcer stage codes, code assignment may be based on medical record documentation from clinicians who are not the patient's provider (ie, physician or other qualified healthcare practitioner legally accountable for establishing the patient's diagnosis), since this information is typically documented by other clinicians involved in the care of the patient (eg, a dietitian often documents the BMI and nurses often document the pressure ulcer stages). However, the associated diagnosis (such as overweight, obesity, or pressure ulcer) must be documented by the patient's provider. If there is conflicting medical record documentation, either from the same clinician or different clinicians, the patient's attending provider should be queried for clarification.

For social determinants of health, such as information found in categories Z55–Z65, Persons with potential health hazards related to socioeconomic and psychosocial circumstances, code assignment may be based on medical record documentation from clinicians involved in the care of the patient who are not the patient's provider since this information represents social information, rather than medical diagnoses. **Patient self-reported documentation may also be used to assign codes for social determinants of health, as long as the patient self-reported information is signed-off by and incorporated into the health record by either a clinician or provider.**

The BMI, coma scale, NIHSS codes and categories Z55–Z65 should only be reported as secondary diagnoses.

15. **Syndromes**

Follow the Alphabetic Index guidance when coding syndromes. In the absence of Alphabetic Index guidance, assign codes for the documented manifestations of the syndrome. Additional codes for manifestations that are not an integral part of the disease process may also be assigned when the condition does not have a unique code.

16. **Documentation of Complications of Care**

Code assignment is based on the provider's documentation of the relationship between the condition and the care or procedure. The guideline extends to any complications of care, regardless of the chapter the code is located in. It is important to note that not all conditions that occur during or following medical care or surgery are classified as complications. There must be a cause-and-effect relationship between the care provided and the condition, and an indication in the documentation that it is a complication. Query the provider for clarification, if the complication is not clearly documented.

17. **Borderline Diagnosis**

If the provider documents a "borderline" diagnosis at the time of discharge, the diagnosis is coded as confirmed, unless the classification provides a specific entry (eg, borderline diabetes). If a borderline condition has a specific index entry in *ICD-10-CM*, it should be coded as such. Since borderline conditions are not uncertain diagnoses, no distinction is made between the care setting (inpatient versus outpatient). Whenever the documentation is unclear regarding a borderline condition, coders are encouraged to query for clarification.

18. **Use of Sign/Symptom/Unspecified Codes**

Sign/symptom and "unspecified" codes have acceptable, even necessary, uses. While specific diagnosis codes should be reported when they are supported by the available medical record documentation and clinical knowledge of the patient's health condition, there are instances when signs/symptoms or unspecified codes are the best choices for accurately reflecting the healthcare encounter. Each health care encounter should be coded to the level of certainty known for that encounter.

If a definitive diagnosis has not been established by the end of the encounter, it is appropriate to report codes for sign(s) and/or symptom(s) in lieu of a definitive diagnosis. When sufficient clinical information isn't known or available about a particular health condition to assign a more specific code, it is acceptable to report the appropriate "unspecified" code (eg, a diagnosis of pneumonia has been determined, but not the specific type). Unspecified codes should be reported when they are the codes that most accurately reflect what is known about the patient's condition at the time of that particular encounter. It would be inappropriate to select a specific code that is not supported by the medical record documentation or conduct medically unnecessary diagnostic testing in order to determine a more specific code.

19. **Coding for Healthcare Encounters in Hurricane Aftermath**

a. **Use of External Cause of Morbidity Codes**

An external cause of morbidity code should be assigned to identify the cause of the injury(ies) incurred as a result of the hurricane. The use of external cause of morbidity codes is supplemental to the application of *ICD-10-CM* codes. External cause of morbidity codes are never to be recorded as a principal diagnosis (first-listed in non-inpatient settings). The appropriate injury code should be sequenced before any external cause codes. The external cause of morbidity codes capture how the injury or health condition happened (cause), the intent (unintentional or accidental; or intentional, such as suicide or assault), the place where the event occurred, the activity of the patient at the time of the event, and the person's status (e.g., civilian, military). They should not be assigned for encounters to treat hurricane victims' medical conditions when no injury, adverse effect or poisoning is involved. External cause of morbidity codes should be assigned for each encounter for care and treatment of the injury. External cause of morbidity codes may be assigned in all health care settings. For the purpose of capturing complete and accurate *ICD-10-CM* data in the aftermath of the hurricane, a healthcare setting should be considered as any location where medical care is provided by licensed healthcare professionals.

b. Sequencing of External Causes of Morbidity Codes

Codes for cataclysmic events, such as a hurricane, take priority over all other external cause codes except child and adult abuse and terrorism and should be sequenced before other external cause of injury codes. Assign as many external cause of morbidity codes as necessary to fully explain each cause. For example, if an injury occurs as a result of a building collapse during the hurricane, external cause codes for both the hurricane and the building collapse should be assigned, with the external causes code for hurricane being sequenced as the first external cause code. For injuries incurred as a direct result of the hurricane, assign the appropriate code(s) for the injuries, followed by the code X37.0-, Hurricane (with the appropriate 7th character), and any other applicable external cause of injury codes. Code X37.0- also should be assigned when an injury is incurred as a result of flooding caused by a levee breaking related to the hurricane. Code X38.-, Flood (with the appropriate 7th character), should be assigned when an injury is from flooding resulting directly from the storm. Code X36.0.-, Collapse of dam or man-made structure, should not be assigned when the cause of the collapse is due to the hurricane. Use of code X36.0- is limited to collapses of man-made structures due to earth surface movements, not due to storm surges directly from a hurricane.

c. Other External Causes of Morbidity Code Issues

For injuries that are not a direct result of the hurricane, such as an evacuee that has incurred an injury as a result of a motor vehicle accident, assign the appropriate external cause of morbidity code(s) to describe the cause of the injury, but do not assign code X37.0-, Hurricane. If it is not clear whether the injury was a direct result of the hurricane, assume the injury is due to the hurricane and assign code X37.0-, Hurricane, as well as any other applicable external cause of morbidity codes. In addition to code X37.0-, Hurricane, other possible applicable external cause of morbidity codes include:

W54.0-, Bitten by dog

X30-, Exposure to excessive natural heat

X31-, Exposure to excessive natural cold

X38-, Flood

d. Use of Z codes

Z codes (other reasons for healthcare encounters) may be assigned as appropriate to further explain the reasons for presenting for healthcare services, including transfers between healthcare facilities. The *ICD-10-CM Official Guidelines for Coding and Reporting* identify which codes maybe assigned as principal or first-listed diagnosis only, secondary diagnosis only, or principal/first-listed or secondary (depending on the circumstances). Possible applicable Z codes include:

Z59.0, Homelessness

Z59.1, Inadequate housing

Z59.5, Extreme poverty

Z75.1, Person awaiting admission to adequate facility elsewhere

Z75.3, Unavailability and inaccessibility of health-care facilities

Z75.4, Unavailability and inaccessibility of other helping agencies

Z76.2, Encounter for health supervision and care of other healthy infant and child

Z99.12, Encounter for respirator [ventilator] dependence during power failure

The external cause of morbidity codes and the Z codes listed above are not an all-inclusive list. Other codes may be applicable to the encounter based upon the documentation. Assign as many codes as necessary to fully explain each healthcare encounter. Since patient history information may be very limited, use any available documentation to assign the appropriate external cause of morbidity and Z codes.

C. Chapter-Specific Coding Guidelines

Please refer to each chapter for information on specific guidelines.

Section II. Selection of Principle Diagnosis

Excluded as not relevant to provider-based coding. Refer to the full *ICD-10-CM* manual if needed.

Section III. Reporting Additional Diagnoses

Excluded as not relevant to provider-based coding. Refer to the full *ICD-10-CM* manual if needed.

Section IV. Diagnostic Coding and Reporting Guidelines for Outpatient Services

These coding guidelines for outpatient diagnoses have been approved for use by hospitals/providers in coding and reporting hospital-based outpatient services and provider-based office visits.

Information about the use of certain abbreviations, punctuation, symbols, and other conventions used in the *ICD-10-CM* Tabular List (code numbers and titles), can be found in Section IA of these guidelines, under "Conventions Used in the Tabular List." Section I.B. contains general guidelines that apply to the entire classification. Section I.C. contains chapter-specific guidelines that correspond to the chapters as they are arranged in the classification. Information about the correct sequence to use in finding a code is also described in Section I.

The terms "encounter" and "visit" are often used interchangeably when describing outpatient service contacts and, therefore, appear together in these guidelines without distinguishing one from the other.

Though the conventions and general guidelines apply to all settings, coding guidelines for outpatient and provider reporting of diagnoses will vary in a number of instances from those for inpatient diagnoses, recognizing that:

A. Selection of first-listed condition

In the outpatient setting, the term "first-listed diagnosis" is used in lieu of "principal diagnosis."

In determining the first-listed diagnosis, the coding conventions of *ICD-10-CM*, as well as the general and disease specific guidelines, take precedence over the outpatient guidelines.

Diagnoses are often not established at the time of the initial encounter/visit. It may take two or more visits before the diagnosis is confirmed.

The most critical rule is to begin the search for the correct code assignment through the Alphabetic Index. Never search initially in the Tabular List, as this will lead to coding errors.

1. Outpatient Surgery

When a patient presents for outpatient surgery (same day surgery), code the reason for the surgery as the first-listed diagnosis (reason for the encounter), even if the surgery is not performed due to a contraindication.

2. Observation Stay

When a patient is admitted for observation for a medical condition, assign a code for the medical condition as the first-listed diagnosis.

When a patient presents for outpatient surgery and develops complications requiring admission to observation, code the reason for the surgery as the first reported diagnosis (reason for the encounter), followed by codes for the complications as secondary diagnoses.

B. Codes from A00.0 through T88.9, Z00 – Z99

The appropriate code(s) from A00.0 through T88.9, Z00 – Z99 must be used to identify diagnoses, symptoms, conditions, problems, complaints, or other reason(s) for the encounter/visit.

C. Accurate reporting of *ICD-10-CM* diagnosis codes

For accurate reporting of *ICD-10-CM* diagnosis codes, the documentation should describe the patient's condition, using terminology which includes specific diagnoses, as well as symptoms, problems, or reasons for the encounter. There are *ICD-10-CM* codes to describe all of these.

D. Codes that describe symptoms and signs

Codes that describe symptoms and signs, as opposed to diagnoses, are acceptable for reporting purposes when a diagnosis has not been established (confirmed) by the provider. Chapter 18 of *ICD-10-CM*, Symptoms, Signs, and Abnormal Clinical and Laboratory Findings Not Elsewhere Classified (codes R00 – R99) contains many, but not all codes for symptoms.

E. Encounters for circumstances other than a disease or injury

ICD-10-CM provides codes to deal with encounters for circumstances other than a disease or injury. The Factors Influencing Health Status and Contact with Health Services codes (Z00 – Z99) are provided to deal with occasions when circumstances other than a disease or injury are recorded as diagnosis or problems.

See Chapter 21, *Factors influencing health status and contact with health services.*

F. Level of Detail in Coding

1. *ICD-10-CM* codes with 3, 4, 5, 6, or 7 characters

ICD-10-CM is composed of codes with 3, 4, 5, 6, or 7 characters. Codes with three characters are included in *ICD-10-CM* as the heading of a category of codes that may be further subdivided by the use of fourth, fifth, sixth, or seventh characters to provide greater specificity.

2. **Use of full number of characters required for a code**

   A three-character code is to be used only if it is not further subdivided. A code is invalid if it has not been coded to the full number of characters required for that code, including the 7th character, if applicable.

G. *ICD-10-CM* **code for the diagnosis, condition, problem, or other reason for encounter/visit**

   List first the *ICD-10-CM* code for the diagnosis, condition, problem, or other reason for encounter/visit shown in the medical record to be chiefly responsible for the services provided. List additional codes that describe any coexisting conditions. In some cases, the first-listed diagnosis may be a symptom when a diagnosis has not been established (confirmed) by the **provider**.

H. **Uncertain diagnosis**

   <u>Do not code</u> diagnoses documented as "probable," "suspected," "questionable," "rule out," or "working diagnosis" or other similar terms indicating uncertainty. Rather, code the condition(s) to the highest degree of certainty for that encounter/visit, such as symptoms, signs, abnormal test results, or other reason for the visit.

I. **Chronic diseases**

   Chronic diseases treated on an ongoing basis may be coded and reported as many times as the patient receives treatment and care for the condition(s)

J. **Code all documented conditions that coexist**

   Code all documented conditions that coexist at the time of the encounter/visit, and require or affect patient care treatment or management. Do not code conditions that were previously treated and no longer exist. However, history codes (categories Z80–Z87) may be used as secondary codes if the historical condition or family history has an impact on current care or influences treatment.

K. **Patients receiving diagnostic services only**

   For patients receiving diagnostic services only during an encounter/visit, sequence first the diagnosis, condition, problem, or other reason for encounter/visit shown in the medical record to be chiefly responsible for the outpatient services provided during the encounter/visit. Codes for other diagnoses (eg, chronic conditions) may be sequenced as additional diagnoses.

   For encounters for routine laboratory/radiology testing in the absence of any signs, symptoms, or associated diagnosis, assign Z01.89, Encounter for other specified special examinations. If routine testing is performed during the same encounter as a test to evaluate a sign, symptom, or diagnosis, it is appropriate to assign both the Z code and the code describing the reason for the non-routine test.

   For outpatient encounters for diagnostic tests that have been interpreted by a physician, and the final report is available at the time of coding, code any confirmed or definitive diagnosis(es) documented in the interpretation. Do not code related signs and symptoms as additional diagnoses.

   Please note: This differs from the coding practice in the hospital inpatient setting regarding abnormal findings on test results.

L. **Patients receiving therapeutic services only**

   For patients receiving therapeutic services only during an encounter/visit, sequence first the diagnosis, condition, problem, or other reason for encounter/visit shown in the medical record to be chiefly responsible for the outpatient services provided during the encounter/visit. Codes for other diagnoses (eg, chronic conditions) may be sequenced as additional diagnoses.

   The only exception to this rule is that when the primary reason for the admission/encounter is chemotherapy or radiation therapy. In this case, the appropriate Z code for the service is listed first, and the diagnosis or problem for which the service is being performed is listed second.

M. **Patients receiving preoperative evaluations only**

   For patients receiving preoperative evaluations only, sequence first a code from subcategory Z01.81, Encounter for pre-procedural examinations, to describe the pre-op consultations. Assign a code for the condition to describe the reason for the surgery as an additional diagnosis. Code also any findings related to the pre-op evaluation.

N. **Ambulatory surgery**

   For ambulatory surgery, code the diagnosis for which the surgery was performed. If the postoperative diagnosis is known to be different from the preoperative diagnosis at the time the diagnosis is confirmed, select the postoperative diagnosis for coding, since it is the most definitive.

O. **Routine outpatient prenatal visits**

   See Chapter 15, *Pregnancy, childbirth and the puerperium.*

P.   Encounters for general medical examinations with abnormal findings

The subcategories for encounters for general medical examinations, Z00.0-, provide codes for with and without abnormal findings. Should a general medical examination result in an abnormal finding, the code for general medical examination with abnormal finding should be assigned as the first-listed diagnosis. A secondary code for the abnormal finding should also be coded.

Q.   Encounters for routine health screenings

See Chapter 21, *Factors influencing health status and contact with health services, Screening*

Alphabetic Index

Instructions are listed in *italic font*. The "*see*" instruction indicates it is necessary to reference another term while "*see also*" instruction indicates another main term may provide additional entries. It is not necessary to follow a "*see also*" instruction when the current entry directs to a code for the condition. "*Code*" or "*Code to*" directs to the appropriate reference for a condition.

Punctuation

[ ]—used to identify manifestation codes

( )—enclose nonessential words that do not affect code assignment

:—the colon identifies that a term is incomplete and requires additional modifying terms

- —the hyphen indicates additional characters are found in the tabular list

A

Aarskog's syndrome Q87.19

Abandonment—*see* Maltreatment

Abasia (-astasia) (hysterical) F44.4

Abderhalden-Kaufmann-Lignac syndrome (cystinosis) E72.04

Abdomen, abdominal—*see also* Disease, diseased
- acute R10.0
- angina K55.1
- muscle deficiency syndrome Q79.4

Abdominalgia—*see* Pain(s), abdominal

Abduction contracture, hip or other joint—*see* Contraction, joint

Aberrant (congenital)—*see also* Malposition, congenital
- artery (peripheral) Q27.8
  - eye Q15.8
  - pulmonary Q25.79
  - retina Q14.1
- endocrine gland NEC Q89.2
- hepatic duct Q44.5
- parathyroid gland Q89.2
- pituitary gland Q89.2
- thymus (gland) Q89.2
- thyroid gland Q89.2

Abiotrophy R68.89

Ablepharia, ablepharon Q10.3

Abnormal, abnormality, abnormalities—*see also* Anomaly
- auditory perception H93.29-
- autosomes Q99.9
- basal metabolic rate R94.8
- bleeding time R79.1
- blood gas level R79.81
- blood pressure
  - elevated R03.0
- brain scan R94.02
- caloric test R94.138
- chemistry, blood R79.9
  - C-reactive protein R79.82
  - drugs—*see* Findings, abnormal, in blood
  - gas level R79.81
  - pancytopenia D61.818
  - PTT R79.1
- chest sounds (friction) (rales) R09.89
- chromosome, chromosomal Q99.9
  - sex Q99.8
    - female phenotype Q97.9
    - male phenotype Q98.9
- clinical findings NEC R68.89
- coagulation D68.9
  - newborn, transient P61.6
  - profile R79.1
  - time R79.1
- cortisol-binding globulin E27.8
- creatinine clearance R94.4
- development, developmental Q89.9
  - central nervous system Q07.9
- diagnostic imaging
  - abdomen, abdominal region NEC R93.5
  - bladder R93.41
  - coronary circulation R93.1
  - head R93.0
  - heart R93.1

Abnormal, abnormality, abnormalities, *continued*
- kidney R93.42-
- lung (field) R91.8
- musculoskeletal system NEC R93.7
- renal pelvis R93.41
- retroperitoneum R93.5
- site specified NEC R93.89
- skull R93.0
- testis R93.81-
- ureter R93.41
- urinary organs, specified R93.49
- echocardiogram R93.1
- electrocardiogram [ECG] [EKG] R94.31
- electroencephalogram [EEG] R94.01
- electrolyte—*see* Imbalance, electrolyte
- electromyogram [EMG] R94.131
- electro-oculogram [EOG] R94.110
- electrophysiological intracardiac studies R94.39
- electroretinogram [ERG] R94.111
- feces (color) (contents) (mucus) R19.5
- function studies
  - auditory R94.120
  - bladder R94.8
  - brain R94.09
  - cardiovascular R94.30
  - ear R94.128
  - endocrine NEC R94.7
  - eye NEC R94.118
  - kidney R94.4
  - liver function test R94.5
  - nervous system
    - central NEC R94.09
    - peripheral NEC R94.138
  - pancreas R94.8
  - placenta R94.8
  - pulmonary R94.2
  - special senses NEC R94.128
  - spleen R94.8
  - thyroid R94.6
  - vestibular R94.121
- gait—*see* Gait abnormality
  - hysterical F44.4
- globulin R77.1
  - cortisol-binding E27.8
- heart
  - rate R00.9
    - specified NEC R00.8
  - shadow R93.1
- hemoglobin (disease) (*see also* Disease, hemoglobin) D58.2
  - trait—*see* Trait, hemoglobin, abnormal
- kidney function test R94.4
- loss of
  - weight R63.4
- Mantoux test R76.11
- movement (disorder)—*see also* Disorder, movement
  - involuntary R25.9
    - spasm R25.2
    - tremor R25.1
- neonatal screening P09
- oculomotor study R94.113
- palmar creases Q82.8
- partial thromboplastin time (PTT) R79.1
- percussion, chest (tympany) R09.89
- phonocardiogram R94.39
- plasma
  - protein R77.9
    - specified NEC R77.8
  - viscosity R70.1
- posture R29.3
- prothrombin time (PT) R79.1
- pulmonary
  - artery, congenital Q25.79
  - function, newborn P28.89
  - test results R94.2
- pulsations in neck R00.2
- red blood cell(s) (morphology) (volume) R71.8
- renal function test R94.4
- response to nerve stimulation R94.130
- retinal correspondence H53.31
- retinal function study R94.111
- rhythm, heart—*see also* Arrhythmia
- saliva—*see* Abnormal, specimen

Abnormal, abnormality, abnormalities, *continued*
- scan
  - kidney R94.4
  - liver R93.2
  - thyroid R94.6
- serum level (of)
  - acid phosphatase R74.8
  - alkaline phosphatase R74.8
  - amylase R74.8
  - enzymes R74.9
    - specified NEC R74.8
  - lipase R74.8
  - triacylglycerol lipase R74.8
- sinus venosus Q21.1
- specimen
  - specified organ, system and tissue NOS R89.9
- sputum (amount) (color) (odor) R09.3
- stool (color) (contents) (mucus) R19.5
  - bloody K92.1
  - guaiac positive R19.5
- transport protein E88.09
- tumor marker NEC R97.8
- urination NEC R39.198
- urine (constituents) R82.90
  - cytological and histological examination R82.89
  - glucose R81
  - hemoglobin R82.3
  - microbiological examination (positive culture) R82.79
  - pyuria R82.81
  - specified substance NEC R82.998
- vectorcardiogram R94.39
- visually evoked potential (VEP) R94.112
- white blood cells D72.9
  - specified NEC D72.89
- X-ray examination—*see* Abnormal, diagnostic imaging

Abnormity (any organ or part)—*see* Anomaly

Abocclusion M26.29
- hemolytic disease (newborn) P55.1

Abortion (complete) (spontaneous) O03.9
- incomplete (spontaneous) O03.4
- missed O02.1
- spontaneous—*see* Abortion (complete) (spontaneous)
  - threatened O20.0
- threatened (spontaneous) O20.0
- tubal O00.10-
  - with intrauterine pregnancy O00.11

Abramov-Fiedler myocarditis (acute isolated myocarditis) I40.1

Abrasion T14.8
- abdomen, abdominal (wall) S30.811
- alveolar process S00.512
- ankle S90.51-
- antecubital space—*see* Abrasion, elbow
- anus S30.817
- arm (upper) S40.81-
- auditory canal—*see* Abrasion, ear
- auricle—*see* Abrasion, ear
- axilla—*see* Abrasion, arm
- back, lower S30.810
- breast S20.11-
- brow S00.81
- buttock S30.810
- calf—*see* Abrasion, leg
- canthus—*see* Abrasion, eyelid
- cheek S00.81
  - internal S00.512
- chest wall—*see* Abrasion, thorax
- chin S00.81
- clitoris S30.814
- cornea S05.0-
- costal region—*see* Abrasion, thorax
- dental K03.1
- digit(s)
  - foot—*see* Abrasion, toe
  - hand—*see* Abrasion, finger
- ear S00.41-
- elbow S50.31-
- epididymis S30.813
- epigastric region S30.811
- epiglottis S10.11
- esophagus (thoracic)
  - cervical S10.11

Abrasion, *continued*
- eyebrow *S00.21-*
- eyelid S00.21-
- face S00.81
- finger(s) S60.41-
  - index S60.41-
  - little S60.41-
  - middle S60.41-
  - ring S60.41-
- flank S30.811
- foot (except toe(s) alone) S90.81
  - toe—*see* Abrasion, toe
- forearm S50.81-
  - elbow only—*see* Abrasion, elbow
- forehead S00.81
- genital organs, external
  - male S30.815
- groin S30.811
- gum S00.512
- hand S60.51-
- head S00.91
  - ear—*see* Abrasion, ear
  - eyelid—*see* Abrasion, eyelid
  - lip S00.511
  - nose S00.31
  - oral cavity S00.512
  - scalp S00.01
  - specified site NEC S00.81
- heel—*see* Abrasion, foot
- hip S70.21-
- inguinal region S30.811
- interscapular region S20.419
- jaw S00.81
- knee S80.21-
- labium (majus) (minus) S30.814
- larynx S10.11
- leg (lower) S80.81-
  - knee—*see* Abrasion, knee
  - upper—*see* Abrasion, thigh
- lip S00.511
- lower back S30.810
- lumbar region S30.810
- malar region S00.81
- mammary—*see* Abrasion, breast
- mastoid region S00.81
- mouth S00.512
- nail
  - finger—*see* Abrasion, finger
  - toe—*see* Abrasion, toe
- nape S10.81
- nasal S00.31
- neck S10.91
  - specified site NEC S10.81
  - throat S10.11
- nose S00.31
- occipital region S00.01
- oral cavity S00.512
- orbital region—*see* Abrasion, eyelid
- palate S00.512
- palm—*see* Abrasion, hand
- parietal region S00.01
- pelvis S30.810
- penis S30.812
- perineum
  - female S30.814
  - male S30.810
- periocular area—*see* Abrasion, eyelid
- phalanges
  - finger—*see* Abrasion, finger
  - toe—*see* Abrasion, toe
- pharynx S10.11
- pinna—*see* Abrasion, ear
- popliteal space—*see* Abrasion, knee
- prepuce S30.812
- pubic region S30.810
- pudendum
  - female S30.816
  - male S30.815
- sacral region S30.810
- scalp S00.01
- scapular region—*see* Abrasion, shoulder
- scrotum S30.813
- shin—*see* Abrasion, leg

Abrasion, *continued*
- shoulder S40.21
- skin NEC T14.8
- sternal region S20.319
- submaxillary region S00.81
- submental region S00.81
- subungual
  - finger(s)—*see* Abrasion, finger
  - toe(s)—*see* Abrasion, toe
- supraclavicular fossa S10.81
- supraorbital S00.81
- temple S00.81
- temporal region S00.81
- testis S30.813
- thigh S70.31-
- thorax, thoracic (wall) S20.91
  - back S20.41-
  - front S20.31-
- throat S10.11
- thumb S60.31-
- toe(s) (lesser) S90.41-
  - great S90.41-
- tongue S00.512
- tooth, teeth (dentifrice) (habitual) (hard tissues) (occupational) (ritual) (traditional) K03.1
- trachea S10.11
- tunica vaginalis S30.813
- tympanum, tympanic membrane—*see* Abrasion, ear
- uvula S00.512
- vagina S30.814
- vocal cords S10.11
- vulva S30.814
- wrist S60.81-

Abscess (connective tissue) (embolic) (fistulous) (metastatic) (multiple) (pernicious) (pyogenic) (septic) L02.91
- abdomen, abdominal
  - cavity K65.1
  - wall L02.211
- abdominopelvic K65.1
- accessory sinus—*see* Sinusitis
- adrenal (capsule) (gland) E27.8
- alveolar K04.7
- anorectal K61.2
- anus K61.0
- apical (tooth) K04.7
- appendix K35.33
- areola (acute) (chronic) (nonpuerperal) N61.1
- axilla (region) L02.41
  - lymph gland or node L04.2
- back (any part, except buttock) L02.212
- Bartholin's gland N75.1
- brain (any part) (cystic) (otogenic) G06.0
  - newborn P39.0
- breast (acute) (chronic) (nonpuerperal) N61.1
  - newborn P39.0
- buccal cavity K12.2
- buttock L02.31
- cecum K35.33
- cerebellum, cerebellar G06.0
  - sequelae G09
- cerebral (embolic) G06.0
  - sequelae G09
- cervical (meaning neck) L02.11
  - lymph gland or node L04.0
- cheek (external) L02.01
  - inner K12.2
- chest J86.9
  - with fistula J86.0
  - wall L02.213
- chin L02.01
- circumtonsillar J36
- colostomy K94.02
- cranium G06.0
- dental K04.7
- dentoalveolar K04.7
- ear (middle)—*see also* Otitis, media
  - acute—*see* Otitis, media
  - external H60.0-
- epididymis N45.4
- epidural G06.2
  - brain G06.0
  - spinal cord G06.1
- erysipelatous—*see* Erysipelas

Abscess, *continued*
- esophagus K20.80
- ethmoid (bone) (chronic) (sinus) J32.2
- extradural G06.2
  - brain G06.0
    - sequelae G09
  - spinal cord G06.1
- eyelid H00.03-
- face (any part, except ear, eye and nose) L02.01
- foot L02.61-
- forehead L02.01
- frontal sinus (chronic) J32.1
- gallbladder K81.0
- gluteal (region) L02.31
- groin L02.214
- hand L02.51-
  - head NEC L02.811 part, except ear, eye and nose) L02.01
- horseshoe K61.31
- heel—*see* Abscess, foot
- ileocecal K35.33
- iliac (region) L02.214
  - fossa K35.33
- inguinal (region) L02.214
  - lymph gland or node L04.1
- intersphincteric K61.4
- intracranial G06.0
- intratonsillar J36
- knee—*see also* Abscess, lower limb
  - joint M00.9
- lateral (alveolar) K04.7
- lingual K14.0
  - tonsil J36
- lip K13.0
- loin (region) L02.211
- lower limb L02.41
- lumbar (tuberculous) A18.01
  - nontuberculous L02.212
- lymph, lymphatic, gland or node (acute)—*see also* Lymphadenitis, acute
  - mesentery I88.0
- marginal, anus K61.0
- maxilla, maxillary M27.2
  - molar (tooth) K04.7
  - premolar K04.7
  - sinus (chronic) J32.0
- mons pubis L02.215
- mouth (floor) K12.2
- myocardium I40.0
- nasal J32.9
- navel L02.216
  - newborn P38.9
    - with mild hemorrhage P38.1
    - without hemorrhage P38.9
- neck (region) L02.11
  - lymph gland or node L04.0
- nipple N61.1
- nose (external) (fossa) (septum) J34.0
  - sinus (chronic)—*see* Sinusitis
- operative wound T81.43
- otogenic G06.0
- palate (soft) K12.2
  - hard M27.2
- parapharyngeal J39.0
- pararectal K61.1
- parietal region (scalp) L02.811
- parotid (duct) (gland) K11.3
  - region K12.2
- pectoral (region) L02.213
- perianal K61.0
- periapical K04.7
- periappendicular K35.33
- pericardial I30.1
- pericecal K35.33
- perineum, perineal (superficial) L02.215
  - urethra N34.0
- periodontal (parietal)
  - apical K04.7
- peripharyngeal J39.0
- peripleuritic J86.9
  - with fistula J86.0
- perirectal K61.1

Abscess, *continued*
- peritoneum, peritoneal (perforated) (ruptured) K65.1
  - with appendicitis K35.33
  - postoperative T81.43
- peritonsillar J36
- perityphlic K35.33
- phagedenic NOS L02.91
  - pituitary (gland) E23.6
- pleura J86.9
  - with fistula J86.0
- pilonidal L05.01
- postcecal K35.33
  - postoperative (any site) T81.43
- postnasal J34.0
- postpharyngeal J39.0
- posttonsillar J36
- rectum K61.1
- retropharyngeal J39.0
- root, tooth K04.7
- rupture (spontaneous) NOS L02.91
- scalp (any part) L02.811
- scrofulous (tuberculous) A18.2
- septal, dental K04.7
- sinus (accessory) (chronic) (nasal)—*see also* Sinusitis
  - intracranial venous (any) G06.0
- specified site NEC L02.818
- sphenoidal (sinus) (chronic) J32.3
- stitch T81.41
- subarachnoid G06.2
  - brain G06.0
  - spinal cord G06.1
- subcecal K35.33
- subcutaneous—*see also* Abscess, by site
- subdural G06.2
  - brain G06.0
    - sequelae G09
  - spinal cord G06.1
- subgaleal L02.811
- sublingual K12.2
  - gland K11.3
- submandibular (region) (space) (triangle) K12.2
  - gland K11.3
- submaxillary (region) L02.01
  - gland K11.3
- submental L02.01
  - gland K11.3
- supralevator K61.5
- suprarenal (capsule) (gland) E27.8
- temple L02.01
- temporal region L02.01
- temporosphenoidal G06.0
- testes N45.4
- thorax J86.9
  - with fistula J86.0
- thyroid (gland) E06.0
- tongue (staphylococcal) K14.0
- tonsil(s) (lingual) J36
- tonsillopharyngeal J36
- tooth, teeth (root) K04.7
- trunk L02.219
  - abdominal wall L02.211
  - back L02.212
  - chest wall L02.213
  - groin L02.214
  - perineum L02.215
  - umbilicus L02.216
- umbilicus L02.216
- upper
  - limb L02.41-
- uvula K12.2
- vermiform appendix K35.33
- vulvovaginal gland N75.1
- wound T81.49

Absence (of) (organ or part) (complete or partial)
- albumin in blood E88.09
- alimentary tract (congenital) Q45.8
  - upper Q40.8
- anus (congenital) Q42.3
  - with fistula Q42.2
- aorta (congenital) Q25.41
- appendix, congenital Q42.8

Absence, *continued*
- artery (congenital) (peripheral) Q27.8
  - pulmonary Q25.79
  - umbilical Q27.0
- atrial septum (congenital) Q21.1
- auditory canal (congenital) (external) Q16.1
- auricle (ear), congenital Q16.0
- bile, biliary duct, congenital Q44.5
- canaliculus lacrimalis, congenital Q10.4
- cervix (with uterus) congenital Q51.5
- cilia (congenital) Q10.3
- corpus callosum Q04.0
- digestive organ(s) or tract, congenital Q45.8
  - acquired NEC Z90.49
  - upper Q40.8
- ear, congenital Q16.9
  - acquired H93.8-
  - auricle Q16.0
  - external Q16.0
  - inner Q16.5
  - lobe, lobule Q17.8
  - middle, except ossicles Q16.4
    - ossicles Q16.3
- endocrine gland (congenital) NEC Q89.2
  - acquired E89.89
- eustachian tube (congenital) Q16.2
- eye (acquired)
  - congenital Q11.1
  - muscle (congenital) Q10.3
- eyelid (fold) (congenital) Q10.3
- family member (causing problem in home) NEC (*see also* Disruption, family) Z63.32
- fibrinogen (congenital) D68.2
  - acquired D65
- gallbladder (acquired) Z90.49
  - congenital Q44.0
- gamma globulin in blood D80.1
  - hereditary D80.0
- genital organs
  - acquired (female) (male) Z90.79
  - female, congenital Q52.8
    - external Q52.71
    - internal NEC Q52.8
  - male, congenital Q55.8
- genitourinary organs, congenital NEC
  - female Q52.8
  - male Q55.8
- ileum (acquired) Z90.49
  - congenital Q41.2
- incus (acquired)
  - congenital Q16.3
- inner ear, congenital Q16.5
- intestine (acquired) (small) Z90.49
  - congenital Q41.9
    - specified NEC Q41.8
  - large Z90.49
    - congenital Q42.9
      - specified NEC Q42.8
- iris, congenital Q13.1
- jejunum (acquired) Z90.49
  - congenital Q41.1
- kidney(s) (acquired) Z90.5
  - congenital
    - bilateral Q60.1
    - unilateral Q60.0
- labyrinth, membranous Q16.5
- lens (acquired)—*see also* Aphakia
  - congenital Q12.3
- muscle (congenital) (pectoral) Q79.8
  - ocular Q10.3
- organ
  - or site, congenital NEC Q89.8
    - acquired NEC Z90.89
- osseous meatus (ear) Q16.4
- parathyroid gland (acquired) E89.2
  - congenital Q89.2
- pituitary gland (congenital) Q89.2
  - acquired E89.3
- punctum lacrimale (congenital) Q10.4
- rectum (congenital) Q42.1
  - with fistula Q42.0
  - acquired Z90.49
- respiratory organ NOS Q34.9

Absence, *continued*
- scrotum, congenital Q55.29
- septum
  - atrial (congenital) Q21.1
- skull bone (congenital) Q75.8
  - with
    - anencephaly Q00.0
    - encephalocele—*see* Encephalocele
    - hydrocephalus Q03.9
      - with spina bifida—*see* Spina bifida, by site, with hydrocephalus
    - microcephaly Q02
- teeth, tooth (congenital) K00.0
  - acquired (complete) K08.109
    - class I K08.101
    - class II K08.102
    - class III K08.103
    - class IV K08.104
    - due to
      - caries K08.139
        - class I K08.131
        - class II K08.132
        - class III K08.133
        - class IV K08.134
      - periodontal disease K08.129
        - class I K08.121
        - class II K08.122
        - class III K08.123
        - class IV K08.124
      - specified NEC K08.199
        - class I K08.191
        - class II K08.192
        - class III K08.193
        - class IV K08.194
      - trauma K08.119
        - class I K08.111
        - class II K08.112
        - class III K08.113
        - class IV K08.114
    - partial K08.409
      - class I K08.401
      - class II K08.402
      - class III K08.403
      - class IV K08.404
      - due to
        - caries K08.439
          - class I K08.431
          - class II K08.432
          - class III K08.433
          - class IV K08.434
        - periodontal disease K08.429
          - class I K08.421
          - class II K08.422
          - class III K08.423
          - class IV K08.424
        - specified NEC K08.499
          - class I K08.491
          - class II K08.492
          - class III K08.493
          - class IV K08.494
        - trauma K08.419
          - class I K08.411
          - class II K08.412
          - class III K08.413
          - class IV K08.414
- testes (congenital) Q55.0
  - acquired Z90.79
- thymus gland Q89.2
- thyroid (gland) (acquired) E89.0
  - cartilage, congenital Q31.8
  - congenital E03.1
  - tricuspid valve Q22.4
- transverse aortic arch, congenital Q25.49
- umbilical artery, congenital Q27.0
- uterus congenital Q51.0

Absorption
- carbohydrate, disturbance K90.49
- chemical—*see* Table of Drugs and Chemicals
  - through placenta (newborn) P04.9
    - environmental substance P04.6
    - nutritional substance P04.5
    - obstetric anesthetic or analgesic drug P04.0

Absorption, *continued*
- drug NEC—*see* Table of Drugs and Chemicals
  - addictive
    - through placenta (newborn) (*see also* newborn, affected by, maternal use of) P04.40
      - ~ cocaine P04.41
      - ~ hallucinogens P04.42
      - ~ specified drug NEC P04.49
  - medicinal
    - through placenta (newborn) P04.19
  - through placenta (newborn) P04.19
    - obstetric anesthetic or analgesic drug P04.0
- fat, disturbance K90.49
  - pancreatic K90.3
- noxious substance—*see* Table of Drugs and Chemicals
- protein, disturbance K90.49
- starch, disturbance K90.49
- toxic substance—*see* Table of Drugs and Chemicals

Abstinence symptoms, syndrome
- alcohol F10.239
- cocaine F14.23
- neonatal P96.1
- nicotine—*see* Dependence, drug, nicotine
- stimulant NEC F15.93
  - with dependence F15.23

Abuse
- alcohol (nondependent) F10.10
  - in remission (early) (sustained) F10.11
  - with
    - intoxication F10.129
      - ~ with delirium F10.121
      - ~ uncomplicated F10.120
    - withdrawal F10.139
      - ~ with
        - ◊ perceptual disturbance F10.132
      - delirium F10.131
      - uncomplicated F10.130
  - counseling and surveillance Z71.41
- amphetamine (or related substance)—*see also* Abuse, drug, stimulant NEC
  - stimulant NEC F15.10
    - with
      - ~ intoxication F15.129
        - ◊ with
          - » delirium F15.121
          - » perceptual disturbance F15.122
- analgesics (non-prescribed) (over the counter) F55.8
- antacids F55.0
- anxiolytic—*see* Abuse, drug, sedative
- barbiturates—*see* Abuse, drug, sedative
- caffeine—*see* Abuse, drug, stimulant NEC
- cannabis, cannabinoids—*see* Abuse, drug, cannabis
- child—*see* Maltreatment, child
- cocaine—*see* Abuse, drug, cocaine
- drug NEC (nondependent) F19.10
  - amphetamine type—*see* Abuse, drug, stimulant NEC
  - anxiolytics—*see* Abuse, drug, sedative
  - barbiturates—*see* Abuse, drug, sedative
  - caffeine—*see* Abuse, drug, stimulant NEC
  - cannabis F12.10
    - in remission (early) (sustained) F12.11
  - cocaine F14.10
    - in remission (early) (sustained) F14.11
    - with
      - ~ intoxication F14.129
        - ◊ uncomplicated F14.120
  - counseling and surveillance Z71.51
  - herbal or folk remedies F55.1
  - hormones F55.3
  - hashish—*see* Abuse, drug, cannabis
  - inhalant F18.10
    - in remission (early) (sustained) F18.11
  - laxatives F55.2
  - opioid F11.10
    - in remission (early) (sustained) F11.11
  - PCP (phencyclidine) (or related substance)—*see* Abuse, drug, hallucinogen
  - psychoactive NEC F19.10
  - sedative, hypnotic, or anxiolytic F13.10
    - in remission (early) (sustained) F13.11
  - solvent—*see* Abuse, drug, inhalant
  - steroids F55.3

Abuse, *continued*
- stimulant NEC F15.10
  - in remission (early) (sustained) F15.11
  - with
    - intoxication F15.129
      - ◊ uncomplicated F15.120
      - ◊ vitamins F55.4
- hallucinogens F16.1-
- hashish—*see* Abuse, drug, cannabis
- herbal or folk remedies F55.1
- hormones F55.3
- inhalant F18.1-
- laxatives F55.2
- marijuana—*see* Abuse, drug, cannabis
- PCP (phencyclidine) (or related substance) F16.1-
- physical (adult) (child)—*see* Maltreatment
- psychoactive substance F19.1-
- psychological (adult) (child)—*see* Maltreatment
- sexual—*see* Maltreatment
- solvent—*see* Abuse, drug, inhalant

Acalculia R48.8
- developmental F81.2

Acanthamebiasis (with) B60.10
- conjunctiva B60.12
- keratoconjunctivitis B60.13
- meningoencephalitis B60.11
- other specified B60.19

Acanthosis (acquired) (nigricans) L83
- benign Q82.8
- congenital Q82.8
- seborrheic L82.1
  - inflamed L82.0
- tongue K14.3

Acardia, acardius Q89.8

Acardiacus amorphus Q89.8

Acariasis B88.0
- scabies B86

Acarodermatitis (urticarioides) B88.0

Acathisia (drug induced) G25.71

Accelerated atrioventricular conduction I45.6

Accessory (congenital)
- atrioventricular conduction I45.6
- auditory ossicles Q16.3
- biliary duct or passage Q44.5
- carpal bones Q74.0
- cusp
  - pulmonary Q22.3
- cystic duct Q44.5
- endocrine gland NEC Q89.2
- eye muscle Q10.3
- eyelid Q10.3
- face bone(s) Q75.8
- finger(s) Q69.0
- foreskin N47.8
- frontonasal process Q75.8
- gallbladder Q44.1
- genital organ(s)
  - female Q52.8
    - external Q52.79
    - internal NEC Q52.8
  - male Q55.8
- genitourinary organs NEC Q89.8
  - female Q52.8
  - male Q55.8
- hallux Q69.2
- heart Q24.8
  - valve, NEC Q24.8
    - pulmonary Q22.3
- hepatic ducts Q44.5
- lacrimal canal Q10.6
- liver Q44.7
  - duct Q44.5
- navicular of carpus Q74.0
- nipple Q83.3
- parathyroid gland Q89.2
- pituitary gland Q89.2
- prepuce N47.8
- sesamoid bones Q74.8
  - foot Q74.2
  - hand Q74.0

Accessory, *continued*
- skin tags Q82.8
- tarsal bones Q74.2
- thumb Q69.1
- thymus gland Q89.2
- thyroid gland Q89.2
- toes Q69.2
- uterus Q51.28
- valve, heart
  - pulmonary Q22.3

See also the *ICD-10-CM* External Cause of Injuries Table for codes describing accident details.

Accident
- birth—*see* Birth, injury
- cerebrovascular (embolic) (ischemic) (thrombotic) I63.9
  - old (without sequelae) Z86.73

Accretio cordis (nonrheumatic) I31.0

Acculturation difficulty Z60.3

Acephalobrachia monster Q89.8

Acephalochirus monster Q89.8

Acephalogaster Q89.8

Acephalostomus monster Q89.8

Acephalothorax Q89.8

Acetonemia R79.89
- in Type 1 diabetes E10.10
  - with coma E10.11

Achalasia (cardia) (esophagus) K22.0
- congenital Q39.5
- pylorus Q40.0

Achlorhydria, achlorhydric (neurogenic) K31.83
- anemia D50.8
- psychogenic F45.8

Achroma, cutis L80

Achromia parasitica B36.0

Achondrogenesis Q77.0

Achondroplasia (osteosclerosis congenita) Q77.4

Achylia gastrica K31.89
- psychogenic F45.8

Acid
- peptic disease K30
- stomach K30
  - psychogenic F45.8

Acidemia E87.2
- metabolic (newborn) P19.9
  - first noted before onset of labor P19.0
  - first noted during labor P19.1
  - noted at birth P19.2

Acidity, gastric (high) K30
- psychogenic F45.8

Acidocytopenia—*see* Agranulocytosis

Acidocytosis D72.10

Acidosis (lactic) (respiratory) E87.2
- in Type 1 diabetes E10.10
  - with coma E10.11
- metabolic NEC E87.2
  - hyperchlorimic, of newborn P74.421
- mixed metabolic and respiratory, newborn P84
- newborn P84

Aciduria
- 4-hydroxybutyric E72.81
- gamma-hydroxybutyric E72.81
- glutaric (type I)
  - type II E71.313
  - type III E71.5-

Acladiosis (skin) B36.0

Acleistocardia Q21.1

Acne L70.9
- artificialis L70.8
- atrophica L70.2
- cachecticorum (Hebra) L70.8
- conglobata L70.1
- cystic L70.0
- excoriée des jeunes filles L70.5
- frontalis L70.2
- indurata L70.0
- infantile L70.4

Acne, *continued*
- lupoid L70.2
- necrotic, necrotica (miliaris) L70.2
- neonatal L70.4
- nodular L70.0
- occupational L70.8
- picker's L70.5
- pustular L70.0
- rodens L70.2
- specified NEC L70.8
- tropica L70.3
- varioliformis L70.2
- vulgaris L70.0

Acquired—*see also* Disease, diseased
- immunodeficiency syndrome (AIDS) B20

Acroasphyxia, chronic I73.89

Acrocephalopolysyndactyly Q87.0

Acrocephalosyndactyly Q87.0

Acrochondrohyperplasia—*see* Syndrome, Marfan's

Acrocyanosis I73.89
- newborn P28.2
  - meaning transient blue hands and feet—omit code

Acrodermatitis
- infantile papular L44.4

Acromegaly, acromegalia E22.0

Acronyx L60.0

Acroparesthesia (simple) (vasomotor) I73.89

Action, heart
- disorder I49.9
- irregular I49.9
  - psychogenic F45.8

Activation
- mast cell (disorder) (syndrome) D89.40
  - idiopathic D89.42
  - monoclonal D89.41
  - secondary D89.43
  - specified type NEC D89.49

Active—*see* Disease, diseased

Acute—*see also* Disease, diseased
- abdomen R10.0
- gallbladder—*see* Cholecystitis, acute

Acyanotic heart disease (congenital) Q24.9

Adair-Dighton syndrome (brittle bones and blue sclera, deafness) Q78.0

Adamantinoma
- long bones C40.9-
  - lower limb C40.2-
  - upper limb C40.0-
- malignant C41.1
  - jaw (bone) (lower) C41.1
    - upper C41.0
- tibial C40.2-

Adams-Stokes (-Morgagni) disease or syndrome I45.9

Adaption reaction—*see* Disorder, adjustment

Addiction (*see also* Dependence) F19.20
- alcohol, alcoholic (ethyl) (methyl) (wood) (without remission) F10.20
  - with remission F10.21
- drug—*see* Dependence, drug
- ethyl alcohol (without remission) F10.20
  - with remission F10.21
- ethyl alcohol (without remission) F10.20
  - with remission F10.21
- methylated spirit (without remission) F10.20
  - with remission F10.21
- tobacco—*see* Dependence, drug, nicotine

Addisonian crisis E27.2

Addison's
- anemia (pernicious) D51.0
- disease (bronze) or syndrome E27.1

Addison-Schilder complex E71.528

Additional—*see also* Accessory
- chromosome(s) Q99.8
  - sex—*see* Abnormal, chromosome, sex
  - 21—*see* Trisomy, 21

Adduction contracture, hip or other joint—*see* Contraction, joint

Adenitis—*see also* lymphadenitis
- acute, unspecified site L04.9
- axillary I88.9
  - acute L04.2
  - chronic or subacute I88.1
- cervical I88.9
  - acute L04.0
  - chronic or subacute I88.1
- chronic, unspecified site I88.1
- due to Pasteurella multocida (p. septica) A28.0
- gangrenous L04.9
- groin I88.9
  - acute L04.1
  - chronic or subacute I88.1
- inguinal I88.9
  - acute L04.1
  - chronic or subacute I88.1
- lymph gland or node, except mesenteric I88.9
  - acute—*see* Lymphadenitis, acute
  - chronic or subacute I88.1
- mesenteric (acute) (chronic) (nonspecific) (subacute) I88.0
- scrofulous (tuberculous) A18.2
- strumous, tuberculous A18.2
- subacute, unspecified site I88.1

Adenocarcinoma—*see also* Neoplasm, malignant, by site in Table of Neoplasms in the complete *ICD-10-CM* manual
- renal cell C64-

Adenoiditis (chronic) J35.02
- with tonsillitis J35.03
- acute J03.90
  - recurrent J03.91
  - specified organism NEC J03.80
    - recurrent J03.81
  - staphylococcal J03.80
    - recurrent J03.81
  - streptococcal J03.00
    - recurrent J03.01

Adenoma—*see also* Neoplasm, benign, by site in Table of Neoplasms in the complete *ICD-10-CM* manual
- apocrine
  - breast D24-
  - specified site NEC—*see* Neoplasm, skin, benign, by site in Table of Neoplasms in the complete *ICD-10-CM* manual
  - unspecified site D23.9
- ceruminous D23.2-

Adenomatosis
- endocrine (multiple) E31.20
  - single specified site—*see* Neoplasm, uncertain behavior, by site in Table of Neoplasms in the complete *ICD-10-CM* manual
- specified site—*see* Neoplasm, benign, by site in Table of Neoplasms in the complete *ICD-10-CM* manual
- unspecified site D12.6

Adenomatous
- goiter (nontoxic) E04.9
  - with hyperthyroidism—*see* Hyperthyroidism, with, goiter
  - toxic—*see* Hyperthyroidism, with, goiter

Adenopathy (lymph gland) R59.9
- generalized R59.1

Adenosclerosis I88.8

Adenovirus, as cause of disease classified elsewhere B97.0

Adherent—*see also* Adhesions
- labia (minora) N90.89
- pericardium (nonrheumatic) I31.0
  - rheumatic I09.2
- scar (skin) L90.5
- tendon in scar L90.5

Adhesions, adhesive (postinfective)
- cardiac I31.0
  - rheumatic I09.2
- cervicovaginal N88.1
  - congenital Q52.8
- conjunctiva congenital Q15.8

Adhesions, adhesive, *continued*
- joint—*see* Ankylosis
  - temporomandibular M26.61-
- labium (majus) (minus), congenital Q52.5
- meninges (cerebral) (spinal) G96.12
  - congenital Q07.8
  - tuberculous (cerebral) (spinal) A17.0
- nasal (septum) (to turbinates) J34.89
- pericardium (nonrheumatic) I31.0
  - focal I31.8
  - rheumatic I09.2
- preputial, prepuce N47.5
- temporomandibular M26.61-
- vagina (chronic) N89.5

Adiponecrosis neonatorum P83.88

Adiposis—*see also* Obesity
- cerebralis E23.6
- adiposogenital dystrophy E23.6

Admission (for)—*see also* Encounter (for)
- aftercare (*see also* Aftercare) Z51.89
  - radiation therapy (antineoplastic) Z51.0
- attention to artificial opening (of) Z43.9
  - artificial vagina Z43.7
    - colostomy Z43.3
    - cystostomy Z43.5
    - enterostomy Z43.4
    - gastrostomy Z43.1
    - ileostomy Z43.2
    - jejunostomy Z43.4
    - nephrostomy Z43.6
    - specified site NEC Z43.8
      - ~ intestinal tract Z43.4
      - ~ urinary tract Z43.6
    - tracheostomy Z43.0
    - ureterostomy Z43.6
    - urethrostomy Z43.6
- change of
  - dressing (nonsurgical) Z48.00
  - surgical dressing Z48.01
- circumcision, ritual or routine (in absence of diagnosis) Z41.2
- counseling—*see also* Counseling
  - dietary Z71.3
  - HIV Z71.7
  - human immunodeficiency virus Z71.7
  - non-attending third party Z71.0
  - procreative management NEC Z31.69
  - travel Z71.84
- desensitization to allergens Z51.6
- dietary surveillance and counseling Z71.3
- ear piercing Z41.3
- examination at health care facility (adult) (*see also* Examination) Z00.00
  - with abnormal findings Z00.01
  - ear Z01.10
    - with abnormal findings NEC Z01.118
  - eye Z01.00
    - with abnormal findings Z01.01
    - after failed exam Z01.02-
  - hearing Z01.10
    - infant or child (over 28 days old) Z00.129
      - ~ with abnormal findings Z00.121
    - with abnormal findings NEC Z01.118
  - vision Z01.00
    - infant or child (over 28 days old) Z00.129
      - ~ with abnormal findings Z00.121
    - with abnormal findings Z01.01
    - after failed exam Z01.02-
- followup examination Z09
- intrauterine device management Z30.431
  - initial prescription Z30.014
- prophylactic (measure)—*see also* Encounter, prophylactic measure
  - vaccination Z23
- radiation therapy (antineoplastic) Z51.0
- removal of
  - dressing (nonsurgical) Z48.00
  - implantable subdermal contraceptive Z30.46
  - intrauterine contraceptive device Z30.432
  - staples Z48.02
  - surgical dressing Z48.01
  - sutures Z48.02

Admission (for), *continued*
- sensitivity test—*see also* Test, skin
  – allergy NEC Z01.82
  – Mantoux Z11.1
- vision examination Z01.00
  – with abnormal findings Z01.01
  – after failed exam Z01.02-

Adolescent X-linked adrenoleukodystrophy E71.521

Adrenal (gland)—*see* Disease, diseased

Adrenalitis, adrenitis E27.8
- autoimmune E27.1

Adrenogenital syndrome E25.9
- congenital E25.0
- salt loss E25.0

Adrenogenitalism, congenital E25.0

Adrenoleukodystrophy E71.529
- neonatal E71.511
- Xlinked E71.529
  – Addison only phenotype E71.528
  – Addison-Schilder E71.528
  – adolescent E71.521
  – adrenomyeloneuropathy E71.522
  – childhood cerebral E71.520
  – other specified E71.528

Adrenomyeloneuropathy E71.522

Adverse effect—*see* Table of Drugs and Chemicals, categories T36 – T50, with 6th character 5

Aerodermectasia
- subcutaneous (traumatic) T79.7

Aerophagy, aerophagia (psychogenic) F45.8

Afibrinogenemia (*see also* Defect, coagulation) D68.8
- acquired D65
- congenital D68.2

Aftercare (*see also* Care) Z51.89
- following surgery (for) (on)
  – attention to
    ▪ dressings (nonsurgical) Z48.00
      ~ surgical Z48.01
    ▪ sutures Z48.02
  – circulatory system Z48.812
  – digestive system Z48.815
  – genitourinary system Z48.816
  – nervous system Z48.811
  – oral cavity Z48.814—respiratory system Z48.813
  – sense organs Z48.810
  – skin and subcutaneous tissue Z48.817
  – specified body system
    ▪ circulatory Z48.812
    ▪ digestive Z48.815
    ▪ genitourinary Z48.816
    ▪ nervous Z48.811
    ▪ oral cavity Z48.814
    ▪ respiratory Z48.813
    ▪ sense organs Z48.810
    ▪ skin and subcutaneous tissue Z48.817
    ▪ teeth Z48.814
  – spinal Z47.89
  – teeth Z48.814
- fracture *code to* fracture with seventh character D
- involving
  – removal of
    ▪ dressings (nonsurgical) Z48.00
    ▪ staples Z48.02
    ▪ surgical dressings Z48.01
    ▪ sutures Z48.02

Agammaglobulinemia (acquired) (secondary) (nonfamilial) D80.1
- with
  – immunoglobulin-bearing B-lymphocytes D80.1
  – lymphopenia D81.9
- common variable (CVAgamma) D80.1
- lymphopenic D81.9

Aganglionosis (bowel) (colon) Q43.1

Agenesis
- alimentary tract (complete) (partial) NEC Q45.8
  – upper Q40.8
- anus, anal (canal) Q42.3
  – with fistula Q42.2
- aorta Q25.41

Agenesis, *continued*
- appendix Q42.8
- artery (peripheral) Q27.9
  – pulmonary Q25.79
  – umbilical Q27.0
- auditory (canal) (external) Q16.1
- auricle (ear) Q16.0
- bile duct or passage Q44.5
- bone Q79.9
- breast (with nipple present) Q83.8
  – with absent nipple Q83.0
- canaliculus lacrimalis Q10.4
- cartilage Q79.9
- cecum Q42.8
- cervix Q51.5
- cilia Q10.3
- clavicle Q74.0
- colon Q42.9
  – specified NEC Q42.8
- corpus callosum Q04.0
- digestive organ(s) or tract (complete) (partial) NEC Q45.8
  – upper Q40.8
- ear Q16.9
  – auricle Q16.0
  – lobe Q17.8
- endocrine (gland) NEC Q89.2
- eustachian tube Q16.2
- eye Q11.1
  – adnexa Q15.8
- eyelid (fold) Q10.3
- face
  – bones NEC Q75.8
- gallbladder Q44.0
- heart Q24.8
  – valve, NEC Q24.8
    ▪ pulmonary Q22.0
- intestine (small) Q41.9
  – large Q42.9
    ▪ specified NEC Q42.8
- iris (dilator fibers) Q13.1
- genitalia, genital (organ(s))
  – female Q52.8
    ▪ external Q52.71
    ▪ internal NEC Q52.8
  – male Q55.8
- incus Q16.3
- labyrinth, membranous Q16.5
- lacrimal apparatus Q10.4
- lens Q12.3
- muscle Q79.8
  – eyelid Q10.3
  – ocular Q15.8
- parathyroid (gland) Q89.2
- pelvic girdle (complete) (partial) Q74.2
- pituitary (gland) Q89.2
- punctum lacrimale Q10.4
- rectum Q42.1
  – with fistula Q42.0
- roof of orbit Q75.8
- round ligament Q52.8
- scapula Q74.0
- scrotum Q55.29
- septum
  – atrial Q21.1
- shoulder girdle (complete) (partial) Q74.0
- skull (bone) Q75.8
  – with
    ▪ anencephaly Q00.0
    ▪ encephalocele—*see* Encephalocele
    ▪ hydrocephalus Q03.9
      ~ with spina bifida—*see* Spina bifida, by site, with hydrocephalus
    ▪ microcephaly Q02
- spinal cord Q06.0
- testicle Q55.0
- thymus (gland) Q89.2
- thyroid (gland) E03.1
  – cartilage Q31.8
  – uterus Q51.0

Aglossia-adactylia syndrome Q87.0

Agnosia (body image) (other senses) (tactile) R48.1
- developmental F88

Agnosia, *continued*
- verbal R48.1
  – auditory R48.1
    ▪ developmental F80.2
  – developmental F80.2

Agranulocytosis (chronic) (cyclical) (genetic) (infantile) (periodic) (pernicious) (*see also* Neutropenia) D70.9
- congenital D70.0
- cytoreductive cancer chemotherapy sequela D70.1
- drug-induced D70.2
  – due to cytoreductive cancer chemotherapy D70.1
- due to infection D70.3
- secondary D70.4
  – drug-induced D70.2
    ▪ due to cytoreductive cancer chemotherapy D70.1

Agraphia (absolute) R48.8
- with alexia R48.0
- developmental F81.81

Ague (dumb)—*see* Malaria

Ahumada-del Castillo syndrome E23.0

AIDS (related complex) B20

AIPHI (acute idiopathic pulmonary hemorrhage in infants (over 28 days old)) R04.81

Air
- anterior mediastinum J98.2
- hunger, psychogenic F45.8
- sickness T75.3

Airplane sickness T75.3

Akathisia (drug-induced) (treatment-induced) G25.71
- neuroleptic induced (acute) G25.71

Alactasia, congenital E73.0

Albuminuria, albuminuric (acute) (chronic) (subacute) (*see also* Proteinuria) R80.9
- orthostatic R80.2
- postural R80.2
- scarlatinal A38.8

Alcohol, alcoholic, alcohol-induced
- addiction (without remission) F10.20
  – with remission F10.21
- counseling and surveillance Z71.41
  – family member Z71.42
- intoxication (acute) (without dependence) F10.129
  – with
    ▪ delirium F10.121
    ▪ dependence F10.229
      ~ with delirium F10.221
      ~ uncomplicated F10.220
    ▪ uncomplicated F10.120

Alcoholism (chronic) (without remission) F10.20
- with
  – psychosis—*see* Psychosis
  – remission F10.21

Alder (-Reilly) anomaly or syndrome (leukocyte granulation) D72.0

Aldrich (-Wiskott) syndrome (eczema-thrombocytopenia) D82.0

Aleukia
- congenital D70.0
- hemorrhagica D61.9
  – congenital D61.09

Alexia R48.0
- developmental F81.0
- secondary to organic lesion R48.0

Alkalosis E87.3
- metabolic E87.3
  – of newborn P74.41

Allergy, allergic (reaction) (to) T78.40
- air-borne substance NEC (rhinitis) J30.89
- anaphylactic reaction or shock T78.2
- angioneurotic edema T78.3
- animal (dander) (epidermal) (hair) (rhinitis) J30.81
- bee sting (anaphylactic shock)—*see* Table of Drugs and Chemicals, by animal or substance, poisoning
- biological—*see* Allergy, drug
- colitis K52.29
  – food protein-induced K52.22
- dander (animal) (rhinitis) J30.81
- dandruff (rhinitis) J30.81

Allergy, allergic, *continued*
- desensitization to allergens, encounter for Z51.6
- drug, medicament & biological (any) (external) (internal) T78.40
  - correct substance properly administered—*see* Table of Drugs and Chemicals, by drug, adverse effect
  - wrong substance given or taken NEC (by accident)—*see* Table of Drugs and Chemicals, by drug, poisoning
- due to pollen J30.1
- dust (house) (stock) (rhinitis) J30.89
  - with asthma—*see* Asthma, allergic extrinsic
- eczema—*see* Dermatitis, contact, allergic
- epidermal (animal) (rhinitis) J30.81
- feathers (rhinitis) J30.89
- food (any) (ingested) NEC T78.1
  - anaphylactic shock—*see* Shock, anaphylactic, due to food
  - dermatitis—*see* Dermatitis, due to, food
  - dietary counseling and surveillance Z71.3
  - in contact with skin L23.6
  - rhinitis J30.5
  - status (without reaction) Z91.018
    - eggs Z91.012
    - milk products Z91.011
    - peanuts Z91.010
    - seafood Z91.013
    - specified NEC Z91.018
- gastrointestinal K52.29
  - food protein-induced K52.22
  - meaning colitis or gastroenteritis K52.59
  - meaning other adverse food reaction NEC T78.1
- grain J30.1
- grass (hay fever) (pollen) J30.1
  - asthma—*see* Asthma, allergic extrinsic
- hair (animal) (rhinitis) J30.81
- history (of)—*see* History, family of, allergy
- horse serum—*see* Allergy, serum
- inhalant (rhinitis) J30.89
  - pollen J30.1
- kapok (rhinitis) J30.89
- medicine—*see* Allergy, drug
- milk protein Z91.011
  - anaphylactic reaction T78.07
  - dermatitis L27.2
  - enterocolitis syndrome K52.21
  - enteropathy K52.22
  - gastroenteritis K52.29
  - gastroesophageal reflux (*see also* Reaction, adverse, food) K21.9
    - with esophagitis K21.0-
  - proctocolitis K52.82
  - nasal, seasonal due to pollen J30.1
- pollen (any) (hay fever) J30.1
  - asthma—*see* Asthma, allergic extrinsic
- primrose J30.1
- primula J30.1
- purpura D69.0
- ragweed (hay fever) (pollen) J30.1
  - asthma—*see* Asthma, allergic extrinsic
- rose (pollen) J30.1
- seasonal NEC J30.2
- Senecio jacobae (pollen) J30.1
- serum (*see also* Reaction, serum) T80.69
  - anaphylactic shock T80.59
- shock (anaphylactic) T78.2
  - due to
    - administration of blood and blood products T80.51
    - immunization T80.52
    - serum NEC T80.59
    - vaccination T80.52
- specific NEC T78.49
- tree (any) (hay fever) (pollen) J30.1
  - asthma—*see* Asthma, allergic extrinsic
- upper respiratory J30.9
- urticaria L50.0
- vaccine—*see* Allergy, serum
- wheat—*see* Allergy, food

Alopecia (hereditaria) (seborrheica) L65.9
- due to cytotoxic drugs NEC L65.8
- postinfective NEC L65.8
- specified NEC L65.8

Alport syndrome Q87.81

ALTE (apparent life threatening event) **in newborn and infant** R68.13

Alteration (of), Altered
- mental status R41.82
- pattern of family relationships affecting child Z62.898

Alymphocytosis D72.810
- thymic (with immunodeficiency) D82.1

Alymphoplasia, thymic D82.1

Amastia (with nipple present) Q83.8
- with absent nipple Q83.0

Amaurosis (acquired) (congenital)—*see also* Blindness
- hysterical F44.6
- Leber's congenital H35.50

Ambiguous genitalia Q56.4

Amblyopia (congenital) (ex anopsia) (partial) (suppression) H53.00-
- anisometropic—*see* Amblyopia
- hysterical F44.6
- suspect H53.04-

Amebiasis
- acute A06.0
- intestine A06.0

Ameloblastoma—*see also* Cyst
- long bones C40.9-
  - lower limb C40.2-
  - upper limb C40.0-
- malignant C41.1
  - jaw (bone) (lower) C41.1
    - upper C41.0
- tibial C40.2-

Amenorrhea N91.2

Amsterdam dwarfism Q87.19

Amyelia Q06.0

Amygdalitis—*see* Tonsillitis

Amygdalolith J35.8

Amyotonia M62.89
- congenita G70.2

Anacidity, gastric K31.83
- psychogenic F45.8

Anaerosis of newborn P28.89

Analbuminemia E88.09

Anaphylactic
- purpura D69.0
- shock or reaction—*see* Shock, anaphylactic

Anaphylactoid shock or reaction—*see* Shock, anaphylactic

Anaphylaxis—*see* Shock, anaphylactic

Anarthria R47.1

Anasarca R60.1
- renal N04.9

Anastomosis
- arteriovenous ruptured brain I60.8-
  - intracerebral I61.8
  - intraparenchymal I61.8
  - intraventricular I61.5
  - subarachnoid I60.8-

Android pelvis Q74.2

Anemia (essential) (general) (hemoglobin deficiency) (infantile) (primary) (profound) D64.9
- achlorhydric D50.8
- aplastic D61.9
  - congenital D61.09
  - drug-induced D61.1
  - due to
    - drugs D61.1
    - external agents NEC D61.2
    - infection D61.2
    - radiation D61.2
    - red cell (pure) D60.9
      - ~ chronic D60.0
      - ~ specified type NEC D60.8
      - ~ transient D60.1
  - idiopathic D61.3
  - red cell (pure) D60.9
    - chronic D60.0
    - congenital D61.01

Anemia, *continued*
- specified type NEC D61.89
- toxic D61.2
- aregenerative
  - congenital D61.09
- atypical D64.9
- Baghdad spring D55.0
- blood loss (chronic) D50.0
  - acute D62
- chlorotic D50.8
- chronic
  - hemolytic D58.9
    - idiopathic D59.9
- chronica congenita aregenerativa D61.09
- congenital P61.4
  - aplastic D61.09
  - Heinz body D58.2
  - spherocytic D58.0
- Cooley's (erythroblastic) D56.1
- deficiency D53.9
  - enzyme D55.9
    - drug-induced (hemolytic) D59.2
    - glucose-6-phosphate dehydrogenase (G6PD) with anemia D55.0
  - folate D52.9
    - dietary D52.0
    - drug-induced D52.1
  - folic acid D52.9
    - dietary D52.0
    - drug-induced D52.1
  - glucose-6-phosphate dehydrogenase
    - with anemia D55.0
  - G6PD with anemia D55.0
  - nutritional D53.9
    - with
      - ~ poor iron absorption D50.8
- Diamond-Blackfan (congenital hypoplastic) D61.01
- due to (in) (with)
  - antineoplastic chemotherapy D64.81
  - blood loss (chronic) D50.0
    - acute D62
  - chemotherapy, antineoplastic D64.81
  - chronic disease classified elsewhere NEC D63.8
  - chronic kidney disease D63.1
  - end stage renal disease D63.1
  - hemorrhage (chronic) D50.0
    - acute D62
  - loss of blood (chronic) D50.0
    - acute D62
  - myxedema E03.9 *[D63.8]*
  - prematurity P61.2
- Dyke-Young type (secondary) (symptomatic) D59.19
- enzyme-deficiency, drug-induced D59.2
- erythroblastic
  - familial D56.1
  - newborn (*see also* Disease, hemolytic) P55.9
  - of childhood D56.1
- erythropoietin-resistant anemia (EPO resistant anemia) D63.1
- familial erythroblastic D56.1
- Fanconi's (congenital pancytopenia) D61.09
- favism D55.0
- glucose-6-phosphate dehydrogenase (G6PD) deficiency D55.0
  - with anemia D55.0
  - without anemia D75.A
- Heinz body, congenital D58.2
- hemolytic D58.9
  - acquired D59.9
    - autoimmune NEC D59.19
      - ~ acute D59.9
      - ~ Lederer's D59.19
  - autoimmune D59.10
    - cold D59.12
    - mixed D59.13
    - warm D59.11
  - cold type (primary) (secondary) (symptomatic) D59.12
  - mixed type (primary) (secondary) (symptomatic) D59.13

Anemia, *continued*
- nonspherocytic
  - congenital or hereditary NEC D55.8
    - ~ glucose-6-phosphate dehydrogenase deficiency with anemia D55.0
    - ~ glucose-6-phosphate dehydrogenase deficiency without anemia D75.A
  - primary
    - autoimmune
      - ~ cold type D59.12
      - ~ mixed type D59.13
      - ~ warm type D59.11
  - secondary D59.4
    - autoimmune D59.1
    - autoimmune
    - cold type D59.12
    - mixed type D59.13
    - warm type D59.11
    - autoimmune
      - ~ cold type D59.12
      - ~ mixed type D59.13
      - ~ warm type D59.11
  - warm type (primary) (secondary) (symptomatic) D59.11
- hemorrhagic (chronic) D50.0
  - acute D62
- Herrick's D57.1
- hookworm B76.9 [D63.8]
- hypochromic (idiopathic) (microcytic) (normoblastic) D50.9
  - due to blood loss (chronic) D50.0
    - acute D62
- hypoplasia, red blood cells D61.9
  - congenital or familial D61.01
- hypoplastic (idiopathic) D61.9
  - congenital or familial (of childhood) D61.01
- hypoproliferative (refractive) D61.9
- idiopathic D64.9
- iron deficiency D50.9
  - secondary to blood loss (chronic) D50.0
    - acute D62
  - specified type NEC D50.8
- Joseph-Diamond-Blackfan (congenital hypoplastic) D61.01
- leukoerythroblastic D61.82
- malarial (*see also* Malaria) B54 [D63.8]
- marsh (*see also* Malaria) B54 [D63.8]
- Mediterranean (with other hemoglobinopathy) D56.9
- microcytic (hypochromic) D50.9
  - due to blood loss (chronic) D50.0
    - acute D62
  - familial D56.8
- microdrepanocytosis D57.40
- microelliptopoikilocytic (RiettiGreppi Micheli) D56.9
- myelofibrosis D75.81
- myelophthisic D61.82
- myeloproliferative D47.Z9
- newborn P61.4
  - due to
    - ABO (antibodies, isoimmunization, maternal/fetal incompatibility) P55.1
    - Rh (antibodies, isoimmunization, maternal/fetal incompatibility) P55.0
  - following fetal blood loss P61.3
  - posthemorrhagic (fetal) P61.3
- normocytic (infectional) D64.9
  - due to blood loss (chronic) D50.0
    - acute D62
  - myelophthisic D61.82
- nutritional (deficiency) D53.9
  - with
    - poor iron absorption D50.8
- of prematurity P61.2
- paludal (*see also* Malaria) B54 [D63.8]
- posthemorrhagic (chronic) D50.0
  - acute D62
  - newborn P61.3
- postoperative (postprocedural)
  - due to (acute) blood loss D62
    - chronic blood loss D50.0
  - specified NEC D64.9

Anemia, *continued*
- progressive D64.9
  - malignant D51.0
  - pernicious D51.0
- pure red cell D60.9
  - congenital D61.01
- Rietti-Greppi-Micheli D56.9
- secondary to
  - blood loss (chronic) D50.0
    - acute D62
  - hemorrhage (chronic) D50.0
    - acute D62
- semiplastic D61.89
- sickle-cell—*see* Disease, sickle-cell
- sideropenic (refractory) D50.9
  - due to blood loss (chronic) D50.0
    - acute D62
- syphilitic (acquired) (late) A52.79 [D63.8]
- thalassemia D56.9
- thrombocytopenic—*see* Thrombocytopenia
- toxic D61.2
- tuberculous A18.89 [D63.8]
- Witts' (achlorhydric anemia) D50.8

Anesthesia, anesthetic R20.0
- dissociative F44.6
- functional (hysterical) F44.6
- hysterical F44.6
- testicular N50.9

Aneurysm (anastomotic) (artery) (cirsoid) (diffuse) (false) (fusiform) (multiple) (saccular)
- aorta, aortic (nonsyphilitic) I71.9
  - congenital Q25.4
  - root Q25.43
  - sinus Q25.43
  - valve (heart) (*see also* Endocarditis, aortic) I35.8
- arteriovenous (congenital)—*see also* Malformation, arteriovenous
  - brain Q28.2
    - ruptured I60.8-
      - ~ intracerebral I61.8
      - ~ intraparenchymal I61.8
      - ~ intraventricular I61.5
      - ~ subarachnoid I60.8-
- berry (congenital) (nonruptured) I67.1
  - ruptured I60.7
- brain I67.1
  - arteriovenous (congenital) (nonruptured) Q28.2
    - acquired I67.1
      - ~ ruptured I60.8-
    - ruptured I60.8-
  - berry (congenital) (nonruptured) I67.1
    - ruptured (*see also* Hemorrhage, intracranial, subarachnoid) I60.7
  - congenital Q28.3
    - ruptured I60.7
  - meninges I67.1
    - ruptured I60.8-
  - miliary (congenital) (nonruptured) I67.1
    - ruptured (*see also* Hemorrhage, intracranial, subarachnoid) I60.7
  - mycotic I33.0ruptured into brain I60.0-
- cavernous sinus I67.1
  - arteriovenous (congenital) (nonruptured) Q28.3
    - ruptured I60.8-
- circle of Willis I67.1
  - congenital Q28.3
    - ruptured I60.6
  - ruptured I60.6
- congenital (peripheral) Q27.8
  - brain Q28.3
    - ruptured I60.7
  - pulmonary Q25.79
- ductus arteriosus Q25.0
- endocardial, infective (any valve) I33.0
- infective
  - endocardial (any valve) I33.0
- mycotic
  - endocardial (any valve) I33.0
  - ruptured, brain—*see* Hemorrhage, intracerebral, subarachnoid
- patent ductus arteriosus Q25.0

Aneurysm, *continued*
- pulmonary I28.1
  - arteriovenous Q25.72
- tricuspid (heart) (valve) I07.8

Angelman syndrome Q93.51

Anger R45.4

Angina (attack) (cardiac) (chest) (heart) (pectoris) (syndrome) (vasomotor) I20.9
- aphthous B08.5
- croupous J05.0
- exudative, chronic J37.0
- Ludovici K12.2
- Ludwig's K12.2
- membranous J05.0
- monocytic—*see* Mononucleosis, infectious
- phlegmonous J36
- tonsil J36
- trachealis J05.0

Angioedema (allergic) (any site) (with urticaria) T78.3
- episodic, with eosinophilia D72.118

Angioendothelioma—*see* Neoplasm, uncertain behavior, by site in Table of Neoplasms in the complete *ICD-10-CM* manual
- benign D18.00
  - skin D18.01
  - specified site NEC D18.09
- bone—*see* Neoplasm, bone, malignant in Table of Neoplasms in the complete *ICD-10-CM* manual
- Ewing's—*see* Neoplasm, bone, malignant in Table of Neoplasms in the complete *ICD-10-CM* manual

Angiohemophilia (A) (B) D68.0

Angioma—*see also* Hemangioma, by site
- capillary I78.1
- hemorrhagicum hereditaria I78.0
- malignant—*see* Neoplasm, connective tissue, malignant in Table of Neoplasms in the complete *ICD-10-CM* manual
- plexiform D18.00
  - skin D18.01
  - specified site NEC D18.09
- senile I78.1
- skin D18.01
- specified site NEC D18.09
- spider I78.1
- stellate I78.1

Angiomatosis Q82.8
- encephalotrigeminal Q85.8
- hemorrhagic familial I78.0
- hereditary familial I78.0

Angioneurosis F45.8

Angioneurotic edema (allergic) (any site) (with urticaria) T78.3

Angiopathia, angiopathy I99.9
- peripheral I73.9
  - specified type NEC I73.89

Angiospasm (peripheral) (traumatic) (vessel) I73.9
- cerebral G45.9

Angulation
- femur (acquired)—*see also* Deformity, limb, specified type NEC, thigh
  - congenital Q74.2
- tibia (acquired)—*see also* Deformity, limb, specified type NEC, lower leg
  - congenital Q74.2
- wrist (acquired)—*see also* Deformity, limb, specified type NEC, forearm
  - congenital Q74.0

Angulus infectiosus (lips) K13.0

Anhydration, anhydremia E86.0
- with
  - hypernatremia E87.0
  - hyponatremia E87.1

Anhydremia E86.0
- with
  - hypernatremia E87.0
  - hyponatremia E87.1

Aniridia (congenital) Q13.1

Anisocoria (pupil) H57.02
- congenital Q13.2

Ankyloblepharon (eyelid) (acquired)
- filiforme (adnatum) (congenital) Q10.3
- total Q10.3

Ankyloglossia Q38.1

Ankylosis (fibrous) (osseous) (joint) M24.60
- jaw (temporomandibular) M26.61-
- specified site NEC M24.69
- temporomandibular M26.61-

Anodontia (complete) (partial) (vera) K00.0
- acquired K08.10

Anomaly, anomalous (congenital) (unspecified type) Q89.9
- Alder (-Reilly) (leukocyte granulation) D72.0
- alimentary tract Q45.9
  - upper Q40.9
- ankle (joint) Q74.2
- aorta (arch) NEC Q25.40
  - absence and aplasia Q25.41
  - aneurysm (congenital) Q25.43
  - coarctation (preductal) (postductal) Q25.1
  - dilation (congenital) Q25.44
  - double arch Q25.45
  - hypoplasia Q25.42
  - right aortic arch Q25.47
  - tortuous arch Q25.46
- aqueduct of Sylvius Q03.0
  - with spina bifida—*see* Spina bifida, with hydrocephalus
- arm Q74.0
- artery (peripheral) Q27.9
  - eye Q15.8
  - pulmonary NEC Q25.79
  - retina Q14.1
  - subclavian Q27.8
    - origin Q25.48
  - umbilical Q27.0
- atrial
  - septa Q21.1
- atrioventricular
  - excitation I45.6
  - septum Q21.0
- Axenfeld's Q15.0
- biliary duct or passage Q44.5
- bladder Q64.70
  - absence Q64.5
  - diverticulum Q64.6
  - exstrophy Q64.10
    - cloacal Q64.12
    - extroversion Q64.19
    - specified type NEC Q64.19
    - supravesical fissure Q64.11
  - neck obstruction Q64.31
  - specified type NEC Q64.79
- bone Q79.9
  - arm Q74.0
  - leg Q74.2
  - pelvic girdle Q74.2
  - shoulder girdle Q74.0
  - skull Q75.9
    - with
      - anencephaly Q00.0
      - encephalocele—*see* Encephalocele
      - hydrocephalus Q03.9
        - with spina bifida—*see* Spina bifida, by site, with hydrocephalus
      - microcephaly Q02
- broad ligament Q50.6
- bursa Q79.9
- canthus Q10.3
- cardiac Q24.9
- carpus Q74.0
- caruncle, lacrimal Q10.6
- cervix Q51.9
- cheek Q18.9
- chin Q18.9
- chromosomes, chromosomal Q99.9
  - D (1)—*see* condition, chromosome 13
  - E (3)—*see* condition, chromosome 18
  - G—*see* condition, chromosome 21
  - sex
    - female phenotype Q97.8
    - gonadal dysgenesis (pure) Q99.1
    - Klinefelter's Q98.4

Anomaly, *continued*
  - male phenotype Q98.9
  - Turner's Q96.9
  - specified NEC Q99.8
- cilia Q10.3
- clavicle Q74.0
- common duct Q44.5
- communication
  - left ventricle with right atrium Q21.0
- connection
  - pulmonary venous Q26.4
    - partial Q26.3
    - total Q26.2
- cystic duct Q44.5
- dental
  - arch relationship M26.20
  - specified NEC M26.29
- dentofacial M26.9
  - dental arch relationship M26.20
    - specified NEC M26.29
  - jaw size M26.00
    - mandibular
      - hypoplasia M26.04
  - malocclusion M26.4
    - dental arch relationship NEC M26.29
  - specified type NEC M26.89
  - temporomandibular joint M26.60-
    - adhesions M26.61-
    - ankylosis M26.61-
    - arthralgia M26.62-
    - articular disc M26.63-
    - specified type NEC M26.69
- dermatoglyphic Q82.8
- digestive organ(s) or tract Q45.9
  - lower Q43.9
  - upper Q40.9
- ductus
  - arteriosus Q25.0
  - botalli Q25.0
- ear (external) Q17.9
- elbow Q74.0
- endocrine gland NEC Q89.2
- eye Q15.9
  - anterior segment Q13.9
    - specified NEC Q13.89
  - posterior segment Q14.9
    - specified NEC Q14.8
  - ptosis (eyelid) Q10.0
  - specified NEC Q15.8
- eyelid Q10.3
  - ptosis Q10.0
- face Q18.9
- fallopian tube Q50.6
- fascia Q79.9
- femur NEC Q74.2
- fibula NEC Q74.2
- finger Q74.0
- flexion (joint) NOS Q74.9
  - hip or thigh Q65.89
- foot NEC Q74.2
  - varus (congenital) Q66.3-
- foramen
  - Botalli Q21.1
  - ovale Q21.1
- forearm Q74.0
- forehead Q75.8
- gastrointestinal tract Q45.9
- gallbladder (position) (shape) (size) Q44.1
- genitalia, genital organ(s) or system
  - female Q52.9
    - external Q52.70
    - internal Q52.9
  - male Q55.9
    - hydrocele P83.5
    - specified NEC Q55.8
- genitourinary NEC
  - female Q52.9
  - male Q55.9
- Gerbode Q21.0
- granulation or granulocyte, genetic (constitutional) (leukocyte) D72.0
- gyri Q07.9
- hand Q74.0

Anomaly, *continued*
- heart Q24.9
  - patent ductus arteriosus (Botalli) Q25.0
  - septum Q21.9
    - auricular Q21.1
    - interatrial Q21.1
    - interventricular Q21.0
      - with pulmonary stenosis or atresia, dextraposition of aorta and hypertrophy of right ventricle Q21.3
    - specified NEC Q21.8
    - ventricular Q21.0
      - with pulmonary stenosis or atresia, dextraposition of aorta and hypertrophy of right ventricle Q21.3
  - tetralogy of Fallot Q21.3
  - valve NEC Q24.8
    - aortic
      - stenosis Q23.0
    - pulmonary Q22.3
      - stenosis Q22.1
- heel NEC Q74.2
- Hegglin's D72.0
- hepatic duct Q44.5
- hip NEC Q74.2
- humerus Q74.0
- hydatid of Morgagni
  - female Q50.5
  - male (epididymal) Q55.4
    - testicular Q55.29
- hypersegmentation of neutrophils, hereditary D72.0
- hypophyseal Q89.2
- ilium NEC Q74.2
- integument Q84.9
- ischium NEC Q74.2
- joint Q74.9
- Jordan's D72.0
- lens Q12.9
- leukocytes, genetic D72.0
  - granulation (constitutional) D72.0
- ligament Q79.9
  - broad Q50.6
  - round Q52.8
- limb Q74.9
  - lower NEC Q74.2
    - reduction deformity—*see* Defect, reduction, limb, lower
  - upper Q74.0
- liver Q44.7
  - duct Q44.5
- lower limb NEC Q74.2
- May (-Hegglin) D72.0
- meningeal bands or folds Q07.9
  - constriction of Q07.8
  - spinal Q06.9
- meninges Q07.9
  - cerebral Q04.8
  - spinal Q06.9
- meningocele Q05.9
- mesentery Q45.9
- metacarpus Q74.0
- metatarsus NEC Q74.2
- multiple NEC Q89.7
- muscle Q79.9
- musculoskeletal system, except limbs Q79.9
- neck (any part) Q18.9
- nerve Q07.9
  - acoustic Q07.8
  - optic Q07.8
- nervous system (central) Q07.9
- omphalomesenteric duct Q43.0
- origin
  - artery
    - pulmonary Q25.79
- ovary Q50.39
- oviduct Q50.6
- parathyroid gland Q89.2
- Pelger-Huët (hereditary hyposegmentation) D72.0
- pelvic girdle NEC Q74.2
- pelvis (bony) NEC Q74.2
- penis (glans) Q55.69
- pigmentation L81.9
  - congenital Q82.8

Anomaly, *continued*
- pituitary (gland) Q89.2
- prepuce Q55.69
- pulmonary Q33.9
  - artery NEC Q25.79
  - valve Q22.3
    - stenosis Q22.1
  - venous connection Q26.4
    - partial Q26.3
    - total Q26.2
- radius Q74.0
- respiratory system Q34.9
  - specified NEC Q34.8
- rotation
  - hip or thigh Q65.89
- round ligament Q52.8
- sacroiliac (joint) NEC Q74.2
- scapula Q74.0
- sex chromosomes NEC—*see also* Anomaly, chromosomes
  - female phenotype Q97.8
  - male phenotype Q98.9
- shoulder Q74.0
- simian crease Q82.8
- sinus of Valsalva Q25.49
- skull Q75.9
  - with
    - anencephaly Q00.0
    - encephalocele—*see* Encephalocele
    - hydrocephalus Q03.9
      - ~ with spina bifida—*see* Spina bifida, by site, with hydrocephalus
    - microcephaly Q02
- specified organ or site NEC Q89.8
- tarsus NEC Q74.2
- tendon Q79.9
- thigh NEC Q74.2
- thumb Q74.0
- thymus gland Q89.2
- thyroid (gland) Q89.2
  - cartilage Q31.8
- tibia NEC Q74.2
- toe NEC Q74.2
- tooth, teeth K00.9
  - eruption K00.6
- tragus Q17.9
- ulna Q74.0
- umbilical artery Q27.0
- upper limb Q74.0
- ureter Q62.8
  - obstructive NEC Q62.39
    - orthotopic ureterocele Q62.31
- urinary tract Q64.9
- uterus Q51.9
- ventricular
  - septa Q21.0
- vitelline duct Q43.0
- wrist Q74.0

Anonychia (congenital) Q84.3
- acquired L60.8

Anorchia, anorchism, anorchidism Q55.0

Anorexia R63.0
- nervosa F50.00
  - atypical F50.9
  - binge-eating type with purging F50.02
  - restricting type F50.01

Anosmia R43.0
- hysterical F44.6

Anovulatory cycle N97.0

Anoxemia R09.02
- newborn P84

Anoxia (pathological) R09.02
- cerebral G93.1
  - newborn P84
- due to
  - drowning T75.1
  - high altitude T70.29
- intrauterine P84
- newborn P84

Anteversion
- femur (neck), congenital Q65.89

Anthrax
- with pneumonia A22.1
- cutaneous A22.0
- colitis A22.2
- gastrointestinal A22.2
- inhalation A22.1
- intestinal A22.2
- pulmonary A22.1
- respiratory A22.1

Anthropoid pelvis Q74.2

Antibody
- antiphospholipid R76.0
  - with
    - hemorrhagic disorder D68.312
    - hypercoagulable state D68.61

Anticardiolipin syndrome D68.61

Anticoagulant, circulating (intrinsic)—*see also* Disorder, hemorrhagic D68.318
- drug-induced (extrinsic)—*see also* Disorder, hemorrhagic D68.32
- iatrogenic D68.32

Antidiuretic hormone syndrome E22.2

Antiphospholipid
- antibody
  - with hemorrhagic disorder D68.312
  - syndrome D68.61

Antisocial personality F60.2

Antritis J32.0
- maxilla J32.0
  - acute J01.00
    - recurrent J01.01

Anuria R34
- postrenal N13.8

Anusitis K62.89

Anxiety F41.9
- depression F41.8
- episodic paroxysmal F41.0
- hysteria F41.8
- panic type F41.0
- separation, abnormal (of childhood) F93.0
- social F40.1-
- specified NEC F41.8

Aorta (aortic arch) anomaly Q25.4-

Apepsia K30
- psychogenic F45.8

Apertognathia M26.09

Apert's syndrome Q87.0

Aphagia R13.0
- psychogenic F50.9

Aphakia (acquired) (postoperative) H27.0-
- congenital Q12.3

Aphasia (amnestic) (global) (nominal) (semantic) (syntactic)
- developmental (receptive type) F80.2
  - expressive type F80.1
  - Wernicke's F80.2
- sensory F80.2
- Wernicke's F80.2

Aphonia (organic) R49.1
- hysterical F44.4
- psychogenic F44.4

Aphthae, aphthous—*see also* Disease, diseased
- Bednar's K12.0
- cachectic K14.0
- oral (recurrent) K12.0
- stomatitis (major) (minor) K12.0
- thrush B37.0
- ulcer (oral) (recurrent) K12.0

Aplasia—*see also* Agenesis
- abdominal muscle syndrome Q79.4
- aorta (congenital) Q25.41
- bone marrow (myeloid) D61.9
  - congenital D61.01
- cervix (congenital) Q51.5
- congenital pure red cell D61.01
- corpus callosum Q04.0
- erythrocyte congenital D61.01
- gallbladder, congenital Q44.0
- parathyroid-thymic D82.1

Aplasia, *continued*
- red cell (with thymoma) D60.9
  - acquired D60.9
    - due to drugs D60.9
  - chronic D60.0
  - congenital D61.01
  - constitutional D61.01
  - due to drugs D60.9
  - hereditary D61.01
  - of infants D61.01
  - primary D61.01
  - pure D61.01
    - due to drugs D60.9
    - transient D60.1
- round ligament Q52.8
- testicle Q55.0
- thymic, with immunodeficiency D82.1
- thyroid (congenital) (with myxedema) E03.1
- uterus Q51.0

Apnea, apneic (of) (spells) R06.81
- newborn NEC P28.4
  - obstructive P28.4
  - sleep (central) (obstructive) (primary) P28.3
- prematurity P28.4
- sleep G47.30
  - central (primary) G47.31
    - idiopathic G47.31
    - in conditions classified elsewhere G47.37
  - obstructive (adult) (pediatric) G47.33
    - hypopnea G47.33
  - primary central G47.31
  - specified NEC G47.39

Apneumatosis, newborn P28.0

Apophysitis (bone)—*see also* Osteochondropathy
- juvenile M92.9

Apoplexia, apoplexy, apoplectic
- heat T67.01

Appendage
- testicular (organ of Morgagni) Q55.29

Appendicitis (pneumococcal) (retrocecal) K37
- with
  - gangrene K35.891
  - perforation NOS K35.32
  - peritoneal abscess K35.33
  - peritonitis NEC K35.33
    - generalized (with perforation or rupture) K35.20
    - with abscess K35.21
    - localized K35.30
      - ~ with
        - ◊ gangrene K35.31
        - ◊ perforation K35.32
          - » and abscess K35.33
    - rupture K35.32
- acute (catarrhal) (fulminating) (gangrenous) (obstructive) (retrocecal) (suppurative) K35.80
  - with
    - gangrene K35.891
    - peritoneal abscess K35.33
    - peritonitis NEC K35.33
      - ~ generalized (with perforation or rupture) K35.20
        - ◊ with abscess K35.21
      - ~ localized K35.30
        - ◊ with
          - » gangrene K35.31
          - » perforation K35.32
            - ❖ and abscess K35.33
  - specified NEC K35.890
    - with gangrene K35.891
- ruptured NOS (with local peritonitis) K35.32

Appendicopathia oxyurica B80

Appendix, appendicular—*see also* Disease, diseased
- Morgagni
  - female Q50.5
  - male (epididymal) Q55.4
    - testicular Q55.29
- testis Q55.29

Appetite
- depraved—*see* Pica
- excessive R63.2

Appetite, *continued*
- lack or loss (*see also* Anorexia) R63.0
  - nonorganic origin F50.89
  - psychogenic F50.89
- perverted (hysterical)—*see* Pica

Apprehensiveness, abnormal F41.9

ARC (AIDS-related complex) B20

Arch
- aortic Q25.49
- bovine Q25.49

Arcuate uterus Q51.810

Arcuatus uterus Q51.810

Arnold-Chiari disease, obstruction or syndrome (type II) Q07.00
- with
  - hydrocephalus Q07.02
    - with spina bifida Q07.03
  - spina bifida Q07.01
    - with hydrocephalus Q07.03
- type III—*see* Encephalocele
- type IV Q04.8

Arousals, confusional G47.51

Arrest, arrested
- cardiac I46.9
  - due to
    - cardiac condition I46.2
    - specified condition NEC I46.8
  - newborn P29.81
  - postprocedural I97.12-
- development or growth
  - child R62.50
- epiphyseal
  - complete
    - femur M89.15-
    - humerus M89.12-
    - tibia M89.16-
    - ulna M89.13-
  - forearm M89.13-
    - specified NEC M89.13-
    - ulna—*see* Arrest, epiphyseal, by type, ulna
  - lower leg M89.16-
    - specified NEC M89.168
    - tibia—*see* Arrest, epiphyseal, by type, tibia
  - partial
    - femur M89.15-
    - humerus M89.12-
    - tibia M89.16-
    - ulna M89.13-
  - specified NEC M89.18
- growth plate—*see* Arrest, epiphyseal
- physeal—*see* Arrest, epiphyseal
- respiratory R09.2
  - newborn P28.81

Arrhythmia (auricle) (cardiac) (juvenile) (nodal) (reflex) (supraventricular) (transitory) (ventricle) I49.9
- block I45.9
- newborn
  - bradycardia P29.12
  - occurring before birth P03.819
    - before onset of labor P03.810
    - during labor P03.811
  - tachycardia P29.11
- psychogenic F45.8
- sinus I49.8
- vagal R55

Arrillaga-Ayerza syndrome (pulmonary sclerosis with pulmonary hypertension) I27.0

Arsenical pigmentation L81.8
- from drug or medicament—*see* Table of Drugs and Chemicals

Arteriosclerosis, arteriosclerotic (diffuse) (obliterans) (of) (senile) (with calcification) I70.90
- pulmonary (idiopathic) I27.0

Arteritis I77.6
- cerebral I67.7
  - in
    - systemic lupus erythematosus M32.19
- coronary (artery) I25.89
  - rheumatic I01.8
    - chronic I09.89

Artery, arterial—*see also* Disease, diseased
- single umbilical Q27.0

Arthralgia (allergic)—*see also* Pain, joint
- temporomandibular M26.62-

Arthritis, arthritic (acute) (chronic) (nonpyogenic) (subacute) M19.9-
- due to or associated with
  - acromegaly (*see also* subcategory M14.8-) E22.0
  - bacterial disease (*see also* subcategory M01) A49.9
  - erysipelas (*see also* category M01) A46
  - erythema
    - nodosum L52
  - hemophilia D66 [M36.2]
  - Henoch- (Schönlein) purpura D69.0 [M36.4]
  - human parvovirus (*see also* category M01) B97.6
  - Lyme disease A69.23
  - rat bite fever (*see also* M01) A25.1
  - serum sickness (*see also* Reaction, serum) T80.69
- in (due to)
  - acromegaly (*see also* subcategory M14.8-) E22.0
  - endocrine disorder NEC (*see also* subcategory M14.8-) E34.9
  - enteritis, infectious NEC (*see also* category M01) A09
  - erythema
    - multiforme (*see also* subcategory M14.8-) L51.9
    - nodosum (*see also* subcategory M14.8-) L52
  - hemochromatosis (*see also* subcategory M14.8-) E83.118
  - hemoglobinopathy NEC D58.2 [M36.3]
  - hemophilia NEC D66 [M36.2]
  - Hemophilus influenzae M00.8- [B96.3]
  - Henoch (-Schönlein)purpura D69.0 [M36.4]
  - hypogammaglobulinemia (*see also* subcategory M14.8-) D80.1
  - hypothyroidism NEC (*see also* subcategory M14.8-) E03.9
  - infection—*see* Arthritis, pyogenic or pyemic
  - infectious disease NEC—*see* category M01
  - Lyme disease A69.23
  - metabolic disorder NEC (*see also* subcategory M14.8-) E88.9
  - respiratory disorder NEC (*see also* subcategory M14.8-) J98.9
  - Salmonella (arizonae) (choleraesuis) (typhimurium) A02.23
    - specified organism NEC (*see also* category M01) A08.8
  - sarcoidosis D86.86
  - thalassemia NEC D56.9 [M36.3]
- juvenile M08.90
  - with systemic onset—*see* Still's disease
  - ankle M08.97-
  - elbow M08.92-
  - foot joint M08.97-
  - hand joint M08.94-
  - hip M08.95-
  - knee M08.96-
  - multiple site M08.99
  - pauciarticular M08.40
    - ankle M08.47-
    - elbow M08.42-
    - foot joint M08.47-
    - hand joint M08.44-
    - hip M08.45-
    - knee M08.46-
    - shoulder M08.41-
    - specified site NEC M08.4A
    - vertebrae M08.48
    - wrist M08.43-
  - rheumatoid—*see* Arthritis, rheumatoid, juvenile
  - shoulder M08.91-
  - specified site NEC M08.9A
  - vertebra M08.98
  - specified type NEC M08.8-
    - ankle M08.87-
    - elbow M08.82-
    - foot joint M08.87-
    - hand joint M08.84-
    - hip M08.85-
    - knee M08.86-
    - multiple site M08.89
    - shoulder M08.81-

Arthritis, arthritic, *continued*
    - specified joint NEC M08.88
    - vertebrae M08.88
    - wrist M08.83-
  - wrist M08.93-
- pneumococcal M00.10
  - ankle M00.17-
  - elbow M00.12-
  - foot joint M00.17-
  - hand joint M00.14-
  - hip M00.15-
  - knee M00.16-
  - multiple site M00.19
  - shoulder M00.11-
  - vertebra M00.18
  - wrist M00.13-
- pyogenic or pyemic (any site except spine) M00.9
  - bacterial NEC M00.80
    - ankle M00.87-
    - elbow M00.82-
    - foot joint M00.87-
    - hand joint M00.84-
    - hip M00.85-
    - knee M00.86-
    - multiple site M00.89
    - shoulder M00.81-
    - vertebra M00.88
    - wrist M00.83-
  - pneumococcal—*see* Arthritis, pneumococcal
  - spine—*see* Spondylopathy, infective
  - staphylococcal—*see* Arthritis, staphylococcal
  - streptococcal—*see* Arthritis, streptococcal NEC
    - pneumococcal—*see* Arthritis, pneumococcal
- rheumatoid M06.9
  - juvenile (with or without rheumatoid factor) M08.00
    - ankle M08.07-
    - elbow M08.02-
    - foot joint M08.07-
    - hand joint M08.04-
    - hip M08.05-
    - knee M08.06-
    - multiple site M08.09
    - shoulder M08.01-
    - vertebra M08.08
    - wrist M08.03-
- septic (any site except spine)—*see* Arthritis, pyogenic or pyemic
- staphylococcal M00.00
  - ankle M00.07-
  - elbow M00.02-
  - foot joint M00.07-
  - hand joint M00.04-
  - hip M00.05-
  - knee M00.06-
  - multiple site M00.09
  - shoulder M00.01-
  - vertebra M00.08
  - wrist M00.03-
- streptococcal NEC M00.20
  - ankle M00.27-
  - elbow M00.22-
  - foot joint M00.07-
  - hand joint M00.24-
  - hip M00.25-
  - knee M00.26-
  - multiple site M00.29
  - shoulder M00.21-
  - vertebra M00.28
  - wrist M00.23-
- suppurative—*see* Arthritis, pyogenic or pyemic
- temporomandibular M26.64-

Arthrodysplasia Q74.9

Arthrogryposis (congenital) Q68.8
- multiplex congenita Q74.3

Arthropathy (*see also* Arthritis) M12.9
- hemophilic NEC D66 [M36.2]
- in (due to)
  - acromegaly E22.0 [M14.8-]
  - blood disorder NOS D75.9 [M36.3]
  - endocrine disease NOS E34.9 [M14.8-]

Arthropathy, *continued*
- – erythema
  - ◼ multiforme L51.9 [M14.8-]
  - ◼ nodosum L52 [M14.8-]
  - – hemochromatosis E83.118 [M14.8-]
  - – hemoglobinopathy NEC D58.2 [M36.3]
  - – hemophilia NEC D66 [M36.2]
  - – Henoch-Schönlein purpura D69.0 [M36.4]
  - – hypothyroidism E03.9 [M14.8-]
  - – infective endocarditis I33.0 [M12.8-]
  - – metabolic disease NOS E88.9 [M14.8-]
  - – neoplastic disease NOS (*see also* Table of Neoplasms in the complete *ICD-10-CM* manual) D49.9 [M36.1]
  - – nutritional deficiency (*see also* subcategory M14.8-) E63.9
  - – sarcoidosis D86.86
  - – thyrotoxicosis (*see also* subcategory M14.8-) E05.90
  - – ulcerative colitis K51.90 [M07.6-]
  - – viral hepatitis (postinfectious) NEC B19.9 [M12.8-]
  - – Whipple's disease (*see also* subcategory M14.8-) K90.81
- • postinfectious NEC B99 [M12.8-]
  - – in (due to)
    - ◼ viral hepatitis NEC B19.9 [M12.8-]
- • temporomandibular joint M26.65-
- • traumatic M12.50
  - – ankle M12.57-
  - – elbow M12.52-
  - – foot joint M12.57-
  - – hand joint M12.54-
  - – hip M12.55-
  - – knee M12.56-
  - – multiple site M12.59
  - – shoulder M12.51-
  - – specified joint NEC M12.58
  - – vertebrae M12.58
  - – wrist M12.53-

Artificial
- • opening status (functioning) (without complication) Z93.9
  - – gastrostomy Z93.1

Ascariasis B77.9
- • with
  - – complications NEC B77.89
  - – intestinal complications B77.0
  - – pneumonia, pneumonitis B77.81

Ascites (abdominal) R18.8
- • cardiac I50.9
- • heart I50.9
- • malignant R18.0
- • pseudochylous R18.8

Asocial personality F60.2

Aspartylglucosaminuria E77.1

Asperger's disease or syndrome F84.5

Asphyxia, asphyxiation (by) R09.01
- • antenatal P84
- • birth P84
- • bunny bag—*see* Asphyxia, due to, mechanical threat to breathing, trapped in bed clothes
- • drowning T75.1
- • gas, fumes, or vapor—*see* Table of Drugs and Chemicals
- • inhalation—*see* Inhalation
- • intrauterine P84
- • newborn P84
- • pathological R09.01
- • postnatal P84
  - – mechanical—*see* Asphyxia, due to, mechanical threat to breathing
- • prenatal P84
- • reticularis R23.1
- • strangulation—*see* Asphyxia, due to, mechanical threat to breathing
- • submersion T75.1
- • traumatic T71.9
  - – due to
    - ◼ foreign body (in)—*see* Foreign body, respiratory tract, causing, asphyxia

Asphyxia, asphyxiation, *continued*
- ◼ low oxygen content of ambient air T71.2-
  - ~ due to
    - ◊ being trapped in
      - » low oxygen environment T71.29
        - ❖ in car trunk T71.221
          - ★ circumstances undetermined T71.224
          - ★ done with intent to harm by
            - ✓ another person T71.223
            - ✓ self T71.222
        - ❖ in refrigerator T71.231
          - ★ circumstances undetermined T71.234
          - ★ done with intent to harm by
            - ✓ another person T71.233
            - ✓ self T71.232
    - ◊ cave-in T71.21
  - ◼ mechanical threat to breathing (accidental) T71.191
    - ~ circumstances undetermined T71.194
    - ~ done with intent to harm by
      - ◊ another person T71.193
      - ◊ self T71.192
    - ~ hanging T71.161
      - ◊ circumstances undetermined T71.164
      - ◊ done with intent to harm by
        - » another person T71.163
        - » self T71.162
    - ~ plastic bag T71.121
      - ◊ circumstances undetermined T71.124
      - ◊ done with intent to harm by
        - » another person T71.123
        - » self T71.122
    - ~ smothering
      - ◊ in furniture T71.151
        - » circumstances undetermined T71.154
        - » done with intent to harm by
          - ❖ another person T71.153
          - ❖ self T71.152
      - ◊ under
        - » another person's body T71.141
          - ❖ circumstances undetermined T71.144
          - ❖ done with intent to harm T71.143
        - » pillow T71.111
          - ❖ circumstances undetermined T71.114
          - ❖ done with intent to harm by
            - ★ another person T71.113
            - ★ self T71.112
    - ~ trapped in bed clothes T71.131
      - ◊ circumstances undetermined T71.134
      - ◊ done with intent to harm by
        - » another person T71.133
        - » self T71.132
- • vomiting, vomitus—*see* Foreign body, respiratory tract, causing, asphyxia

Aspiration
- • amniotic (clear) fluid (newborn) P24.10
  - – with
    - ◼ pneumonia (pneumonitis) P24.11
    - ◼ respiratory symptoms P24.11
- • blood
  - – newborn (without respiratory symptoms) P24.20
    - ◼ with
      - ~ pneumonia (pneumonitis) P24.21
      - ~ respiratory symptoms P24.21
  - – specified age NEC—*see* Foreign body, respiratory tract
- • bronchitis J69.0
- • food or foreign body (with asphyxiation)—*see* Asphyxia
- • liquor (amnii) (newborn) P24.10
  - – with
    - ◼ pneumonia (pneumonitis) P24.11
    - ◼ respiratory symptoms P24.11
- • meconium (newborn) (without respiratory symptoms) P24.00
  - – with
    - ◼ pneumonitis (pneumonitis) P24.01
    - ◼ respiratory symptoms P24.01
- • milk (newborn) (without respiratory symptoms) P24.30
  - – with
    - ◼ pneumonia (pneumonitis) P24.31
    - ◼ respiratory symptoms P24.31
  - – specified age NEC—*see* Foreign body, respiratory tract

Aspiration, *continued*
- • mucus—*see also* Foreign body, by site
  - – newborn P24.10
    - ◼ with
      - ~ pneumonia (pneumonitis) P24.11
      - ~ respiratory symptoms P24.11
- • neonatal P24.9
  - – specific NEC (without respiratory symptoms) P24.80
    - ◼ with
      - ~ pneumonia (pneumonitis) P24.81
      - ~ respiratory symptoms P24.81
- • newborn P24.9
  - – specific NEC (without respiratory symptoms) P24.80
    - ◼ with
      - ~ pneumonia (pneumonitis) P24.81
      - ~ respiratory symptoms P24.81
- • pneumonia J69.0
- • pneumonitis J69.0
- • syndrome of newborn—*see* Aspiration, by substance, with pneumonia
- • vernix caseosa (newborn) P24.80
  - – with
    - ◼ pneumonia (pneumonitis) P24.81
    - ◼ respiratory symptoms P24.81
- • vomitus—*see also* Foreign body, respiratory tract
  - – newborn (without respiratory symptoms) P24.30
    - ◼ with
      - ~ pneumonia (pneumonitis) P24.31
      - ~ respiratory symptoms P24.31

Asplenia (congenital) Q89.01

Astasia (-abasia) (hysterical) F44.4

Asthenia, asthenic R53.1
- • cardiac (*see also* Failure, heart) I50.9
  - – psychogenic F45.8
- • cardiovascular (*see also* Failure, heart) I50.9
  - – psychogenic F45.8
- • heart (*see also* Failure, heart) I50.9
  - – psychogenic F45.8
- • hysterical F44.4
- • myocardial (*see also* Failure, heart) I50.9
  - – psychogenic F45.8
- • nervous F48.8
- • neurocirculatory F45.8

Asthenopia
- • hysterical F44.6
- • psychogenic F44.6

Asthma, asthmatic (bronchial) (catarrh) (spasmodic) J45.909
- • with
  - – exacerbation (acute) J45.901
  - – hay fever—*see* Asthma, allergic extrinsic
  - – rhinitis, allergic—*see* Asthma, allergic extrinsic
  - – status asthmaticus J45.902
- • allergic extrinsic J45.909
  - – with
    - ◼ exacerbation (acute) J45.901
    - ◼ status asthmaticus J45.902
- • atopic—*see* Asthma, allergic extrinsic
- • childhood J45.909
  - – with
    - ◼ exacerbation (acute) J45.901
    - ◼ status asthmaticus J45.902
- • cough variant J45.991
- • detergent J69.8
- • due to
  - – detergent J69.8
- • extrinsic, allergic—*see* Asthma, allergic extrinsic
- • hay—*see* Asthma, allergic extrinsic
- • idiosyncratic—*see* Asthma, nonallergic
- • intermittent (mild) J45.20
  - – with
    - ◼ exacerbation (acute) J45.21
    - ◼ status asthmaticus J45.22
- • intrinsic, nonallergic—*see* Asthma, nonallergic
- • late onset J45.909
  - – with
    - ◼ exacerbation (acute) J45.901
    - ◼ status asthmaticus J45.902
- • mild intermittent J45.20
  - – with
    - ◼ exacerbation (acute) J45.21
    - ◼ status asthmaticus J45.22

Asthma, asthmatic, *continued*
- mild persistent J45.30
  - with
    - exacerbation (acute) J45.31
    - status asthmaticus J45.32
- mixed J45.909
  - with
    - exacerbation (acute) J45.901
    - status asthmaticus J45.902
- moderate persistent J45.40
  - with
    - exacerbation (acute) J45.41
    - status asthmaticus J45.42
- nervous—*see* Asthma, nonallergic
- nonallergic (intrinsic) J45.909
  - with
    - exacerbation (acute) J45.901
    - status asthmaticus J45.902
- persistent
  - mild J45.30
    - with
      - ~ exacerbation (acute) J45.31
      - ~ status asthmaticus J45.32
  - moderate J45.40
    - with
      - ~ exacerbation (acute) J45.41
      - ~ status asthmaticus J45.42
  - severe J45.50
    - with
      - ~ exacerbation (acute) J45.51
      - ~ status asthmaticus J45.52
- predominantly allergic J45.909
- severe persistent J45.50
  - with
    - exacerbation (acute) J45.51
    - status asthmaticus J45.52
- specified NEC J45.998

Astroblastoma
- specified site—*see* Neoplasm, malignant, by site in Table of Neoplasms in the complete *ICD-10-CM* manual
- unspecified site C71.9

Astrocytoma (cystic)
- anaplastic
  - specified site—*see* Neoplasm, malignant, by site in Table of Neoplasms in the complete *ICD-10-CM* manual
  - unspecified site C71.9
- fibrillary
  - specified site—*see* Neoplasm, malignant, by site in Table of Neoplasms in the complete *ICD-10-CM* manual
  - unspecified site C71.9
- fibrous
  - specified site—*see* Neoplasm, malignant, by site in Table of Neoplasms in the complete *ICD-10-CM* manual
  - unspecified site C71.9
- gemistocytic
  - specified site—*see* Neoplasm, malignant, by site in Table of Neoplasms in the complete *ICD-10-CM* manual
  - unspecified site C71.9
- juvenile
  - specified site—*see* Neoplasm, malignant, by site in Table of Neoplasms in the complete *ICD-10-CM* manual
  - unspecified site C71.9
- pilocytic
  - specified site—*see* Neoplasm, malignant, by site in Table of Neoplasms in the complete *ICD-10-CM* manual
  - unspecified site C71.9
- piloid
  - specified site—*see* Neoplasm, malignant, by site in Table of Neoplasms in the complete *ICD-10-CM* manual
  - unspecified site C71.9
- protoplasmic
  - specified site—*see* Neoplasm, malignant, by site in Table of Neoplasms in the complete *ICD-10-CM* manual
  - unspecified site C71.9

Astrocytoma (cystic), *continued*
- unspecified site C71.9

Astroglioma
- specified site—*see* Neoplasm, malignant, by site in Table of Neoplasms in the complete *ICD-10-CM* manual
- unspecified site C71.9

Asymmetrical face Q67.0

At risk
- for
  - dental caries Z91.849
    - high Z91.843
    - low Z91.841
    - moderate Z91.842
  - falling Z91.81

Ataxia, ataxy, ataxic R27.0
- autosomal recessive Friedreich G11.11
- cerebellar (hereditary) G11.9
  - with defective DNA repair G11.3
  - early-onset G11.10
  - in
    - myxedema E03.9 *[G13.2]*
    - neoplastic disease (*see also* Table of Neoplasms in the complete *ICD-10-CM* manual) D49.9 *[G32.81]*
    - specified disease NEC G32.81
  - late-onset (Marie's) G11.2
  - with
    - essential tremor G11.19
    - myoclonus [Hunt's ataxia] G11.19
    - retained tendon reflexes G11.19
- Friedreich's (heredofamilial) (cerebellar) (spinal) G11.11
- gait R26.0
  - hysterical F44.4
- gluten M35.9 *[G32.81]*
  - with celiac disease K90.0 *[G32.81]*
- hereditary G11.9
  - cerebellar—*see* Ataxia, cerebellar
  - spinal (Friedreich's) G11.11
- heredofamilial—*see* Ataxia, hereditary
- Hunt's G11.19
- hysterical F44.4
- Marie's (cerebellar) (heredofamilial) (late-onset) G11.2
- nonorganic origin F44.4
- nonprogressive, congenital G11.0
- psychogenic F44.4
- SangerBrown's (hereditary) G11.2
- spinal
  - hereditary (Friedreich's) G11.11
- spinocerebellar, Xlinked recessive G11.11
- telangiectasia (LouisBar) G11.3

Ataxia-telangiectasia (Louis-Bar) G11.3

Atelectasis (massive) (partial) (pressure) (pulmonary) J98.11
- newborn P28.10
  - due to resorption P28.11
  - partial P28.19
  - primary P28.0
  - secondary P28.19
- primary (newborn) P28.0

Atelocardia Q24.9

Atheroma, atheromatous (*see also* Arteriosclerosis) I70.90
- aorta, aortic I70.0
  - valve (*see also* Endocarditis, aortic) I35.8
- pulmonary valve (heart) (*see also* Endocarditis, pulmonary) I37.8
- tricuspid (heart) (valve) I36.8
- valve, valvular—*see* Endocarditis

Athlete's
- foot B35.3
- heart I51.7

Athyrea (acquired)—*see also* Hypothyroidism
- congenital E03.1

Atonia, atony, atonic
- capillary I78.8
- congenital P94.2
- intestine K59.89
  - psychogenic F45.8
- stomach K31.89
  - neurotic or psychogenic F45.8
- uterus (during labor)
  - without hemorrhage O75.89

Atransferrinemia, congenital E88.09

Atresia, atretic
- alimentary organ or tract NEC Q45.8
  - upper Q40.8
- ani, anus, anal (canal) Q42.3
  - with fistula Q42.2
- aortic (orifice) (valve) Q23.0
  - congenital with hypoplasia of ascending aorta and defective development of left ventricle (with mitral stenosis) Q23.4
  - in hypoplastic left heart syndrome Q23.4
- aqueduct of Sylvius Q03.0
  - with spina bifida—*see* Spina bifida, with hydrocephalus
- artery NEC Q27.8
  - umbilical Q27.0
- bile duct (common) (congenital) (hepatic) Q44.2
  - acquired—*see* Obstruction, bile duct
- cecum Q42.8
- cervix (acquired) N88.2
  - congenital Q51.828
- choana Q30.0
- colon Q42.9
  - specified NEC Q42.8
- common duct Q44.2
- cystic duct Q44.2
  - acquired K82.8
    - with obstruction K82.0
- digestive organs NEC Q45.8
- esophagus Q39.0
  - with tracheoesophageal fistula Q39.1
- fallopian tube (congenital) Q50.6
  - acquired N97.1
- follicular cyst N83.0-
- foramen of
  - Luschka Q03.1
    - with spina bifida—*see* Spina bifida, with hydrocephalus
  - Magendie Q03.1
    - with spina bifida—*see* Spina bifida, with hydrocephalus
- gallbladder Q44.1
- genital organ
  - external
    - female Q52.79
    - male Q55.8
  - internal
    - female Q52.8
    - male Q55.8
- gullet Q39.0
  - with tracheoesophageal fistula Q39.1
- hymen Q52.3
  - acquired (postinfective) N89.6
- intestine (small) Q41.9
  - large Q42.9
    - specified NEC Q42.8
- iris, filtration angle Q15.0
- mitral valve Q23.2
  - in hypoplastic left heart syndrome Q23.4
- nares (anterior) (posterior) Q30.0
- nose, nostril Q30.0
  - acquired J34.89
- organ or site NEC Q89.8
- oviduct (congenital) Q50.6
  - acquired N97.1
- rectum Q42.1
  - with fistula Q42.0
- ureter Q62.10
  - pelvic junction Q62.11
  - vesical orifice Q62.12
- ureteropelvic junction Q62.11
- ureterovesical orifice Q62.12
- uterus Q51.818
  - acquired N85.8
- vagina (congenital) Q52.4
  - acquired (postinfectional) (senile) N89.5
- vein NEC Q27.8
  - pulmonary Q26.4
    - partial Q26.3
    - total Q26.2

Atrophy, atrophic (of)
- adrenal (capsule) (gland) E27.49
  - primary (autoimmune) E27.1
- buccal cavity K13.79

Atrophy, atrophic, *continued*
- facioscapulohumeral (Landouzy-Déjérine) G71.02
- hemifacial Q67.4
  - Romberg G51.8
- Landouzy-Déjérine G71.02
- laryngitis, infective J37.0
- lip K13.0
- muscle, muscular (diffuse) (general) (idiopathic) (primary)
  - infantile spinal G12.0
  - progressive (bulbar) G12.21
    - infantile (spinal) G12.0
    - spinal G12
      ~ infantile G12.0
  - pseudohypertrophic G71.02
  - spinal G12.9
    - infantile, type I (Werdnig-Hoffmann) G12.0
- nail L60.3
- pseudohypertrophic (muscle) G71.0
- rhinitis J31.0
- scar L90.5
- suprarenal (capsule) (gland) E27.49
  - primary E27.1
- systemic affecting central nervous system
  - in
    - myxedema E03.9 *[G13.2]*
    - neoplastic disease (*see also* Table of Neoplasms in the complete *ICD-10-CM* manual) D49.9 *[G13.1]*
    - specified disease NEC G13.8
- testes N50.0
- thyroid (gland) (acquired) E03.4
  - with cretinism E03.1
  - congenital (with myxedema) E03.1
- turbinate J34.89
- WerdnigHoffmann G12.0

Attack, attacks
- AdamsStokes I45.9
- benign shuddering G25.83
- cyanotic, newborn P28.2
- drop NEC R55
- epileptic—*see* Epilepsy
- hysterical F44.9
- panic F41.0
- shuddering, benign G25.83
- StokesAdams I45.9
- syncope R55
- transient ischemic (TIA) G45.9
  - specified NEC G45.8
- unconsciousness R55
  - hysterical F44.89
- vasomotor R55
- vasovagal (paroxysmal) (idiopathic) R55
- without alteration of consciousness—*see* Epilepsy, syndromes, localization-related, symptomatic, with simple partial seizure

Attention (to)
- artificial
  - opening (of) Z43.9
    - digestive tract NEC Z43.4
      ~ stomach Z43.1
    - specified NEC Z43.8
    - trachea Z43.0
    - urinary tract NEC Z43.6
      ~ cystostomy Z43.5
      ~ nephrostomy Z43.6
      ~ ureterostomy Z43.6
      ~ urethrostomy Z43.6
- colostomy Z43.3
- cystostomy Z43.5
- deficit disorder or syndrome F98.8
  - with hyperactivity—*see* Disorder, attention-deficit hyperactivity
- gastrostomy Z43.1
- ileostomy Z43.2
- jejunostomy Z43.4
- nephrostomy Z43.6
- surgical dressings Z48.01
- sutures Z48.02
- tracheostomy Z43.0
- ureterostomy Z43.6
- urethrostomy Z43.6

Austin Flint murmur (aortic insufficiency) I35.1

Autism, autistic (childhood) (infantile) F84.0
- atypical F84.9
- spectrum disorder F84.0

Autoerythrocyte sensitization (syndrome) D69.2

Autographism L50.3

Autoimmune
- disease (systemic) M35.9
- lymphoproliferative syndrome *[ALPS]* D89.82
- thyroiditis E06.3

Automatism G93.89
- with temporal sclerosis G93.81
- epileptic—*see* Epilepsy, localization-related, symptomatic, with complex partial seizures
- paroxysmal, idiopathic—*see* Epilepsy, localization-related, symptomatic, with complex partial seizures

Autosensitivity, erythrocyte D69.2

Aversion
- oral R63.3
  - newborn P92.-
  - nonorganic origin F98.2

Avitaminosis (multiple) (*see also* Deficiency, vitamin) E56.9
- D E55.9
  - with rickets E55.0

AVNRT (atrioventricular nodal re-entrant tachycardia) I47.1

AVRT (atrioventricular nodal re-entrant tachycardia) I47.1

Avulsion (traumatic)
- spleen S36.032

Awareness of heart beat R00.2

Axenfeld's
- anomaly or syndrome Q15.0

Ayerza's disease or syndrome (pulmonary artery sclerosis with pulmonary hypertension) I27.0

Azotemia R79.89
- meaning uremia N19

B

Babesiosis B60.00
- due to
  - Babesia
    - divergens B60.03
    - duncani B60.02
    - KO-1 B60.09
    - microti B60.01
    - MO-1 B60.03
    - species
      ~ unspecified B60.00
    - venatorum B60.09
  - specified NEC B60.09

Babington's disease (familial hemorrhagic telangiectasia) I78.0

Baby
- crying constantly R68.11
- floppy (syndrome) P94.2

Bacilluria R82.71

Bacillus
- coli infection (*see also* Escherichia coli) B96.20
- Shiga's A03.0
- suipestifer infection—*see* Infection, salmonella

Backache (postural) M54.9
- sacroiliac M53.3

Backward reading (dyslexia) F81.0

Bacteremia R78.81
- with sepsis—*see* Sepsis

Bacterium, bacteria, bacterial
- agent NEC, as cause of disease classified elsewhere B96.89
- in blood—*see* Bacteremia
- in urine R82.71

Bacteriuria, bacteruria R82.71
- asymptomatic R82.71
- urinary tract infection N39.0

Baelz's disease (cheilitis glandularis apostematosa) K13.0

Baerensprung's disease (eczema marginatum) B35.6

Balanitis (circinata) (erosiva) (gangrenosa) (phagedenic) (vulgaris) N48.1
- candidal B37.42

Balanoposthitis N47.6

Band(s)
- gallbladder (congenital) Q44.1
- vagina N89.5

Bandemia D72.825

Bannister's disease T78.3

Bartonellosis A44.9
- cutaneous A44.1
- mucocutaneous A44.1
- specified NEC A44.8
- systemic A44.0

Barton's fracture S52.56-

Basophilia D72.824

Basophilism (cortico-adrenal) (Cushing's) (pituitary) E24.0

Bateman's
- disease B08.1
- purpura (senile) D69.2

Bathing cramp T75.1

Battle exhaustion F43.0

Beach ear—*see* Swimmer's, ear

Beat(s)
- atrial, premature I49.1
- premature I49.40
  - atrial I49.1
  - auricular I49.1
  - supraventricular I49.1

Becker's
- disease
  - myotonia congenita, recessive form G71.12
- dystrophy G71.01

Beckwith-Wiedemann syndrome Q87.3

Bedbug bite(s)—*see* Bite(s), by site, superficial, insect

Bedclothes, asphyxiation or suffocation by—*see* Asphyxia, traumatic

Bednar's
- aphthae K12.0

Bedwetting—*see* Enuresis

Bee sting (with allergic or anaphylactic shock)—*see* Table of Drugs and Chemicals, by animal or substance, poisoning

Behavior
- drug seeking Z76.5
- self-damaging (lifestyle) Z72.89

Bell's
- palsy, paralysis G51.0
  - infant or newborn P11.3

Bence Jones albuminuria or proteinuria NEC R80.3

Bennett's fracture (displaced) S62.21-

Bent
- back (hysterical) F44.4
- nose M95.0
  - congenital Q67.4

Bereavement (uncomplicated) Z63.4

Bergeron's disease (hysterical chorea) F44.4

Besnier's
- lupus pernio D86.3
- prurigo L20.0

Best's disease H35.50

Betalipoproteinemia, broad or floating E78.2

Betting and gambling Z72.6

Bicornate or bicornis uterus Q51.3

Bifid (congenital)
- scrotum Q55.29
- toe NEC Q74.2
- uterus Q51.3
- uvula Q35.7

Bifurcation (congenital)
- gallbladder Q44.1

Bilharziasis—*see also* Schistosomiasis
- cutaneous B65.3

Bilirubin metabolism disorder E80.7
- specified NEC E80.6

Biparta, bipartite
- carpal scaphoid Q74.0

Bird
- face Q75.8

Birth
- injury NOS P15.9
  – brachial plexus NEC P14.3
  – cerebral hemorrhage P10.1
  – eye P15.3
  – fracture
    ▪ clavicle P13.4
    ▪ skull P13.0
  – laceration
    ▪ brain P10.1
    ▪ by scalpel P15.8
  – nerve
    ▪ brachial plexus P14.3
    ▪ facial P11.3
  – paralysis
    ▪ facial nerve P11.3
  – scalp P12.9
  – scalpel wound P15.8
  – specified type NEC P15.8
  – skull NEC P13.1
    ▪ fracture P13.0
- shock, newborn P96.89
- weight
  – low (2499 grams or less)—*see* Low, birthweight
    ▪ extremely (999 grams or less)—*see* Low, birthweight, extreme
  – 4000 grams to 4499 grams P08.1
  – 4500 grams or more P08.0

Birthmark Q82.5

Bisalbuminemia E88.09

Bite(s) (animal) (human)
- abdomen, abdominal
  – wall S31.159
    ▪ epigastric region S31.152
    ▪ left
      ~ lower quadrant S31.154
      ~ upper quadrant S31.151
    ▪ periumbilic region S31.155
    ▪ right
      ~ lower quadrant S31.153
      ~ upper quadrant S31.150
    ▪ superficial NEC S30.871
      ~ insect S30.861
- amphibian (venomous)—*see* Table of Drugs and Chemicals, by animal or substance, poisoning
- animal—*see also* Bite
  – venomous—*see* Table of Drugs and Chemicals, by animal or substance, poisoning
- ankle S91.05-
  – superficial NEC S90.57-
    ▪ insect S90.56-
- antecubital space—*see* Bite, elbow
- anus S31.835
  – superficial NEC S30.877
    ▪ insect S30.867
- arm (upper) S41.15-
  – lower—*see* Bite, forearm
  – superficial NEC S40.87-
    ▪ insect S40.86-
- arthropod NEC—*see* Table of Drugs and Chemicals, by animal or substance
- auditory canal (external) (meatus)—*see* Bite, ear
- auricle, ear—*see* Bite, ear
- axilla—*see* Bite, arm
- back—*see also* Bite, thorax, superficial, back
  – lower S31.050
    ▪ superficial NEC S30.870
      ~ insect S30.860
- bedbug—*see* Bite(s), by site, superficial, insect
- breast
  – superficial NEC S20.17-
    ▪ insect S20.16-
- brow—*see* Bite, head, specified site NEC
- buttock S31.8-
  – left S31.825
  – right S31.815
  – superficial NEC S30.870
    ▪ insect S30.860
- calf—*see* Bite, leg

Bite(s), *continued*
- canaliculus lacrimalis—*see* Bite, eyelid
- canthus, eye—*see* Bite, eyelid
- centipede—*see* Table of Drugs and Chemicals, by animal or substance, poisoning
- cheek (external) S01.45-
  – internal—*see* Bite, oral cavity
  – superficial NEC S00.87
    ▪ insect S00.86
- chest wall—*see* Bite, thorax
- chigger B88.0
- chin—*see* Bite, head, specified site NEC
- clitoris—*see* Bite, vulva
- costal region—*see* Bite, thorax
- digit(s)
  – hand—*see* Bite, finger
  – toe—*see* Bite, toe
- ear (canal) (external) S01.35-
  – superficial NEC S00.47-
    ▪ insect S00.46-
- elbow S51.05-
  – superficial NEC S50.37-
    ▪ insect S50.36-
- epididymis—*see* Bite, testis
- epigastric region—*see* Bite, abdomen
- epiglottis—*see* Bite, neck, specified site NEC
- esophagus, cervical
  – superficial NEC S10.17
    ▪ insect S10.16
- eyebrow—*see* Bite, eyelid
- eyelid S01.15-
  – superficial NEC S00.27-
    ▪ insect S00.26-
- face NEC—*see* Bite, head, specified site NEC
- finger(s) S61.25-
  – with
    ▪ damage to nail S61.35-
  – index S61.25-
    ▪ with
      ~ damage to nail S61.35-
    ▪ left S61.251
      ~ with
        ◊ damage to nail S61.351
    ▪ right S61.250
      ~ with
        ◊ damage to nail S61.350
    ▪ superficial NEC S60.47-
      ~ insect S60.46-
  – little S61.25-
    ▪ with
      ~ damage to nail S61.35-
    ▪ superficial NEC S60.47-
      ~ insect S60.46-
  – middle S61.25-
    ▪ with
      ~ damage to nail S61.35-
    ▪ superficial NEC S60.47-
      ~ insect S60.46-
  – ring S61.25-
    ▪ with
      ~ damage to nail S61.35-
    ▪ superficial NEC S60.47-
      ~ insect S60.46-
  – superficial NEC S60.47-
    ▪ insect S60.46-
  – thumb—*see* Bite, thumb
- flank—*see* Bite, abdomen, wall
- flea—*see* Bite, superficial, insect
- foot (except toe(s) alone) S91.35-
  – superficial NEC S90.87-
    ▪ insect S90.86-
  – toe—*see* Bite, toe
- forearm S51.85-
  – elbow only—*see* Bite, elbow
  – superficial NEC S50.87-
    ▪ insect S50.86-
- forehead—*see* Bite, head, specified site NEC
- genital organs, external
  – female
    ▪ superficial NEC S30.876
      ~ insect S30.866
    ▪ vagina and vulva—*see* Bite, vulva

Bite(s), *continued*
- male
  ▪ penis—*see* Bite, penis
  ▪ scrotum—*see* Bite, scrotum
  ▪ superficial NEC S30.875
    ~ insect S30.865
  ▪ testes—*see* Bite, testis
- groin—*see* Bite, abdomen, wall
- gum—*see* Bite, oral cavity
- hand S61.45-
  – finger—*see* Bite, finger
  – superficial NEC S60.57-
    ▪ insect S60.56-
  – thumb—*see* Bite, thumb
- head (*code to* Bite of specific site for cheek, ear, eyelid, lip, nose, oral cavity, or scalp) S01.95
  – specified site NEC S01.85
    ▪ superficial NEC S00.87
      ~ insect S00.86
  – superficial NEC S00.97
    ▪ insect S00.96
  – temporomandibular area—*see* Bite, cheek
- heel—*see* Bite, foot
- hip S71.05-
  – superficial NEC S70.27-
    ▪ insect S70.26-
- hymen S31.45
- hypochondrium—*see* Bite, abdomen, wall
- hypogastric region—*see* Bite, abdomen, wall
- inguinal region—*see* Bite, abdomen, wall
- insect—*see* Bite, by site, superficial, insect
- instep—*see* Bite, foot
- interscapular region—*see* Bite, thorax, superficial, back
- jaw—*see* Bite, head, specified site NEC
- knee S81.05-
  – superficial NEC S80.27-
    ▪ insect S80.26-
- labium (majus) (minus)—*see* Bite, vulva
- lacrimal duct—*see* Bite, eyelid
- larynx
  – superficial NEC S10.17
    ▪ insect S10.16
- leg (lower) (*code to* Bite of specific site for ankle, foot, knee, upper leg/thigh, or toe) S81.85-
  – superficial NEC S80.87-
    ▪ insect S80.86-
- lip S01.551
  – superficial NEC S00.571
    ▪ insect S00.561
- lizard (venomous)—*see* Table of Drugs and Chemicals, by animal or substance, poisoning
- loin—*see* Bite, abdomen, wall
- lower back—*see* Bite, back, lower
- lumbar region—*see* Bite, back, lower
- malar region—*see* Bite, head, specified site NEC
- mammary—*see* Bite, breast
- marine animals (venomous)—*see* Table of Drugs and Chemicals, by animal or substance, poisoning
- mastoid region—*see* Bite, head, specified site NEC
- mouth—*see* Bite, oral cavity
- nail
  – finger—*see* Bite, finger
  – toe—*see* Bite, toe
- nape—*see* Bite, neck, specified site NEC
- nasal (septum) (sinus)—*see* Bite, nose
- nasopharynx—*see* Bite, head, specified site NEC
- neck (*code to* Bite by specific site for esophagus, larynx, pharynx, or trachea) S11.95
  – involving
  – specified site NEC S11.85
    ▪ superficial NEC S10.87
      ~ insect S10.86
  – superficial NEC S10.97
    ▪ insect S10.96
  – throat S11.85
    ▪ superficial NEC S10.17
      ~ insect S10.16
- nose (septum) (sinus) S01.25
  – superficial NEC S00.37
    ▪ insect S00.36
- occipital region—*see* Bite, scalp

Bite(s), *continued*
- oral cavity S01.552
  - superficial NEC S00.572
    - insect S00.562
- orbital region—*see* Bite, eyelid
- palate—*see* Bite, oral cavity
- palm—*see* Bite, hand
- parietal region—*see* Bite, scalp
- pelvis S31.050
  - superficial NEC S30.870
    - insect S30.860
- penis S31.25
  - superficial NEC S30.872
    - insect S30.862
- perineum
  - female—*see* Bite, vulva
  - male—*see* Bite, pelvis
- periocular area (with or without lacrimal passages)—*see* Bite, eyelid
- phalanges
  - finger—*see* Bite, finger
  - toe—*see* Bite, toe
- pharynx
  - superficial NEC S10.17
    - insect S10.16
- pinna—*see* Bite, ear
- poisonous—*see* Table of Drugs and Chemicals, by animal or substance, poisoning
- popliteal space—*see* Bite, knee
- prepuce—*see* Bite, penis
- pubic region—*see* Bite, abdomen, wall
- rectovaginal septum—*see* Bite, vulva
- red bug B88.0
- reptile NEC—*see* Table of Drugs and Chemicals, by animal or substance, poisoning
  - nonvenomous—*see* Bite, by site
  - snake—*see* Table of Drugs and Chemicals, by animal or substance, poisoning
- sacral region—*see* Bite, back, lower
- sacroiliac region—*see* Bite, back, lower
- salivary gland—*see* Bite, oral cavity
- scalp S01.05
  - superficial NEC S00.07
    - insect S00.06
- scapular region—*see* Bite, shoulder
- scrotum S31.35
  - superficial NEC S30.873
    - insect S30.863
- sea-snake (venomous)—*see* Table of Drugs and Chemicals, by animal or substance, poisoning
- shin—*see* Bite, leg
- shoulder S41.05-
  - superficial NEC S40.27-
    - insect S40.26-
- snake—*see* Table of Drugs and Chemicals, by animal or substance, poisoning
  - nonvenomous—*see* Bite, by site
- spermatic cord—*see* Bite, testis
- spider (venomous)—*see* Table of Drugs and Chemicals, by animal or substance, poisoning
  - nonvenomous—*see* Bite, by site, superficial, insect
- sternal region—*see* Bite, thorax, superficial, front
- submaxillary region—*see* Bite, head, specified site NEC
- submental region—*see* Bite, head, specified site NEC
- subungual
  - finger(s)—*see* Bite, finger
  - toe—*see* Bite, toe
- superficial—*see* Bite, by site, superficial
- supraclavicular fossa S11.85
- supraorbital—*see* Bite, head, specified site NEC
- temple, temporal region—*see* Bite, head, specified site NEC
- temporomandibular area—*see* Bite, cheek
- testis S31.35
  - superficial NEC S30.873
    - insect S30.863
- thigh S71.15-
  - superficial NEC S70.37-
    - insect S70.36-
- thorax, thoracic (wall) S21.95
  - breast—*see* Bite, breast

Bite(s), *continued*
- superficial NEC S20.97
  - back S20.47-
  - front S20.37-
  - insect S20.96
    - back S20.46-
    - front S20.36-
- throat—*see* Bite, neck, throat
- thumb S61.05-
  - with
    - damage to nail S61.15-
  - superficial NEC S60.37-
    - insect S60.36-
- thyroid
  - superficial NEC S10.87
    - insect S10.86
- toe(s) S91.15-
  - with
    - damage to nail S91.25-
  - great S91.15-
    - with
      - damage to nail S91.25-
  - lesser S91.15-
    - with
      - damage to nail S91.25-
  - superficial NEC S90.47-
    - great S90.47-
    - insect S90.46-
      - great S90.46-
- tongue S01.552
- trachea
  - superficial NEC S10.17
    - insect S10.16
- tunica vaginalis—*see* Bite, testis
- tympanum, tympanic membrane—*see* Bite, ear
- umbilical region S31.155
- uvula—*see* Bite, oral cavity
- vagina—*see* Bite, vulva
- venomous—*see* Table of Drugs and Chemicals, by animal or substance, poisoning
- vulva S31.45
  - superficial NEC S30.874
    - insect S30.864
- wrist S61.55-
  - superficial NEC S60.87-
    - insect S60.86-

Biting, cheek or lip K13.1

Biventricular failure (heart) I50.9

Blackfan-Diamond anemia or syndrome (congenital hypoplastic anemia) D61.01

Blackhead L70.0

Blackout R55

Blastomycosis, blastomycotic B40.9
- cutaneous B40.3
- disseminated B40.7
- generalized B40.7
- North American B40.9
- primary pulmonary B40.0
- pulmonary
  - acute B40.0
  - chronic B40.1
  - skin B40.3
  - specified NEC B40.89

Bleeding—*see also* Hemorrhage
- anal K62.5
- anovulatory N97.0
- gastrointestinal K92.2
- intermenstrual (regular) N92.3
  - irregular N92.1
- irregular N92.6
- nipple N64.59
- nose R04.0
- ovulation N92.3
- pre-pubertal vaginal N93.1
- puberty (excessive, with onset of menstrual periods) N92.2
- rectum, rectal K62.5
  - newborn P54.2
- tendencies—*see* Defect, coagulation
- uterus, uterine NEC N93.9
  - dysfunctional or functional N93.8

Bleeding, *continued*
- vagina, vaginal (abnormal) N93.9
  - dysfunctional or functional N93.8
  - newborn P54.6
  - pre-pubertal N93.1
- vicarious N94.89

Blennorrhea (acute) (chronic)—*see also* Gonorrhea
- inclusion (neonatal) (newborn) P39.1
- lower genitourinary tract (gonococcal) A54.00
- neonatorum (gonococcal ophthalmia) A54.31

Blepharitis (angularis) (ciliaris) (eyelid) (marginal) (nonulcerative) H01.00-
- left H01.006
  - lower H01.005
  - upper H01.004
  - upper and lower H01.00B
- right H01.003
  - lower H01.002
  - upper H01.001
  - upper and lower H01.00A

Blepharochalasis H02.3-
- congenital Q10.0

Blepharoconjunctivitis H10.50-

Blepharoptosis H02.40-
- congenital Q10.0

Blindness (acquired) (congenital) (both eyes) H54.0X
- emotional (hysterical) F44.6
- hysterical F44.6
- one eye (other eye normal) H54.4-
  - left (normal vision on right) H54.42-
    - low vision on right H54.12-
  - right (normal vision on left) H54.41-
    - low vision on left H54.11-
- sac, fallopian tube (congenital) Q50.6
- word (developmental) F81.0
  - acquired R48.0
  - secondary to organic lesion R48.0

Blister (nonthermal)
- abdominal wall S30.821
- alveolar process S00.522
- ankle S90.52-
- antecubital space—*see* Blister, elbow
- anus S30.827
- arm (upper) S40.82-
- auditory canal—*see* Blister, ear
- auricle—*see* Blister, ear
- axilla—*see* Blister, arm
- back, lower S30.820
- beetle dermatitis L24.89
- breast S20.12-
- brow S00.82
- calf—*see* Blister, leg
- canthus—*see* Blister, eyelid
- cheek S00.82
  - internal S00.522
- chest wall—*see* Blister, thorax
- chin S00.82
- costal region—*see* Blister, thorax
- digit(s)
  - foot—*see* Blister, toe
  - hand—*see* Blister, finger
- due to burn—*see* Burn, by site, second degree
- ear S00.42-
- elbow S50.32-
- epiglottis S10.12
- esophagus, cervical S10.12
- eyebrow—*see* Blister, eyelid
- eyelid S00.22-
- face S00.82
- fever B00.1
- finger(s) S60.42-
  - index S60.42-
  - little S60.42-
  - middle S60.42-
  - ring S60.42-
- foot (except toe(s) alone) S90.82-
  - toe—*see* Blister, toe
- forearm S50.82-
  - elbow only—*see* Blister, elbow
- forehead S00.82
- fracture omit code

Blister, *continued*
- genital organ
  - female S30.826
  - male S30.825
- gum S00.522
- hand S60.52-
- head S00.92
  - ear—*see* Blister, ear
  - eyelid—*see* Blister, eyelid
  - lip S00.521
  - nose S00.32
  - oral cavity S00.522
  - scalp S00.02
  - specified site NEC S00.82
- heel—*see* Blister, foot
- hip S70.22-
- interscapular region S20.429
- jaw S00.82
- knee S80.22-
- larynx S10.12
- leg (lower) S80.82-
  - knee—*see* Blister, knee
  - upper—*see* Blister, thigh
- lip S00.521
- malar region S00.82
- mammary—*see* Blister, breast
- mastoid region S00.82
- mouth S00.522
- multiple, skin, nontraumatic R23.8
- nail
  - finger—*see* Blister, finger
  - toe—*see* Blister, toe
- nasal S00.32
- neck S10.92
  - specified site NEC S10.82
  - throat S10.12
- nose S00.32
- occipital region S00.02
- oral cavity S00.522
- orbital region—*see* Blister, eyelid
- palate S00.522
- palm—*see* Blister, hand
- parietal region S00.02
- pelvis S30.820
- penis S30.822
- periocular area—*see* Blister, eyelid
- phalanges
  - finger—*see* Blister, finger
  - toe—*see* Blister, toe
- pharynx S10.12
- pinna—*see* Blister, ear
- popliteal space—*see* Blister, knee
- scalp S00.02
- scapular region—*see* Blister, shoulder
- scrotum S30.823
- shin—*see* Blister, leg
- shoulder S40.22-
- sternal region S20.32-
- submaxillary region S00.82
- submental region S00.82
- subungual
  - finger(s)—*see* Blister, finger
  - toe(s)—*see* Blister, toe
- supraclavicular fossa S10.82
- supraorbital S00.82
- temple S00.82
- temporal region S00.82
- testis S30.823
- thermal—*see* Burn, second degree, by site
- thigh S70.32-
- thorax, thoracic (wall) S20.92
  - back S20.42-
  - front S20.32-
- throat S10.12
- thumb S60.32-
- toe(s) S90.42-
  - great S90.42-
- tongue S00.522
- trachea S10.12
- tympanum, tympanic membrane—*see* Blister, ear
- upper arm—*see* Blister, arm (upper)
- uvula S00.522

Blister, *continued*
- vagina S30.824
- vocal cords S10.12
- vulva S30.824
- wrist S60.82-

Bloating R14.0

Block, blocked
- arrhythmic I45.9
- atrioventricular (incomplete) (partial) I44.30
  - with atrioventricular dissociation I44.2
  - complete I44.2
    - congenital Q24.6
  - congenital Q24.6
  - first degree I44.0
  - second degree (types I and II) I44.1
  - specified NEC I44.39
  - third degree I44.2
  - types I and II I44.1
- cardiac I45.9
- conduction I45.9
  - complete I44.2
- foramen Magendie (acquired) G91.1
  - congenital Q03.1
    - with spina bifida—*see* Spina bifida, with hydrocephalus
- heart I45.9
  - complete (atrioventricular) I44.2
  - congenital Q24.6
  - first degree (atrioventricular) I44.0
  - second degree (atrioventricular) I44.1
  - third degree (atrioventricular) I44.2
- Mobitz (types I and II) I44.1
- portal (vein) I81
- second degree (types I and II) I44.1
- third degree I44.2
- Wenckebach (types I and II) I44.1

Blocq's disease F44.4

Blood
- constituents, abnormal R78.9
- disease D75.9
- in
  - feces K92.1
    - occult R19.5
  - urine—*see* Hematuria
- occult in feces R19.5
- pressure
  - decreased, due to shock following injury T79.4
  - examination only Z01.30
  - high—*see* Hypertension
    - borderline R03.0
    - incidental reading, without diagnosis of hypertension R03.0
- transfusion
  - reaction or complication—*see* Complications, transfusion
- type Z67-

Blood-forming organs, disease D75.9

Bloom (-Machacek) (-Torre) syndrome Q82.8

Blount disease or osteochondrosis M92.51-

Blue
- baby Q24.9
- dot cataract Q12.0
  - sclera Q13.5

Blurring, visual H53.8

Blushing (abnormal) (excessive) R23.2

BMI—*see* Body, mass index

Boarder, hospital NEC Z76.4
- healthy infant or child Z76.2
  - foundling Z76.1

Blue
- baby Q24.9
- dot cataract Q12.0
- sclera Q13.5
  - with fragility of bone and deafness Q78.0

Boder-Sedgwick syndrome (ataxia-telangiectasia) G11.3

Body, bodies
- mass index (BMI)
  - adult Z68-
  - pediatric

Body, bodies, *continued*
  - 5th percentile to less than 85th percentile for age Z68.52
  - 85th percentile to less than 95th percentile for age Z68.53
  - greater than or equal to ninety-fifth percentile for age Z68.54
  - less than fifth percentile for age Z68.51
- rocking F98.4

Boeck's
- disease or sarcoid—*see* Sarcoidosis
- lupoid (miliary) D86.3

Bonnevie-Ullrich syndrome Q87.19

Borderline
- diabetes mellitus (prediabetes) R73.03
- hypertension R03.0
- personality F60.3

Botalli, ductus (patent) (persistent) Q25.0

Botulism (foodborne intoxication) A05.1
- infant A48.51
- non-foodborne A48.52
- wound A48.52

Bouillaud's disease or syndrome (rheumatic heart disease) I01.9

Bourneville's disease Q85.1

Bowleg(s) (acquired) M21.16-
- congenital Q68.5

Brachycardia R00.1

Bradycardia (sinoatrial) (sinus) (vagal) R00.1
- neonatal P29.12
- tachycardia syndrome I49.5

Bradypnea R06.89

Bradytachycardia I49.5

Brailsford's disease or osteochondrosis—*see* Osteochondrosis, juvenile, radius

Brain—*see also* Disease, diseased
- death G93.82
- syndrome—*see* Syndrome, brain

Brash (water) R12

BRBPR K62.5

Breast—*see also* Disease, diseased
- buds E30.1
  - in newborn P96.89
- nodule N63.0

Breath
- foul R19.6
- holder, child R06.89
- holding spell R06.89
- shortness R06.02

Breathing
- labored—*see* Hyperventilation
- mouth R06.5
- periodic R06.3
  - high altitude G47.32

Breathlessness R06.81

Brennemann's syndrome I88.0

Bright red blood per rectum (BRBPR) K62.5

Briquet's disorder or syndrome F45.0

Brissaud's
- infantilism or dwarfism E23.0
- motor-verbal tic F95.2

Brittle
- bones disease Q78.0
- nails L60.3

Broad—*see also* Disease, diseased
- beta disease E78.2

Broad- or floating-betalipoproteinemia E78.2

Broken
- arm (meaning upper limb)—*see* Fracture, arm
- bone—*see* Fracture
- leg (meaning lower limb)—*see* Fracture, leg
- nose S02.2-
- tooth, teeth—*see* Fracture, tooth

Bromidism, bromism G92
- due to
  - correct substance properly administered—*see* Table of Drugs and Chemicals, by drug, adverse effect
  - overdose or wrong substance given or taken—*see* Table of Drugs and Chemicals, by drug, poisoning

Bronchiolitis (acute) (infective) (subacute) J21.9
- with
  - bronchospasm or obstruction J21.9
  - influenza, flu or grippe—*see* Influenza, with, respiratory manifestations NEC
- due to
  - external agent—*see* Bronchitis, acute, due to
  - human metapneumovirus J21.1
  - respiratory syncytial virus (RSV) J21.0
  - specified organism NEC J21.8
- influenzal—*see* Influenza, with, respiratory manifestations NEC

Bronchitis (diffuse) (fibrinous) (hypostatic) (infective) (membranous) J40
- with
  - influenza, flu or grippe—*see* Influenza, with, respiratory manifestations NEC
  - tracheitis (l5 years of age and above) J40
    - acute or subacute J20.9
    - under l5 years of age J20.9
- acute or subacute (with bronchospasm or obstruction) J20.9
  - due to
    - Haemophilus influenzae J20.1
    - Mycoplasma pneumoniae J20.0
    - specified organism NEC J20.8
    - Streptococcus J20.2
    - virus
      ~ coxsackie J20.3
      ~ echovirus J20.7
      ~ parainfluenza J20.4
      ~ respiratory syncytial (RSV) J20.5
      ~ rhinovirus J20.6
  - viral NEC J20.8
- allergic (acute) J45.909
  - with
    - exacerbation (acute) J45.901
    - status asthmaticus J45.902
- asthmatic J45.9
- catarrhal (l5 years of age and above) J40
  - acute—*see* Bronchitis, acute
  - under l5 years of age J20.9
- chronic J42
- mucopurulent
  - acute or subacute J20.9
- pneumococcal, acute or subacute J20.2
- viral NEC, acute or subacute (*see also* Bronchitis, acute) J20.8

Bronchoalveolitis J18.0

Bronchocele meaning goiter E04.0

Bronchomycosis NOS B49 *[J99]*
- candidal B37.1

Bronchorrhea J98.09
- acute J20.9

Bronchospasm (acute) J98.01
- with
  - bronchiolitis, acute J21.9
  - bronchitis, acute (conditions in J20)—*see* Bronchitis, acute
- due to external agent—*see* Disease, diseased, respiratory, acute, due to
- exercise induced J45.990

Bronze baby syndrome P83.88

Bruck-de Lange disease Q87.19

BRUE (brief resolved unexplained event) R68.13

Brugsch's syndrome Q82.8

Bruise (skin surface intact)—*see also* Contusion
- with
  - open wound—*see* Wound, open
- internal organ—*see* Injury, by site
- newborn P54.5
- scalp, due to birth injury, newborn P12.3

Bruit (arterial) R09.89
- cardiac R01.1

Bruxism
- psychogenic F45.8

Bubo I88.8
- indolent (nonspecific) I88.8
- inguinal (nonspecific) I88.8
  - infective I88.8
- scrofulous (tuberculous) A18.2
- syphilitic (primary) A51.0

Buds
- breast E30.1
  - in newborn P96.89

Bulimia (nervosa) F50.2
- atypical F50.9
- normal weight F50.9

Bulky
- stools R19.5

Bunion M21.61-
- tailor's M21.62-

Bunionette M21.62-

Buphthalmia, buphthalmos (congenital) Q15.0

Buried
- penis (congenital) Q55.64

Burkitt
- cell leukemia C91.0-
- lymphoma (malignant) C83.7-
  - small noncleaved, diffuse C83.7-
  - spleen C83.77
  - undifferentiated C83.7-
- tumor C83.7-
- type
  - acute lymphoblastic leukemia C91.0-
  - undifferentiated C83.7-

Burn (electricity) (flame) (hot gas, liquid or hot object) (radiation) (steam) (thermal) T30.0
- abdomen, abdominal (muscle) (wall) T21.02
  - first degree T21.12
  - second degree T21.22
  - third degree T21.32
- above elbow T22.03-
  - first degree T22.13-
  - left T22.032
    - first degree T22.132
    - second degree T22.232
    - third degree T22.332
  - right T22.031
    - first degree T22.131
    - second degree T22.231
    - third degree T22.331
  - second degree T22.23-
  - third degree T22.33-
- acid (caustic) (external) (internal)—*see* Corrosion, by site
- alimentary tract
  - esophagus T28.1
  - mouth T28.0
  - pharynx T28.0
- alkaline (caustic) (external) (internal)—*see* Corrosion, by site
- ankle T25.01-
  - first degree T25.11-
  - left T25.012
    - first degree T25.112
    - second degree T25.212
    - third degree T25.312
  - multiple with foot—*see* Burn, lower, limb, multiple sites, ankle and foot
  - right T25.011
    - first degree T25.111
    - second degree T25.211
    - third degree T25.311
  - second degree T25.21-
  - third degree T25.31-
- anus—*see* Burn, buttock
- arm (lower) (upper)—*see* Burn, upper limb
- axilla T22.04-
  - first degree T22.14-
  - left T22.042
    - first degree T22.142
    - second degree T22.242
    - third degree T22.342

Burn, *continued*
- right T22.041
  - first degree T22.141
  - second degree T22.241
  - third degree T22.341
- second degree T22.24-
- third degree T22.34-
- back (lower) T21.04
  - first degree T21.14
  - second degree T21.24
  - third degree T21.34
  - upper T21.03
    - first degree T21.13
    - second degree T21.23
    - third degree T21.33
- blisters *code as* Burn, second degree, by site
- breast(s)—*see* Burn, chest wall
- buttock(s) T21.05
  - first degree T21.15
  - second degree T21.25
  - third degree T21.35
- calf T24.03-
  - first degree T24.13-
  - left T24.032
    - first degree T24.132
    - second degree T24.232
    - third degree T24.332
  - right T24.031
    - first degree T24.131
    - second degree T24.231
    - third degree T24.331
  - second degree T24.23-
  - third degree T24.33-
- canthus (eye)—*see* Burn, eyelid
- caustic acid or alkaline—*see* Corrosion, by site
- cheek T20.06
  - first degree T20.16
  - second degree T20.26
  - third degree T20.36
- chemical (acids) (alkalines) (caustics) (external) (internal)—*see* Corrosion, by site
- chest wall T21.01
  - first degree T21.11
  - second degree T21.21
  - third degree T21.31
- chin T20.03
  - first degree T20.13
  - second degree T20.23
  - third degree T20.33
- conjunctiva (and cornea)—*see* Burn, cornea
- cornea (and conjunctiva) T26.1- (see complete *ICD-10-CM* Manual)
- corrosion (external) (internal)—*see* Corrosion, by site
- deep necrosis of underlying tissue *code as* Burn, third degree, by site
- dorsum of hand T23.069
  - first degree T23.16-
  - left T23.062
    - first degree T23.162
    - second degree T23.262
    - third degree T23.362
  - right T23.061
    - first degree T23.161
    - second degree T23.261
    - third degree T23.361
  - second degree T23.26-
  - third degree T23.36-
- due to ingested chemical agent—*see* Corrosion, by site
- ear (auricle) (external) (canal) T20.01
  - first degree T20.11
  - second degree T20.21
  - third degree T20.31
- elbow T22.02-
  - first degree T22.12-
  - left T22.022
    - first degree T22.122
    - second degree T22.222
    - third degree T22.322
  - right T22.021
    - first degree T22.121
    - second degree T22.221
    - third degree T22.321

Burn, *continued*
- – second degree T22.22-
- – third degree T22.32-
- • epidermal loss *code as* Burn, second degree, by site
- • erythema, erythematous *code as* Burn, first degree, by site
- • esophagus T28.1
- • extent (percentage of body surface)
  - – less than 10 percent T31.0
  - – 10 –19 percent T31.10
    - ■ with 0 – 9 percent third degree burns T31.10
    - ■ with 10 –19 percent third degree burns T31.11
- • extremity—*see* Burn, limb
- • eye(s) and adnexa T26.4- (see complete *ICD-10-CM* Manual)
- • eyelid(s) T26.0- (See complete *ICD-10-CM* Manual for codes)
- • face—*see* Burn, head
- • finger T23.029
  - – first degree T23.12-
  - – left T23.022
    - ■ first degree T23.122
    - ■ second degree T23.222
    - ■ third degree T23.322
  - – multiple sites (without thumb) T23.03-
    - ■ with thumb T23.04-
      - ~ first degree T23.14-
      - ~ left T23.042
        - ◊ first degree T23.142
        - ◊ second degree T23.242
        - ◊ third degree T23.342
      - ~ right T23.041
        - ◊ first degree T23.141
        - ◊ second degree T23.241
        - ◊ third degree T23.341
      - ~ second degree T23.24-
      - ~ third degree T23.34-
    - ■ first degree T23.13-
    - ■ left T23.032
      - ~ first degree T23.132
      - ~ second degree T23.232
      - ~ third degree T23.332
    - ■ right T23.031
      - ~ first degree T23.131
      - ~ second degree T23.231
      - ~ third degree T23.331
    - ■ second degree T23.23-
    - ■ third degree T23.33-
  - – right T23.021
    - ■ first degree T23.121
    - ■ second degree T23.221
    - ■ third degree T23.321
  - – second degree T23.22-
  - – third degree T23.32-
- • flank—*see* Burn, abdomen, abdominal (muscle) (wall)
- • foot T25.02-
  - – first degree T25.12-
  - – left T25.022
    - ■ first degree T25.122
    - ■ second degree T25.222
    - ■ third degree T25.322
  - – multiple with ankle—*see* Burn, lower, limb, multiple sites
  - – right T25.021
    - ■ first degree T25.121
    - ■ second degree T25.221
    - ■ third degree T25.321
  - – second degree T25.22-
  - – third degree T25.32-
- • forearm T22.01-
  - – first degree T22.11-
  - – left T22.012
    - ■ first degree T22.112
    - ■ second degree T22.212
    - ■ third degree T22.312
  - – right T22.011
    - ■ first degree T22.111
    - ■ second degree T22.211
    - ■ third degree T22.311
  - – second degree T22.219
  - – third degree T22.319

Burn, *continued*
- • forehead T20.06
  - – first degree T20.16
  - – second degree T20.26
  - – third degree T20.36
- • fourth degree *code as* Burn, third degree, by site
- • friction—*see* Burn, by site
- • from swallowing caustic or corrosive substance NEC—*see* Corrosion, by site
- • full thickness skin loss *code as* Burn, third degree, by site
- • genital organs
  - – external
    - ■ female T21.07
      - ~ first degree T21.17
      - ~ second degree T21.27
      - ~ third degree T21.37
    - ■ male T21.06
      - ~ first degree T21.16
      - ~ second degree T21.26
      - ~ third degree T21.36
- • groin—*see* Burn, abdomen, abdominal (muscle) (wall)
- • hand(s) T23.009
  - – back—*see* Burn, dorsum of hand
  - – finger—*see* Burn, finger
  - – first degree T23.10-
  - – left T23.002
    - ■ first degree T23.102
    - ■ second degree T23.202
    - ■ third degree T23.302
  - – multiple sites with wrist T23.09-
    - ■ first degree T23.19-
    - ■ left T23.092
      - ~ first degree T23.192
      - ~ second degree T23.292
      - ~ third degree T23.392
    - ■ right T23.091
      - ~ first degree T23.191
      - ~ second degree T23.291
      - ~ third degree T23.391
    - ■ second degree T23.29-
    - ■ third degree T23.39-
  - – palm—*see* Burn, palm
  - – right T23.001
    - ■ first degree T23.101
    - ■ second degree T23.201
    - ■ third degree T23.301
  - – second degree T23.20-
  - – third degree T23.30-
  - – thumb—*see* Burn, thumb
- • head (and face) (and neck) (*Code by* Burn to specific site for cheek, chin, ear, eye, forehead, lip, neck, nose, or scalp) T20.00
  - – first degree T20.10
  - – multiple sites T20.09
    - ■ first degree T20.19
    - ■ second degree T20.29
    - ■ third degree T20.39
  - – second degree T20.20
  - – third degree T20.30
- • hip(s)—*see* Burn, thigh
- • inhalation—*see* Burn, respiratory tract
  - – caustic or corrosive substance (fumes)—*see* Corrosion
- • internal organ(s)
  - – esophagus T28.1
  - – from caustic or corrosive substance (swallowing) NEC—*see* Corrosion, by site
  - – mouth T28.0
  - – pharynx T28.0
- • interscapular region—*see* Burn, back, upper
- • knee T24.02-
  - – first degree T24.12-
  - – left T24.022
    - ■ first degree T24.122
    - ■ second degree T24.222
    - ■ third degree T24.322
  - – right T24.021
    - ■ first degree T24.121
    - ■ second degree T24.221
    - ■ third degree T24.321
  - – second degree T24.22-
  - – third degree T24.32-

Burn, *continued*
- • labium (majus) (minus)—*see* Burn, genital organs, external, female
- • lacrimal apparatus, duct, gland or sac—*see* Burn, eye, specified site NEC
- • larynx T27.0- (See complete *ICD-10-CM* Manual for codes)
  - – with lung T27.1-
- • leg(s) (lower) (upper)—*see* Burn, lower, limb
- • lightning—*see* Burn, by site
- • limb(s)
  - – lower (except ankle or foot alone)—*see* Burn, lower, limb
  - – upper—*see* Burn, upper limb
- • lip(s) T20.02
  - – first degree T20.12
  - – second degree T20.22
  - – third degree T20.32
- • lower
  - – back—*see* Burn, back
  - – limb T24.00- (*Code to* Burn by specific site for ankle, calf, foot, thigh, knee)
    - ■ first degree T24.109
    - ■ left T24.002
      - ~ first degree T24.102
      - ~ second degree T24.202
      - ~ third degree T24.302
    - ■ multiple sites, except ankle and foot T24.099
      - ~ ankle and foot T25.09-
        - ◊ first degree T25.19-
        - ◊ left T25.092
          - » first degree T25.192
          - » second degree T25.292
          - » third degree T25.392
        - ◊ right T25.091
          - » first degree T25.191
          - » second degree T25.291
          - » third degree T25.391
        - ◊ second degree T25.29-
        - ◊ third degree T25.39-
      - ~ first degree T24.19-
      - ~ left T24.092
        - ◊ first degree T24.192
        - ◊ second degree T24.292
        - ◊ third degree T24.392
      - ~ right T24.091
        - ◊ first degree T24.191
        - ◊ second degree T24.291
        - ◊ third degree T24.391
      - ~ second degree T24.29-
      - ~ third degree T24.39-
    - ■ right T24.001
      - ~ first degree T24.101
      - ~ second degree T24.201
      - ~ third degree T24.301
    - ■ second degree T24.20-
    - ■ thigh—*see* Burn, thigh
    - ■ third degree T24.30-
    - ■ toe—*see* Burn, toe
- • mouth T28.0
- • neck T20.07
  - – first degree T20.17
  - – second degree T20.27
  - – third degree T20.37
- • nose (septum) T20.04
  - – first degree T20.14
  - – second degree T20.24
  - – third degree T20.34
- • ocular adnexa—*see* Burn, eye
- • orbit region—*see* Burn, eyelid
- • palm T23.059
  - – first degree T23.15-
  - – left T23.052
    - ■ first degree T23.152
    - ■ second degree T23.252
    - ■ third degree T23.352
  - – right T23.051
    - ■ first degree T23.151
    - ■ second degree T23.251
    - ■ third degree T23.351
  - – second degree T23.25-
  - – third degree T23.35-

Burn, *continued*
- partial thickness *code as* Burn, unspecified degree, by site
- pelvis—*see* Burn, trunk
- penis—*see* Burn, genital organs, external, male
- perineum
  - female—*see* Burn, genital organs, external, female
  - male—*see* Burn, genital organs, external, male
- periocular area—*see* Burn, eyelid
- pharynx T28.0
- respiratory tract T27.- (See complete *ICD-10-CM* Manual for codes)
- scalp T20.05
  - first degree T20.15
  - second degree T20.25
  - third degree T20.35
- scapular region T22.06-
  - first degree T22.16-
  - left T22.062
    - first degree T22.162
    - second degree T22.262
    - third degree T22.362
  - right T22.061
    - first degree T22.161
    - second degree T22.261
    - third degree T22.361
  - second degree T22.26-
  - third degree T22.36-
- scrotum—*see* Burn, genital organs, external, male
- shoulder T22.05-
  - first degree T22.15-
  - left T22.052
    - first degree T22.152
    - second degree T22.252
    - third degree T22.352
  - right T22.051
    - first degree T22.151
    - second degree T22.251
    - third degree T22.351
  - second degree T22.25-
  - third degree T22.35-
- temple—*see* Burn, head
- testis—*see* Burn, genital organs, external, male
- thigh T24.01-
  - first degree T24.11-
  - left T24.012
    - first degree T24.112
    - second degree T24.212
    - third degree T24.312
  - right T24.011
    - first degree T24.111
    - second degree T24.211
    - third degree T24.311
  - second degree T24.21-
  - third degree T24.31-
- thorax (external)—*see* Burn, trunk
- throat (meaning pharynx) T28.0
- thumb(s) T23.01-
  - first degree T23.11-
  - left T23.012
    - first degree T23.112
    - second degree T23.212
    - third degree T23.312
  - multiple sites with fingers T23.04-
    - first degree T23.14-
    - left T23.042
      - ~ first degree T23.142
      - ~ second degree T23.242
      - ~ third degree T23.342
    - right T23.041
      - ~ first degree T23.141
      - ~ second degree T23.241
      - ~ third degree T23.341
    - second degree T23.24-
    - third degree T23.34-
  - right T23.011
    - first degree T23.111
    - second degree T23.211
    - third degree T23.311
  - second degree T23.21-
  - third degree T23.31-

Burn, *continued*
- toe T25.039
  - first degree T25.139
  - left T25.032
    - first degree T25.132
    - second degree T25.232
    - third degree T25.332
  - right T25.031
    - first degree T25.131
    - second degree T25.231
    - third degree T25.331
  - second degree T25.23-
  - third degree T25.33-
- tongue T28.0
- tonsil(s) T28.0
- trachea T27.- (See complete *ICD-10-CM* Manual for codes)
- trunk T21.00 *(Code to Burn by specific site for abdominal wall, buttock, upper limb, back, chest wall, genital organs, or scapular region)*
  - first degree T21.10
  - second degree T21.20
  - specified site NEC T21.09
    - first degree T21.19
    - second degree T21.29
    - third degree T21.39
  - third degree T21.30
- unspecified site with extent of body surface involved specified
  - less than 10 percent T31.0
  - 10 –19 percent (0 – 9 percent third degree) T31.10
    - with 10 –19 percent third degree T31.11
- upper limb *(Code to Burn by specific site for above elbow, axilla, elbow, forearm, hand, scapular region, shoulder, upper back, or wrist)* T22.00
  - first degree T22.10
  - multiple sites T22.09-
    - first degree T22.19-
    - left T22.092
      - ~ first degree T22.192
      - ~ second degree T22.292
      - ~ third degree T22.392
    - right T22.091
      - ~ first degree T22.191
      - ~ second degree T22.291
      - ~ third degree T22.391
    - second degree T22.29-
    - third degree T22.39-
  - second degree T22.20
  - third degree T22.3-
- vulva—*see* Burn, genital organs, external, female
- wrist T23.07-
  - first degree T23.17-
  - left T23.072
    - first degree T23.172
    - second degree T23.272
    - third degree T23.372
  - multiple sites with hand T23.09-
    - first degree T23.19-
    - left T23.092
      - ~ first degree T23.192
      - ~ second degree T23.292
      - ~ third degree T23.392
    - right T23.091
      - ~ first degree T23.191
      - ~ second degree T23.291
      - ~ third degree T23.391
    - second degree T23.29-
    - third degree T23.39-
  - right T23.071
    - first degree T23.171
    - second degree T23.271
    - third degree T23.371
  - second degree T23.27-
  - third degree T23.37-

Burnett's syndrome E83.52

Bursitis M71.9
- hip NEC M70.7-
  - trochanteric M70.6-
- radiohumeral M77.8

Bursitis, *continued*
- specified NEC M71.50
  - ankle M71.57-
  - due to use, overuse or pressure—*see* Disorder
  - elbow M71.52-
  - foot M71.57-
  - hand M71.54-
  - hip M71.55-
  - knee M71.56-
  - specified site NEC M71.58
  - tibial collateral M76.4-
  - wrist M71.53-

C

Cachexia R64
- dehydration E86.0
  - with
    - hypernatremia E87.0
    - hyponatremia E87.1
    - hypophyseal E23.0
    - hypopituitary E23.0
    - pituitary E23.0
    - Simmonds' E23.0

CADASIL (cerebral autosomal dominate arteriopathy with subcortical infarcts and leukocephalopathy) I67.850

Café au lait spots L81.3

Caked breast (puerperal, postpartum) O92.79

Calciferol (vitamin D) deficiency E55.9
- with rickets E55.0

Calcification
- adrenal (capsule) (gland) E27.49
- cerebral (cortex) G93.89
- choroid plexus G93.89
- kidney N28.89
  - tuberculous B90.9
- lymph gland or node (postinfectional) I89.8
  - tuberculous B90.8
- pericardium *(see also* Pericarditis) I31.1
- pleura
  - tuberculous NEC B90.9
- subcutaneous L94.2
- suprarenal (capsule) (gland) E27.49

Calcinosis (interstitial) (tumoral) (universalis) E83.59
- circumscripta (skin) L94.2
- cutis L94.2

Calciuria 82.994

Calculus, calculi, calculous
- biliary—*see also* Calculus, gallbladder
  - specified NEC K80.80
    - with obstruction K80.81
- bilirubin, multiple—*see* Calculus, gallbladder
- bladder (encysted) (impacted) (urinary) (diverticulum) N21.0
- gallbladder K80.20
  - with
    - bile duct calculus—*see* Calculus, gallbladder, with, bile duct calculus
    - cholecystitis K80.10
      - ~ with obstruction K80.11
      - ~ acute K80.00
        - ◊ with
          - » chronic cholecystitis K80.12
            - ❖ with obstruction K80.13
          - » obstruction K80.01
      - ~ chronic K80.10
        - ◊ with
          - » acute cholecystitis K80.12
            - ❖ with obstruction K80.13
          - » obstruction K80.11
      - ~ specified NEC K80.18
        - ◊ with obstruction K80.19
    - obstruction K80.21
- intestinal (impaction) (obstruction) K56.49
- kidney (impacted) (multiple) (pelvis) (recurrent) (staghorn) N20.0
  - with calculus, ureter N20.2
  - congenital Q63.8
- nose J34.89
- pyelitis (impacted) (recurrent) N20.0
  - with hydronephrosis N13.6

Calculus, calculi, calculous, *continued*
- pyelonephritis (impacted) (recurrent)—*see* category N20
  - with hydronephrosis N13.2
- tonsil J35.8
- ureter (impacted) (recurrent) N20.1
  - with calculus, kidney N20.2
    - with hydronephrosis N13.6
      ~ with infection N13.6
      ~ ureteropelvic junction N20.1
- urethra (impacted) N21.1
- urinary (duct) (impacted) (passage) (tract) N20.9
  - with hydronephrosis N13.2
    - with infection N13.6
- vagina N89.8
- xanthine E79.8 [N22]

California
- encephalitis A83.5

Callositas, callosity (infected) L84

Callus (infected) L84

CALME (Childhood asymmetric labium majus enlargement) N90.61

Calorie deficiency or malnutrition (*see also* Malnutrition) E46

Calvé-Perthes disease M91.1-

Camptocormia (hysterical) F44.4

Canal—*see also* Disease, diseased
- atrioventricular common Q21.2

Candidiasis, candidal B37.9
- balanitis B37.42
- bronchitis B37.1
- cheilitis B37.83
- congenital P37.5
- cystitis B37.41
- disseminated B37.7
- endocarditis B37.6
- enteritis B37.82
- esophagitis B37.81
- intertrigo B37.2
- lung B37.1
- meningitis B37.5
- mouth B37.0
- nails B37.2
- neonatal P37.5
- onychia B37.2
- oral B37.0
- osteomyelitis B37.89
- otitis externa B37.84
- paronychia B37.2
- perionyxis B37.2
- pneumonia B37.1
- proctitis B37.82
- pulmonary B37.1
- pyelonephritis B37.49
- sepsis B37.7
- skin B37.2
- specified site NEC B37.89
- stomatitis B37.0
- systemic B37.7
- urethritis B37.41
- urogenital site NEC B37.49
- vagina B37.3
- vulva B37.3
- vulvovaginitis B37.3

Canker (mouth) (sore) K12.0
- rash A38.9

Caput
- crepitus Q75.8

Carbuncle L02.93
- abdominal wall L02.231
- anus K61.0
- axilla L02.43-
- back (any part) L02.232
- breast N61.1
- buttock L02.33
- cheek (external) L02.03
- chest wall L02.233
- chin L02.03
- face NEC L02.03
- finger L02.53-
- flank L02.231

Carbuncle, *continued*
- foot L02.63-
- forehead L02.03
- gluteal (region) L02.33
- groin L02.234
- hand L02.53-
- head NEC L02.831
- heel L02.63-
- hip L02.43-
- knee L02.43-
- lower limb L02.43-
- navel L02.236
- neck L02.13
- nose (external) (septum) J34.0
- partes posteriores L02.33
- pectoral region L02.233
- perineum L02.235
- pinna—*see* Abscess, ear, external
- scalp L02.831
- specified site NEC L02.838
- temple (region) L02.03
- thumb L02.53-
- toe L02.63-
- trunk L02.239
  - abdominal wall L02.231
  - back L02.232
  - chest wall L02.233
  - groin L02.234
  - perineum L02.235
  - umbilicus L02.236
- umbilicus L02.236
- upper limb L02.43-
- urethra N34.0
- vulva N76.4

Carcinoma (malignant)—*see also* Neoplasm, by site, malignant in the Table of Neoplasms in the complete *ICD-10-CM* manual.
- Merkel cell C4A.-
- renal cell C64-

Cardiac—*see also* Disease, diseased
- death, sudden—*see* Arrest, cardiac
- pacemaker
  - in situ Z95.0
  - management or adjustment Z45.018
- tamponade I31.4

Cardiochalasia K21.9

Cardiomegaly—*see also* Hypertrophy, cardiac
- congenital Q24.8
- idiopathic I51.7

Cardiomyopathy (familial) (idiopathic) I42.9
- constrictive NOS I42.5
- due to
  - Friedreich's ataxia G11.11
  - progressive muscular dystrophy G71.0
- hypertrophic (nonobstructive) I42.2
  - obstructive I42.1
    - congenital Q24.8
- in
  - sarcoidosis D86.85
- metabolic E88.9 [I43]
  - thyrotoxic E05.90 [I43]
    - with thyroid storm E05.91 [I43]
- nutritional E63.9 [I43]
- restrictive NEC I42.5
- secondary I42.9
- specified NEC I42.8
- thyrotoxic E05.90 [I43]
  - with thyroid storm E05.91 [I43]

Cardiopathia nigra I27.0

Cardiopathy
- idiopathic I42.9
- mucopolysaccharidosis E76.3 [I52]

Cardiosymphysis I31.0

Care (of) (for) (following)
- family member (handicapped) (sick)
  - unavailable, due to
    - absence (person rendering care) (sufferer) Z74.2
    - inability (any reason) of person rendering care Z74.2
- foundling Z76.1

Care, *continued*
- palliative Z51.5
- unavailable, due to
  - absence of person rendering care Z74.2
  - inability (any reason) of person rendering care Z74.2
- well baby Z76.2

Caries
- dental K02.9

Carnitine insufficiency E71.40

Carpenter's syndrome Q87.0

Carrier (suspected) **of**
- bacterial disease NEC Z22.39
  - diphtheria Z22.2
  - intestinal infectious NEC Z22.1
    - typhoid Z22.0
  - meningococcal Z22.31
  - sexually transmitted Z22.4
  - specified NEC Z22.39
  - staphylococcal (Methicillin susceptible) Z22.321
    - Methicillin resistant Z22.322
  - streptococcal Z22.338
    - group B Z22.330
- genetic Z14.8
  - cystic fibrosis Z14.1
  - hemophilia A (asymptomatic) Z14.01
    - symptomatic Z14.02
- gonorrhea Z22.4
- HAA (hepatitis Australian-antigen) Z22.5
- HB (c)(s)-AG Z22.5
- hepatitis (viral) Z22.5
  - Australia-antigen (HAA) Z22.5
  - B surface antigen (HBsAg) Z22.5
  - C Z22.5
  - specified NEC Z22.5
- infectious organism Z22.9
  - specified NEC Z22.8
- meningococci Z22.31
- serum hepatitis—*see* Carrier, hepatitis
- staphylococci (Methicillin susceptible) Z22.321
  - Methicillin resistant Z22.322
- streptococci Z22.338
  - group B Z22.330
- syphilis Z22.4
- venereal disease Z22.4

Car sickness T75.3

Caruncle (inflamed)
- myrtiform N89.8

Caseation lymphatic gland (tuberculous) A18.2

Casts in urine R82.998

Cat
- cry syndrome Q93.4

Cataract (cortical) (immature) (incipient) H26.9
- anterior
  - and posterior axial embryonal Q12.0
  - pyramidal Q12.0
- blue Q12.0
- central Q12.0
- cerulean Q12.0
- congenital Q12.0
- coraliform Q12.0
- coronary Q12.0
- crystalline Q12.0
- in
  - hypoparathyroidism E20.9 [H28]
  - nutritional disease E63.9 [H28]
- infantile—*see* Cataract, presenile
- juvenile—*see* Cataract, presenile
- nuclear
  - embryonal Q12.0
- presenile H26.00-
- zonular (perinuclear) Q12.0

Cataracta—*see also* Cataract
- centralis pulverulenta Q12.0
- cerulea Q12.0
- congenita Q12.0
- coralliformis Q12.0
- coronaria Q12.0
- membranacea
  - congenita Q12.0

Catarrh, catarrhal (acute) (febrile) (infectious) (inflammation) (see also Disease, diseased) J00
- chronic J31.0
- gingivitis K05.00
  - plaque induced K05.00
- larynx, chronic J37.0
- liver B15.9
- middle ear, chronic H65.2-
- mouth K12.1
- nasal (chronic)—see Rhinitis
- nasopharyngeal (chronic) J31.1
  - acute J00
- pulmonary—see Bronchitis
- spring (eye) (vernal)—see Conjunctivitis, acute, atopic
- summer (hay)—see Fever, hay
- throat J31.2
- tubotympanal—see also Otitis, media, acute, subacute, nonsupparative NEC
  - chronic H65.2-

Catatonic
- stupor R40.1

Cat-scratch disease or fever A28.1

Cavovarus foot, congenital Q66.1-

Cavus foot (congenital) Q66.7-

CDKL5 (Cyclin-Dependent Kinase-Like 5 Deficiency Disorder) G40.42

Cecitis K52.9
- with perforation, peritonitis, or rupture K65.8

Cecoureterocele Q62.32

Celiac
- disease (with steatorrhea) K90.0
- infantilism K90.0

Cells (see Disease, diseased)
- in urine R82.998

Cellulitis (diffuse) (phlegmonous) (septic) (suppurative) L03.90
- abdominal wall L03.311
- ankle L03.11-
- anus K61.0
- axilla L03.11-
- back (any part) L03.312
- breast (acute) (nonpuerperal) N61.0
  - nipple N61.0
- buttock L03.317
- cervical (meaning neck) L03.221
- cheek (external) L03.211
  - internal K12.2
- chest wall L03.313
- chronic L03.90
- drainage site (following operation) T81.49
- ear (external) H60.1-
- erysipelatous—see Erysipelas
- face NEC L03.211
- finger (intrathecal) (periosteal) (subcutaneous) (subcuticular) L03.01-
- foot L03.11-
- gangrenous—see Gangrene
- gluteal (region) L03.317
- groin L03.314
- head NEC L03.811
  - face (any part, except ear, eye and nose) L03.211
- jaw (region) L03.211
- knee L03.11-
- lip K13.0
- lower limb L03.11-
  - toe—see Cellulitis, toe
- mouth (floor) K12.2
- multiple sites, so stated L03.90
- navel L03.316
  - newborn P38.9
    - with mild hemorrhage P38.1
    - without hemorrhage P38.9
- neck (region) L03.221
- nose (septum) (external) J34.0
- orbit, orbital H05.01-
  - periorbital L03.213
- palate (soft) K12.2
- pectoral (region) L03.313

Cellulitis, continued
- pelvis, pelvic (chronic)
  - female (see also Disease, pelvis, inflammatory) N73.2
    - acute N73.0
  - male K65.0
- perineal, perineum L03.315
- periorbital L03.213
- perirectal K61.1peritonsillar J36
- preseptal L03.213
- rectum K61.1
- scalp (any part) L03.811
- specified site NEC L03.818
- submandibular (region) (space) (triangle) K12.2
  - gland K11.3
- submaxillary (region) K12.2
  - gland K11.3
- toe (intrathecal) (periosteal) (subcutaneous) (subcuticular) L03.03
- tonsil J36
- trunk L03.319
  - abdominal wall L03.311
  - back (any part) L03.312
  - buttock L03.317
  - chest wall L03.313
  - groin L03.314
  - perineal, perineum L03.315
  - umbilicus L03.316
- umbilicus L03.316
- upper limb L03.11-
  - axilla L03.11-
  - finger L03.01-
  - thumb L03.01-
- vaccinal T88.0

Central auditory processing disorder H93.25

Cephalematoma, cephalhematoma (calcified)
- newborn (birth injury) P12.0

Cephalgia, cephalalgia—see also Headache
- histamine G44.009
  - intractable G44.001
  - not intractable G44.009

Cerumen (accumulation) (impacted) H61.2-

Cervicalgia M54.2

Cervicitis (acute) (chronic) (nonvenereal) (senile (atrophic)) (subacute) (with ulceration) N72
- chlamydial A56.09
- gonococcal A54.03
- trichomonal A59.09

Cervicocolpitis (emphysematosa) (see also Cervicitis) N72

Cestode infestation B71.9
- specified type NEC B71.8

Cestodiasis B71.9

Chafing L30.4

Chalasia (cardiac sphincter) K21.9

Chalazion H00.10
- left H00.16
  - lower H00.15
  - upper H00.14
- right H00.13
  - lower H00.12
  - upper H00.11

Chancre (any genital site) (hard) (hunterian) (mixed) (primary) (seronegative) (seropositive) (syphilitic) A51.0
- conjunctiva NEC A51.2
- extragenital A51.2
- eyelid A51.2
- lip A51.2
- nipple A51.2
- palate, soft A51.2
- soft
  - palate A51.2
- urethra A51.0

Change(s) (in) (of)—see also Removal
- circulatory I99.9
- contraceptive device Z30.433
- dressing (nonsurgical) Z48.00
  - surgical Z48.01

Change(s), continued
- hypertrophic
  - nasal sinus J34.89
  - turbinate, nasal J34.3
  - upper respiratory tract J39.8
- mental status R41.82
- sacroiliac joint M53.3
- skin R23.9
  - acute, due to ultraviolet radiation L56.9
    - specified NEC L56.8
  - cyanosis R23.0
  - flushing R23.2
  - pallor R23.1
  - petechiae R23.3
  - specified change NEC R23.8
  - swelling—see Mass, localized
- vascular I99.9
- voice R49.9
  - psychogenic F44.4

CHARGE association Q89.8

Charley-horse (quadriceps) M62.831
- traumatic (quadriceps) S76.11-

Checking (of)
- implantable subdermal contraceptive Z30.46
- intrauterine contraceptive device Z30.431

Cheese itch B88.0

Cheilitis (acute) (angular) (catarrhal) (chronic) (exfoliative) (gangrenous) (glandular) (infectional) (suppurative) (ulcerative) (vesicular) K13.0
- actinic (due to sun) L56.8
  - other than from sun L56.9
- candidal B37.83

Cheilodynia K13.0

Cheiloschisis—see Cleft, lip

Cheilosis (angular) K13.0

Cheiropompholyx L30.1

Chemotherapy (session) (for)
- cancer Z51.11
- neoplasm Z51.11

Cheyne-Stokes breathing (respiration) R06.3

Chickenpox—see Varicella

Chigger (infestation) B88.0

Child
- custody dispute Z65.3

Childhood
- cerebral X-linked adrenoleukodystrophy E71.520
- period of rapid growth Z00.2

Chill(s) R68.83
- with fever R50.9
- congestive in malarial regions B54
- without fever R68.83

Chinese dysentery A03.9

Chlamydia, chlamydial A74.9
- cervicitis A56.09
- conjunctivitis A74.0
- cystitis A56.01
- endometritis A56.11
- epididymitis A56.19
- female
  - pelvic inflammatory disease A56.11
  - pelviperitonitis A56.11
- orchitis A56.19
- peritonitis A74.81
- pharyngitis A56.4
- proctitis A56.3
- salpingitis A56.11
- sexually-transmitted infection NEC A56.8
- specified NEC A74.89
- urethritis A56.01
- vulvovaginitis A56.02

Chlamydiosis—see Chlamydia

Chlorotic anemia D50.8

Cholecystitis K81.9
- with
  - gangrene of gallbladder K82.A1
  - perforation of gallbladder K82.A2
- acute (emphysematous) (gangrenous) (suppurative) K81.0

Cholecystitis, *continued*
- with
  - calculus, stones in
    - ~ cystic duct—*see* Calculus, gallbladder, with, cholecystitis, acute
    - ~ gallbladder—*see* Calculus, gallbladder, with, cholecystitis, acute
  - choledocholithiasis—*see* Calculus, gallbladder, with, cholecystitis, acute
  - cholelithiasis—*see* Calculus, gallbladder, with, cholecystitis, acute
  - chronic cholecystitis K81.2
    - ~ with gallbladder calculus K80.12
    - ◊ with obstruction K80.13
- chronic K81.1
  - with acute cholecystitis K81.2
    - with gallbladder calculus K80.12
    - ~ with obstruction K80.13
- emphysematous (acute)—*see* Cholecystitis, acute
- gangrenous—*see* Cholecystitis, acute
- suppurative—*see* Cholecystitis, acute

Choking sensation R09.89

Cholesteremia E78.0

Cholesterol
- elevated (high) E78.00
  - with elevated (high) triglycerides E78.2
  - screening for Z13.220

Cholesterolemia (essential) (pure) E78.00
- familial E78.01
- hereditary E78.01

Chondritis M94.8X-
- costal (Tietze's) M94.0
- patella, posttraumatic M22.4-

Chondrodysplasia Q78.9
- with hemangioma Q78.4
- calcificans congenita Q77.3
- fetalis Q77.4
- metaphyseal (Jansen's) (McKusick's) (Schmid's) Q78.8
- punctata Q77.3

Chondrodystrophy, chondrodystrophia (familial) (fetalis) (hypoplastic) Q78.9
- calcificans congenita Q77.3
- myotonic (congenital) G71.13
- punctata Q77.3

Chondroectodermal dysplasia Q77.6

Chondrogenesis imperfecta Q77.4

Chondromalacia (systemic) M94.2-
- knee M94.26-
  - patella M22.4-

Chondro-osteodysplasia (Morquio-Brailsford type) E76.219

Chondro-osteodystrophy E76.29

Chondropathia tuberosa M94.0

Chordee (nonvenereal) N48.89
- congenital Q54.4

Chorea (chronic) (gravis) (posthemiplegic) (senile) (spasmodic) G25.5
- drug-induced G25.4
- hysterical F44.4
- progressive G25.5
- with
  - heart involvement I02.0
    - active or acute (conditions in I01-) I02.0
    - rheumatic I02.9
      - ~ with valvular disorder I02.0
  - rheumatic heart disease (chronic) (inactive) (quiescent)—*code to* rheumatic heart condition involved

Choreoathetosis (paroxysmal) G25.5

Chorioretinitis
- in (due to)
  - toxoplasmosis (acquired) B58.01
    - congenital (active) P37.1 *[H32]*

Chromophytosis B36.0

Chylopericardium I31.3
- acute I30.9

Cicatricial (deformity)—*see* Cicatrix

Cicatrix (adherent) (contracted) (painful) (vicious) (*see also* Scar) L90.5
- adenoid (and tonsil) J35.8
- anus K62.89
- brain G93.89
- mouth K13.79
- muscle M62.89
  - with contracture—*see* Contraction, muscle NEC
- palate (soft) K13.79
- rectum K62.89
- skin L90.5
  - postinfective L90.5
  - specified site NEC L90.5
  - tuberculous B90.8
- tonsil (and adenoid) J35.8
- tuberculous NEC B90.9
- vagina N89.8
  - postoperative N99.2
- wrist, constricting (annular) L90.5

CINCA (chronic infantile neurological, cutaneous and articular syndrome) M04.2

Circulation
- failure (peripheral) R57.9
  - newborn P29.89
- fetal, persistent P29.38

Circumcision (in absence of medical indication) (ritual) (routine) Z41.2

Cirrhosis, cirrhotic (hepatic) (liver) K74.60
- due to
  - xanthomatosis E78.2
- fatty K76.0
- liver K74.60
  - congenital P78.81
- pigmentary E83.110
- xanthomatous (biliary) K74.5
  - due to xanthomatosis (familial) (metabolic) (primary) E78.2

Clam digger's itch B65.3

Clammy skin R23.1

Clark's paralysis G80.9

Claudication, intermittent I73.9
- cerebral (artery) G45.9

Clavus (infected) L84

Clawfoot (congenital) Q66.89
- acquired M21.53-

Clawtoe (congenital) Q66.89
- acquired M20.5X-

Cleft (congenital)—*see also* Imperfect, closure
- foot Q72.7
- hand Q71.6
- lip (unilateral) Q36.9
  - with cleft palate Q37.9
    - hard Q37.1
      - ~ with soft Q37.5
    - soft Q37.3
      - ~ with hard Q37.5
  - bilateral Q36.0
    - with cleft palate Q37.8
      - hard Q37.0
        - ◊ with soft Q37.4
      - ~ soft Q37.2
        - ◊ with hard Q37.4
  - median Q36.1
- palate Q35.9
  - with cleft lip (unilateral) Q37.9
    - bilateral Q37.8
  - hard Q35.1
    - with
      - ~ cleft lip (unilateral) Q37.1
        - ◊ bilateral Q37.0
      - ~ soft Q35.5
        - ◊ with cleft lip (unilateral) Q37.5
          - » bilateral Q37.4
  - medial Q35.5
  - soft Q35.3
    - with
      - ~ cleft lip (unilateral) Q37.3
        - ◊ bilateral Q37.2

Cleft, *continued*
  - ~ hard Q35.5
    - ◊ with cleft lip (unilateral) Q37.5
      - » bilateral Q37.4
- penis Q55.69
- scrotum Q55.29
- uvula Q35.7

Cleidocranial dysostosis Q74.0

Clicking hip (newborn) R29.4

Closed bite M26.29

Closure
- congenital, nose Q30.0
- foramen ovale, imperfect Q21.1
- hymen N89.6
- interauricular septum, defective Q21.1
- interventricular septum, defective Q21.0
- lacrimal duct—*see also* Stenosis, lacrimal, duct
  - congenital Q10.5
- nose (congenital) Q30.0
  - acquired M95.0
- vagina N89.5

Clot (blood)—*see also* Embolism
- artery (obstruction) (occlusion)—*see* Embolism
- circulation I74.9

Clouded state R40.1
- epileptic—*see* Epilepsy, specified NEC
- paroxysmal—*see* Epilepsy, specified NEC

Cloudy antrum, antra J32.0

Clubfoot (congenital) Q66.89
- acquired M21.54-
- equinovarus Q66.0-
- paralytic M21.54-

Clubhand (congenital) (radial) Q71.4-
- acquired M21.51-

Clumsiness, clumsy child syndrome F82

Cluttering F80.81

Coagulopathy—*see also* Defect, coagulation
- consumption D65
- intravascular D65
  - newborn P60

Coalition
- calcaneo-scaphoid Q66.89
- tarsal Q66.89

Coarctation
- aorta (preductal) (postductal) Q25.1
- pulmonary artery Q25.71

Coccydynia, coccygodynia M53.3

Cockayne's syndrome Q87.19

Cock's peculiar tumor L72.3

Cold J00
- with influenza, flu, or grippe—*see* Influenza, with, respiratory manifestations NEC
- agglutinin disease or hemoglobinuria (chronic) D59.12
- bronchial—*see* Bronchitis
- chest—*see* Bronchitis
- common (head) J00
- head J00
- on lung—*see* Bronchitis
- rose J30.1
- virus J00
- sensitivity, auto-immune D59.12
- symptoms J00

Colibacillosis A49.8
- as the cause of other disease (*see also* Escherichia coli) B96.20
- generalized A41.50

Colic (bilious) (infantile) (intestinal) (recurrent) (spasmodic) R10.83
- abdomen R10.83
  - psychogenic F45.8
- hysterical F45.8
- kidney N23
- mucous K58.9
  - with constipation K58.1
  - with diarrhea K58.0
  - mixed K58.2
  - other K58.8
  - psychogenic F54

Colic, *continued*
- nephritic N23
- psychogenic F45.8
- renal N23
- ureter N23
- uterus NEC N94.89
  - menstrual—*see* Dysmenorrhea

Colitis (acute) (catarrhal) (chronic) (noninfective) (hemorrhagic) (*see also* Enteritis) K52.9
- allergic K52.29
  - with
    - food protein-induced enterocolitis syndrome K52.21
    - proctocolitis K52.82
- amebic (acute) (*see also* Amebiasis) A06.0
- anthrax A22.2
- C. difficile
  - not specified as recurrent A04.72
  - recurrent A04.71
- collagenous K52.831
- cystica superficialis K52.89
- dietary counseling and surveillance (for) Z71.3
- dietetic K52.29
- eosinophilic K52.82
- food hypersensitivity K52.29
- giardial A07.1
- granulomatous—*see* Enteritis, regional, large intestine
- infectious—*see* Enteritis, infectious
- indeterminate, so stated K52.3
- left sided K51.50
  - with
    - abscess K51.514
    - complication K51.519
      - ~ specified NEC K51.518
    - fistula K51.513
    - obstruction K51.512
    - rectal bleeding K51.511
- lymphocytic K52.832
- microscopic, other K52.838
  - unspecified K52.839
- noninfective K52.9
  - specified NEC K52.89
- septic—*see* Enteritis, infectious
- spastic K58.9
  - with constipation K58.1
  - with diarrhea K58.0
  - mixed K58.2
  - other K58.8
  - psychogenic F54
- staphylococcal A04.8
  - foodborne A05.0
- ulcerative (chronic) K51.90
  - with
    - complication K51.919
      - ~ abscess K51.914
      - ~ fistula K51.913
      - ~ obstruction K51.912
      - ~ rectal bleeding K51.911
      - ~ specified complication NEC K51.918
  - enterocolitis—*see* Pancolitis, ulcerative
  - ileocolitis—*see* Ileocolitis, ulcerative
  - mucosal proctocolitis—*see* Rectosigmoiditis, ulcerative
  - proctitis—*see* Proctitis, ulcerative
  - pseudopolyposis—*see* Polyp, colon, inflammatory
  - psychogenic F54
  - rectosigmoiditis—*see* Rectosigmoiditis, ulcerative
  - specified type NEC K51.80
    - with
      - ~ complication K51.819
        - ◊ abscess K51.814
        - ◊ fistula K51.813
        - ◊ obstruction K51.812
        - ◊ rectal bleeding K51.811
        - ◊ specified complication NEC K51.818

Collagenosis, collagen disease (nonvascular) (vascular) M35.9
- specified NEC M35.8

Collapse R55
- adrenal E27.2
- cardiorespiratory R57.0

Collapse, *continued*
- cardiovascular R57.0
  - newborn P29.89
- circulatory (peripheral) R57.9
- during or
  - resulting from a procedure, not elsewhere classified T81.10
- general R55
- neurocirculatory F45.8
- postoperative T81.10
- valvular—*see* Endocarditis
- vascular (peripheral) R57.9
  - newborn P29.89

Colles' fracture S52.53-

Collet (-Sicard) syndrome G52.7

Collodion baby Q80.2

Coloboma (iris) Q13.0
- eyelid Q10.3
- fundus Q14.8
- lens Q12.2
- optic disc (congenital) Q14.2

Colonization
- MRSA (Methicillin resistant Staphylococcus aureus) Z22.322
- MSSA (Methicillin susceptible Staphylococcus aureus) Z22.321
- status—*see* Carrier (suspected) of

Colostomy
- attention to Z43.3
- fitting or adjustment Z46.89
- malfunctioning K94.03
- status Z93.3

Coma R40.20
- with
  - motor response (none) R40.231
    - abnormal R40.233
    - extension R40.232
    - flexion withdrawal R40.234
    - localizes pain R40.235
    - obeys commands R40.236
    - score of
      - ~ 1 R40.231
      - ~ 2 R40.232
      - ~ 3 R40.233
      - ~ 4 R40.234
      - ~ 5 R40.235
      - ~ 6 R40.236
  - opening of eyes (never) R40.211
    - in response to
      - ~ pain R40.212
      - ~ sound R40.213
    - score of
      - ~ 1 R40.211
      - ~ 2 R40.212
      - ~ 3 R40.213
      - ~ 4 R40.214
    - spontaneous R40.214
  - verbal response (none) R40.221
    - confused conversation R40.224
    - inappropriate words R40.223
    - incomprehensible words R40.222
    - oriented R40.225
    - score of
      - ~ 1 R40.221
      - ~ 2 R40.222
      - ~ 3 R40.223
      - ~ 4 R40.224
      - ~ 5 R40.225
- hyperosmolar (diabetic)—*see* Diabetes
- hypoglycemic (diabetic)—*see* Diabetes
  - nondiabetic E15
- in diabetes—*see* Diabetes
- insulin-induced—*see* Diabetes, coma
- newborn P91.5
- persistent vegetative state R40.3
- specified NEC, without documented Glasgow coma scale score, or with partial Glasgow coma scale score reported R40.244

Comatose—*see* Coma

Comedo, comedones (giant) L70.0

Common
- arterial trunk Q20.0
- atrioventricular canal Q21.2
- atrium Q21.1
- cold (head) J00
- truncus (arteriosus) Q20.0

Communication
- between
  - pulmonary artery and pulmonary vein, congenital Q25.72
- congenital between uterus and digestive or urinary tract Q51.7
- disorder
  - social pragmatic F80.82

Complaint—*see also* Disease
- bowel, functional K59.9
  - psychogenic F45.8
- intestine, functional K59.9
  - psychogenic F45.8
- kidney—*see* Disease, renal

Complex
- Addison-Schilder E71.528
- Costen's M26.69
- Eisenmenger's (ventricular septal defect) I27.83
- Schilder-Addison E71.528

Complication(s) (from) (of)
- arteriovenous
  - fistula, surgically created T82.9
    - infection or inflammation T82.7
  - shunt, surgically created T82.9
    - infection or inflammation T82.7
  - vascular (counterpulsation) T82.9
    - infection or inflammation T82.7
- cardiac—*see also* Disease, heart
  - device, implant or graft T82.9
    - infection or inflammation T82.7
- cardiovascular device, graft or implant T82.9
  - infection or inflammation T82.7
- catheter (device) NEC—*see also* Complications, prosthetic device or implant
  - cystostomy T83.9
    - infection and inflammation T83.510
    - mechanical
      - ~ obstruction T83.090
      - ~ perforation T83.090
      - ~ protrusion T83.090
      - ~ specified NEC T83.090
  - dialysis (vascular) T82.9
    - infection and inflammation T82.7
  - intravenous infusion T82.9
    - infection or inflammation T82.7
  - urethral T83.9
    - indwelling
      - ~ infection and inflammation T83.511
      - ~ specified complication NEC T83.091
    - infection and inflammation T83.511
    - obstruction (mechanical)
    - perforation T83.091
    - protrusion T83.091
    - specified type NEC T83.091
  - urinary NEC
    - infection and inflammation T83.518
    - specified complication NEC T83.098
- circulatory system I99.8
  - postprocedural I97.89
    - following cardiac surgery I97.19-
      - ~ postcardiotomy syndrome I97.0
    - postcardiotomy syndrome I97.0
- delivery (*see also* Complications, obstetric) O75.9
  - specified NEC O75.89
- extracorporeal circulation T80.90
- gastrointestinal K92.9
  - postoperative
    - malabsorption NEC K91.2
- gastrostomy (stoma) K94.20
  - hemorrhage K94.21
  - infection K94.22
  - malfunction K94.23
  - mechanical K94.23
  - specified complication NEC K94.29
- genitourinary
  - device or implant T83.9

Complication(s), *continued*
- ▪ urinary system T83.9
  - ~ infection or inflammation T83.598
    - ◊ indwelling urethral catheter T83.511
- • graft (bypass) (patch)—*see also* Complications, prosthetic device or implant
  - – urinary organ
    - ▪ infection and inflammation T83.598
      - ~ indwelling urethral catheter T83.511
- • infusion (procedure) T80.90
  - – infection T80.29
  - – sepsis T80.29
  - – serum reaction (*see also* Reaction, serum) T80.69
    - ▪ anaphylactic shock (*see also* Shock, anaphylactic) T80.59
- • injection (procedure) T80.90
  - – drug reaction—*see* Reaction, drug
  - – infection T80.29
  - – sepsis T80.29
- • labor O75.9
  - – specified NEC O75.89
- • metabolic E88.9
  - – postoperative E89.89
    - ▪ specified NEC E89.89
- • obstetric O75.9
  - – specified NEC O75.89
- • perfusion NEC T80.90
- • postprocedural—*see also* Complications, surgical procedure
  - – cardiac arrest
    - ▪ following cardiac surgery I97.120
    - ▪ following other surgery I97.121
  - – cardiac functional disturbance NEC
    - ▪ following cardiac surgery I97.190
    - ▪ following other surgery I97.191
  - – cardiac insufficiency
    - ▪ following cardiac surgery I97.110
    - ▪ following other surgery I97.111
  - – heart failure
    - ▪ following cardiac surgery I97.130
    - ▪ following other surgery I97.131
  - – hemorrhage (hematoma) (of)
    - ▪ genitourinary organ or structure
      - ~ following procedure on genitourinary organ or structure N99.820
  - – specified NEC
    - ▪ respiratory system J95.89
- • prosthetic device or implant T85
  - – mechanical NEC T85.698
    - ▪ ventricular shunt
      - ~ breakdown T85.01
      - ~ displacement T85.02
      - ~ leakage T85.03
      - ~ malposition T85.02
      - ~ obstruction T85.09
      - ~ perforation T85.09
      - ~ protrusion T85.09
      - ~ specified NEC T85.09
- • respiratory system J98.9
  - – postoperative J95.89
    - ▪ air leak J95.812
    - ▪ specified NEC J95.89
- • surgical procedure (on) T81.9
  - – malabsorption (postsurgical) NEC K91.2
  - – postcardiotomy syndrome I97.0
  - – postcommissurotomy syndrome I97.0
  - – postvalvulotomy syndrome I97.0
  - – shock (hypovolemic) T81.19
  - – stitch abscess T81.41
  - – wound infection T81.49
  - – transfusion (blood) (lymphocytes) (plasma) T80.92
- • transfusion (blood) (lymphocytes) (plasma) T80.92
  - – circulatory overload E87.71
  - – febrile nonhemolytic transfusion reaction R50.84
  - – hemochromatosis E83.111
  - – hemolytic reaction (antigen unspecified) T80.919
  - – incompatibility reaction (antigen unspecified) T80.919
    - ▪ acute (antigen unspecified) T80.910
    - ▪ delayed (antigen unspecified) T80.911
    - ▪ delayed serologic (DSTR) T80.89
  - – infection T80.29
    - ▪ acute T80.22
  - – reaction NEC T80.89

Complication(s), *continued*
- – sepsis T80.29
- – shock T80.89
- • transplant T86.90
  - – bone marrow T86.00
    - ▪ failure T86.02
    - ▪ rejection T86.01
  - – failure T86.-
  - – heart T86.2-
    - ▪ with lung T86.30
    - ▪ cardiac allograft vasculopathy T86.290
      - ~ failure T86.32
      - ~ rejection T86.31
    - ▪ failure T86.22
    - ▪ rejection T86.21
  - – infection T86.-
  - – kidney T86.10
    - ▪ failure T86.12
    - ▪ rejection T86.11
  - – liver T86.4-
    - ▪ failure T86.42
    - ▪ rejection T86.41
  - – lung T86.81-
    - ▪ with heart T86.30
      - ~ failure T86.32
      - ~ rejection T86.31
    - ▪ failure T86.811
    - ▪ rejection T86.810
  - – malignant neoplasm C80.2
  - – peripheral blood stem cells T86.5
  - – post-transplant lymphoproliferative disorder (PTLD) D47.Z1
  - – rejection T86. -
  - – specified
    - ▪ type NEC T86.-
  - – stem cell (from peripheral blood) (from umbilical cord) T86.5
  - – umbilical cord stem cells T86.5
- • vaccination T88.1-
  - – anaphylaxis NEC T80.52-
  - – cellulitis T88.0-
  - – encephalitis or encephalomyelitis G04.02
  - – infection (general) (local) NEC T88.0-
    - ▪ meningitis G03.8
  - – myelitis G04.89
  - – protein sickness T80.62-
  - – rash T88.1-
  - – reaction (allergic) T88.1-
    - ▪ serum T80.62-
  - – sepsis T88.0-
  - – serum intoxication, sickness, rash, or other serum reaction NEC T80.62-
    - ▪ anaphylactic shock T80.52-
  - – shock (allergic) (anaphylactic) T80.52-
  - – vaccinia (generalized) (localized) T88.1-
- • vascular I99.9
  - – device or implant T82.9
    - ▪ infection or inflammation T82.7
- • ventricular (communicating) shunt (device) T85-
  - – mechanical
    - ▪ breakdown T85.01
    - ▪ displacement T85.02
    - ▪ leakage T85.03
    - ▪ malposition T85.02
    - ▪ obstruction T85.09
    - ▪ perforation T85.09
    - ▪ protrusion T85.09
    - ▪ specified NEC T85.09

Compression
- • facies Q67.1
- • with injury *code by* Nature of injury
- • laryngeal nerve, recurrent G52.2
  - – with paralysis of vocal cords and larynx J38.00
    - ▪ bilateral J38.02
    - ▪ unilateral J38.01
- • nerve (*see also* Disorder, nerve) G58.9
  - – root or plexus NOS (in) G54.9
    - ▪ neoplastic disease (*see also* Table of Neoplasms in the complete *ICD-10-CM* manual) D49.9 [G55]

Compulsion, compulsive
- • neurosis F42.8
- • personality F60.5

Compulsion, compulsive, *continued*
- • states F42.9
- • swearing F42.8
  - – in Gilles de la Tourette's syndrome F95.2
- • tics and spasms F95.9

Concato's disease (pericardial polyserositis) A19.9
- • nontubercular I31.1
- • pleural—*see* Pleurisy, with, effusion

Concealed penis Q55.64

Concretio cordis I31.1
- • rheumatic I09.2

Concretion—*see also* Calculus
- • prepuce (male) N47.8
- • tonsil J35.8

Concussion (brain) (cerebral) (current) S06.0X-
- • syndrome F07.81
- • with
  - – loss of consciousness of 30 minutes or less S06.0X1
  - – loss of consciousness of unspecified duration S06.0X9
- • without loss of consciousness S06.0X0

Condition—*see* Disease

Conditions arising in the perinatal period—*see* Newborn, affected by

Conduct disorder—*see* Disorder, conduct

Condyloma A63.0
- • acuminatum A63.0
- • gonorrheal A54.09
- • latum A51.31
- • syphilitic A51.31
  - – congenital A50.07
- • venereal, syphilitic A51.31

Conflagration—*see also* Burn
- • asphyxia (by inhalation of gases, fumes or vapors) *see* Table of Drugs and Chemicals

Conflict (with)—*see also* Discord
- • family Z73.9
- • marital Z63.0
  - – involving divorce or estrangement Z63.5
- • parent-child Z62.820
  - – parent-adopted child Z62.821
  - – parent-biological child Z62.820
  - – parent-foster child Z62.822

Confusional arousals G47.51

Congestion, congestive
- • brain G93.89
- • breast N64.59
- • catarrhal J31.0
- • chest R09.89
- • glottis J37.0
- • larynx J37.0
- • lung R09.89
  - – active or acute—*see* Pneumonia

Conjunctivitis (staphylococcal) (streptococcal) NOS H10.9
- • acute H10.3-
  - – atopic H10.1-
  - – chemical H10.21-
  - – mucopurulent H10.02-
    - ▪ viral—*see* Conjunctivitis, viral
  - – toxic H10.21-
- • blennorrhagic (gonococcal) (neonatorum) A54.31
- • chemical (acute) H10.21-
- • chlamydial A74.0
  - – neonatal P39.1
- • epidemic (viral) B30.9
- • gonococcal (neonatorum) A54.31
- • in (due to)
  - – Chlamydia A74.0
  - – gonococci A54.31
  - – rosacea H10.82-
- • inclusion A74.0
- • infantile P39.1
  - – gonococcal A54.31
- • neonatal P39.1
  - – gonococcal A54.31
- • viral B30.9

Conradi (-Hunermann) disease Q77.3

Conscious simulation (of illness) Z76.5

Consecutive—*see* Disease, diseased

Consolidation lung (base)—*see* Pneumonia, lobar
Constipation (atonic) (neurogenic) (simple) (spastic) K59.00
- chronic K59.09
  - idiopathic K59.04
- drug-induced K59.03
- functional K59.04
- outlet dysfunction K59.02
- psychogenic F45.8
- slow transit K59.01
- specified NEC K59.09

Constriction—*see also* Stricture
- external
  - abdomen, abdominal (wall) S30.841
  - alveolar process S00.542
  - ankle S90.54-
  - antecubital space S50.84-
  - arm (upper) S40.84-
  - auricle S00.44-
  - axilla S40.84-
  - back, lower S30.840
  - breast S20.14-
  - brow S00.84
  - buttock S30.840
  - calf S80.84-
  - canthus S00.24-
  - cheek S00.84
    - internal S00.542
  - chest wall—*see* Constriction, external, thorax
  - chin S00.84
  - clitoris S30.844
  - costal region—*see* Constriction, external, thorax
  - digit(s)
    - foot—*see* Constriction, external, toe
    - hand—*see* Constriction, external, finger
  - ear S00.44-
  - elbow S50.34-
  - epididymis S30.843
  - epigastric region S30.841
  - esophagus, cervical S10.14
  - eyebrow S00.24-
  - eyelid S00.24-
  - face S00.84
  - finger(s) S60.44-
    - index S60.44-
    - little S60.44-
    - middle S60.44-
    - ring S60.44-
  - flank S30.841
  - foot (except toe(s) alone) S90.84-
    - toe—*see* Constriction, external, toe
  - forearm S50.84-
    - elbow only S50.34-
  - forehead S00.84
  - genital organs, external
    - female S30.846
    - male S30.845
  - groin S30.841
  - gum S00.542
  - hand S60.54-
  - head S00.94
    - ear S00.44-
    - eyelid S00.24-
    - lip S00.541
    - nose S00.34
    - oral cavity S00.542
    - scalp S00.04
    - specified site NEC S00.84
  - heel S90.84-
  - hip S70.24-
  - inguinal region S30.841
  - interscapular region S20.449
  - jaw S00.84
  - knee S80.24-
  - labium (majus) (minus) S30.844
  - larynx S10.14
  - leg (lower) S80.84-
    - knee S80.24-
    - upper S70.34-
  - lip S00.541
  - lower back S30.840
  - lumbar region S30.840
  - malar region S00.84

Constriction, *continued*
- mammary S20.14-
- mastoid region S00.84
- mouth S00.542
- nail
  - finger—*see* Constriction, external, finger
  - toe—*see* Constriction, external, toe
- nasal S00.34
- neck S10.94
  - specified site NEC S10.84
  - throat S10.14
- nose S00.34
- occipital region S00.04
- oral cavity S00.542
- orbital region S00.24-
- palate S00.542
- palm S60.54-
- parietal region S00.04
- pelvis S30.840
- penis S30.842
- perineum
  - female S30.844
  - male S30.840
- periocular area S00.24-
- phalanges
  - finger—*see* Constriction, external, finger
  - toe—*see* Constriction, external, toe
- pharynx S10.14
- pinna S00.44-
- popliteal space S80.24-
- prepuce S30.842
- pubic region S30.840
- pudendum
  - female S30.846
  - male S30.845
- sacral region S30.840
- scalp S00.04
- scapular region S40.24-
- scrotum S30.843
- shin S80.84-
- shoulder S40.24-
- sternal region S20.349
- submaxillary region S00.84
- submental region S00.84
- subungual
  - finger(s)—*see* Constriction, external, finger
  - toe(s)—*see* Constriction, external, toe
- supraclavicular fossa S10.84
- supraorbital S00.84
- temple S00.84
- temporal region S00.84
- testis S30.843
- thigh S70.34-
- thorax, thoracic (wall) S20.94
  - back S20.44-
  - front S20.34-
- throat S10.14
- thumb S60.34-
- toe(s) (lesser) S90.44-
  - great S90.44-
- tongue S00.542
- trachea S10.14
- tunica vaginalis S30.843
- uvula S00.542
- vagina S30.844
- vulva S30.844
- wrist S60.84-
- prepuce (acquired) (congenital) N47.1
- pylorus (adult hypertrophic) K31.1
  - congenital or infantile Q40.0
  - newborn Q40.0

Constrictive—*see* Disease, diseased
Consultation
- medical—*see* Counseling
- specified reason NEC Z71.89
- without complaint or sickness Z71.9
  - specified reason NEC Z71.89

Consumption—*see* Tuberculosis
Contact (with)—*see also* Exposure (to)
- AIDS virus Z20.6
- anthrax Z20.810
- aromatic amines Z77.020

Contact, *continued*
- arsenic Z77.010
- asbestos Z77.090
- bacterial disease NEC Z20.818
- body fluids (potentially hazardous) Z77.21
- benzene Z77.021
- chemicals (chiefly nonmedicinal) (hazardous) NEC Z77.098
- chromium compounds Z77.018
- communicable disease Z20.9
  - bacterial NEC Z20.818
  - specified NEC Z20.89
  - viral NEC Z20.828
  - Zika virus Z20.821
- dyes Z77.098
- Escherichia coli (E. coli) Z20.01
- German measles Z20.4
- gonorrhea Z20.2
- hazardous metals NEC Z77.018
- hazardous substances NEC Z77.29
- hazards in the physical environment NEC Z77.128
- hazards to health NEC Z77.9
- HIV Z20.6
- HTLV-III/LAV Z20.6
- human immunodeficiency virus Z20.6
- infection Z20.9
  - specified NEC Z20.89
- intestinal infectious disease NEC Z20.09
  - Escherichia Coli (E. coli) Z20.01
- lead Z77.011
- meningococcus Z20.811
- mold (toxic) Z77.120
- nickel dust Z77.018
- poliomyelitis Z20.89
- rabies Z20.3
- rubella Z20.4
- sexually-transmitted disease Z20.2
- smallpox (laboratory) Z20.89
- syphilis Z20.2
- tuberculosis Z20.1
- varicella Z20.820
- venereal disease Z20.2
- viral disease NEC Z20.828
- viral hepatitis Z20.5
- Zika virus Z20.821

Contamination, food—*see* Intoxication, foodborne
Contraception, contraceptive
- advice Z30.09
- counseling Z30.09
- device (intrauterine) (in situ) Z97.5
  - checking Z30.431
  - in place Z97.5
  - initial prescription Z30.014
    - barrier Z30.018
    - diaphragm Z30.018
    - subdermal implantable Z30.017
    - transdermal patch hormonal Z30.016
    - vaginal ring hormonal Z30.015
  - maintenance Z30.40
    - barrier Z30.49
    - diaphragm Z30.49
    - subdermal implantable Z30.46
    - transdermal patch hormonal Z30.45
    - vaginal ring hormonal Z30.44
  - reinsertion Z30.433
  - removal Z30.432
  - replacement Z30.433
- emergency (postcoital) Z30.012
- initial prescription Z30.019
  - injectable Z30.013
  - intrauterine device Z30.014
  - pills Z30.011
  - postcoital (emergency) Z30.012
  - specified type NEC Z30.018
  - subdermal implantable Z30.019
- maintenance Z30.40
  - examination Z30.8
  - injectable Z30.42
  - intrauterine device Z30.431
  - pills Z30.41
  - specified type NEC Z30.49
  - subdermal implantable Z30.46

Contraception, contraceptive, *continued*
- – transdermal patch Z30.45
- – vaginal ring Z30.44
- • management Z30.9
- – specified NEC Z30.8
- • postcoital (emergency) Z30.012
- • prescription Z30.019
- – repeat Z30.40
- • surveillance (drug)—*see* Contraception, maintenance

Contraction(s), contracture, contracted
- • Achilles tendon—*see also* Short, tendon, Achilles
- – congenital Q66.89
- • bladder N32.89
- – neck or sphincter N32.0
- • congenital Q65.89
- – hysterical F44.4
- – knee M24.56-
- – shoulder M24.51-
- – wrist M24.53-
- • hip Q65.89
- – elbow M24.52-
- – foot joint M24.57-
- – hand joint M24.54-
- – hip M24.55-
- • hourglass
- – bladder N32.89
  - ■ congenital Q64.79
- – gallbladder K82.0
  - ■ congenital Q44.1
- – stomach K31.89
  - ■ congenital Q40.2
  - ■ psychogenic F45.8
- • hysterical F44.4
- • joint (abduction) (acquired) (adduction) (flexion) (rotation) M24.5-
- – ankle M24.57-
- – congenital NEC Q68.8
- • muscle (postinfective) (postural) NEC M62.40
- – with contracture of joint—*see* Contraction, joint
- – congenital Q79.8
  - ■ sternocleidomastoid Q68.0
- – hysterical F44.4
- – posttraumatic—*see* Strabismus, paralytic
- – psychogenic F45.8
  - ■ conversion reaction F44.4
- – psychogenic F45.8
  - ■ conversion reaction F44.4
- • premature
- – atrium I49.1
- – supraventricular I49.1
- • pylorus NEC—*see also* Pylorospasm
- – psychogenic F45.8
- • sternocleidomastoid (muscle), congenital Q68.0
- • stomach K31.89
- – hourglass K31.89
  - ■ congenital Q40.2
  - ■ psychogenic F45.8
- – psychogenic F45.8
- • tendon (sheath) M62.40
- – ankle M62.47-
- – foot M62.47-
- – forearm M62.43-
- – hand M62.44-
- – lower leg M62.46-
- – multiple sites M62.49
- – neck M62.48
- – pelvic region M62.45-
- – shoulder region M62.41-
- – specified site NEC M62.48
- – thigh M62.45-
- – thorax M62.48
- – trunk M62.48
- – upper arm M62.42-
- • urethra—*see also* Stricture, urethra
- – orifice N32.0
- • vagina (outlet) N89.5
- • vesical N32.89
- – neck or urethral orifice N32.0

Contusion (skin surface intact) T14.8
- • abdomen, abdominal (muscle) (wall) S30.1
- • adnexa, eye NEC S05.8X-
- • alveolar process S00.532

Contusion, *continued*
- • ankle S90.0-
- • antecubital space S50.1-
- • anus S30.3
- • arm (upper) S40.02-
- – lower (with elbow) S50.1-
- • auditory canal S00.43-
- • auricle S00.43-
- • axilla S40.02-
- • back S20.22-
- – lower S30.0
- • bone NEC T14.8
- • brainstem S06.38-
- • breast S20.0-
- • brow S00.83
- • buttock S30.0
- • canthus, eye S00.1-
- • cauda equina S34.3
- • cerebellar, traumatic S06.37-
- • cheek S00.83
- – internal S00.532
- • chest (wall)—*see* Contusion, thorax
- • chin S00.83
- • clitoris S30.23
- • conus medullaris (spine) S34.139
- • corpus cavernosum S30.21
- • costal region—*see* Contusion, thorax
- • ear S00.43-
- • elbow S50.0-
- – with forearm S50.1-
- • epididymis S30.22
- • epigastric region S30.1
- • epiglottis S10.0
- • esophagus (thoracic)
- – cervical S10.0
- • eyebrow S00.1-
- • eyelid (and periocular area) S00.1-
- • face NEC S00.83
- • femoral triangle S30.1
- • finger(s) S60.00
- – with damage to nail (matrix) S60.1-
- – index S60.02-
  - ■ with damage to nail S60.12-
- – little S60.05-
  - ■ with damage to nail S60.15-
- – middle S60.03-
  - ■ with damage to nail S60.13-
- – ring S60.04-
  - ■ with damage to nail S60.14-
- – thumb—*see* Contusion, thumb
- • flank S30.1
- • foot (except toe(s) alone) S90.3-
- – toe—*see* Contusion, toe
- • forearm S50.1-
- – elbow only S50.0-
- • forehead S00.83
- • genital organs, external
- – female S30.202
- – male S30.201
- • groin S30.1
- • gum S00.532
- • hand S60.22-
- – finger(s)—*see* Contusion, finger
- – wrist S60.21-
- • head S00.93
- – ear S00.43-
- – eyelid S00.1-
- – lip S00.531
- – nose S00.33
- – oral cavity S00.532
- – scalp S00.03
- – specified part NEC S00.83
- • heel S90.3-
- • hip S70.0-
- • iliac region S30.1
- • inguinal region S30.1
- • interscapular region S20.229
- • intra-abdominal organ S36.92
- – refer to specific organ under contusion
- • jaw S00.83
- • kidney S37.01-
- – major (greater than 2 cm) S37.02-
- – minor (less than 2 cm) S37.01-

Contusion, *continued*
- • knee S80.0-
- • labium (majus) (minus) S30.23
- • lacrimal apparatus, gland or sac S05.8X-
- • larynx S10.0
- • leg (lower) S80.1-
- – knee S80.0-
- • lip S00.531
- • lower back S30.0
- • lumbar region S30.0
- • lung S27.329
- – bilateral S27.322
- – unilateral S27.321
- • malar region S00.83
- • mastoid region S00.83
- • mouth S00.532
- • muscle—*see* Contusion, by site
- • nail
- – finger—*see* Contusion, finger, with damage to nail
- – toe—*see* Contusion, toe, with damage to nail
- • nasal S00.33
- • neck S10.93
- – specified site NEC S10.83
- – throat S10.0
- • nerve—*see* Injury, nerve
- • newborn P54.5
- • nose S00.33
- • occipital
- – region (scalp) S00.03
- • palate S00.532
- • parietal
- – region (scalp) S00.03
- – kidney—*see* Contusion, kidney
- • pelvis S30.0
- • penis S30.21
- • perineum
- – female S30.23
- – male S30.0
- • periocular area S00.1-
- • pharynx S10.0
- • pinna S00.43-
- • popliteal space S80.0-
- • prepuce S30.21
- • pubic region S30.1
- • pudendum
- – female S30.202
- – male S30.201
- • quadriceps femoris S70.1-
- • rectum S36.62
- • sacral region S30.0
- • scalp S00.03
- – due to birth injury P12.3
- • scapular region S40.01-
- • scrotum S30.22
- • shoulder S40.01-
- • skin NEC T14.8
- • spermatic cord S30.22
- • spinal cord—*see* Injury, spinal cord, by region
- – cauda equina S34.3
- – conus medullaris S34.139
- • spleen S36.02-
- – major S36.021
- – minor S36.020
- • sternal region S20.219
- • stomach S36.32
- • subcutaneous NEC T14.8
- • submaxillary region S00.83
- • submental region S00.83
- • subperiosteal NEC T14.8
- • subungual
- – finger—*see* Contusion, finger, with damage to nail
- – toe—*see* Contusion, toe, with damage to nail
- • supraclavicular fossa S10.83
- • supraorbital S00.83
- • temple (region) S00.83
- • testis S30.22
- • thigh S70.1-
- • thorax (wall) S20.20
- – back S20.22-
- – front S20.21-
- • throat S10.0
- • thumb S60.01-
- – with damage to nail S60.11-

Contusion, *continued*
- toe(s) (lesser) S90.12-
  - with damage to nail S90.22-
  - great S90.11-
    - with damage to nail S90.21-
    - specified type NEC S90.221
- tongue S00.532
- trachea (cervical) S10.0
- tunica vaginalis S30.22
- tympanum, tympanic membrane S00.43-
- uvula S00.532
- vagina S30.23
- vocal cord(s) S10.0
- vulva S30.23
- wrist S60.21-

Conversion hysteria, neurosis or reaction F44.9

Converter, tuberculosis (test reaction) R76.11

Convulsions (idiopathic) (*see also* Seizure(s)) R56.9
- febrile R56.00
  - with status epilepticus G40.901
  - complex R56.01
    - with status epilepticus G40.901
  - simple R56.00
- infantile P90
  - epilepsy—*see* Epilepsy
- myoclonic G25.3
- neonatal, benign (familial)—*see* Epilepsy, generalized, idiopathic
- newborn P90
- post traumatic R56.1
- recurrent R56.9
- scarlatinal A38.8

Convulsive—*see also* Convulsions

Cooley's anemia D56.1

Copra itch B88.0

Coprophagy F50.89

Cor
- pulmonale (chronic) I27.81
- triloculare Q20.8
  - biventriculare Q21.1

Corbus' disease (gangrenous balanitis) N48.1

Corn (infected) L84

Cornelia de Lange syndrome Q87.19

Cornual gestation or pregnancy O00.8-

Coronavirus (Infection)
- as cause of diseases classified elsewhere B97.29
- coronavirus-19 U07.1
- COVID-19 U07.1
- SARS-associated B97.21

Corrosion (injury) (acid) (caustic) (chemical) (lime) (external) (internal) T30.4
- extent (percentage of body surface)
  - less than 10 percent T32.0

Coryza (acute) J00
- with grippe or influenza—*see* Influenza, with, respiratory manifestations NEC

Costen's syndrome or complex M26.69

Costochondritis M94.0

Cot death R99

Cough (affected) (chronic) (epidemic) (nervous) R05
- with hemorrhage—*see* Hemoptysis
- bronchial R05
  - with grippe or influenza—*see* Influenza, with, respiratory manifestations NEC
- functional F45.8
- hysterical F45.8
- laryngeal, spasmodic R05
- psychogenic F45.8

Counseling (for) Z71.9
- abuse NEC
  - perpetrator Z69.82
  - victim Z69.81
- alcohol abuser Z71.41
  - family Z71.42
- child abuse
  - non-parental
    - perpetrator Z69.021
    - victim Z69.020

Counseling, *continued*
- parental
  - perpetrator Z69.011
  - victim Z69.010
- contraceptive Z30.09
- dietary Z71.3
- drug abuser Z71.51
  - family member Z71.52
- exercise Z71.82
- family Z71.89
- for non-attending third party Z71.0
  - related to sexual behavior or orientation Z70.2
- genetic
  - nonprocreative Z71.83
  - procreative NEC Z31.5
- health (advice) (education) (instruction)—*see* Counseling
- human immunodeficiency virus (HIV) Z71.7
- insulin pump use Z46.81
- medical (for) Z71.9
  - human immunodeficiency virus (HIV) Z71.7
  - on behalf of another Z71.0
  - specified reason NEC Z71.89
- natural family planning
  - to avoid pregnancy Z30.02
- perpetrator (of)
  - abuse NEC Z69.82
  - child abuse
    - non-parental Z69.021
    - parental Z69.011
  - rape NEC Z69.82
  - spousal abuse Z69.12
- procreative NEC Z31.69
- rape victim Z69.81
- safety for (international) travel Z71.84
- specified reason NEC Z71.89
- spousal abuse (perpetrator) Z69.12
  - victim Z69.11
- substance abuse Z71.89
  - alcohol Z71.41
  - drug Z71.51
  - tobacco Z71.6
- tobacco use Z71.6
- travel (international) Z71.84
- use (of)
  - insulin pump Z46.81
- victim (of)
  - abuse Z69.81
  - child abuse
    - by parent Z69.010
    - non-parental Z69.020
  - rape NEC Z69.81

Coxsackie (virus) (infection) B34.1
- as cause of disease classified elsewhere B97.11
- enteritis A08.3
- meningitis (aseptic) A87.0
- pharyngitis B08.5

Crabs, meaning pubic lice B85.3

Crack baby P04.41

Cracked tooth K03.81

Cradle cap L21.0

Cramp(s) R25.2
- abdominal—*see* Pain, abdominal
- bathing T75.1
- colic R10.83
- due to immersion T75.1
- fireman T67.2
- heat T67.2
- immersion T75.1
- intestinal—*see* Pain, abdominal
  - psychogenic F45.8
- limb (lower) (upper) NEC R25.2
  - sleep related G47.62
- muscle (limb) (general) R25.2
  - due to immersion T75.1
  - psychogenic F45.8
- salt-depletion E87.1
- stoker's T67.2
- swimmer's T75.1

Craniocleidodysostosis Q74.0

Craniofenestria (skull) Q75.8

Craniolacunia (skull) Q75.8

Cranioschisis Q75.8

Crepitus
- caput Q75.8
- joint—*see* Derangement, joint, specified type NEC

Crib death R99

Cribriform hymen Q52.3

Cri-du-chat syndrome Q93.4

Crigler-Najjar disease or syndrome E80.5

Crisis
- abdomen R10.0
- acute reaction F43.0
- addisonian E27.2
- adrenal (cortical) E27.2
- celiac K90.0
- Dietl's N13.8
- emotional—*see also* Disorder, adjustment
  - acute reaction to stress F43.0
  - specific to childhood and adolescence F93.8
- oculogyric H51.8
  - psychogenic F45.8
- psychosexual identity F64.2
- sickle-cell D57.00
  - with
    - acute chest syndrome D57.01
    - cerebral vascular involvement D57.03
    - crisis (painful) D57.00
      - with complication specified NEC D57.09
    - splenic sequestration D57.02
    - vasoocclusive pain D57.00
- state (acute reaction) F43.0

Crocq's disease (acrocyanosis) I73.89

Crohn's disease—*see* Enteritis, regional

Crooked septum, nasal J34.2

Croup, croupous (catarrhal) (infectious) (inflammatory) (nondiphtheritic) J05.0
- bronchial J20.9

Crush, crushed, crushing T14.8
- ankle S97.0-
- arm (upper) (and shoulder) S47.- (See complete *ICD-10-CM* Manual for codes)
- finger(s) S67.1-
  - with hand (and wrist) S67.2-
  - index S67.19-
  - little S67.19-
  - middle S67.19-
  - ring S67.19-
  - thumb—*see* Crush, thumb
- foot S97.8-
  - toe—*see* Crush, toe
- hand (except fingers alone) S67.2-
  - with wrist S67.4-
- thumb S67.0-
  - with hand (and wrist) S00.44-
- toe(s) S97.10-
  - great S97.11-
  - lesser S97.12-
- wrist S67.3-
  - with hand S67.4-

Crusta lactea L21.0

Crying (constant) (continuous) (excessive)
- child, adolescent, or adult R45.83
- infant (baby) (newborn) R68.11

Cryptitis (anal) (rectal) K62.89

Cryptopapillitis (anus) K62.89

Cryptophthalmos Q11.2
- syndrome Q87.0

Cryptorchid, cryptorchism, cryptorchidism Q53.9
- bilateral Q53.20
  - abdominal Q53.211
  - perineal Q53.22
- unilateral Q53.10
  - abdominal Q53.111
  - perineal Q53.12

Cryptosporidiosis A07.2
- hepatobiliary B88.8
- respiratory B88.8

Crystalluria R82.998

Cubitus
- congenital Q68.8
- valgus (acquired) M21.0-
  - congenital Q68.8
- varus (acquired) M21.1-
  - congenital Q68.8

Cultural deprivation or shock Z60.3

Curvature
- organ or site, congenital NEC—*see* Distortion
- penis (lateral) Q55.61
- Pott's (spinal) A18.01
- radius, idiopathic, progressive (congenital) Q74.0
- spine (acquired) (angular) (idiopathic) (incorrect) (postural)
  - congenital Q67.5
  - due to or associated with
    - osteitis
      - ~ deformans M88.88
      - ~ tuberculosis (Pott's curvature) A18.01
  - tuberculous A18.01

Cushingoid due to steroid therapy E24.2
- correct substance properly administered—*see* Table of Drugs and Chemicals, by drug, adverse effect
- overdose or wrong substance given or taken—*see* Table of Drugs and Chemicals, by drug, poisoning

Cushing's
- syndrome or disease E24.9
  - drug-induced E24.2
  - iatrogenic E24.2
  - pituitary-dependent E24.0
  - specified NEC E24.8
- ulcer—*see* Ulcer, peptic, acute

Cutaneous—*see also* Disease, diseased
- hemorrhage R23.3

Cutis—*see also* Disease, diseased
- hyperelastica Q82.8
- osteosis L94.2
- verticis gyrata Q82.8
  - acquired L91.8

Cyanosis R23.0
- due to
  - patent foramen botalli Q21.1
  - persistent foramen ovale Q21.1
- enterogenous D74.8

Cyanotic heart disease I24.9
- congenital Q24.9

Cycle
- anovulatory N97.0
- menstrual, irregular N92.6

Cyclical vomiting, in migraine (*see also* Vomiting, cyclical) G43.A0
- psychogenic F50.89

Cyclical vomiting syndrome unrelated to migraine R11.15

Cycloid personality F34.0

Cyclopia, cyclops Q87.0

Cyclopism Q87.0

Cyclothymia F34.0

Cyclothymic personality F34.0

Cylindruria R82.998

Cynanche
- tonsillaris J36

Cyst (colloid) (mucous) (simple) (retention)
- adenoid (infected) J35.8
- antrum J34.1
- anus K62.89
- arachnoid, brain (acquired) G93.0
  - congenital Q04.6
- Baker's M71.2-
  - choroid plexus Q04.6
- Bartholin's gland N75.0
- bone (local) NEC M85.60
  - specified type NEC M85.60
    - ankle M85.67-
    - foot M85.67-
    - forearm M85.63-
    - hand M85.64-
    - jaw M27.40
      - ~ developmental (nonodontogenic) K09.1
        - ◊ odontogenic K09.0

Cyst, *continued*
  - lower leg M85.66-
  - multiple site M85.69
  - neck M85.68
  - rib M85.68
  - shoulder M85.61-
  - skull M85.68
  - specified site NEC M85.68
  - thigh M85.65-
  - toe M85.67-
  - upper arm M85.62-
  - vertebra M85.68
- brain (acquired) G93.0
  - congenital Q04.6
  - third ventricle (colloid), congenital Q04.6
- breast (benign) (blue dome) (pedunculated) (solitary) N60.0-
- canal of Nuck (female) N94.89
  - congenital Q52.4
- choledochus, congenital Q44.4
- common (bile) duct
  - congenital NEC Q89.8
  - fallopian tube Q50.4
  - kidney Q61.00
    - more than one (multiple) Q61.02
    - specified as polycystic Q61.3
      - ~ infantile type NEC Q61.19
  - ovary Q50.1
  - oviduct Q50.4
- congenital NEC Q89.8
  - kidney Q61.00
    - more than one (multiple) Q61.02
      - ~ specified as polycystic Q61.3
        - ◊ infantile type NEC Q61.19
          - » collecting duct dilation Q61.11
    - solitary Q61.01
  - prepuce Q55.69
  - thymus (gland) Q89.2
- corpus
  - albicans N83.29-
  - luteum (hemorrhagic) (ruptured) N83.1-
- craniobuccal pouch E23.6
- craniopharyngeal pouch E23.6
- Dandy-Walker Q03.1
  - with spina bifida—*see* Spina bifida
- dental (root) K04.8
  - developmental K09.0
  - eruption K09.0
  - primordial K09.0
- dentigerous (mandible) (maxilla) K09.0
- dermoid—*see* Neoplasm, benign, by site in Table of Neoplasms in the complete *ICD-10-CM* manual
  - implantation
    - vagina N89.8
- developmental K09.1
  - odontogenic K09.0
- dura (cerebral) G93.0
  - spinal G96.198
- epoophoron Q50.5
- eruption K09.0
- ethmoid sinus J34.1
- eye NEC H57.89
- eyelid (sebaceous) H02.82-
  - infected—*see* Hordeolum
  - left H02.826
    - lower H02.825
    - upper H02.824
  - right H02.823
    - lower H02.822
    - upper H02.821
- fallopian tube N83.8
  - congenital Q50.4
- follicle (graafian) (hemorrhagic) N83.0-
- follicular (atretic) (hemorrhagic) (ovarian) N83.0-
  - dentigerous K09.0
  - odontogenic K09.0
  - skin L72.9
    - specified NEC L72.8
- frontal sinus J34.1
- gingiva K09.0
- graafian follicle (hemorrhagic) N83.0-
- granulosal lutein (hemorrhagic) N83.1-

Cyst, *continued*
- hemangiomatous D18.00
  - skin D18.01
  - specified site NEC D18.09
- hydatid (*see also* Echinococcus)
  - Morgagni
    - male (epididymal) Q55.4
    - ~ testicular Q55.29
- hymen N89.8
  - embryonic Q52.4
- hypophysis, hypophyseal (duct) (recurrent) E23.6
  - cerebri E23.6
- implantation (dermoid)
  - vagina N89.8
- intrasellar E23.6
- jaw (bone) M27.40
  - developmental (odontogenic) K09.0
- kidney (acquired) N28.1
  - congenital Q61.00
  - more than one (multiple) Q61.02
    - specified as polycystic Q61.3
      - ~ infantile type (autosomal recessive) NEC Q61.19
        - ◊ collecting duct dilation Q61.11
  - simple N28.1
  - solitary (single) Q61.01
    - acquired N28.1
- lateral periodontal K09.0
- lens H27.8
  - congenital Q12.8
- lip (gland) K13.0
- lutein N83.1-
- mandible M27.40
  - dentigerous K09.0
- maxilla M27.40
  - dentigerous K09.0
- meninges (cerebral) G93.0
  - spinal G96.19-
- Morgagni (hydatid)
  - male (epididymal) Q55.4
    - testicular Q55.29
- Müllerian duct Q50.4
  - appendix testis Q55.29
  - cervix Q51.6
  - fallopian tube Q50.4
  - female Q50.4
  - male Q55.29
- nerve root
  - cervical G96.191
  - lumbar G96.191
  - sacral G96.191
  - thoracic G96.191
- nervous system NEC G96.89
- nose (turbinates) J34.1
  - sinus J34.1
- odontogenic, developmental K09.0
- omentum (lesser) congenital Q45.8
- ovary, ovarian (twisted) N83.20-
  - adherent N83.20-
  - corpus
    - albicans N83.29-
    - luteum (hemorrhagic) N83.1-
  - developmental Q50.1
  - due to failure of involution NEC N83.20-
  - follicular (graafian) (hemorrhagic) N83.0-
  - hemorrhagic N83.20-
  - retention N83.29-
  - serous N83.20-
  - specified NEC N83.29-
  - theca lutein (hemorrhagic) N83.1-
- paramesonephric duct Q50.4
  - female Q50.4
  - male Q55.29
- paranephric N28.1
- paraphysis, cerebri, congenital Q04.6
- paroophoron Q50.5
- parovarian Q50.5
- pericardial (congenital) Q24.8
  - acquired (secondary) I31.8
- pericoronal K09.0
- periodontal K04.8
  - lateral K09.0
- perineural G96.191
- peripelvic (lymphatic) N28.1

Cyst, *continued*
- periventricular, acquired, newborn P91.1
- pilar L72.11
- pilonidal (infected) (rectum) L05.91
  - with abscess L05.01
- pituitary (duct) (gland) E23.6
- porencephalic Q04.6
  - acquired G93.0
- prepuce N47.4
  - congenital Q55.69
- primordial (jaw) K09.0
- Rathke's pouch E23.6
- rectum (epithelium) (mucous) K62.89
- renal—*see* Cyst, kidney
- retention (ovary) N83.29-
- sebaceous (duct) (gland) L72.3
  - eyelid—*see* Cyst, eyelid
  - genital organ NEC
    - female N94.89
    - male N50.89
  - scrotum L72.3
- serous (ovary) N83.20-
- sinus (accessory) (nasal) J34.1
- skin L72.9
  - sebaceous L72.3
- solitary
  - bone—*see* Cyst, bone
  - jaw M27.40
  - kidney N28.1
- sphenoid sinus J34.1
- spinal meninges G96.198
- subdural (cerebral) G93.0
  - spinal cord G96.198
- Tarlov G96.191
- testis N44.2
  - tunica albuginea N44.1
- theca lutein (ovary) N83.1-
- thyroglossal duct (infected) (persistent) Q89.2
- thyrolingual duct (infected) (persistent) Q89.2
- tonsil J35.8
- trichilemmal (proliferating) L72.12
- trichodermal L72.12
- turbinate (nose) J34.1
- vagina, vaginal (implantation) (inclusion) (squamous cell) (wall) N89.8
  - embryonic Q52.4
- wolffian
  - female Q50.5
  - male Q55.4

Cystic—*see also* Disease, diseased
- corpora lutea (hemorrhagic) N83.1-
- kidney (congenital) Q61.9
  - infantile type NEC Q61.19
    - collecting duct dilatation Q61.11
  - medullary Q61.5
- ovary N83.20-

Cysticerosis, cysticerciasis B69.9
- with
  - epileptiform fits B69.0
- brain B69.0
- central nervous system B69.0
- cerebral B69.0
- specified NEC B69.89

Cystinosis (malignant) E72.04

Cystitis (exudative) (hemorrhagic) (septic) (suppurative) N30.90
- acute N30.00
  - with hematuria N30.01
  - of trigone N30.00
    - with hematuria N30.31
- blennorrhagic (gonococcal) A54.01
- chlamydial A56.01
- gonococcal A54.01
- trichomonal A59.03

Cystoma—*see also* Neoplasm, benign, by site in Table of Neoplasms in the complete *ICD-10-CM* manual
- simple (ovary) N83.29-

Cytomegalic inclusion disease
- congenital P35.1

Cytomegalovirus infection B25.9

Cytopenia D75.9

D

Da Costa's syndrome F45.8

Dacryocystitis
- neonatal P39.1

Dacryostenosis—*see also* Stenosis, lacrimal
- congenital Q10.5

Dactylitis
- bone—*see* Osteomyelitis
- sickle-cell D57.00
  - Hb C D57.219
  - Hb SS D57.00
  - specified NEC D57.819
- skin L08.9
- tuberculous A18.03

Dactylosymphysis Q70.9
- fingers—*see* Syndactylism, complex, fingers
- toes—*see* Syndactylism, complex, toes

Damage
- brain (nontraumatic) G93.9
  - anoxic, hypoxic G93.1
  - child NEC G80.9
  - due to birth injury P11.2
- cerebral NEC—*see* Damage, brain
- eye, birth injury P15.3
- lung
  - dabbing (related) U07.0
  - electronic cigarette (related) U07.0
  - vaping (associated) (device) (product) (use) U07.0
- organ
  - dabbing (related) U07.0
  - electronic cigarette (related) U07.0
  - vaping (device) (product) (use) (associated) U07.0
- vascular I99.9

Dandruff L21.0

Dandy-Walker syndrome Q03.1
- with spina bifida—*see* Spina bifida

Danlos' syndrome Q79.60
- classical Ehlers-Danlos syndrome Q79.61
- hypermobile Ehlers-Danlos syndrome Q79.62
- other Ehlers-Danlos syndromes Q79.69
- vascular Ehlers-Danlos syndrome Q79.63

Darier (-White) disease (congenital) Q82.8
- meaning erythema annulare centrifugum L53.1

Darier-Roussy sarcoid D86.3

De la Tourette's syndrome F95.2

De Lange's syndrome Q87.19

De Morgan's spots (senile angiomas) I78.1

De Toni-Fanconi (-Debré) syndrome E72.09
- with cystinosis E72.04

Dead
- fetus, retained (mother) O36.4
  - early pregnancy O02.1

Deaf-mutism (acquired) (congenital) NEC H91.3
- hysterical F44.6

Deafness (acquired) (complete) (hereditary) (partial) H91.9-
- with blue sclera and fragility of bone Q78.0
- central—*see* Deafness, sensorineural
- conductive H90.2
  - and sensorineural, mixed H90.8
    - bilateral H90.6
  - bilateral H90.0
  - unilateral H90.1-
    - with restrictive hearing on contralateral side H90.A-
- congenital H90.5
  - with blue sclera and fragility of bone Q78.0
- emotional (hysterical) F44.6
- functional (hysterical) F44.6
- high frequency H91.9-
- hysterical F44.6
- low frequency H91.9-
- mixed conductive and sensorineural H90.8
  - bilateral H90.6
  - unilateral H90.7-
- nerve—*see* Deafness, sensorineural
- neural—*see* Deafness, sensorineural
- noise-induced—*see also* subcategory H83.3
- psychogenic (hysterical) F44.6

Deafness, *continued*
- sensorineural H90.5
  - and conductive, mixed H90.8
    - bilateral H90.6
  - bilateral H90.3
  - unilateral H90.4-
- sensory—*see* Deafness, sensorineural
- word (developmental) H93.25

Death (cause unknown) (of) (unexplained) (unspecified cause) R99
- brain G93.82
- cardiac (sudden) (with successful resuscitation)—*code to* underlying disease
  - family history of Z82.41
  - personal history of Z86.74
- family member (assumed) Z63.4

Debility (chronic) (general) (nervous) R53.81
- congenital or neonatal NOS P96.9
- nervous R53.81

Débove's disease (splenomegaly) R16.1

Decalcification
- teeth K03.89

Decrease(d)
- absolute neutrophil count—*see* Neutropenia
- blood
  - platelets—*see* Thrombocytopenia
  - pressure R03.1
    - due to shock following
      - ~ injury T79.4
      - ~ operation T81.19
- function
  - ovary in hypopituitarism E23.0
  - pituitary (gland) (anterior) (lobe) E23.0
    - posterior (lobe) E23.0
- hematocrit R71.0
- hemoglobin R71.0
- leukocytes D72.819
  - specified NEC D72.818
- lymphocytes D72.810
- respiration, due to shock following injury T79.4
- tolerance
  - fat K90.49
  - glucose R73.09
  - salt and water E87.8
- vision NEC H54.7
- white blood cell count D72.819
  - specified NEC D72.818

Defect, defective Q89.9
- 3-beta-hydroxysterioid dehydrogenase E25.0
- 11-hydroxylase E25.0
- 21-hydroxylase E25.0
- atrial septal (ostium secundum type) Q21.1
  - ostium primum type Q21.2
- atrioventricular
  - canal Q21.2
  - septum Q21.2
- auricular septal Q21.1
- bilirubin excretion NEC E80.6
- bulbar septum Q21.0
- cell membrane receptor complex (CR3) D71
- circulation I99.9
  - congenital Q28.9
  - newborn Q28.9
- coagulation (factor) (*see also* Deficiency) D68.9
  - newborn, transient P61.6
- conduction (heart) I45.9
  - bone—*see* Deafness, conductive
- coronary sinus Q21.1
- cushion, endocardial Q21.2
- degradation, glycoprotein E77.1
- diaphragm
  - with elevation, eventration or hernia—*see* Hernia, diaphragm
  - congenital Q79.1
    - with hernia Q79.0
    - gross (with hernia) Q79.0
- extensor retinaculum M62.89
- filling
  - bladder R93.41
  - kidney R93.42-
  - renal pelvis R93.41

Defect, defective, *continued*
- – ureter R93.41
- – urinary organs, specified NEC R93.49
- • GABA (gamma aminobutyric acid) metabolic E72.81
- • Gerbode Q21.0
- • glucose transport, blood-brain barrier E74.810
- • glycoprotein degradation E77.1
- • interatrial septal Q21.1
- • interauricular septal Q21.1
- • interventricular septal Q21.0
  - – with dextroposition of aorta, pulmonary stenosis and hypertrophy of right ventricle Q21.3
  - – in tetralogy of Fallot Q21.3
- • learning (specific)—*see* Disorder, learning
- • lymphocyte function antigen-1 (LFA-1) D84.0
- • lysosomal enzyme, post-translational modification E77.0
- • modification, lysosomal enzymes, post-translational E77.0
- • obstructive, congenital
  - – ureter Q62.39
    - ▪ orthotopic ureterocele Q62.31
- • osteochondral NEC—*see also* Deformity M95.8
- • ostium
  - – primum Q21.2
  - – secundum Q21.1
- • platelets, qualitative D69.1
  - – constitutional D68.0
- • reduction
  - – limb
    - ▪ lower Q72.9-
      - ~ longitudinal
        - ◊ femur Q72.4-
        - ◊ fibula Q72.6-
        - ◊ tibia Q72.5-
      - ~ specified type NEC Q72.89-
    - ▪ upper Q71.9-
      - ~ longitudinal
        - ◊ radius Q71.4-
        - ◊ ulna Q71.5-
      - ~ specified type NEC Q71.89-
- • respiratory system, congenital Q34.9
- • septal (heart) NOS Q21.9
  - – atrial Q21.1
  - – ventricular (*see also* Defect, ventricular septal) Q21.0
- • sinus venosus Q21.1
- • speech R47.9
  - – developmental F80.9
  - – specified NEC R47.89
- • vascular (local) I99.9
  - – congenital Q27.9
- • ventricular septal Q21.0
  - – in tetralogy of Fallot Q21.3
- • vision NEC H54.7

Defibrination (syndrome) D65
- • newborn P60

Deficiency, deficient
- • 3-beta-hydroxysterioid dehydrogenase E25.0
- • 11-hydroxylase E25.0
- • 21-hydroxylase E25.0
- • AADC (aromatic L-amino acid decarboxylase) E70.81
- • abdominal muscle syndrome Q79.4
- • adenosine deaminase (ADA) D81.30
  - – deaminase 2 D81.32
  - – other adenosine deaminase D81.39
  - – severe combined immunodeficiency due to adenosine deaminase deficiency D81.31
    - ▪ type 1 (without SCID) (without severe combined immunodeficiency) D81.39
    - ▪ type 2 D81.32
- • anti-hemophilic
  - – factor (A) D66
    - ▪ B D67
    - ▪ C D68.1
  - – globulin (AHG) NEC D66
- • antidiuretic hormone E23.2
- • aromatic L-amino acid decarboxylase (AADC) E70.81
- • attention (disorder) (syndrome) F98.8
  - – with hyperactivity—*see* Disorder, attention-deficit hyperactivity
- • beta-glucuronidase E76.29
- • calcium (dietary) E58

Deficiency, deficient, *continued*
- • carnitine E71.40
  - – due to
    - ▪ hemodialysis E71.43
    - ▪ inborn errors of metabolism E71.42
    - ▪ Valproic acid therapy E71.43
  - – iatrogenic E71.43
  - – muscle palmityltransferase E71.314
  - – primary E71.41
  - – secondary E71.448
- • cell membrane receptor complex (CR3) D71
- • central nervous system G96.89
- • clotting (blood) (*see also* Deficiency) D68.9
- • coagulation NOS D68.9
- • combined glucocorticoid and mineralocorticoid E27.49
- • corticoadrenal E27.40
  - – primary E27.1
- • dehydrogenase
  - – long chain/very long chain acyl CoA E71.310
  - – medium chain acyl CoA E71.311
  - – short chain acyl CoA E71.312
- • diet E63.9
- • disaccharidase E73.9
- • enzymes, circulating NEC E88.09
- • essential fatty acid (EFA) E63.0
- • factor—*see also* Deficiency
  - – IX (congenital) (functional) (hereditary) (with functional defect) D67
  - – VIII (congenital) (functional) (hereditary) (with functional defect) D66
    - ▪ with vascular defect D68.0
  - – XI (congenital) (hereditary) D68.1
- • fibrinogen (congenital) (hereditary) D68.2
  - – acquired D65
- • GABA (gamma aminobutyric acid) metabolic E72.81
- • GABA-T (gamma aminobutyric acid) metabolic E72.81
- • gammaglobulin in blood D80.1
  - – hereditary D80.0
- • glucocorticoid E27.49
  - – mineralocorticoid E27.49
- • glucose-6-phosphate dehydrogenase (G6PD) with anemia D55.0
- • glucose-6-phosphate dehydrogenase (G6PD) without anemia D75.A
- • glucose transporter protein type 1 E74.810
- • glucuronyl transferase E80.5
- • Glut1 E74.810
- • gonadotropin (isolated) E23.0
- • growth hormone (idiopathic) (isolated) E23.0
- • hearing—*see* Deafness
- • high grade F70
- • hemoglobin D64.9
- • hormone
  - – anterior pituitary (partial) NEC E23.0
    - ▪ growth E23.0
  - – growth (isolated) E23.0
  - – pituitary E23.0
- • hypoxanthine- (guanine)-phosphoribosyltransferase (HG-PRT) (total H-PRT) E79.1
- • immunity D84.9
  - – cell-mediated D84.89
    - ▪ with thrombocytopenia and eczema D82.0
  - – combined D81.9
- • kappa-light chain D80.8
- • lacrimal fluid (acquired)—*see also* Syndrome
  - – congenital Q10.6
- • lactase
  - – congenital E73.0
  - – secondary E73.1
- • menadione (vitamin K) E56.1
  - – newborn P53
- • mineralocorticoid E27.49
  - – with glucocorticoid E27.49
- • moral F60.2
- • multiple sulfatase (MSD) E75.26
  - – *Add-* succinic semialdehyde dehydrogenase E72.81
  - – *Revise from-* sulfatase E75.29
  - – *Revise to-* sulfatase E75.26
- • muscle
  - – carnitine (palmityltransferase) E71.314
- • NADH diaphorase or reductase (congenital) D74.0
- • NADH-methemoglobin reductase (congenital) D74.0

Deficiency, deficient, *continued*
- • natrium E87.1
- • parathyroid (gland) E20.9
- • phosphoenolpyruvate carboxykinase E74.4
- • phosphomannomutuse E74.818
- • phosphomannose isomerase E74.818
- • phosphomannosyl mutase E74.818
- • pituitary hormone (isolated) E23.0
- • plasma thromboplastin
  - – antecedent (PTA) D68.1
  - – component (PTC) D67
- • plasminogen (type 1) (type 2) E88.02
- • platelet NEC D69.1
  - – constitutional D68.0
- • protein (*see also* Malnutrition) E46
- • pseudocholinesterase E88.09
- • PTA (plasma thromboplastin antecedent) D68.1
- • pyruvate
  - – carboxylase E74.4
  - – dehydrogenase E74.4
- • salt E87.1
- • secretion
  - – urine R34
- • short stature homeobox gene (SHOX)
  - – with
    - ▪ dyschondrosteosis Q78.8
    - ▪ short stature (idiopathic) E34.3
    - ▪ Turner's syndrome Q96.9
- • sodium (Na) E87.1
- • thrombokinase D68.2
  - – newborn P53
- • vascular I99.9
- • vasopressin E23.2
- • vitamin (multiple) NOS E56.9
  - – K E56.1
    - ▪ of newborn P53

Deficit—*see also* Deficiency
- • attention and concentration R41.840
  - – disorder—*see* Attention, deficit
- • concentration R41.840
- • oxygen R09.02

Deflection
- • radius M21.83-
- • septum (acquired) (nasal) (nose) J34.2
- • spine—*see* Curvature, spine
- • turbinate (nose) J34.2

Defluvium
- • capillorum—*see* Alopecia
- • unguium L60.8

Deformity Q89.9
- • abdominal wall
  - – acquired M95.8
  - – congenital Q79.59
- • alimentary tract, congenital Q45.9
  - – upper Q40.9
- • anus (acquired) K62.89
  - – congenital Q43.9
- • aorta (arch) (congenital) Q25.40
- • aortic
  - – cusp or valve (congenital) Q23.8
    - ▪ acquired (*see also* Endocarditis, aortic) I35.8
- • artery (congenital) (peripheral) NOS Q27.9
  - – umbilical Q27.0
- • atrial septal Q21.1
- • bile duct (common) (congenital) (hepatic) Q44.5
  - – acquired K83.8
- • biliary duct or passage (congenital) Q44.5
  - – acquired K83.8
- • bladder (neck) (trigone) (sphincter) (acquired) N32.89
  - – congenital Q64.79
- • bone (acquired) NOS M95.9
  - – congenital Q79.9
- • brain (congenital) Q04.9
  - – acquired G93.89
- • bursa, congenital Q79.9
- • cerebral, acquired G93.89
  - – congenital Q04.9
- • cheek (acquired) M95.2
  - – congenital Q18.9
- • chin (acquired) M95.2
  - – congenital Q18.9

Deformity, *continued*
- choroid (congenital) Q14.3
  - plexus Q07.8
    - acquired G96.198
- clavicle (acquired) M95.8
  - congenital Q68.8
- cystic duct (congenital) Q44.5
  - acquired K82.8
- Dandy-Walker Q03.1
  - with spina bifida—*see* Spina bifida
- diaphragm (congenital) Q79.1
  - acquired J98.6
- digestive organ NOS Q45.9
- ductus arteriosus Q25.0
- ear (acquired) H61.1-
  - congenital (external) Q17.9
- ectodermal (congenital) NEC Q84.9
- endocrine gland NEC Q89.2
- eye, congenital Q15.9
- face (acquired) M95.2
  - congenital Q18.9
- flexion (joint) (acquired) (*see also* Deformity, limb, flexion) M21.20
  - congenital NOS Q74.9
  - hip Q65.89
- foot (acquired)—*see also* Deformity, limb, lower leg
  - cavovarus (congenital) Q66.1-
  - congenital NOS Q66.9-
    - specified type NEC Q66.89
  - specified type NEC M21.6X-
  - valgus (congenital) Q66.6
    - acquired M21.07-
  - varus (congenital) NEC Q66.3-
    - acquired M21.17-
- forehead (acquired) M95.2
  - congenital Q75.8
- frontal bone (acquired) M95.2
  - congenital Q75.8
- gallbladder (congenital) Q44.1
  - acquired K82.8
- gastrointestinal tract (congenital) NOS Q45.9
  - acquired K63.89
- genitalia, genital organ(s) or system NEC
  - female (congenital) Q52.9
    - acquired N94.89
    - external Q52.70
  - male (congenital) Q55.9
    - acquired N50.89
- head (acquired) M95.2
  - congenital Q75.8
- heart (congenital) Q24.9
  - septum Q21.9
    - auricular Q21.1
    - ventricular Q21.0
- hepatic duct (congenital) Q44.5
  - acquired K83.8
- humerus (acquired) M21.82-
  - congenital Q74.0
- hypophyseal (congenital) Q89.2
- ilium (acquired) M95.5
  - congenital Q74.2
- integument (congenital) Q84.9
- ischium (acquired) M95.5
  - congenital Q74.2
- ligament (acquired)—*see* Disorder
  - congenital Q79.9
- limb (acquired) M21.90
  - congenital Q38.0
  - congenital, except reduction deformity Q74.9
  - flat foot M21.4-
  - flexion M21.20
    - ankle M21.27-
    - elbow M21.22-
    - finger M21.24-
    - hip M21.25-
    - knee M21.26-
    - shoulder M21.21-
    - toe M21.27-
    - wrist M21.23-
  - foot
    - drop M21.37-
    - flat—*see* Deformity, limb, flat foot
    - specified NEC M21.6X-

Deformity, *continued*
- forearm M21.93-
- hand M21.94-
- lower leg M21.96-
- specified type NEC M21.80
  - forearm M21.83-
  - lower leg M21.86-
  - thigh M21.85-
    - unequal length M21.70
  - thigh M21.95-
  - upper arm M21.82-
- lip (acquired) NEC K13.0
- liver (congenital) Q44.7
  - acquired K76.89
- Madelung's (radius) Q74.0
- meninges or membrane (congenital) Q07.9
  - cerebral Q04.8
    - acquired G96.198
  - spinal cord (congenital) G96.198
    - acquired G96.198
- metacarpus (acquired)—*see* Deformity, limb, forearm
  - congenital Q74.0
- mitral (leaflets) (valve) I05.8
  - parachute Q23.2
  - stenosis, congenital Q23.2
- mouth (acquired) K13.79
  - congenital Q38.6
- multiple, congenital NEC Q89.7
- muscle (acquired) M62.89
  - congenital Q79.9
    - sternocleidomastoid Q68.0
- musculoskeletal system (acquired) M95.9
  - congenital Q79.9
  - specified NEC M95.8
- nail (acquired) L60.8
  - congenital Q84.6
- nasal—*see* Deformity, nose
- neck (acquired) M95.3
  - congenital Q18.9
    - sternocleidomastoid Q68.0
- nervous system (congenital) Q07.9
- nose (acquired) (cartilage) M95.0
  - bone (turbinate) M95.0
  - congenital Q30.9
    - bent or squashed Q67.4
  - septum (acquired) J34.2
    - congenital Q30.8
- ovary (congenital) Q50.39
- parathyroid (gland) Q89.2
- pelvis, pelvic (bony) M95.5
  - congenital Q74.2
- penis (glans) (congenital) Q55.69
  - acquired N48.89
- pinna, acquired H61.1-
  - congenital Q17.9
- pituitary (congenital) Q89.2
  - posture—*see* Dorsopathy
- prepuce (congenital) Q55.69
  - acquired N47.8
- rectum (congenital) Q43.9
  - acquired K62.89
- respiratory system (congenital) Q34.9
- rotation (joint) (acquired)—*see* Deformity, limb, specified site NEC
  - congenital Q74.9
  - hip M21.85-
    - congenital Q65.89
- sacroiliac joint (congenital) Q74.2
- septum, nasal (acquired) J34.2
- scapula (acquired) M95.8
  - congenital Q68.8
- shoulder (joint) (acquired) M21.92-
  - congenital Q74.0
- skull (acquired) M95.2
  - congenital Q75.8
    - with
      - anencephaly Q00.0
      - encephalocele—*see* Encephalocele
      - hydrocephalus Q03.9
        - ◊ with spina bifida—*see* Spina bifida, by site, with hydrocephalus
      - microcephaly Q02

Deformity, *continued*
- spinal
  - nerve root (congenital) Q07.9
- Sprengel's (congenital) Q74.0
- sternocleidomastoid (muscle), congenital Q68.0
- thymus (tissue) (congenital) Q89.2
- thyroid (gland) (congenital) Q89.2
- toe (acquired) M20.6-
  - congenital Q66.9-
  - hallux valgus M20.1-
- tricuspid (leaflets) (valve) I07.8
  - atresia or stenosis Q22.4
  - Ebstein's Q22.5
- trunk (acquired) M95.8
  - congenital Q89.9
- urachus (congenital) Q64.4
- urinary tract (congenital) Q64.9
  - urachus Q64.4
- vagina (acquired) N89.8
  - congenital Q52.4
- valgus NEC M21.00
  - knee M21.06-
- varus NEC M21.10
  - knee M21.16-
- vesicourethral orifice (acquired) N32.89
  - congenital NEC Q64.79
  - wrist drop M21.33-

Degeneration, degenerative
- brain (cortical) (progressive) G31.9
  - childhood G31.9
    - specified NEC G31.89
  - cystic G31.89
    - congenital Q04.6
  - in
    - congenital hydrocephalus Q03.9
      - with spina bifida—*see also* Spina bifida
    - Hunter's syndrome E76.1
- cerebrovascular I67.9
  - due to hypertension I67.4
- cortical (cerebellar) (parenchymatous) G31.89
- cutis L98.8
- extrapyramidal G25.9
- fatty
  - liver NEC K76.0
- intervertebral disc NOS
  - sacrococcygeal region M53.3
- kidney N28.89
  - cystic, congenital Q61.9
  - fatty N28.89
  - polycystic Q61.3
    - infantile type (autosomal recessive) NEC Q61.19
      - collecting duct dilatation Q61.11
- muscle (fatty) (fibrous) (hyaline) (progressive) M62.89
  - heart—*see* Degeneration, myocardial
- myocardial, myocardium (fatty) (hyaline) (senile) I51.5
  - with rheumatic fever (conditions in I00) I09.0
    - active, acute or subacute I01.2
      - with chorea I02.0
    - inactive or quiescent (with chorea) I09.0
- nasal sinus (mucosa) J32.9
  - frontal J32.1
  - maxillary J32.0
- nervous system G31.9
  - fatty G31.89
  - specified NEC G31.89
- ovary N83.8
  - cystic N83.20-
  - microcystic N83.20-
- pituitary (gland) E23.6
- pulmonary valve (heart) I37.8
- sinus (cystic)—*see also* Sinusitis
- skin L98.8
  - colloid L98.8
- spinal (cord) G31.89
  - familial NEC G31.89
  - fatty G31.89
- tricuspid (heart) (valve) I07.9
- turbinate J34.89

Deglutition
- paralysis R13.0
  - hysterical F44.4
- pneumonia J69.0

Dehiscence (of)
- closure
  - laceration (internal) (external) T81.33
  - traumatic laceration (external) (internal) T81.33
- traumatic injury wound repair T81.33
- wound T81.30
  - traumatic repair T81.33

Dehydration E86.0
- hypertonic E87.0
- hypotonic E87.1
- newborn P74.1

Delay, delayed
- closure, ductus arteriosus (Botalli) P29.38
- conduction (cardiac) (ventricular) I45.9
- development R62.50
  - intellectual (specific) F81.9
  - language F80.9
    - due to hearing loss F80.4
  - learning F81.9
  - pervasive F84.9
  - physiological R62.50
    - specified stage NEC R62.0
  - reading F81.0
  - sexual E30.0
  - speech F80.9
    - due to hearing loss F80.4
  - spelling F81.81
- gastric emptying K30
- menarche E30.0
- milestone R62.0
- passage of meconium (newborn) P76.0
- primary respiration P28.9
- puberty (constitutional) E30.0
- separation of umbilical cord P96.82
- sexual maturation, female E30.0
- sleep phase syndrome G47.21
- vaccination Z28.9

Deletion(s)
- autosome Q93.9
  - identified by fluorescence in situ hybridization (FISH) Q93.89
  - identified by in situ hybridization (ISH) Q93.89
- chromosome
  - seen only at prometaphase Q93.89
  - part of NEC Q93.59
  - short arm
    - 5p Q93.4
    - 22q11.2 Q93.81
  - specified NEC Q93.89
- microdeletions NEC Q93.88

Delinquency (juvenile) (neurotic) F91.8
- group Z72.810

Delinquent immunization status Z28.3

Delirium, delirious (acute or subacute) (not alcohol- or drug-induced) (with dementia) R41.0
- exhaustion F43.0

Delivery (childbirth) (labor)
- cesarean (for)
  - fetal-maternal hemorrhage O43.01-
  - placental insufficiency O36.51-
  - placental transfusion syndromes
    - fetomaternal O43.01-
    - fetus to fetus O43.02-
    - maternofetal O43.01-
  - pre-eclampsia O14.9-
    - mild O14.0-
    - moderate O14.0-
    - severe
      - with hemolysis, elevated liver enzymes and low platelet count (HELLP) O14.2-
- complicated O75.9
  - by
    - premature rupture, membranes (*see also* Pregnancy, complicated by, premature rupture of membranes) O42.90
- missed (at or near term) O36.4

Dementia (degenerative (primary)) (old age) (persisting)
- in (due to)
  - hypercalcemia E83.52 *[F02.80]*
    - with behavioral disturbance E83.52 *[F02.81]*
  - hypothyroidism, acquired E03.9 *[F02.80]*

Dementia, *continued*
  - with behavioral disturbance E03.9 *[F02.81]*
  - due to iodine deficiency E01.8 *[F02.80]*
    - with behavioral disturbance E01.8 *[F02.81]*

Demodex folliculorum (infestation) B88.0

Demyelination, demyelinization
- central nervous system G37.9
  - specified NEC G37.8
- corpus callosum (central) G37.1
- disseminated, acute G36.9
  - specified NEC G36.8
- global G35
- in optic neuritis G36.0

Dentia praecox K00.6

Dentigerous cyst K09.0

Dentin
- sensitive K03.89

Dentition (syndrome) K00.7
- delayed K00.6
- difficult K00.7
- precocious K00.6
- premature K00.6
- retarded K00.6

Dependence (on) (syndrome) F19.20
- with remission F19.21
- alcohol (ethyl) (methyl) (without remission) F10.20
  - with
    - anxiety disorder F10.280
    - intoxication F10.229
      - with delirium F10.221
      - uncomplicated F10.220
  - counseling and surveillance Z71.41
- amphetamine(s) (type)—*see* Dependence, drug, stimulant NEC
- benzedrine—*see* Dependence, drug, stimulant NEC
- bhang—*see* Dependence, drug, cannabis
- caffeine—*see* Dependence, drug, stimulant NEC
- cannabis (sativa) (indica) (resin) (derivatives) (type)—F12.20
  - withdrawal F12.23
- coca (leaf) (derivatives)—*see* Dependence, drug, cocaine
- cocaine—*see* Dependence, drug, cocaine
- combinations of drugs F19.20
- dagga—*see* Dependence, drug, cannabis
- dexamphetamine—*see* Dependence, drug, stimulant NEC
- dexedrine—*see* Dependence, drug, stimulant NEC
- dextro-nor-pseudo-ephedrine—*see* Dependence, drug, stimulant NEC
- diazepam—*see* Dependence, drug
- drug NEC F19.20
  - cannabis F12.20
    - with
      - intoxication F12.229
        - uncomplicated F12.220
    - in remission F12.21
  - cocaine F14.20
    - with
      - intoxication F14.229
        - uncomplicated F14.220
      - withdrawal F14.23
    - in remission F14.21
    - withdrawal symptoms in newborn P96.1
  - counseling and surveillance Z71.51
  - inhalant F18.20
    - with
      - intoxication F18.229
        - uncomplicated F18.220
    - in remission F18.21
  - nicotine F17.200
    - with disorder F17.209
      - in remission F17.201
      - specified disorder NEC F17.208
      - withdrawal F17.203
    - chewing tobacco F17.220
      - with disorder F17.229
        - in remission F17.221
        - specified disorder NEC F17.228
        - withdrawal F17.223

Dependence, *continued*
    - cigarettes F17.210
      - with disorder F17.219
        - in remission F17.211
        - specified disorder NEC F17.218
    - specified product NEC F17.290
      - with disorder F17.299
        - in remission F17.291
        - specified disorder NEC F17.298
        - withdrawal F17.293
  - psychoactive NEC F19.20
  - sedative, anxiolytic or hypnotic F13.-
  - stimulant NEC F15.20
    - with
      - intoxication F15.229
        - uncomplicated F15.220
      - withdrawal F15.23
    - in remission F15.21
- ethyl
  - alcohol (without remission) F10.20
    - with remission F10.21
- ganja—*see* Dependence, drug, cannabis
- glue (airplane) (sniffing)—*see* Dependence, drug, inhalant
- hashish—*see* Dependence, drug, cannabis
- hemp—*see* Dependence, drug, cannabis
- Indian hemp—*see* Dependence, drug, cannabis
- inhalants—*see* Dependence, drug, inhalant
- maconha—*see* Dependence, drug, cannabis
- marijuana—*see* Dependence, drug, cannabis
- methyl
  - alcohol (without remission) F10.20
    - with remission F10.21
- nicotine—*see* Dependence, drug, nicotine
- on
  - assistance with personal care Z74.1
  - care provider (because of) Z74.9
    - no other household member able to render care Z74.2
  - machine Z99.89
    - enabling NEC Z99.89
    - specified type NEC Z99.89
  - renal dialysis (hemodialysis) (peritoneal) Z99.2
  - respirator Z99.11
  - ventilator Z99.11
  - wheelchair Z99.3
- oxygen (long-term) (supplemental) Z99.81
- PCP (phencyclidine) (*see also* Abuse, drug) F16.20
- phencyclidine (PCP) (and related substances) (*see also* Abuse, drug) F16.20
- phenmetrazine—*see* Dependence, drug, stimulant NEC
- polysubstance F19.20
- psychostimulant NEC—*see* Dependence, drug, stimulant NEC
- sedative, anxiolytic or hypnotic F13.-
- specified drug NEC—*see* Dependence, drug
- stimulant NEC—*see* Dependence, drug, stimulant NEC
- substance NEC—*see* Dependence, drug
- supplemental oxygen Z99.81
- tobacco—*see* Dependence, drug, nicotine
  - counseling and surveillance Z71.6
- volatile solvents—*see* Dependence, drug, inhalant

Depletion
- extracellular fluid E86.9
- plasma E86.1
- salt or sodium E87.1
  - causing heat exhaustion or prostration T67.4
  - nephropathy N28.9
- volume NOS E86.9

Depolarization, premature I49.40
- atrial I49.1
- specified NEC I49.49

Deposit
- bone in Boeck's sarcoid D86.89

Depression (acute) (mental) F32.9
- anaclitic—*see* Disorder, adjustment
- anxiety F41.8
  - persistent F34.1
- atypical (single episode) F32.89
- basal metabolic rate R94.8
- bone marrow D75.89
- central nervous system R09.2

Depression, *continued*
- cerebral R29.818
  - newborn P91.4
- major F32.9
- medullary G93.89
- nervous F34.1
- neurotic F34.1
- psychogenic (reactive) (single episode) F32.9
- psychoneurotic F34.1
- reactive (psychogenic) (single episode) F32.9
  - psychotic (single episode) F32.3
- recurrent—*see* Disorder, depressive, recurrent
- respiratory center G93.89
- situational F43.21
- skull Q67.4
- specified NEC (single episode) F32.89

Deprivation
- cultural Z60.3
- emotional NEC Z65.8
  - affecting infant or child—*see* Maltreatment, child, psychological
- social Z60.4
  - affecting infant or child—*see* Maltreatment, child, psychological abuse

De Quervain's
- syndrome E34.51
- thyroiditis (subacute granulomatous thyroiditis) E06.1

Derangement
- joint (internal) M24.9
  - ankylosis—*see* Ankylosis
  - specified type NEC M24.8-
    - ankle M24.87-
    - elbow M24.82-
    - foot joint M24.87-
    - hand joint M24.84-
    - hip M24.85-
    - shoulder M24.81-
  - temporomandibular M26.69

Dermatitis (eczematous) L30.9
- acarine B88.0
- ammonia L22
- arsenical (ingested) L27.8
- artefacta L98.1
  - psychogenic F54
- atopic L20.9
  - psychogenic F54
  - specified NEC L20.89
- cercarial B65.3
- contact (occupational) L25.9
  - allergic L23.9
    - due to
      - ~ adhesives L23.1
      - ~ cement L24.5
      - ~ chemical products NEC L23.5
      - ~ chromium L23.0
      - ~ cosmetics L23.2
      - ~ dander (cat) (dog) L23.81
      - ~ drugs in contact with skin L23.3
      - ~ dyes L23.4
      - ~ food in contact with skin L23.6
      - ~ hair (cat) (dog) L23.81
      - ~ insecticide L23.5
      - ~ metals L23.0
      - ~ nickel L23.0
      - ~ plants, non-food L23.7
      - ~ plastic L23.5
      - ~ rubber L23.5
      - ~ specified agent NEC L23.89
  - due to
    - dander (cat) (dog) L23.81
    - hair (cat) (dog) L23.81
- contusiformis L52
- desquamative L30.8
- diabetic—*see* E08-E13 with .620
- diaper L22
- due to
  - adhesive(s) (allergic) (contact) (plaster) L23.1
  - alcohol (irritant) (skin contact) L24.2
    - taken internally L27.8
  - alkalis (contact) (irritant) L24.5
  - arsenic (ingested) L27.8
  - cereal (ingested) L27.2

Dermatitis, *continued*
- chemical(s) NEC L25.3
  - taken internally L27.8
- coffee (ingested) L27.2
- cosmetics (contact) L25.0
  - allergic L23.2
- dander (cat) (dog) L23.81
- Demodex species B88.0
- Dermanyssus gallinae B88.0
- drugs and medicaments (generalized) (internal use) L27.0
  - in contact with skin L25.1
    - ~ allergic L23.3
  - localized skin eruption L27.1
  - specified substance—*see* Table of Drugs and Chemicals
- dyes (contact) L25.2
  - allergic L23.4
- fish (ingested) L27.2
- flour (ingested) L27.2
- food (ingested) L27.2
  - in contact with skin L25.4
- fruit (ingested) L27.2
- furs (allergic) (contact) L23.81
- hair (cat) (dog) L23.81
- infrared rays
- ingestion, ingested substance L27.9
  - chemical NEC L27.8
  - drugs and medicaments—*see* Dermatitis, due to, drugs and medicaments
  - food L27.2
  - specified NEC L27.8
- insecticide in contact with skin L24.5
- internal agent L27.9
  - drugs and medicaments (generalized)—*see* Dermatitis, due to, drugs and medicaments
  - food L27.2
- irradiation—*see* Dermatitis, due to, radiation
- lacquer tree (allergic) (contact) L23.7
- light (sun) NEC
  - acute L56.8
- Lyponyssoides sanguineus B88.0
- milk (ingested) L27.2
- petroleum products (contact) (irritant) (substances in T52.0) L24.2
- plants NEC (contact) L25.5
  - allergic L23.7
- plasters (adhesive) (any) (allergic) (contact) L23.1
- primrose (allergic) (contact) L23.7
- primula (allergic) (contact) L23.7
- radiation
  - nonionizing (chronic exposure)
  - sun NEC
    - ~ acute L56.8
- ragweed (allergic) (contact) L23.7
- Rhus (allergic) (contact) (diversiloba) (radicans) (toxicodendron) (venenata) (verniciflua) L23.7
- Senecio jacobaea (allergic) (contact) L23.7
- solvents (contact) (irritant) (substances in categories T52) L24.2
- specified agent NEC (contact) L25.8
  - allergic L23.89
- sunshine NEC
  - acute L56.8
- ultraviolet rays (sun NEC) (chronic exposure)
  - acute L56.8
- vaccine or vaccination L27.0
  - specified substance—*see* Table of Drugs and Chemicals
- dyshydrotic L30.1
- dysmenorrheica N94.6
- exfoliative, exfoliativa (generalized) L26
  - neonatorum L00
- eyelid
  - allergic H01.11-
    - left H01.116
      - ~ lower H01.115
      - ~ upper H01.114
    - right H01.113
      - ~ lower H01.112
      - ~ upper H01.111
  - due to
    - Demodex species B88.0

Dermatitis, *continued*
- facta, factitia, factitial L98.1
  - psychogenic F54
- flexural NEC L20.82
- friction L30.4
- gangrenosa, gangrenous infantum L08.0
- harvest mite B88.0
- infectious eczematoid L30.3
- infective L30.3
- irritant—*see* Dermatitis, contact
- Jacquet's (diaper dermatitis) L22
- Leptus B88.0
- mite B88.0
- napkin L22
- purulent L08.0
- pyococcal L08.0
- pyogenica L08.0
- Ritter's (exfoliativa) L00
- schistosome B65.3
- seborrheic L21.9
  - infantile L21.1
  - specified NEC L21.8
- sensitization NOS L23.9
- septic L08.0
- suppurative L08.0
- traumatic NEC L30.4
- ultraviolet (sun) (chronic exposure)
  - acute L56.8

Dermatographia L50.3

Dermatolysis (exfoliativa) (congenital) Q82.8

Dermatomegaly NEC Q82.8

Dermatomycosis B36.9
- furfuracea B36.0
- specified type NEC B36.8

Dermatomyositis (acute) (chronic)—*see also* Dermatopolymyositis
- in (due to) neoplastic disease (*see also* Table of Neoplasms in the complete *ICD-10-CM* manual) D49.9 [M36.0]
- juvenile M33.00
  - with
    - myopathy M33.02
    - respiratory involvement M33.01
    - specified organ involvement NEC M33.09
  - without myopathy M33.03
- specified NEC M33.10
  - with
    - myopathy M33.12
    - respiratory involvement M33.11
    - specified organ involvement NEC M33.19
  - without myopathy M33.13

Dermatoneuritis of children—*see* Poisoning

Dermatophytosis (epidermophyton) (infection) (Microsporum) (tinea) (Trichophyton) B35.9
- beard B35.0
- body B35.4
- capitis B35.0
- corporis B35.4
- deep-seated B35.8
- disseminated B35.8
- foot B35.3
- granulomatous B35.8
- groin B35.6
- hand B35.2
- nail B35.1
- perianal (area) B35.6
- scalp B35.0
- specified NEC B35.8

Dermatopolymyositis M33.90
- with
  - myopathy M33.92
  - respiratory involvement M33.91
  - specified organ involvement NEC M33.99
- juvenile M33.00
  - with
    - myopathy M33.02
    - respiratory involvement M33.01
    - specified organ involvement NEC M33.09
- without myopathy M33.93

Dermatopolyneuritis—*see* Poisoning

Dermatorrhexis (Ehlers-Danos) Q79.60

Dermatosis L98.9
- factitial L98.1
- menstrual NEC L98.8

Dermophytosis—see Dermatophytosis

Despondency F32.9

Destruction, destructive—see also Damage
- joint—see also Derangement, joint, specified type NEC
  - sacroiliac M53.3
- rectal sphincter K62.89
- septum (nasal) J34.89

Detergent asthma J69.8

Deterioration
- general physical R53.81

Development
- abnormal, bone Q79.9
- arrested R62.50
  - bone—see Arrest, development or growth, bone
  - child R62.50
  - due to malnutrition E45
- defective, congenital—see also Anomaly, by site
  - left ventricle Q24.8
    - in hypoplastic left heart syndrome Q23.4
- delayed (see also Delay, development) R62.50
  - arithmetical skills F81.2
  - language (skills) (expressive) F80.1
  - learning skill F81.9
  - mixed skills F88
  - motor coordination F82
  - reading F81.0
  - specified learning skill NEC F81.89
  - speech F80.9
  - spelling F81.81
  - written expression F81.81
- imperfect, congenital—see also Anomaly, by site
  - heart Q24.9
  - lungs Q33.6
- incomplete
  - bronchial tree Q32.4
  - organ or site not listed—see Hypoplasia, by site
  - respiratory system Q34.9
- sexual, precocious NEC E30.1
- tardy, mental (see also Disability, intellectual) F79

Developmental—see Disease, diseased
- testing, infant or child—see Examination, child

Deviation (in)
- midline (jaw) (teeth) (dental arch) M26.29
  - specified site NEC—see Malposition
- nasal septum J34.2
  - congenital Q67.4
- septum (nasal) (acquired) J34.2
  - congenital Q67.4
- sexual transvestism F64.1
- teeth, midline M26.29

Device
- cerebral ventricle (communicating) in situ Z98.2
- drainage, cerebrospinal fluid, in situ Z98.2

Devil's
- pinches (purpura simplex) D69.2

Dextraposition, aorta Q20.3
- in tetralogy of Fallot Q21.3

Dextrocardia (true) Q24.0
- with
  - complete transposition of viscera Q89.3
  - situs inversus Q89.3

Dextrotransposition, aorta Q20.3

Dhobi itch B35.6

Di George's syndrome D82.1

Diabetes, diabetic (mellitus) (sugar) E11.9
- bronzed E83.110
- dietary counseling and surveillance Z71.3
- due to drug or chemical E09.9
  - with
    - amyotrophy E09.44
    - arthropathy NEC E09.618
    - autonomic (poly)neuropathy E09.43
    - cataract E09.36
    - Charcot's joints E09.610
    - chronic kidney disease E09.22

Diabetes, diabetic (mellitus) (sugar), continued
    - circulatory complication NEC E09.59
    - complication E09.8
      ~ specified NEC E09.69
    - dermatitis E09.620
    - foot ulcer E09.621
    - gangrene E09.52
    - gastroparesis E09.43
    - glomerulonephrosis, intracapillary E09.21
    - glomerulosclerosis, intercapillary E09.21
    - hyperglycemia E09.65
    - hyperosmolarity E09.00
      ~ with coma E09.01
    - hypoglycemia E09.649
      ~ with coma E09.641
    - ketoacidosis E09.10
      ~ with coma E09.11
    - kidney complications NEC E09.29
    - Kimmelstiel-Wilson disease E09.21
    - mononeuropathy E09.41
    - myasthenia E09.44
    - necrobiosis lipoidica E09.620
    - nephropathy E09.21
    - neuralgia E09.42
    - neurologic complication NEC E09.49
    - neuropathic arthropathy E09.610
    - neuropathy E09.40
    - ophthalmic complication NEC E09.39
    - oral complication NEC E09.638
    - periodontal disease E09.630
    - peripheral angiopathy E09.51
      ~ with gangrene E09.52
    - polyneuropathy E09.42
    - renal complication NEC E09.29
    - renal tubular degeneration E09.29
    - retinopathy E09.319
      ~ with macular edema E09.311
      ~ nonproliferative E09.329
        ◊ with macular edema E09.321
        ◊ mild E09.329
          » with macular edema E09.321
        ◊ moderate E09.339
          » with macular edema E09.331
        ◊ severe E09.349
          » with macular edema E09.341
      ~ proliferative E09.359
        ◊ with macular edema E09.351
    - skin complication NEC E09.628
    - skin ulcer NEC E09.622
- due to underlying condition E08.9
  - with
    - amyotrophy E08.44
    - arthropathy NEC E08.618
    - autonomic (poly)neuropathy E08.43
    - cataract E08.36
    - Charcot's joints E08.610
    - chronic kidney disease E08.22
    - circulatory complication NEC E08.59
    - complication E08.8
      ~ specified NEC E08.69
    - dermatitis E08.620
    - foot ulcer E08.621
    - gangrene E08.52
    - gastroparesis E08.43
    - glomerulonephrosis, intracapillary E08.21
    - glomerulosclerosis, intercapillary E08.21
    - hyperglycemia E08.65
    - hyperosmolarity E08.00
      ~ with coma E08.01
    - hypoglycemia E08.649
      ~ with coma E08.641
    - ketoacidosis E08.10
      ~ with coma E08.11
    - kidney complications NEC E08.29
    - Kimmelstiel-Wilson disease E08.21
    - mononeuropathy E08.41
    - myasthenia E08.44
    - necrobiosis lipoidica E08.620
    - nephropathy E08.21
    - neuralgia E08.42
    - neurologic complication NEC E08.49
    - neuropathic arthropathy E08.610
    - neuropathy E08.40

Diabetes, diabetic (mellitus) (sugar), continued
    - ophthalmic complication NEC E08.39
    - oral complication NEC E08.638
    - periodontal disease E08.630
    - peripheral angiopathy E08.51
      ~ with gangrene E08.52
    - polyneuropathy E08.42
    - renal complication NEC E08.29
    - renal tubular degeneration E08.29
    - retinopathy E08.319
      ~ with macular edema E08.311
      ~ nonproliferative E08.329
        ◊ with macular edema E08.321
        ◊ mild E08.329
          » with macular edema E08.321
        ◊ moderate E08.339
          » with macular edema E08.331
        ◊ severe E08.349
          » with macular edema E08.341
      ~ proliferative E08.359
        ◊ with macular edema E08.351
    - skin complication NEC E08.628
    - skin ulcer NEC E08.622
- gestational (in pregnancy)
  - affecting newborn P70.0
  - diet controlled O24.410
  - insulin (and diet) controlled O24.414
  - oral hypoglycemic drug controlled O24.415
- inadequately controlled—code to Diabetes, by type, with hyperglycemia
- insipidus E23.2
  - nephrogenic N25.1
  - pituitary E23.2
- insulin dependent—code to type of diabetes
- juvenile-onset—see Diabetes, type 1
- ketosis-prone—see Diabetes, type 1
- latent R73.09
- neonatal (transient) P70.2
- non-insulin dependent—code to type of diabetes
- out of control—code to Diabetes, by type, with hyperglycemia
- poorly controlled—code to Diabetes, by type, with hyperglycemia
- postpancreatectomy—see Diabetes
- postprocedural—see Diabetes
- prediabetes R73.03
- secondary diabetes mellitus NEC—see Diabetes
- steroid-induced—see Diabetes, due to drug or chemical
- type 1 E10.9
  - with
    - amyotrophy E10.44
    - arthropathy NEC E10.618
    - autonomic (poly)neuropathy E10.43
    - cataract E10.36
    - Charcot's joints E10.610
    - chronic kidney disease E10.22
    - circulatory complication NEC E10.59
    - complication E10.8
      ~ specified NEC E10.69
    - dermatitis E10.620
    - foot ulcer E10.621
    - gangrene E10.52
    - gastroparesis E10.43
    - glomerulonephrosis, intracapillary E10.21
    - glomerulosclerosis, intercapillary E10.21
    - hyperglycemia E10.65
    - hypoglycemia E10.649
      ~ with coma E10.641
    - ketoacidosis E10.10
      ~ with coma E10.11
    - kidney complications NEC E10.29
    - Kimmelstiel-Wilson disease E10.21
    - mononeuropathy E10.41
    - myasthenia E10.44
    - necrobiosis lipoidica E10.620
    - nephropathy E10.21
    - neuralgia E10.42
    - neurologic complication NEC E10.49
    - neuropathic arthropathy E10.610
    - neuropathy E10.40
    - ophthalmic complication NEC E10.39
    - oral complication NEC E10.638
    - periodontal disease E10.630

Diabetes, diabetic (mellitus) (sugar), *continued*
- ■ peripheral angiopathy E10.51
  - ~ with gangrene E10.52
- ■ polyneuropathy E10.42
- ■ renal complication NEC E10.29
- ■ renal tubular degeneration E10.29
- ■ retinopathy E10.319
  - ~ with macular edema E10.311
  - ~ nonproliferative E10.329
    - ◊ with macular edema E10.321
    - ◊ mild E10.329
      - » with macular edema E10.321
    - ◊ moderate E10.339
      - » with macular edema E10.331
    - ◊ severe E10.349
      - » with macular edema E10.341
  - ~ proliferative E10.359
    - ◊ with macular edema E10.351
- ■ skin complication NEC E10.628
- ■ skin ulcer NEC E10.622
- • type 2 E11.9
  - – with
    - ■ amyotrophy E11.44
    - ■ arthropathy NEC E11.618
    - ■ autonomic (poly)neuropathy E11.43
    - ■ cataract E11.36
    - ■ Charcot's joints E11.610
    - ■ chronic kidney disease E11.22
    - ■ circulatory complication NEC E11.59
    - ■ complication E11.8
      - ~ specified NEC E11.69
    - ■ dermatitis E11.620
    - ■ foot ulcer E11.621
    - ■ gangrene E11.52
    - ■ gastroparesis E11.43
    - ■ glomerulonephrosis, intracapillary E11.21
    - ■ glomerulosclerosis, intercapillary E11.21
    - ■ hyperglycemia E11.65
    - ■ hyperosmolarity E11.00
      - ~ with coma E11.01
    - ■ hypoglycemia E11.649
      - ~ with coma E11.641
    - ■ ketoacidosis E11.10
      - ~ with coma E11.11
    - ■ kidney complications NEC E11.29
    - ■ Kimmelstiel-Wilson disease E11.21
    - ■ mononeuropathy E11.41
    - ■ myasthenia E11.44
    - ■ necrobiosis lipoidica E11.620
    - ■ nephropathy E11.21
    - ■ neuralgia E11.42
    - ■ neurologic complication NEC E11.49
    - ■ neuropathic arthropathy E11.610
    - ■ neuropathy E11.40
    - ■ ophthalmic complication NEC E11.39
    - ■ oral complication NEC E11.638
    - ■ periodontal disease E11.630
    - ■ peripheral angiopathy E11.51
      - ~ with gangrene E11.52
    - ■ polyneuropathy E11.42
    - ■ renal complication NEC E11.29
    - ■ renal tubular degeneration E11.29
    - ■ retinopathy E11.319
      - ~ with macular edema E11.311
      - ~ nonproliferative E11.329
        - ◊ with macular edema E11.321
        - ◊ mild E11.329
          - » with macular edema E11.321
        - ◊ moderate E11.339
          - » with macular edema E11.331
        - ◊ severe E11.349
          - » with macular edema E11.341
      - ~ proliferative E11.359
        - ◊ with macular edema E11.351
    - ■ skin complication NEC E11.628
    - ■ skin ulcer NEC E11.622

Diagnosis deferred R69

Dialysis (intermittent) (treatment)
- • noncompliance (with) Z91.15
- • renal (hemodialysis) (peritoneal), status Z99.2

Diamond-Blackfan anemia (congenital hypoplastic) D61.01

Diamond-Gardener syndrome (autoerythrocyte sensitization) D69.2

Diaper rash L22

Diaphoresis (excessive) R61

Diaphragmatitis, diaphragmitis J98.6

Diarrhea, diarrheal (disease) (infantile) (inflammatory) R19.7
- • allergic K52.29
- • amebic (*see also* Amebiasis) A06.0
  - – acute A06.0
- • cachectic NEC K52.89
- • chronic (noninfectious) K52.9
- • dietetic K52.29
- • due to
  - – Campylobacter A04.5
  - – C. difficile A04.7-
  - – Escherichia coli A04.4
    - ■ enteroaggregative A04.4
    - ■ enterohemorrhagic A04.3
    - ■ enteropathogenic A04.0
    - ■ enterotoxigenic A04.1
    - ■ specified NEC A04.4
  - – food hypersensitivity K52.29
  - – specified organism NEC A08.8
    - ■ bacterial A04.8
    - ■ viral A08.39
- • dysenteric A09
- • endemic A09
- • epidemic A09
- • functional K59.1
  - – following gastrointestinal surgery K91.89
  - – psychogenic F45.8
- • Giardia lamblia A07.1
- • giardial A07.1
- • infectious A09
- • mite B88.0
- • neonatal (noninfectious) P78.3
- • nervous F45.8
- • noninfectious K52.9
- • psychogenic F45.8
- • specified
  - – bacterial A04.8
  - – virus NEC A08.39

Diastasis
- • cranial bones M84.88
  - – congenital NEC Q75.8
- • joint (traumatic)—*see* Dislocation

Diathesis
- • hemorrhagic (familial) D69.9
  - – newborn NEC P53

Didymytis N45.1
- • with orchitis N45.3

Dietary
- • surveillance and counseling Z71.3

Dietl's crisis N13.8

Difficult, difficulty (in)
- • acculturation Z60.3
- • feeding R63.3
  - – newborn P92.9
    - ■ breast P92.5
    - ■ specified NEC P92.8
  - – nonorganic (infant or child) F98.29
- • reading (developmental) F81.0
  - – secondary to emotional disorders F93.9
- • spelling (specific) F81.81
  - – with reading disorder F81.89
  - – due to inadequate teaching Z55.8
- • swallowing—*see* Dysphagia
- • walking R26.2

DiGeorge's syndrome (thymic hypoplasia) D82.1

Dilatation
- • aorta (congenital) Q25.44
- • bladder (sphincter) N32.89
  - – congenital Q64.79
- • colon K59.39
  - – congenital Q43.1
  - – psychogenic F45.8
  - – toxic K59.31
- • common duct (acquired) K83.8
  - – congenital Q44.5

Dilatation, *continued*
- • cystic duct (acquired) K82.8
  - – congenital Q44.5
- • ileum K59.89
  - – psychogenic F45.8
- • jejunum K59.89
  - – psychogenic F45.8
- • Meckel's diverticulum (congenital) Q43.0
- • rectum K59.39
- • sphincter ani K62.89
- • stomach K31.89
  - – acute K31.0
  - – psychogenic F45.8
- • vesical orifice N32.89

Dilated, dilation—*see* Dilatation

Diminished, diminution
- • hearing (acuity)—*see* Deafness
- • sense or sensation (cold) (heat) (tactile) (vibratory) R20.8
- • vision NEC H54.7

Dimitri-Sturge-Weber disease Q85.8

Dimple
- • congenital, sacral Q82.6
  - – parasacral Q82.6
- • parasacral, pilonidal or postanal—*see* Cyst, pilonidal

Diphallus Q55.69

Diphtheria, diphtheritic (gangrenous) (hemorrhagic) A36.9
- • carrier Z22.2

Diplegia (upper limbs) G83.0
- • lower limbs G82.20

Dipsomania F10.20
- • with
  - – remission F10.21

Dirt-eating child F98.3

Disability, disabilities
- • intellectual F79
  - – with
    - ■ autistic features F84.9
  - – mild (I.Q.50 – 69) F70
  - – moderate (I.Q.35 – 49) F71
  - – profound (I.Q. under 20) F73
  - – severe (I.Q.20 – 34) F72
  - – specified level NEC F78
- • knowledge acquisition F81.9
- • learning F81.9
- • limiting activities Z73.6
- • spelling, specific F81.81

Disappearance of family member Z63.4

Discharge (from)
- • abnormal finding in—*see* Abnormal, specimen
- • breast (female) (male) N64.52
- • diencephalic autonomic idiopathic—*see* Epilepsy, specified NEC
- • ear—*see also* Otorrhea
- • excessive urine R35.8
- • nipple N64.52
- • penile R36.9
- • postnasal R09.82
- • urethral R36.9
  - – without blood R36.0
- • vaginal N89.8

Discoloration
- • nails L60.8

Discord (with)
- • family Z63.8

Discordant connection
- • ventriculoarterial Q20.3

Discrepancy
- • leg length (acquired)—*see* Deformity, limb, unequal length
  - – congenital—*see* Defect, reduction, limb, lower

Disease, diseased—*see also* Syndrome
- • acid-peptic K30
- • Adams-Stokes (-Morgagni) (syncope with heart block) I45.9
- • adenoids (and tonsils) J35.9
- • airway
  - – reactive—*see* Asthma
- • alligator-skin Q80.9

Disease, diseased, *continued*
- angiospastic I73.9
  - cerebral G45.9
- anus K62.9
  - specified NEC K62.89
- aortic (heart) (valve) I35.9
  - rheumatic I06.9
- autoimmune (systemic) NOS M35.9
  - hemolytic D59.1
    - cold type (primary) (secondary) (symptomatic) D59.12
    - drug-induced D59.0
    - mixed type (primary) (secondary) (symptomatic) D59.13
    - warm type (primary) (secondary) (symptomatic) D59.11
  - thyroid E06.3
- autoinflammatory M04.9
  - NOD2-associated M04.8
- Ayerza's (pulmonary artery sclerosis with pulmonary hypertension) I27.0
- Babington's (familial hemorrhagic telangiectasia) I78.0
- Baelz's (cheilitis glandularis apostematosa) K13.0
- Bannister's T78.3
- basal ganglia G25.9
  - specified NEC G25.89
- Bateman's B08.1
- Becker
  - myotonia congenita G71.12
- bladder N32.9
  - specified NEC N32.89
- bleeder's D66
- blood D75.9
  - vessel I99.9
- Blount M92.51-
- Bouillaud's (rheumatic heart disease) I01.9
- Bourneville (-Brissaud) (tuberous sclerosis) Q85.1
- bowel K63.9
  - functional K59.9
    - psychogenic F45.8
- brain G93.9
  - parasitic NEC B71.9 *[G94]*
  - specified NEC G93.89
- broad
  - beta E78.2
- bronze Addison's E27.1
- cardiopulmonary, chronic I27.9
- cardiovascular (atherosclerotic) I25.10
- celiac (adult) (infantile) K90.0
- cerebrovascular I67.9
  - acute I67.89
  - hereditary NEC I67.858
  - specified NEC I67.89
- chigo, chigoe B88.1
- childhood granulomatous D71
- chlamydial A74.9
  - specified NEC A74.89
- cold
  - agglutinin or hemoglobinuria D59.12
  - hemagglutinin (chronic) D59.12
- collagen NOS (nonvascular) (vascular) M35.9
  - specified NEC M35.8
- colon K63.9
  - functional K59.9
    - congenital Q43.2
- Concato's (pericardial polyserositis) A19.9
  - nontubercular I31.1
  - pleural—*see* Pleurisy, with, effusion
- congenital Q07.9
  - nonautoimmune hemolytic D59.4
- conjunctiva H11.9
  - chlamydial A74.0
  - viral B30.9
- connective tissue, systemic (diffuse) M35.9
  - in (due to)
    - hypogammaglobulinemia D80.1 *[M36.8]*
  - specified NEC M35.8
  - COVID-19 U07.1
- Crocq's (acrocyanosis) I73.89
- cystic
  - kidney, congenital Q61.9
- cytomegalic inclusion (generalized) B25.9
  - congenital P35.1

Disease, diseased, *continued*
- cytomegaloviral B25.9
- Débove's (splenomegaly) R16.1
- de Quervain's (tendon sheath) M65.4
  - thyroid (subacute granulomatous thyroiditis) E06.1
- diaphorase deficiency D74.0
- diaphragm J98.6
- diarrheal, infectious NEC A09
- disruptive F91.9
  - mood dysregulation F34.81
  - specified NEC F91.8
- disruptive behavior F91.9
- Duchenne-Griesinger G71.01
- Duchenne's
  - muscular dystrophy G71.01
  - pseudohypertrophy, muscles G71.01
- Dupré's (meningism) R29.1
- dysmorphic body F45.22
- Eddowes' (brittle bones and blue sclera) Q78.0
- Edsall's T67.2
- Eichstedt's (pityriasis versicolor) B36.0
- Eisenmenger's (irreversible) I27.83
- Ellis-van Creveld (chondroectodermal dysplasia) Q77.6
- end stage renal (ESRD) N18.6
- English (rickets) E55.0
- Erb (-Landouzy) G71.02
- esophagus K22.9
  - functional K22.4
  - psychogenic F45.8
- eustachian tube—*see* Disorder, eustachian tube
- facial nerve (seventh) G51.9
  - newborn (birth injury) P11.3
- Fanconi's (congenital pancytopenia) D61.09
- fascia NEC—*see also* Disorder, muscle
  - inflammatory—*see* Myositis
  - specified NEC M62.89
- Fede's K14.0
- female pelvic inflammatory (*see also* Disease, pelvis, inflammatory) N73.9
- fifth B08.3
- Fothergill's
  - scarlatina anginosa A38.9
- Friedreich's
  - combined systemic or ataxia G11.11
  - myoclonia G25.3
- frontal sinus—*see* Sinusitis, frontal
- fungus NEC B49
- Gaisböck's (polycythemia hypertonica) D75.1
- gastroesophageal reflux (GERD) K21.9
  - with esophagitis K21.0-
- gastrointestinal (tract) K92.9
  - functional K59.9
    - psychogenic F45.8
  - specified NEC K92.89
- Gee (-Herter) (-Heubner) (-Thaysen) (nontropical sprue) K90.0
- genital organs
  - female N94.9
  - male N50.9
- Gibert's (pityriasis rosea) L42
- Gilles de la Tourette's (motor-verbal tic) F95.2
- Goldstein's (familial hemorrhagic telangiectasia) I78.0
- graft-versus-host (GVH) D89.813
  - acute D89.810
  - acute on chronic D89.812
  - chronic D89.811
- granulomatous (childhood) (chronic) D71
- Grisel's M43.6
- Gruby's (tinea tonsurans) B35.0
- Guinon's (motor-verbal tic) F95.2
  - follicles L73.9
    - specified NEC L73.8
- Hamman's (spontaneous mediastinal emphysema) J98.2
- hand, foot, and mouth B08.4
- heart (organic) I51.9
  - with
    - pulmonary edema (acute) (*see also* Failure, ventricular, left) I50.1
    - rheumatic fever (conditions in I00)
      - active I01.9
        - with chorea I02.0
        - specified NEC I01.8

Disease, diseased, *continued*
  - inactive or quiescent (with chorea) I09.9
    - specified NEC I09.89
  - aortic (valve) I35.9
  - black I27.0
  - congenital Q24.9
    - cyanotic Q24.9
    - specified NEC Q24.8
  - fibroid—*see* Myocarditis
  - functional I51.89
    - psychogenic F45.8
  - hyperthyroid (*see also* Hyperthyroidism) E05.90 [I43]
    - with thyroid storm E05.91 [I43]
  - kyphoscoliotic I27.1
  - mitral I05.9
    - specified NEC I0
  - psychogenic (functional) F45.8
  - pulmonary (chronic) I27.9
    - in schistosomiasis B65.9 *[I52]*
    - specified NEC I27.89
  - rheumatic (chronic) (inactive) (old) (quiescent) (with chorea) I09.9
    - active or acute I01.9
      - with chorea (acute) (rheumatic) (Sydenham's) I02.0
  - thyrotoxic (*see also* Thyrotoxicosis) E05.90 [I43]
    - with thyroid storm E05.91 [I43]
- Hebra's
  - pityriasis
    - maculata et circinata L42
- hemoglobin or Hb
  - abnormal (mixed) NEC D58.2
    - with thalassemia D56.9
  - AS genotype D57.3
  - Bart's D56.0
  - C (Hb-C) D58.2
    - with other abnormal hemoglobin NEC D58.2
    - elliptocytosis D58.1
    - Hb-S D57.2-
    - sickle-cell D57.2-
    - thalassemia D56.8
  - Constant Spring D58.2
  - D (Hb-D) D58.2
  - E (Hb-E) D58.2
  - E-beta thalassemia D56.5
  - elliptocytosis D58.1
  - H (Hb-H) (thalassemia) D56.0
    - with other abnormal hemoglobin NEC D56.9
    - Constant Spring D56.0
  - I thalassemia D56.9
  - M D74.0
  - S or SS D57.1
    - with
      - acute chest syndrome D57.01
      - cerebral vascular involvement D57.03
      - crisis (painful) D57.00
        - with complication specified NEC D57.09
      - splenic sequestration D57.02
      - vasoocclusive pain D57.00
    - beta plus D57.44
      - with
        - acute chest syndrome D57.451
        - cerebral vascular involvement D57.453
        - crisis D57.459
          - with specified complication NEC D57.458
        - splenic sequestration D57.452
          - vasoocclusive pain D57.459
      - without crisis D57.44
    - beta zero D57.42
      - with
        - acute chest syndrome D57.431
        - cerebral vascular involvement D57.433
        - crisis D57.439
          - with specified complication NEC D57.438
        - splenic sequestration D57.432
        - vasoocclusive pain D57.439
      - without crisis D57.42
  - SC D57.2-
  - SD D57.8-
  - SE D57.8-
  - spherocytosis D58.0
  - unstable, hemolytic D58.2

Disease, diseased, *continued*
- hemolytic (newborn) P55.9
  - autoimmune D59.10
    - cold type (primary) (secondary) (symptomatic) D59.12
    - mixed type (primary) (secondary) (symptomatic) D59.13
    - warm type (primary) (secondary) (symptomatic) D59.11
    - drug-induced D59.0
  - due to or with
    - incompatibility
      - ABO (blood group) P55.1
      - blood (group) (Duffy) (K) (Kell) (Kidd) (Lewis) (M) (S) NEC P55.8
- hemorrhagic D69.9
  - newborn P53
- Henoch (-Schönlein) (purpura nervosa) D69.0
- hepatic—*see* Disease, liver
- Herter (-Gee) (-Heubner) (nontropical sprue) K90.0
- Heubner-Herter (nontropical sprue) K90.0
- high fetal gene or hemoglobin thalassemia D56.9
- hip (joint) M25.9
  - congenital Q65.89
  - suppurative M00.9
- host-versus-graft D89.813
  - acute D89.810
  - acute on chronic D89.812
  - chronic D89.811
- human immunodeficiency virus (HIV) B20
- hyaline (diffuse) (generalized)
  - membrane (lung) (newborn) P22.0
- hypophysis E23.7
- I-cell E77.0
- immune D89.9
- inclusion B25.9
  - salivary gland B25.9
- infectious, infective B99.9
  - congenital P37.9
    - specified NEC P37.8
    - viral P35.9
      - specified type NEC P35.8
  - specified NEC B99.8
- inflammatory
  - prepuce
    - balanoposthitis N47.6
- intestine K63.9
  - functional K59.9
    - psychogenic F45.8
    - specified NEC K59.89
- jigger B88.1
- joint—*see also* Disorder, joint
  - sacroiliac M53.3
- Jourdain's (acute gingivitis) K05.00
  - plaque induced K05.00
- kidney (functional) (pelvis) N28.9
  - chronic N18.9
    - hypertensive—*see* Hypertension, kidney
    - stage 1 N18.1
    - stage 2 (mild) N18.2
    - stage 3 (moderate) N18.30
    - stage 3a N18.31
    - stage 3b N18.32
    - stage 4 (severe) N18.4
    - stage 5 N18.5
  - cystic (congenital) Q61.9
  - in (due to)
  - multicystic Q61.4
  - polycystic Q61.3
    - childhood type NEC Q61.19
      - collecting duct dilatation Q61.11
- Kimmelstiel (-Wilson) (intercapillary polycystic (congenital) glomerulosclerosis)—*see* E08-E13 with .21
- kissing—*see* Mononucleosis, infectious
- Kok Q89.8
- Kostmann's (infantile genetic agranulocytosis) D70.0
- Lenegre's I44.2
- Lev's (acquired complete heart block) I44.2
- lip K13.0
- liver (chronic) (organic) K76.9
  - fatty, nonalcoholic (NAFLD) K76.0
    - gestational alloimmune (GALD) P78.84
- Lobstein's (brittle bones and blue sclera) Q78.0

Disease, diseased, *continued*
- Ludwig's (submaxillary cellulitis) K12.2
- lung J98.4
  - dabbing (related) U07.0
  - electronic cigarette (related) U07.0
  - in
    - sarcoidosis D86.0
    - systemic
      - lupus erythematosus M32.13
  - interstitial J84.9
    - of childhood, specified NEC J84.848
    - specified NEC J84.89
  - vaping (device) (product) (use) (associated) U07.0
- Lutembacher's (atrial septal defect with mitral stenosis) Q21.1
- Lyme A69.20
- lymphoproliferative D47.9
  - specified NEC D47.Z9
  - T-gamma D47.Z9
  - X-linked D82.3
- maple-syrup-urine E71.0
- Marion's (bladder neck obstruction) N32.0
- medullary center (idiopathic) (respiratory) G93.89
- metabolic, metabolism E88.9
  - bilirubin E80.7
  - glycoprotein E77.9
    - specified NEC E77.8
- minicore G71.29
- Minot's (hemorrhagic disease, newborn) P53
- Minot-von Willebrand-Jürgens (angiohemophilia) D68.0
- mitral (valve) I05.9
- Morgagni-Adams-Stokes (syncope with heart block) I45.9
- Morvan's G60.8
- multicore G71.29
- muscle M62.9
  - specified type NEC M62.89
  - tone, newborn P94.9
    - specified NEC P94.8
- myocardium, myocardial (*see also* Degeneration, myocardial) I51.5
  - primary (idiopathic) I42.9
- myoneural G70.9
- nails L60.9
  - specified NEC L60.8
- nasal J34.9
- nemaline body G71.21
- neuromuscular system G70.9
- neutropenic D70.9
- nerve—*see* Disorder, nerve
  - nervous system G98.8 central G96.9
    - specified NEC G96.89
- nose J34.9
- organ
  - dabbing (related) U07.0
  - electronic cigarette (related) U07.0
  - vaping (device) (product) (use) (associated) U07.0
- Osler-Rendu (familial hemorrhagic telangiectasia) I78.0
- ovary (noninflammatory) N83.9
  - cystic N83.20-
  - inflammatory—*see* Salpingo-oophoritis
  - polycystic E28.2
  - specified NEC N83.8
- pancreas K86.9
  - cystic K86.2
  - fibrocystic E84.9
  - specified NEC K86.89
- parasitic B89
  - cerebral NEC B71.9 *[G94]*
  - intestinal NOS B82.9
  - mouth B37.0
  - skin NOS B88.9
  - *specified type*—*see* Infestation
  - tongue B37.0
- pelvis, pelvic
  - gonococcal (acute) (chronic) A54.24
  - inflammatory (female) N73.9
    - acute N73.0
    - chronic N73.1
    - specified NEC N73.8
- Pick's I31.1
- pinworm B80
- pituitary (gland) E23.7

Disease, diseased, *continued*
- Pollitzer's (hidradenitis suppurativa) L73.2
- polycystic
  - kidney or renal Q61.3
    - childhood type NEC Q61.19
      - collecting duct dilatation Q61.11
  - ovary, ovaries E28.2
- prepuce N47.8
  - inflammatory N47.7
    - balanoposthitis N47.6
- Pringle's (tuberous sclerosis) Q85.1
- Puente's (simple glandular cheilitis) K13.0
- pulmonary—*see also* Disease, lung
  - heart I27.9
    - specified NEC I27.89
  - hypertensive (vascular) I27.20
    - primary (idiopathic) I27.0
  - valve I37.9
    - rheumatic I09.89
- rag picker's or rag sorter's A22.1
- rectum K62.9
  - specified NEC K62.89
- renal (functional) (pelvis) (*see also* Disease, kidney) N28.9
  - with
    - edema—*see* Nephrosis
    - glomerular lesion—*see* Glomerulonephritis
      - with edema—*see* Nephrosis
    - interstitial nephritis N12
  - acute N28.9
  - chronic (*see also* Disease, kidney, chronic) N18.9
  - cystic, congenital Q61.9
  - diabetic—*see* E08-E13 with .22
  - end-stage (failure) N18.6
  - fibrocystic (congenital) Q61.8
  - lupus M32.14
  - polycystic (congenital) Q61.3
    - childhood type NEC Q61.19
      - collecting duct dilatation Q61.11
- Rendu-Osler-Weber (familial hemorrhagic telangiectasia) I78.0
- respiratory (tract) J98.9
  - acute or subacute NOS J06.9
    - due to
      - smoke inhalation J70.5
  - newborn P28.9
    - specified type NEC P28.89
  - upper J39.9
    - acute or subacute J06.9
    - streptococcal J06.9
- rickettsial NOS A79.9
  - specified type NEC A79.89
- Riga (-Fede) (cachectic aphthae) K14.0
- Ritter's L00
- Roger's (congenital interventricular septal defect) Q21.0
- Rosenthal's (factor XI deficiency) D68.1
- Rossbach's (hyperchlorhydria) K30
- sacroiliac NEC M53.3
- salivary gland or duct K11.9
  - inclusion B25.9
  - *specified NEC K11.8*
  - virus B25.9
- Schönlein (-Henoch) (purpura rheumatica) D69.0
- scrofulous (tuberculous) A18.2
- scrotum N50.9
- serum NEC (*see also* Reaction, serum) T80.69
- sexually transmitted A64
  - anogenital
    - herpesviral infection—*see* Herpes, anogenital
    - warts A63.0
  - chlamydial infection—*see* Chlamydia
  - gonorrhea—*see* Gonorrhea
  - specified organism NEC A63.8
  - syphilis—*see* Syphilis
  - trichomoniasis—*see* Trichomoniasis
- sickle-cell D57.1
  - with crisis (vasoocclusive pain) D57.00
  - with
    - acute chest syndrome D57.01
    - cerebral vascular involvement D57.03
    - crisis (painful) D57.00
      - with complication specified NEC D57.09

Disease, diseased, *continued*
- ■ splenic sequestration D57.02
- ■ vasoocclusive pain D57.00
- – Hb-C D57.20
  - ■ with
    - ~ acute chest syndrome D57.211
    - ~ cerebral vascular involvement D57.213
    - ~ crisis D57.219
      - ◊ with specified complication NEC D57.218
    - ~ splenic sequestration D57.212
    - ~ vasoocclusive pain D57.219
- – Hb-SD D57.80
  - ■ with
    - ~ acute chest syndrome D57.811
    - ~ cerebral vascular involvement D57.813
    - ~ crisis D57.819
      - ◊ with complication specified NEC D57.818
    - ~ splenic sequestration D57.812
    - ~ vasoocclusive pain D57.819
  - ■ without crisis D57.80
- – Hb-SE D57.80
  - ■ with crisis D57.819
  - ■ with
    - ~ acute chest syndrome D57.811
    - ~ cerebral vascular involvement D57.813
    - ~ crisis D57.819
      - ◊ with complication specified NEC D57.818
    - ~ splenic sequestration D57.812
    - ~ vasoocclusive pain D57.819
  - ■ without crisis D57.80
- – specified NEC D57.80
  - ■ with
    - ~ acute chest syndrome D57.811
    - ~ cerebral vascular involvement D57.813
    - ~ crisis D57.819
      - ◊ with complication specified NEC D57.818
    - ~ splenic sequestration D57.812
    - ~ vasoocclusive pain D57.819
  - ■ without crisis D57.80
- – spherocytosis D57.80
  - ■ with
    - ~ acute chest syndrome D57.811
    - ~ cerebral vascular involvement D57.813
    - ~ crisis D57.819
      - ◊ with complication specified NEC D57.818
    - ~ splenic sequestration D57.812
    - ~ vasoocclusive pain D57.819
  - ■ without crisis D57.80
- – thalassemia D57.40
  - ■ with
    - ~ acute chest syndrome D57.411
    - ~ cerebral vascular involvement D57.413
    - ~ crisis (painful) D57.419
      - ◊ with specified complication NEC D57.418
    - ~ splenic sequestration D57.412
    - ~ vasoocclusive pain D57.419
  - ■ beta plus D57.44
    - ~ with
      - ◊ acute chest syndrome D57.451
      - ◊ cerebral vascular involvement D57.453
      - ◊ crisis D57.459
        - » with specified complication NEC D57.458
      - ◊ splenic sequestration D57.452
      - ◊ vasoocclusive pain D57.459
    - ~ without crisis D57.44
  - ■ beta zero D57.42
    - ~ with
      - ◊ acute chest syndrome D57.431
      - ◊ cerebral vascular involvement D57.433
      - ◊ crisis D57.439
        - » with specified complication NEC D57.438
      - ◊ splenic sequestration D57.432
      - ◊ vasoocclusive pain D57.439
    - ~ without crisis D57.42
- – elliptocytosis D57.8-
- • sixth B08.20
  - – due to human herpesvirus 6 B08.21
  - – due to human herpesvirus 7 B08.22
- • skin L98.9
  - – due to metabolic disorder NEC E88.9 [L99]
  - – specified NEC L98.8
- • slim (HIV) B20
- • South African creeping B88.0

Disease, diseased, *continued*
- • Startle Q89.8
- • Sticker's (erythema infectiosum) B08.3
- • Stokes-Adams (syncope with heart block) I45.9
- • stomach K31.9
  - – functional, psychogenic F45.8
  - – specified NEC K31.89
- • striatopallidal system NEC G25.89
- • testes N50.9
- • thalassemia Hb-S—*see* Disease, sickle-cell, thalassemia
- • Thaysen-Gee (nontropical sprue) K90.0
- • Thomsen G71.12
- • throat J39.2
  - – septic J02.0
- • thyroid (gland) E07.9
  - – heart (*see also* Hyperthyroidism) E05.90 [I43]
    - ■ with thyroid storm E05.91 [I43]
  - – specified NEC E07.89
- • Tietze's M94.0
- • tonsils, tonsillar (and adenoids) J35.9
- • tooth, teeth K08.9
  - – hard tissues K03.9
    - ■ specified NEC K03.89
- • Tourette's F95.2
- • tricuspid I07.9
  - – nonrheumatic I36.9
- • Underwood's (sclerema neonatorum) P83.0
- • urinary (tract) N39.9
  - – bladder N32.9
    - ■ specified NEC N32.89
  - – specified NEC N39.8
- • vagabond's B85.1
- • vagina, vaginal (noninflammatory) N89.9
  - – inflammatory NEC N76.89
  - – specified NEC N89.8
- • vascular I99.9
- • venereal (*see also* Disease, sexually transmitted) A64
  - – chlamydial NEC A56.8
    - ■ anus A56.3
    - ■ genitourinary NOS A56.2
    - ■ pharynx A56.4
    - ■ rectum A56.3
- • viral, virus (*see also* Disease, by type of virus) B34.9
  - – human immunodeficiency (HIV) B20
  - – Powassan A84.81
- • von Willebrand (-Jürgens) (angiohemophilia) D68.0
- • Vrolik's (osteogenesis imperfecta) Q78.0
- • Werdnig-Hoffmann G12.0
- • Werner-Schultz (neutropenic splenomegaly) D73.81
- • white blood cells D72.9
  - – specified NEC D72.89
- • wool sorter's A22.1

Disfigurement (due to scar) L90.5

Dislocation (articular)
- • finger S63.2-
  - – index S63.2-
  - – interphalangeal S63.27-
    - ■ distal S63.29-
      - ~ index S63.29-
      - ~ little S63.29-
      - ~ middle S63.29-
      - ~ ring S63.29-
    - ■ index S63.2-
    - ■ little S63.2-
    - ■ middle S63.2-
    - ■ proximal S63.28-
      - ~ index S63.28-
      - ~ little S63.28-
      - ~ middle S63.28-
      - ~ ring S63.28-
    - ■ ring S63.2-
  - – little S63.2-
  - – metacarpophalangeal S63.26-
    - ■ index S63.26-
    - ■ little S63.26-
    - ■ middle S63.26-
    - ■ ring S63.26-
  - – middle S63.2-
  - – ring S63.2-
  - – thumb—*see* Dislocation

Disease, diseased, *continued*
- • hip S73.0-
  - – congenital (total) Q65.2
    - ■ bilateral Q65.1
    - ■ partial Q65.5
      - ~ bilateral Q65.4
      - ~ unilateral Q65.3-
    - ■ unilateral Q65.0-
- • interphalangeal (joint(s))
  - – finger S63.2-
    - ■ distal S63.29-
      - ~ index S63.29-
      - ~ little S63.29-
      - ~ middle S63.29-
      - ~ ring S63.29-
    - ■ index S63.2-
    - ■ little S63.2-
    - ■ middle S63.2-
    - ■ proximal S63.28-
      - ~ index S63.28-
      - ~ little S63.28-
      - ~ middle S63.28-
      - ~ ring S63.28-
    - ■ ring S63.2-
  - – thumb S63.12-
- • jaw (cartilage) (meniscus) S03.0-
- • knee S83.10-
  - – cap—*see* Dislocation, patella
  - – congenital Q68.2
  - – old M23.8X-
  - – patella—*see* Dislocation, patella
  - – proximal tibia
    - ■ anteriorly S83.11-
    - ■ laterally S83.14-
    - ■ medially S83.13-
    - ■ posteriorly S83.12-
  - – specified type NEC S83.19-
- • lens (complete) H27.10
  - – anterior H27.12-
  - – congenital Q12.1
  - – partial H27.11-
  - – posterior H27.13-
  - – traumatic S05.8X-
- • mandible S03.0-
- • metacarpophalangeal (joint)
  - – finger S63.26-
    - ■ index S63.26-
    - ■ little S63.26-
    - ■ middle S63.26-
    - ■ ring S63.26-
  - – thumb S63.11-
- • partial—*see* Subluxation, by site
- • patella S83.00-
  - – congenital Q74.1
  - – lateral S83.01-
  - – recurrent (nontraumatic) M22.0-
    - ■ incomplete M22.1-
  - – specified type NEC S83.09-
- • sacroiliac (joint) (ligament) S33.2
  - – congenital Q74.2
- • septum (nasal) (old) J34.2
- • temporomandibular S03.0-
- • thumb S63.10-

Disorder (of)—*see also* Disease
- • acute
  - – psychotic—*see* Psychosis, acute
  - – stress F43.0
- • adjustment (grief) F43.20
  - – with
    - ■ anxiety F43.22
      - ~ with depressed mood F43.23
    - ■ conduct disturbance F43.24
      - ~ with emotional disturbance F43.25
    - ■ depressed mood F43.21
      - ~ with anxiety F43.23
    - ■ other specified symptom F43.29
- • adrenogenital E25.9
- • aggressive, unsocialized F91.1
- • alcohol-related
  - – with
    - ■ intoxication F10.929
      - ~ uncomplicated F10.920
- • allergic—*see* Allergy

Disorder, *continued*
- alveolar NEC J84.09
- amino-acid
  - metabolism—*see* Disturbance, metabolism, amino-acid
    - specified NEC E72.89
  - neonatal, transitory P74.8
- anxiety F41.9
  - illness F45.21
  - mixed
    - with depression (mild) F41.8
  - phobic F40.9
    - of childhood F40.8
  - social F40.1-
  - specified NEC F41.8
- aromatic amino-acid metabolism E70.9
  - specified NEC E70.89
- attention-deficit hyperactivity (adolescent) (adult) (child) F90.9
  - combined type F90.2
  - hyperactive type F90.1
  - inattentive type F90.0
  - specified type NEC F90.8
- attention-deficit without hyperactivity (adolescent) (adult) (child) F90.0
- auditory processing (central) H93.25
- autistic F84.0
- autoimmune D89.89
- avoidant
  - restrictive food intake F50.82
- balance
  - acid-base E87.8
    - mixed E87.4
  - electrolyte E87.8
  - fluid NEC E87.8
- beta-amino-acid metabolism E72.89
- bilirubin excretion E80.6
- binge-eating F50.81
- bipolar (I) (type1) F31.9
  - current (or most recent) episode
    - depressed F31.9
      - without psychotic features F31.30
        ◊ mild F31.31
        ◊ moderate F31.32
        ◊ severe (without psychotic features) F31.4
    - hypomanic F31.0
    - manic F31.9
      - without psychotic features F31.10
        ◊ mild F31.11
        ◊ moderate F31.12
        ◊ severe (without psychotic features) F31.13
    - mixed F31.60
      ~ mild F31.61
      ~ moderate F31.62
- bladder N32.9
  - specified NEC N32.89
- bleeding D68.9
- body dysmorphic F45.22
- breast
  - associated with
    - cracked nipple O92.1-
    - galactorrhea O92.6
    - hypogalactia O92.4
    - lactation O92.70
      ~ specified NEC O92.79
    - lactation disorder NEC O92.79
    - pregnancy O92.20
      ~ specified NEC O92.29
    - puerperium O92.20
      ~ specified NEC O92.29
- Briquet's F45.0
- cannabis use
  - due to drug abuse—*see* Abuse, drug, cannabis
  - due to drug dependence—*see* Dependence, drug, cannabis
- carbohydrate
  - metabolism (congenital) E74.9
    - specified NEC E74.89
- carnitine metabolism E71.40
- central auditory processing H93.25
- character NOS F60.9
- coagulation (factor) (*see also* Defect, coagulation) D68.9
  - newborn, transient P61.6

Disorder, *continued*
- coccyx NEC M53.3
- conduct (childhood) F91.9
  - adjustment reaction—*see* Disorder, adjustment
  - adolescent onset type F91.2
  - childhood onset type F91.1
  - depressive F91.8
  - group type F91.2
  - hyperkinetic—*see* Disorder, attention-deficit hyperactivity
  - oppositional defiance F91.3
  - socialized F91.2
  - solitary aggressive type F91.1
  - specified NEC F91.8
  - unsocialized (aggressive) F91.1
- conduction, heart I45.9
- congenital glycosylation (CDG) E74.89
- cornea H18.9
  - due to contact lens H18.82-
  - Cyclin-Dependent Kinase-Like 5 Deficiency (CDKL5) G40.42
- cyclothymic F34.0
- defiant oppositional F91.3
- depressive F32.9
  - major F32.9
    - with psychotic symptoms F32.3
    - in remission (full) F32.5
      ~ partial F32.4
    - recurrent F33.9
    - single episode F32.9
      ~ mild F32.0
      ~ moderate F32.1
      ~ severe (without psychotic symptoms) F32.2
      ◊ with psychotic symptoms F32.3
- developmental F89
  - arithmetical skills F81.2
  - coordination (motor) F82
  - expressive writing F81.81
  - language F80.9
    - expressive F80.1
    - mixed receptive and expressive F80.2
    - receptive type F80.2
    - specified NEC F80.89
  - learning F81.9
    - arithmetical F81.2
    - reading F81.0
  - mixed F88
  - motor coordination or function F82
  - pervasive F84.9
    - specified NEC F84.8
  - phonological F80.0
  - reading F81.0
  - scholastic skills—*see also* Disorder, learning
    - mixed F81.89
  - specified NEC F88
  - speech F80.9
    - articulation F80.0
    - specified NEC F80.89
  - written expression F81.81
- diaphragm J98.6
- digestive (system) K92.9
  - newborn P78.9
    - specified NEC P78.89
  - postprocedural—*see* Complication, gastrointestinal
  - psychogenic F45.8
- disc (intervertebral)
  - with
    - myelopathy
      ~ sacroiliac region M53.3
      ~ sacrococcygeal region M53.3
    - specified NEC
      - sacrococcygeal region M53.3
- disruptive F91.9
  - mood dysregulation F34.81
  - specified NEC F91.8
- dissocial personality F60.2
- dissociative F44.9
  - affecting
    - motor function F44.4
      ~ and sensation F44.7
    - sensation F44.6
      ~ and motor function F44.7

Disorder, *continued*
  - brief reactive F43.0
  - drug induced hemorrhagic D68.32
- drug related
  - abuse—*see* Abuse, drug
  - dependence—*see* Dependence, drug
- dysthymic F34.1
- eating (adult) (psychogenic) F50.9
  - anorexia—*see* Anorexia
  - binge F50.81
  - bulimia F50.2
  - child F98.29
    - pica F98.3
    - rumination disorder F98.21
  - other F50.89
  - pica F50.89
    - childhood F98.3
- electrolyte (balance) NEC E87.8
  - acidosis (metabolic) (respiratory) E87.2
  - alkalosis (metabolic) (respiratory) E87.3
- emotional (persistent) F34.9
  - of childhood F93.9
    - specified NEC F93.8
- esophagus K22.9
  - functional K22.4
  - psychogenic F45.8
- eustachian tube H69.9-
  - specified NEC H69.8-
- factor, coagulation—*see* Defect, coagulation
- fatty acid
  - metabolism E71.30
    - specified NEC E71.39
  - oxidation
    - LCAD E71.310
    - MCAD E71.311
    - SCAD E71.312
    - specified deficiency NEC E71.318
- feeding (infant or child) (*see also* Disorder, eating) R63.3
  - or eating disorder F50.9
  - specified NEC F50.9
- feigned (with obvious motivation) Z76.5
- fibroblastic M72.9
- fluency
  - childhood onset F80.81
  - in conditions classified elsewhere R47.82
- fluid balance E87.8
- follicular (skin) L73.9
  - specified NEC L73.8
- functional polymorphonuclear neutrophils D71
- gamma-glutamyl cycle E72.89
- gastric (functional) K31.9
  - motility K30
  - psychogenic F45.8
  - secretion K30
- gastrointestinal (functional) NOS K92.9
  - newborn P78.9
  - psychogenic F45.8
- gender-identity or -role F64.9
  - childhood F64.2
  - effect on relationship F66
  - of adolescence or adulthood (nontranssexual) F64.0
  - specified NEC F64.8
  - uncertainty F66
- genitourinary system
  - female N94.9
  - male N50.9
  - psychogenic F45.8
- glomerular (in) N05.9
  - disseminated intravascular coagulation D65 [N08]
  - hemolytic-uremic syndrome D59.3
  - Henoch (-Schönlein) purpura D69.0 [N08]
  - sepsis NEC A41. - [N08]
  - subacute bacterial endocarditis I33.0 [N08]
  - systemic lupus erythematosus M32.14
- gluconeogenesis E74.4
- glucose transport E74.819
  - specified NEC E74.818
- glycine metabolism E72.50
  - hyperoxaluria R82.992
    - primary E72.53
- glycoprotein E77.9
  - specified NEC E77.8

Disorder, *continued*
- habit (and impulse) F63.9
  - specified NEC F63.89
- heart action I49.9
- hemorrhagic NEC D69.9
  - drug-induced D68.32
  - due to
    - extrinsic circulating anticoagulants D68.32
    - increase in
      - anti-IIa D68.32
      - anti-Xa D68.32
- hoarding F42.3
- hypochondriacal F45.20
  - body dysmorphic F45.22
- identity
  - dissociative F44.81
  - of childhood F93.8
- immune mechanism (immunity) D89.9
  - specified type NEC D89.89
- integument, newborn P83.9
  - specified NEC P83.88
- intestine, intestinal
  - carbohydrate absorption NEC E74.39
    - postoperative K91.2
  - functional NEC K59.9
  - psychogenic F45.8
- joint M25.9
  - psychogenic F45.8
- lacrimal system H04.9
- lactation NEC O92.79
- language (developmental) F80.9
  - expressive F80.1
  - mixed receptive and expressive F80.2
  - receptive F80.2
- learning (specific) F81.9
  - acalculia R48.8
  - alexia R48.0
  - mathematics F81.2
  - reading F81.0
  - specified NEC F81.89
    - with impairment in
      - mathematics F81.2
      - reading F81.0
      - written expression F81.81
  - spelling F81.81
  - written expression F81.81
- liver K76.9
  - malarial B54 *[K77]*
- lung, interstitial, drug-induced J70.4
  - dabbing (related) U07.0
  - e-cigarette (related) U07.0
  - electronic cigarette (related) U07.0
  - vaping (device) (product) (use) (associated) (related) U07.0
- lymphoproliferative, post-transplant (PTLD) D47.Z1
- meninges, specified type NEC G96.198
- menstrual N92.6
  - psychogenic F45.8
  - specified NEC N92.5
- mental (or behavioral) (nonpsychotic) F99
  - following organic brain damage F07.9
    - postconcussional syndrome F07.81
    - specified NEC F07.89
  - infancy, childhood or adolescence F98.9
  - neurotic—*see* Neurosis
- metabolic, amino acid, transitory, newborn P74.8
- metabolism NOS E88.9
  - amino-acid E72.9
    - aromatic
      - hyperphenylalaninemia E70.1
        - ◊ classical phenylketonuria E70.0
      - other specified E70.89
    - branched chain E71.2
      - maple syrup urine disease E71.0
    - glycine E72.50
      - hyperoxaluria R82.992
        - ◊ primary E72.53
    - other specified E72.8
      - beta-amino acid E72.8
      - gamma-glutamyl cycle E72.8
    - straight-chain E72.8

Disorder, *continued*
- bilirubin E80.7
  - specified NEC E80.6
- calcium E83.50
  - hypercalcemia E83.52
  - hypocalcemia E83.51
  - other specified E83.59
- carbohydrate E74.9
  - specified NEC E74.89
- congenital E88.9
- glutamine E72.89
- glycoprotein E77.9
  - specified NEC E77.8
- mitochondrial E88.40
  - MELAS syndrome E88.41
  - MERRF syndrome (myoclonic epilepsy associated with ragged-red fibers) E88.42
  - other specified E88.49
    - beta-amino acid E72.89
    - gamma-glutamyl cycle E72.89
- plasma protein NEC E88.09
- purine E79.9
- pyrimidine E79.9
- pyruvate E74.4
- serine E72.8
- sodium E87.8
- straight chain E72.89
- threonine E72.89
- micturition NEC R39.198
  - feeling of incomplete emptying R39.14
  - hesitancy R39.11
  - need to immediately re-void R39.191
  - poor stream R39.12
  - position dependent R39.192
  - psychogenic F45.8
  - split stream R39.13
  - straining R39.16
  - urgency R39.15
- mitochondrial metabolism E88.40
- mixed
  - anxiety and depressive F41.8
  - of scholastic skills (developmental) F81.89
  - receptive expressive language F80.2
- mood (affective), unspecified F39
- movement G25.9
  - drug-induced G25.70
    - akathisia G25.71
    - specified NEC G25.79
  - treatment-induced G25.9
  - hysterical F44.4
  - stereotyped F98.4
- muscle M62.9
  - psychogenic F45.8
  - specified type NEC M62.89
  - tone, newborn P94.9
    - specified NEC P94.8
- musculoskeletal system, soft tissue
  - psychogenic F45.8
- myoneural G70.9
  - due to lead G70.1
  - specified NEC G70.89
  - toxic G70.1
- nerve G58.9
  - cranial G52.9
    - multiple G52.7
    - seventh NEC G51.8
    - sixth NEC—*see* Strabismus, paralytic, sixth nerve
  - facial G51.9
    - specified NEC G51.8
- neurodevelopmental F89
  - specified NEC F88
- neurohypophysis NEC E23.3
- neuromuscular G70.9
  - hereditary NEC G71.9
  - specified NEC G70.89
  - toxic G70.1
- neurotic F48.9
  - specified NEC F48.8
- neutrophil, polymorphonuclear D71
- non-rapid eye movement sleep arousal
  - sleep terror type F51.4
  - sleepwalking type F51.3

Disorder, *continued*
- nose J34.9
  - specified NEC J34.89
- obsessive-compulsive F42.9
  - excoriation (skin picking) disorder F42.4
  - hoarding disorder F42.3
  - mixed obsessional thoughts and acts F42.2
  - other F42.8
- oppositional defiant F91.3
- overanxious F41.1
  - of childhood F93.8
- pain
  - with related psychological factors F45.42
  - exclusively related to psychological factors F45.41
- panic F41.0
- parietoalveolar NEC J84.09
- paroxysmal, mixed R56.9
- peroxisomal E71.50
  - biogenesis
    - neonatal adrenoleukodystrophy E71.511
    - specified disorder NEC E71.518
    - Zellweger syndrome E71.510
  - rhizomelic chondrodysplasia punctata E71.540
  - specified form NEC E71.548
    - group 1 E71.518
    - group 2 E71.53
    - group 3 E71.542
  - X-linked adrenoleukodystrophy E71.529
    - adolescent E71.521
    - adrenomyeloneuropathy E71.522
    - childhood E71.520
    - specified form NEC E71.528
  - Zellweger-like syndrome E71.54
- persistent
  - (somatoform) pain F45.41
  - affective (mood) F34.9
- personality (*see also* Personality) F60.9
  - affective F34.0
  - aggressive F60.3
  - amoral F60.2
  - anankastic F60.5
  - antisocial F60.2
  - anxious F60.6
  - asocial F60.2
  - avoidant F60.6
  - borderline F60.3
  - compulsive F60.5
  - cyclothymic F34.0
  - dissocial F60.2
  - emotional instability F60.3
  - expansive paranoid F60.0
  - explosive F60.3
  - histrionic F60.4
  - hysterical F60.4
  - labile F60.3
  - moral deficiency F60.2
  - obsessional F60.5
  - obsessive (-compulsive) F60.5
  - paranoid F60.0
  - pseudosocial F60.2
  - psychopathic F60.2
  - schizoid F60.1
  - type A F60.5
  - unstable (emotional) F60.3
- pervasive, developmental F84.9
- pigmentation L81.9
  - choroid, congenital Q14.3
  - diminished melanin formation L81.6
  - iron L81.8
  - specified NEC L81.8
- pituitary gland E23.7
  - specified NEC E23.6
- polymorphonuclear neutrophils D71
- postconcussional F07.81
- postprocedural (postoperative)—*see* Complications, postprocedural
- post-traumatic stress (PTSD) F43.10
  - acute F43.11
  - chronic F43.12
- premenstrual dysphoric (PMDD) F32.81
- prepuce N47.8

Disorder, *continued*

- psychogenic NOS (*see also* Disease, diseased) F45.9
  - anxiety F41.8
  - appetite F50.9
  - asthenic F48.8
  - cardiovascular (system) F45.8
  - compulsive F42.8
  - cutaneous F54
  - depressive F32.9
  - digestive (system) F45.8
  - dysmenorrheic F45.8
  - dyspneic F45.8
  - endocrine (system) F54
  - eye NEC F45.8
  - feeding—*see* Disorder, eating
  - functional NEC F45.8
  - gastric F45.8
  - gastrointestinal (system) F45.8
  - genitourinary (system) F45.8
  - heart (function) (rhythm) F45.8
  - hyperventilatory F45.8
  - hypochondriacal—*see* Disorder, hypochondriacal
  - intestinal F45.8
  - joint F45.8
  - learning F81.9
  - limb F45.8
  - lymphatic (system) F45.8
  - menstrual F45.8
  - micturition F45.8
  - monoplegic NEC F44.4
  - motor F44.4
  - muscle F45.8
  - musculoskeletal F45.8
  - neurocirculatory F45.8
  - obsessive F42.8
  - organ or part of body NEC F45.8
  - paralytic NEC F44.4
  - phobic F40.9
  - physical NEC F45.8
  - rectal F45.8
  - respiratory (system) F45.8
  - rheumatic F45.8
  - specified part of body NEC F45.8
  - stomach F45.8
- psychomotor NEC F44.4
  - hysterical F44.4
- psychoneurotic—*see also* Neurosis
  - mixed NEC F48.8
- psychophysiologic—*see* Disorder, somatoform
- psychosexual development F66
  - identity of childhood F64.2
- psychosomatic NOS—*see* Disorder, somatoform
  - multiple F45.0
  - undifferentiated F45.1
- psychotic—*see* Psychosis
  - puberty E30.9
  - specified NEC E30.8
- pulmonary (valve)—*see* Endocarditis, pulmonary
- pyruvate metabolism E74.4
- reading R48.0
  - developmental (specific) F81.0
- REM sleep behavior G47.52
- receptive language F80.2
- refraction H52.7
- respiratory function, impaired—*see also* Failure, respiration
  - postprocedural—*see* Complication
  - psychogenic F45.8
- sacrum, sacrococcygeal NEC M53.3
- schizoid of childhood F84.5
- seizure (*see also* Epilepsy) G40.909
- semantic pragmatic F80.89
  - with autism F84.0
- sense of smell R43.1
  - psychogenic F45.8
- separation anxiety, of childhood F93.0
- shyness, of childhood and adolescence F40.10
- sibling rivalry F93.8
- sickle-cell (sickling) (homozygous)—*see* Disease, sickle-cell
  - heterozygous D57.3
  - specified type NEC D57.8-
  - trait D57.3

Disorder, *continued*

- sinus (nasal) J34.9
  - specified NEC J34.89
- skin L98.9
  - hypertrophic L91.9
    - specified NEC L91.8
  - newborn P83.9
    - specified NEC P83.88
  - picking F42.4
- sleep G47.9
  - circadian rhythm G47.20
    - advanced sleep phase type G47.22
    - delayed sleep phase type G47.21
    - free running type G47.24
    - in conditions classified elsewhere G47.27
    - irregular sleep wake type G47.23
    - jet lag type G47.25
    - non-24 hour sleep-wake type G47.24
    - specified NEC G47.29
  - terrors F51.4
  - walking F51.3
- sleep-wake pattern or schedule—*see* Disorder, sleep, circadian rhythm G47.9
- social
  - anxiety (of childhood) F40.10
    - generalized F40.11
  - functioning in childhood F94.9
    - specified NEC F94.8
  - pragmatic F80.82
- somatization F45.0
- somatoform F45.9
  - pain (persistent) F45.41
  - somatization (multiple) (long-lasting) F45.0
  - specified NEC F45.8
  - undifferentiated F45.1
- specific
  - arithmetical F81.2
  - developmental, of motor F82
  - reading F81.0
  - speech and language F80.9
  - spelling F81.81
  - written expression F81.81
- speech R47.9
  - articulation (functional) (specific) F80.0
  - developmental F80.9
  - specified NEC R47.89
- spelling (specific) F81.81
- stereotyped, habit or movement F98.4
- stomach (functional)—*see* Disorder, gastric
- stress F43.9
  - acute F43.0
  - post-traumatic F43.10
    - acute F43.11
    - chronic F43.12
- temperature regulation, newborn P81.9
- thyroid (gland) E07.9
  - function NEC, neonatal, transitory P72.2
  - iodine-deficiency related E01.8
  - specified NEC E07.89
- tic—*see* Tic
- tobacco use
  - mild F17.200
  - moderate or severe F17.200
- tooth K08.9
  - eruption K00.6
- Tourette's F95.2
- trauma and stressor related F43.9
- tubulo-interstitial (in)
  - lymphoma NEC C85.9- [N16]
  - Salmonella infection A02.25
  - sarcoidosis D86.84
  - sepsis A41.9 [N16]
    - streptococcal A40.9 [N16]
  - systemic lupus erythematosus M32.15
  - toxoplasmosis B58.83
  - transplant rejection T86.-- [N16]
- unsocialized aggressive F91.1
- vision, binocular H53.30
  - abnormal retinal correspondence H53.31
  - diplopia H53.2
- white blood cells D72.9
  - specified NEC D72.89

Disorientation R41.0

Displacement, displaced

- acquired traumatic of bone, cartilage, joint, tendon NEC—*see* Dislocation
- bladder (acquired) N32.89
  - congenital Q64.19
- canaliculus (lacrimalis), congenital Q10.6
- fallopian tube (acquired) N83.4-
  - congenital Q50.6
  - opening (congenital) Q50.6
- gallbladder (congenital) Q44.1
- intervertebral disc NEC
  - sacrococcygeal region M53.3
- lachrymal, lacrimal apparatus or duct (congenital) Q10.6
- lens, congenital Q12.1
- macula (congenital) Q14.1
- Meckel's diverticulum Q43.0
- nail (congenital) Q84.6
  - acquired L60.8
- ovary (acquired) N83.4-
  - congenital Q50.39
- oviduct (acquired) N83.4-
  - congenital Q50.6
- sacro-iliac (joint) (congenital) Q74.2
  - current injury S33.2
- uterine opening of oviducts or fallopian tubes Q50.6
- ventricular septum Q21.0

Disproportion

- fiber-type G71.20
  - congenital G71.29

Disruption (of)

- closure of
  - laceration (external) (internal) T81.33
  - traumatic laceration (external) (internal) T81.33
- family Z63.8
  - due to
    - absence of family member due to military deployment Z63.31
    - absence of family member NEC Z63.32
    - alcoholism and drug addiction in family Z63.72
    - bereavement Z63.4
    - death (assumed) or disappearance of family member Z63.4
    - divorce or separation Z63.5
    - drug addiction in family Z63.72
    - stressful life events NEC Z63.79
- wound T81.30
  - traumatic injury repair T81.33
- traumatic injury wound repair T81.33

Dissociation

- auriculoventricular or atrioventricular (AV) (any degree) (isorhythmic) I45.89
  - with heart block I44.2

Dissociative reaction, state F44.9

Distension, distention

- abdomen R14.0
- bladder N32.89
- stomach K31.89
  - acute K31.0
  - psychogenic F45.8

Distortion(s) (congenital)

- bile duct or passage Q44.5
- cervix (uteri) Q51.9
- clavicle Q74.0
- common duct Q44.5
- cystic duct Q44.5
- ear (auricle) (external) Q17.3
  - inner Q16.5
  - middle Q16.4
  - ossicles Q16.3
- endocrine NEC Q89.2
- eustachian tube Q17.8
- eye (adnexa) Q15.8
- face bone(s) NEC Q75.8
- fallopian tube Q50.6
- foot Q66.9-
- genitalia, genital organ(s)
  - female Q52.8
    - external Q52.79
    - internal NEC Q52.8
- hepatic duct Q44.5

Distortion(s), *continued*
- intrafamilial communications Z63.8
- lens Q12.8
- oviduct Q50.6
- parathyroid (gland) Q89.2
- pituitary (gland) Q89.2
- sacroiliac joint Q74.2
- scapula Q74.0
- shoulder girdle Q74.0
- skull bone(s) NEC Q75.8
  - with
    - anencephalus Q00.0
    - encephalocele—*see* Encephalocele
    - hydrocephalus Q03.9
      - ~ with spina bifida—*see* Spina bifida, with hydrocephalus
    - microcephaly Q02
- thymus (gland) Q89.2
- thyroid (gland) Q89.2
- toe(s) Q66.9-

Distress
- abdomen—*see* Pain, abdominal
- acute respiratory R06.03
  - syndrome (adult) (child) J80
- epigastric R10.13
- fetal P84
- gastrointestinal (functional) K30
  - psychogenic F45.8
- intestinal (functional) NOS K59.9
  - psychogenic F45.8
- relationship, with spouse or intimate partner Z63.0
- respiratory R06.03
  - distress syndrome, child J80
  - newborn P22.9
    - specified NEC P22.8
  - orthopnea R06.01
  - psychogenic F45.8
  - shortness of breath R06.02

Disturbance(s)—*see also* Disease
- absorption K90.9
  - calcium E58
  - carbohydrate K90.49
  - fat K90.49
    - pancreatic K90.3
  - protein K90.49
  - starch K90.49
  - vitamin—*see* Deficiency
- acid-base equilibrium E87.8
  - mixed E87.4
- activity and attention (with hyperkinesis)—*see* Disorder, attention-deficit hyperactivity
- assimilation, food K90.9
- blood clotting (mechanism) (*see also* Defect, coagulation) D68.9
- cerebral
  - status, newborn P91.9
    - specified NEC P91.88
- circulatory I99.9
- conduct (*see also* Disorder, conduct) F91.9
  - adjustment reaction—*see* Disorder, adjustment
  - disruptive F91.9
  - hyperkinetic—*see* Disorder, attention-deficit hyperactivity
  - socialized F91.2
  - specified NEC F91.8
  - unsocialized F91.1
- digestive K30
  - psychogenic F45.8
- electrolyte—*see also* Imbalance, electrolyte
  - newborn, transitory P74.49
    - hyperchloremia P74.421
    - hyperchloremic metabolic acidosis P74.421
    - hypochloremia P74.422
    - potassium balance
      - ~ hyperkalemia P74.31
      - ~ hypokalemia P74.32
    - sodium balance
      - ~ hypernatremia P74.21
      - ~ hyponatremia P74.22
    - specified type NEC P74.49

Disturbance(s), *continued*
- emotions specific to childhood and adolescence F93.9
  - endocrine (gland)
  - involving relationship problems F93.8
  - mixed F93.8
  - neonatal, transitory specified P72.8
  - specified NEC F93.8
  - with
    - anxiety and fearfulness NEC F93.8
    - oppositional disorder F91.3
    - sensitivity (withdrawal) F40.10
    - shyness F40.10
    - social withdrawal F40.10
- equilibrium R42
- gait—*see* Gait abnormality
  - hysterical F44.4
  - psychogenic F44.4
- gastrointestinal (functional) K30
  - psychogenic F45.8
- heart, functional (conditions in I44-I50)
  - due to presence of (cardiac) prosthesis I97.19-
  - postoperative I97.89
    - cardiac surgery I97.19-
- keratinization NEC
  - lip K13.0
- metabolism E88.9
  - amino-acid E72.9
    - straight-chain E72.89
  - general E88.9
  - glutamine E72.89
  - neonatal, transitory P74.9
    - calcium and magnesium P71.9
      - ~ specified type NEC P71.8
    - carbohydrate metabolism P70.9
      - ~ specified type NEC P70.8
    - specified NEC P74.8
  - threonine E72.8
- nervous, functional R45.0
- nutritional E63.9
  - nail L60.3
- ocular motion H51.9
  - psychogenic F45.8
- oculogyric H51.8
  - psychogenic F45.8
- oculomotor H51.9
  - psychogenic F45.8
- personality (pattern) (trait) (*see also* Disorder, personality) F60.9
- potassium balance, newborn
  - hyperkalemia P74.31
  - hypokalemia P74.32
- psychomotor F44.4
- rhythm, heart I49.9
- sensation (cold) (heat) (localization) (tactile discrimination) (texture) (vibratory) NEC R20.9
  - hysterical F44.6
- sensory—*see* Disturbance
- situational (transient)—*see also* Disorder, adjustment
  - acute F43.0
- sleep G47.9
  - nonorganic origin F51.9
- smell R43.9
  - and taste (mixed) R43.8
  - anosmia R43.0
  - parosmia R43.1
  - specified NEC R43.8
- sodium balance, newborn
  - hypernatremia P74.21
  - hyponatremia P74.22
- speech R47.9
  - developmental F80.9
  - specified NEC R47.89
- taste R43.9
  - and smell (mixed) R43.8
  - parageusia R43.2
  - specified NEC R43.8
- temperature
  - regulation, newborn P81.9
    - specified NEC P81.8
  - sense R20.8
    - hysterical F44.6
- tooth
  - eruption K00.6

Disturbance(s), *continued*
- vascular I99.9
- vision, visual H53.9
  - specified NEC H53.8
- voice R49.9
  - psychogenic F44.4
  - specified NEC R49.8

Diuresis R35.8

Diverticulum, diverticula (multiple)
- Meckel's (displaced) (hypertrophic) Q43.0
- pericardium (congenital) (cyst) Q24.8
  - acquired I31.8

Division
- glans penis Q55.69

Divorce, causing family disruption Z63.5

Dizziness R42
- hysterical F44.89
- psychogenic F45.8

DNR (do not resuscitate) Z66

Dohle body panmyelopathic syndrome D72.0

Dorsalgia M54.9
- psychogenic F45.41

Dorsopathy M53.9

Double
- albumin E88.09
- aortic arch Q25.45
- uterus Q51.2-

Down syndrome Q90.9

Drinking (alcohol)
- excessive, to excess NEC (without dependence) F10.10
  - habitual (continual) (without remission) F10.20
    - with remission F10.21

Drip, postnasal (chronic) R09.82
- due to
  - allergic rhinitis—*see* Rhinitis, allergic
  - common cold J00
  - nasopharyngitis—*see* Nasopharyngitis
  - other know condition—*code to* condition
  - sinusitis—*see* Sinusitis

Drop (in)
- attack NEC R55
- hematocrit (precipitous) R71.0
- hemoglobin R71.0

Dropped heart beats I45.9

Dropsy, dropsical—*see also* Hydrops
- abdomen R18.8
- brain—*see* Hydrocephalus
- newborn due to isoimmunization P56.0

Drowned, drowning (near) T75.1

Drowsiness R40.0

Drug
- abuse counseling and surveillance Z71.51
- addiction—*see* Dependence
- dependence—*see* Dependence
- habit—*see* Dependence
- harmful use—*see* Abuse, drug
- induced fever R50.2
- overdose—*see* Table of Drugs and Chemicals, by drug, poisoning
- poisoning—*see* Table of Drugs and Chemicals, by drug, poisoning
- resistant organism infection (*see also* Resistant, organism, to, drug) Z16.30
- therapy
  - long term (current) (prophylactic)—*see* Therapy, drug long-term (current) (prophylactic)
  - short term—*omit code*
- wrong substance given or taken in error—*see* Table of Drugs and Chemicals, by drug, poisoning

Drunkenness (without dependence) F10.129
- acute in alcoholism F10.229
- chronic (without remission) F10.20
  - with remission F10.21
- pathological (without dependence) F10.129
  - with dependence F10.229

Dry, dryness—*see also* Disease, diseased
- mouth R68.2
  - due to dehydration E86.0
- nose J34.89

Dubin-Johnson disease or syndrome E80.6

Dubowitz' syndrome Q87.19

Duchenne-Griesinger disease G71.01

Duchenne's
- disease or syndrome
  - muscular dystrophy G71.01
- paralysis
  - birth injury P14.0
  - due to or associated with
    - muscular dystrophy G71.01

Duodenitis (nonspecific) (peptic) K29.80
- with bleeding K29.81

Duplication, duplex—*see also* Accessory
- alimentary tract Q45.8
- biliary duct (any) Q44.5
- cystic duct Q44.5
- digestive organs Q45.8
- frontonasal process Q75.8

Dupré's disease (meningism) R29.1

Dwarfism E34.3
- achondroplastic Q77.4
- congenital E34.3
- constitutional E34.3
- hypochondroplastic Q77.4
- hypophyseal E23.0
- infantile E34.3
- Laron-type E34.3
- Lorain (-Levi) type E23.0
- metatropic Q77.8
- nephrotic-glycosuric (with hypophosphatemic rickets) E72.09
- nutritional E45
- penis Q55.69
- pituitary E23.0
- renal N25.0
- thanatophoric Q77.1

Dysarthria R47.1

Dysbasia R26.2
- hysterical F44.4
- nonorganic origin F44.4
- psychogenic F44.4

Dysbetalipoproteinemia (familial) E78.2

Dyscalculia R48.8
- developmental F81.2

Dyschezia K59.00

Dyscranio-pygo-phalangy Q87.0
- stomach K31.89
  - psychogenic F45.8

Dysentery, dysenteric (catarrhal) (diarrhea) (epidemic) (hemorrhagic) (infectious) (sporadic) (tropical) A09
- amebic (*see also* Amebiasis) A06.0
  - acute A06.0
- arthritis (*see also* category M01) A09
  - bacillary (*see also* category M01) A03.9
- bacillary A03.9
  - arthritis (*see also* category M01)
  - Shigella A03.9
    - boydii A03.2
    - dysenteriae A03.0
    - flexneri A03.1
    - group A A03.0
    - group B A03.1
    - group C A03.2
    - group D A03.3
    - sonnei A03.3
    - specified type NEC A03.8
- candidal B37.82
- Chinese A03.9
- Giardia lamblia A07.1
- Lamblia A07.1
- monilial B37.82
- Salmonella A02.0
- viral (*see also* Enteritis, viral) A08.4

Dysequilibrium R42

Dysesthesia R20.8
- hysterical F44.6

Dysfunction
- autonomic
  - somatoform F45.8
- bladder N31.9
  - neuromuscular NOS N31.9
- bleeding, uterus N93.8
- cerebral G93.89
- colon K59.9
  - psychogenic F45.8
- hypophysis E23.7
- hypothalamic NEC E23.3
- meibomian gland, of eyelid H02.88-
  - left H02.886
    - lower H02.885
    - upper H02.884
    - upper and lower eyelids H02.88B
  - right H02.883
    - lower H02.882
    - upper H02.881
    - upper and lower eyelids H02.88A
- physiological NEC R68.89
  - psychogenic F59
- pituitary (gland) E23.3
- rectum K59.9
  - psychogenic F45.8
- sexual (due to) R37
- sinoatrial node I49.5
- somatoform autonomic F45.8
- temporomandibular (joint) M26.69
  - joint-pain syndrome M26.62-
- ventricular I51.9
  - with congestive heart failure I50.9

Dysgenesis
- gonadal (due to chromosomal anomaly) Q96.9
- renal
  - bilateral Q60.4
  - unilateral Q60.3
- reticular D72.0
- tidal platelet D69.3

Dyshidrosis, dysidrosis L30.1

Dyskeratosis L85.8
- congenital Q82.8

Dyskinesia G24.9
- hysterical F44.4
- nonorganic origin F44.4
- psychogenic F44.4

Dyslalia (developmental) F80.0

Dyslexia R48.0
- developmental F81.0

Dyslipidemia E78.5

Dysmenorrhea (essential) (exfoliative) N94.6
- congestive (syndrome) N94.6
- primary N94.4
- psychogenic F45.8
- secondary N94.5

Dysmetabolic syndrome X E88.81

Dysmorphism (due to)
- alcohol Q86.0

Dysmorphophobia (non-delusional) F45.22

Dysorexia R63.0
- psychogenic F50.89

Dysostosis
- cleidocranial, cleidocranialis Q74.0
- multiplex E76.01

Dyspareunia N94.10
- deep N94.12
- other specified N94.19
- superficial (introital) N94.11

Dyspepsia R10.13
- atonic K30
- functional (allergic) (congenital) (gastrointestinal) (occupational) (reflex) K30
- nervous F45.8
- neurotic F45.8
- psychogenic F45.8

Dysphagia R13.10
- cervical R13.19
- functional (hysterical) F45.8
- hysterical F45.8
- nervous (hysterical) F45.8
- neurogenic R13.19
- oral phase R13.11
- oropharyngeal phase R13.12
- pharyngeal phase R13.13
- pharyngoesophageal phase R13.14
- psychogenic F45.8
- specified NEC R13.19

Dysphagocytosis, congenital D71

Dysphasia
- developmental
  - expressive type F80.1
  - receptive type F80.2

Dysphonia R49.0
- functional F44.4
- hysterical F44.4
- psychogenic F44.4

Dyspituitarism E23.3

Dysplasia—*see also* Anomaly
- acetabular, congenital Q65.89
- alveolar capillary, with vein misalignment J84.843
- anus (histologically confirmed) (mild) (moderate) K62.82
- asphyxiating thoracic (congenital) Q77.2
- brain Q07.9
- bronchopulmonary, perinatal P27.1
- chondroectodermal Q77.6
- colon D12.6
- dystrophic Q77.5
- ectodermal (anhidrotic) (congenital) (hereditary) Q82.4
  - hydrotic Q82.8
- high grade, focal D12.6
- hip, congenital Q65.89
- joint, congenital Q74.8
- kidney Q61.4
  - multicystic Q61.4
- leg Q74.2
- lung, congenital (not associated with short gestation) Q33.6
- oculodentodigital Q87.0
- renal Q61.4
  - multicystic Q61.4
- skin L98.8
- spondyloepiphyseal Q77.7
- thymic, with immunodeficiency D82.1

Dysplasminogenemia E88.02

Dyspnea (nocturnal) (paroxysmal) R06.00
- asthmatic (bronchial) J45.909
  - with
    - exacerbation (acute) J45.901
    - bronchitis J45.909
      ~ with
        ◊ exacerbation (acute) J45.901
        ◊ status asthmaticus J45.902
    - status asthmaticus J45.902
- functional F45.8
- hyperventilation R06.4
- hysterical F45.8
- newborn P28.89
- orthopnea R06.01
- psychogenic F45.8
- shortness of breath R06.02

Dyspraxia R27.8
- developmental (syndrome) F82

Dysproteinemia E88.09

Dysrhythmia
- cardiac I49.9
  - newborn
    - bradycardia P29.12
    - occurring before birth P03.819
      ~ before onset of labor P03.810
      ~ during labor P03.811
    - tachycardia P29.11
  - postoperative I97.89
- cerebral or cortical—*see* Epilepsy

Dyssomnia—*see* Disorder, sleep

Dyssynergia
- cerebellaris myoclonica (Hunt's ataxia) G11.19

Dystocia
- affecting newborn P03.1

Dystonia G24.9
- cervical G24.3
- deformans progressiva G24.1
- drug induced NEC G24.09
  - acute G24.02
  - specified NEC G24.09
- familial G24.1
- idiopathic G24.1
  - familial G24.1
  - nonfamilial G24.2
  - orofacial G24.4
- lenticularis G24.8
- musculorum deformans G24.1
- neuroleptic induced (acute) G24.02
- orofacial (idiopathic) G24.4
- oromandibular G24.4
  - due to drug G24.01
- specified NEC G24.8
- torsion (familial) (idiopathic) G24.1
  - acquired G24.8
  - genetic G24.1
  - symptomatic (nonfamilial) G24.2

Dystonic movements R25.8

Dystrophy, dystrophia
- adiposogenital E23.6
- autosomal recessive, childhood type, muscular dystrophy resembling Duchenne or Becker G71.01
- Becker's type G71.01
- cornea (hereditary) H18.50-
  - endothelial H18.51-
  - epithelial H18.52-
  - granular H18.53-
  - lattice H18.54-
  - macular H18.55-
  - specified type NEC H18.59-
- Duchenne's type G71.01
- Erb's G71.02
- Fuchs' H18.51-
- Gower's muscular G71.01
- infantile neuraxonal G31.89
- Landouzy-Déjérine G71.02
- Leyden-Möbius G71.09
- muscular G71.00
  - autosomal recessive, childhood type, muscular dystrophy resembling Duchenne or Becker G71.01
  - benign (Becker type) G71.01
    - capuloperoneal with early contractures [Emery-Dreifuss] G71.09
  - congenital (hereditary) (progressive) (with specific morphological abnormalities of the muscle fiber) G71.09
  - distal G71.09
  - Duchenne type G71.01
  - Emery-Dreifuss G71.09
  - Erb type G71.02
  - facioscapulohumeral G71.02
  - Gower's G71.01
  - hereditary (progressive) G71.09
  - Landouzy-Déjérine type G71.02
  - limb-girdle G71.09
  - progressive (hereditary) G71.09
  - pseudohypertrophic (infantile) G71.01
  - scapulohumeral G71.02
  - scapuloperoneal G71.09
  - severe (Duchenne type) G71.01
  - specified type NEC G71.09
- nail L60.3
- ocular G71.09
- oculocerebrorenal E72.03
- oculopharyngeal G71.09
- retinal (hereditary) H35.50
  - involving
    - sensory area H35.53
- scapuloperoneal G71.09
- skin NEC L98.8
- thoracic, asphyxiating Q77.2
- unguium L60.3

Dysuria R30.0
- psychogenic F45.8

E

Ear—*see also* Disease, diseased
- piercing Z41.3
- wax (impacted) H61.2-

Earache—*see* subcategory H92.0

Ebola virus disease A98.4

Eccentro-osteochondrodysplasia E76.29

Ecchymosis R58
- newborn P54.5
- spontaneous R23.3
- traumatic—*see* Contusion

Echovirus, as cause of disease classified elsewhere B97.12

Ectasia, ectasis
- annuloaortic I35.8

Ecthyma L08.0
- gangrenosum L08.0

Ectodermosis erosiva pluriorificialis L51.1

Ectopic, ectopia (congenital)
- abdominal viscera Q45.8
  - due to defect in anterior abdominal wall Q79.59
- atrial beats I49.1
- beats I49.49
  - atrial I49.1
- bladder Q64.10
- lens, lentis Q12.1
- testis Q53.00
  - bilateral Q53.02
  - unilateral Q53.01
- thyroid Q89.2
- vesicae Q64.10

Ectropion H02.10-
- cervix N86
  - with cervicitis N72
- congenital Q10.1
- lip (acquired) K13.0
  - congenital Q38.0

Eczema (acute) (chronic) (erythematous) (fissum) (rubrum) (squamous) (*see also* Dermatitis) L30.9
- contact—*see* Dermatitis, contact
- dyshidrotic L30.1
- flexural L20.82
- infantile L20.83
  - intertriginous L21.1
  - seborrheic L21.1
- intertriginous NEC L30.4
  - infantile L21.1
- intrinsic (allergic) L20.84
- marginatum (hebrae) B35.6
- pustular L30.3
- vaccination, vaccinatum T88.1

Eddowes (-Spurway) syndrome Q78.0

Edema, edematous (infectious) (pitting) (toxic) R60.9
- with nephritis—*see* Nephrosis
- allergic T78.3
- angioneurotic (allergic) (any site) (with urticaria) T78.3
- brain (cytotoxic) (vasogenic) G93.6
  - due to birth injury P11.0
  - newborn (anoxia or hypoxia) P52.4
    - birth injury P11.0
- circumscribed, acute T78.3
- conjunctiva H11.42-
- due to
  - salt retention E87.0
- epiglottis—*see* Edema, glottis
- essential, acute T78.3
- eyelid NEC H02.84-
  - left H02.846
    - lower H02.845
    - upper H02.844
  - right H02.843
    - lower H02.842
    - upper H02.841
- generalized R60.1
- glottis, glottic, glottidis (obstructive) (passive) J38.4
  - allergic T78.3

Edema, edematous, *continued*
- intracranial G93.6
- legs R60.0
- localized R60.0
- lower limbs R60.0
- lung J81.1
  - acute J81.0
  - due to
    - high altitude T70.29
    - near drowning T75.1
- newborn P83.30
  - hydrops fetalis—*see* Hydrops, fetalis
  - specified NEC P83.39
- penis N48.89
- periodic T78.3
- Quincke's T78.3
- salt E87.0

Edentulism—*see* Absence, teeth, acquired

Edsall's disease T67.2

Educational handicap Z55.9
- specified NEC Z55.8

Edward's syndrome—*see* Trisomy, 18

Effect, adverse
- abuse—*see* Maltreatment
- altitude (high)—*see* Effect, adverse, high altitude
- biological, correct substance properly administered—*see* Effect, adverse, drugs and medicaments
- blood (derivatives) (serum) (transfusion)—*see* Complications, transfusion
- chemical substance—*see* Table of Drugs and Chemicals
- cold (temperature) (weather)
  - frostbite—*see* Frostbite
- drugs and medicaments T88.7
  - specified drug—*see* Table of Drugs and Chemicals, by drug, adverse effect
  - specified effect—*code to* condition
- electric current, electricity (shock) T75.4
  - burn—*see* Burn
- exposure—*see* Exposure
- external cause NEC T75.89
- foodstuffs T78.1
  - allergic reaction—*see* Allergy, food
    - causing anaphylaxis—*see* Shock, anaphylactic, due to food
  - noxious—*see* Poisoning, food, noxious
- gases, fumes, or vapors
  - specified agent—*see* Table of Drugs and Chemicals
- glue (airplane) sniffing
  - due to drug abuse—*see* Abuse, drug, inhalant
  - due to drug dependence—*see* Dependence, drug, inhalant
- heat—*see* Heat
- high altitude NEC T70.29
  - anoxia T70.29
  - on
    - ears T70.0
    - sinuses T70.1
  - polycythemia D75.1
- hot weather—*see* Heat
- hunger T73.0
- immersion, foot—*see* Immersion
- immunization—*see* Complications, vaccination
- immunological agents—*see* Complications, vaccination
- infusion—*see* Complications, infusion
- lack of care of infants—*see* Maltreatment, child
- medical care T88.9
  - specified NEC T88.8
- medicinal substance, correct, properly administered—*see* Effect, adverse, drugs and medicaments
- motion T75.3
- serum NEC (*see also* Reaction, serum) T80.69
- specified NEC T78.8
- strangulation—*see* Asphyxia, traumatic
- submersion T75.1
- toxic—*see* Table of Drugs and Chemicals, by animal or substance, poisoning
- transfusion—*see* Complications, transfusion
- ultraviolet (radiation) (rays) NOS
  - burn—*see* Burn
  - dermatitis or eczema—*see* Dermatitis, due to, ultraviolet rays
    - acute L56.8

Effect, adverse, *continued*
- vaccine (any)—*see* Complications, vaccination
- whole blood—*see* Complications, transfusion

Effect(s) (of) (from)—*see* Effect, adverse

Effects, late—*see* Sequelae

Effort syndrome (psychogenic) F45.8

Effusion
- brain (serous) G93.6
- bronchial—*see* Bronchitis
- cerebral G93.6
- cerebrospinal—*see also* Meningitis
  - vessel G93.6
- chest—*see* Effusion, pleura
- intracranial G93.6
- joint M25.40
  - ankle M25.47-
  - elbow M25.42-
  - foot joint M25.47-
  - hand joint M25.44-
  - hip M25.45-
  - knee M25.46-
  - shoulder M25.41-
  - specified joint NEC M25.48
  - wrist M25.43-
- malignant pleural J91.0
- pericardium, pericardial (noninflammatory) I31.3
  - acute—*see* Pericarditis, acute
- peritoneal (chronic) R18.8
- pleura, pleurisy, pleuritic, pleuropericardial J90
  - due to systemic lupus erythematosus M32.13
  - in conditions classified elsewhere J91.8
  - malignant J91.0
  - newborn P28.89
- spinal—*see* Meningitis
- thorax, thoracic—*see* Effusion, pleura

Ehlers-Danlos syndrome Q79.60
- classical Ehlers-Danlos syndrome Q79.61
- hypermobile Ehlers-Danlos syndrome Q79.62
- other Ehlers-Danlos syndromes Q79.69
- vascular Ehlers-Danlos syndrome Q79.63

Ehrlichiosis A77.4-

Eichstedt's disease B36.0

Eisenmenger's
- complex or syndrome I27.83
- defect Q21.8

Ekbom's syndrome (restless legs) G25.81

Ekman's syndrome (brittle bones and blue sclera) Q78.0

Elastic skin Q82.8

Elastoma (juvenile) Q82.8

Electric current, electricity, effects (concussion) (fatal) (nonfatal) (shock) T75.4
- burn—*see* Burn

Electrocution T75.4
- from electroshock gun (taser) T75.4

Electrolyte imbalance E87.8

Elevated, elevation
- alanine transaminase (ALT) R74.01
- ALT (alanine transaminase) R74.01
- aspartate transaminase (AST) R74.01
- AST (aspartate transaminase) R74.01
- basal metabolic rate R94.8
- blood pressure—*see also* Hypertension
  - reading (incidental) (isolated) (nonspecific), no diagnosis of hypertension R03.0
- blood sugar R73.9
- body temperature (of unknown origin) R50.9
- C-reactive protein (CRP) R79.82
- cancer antigen 125 [CA 125] R97.1
- carcinoembryonic antigen [CEA] R97.0
- cholesterol E78.00
  - with high triglycerides E78.2
- erythrocyte sedimentation rate R70.0
- fasting glucose R73.01
- finding on laboratory examination—*see* Findings, abnormal, inconclusive, without diagnosis
- glucose tolerance (oral) R73.02
- lactic acid dehydrogenase (LDH) level R74.02
- leukocytes D72.829

Elevated, elevation, *continued*
- lipoprotein a (Lp(a)) level E78.41
- liver function
  - study R94.5
  - test R79.89
    - alkaline phosphatase R74.8
    - aminotransferase R74.01
    - bilirubin R17
    - hepatic enzyme R74.8
    - lactate dehydrogenase R74.02
- lymphocytes D72.820
- scapula, congenital Q74.0
- sedimentation rate R70.0
- SGOT R74.0
- SGPT R74.0
- transaminase level R74.0
- triglycerides E78.1
  - with high cholesterol E78.2
- troponin R77.8
- tumor associated antigens [TAA] NEC R97.8
- tumor specific antigens [TSA] NEC R97.8
- white blood cell count D72.829
  - specified NEC D72.828

Elliptocytosis (congenital) (hereditary) D58.1
- Hb C (disease) D58.1
- hemoglobin disease D58.1
- sickle-cell (disease) D57.8-
  - trait D57.3

Elongated, elongation (congenital)—*see also* Distortion
- bone Q79.9
- cystic duct Q44.5
- frenulum, penis Q55.69
- labia minora (acquired) N90.69

Embolism (multiple) (paradoxical) I74.9
- artery I74.9
- pituitary E23.6
- portal (vein) I81
- pulmonary (acute) (artery) (vein)
  - chronic I27.82
- pyemic (multiple) I76
  - following
  - Hemophilus influenzae A41.3
  - pneumococcal A40.3
    - with pneumonia J13
  - specified organism NEC A41.89
  - staphylococcal A41.2
  - streptococcal A40.9
- renal (artery) N28.0
  - vein I82.3
- vein (acute) I82.90
  - renal I82.3

Embryoma—*see also* Neoplasm, uncertain behavior, by site in Table of Neoplasms in the complete *ICD-10-CM* manual
- kidney C64.-
- malignant—*see also* Neoplasm, malignant, by site in Table of Neoplasms in the complete *ICD-10-CM* manual
  - kidney C64.-

Emesis—*see* Vomiting

Emotional lability R45.86

Emotionality, pathological F60.3

Emphysema
- cellular tissue (traumatic) T79.7
- connective tissue (traumatic) T79.7
- eyelid(s) H02.89
  - traumatic T79.7
- interstitial J98.2
  - congenital P25.0
  - perinatal period P25.0
- laminated tissue T79.7
- mediastinal J98.2
  - newborn P25.2
- subcutaneous (traumatic) T79.7
  - nontraumatic J98.2
- traumatic T79.7

Empyema (acute) (chest) (double) (pleura) (supradiaphragmatic) (thorax) J86.9
- with fistula J86.0
- gallbladder K81.0

Enanthema, viral B09

Encephalomyelitis (*see also* Encephalitis) G04.90
- acute disseminated G04.00
  - infectious G04.01
  - noninfectious G04.81
  - postimmunization G04.02
  - postinfectious G04.01
- acute necrotizing hemorrhagic G04.30
  - postimmunization G04.32
  - postinfectious G04.31
  - specified NEC G04.39
- equine A83.9
  - Eastern A83.2
- in diseases classified elsewhere G05.3
- postchickenpox B01.11
- postinfectious NEC G04.01
- postmeasles B05.0
- postvaccinal G04.02
- postvaricella B01.11

Encephalopathy (acute) G93.40
- acute necrotizing hemorrhagic G04.30
  - postimmunization G04.32
  - postinfectious G04.31
  - specified NEC G04.39
- congenital Q07.9
- due to
  - drugs (*see also* Table of Drugs and Chemicals) G92
- hyperbilirubinemic, newborn P57.9
  - due to isoimmunization (conditions in P55) P57.0
- hypertensive I67.4
- hypoglycemic E16.2
- hypoxic—*see* Damage, brain, anoxic
- hypoxic ischemic P91.60
  - mild P91.61
  - moderate P91.62
  - severe P91.63
- in (due to) (with)
  - birth injury P11.1
  - hyperinsulinism E16.1 [G94]
  - influenza—*see* Influenza, with, encephalopathy
  - lack of vitamin (*see also* Deficiency, vitamin) E56.9 [G32.89]
  - neoplastic disease (*see also* Neoplasm) D49.9 [G13.1]
  - serum (*see also* Reaction, serum) T80.69
  - trauma (postconcussional) F07.81
    - current injury—*see* Injury, intracranial
  - vaccination G04.02
- lead—*see* Poisoning, lead
- metabolic G93.41
  - drug induced G92
  - toxic G92
- neonatal P91.819
  - in diseases classified elsewhere P91.811
- postcontusional F07.81
  - current injury—*see* Injury, intracranial, diffuse
- postradiation G93.89
- toxic G92
  - metabolic G92
- traumatic (postconcussional) F07.81
  - current injury—*see* Injury, intracranial

Encephalocele Q01.9
- frontal Q01.0
- nasofrontal Q01.1
- occipital Q01.2
- specified NEC Q01.8

Encephalomalacia (brain) (cerebellar) (cerebral)—*see* Softening, brain

Encephalomyelitis (*see also* Encephalitis) G04.90
- acute disseminated G04.00
  - infectious G04.01
  - noninfectious G04.81
  - postimmunization G04.02
  - postinfectious G04.01
- acute necrotizing hemorrhagic G04.30
  - postimmunization G04.32
  - postinfectious G04.31
  - specified NEC G04.39
- congenital Q07.9
- due to
  - drugs (*see also* Table of Drugs and Chemicals) G92
- equine A83.9
  - Eastern A83.2

Encephalomyelitis, *continued*
- hyperbilirubinemic, newborn P57.9
  - due to isoimmunization (conditions in P55) P57.0
- hypertensive I67.4
- hypoglycemic E16.2
- hypoxic—*see* Damage, brain, anoxic
- hypoxic ischemic P91.60
  - mild P91.61
  - moderate P91.62
  - severe P91.63
- in diseases classified elsewhere G05.3
- in (due to) (with)
  - birth injury P11.1
  - hyperinsulinism E16.1 [G94]
  - influenza—*see* Influenza, with, encephalopathy
  - lack of vitamin (*see also* Deficiency, vitamin) E56.9 [G32.89]
  - neoplastic disease (*see also* Table of Neoplasms in the complete *ICD-10-CM* manual) D49.9 [G13.1]
  - serum (*see also* Reaction, serum) T80.69
  - trauma (postconcussional) F07.81
    - current injury—*see* Injury, intracranial
  - vaccination G04.02
- lead—*see* Poisoning, lead
- metabolic G93.41
  - drug induced G92
  - toxic G92
- neonatal P91.819
  - in diseases classified elsewhere P91.811
- postchickenpox B01.11
- postcontusional F07.81
  - current injury—*see* Injury, intracranial, diffuse
- postinfectious NEC G04.01
- postmeasles B05.0
- postradiation G93.89
- postvaccinal G04.02
- postvaricella B01.11
  - specified NEC G04.39
- toxic G92
  - metabolic G92
- traumatic (postconcussional) F07.81
  - current injury—*see* Injury, intracranial

Encephalorrhagia—*see* Hemorrhage, intracranial, intracerebral

Encephalosis, posttraumatic F07.81

Encopresis R15.9
- functional F98.1
- nonorganic origin F98.1
- psychogenic F98.1

Encounter (with health service) (for) Z76.89
- administrative purpose only Z02.9
  - examination for
    - adoption Z02.82
    - armed forces Z02.3
    - disability determination Z02.71
    - driving license Z02.4
    - employment Z02.1
    - insurance Z02.6
    - medical certificate NEC Z02.79
    - residential institution admission Z02.2
    - school admission Z02.0
    - sports Z02.5
  - specified reason NEC Z02.89
- aftercare—*see* Aftercare
- check-up—*see* Examination
- chemotherapy for neoplasm Z51.11
- counseling—*see* Counseling
- desensitization to allergens Z51.6
- ear piercing Z41.3
- examination—*see* Examination
- expectant parent(s) (adoptive) pre-birth pediatrician visit Z76.81
- fluoride varnish application Z29.3
- genetic
  - nonprocreative Z71.83
  - procreative counseling Z31.5
  - testing—*see* Test
- hearing conservation and treatment Z01.12
- instruction (in)
  - child care (postpartal) (prenatal) Z32.3
  - natural family planning
    - to avoid pregnancy Z30.02

Encounter, *continued*
- laboratory (as part of a general medical examination) Z00.00
  - with abnormal findings Z00.01
- mental health services (for)
  - abuse NEC
    - perpetrator Z69.82
    - victim Z69.81
  - child abuse/neglect (psychological) (sexual)
    - non-parental
      - perpetrator Z69.021
      - victim Z69.020
    - parental
      - perpetrator Z69.011
      - victim Z69.010
  - spousal or partner abuse (psychological)
    - perpetrator Z69.12
    - victim Z69.11
- observation (for) (ruled out)
  - exposure to (suspected)
    - anthrax Z03.810
    - biological agent NEC Z03.818
- pediatrician visit, by expectant parent(s) (adoptive) Z76.81
- pregnancy
  - supervision of—*see* Pregnancy, supervision of
  - test Z32.00
    - result negative Z32.02
    - result positive Z32.01
- prophylactic measures
  - antivenin Z29.12
  - ear piercing Z41.3
  - fluoride administration Z29.3
  - other specified Z29.8
  - rabies immune globulin Z29.14
  - respiratory syncytial virus (RSV) immune globulin Z29.11
  - Rho(D) immune globulin Z29.13
  - unspecified Z29.9
- radiation therapy (antineoplastic) Z51.0
- radiological (as part of a general medical examination) Z00.00
  - with abnormal findings Z00.01
- repeat cervical smear to confirm findings of recent normal smear following initial abnormal smear Z01.42
- respiratory syncytial virus (RSV) immune globulin administration Z29.11
- suspected condition, ruled out
  - fetal anomaly Z03.73
  - fetal growth Z03.74
- suspected exposure (to), ruled out
  - anthrax Z03.810
  - biological agents NEC Z03.818
- therapeutic drug level monitoring Z51.81
- to determine fetal viability of pregnancy O36.80
- training
  - insulin pump Z46.81
- X-ray of chest (as part of a general medical examination) Z00.00
  - with abnormal findings Z00.01

Endocarditis (chronic) (marantic) (nonbacterial) (thrombotic) (valvular) I38
- with rheumatic fever (conditions in I00)
  - active—*see* Endocarditis, acute, rheumatic
  - inactive or quiescent (with chorea) I09.1
- acute or subacute I33.9
  - infective I33.0
  - rheumatic (aortic) (mitral) (pulmonary) (tricuspid) I01.1
    - with chorea (acute) (rheumatic) (Sydenham's) I02.0
- aortic (heart) (nonrheumatic) (valve) I35.8
  - with
    - mitral disease I08.0
      - with tricuspid (valve) disease I08.3
      - active or acute I01.1
        ◊ with chorea (acute) (rheumatic) (Sydenham's) I02.0
    - rheumatic fever (conditions in I00)
      - active—*see* Endocarditis, acute, rheumatic
      - inactive or quiescent (with chorea) I06.9
    - tricuspid (valve) disease I08.2
      - with mitral (valve) disease I08.3

Endocarditis, *continued*
- acute or subacute I33.9
- arteriosclerotic I35.8
- rheumatic I06.9
  - with mitral disease I08.0
    - with tricuspid (valve) disease I08.3
    - active or acute I01.1
      ◊ with chorea (acute) (rheumatic) (Sydenham's) I02.0
  - active or acute I01.1
    - with chorea (acute) (rheumatic) (Sydenham's) I02.0
  - specified NEC I06.8
  - specified cause NEC I35.8
- atypical verrucous (Libman-Sacks) M32.11
- bacterial (acute) (any valve) (subacute) I33.0
- candidal B37.6
- constrictive I33.0
- due to
  - Serratia marcescens I33.0
- infectious or infective (acute) (any valve) (subacute) I33.0
- lenta (acute) (any valve) (subacute) I33.0
- Libman-Sacks M32.11
- malignant (acute) (any valve) (subacute) I33.0
- mitral (chronic) (double) (fibroid) (heart) (inactive) (valve) (with chorea) I05.9
  - with
    - aortic (valve) disease I08.0
      - with tricuspid (valve) disease I08.3
      - active or acute I01.1
        ◊ with chorea (acute) (rheumatic) (Sydenham's) I02.0
    - rheumatic fever (conditions in I00)
      - active—*see* Endocarditis, acute, rheumatic
      - inactive or quiescent (with chorea) I05.9
  - active or acute I01.1
    - with chorea (acute) (rheumatic) (Sydenham's) I02.0
  - bacterial I33.0
  - nonrheumatic I34.8
    - acute or subacute I33.9
  - specified NEC I05.8
- monilial B37.6
- mycotic (acute) (any valve) (subacute) I33.0
- pneumococcal (acute) (any valve) (subacute) I33.0
- pulmonary (chronic) (heart) (valve) I37.8
  - with rheumatic fever (conditions in I00)
    - active—*see* Endocarditis, acute, rheumatic
    - inactive or quiescent (with chorea) I09.89
      - with aortic, mitral or tricuspid disease I08.8
  - acute or subacute I33.9
    - rheumatic I01.1
      - with chorea (acute) (rheumatic) (Sydenham's) I02.0
  - arteriosclerotic I37.8
  - congenital Q22.2
- purulent (acute) (any valve) (subacute) I33.0
- rheumatic (chronic) (inactive) (with chorea) I09.1
  - active or acute (aortic) (mitral) (pulmonary) (tricuspid) I01.1
    - with chorea (acute) (rheumatic) (Sydenham's) I02.0
- septic (acute) (any valve) (subacute) I33.0
- streptococcal (acute) (any valve) (subacute) I33.0
- subacute—*see* Endocarditis, acute
- suppurative (acute) (any valve) (subacute) I33.0
- toxic I33.9
- tricuspid (chronic) (heart) (inactive) (rheumatic) (valve) (with chorea) I07.9
  - with
    - aortic (valve) disease I08.2
      - mitral (valve) disease I08.3
    - mitral (valve) disease I08.1
      - aortic (valve) disease I08.3
    - rheumatic fever (conditions in I00)
      - active—*see* Endocarditis, acute, rheumatic
      - inactive or quiescent (with chorea) I07.8
  - active or acute I01.1
    - with chorea (acute) (rheumatic) (Sydenham's) I02.0
  - arteriosclerotic I36.8

Endocarditis, *continued*
- nonrheumatic I36.8
  - acute or subacute I33.9
- specified cause, except rheumatic I36.8
- ulcerative (acute) (any valve) (subacute) I33.0
- vegetative (acute) (any valve) (subacute) I33.0
- verrucous (atypical) (nonbacterial) (nonrheumatic) M32.11

Endocardium, endocardial—*see also* Disease, diseased
- cushion defect Q21.2

Endocervicitis—*see also* Cervicitis
- hyperplastic N72

Endometritis (decidual) (nonspecific) (purulent) (senile) (atrophic) (suppurative) N71.9
- acute N71.0
- blennorrhagic (gonococcal) (acute) (chronic) A54.24
- cervix, cervical (with erosion or ectropion)—*see also* Cervicitis
  - hyperplastic N72
- chlamydial A56.11
- gonococcal, gonorrheal (acute) (chronic) A54.24
- hyperplastic N85.00-
  - cervix N72

Engman's disease L30.3

Engorgement
- breast N64.59
  - newborn P83.4
  - puerperal, postpartum O92.79

Enlargement, enlarged—*see also* Hypertrophy
- adenoids J35.2
  - with tonsils J35.3
- gingival K06.1
- labium majus (childhood asymmetric) CALME N90.61
- lymph gland or node R59.9
  - generalized R59.1
  - localized R59.0
- tonsils J35.1
  - with adenoids J35.3
- vestibular aqueduct Q16.5

Enteritis (acute) (diarrheal) (hemorrhagic) (noninfective) K52.9
- aertrycke infection A02.0
- allergic K52.29
  - with
    - eosinophilic gastritis or gastroenteritis K52.81
    - food protein-induced enterocolitis syndrome (FPIES) K52.21
    - food protein-induced enteropathy K52.22
- amebic (acute) A06.0
- bacillary NOS A03.9
- candidal B37.82
- chronic (noninfectious) K52.9
  - ulcerative—*see* Colitis, ulcerative
- Clostridium
  - botulinum (food poisoning) A05.1
  - difficile
    - not specified as recurrent A04.72
    - recurrent A04.71
- coxsackie virus A08.39
- dietetic K52.29
- due to
  - Clostridium difficile A04.7-
  - coxsackie virus A08.39
  - echovirus A08.39
  - enterovirus NEC A08.39
  - food hypersensitivity K52.29
  - torovirus A08.39
- echovirus A08.39
- enterovirus NEC A08.39
- eosinophilic K52.81
- epidemic (infectious) A09
- fulminant (*see also* Ischemia, intestine) K55.019
  - ischemic K55.9
    - acute (*see also* Ischemia, intestine) K55.019
- giardial A07.1
- infectious NOS A09
  - due to
    - Arizona (bacillus) A02.0
    - Campylobacter A04.5

Enteritis, *continued*
  - Escherichia coli A04.4
    - ~ enteroaggregative A04.4
    - ~ enterohemorrhagic A04.3
    - ~ enteropathogenic A04.0
    - ~ enterotoxigenic A04.1
    - ~ specified NEC A04.4
  - enterovirus A08.39
  - specified
    - ~ bacteria NEC A04.8
    - ~ virus NEC A08.39
  - virus NEC A08.4
    - ~ specified type NEC A08.39
- necroticans A05.2
- noninfectious K52.9
- parasitic NEC B82.9
- regional (of) K50.90
  - with
    - complication K50.919
      - ~ abscess K50.914
      - ~ fistula K50.913
      - ~ intestinal obstruction K50.912
      - ~ rectal bleeding K50.911
      - ~ specified complication NEC K50.918
  - large intestine (colon) (rectum) K50.10
    - with
      - ~ complication K50.119
        - ◊ abscess K50.114
        - ◊ fistula K50.113
        - ◊ intestinal obstruction K50.112
        - ◊ rectal bleeding K50.111
        - ◊ small intestine (duodenum) (ileum) (jejunum) involvement K50.80
          - » with
            - ❖ complication K50.819
              - ★ abscess K50.814
              - ★ fistula K50.813
              - ★ intestinal obstruction K50.812
              - ★ rectal bleeding K50.811
              - ★ specified complication NEC K50.818
        - ◊ specified complication NEC K50.118
  - rectum—*see* Enteritis, regional, large intestine
  - small intestine (duodenum) (ileum) (jejunum) K50.00
    - with
      - ~ complication K50.019
        - ◊ abscess K50.014
        - ◊ fistula K50.013
        - ◊ intestinal obstruction K50.012
        - ◊ large intestine (colon) (rectum) involvement K50.80
          - » with
            - ❖ complication K50.819
              - ★ abscess K50.814
              - ★ fistula K50.813
              - ★ intestinal obstruction K50.812
              - ★ rectal bleeding K50.811
              - ★ specified complication NEC K50.818
        - ◊ rectal bleeding K50.011
        - ◊ specified complication NEC K50.018
- rotaviral A08.0
- Salmonella, salmonellosis (arizonae) (choleraesuis) (enteritidis) (typhimurium) A02.0
- septic A09
- staphylococcal A04.8
  - due to food A05.0
- torovirus A08.39
- viral A08.4
  - enterovirus A08.39
  - Rotavirus A08.0
  - specified NEC A08.39
  - virus specified NEC A08.39

Enterobiasis B80

Enterobius vermicularis (infection) (infestation) B80

Enterocolitis (*see also* Enteritis) K52.9
- due to Clostridium difficile A04.7-
- fulminant ischemic (*see also* Ischemia, intestine) K55.059
- hemorrhagic (acute) (*see also* Ischemia, intestine) K55.059
- infectious NEC A09

Enterocolitis, *continued*
- necrotizing
  - due to Clostridium difficile A04.7-
  - in newborn P77.9
    - stage 1 (without pneumatosis, without perforation) P77.1
    - stage 2 (with pneumatosis, without perforation) P77.2
    - stage 3 (with pneumatosis, with perforation) P77.3
  - stage 1 (excluding newborns) K55.31
  - stage 2 (excluding newborns) K55.32
  - stage 3 (excluding newborns) K55.33
  - unspecified K55.30
- noninfectious K52.9
  - newborn—*see* Enterocolitis, necrotizing
- protein-induced syndrome K52.21
- pseudomembranous (newborn) A04.7-

Enteropathy K63.9
- food protein-induced enterocolitis K52.22
- gluten-sensitive
  - celiac K90.0
  - non-celiac K90.41
- protein-losing K90.49

Enterorrhagia K92.2

Enterospasm—*see also* Syndrome, irritable, bowel
- psychogenic F45.8

Enterovirus, as cause of disease classified elsewhere B97.10
- coxsackievirus B97.11
- echovirus B97.12
- other specified B97.19

Enthesopathy (peripheral) M77.9
- ankle and tarsus M77.5
  - specified type NEC—*see* Enthesopathy, foot, specified type NEC
- elbow region M77.8
  - lateral epicondylitis—*see* Epicondylitis, lateral
  - medial epicondylitis—*see* Epicondylitis, medial
- foot NEC M77.9
  - specified type NEC M77.5-
- forearm M77.9
- hand M77.9
- hip —*see* Enthesopathy, lower limb, specified type NEC
- iliac crest spur—*see* Spur, bone, iliac crest
- lateral epicondylitis—*see* Epicondylitis, lateral
- lower limb (excluding foot) M76.9
  - Achilles tendinitis—*see* Tendinitis, Achilles
  - anterior tibial syndrome M76.81-
  - iliac crest spur—*see* Spur, bone, iliac crest
  - iliotibial band syndrome—*see* Syndrome, iliotibial band
  - pelvic region—*see* Enthesopathy, lower limb, specified type NEC
  - posterior tibial syndrome M76.82-
  - specified type NEC M76.89-
  - tibial collateral bursitis—*see* Bursitis, tibial collateral
- medial epicondylitis—*see* Epicondylitis, medial
- metatarsalgia—*see* Metatarsalgia
- multiple sites M77.9
- pelvis M77.9
- posterior tibial syndrome M76.82-
- psoas tendinitis—*see* Tendinitis
- shoulder M77.9
- specified site NEC M77.9
- specified type NEC M77.8
- upper arm M77.9
- wrist and carpus NEC M77.8

Entropion (eyelid) (paralytic)
- congenital Q10.2

Enuresis R32
- functional F98.0
- habit disturbance F98.0
- nocturnal N39.44
  - psychogenic F98.0
- nonorganic origin F98.0
- psychogenic F98.0

Eosinophilia (allergic) (hereditary) (idiopathic) (secondary) D72.10
- familial D72.19
- hereditary D72.19

Eosinophilia, *continued*
- in disease classified elsewhere D72.18
- with
  - angiolymphoid hyperplasia (ALHE) D18.01

Eosinophilia-myalgia syndrome M35.8

Ependymoblastoma
- specified site—*see* Neoplasm, malignant, by site in Table of Neoplasms in the complete *ICD-10-CM* manual
- unspecified site C71.9

Ependymoma (epithelial) (malignant)
- anaplastic
  - specified site—*see* Neoplasm, malignant, by site in Table of Neoplasms in the complete *ICD-10-CM* manual
  - unspecified site C71.9
- benign specified site—*see* Neoplasm, benign, by site in Table of Neoplasms in the complete *ICD-10-CM* manual
- specified site—*see* Neoplasm, malignant, by site in Table of Neoplasms in the complete *ICD-10-CM* manual
- unspecified site C71.9

Ependymopathy G93.89

Epiblepharon (congenital) Q10.3

Epicanthus, epicanthic fold (eyelid) (congenital) Q10.3

Epicondylitis (elbow)
- lateral M77.1-
- medial M77.0-

Epidermodysplasia verruciformis B07.8

Epidermolysis
- bullosa (congenital) Q81.9
  - dystrophica Q81.2
  - letalis Q81.1
  - simplex Q81.0
  - specified NEC Q81.8
- necroticans combustiformis L51.2
  - due to drug—*see* Table of Drugs and Chemicals, by drug

Epididymitis (acute) (nonvenereal) (recurrent) (residual) N45.1
- with orchitis N45.3
- blennorrhagic (gonococcal) A54.23
- chlamydial A56.19
- gonococcal A54.23
- syphilitic A52.76

Epididymo-orchitis (*see also* Epididymitis) N45.3

Epiglottitis, epiglottiditis (acute) J05.10
- with obstruction J05.11
- chronic J37.0

Epilepsia partialis continua (*see also* Kozhevnikof's epilepsy) G40.1-

Epilepsy, epileptic, epilepsia (attack) (cerebral) (convulsion) (fit) (seizure) G40.909
- *Note*: the following terms are to be considered equivalent to intractable: pharmacoresistant (pharmacologically resistant), treatment resistant, refractory (medically) and poorly controlled
- benign childhood with centrotemporal EEG spikes—*see* Epilepsy, localization-related, idiopathic
- benign myoclonic in infancy G40.80-
- childhood
  - with occipital EEG paroxysms—*see* Epilepsy, localization-related, idiopathic
- generalized
  - specified NEC G40.409
    - intractable G40.419
      ~ with status epilepticus G40.411
      ~ without status epilepticus G40.419
    - not intractable G40.409
      ~ with status epilepticus G40.401
      ~ without status epilepticus G40.409
- impulsive petit mal—*see* Epilepsy, juvenile myoclonic
- localization-related (focal) (partial)
- not intractable G40.909
  - with status epilepticus G40.901
  - without status epilepticus G40.909
- on awakening—*see* Epilepsy, generalized, specified NEC
- parasitic NOS B71.9 *[G94]*
- spasms G40.822
  - intractable G40.824
    - with status epilepticus G40.823
    - without status epilepticus G40.824

Epilepsy, epileptic, epilepsia, *continued*
- not intractable G40.822
  - with status epilepticus G40.821
  - without status epilepticus G40.822
- specified NEC G40.802
  - intractable G40.804
    - with status epilepticus G40.803
    - without status epilepticus G40.804
  - not intractable G40.802
    - with status epilepticus G40.801
    - without status epilepticus G40.802
- syndromes
  - generalized
  - localization-related (focal) (partial)
    - idiopathic
      ~ with seizures of localized onset
        ◊ intractable G40.019
          » without status epilepticus G40.019
  - specified NEC G40.802
    - intractable G40.804
      ~ with status epilepticus G40.803
      ~ without status epilepticus G40.804
    - not intractable G40.802
      ~ with status epilepticus G40.801
      ~ without status epilepticus G40.802
- tonic (-clonic)—*see* Epilepsy, generalized, specified NEC

Epiloia Q85.1

Epimenorrhea N92.0

Epipharyngitis—*see* Nasopharyngitis

Epiphysitis—*see also* Osteochondropathy
- juvenile M92.9

Episode
- depressive F32.9
  - major F32.9
    - mild F32.0
    - moderate F32.1
    - severe (without psychotic symptoms) F32.2
      ~ with psychotic symptoms F32.3
  - recurrent F33.9
    - brief F33.8
  - specified NEC F32.89

Epispadias (female) (male) Q64.0

Epistaxis (multiple) R04.0
- hereditary I78.0

Equinovarus (congenital) (talipes) Q66.0-

Equivalent
- convulsive (abdominal)—*see* Epilepsy, specified NEC
- epileptic (psychic)—*see* Epilepsy, localization-related, symptomatic, with complex partial seizures

Erb (-Duchenne) paralysis (birth injury) (newborn) P14.0

Erb-Goldflam disease or syndrome G70.00
- with exacerbation (acute) G70.01
- in crisis G70.01

Erb's
- disease G71.02
- palsy, paralysis (brachial) (birth) (newborn) P14.0
- pseudohypertrophic muscular dystrophy G71.02

Erdheim's syndrome (acromegalic macrospondylitis) E22.0

Erosio interdigitalis blastomycetica B37.2

Erosion
- cervix (uteri) (acquired) (chronic) (congenital) N86
  - with cervicitis N72

Eructation R14.2
- nervous or psychogenic F45.8

Eruption
- drug (generalized) (taken internally) L27.0
  - fixed L27.1
  - in contact with skin—*see* Dermatitis, due to drugs and medicaments
  - localized L27.1
- napkin L22
- skin (nonspecific) R21
  - due to inoculation/vaccination (generalized) (*see also* Dermatitis, due to, vaccine) L27.0
    - localized L27.1
  - feigned L98.1
- tooth, teeth, abnormal (incomplete) (late) (premature) (sequence) K00.6

Erysipelas (gangrenous) (infantile) (newborn) (phlegmonous) (suppurative) A46
- external ear A46 *[H62.4-]*

Erythema, erythematous (infectional) (inflammation) L53.9
- arthriticum epidemicum A25.1
- chronicum migrans (Borrelia burgdorferi) A69.20
- diaper L22
- gluteal L22
- ichthyosiforme congenitum bullous Q80.3
- induratum (nontuberculous) L52
- infectiosum B08.3
- intertrigo L30.4
- marginatum L53.2
  - in (due to) acute rheumatic fever I00
- migrans A26.0
  - chronicum A69.20
  - tongue K14.1
- multiforme (major) (minor) L51.9
  - bullous, bullosum L51.1
  - conjunctiva L51.1
  - specified NEC L51.8
- napkin L22
- neonatorum P83.88
  - toxic P83.1
- nodosum L52
- rash, newborn P83.88
- solare L55.0
- toxic, toxicum NEC L53.0
  - newborn P83.1

Erythremia (acute) C94.0-
- secondary D75.1

Erythroblastopenia (*see also* Aplasia, red cell) D60.9
- congenital D61.01

Erythroblastophthisis D61.09

Erythroblastosis (fetalis) (newborn) P55.9
- due to
  - ABO (antibodies) (incompatibility) (isoimmunization) P55.1

Erythrocyanosis (crurum) I73.89

Erythrocytosis (megalosplenic) (secondary) D75.1
- familial D75.0
- oval, hereditary—*see* Elliptocytosis
- secondary D75.1
- stress D75.1

Erythroderma (secondary) (*see also* Erythema) L53.9
- bullous ichthyosiform, congenital Q80.3
- desquamativum L21.1
- ichthyosiform, congenital (bullous) Q80.3
- neonatorum P83.88
- psoriaticum L40.8

Erythrodysesthesia, palmar plantar (PPE) L27.1

Erythrogenesis imperfecta D61.09

Erythrophagocytosis D75.89

Escherichia coli (E. coli), as cause of disease classified elsewhere B96.20
- non-O157 Shiga toxin-producing (with known O group) B96.22
- non-Shiga toxin-producing B96.29
- O157 with confirmation of Shiga toxin when H antigen is unknown, or is not H7 B96.21
- O157:H- (nonmotile)with confirmation of Shiga toxin B96.21
- O157:H7 with or without confirmation of Shiga toxin-production B96.21
- Shiga toxin-producing (with unspecified O group) (STEC) B96.23
- O157 B96.21
- O157:H7 with or without confirmation of Shiga toxin-production B96.21
  - specified NEC B96.22
- specified NEC B96.29

Esophagitis (acute) (alkaline) (chemical) (chronic) (infectional) (necrotic) (peptic) (postoperative) K20.9-
- candidal B37.81
- due to gastrointestinal reflux disease K21.0-
- eosinophilic K20.0
- reflux K21.0-
- specified NEC K20.80

Estrangement (marital) Z63.5
- parent-child NEC Z62.890

Ethmoiditis (chronic) (nonpurulent) (purulent)—*see also* Sinusitis, ethmoidal
- influenzal—*see* Influenza manifestations NEC

Evaluation (for) (of)
- development state
  - adolescent Z00.3
  - period of
    - delayed growth in childhood Z00.70
      ~ with abnormal findings Z00.71
    - rapid growth in childhood Z00.2
  - puberty Z00.3
- growth and developmental state (period of rapid growth) Z00.2
- period of
  - delayed growth in childhood Z00.70
    - with abnormal findings Z00.71
  - rapid growth in childhood Z00.2
- suspected condition—*see* Observation

Evans syndrome D69.41

Event
- apparent life threatening in newborn and infant (ALTE) R68.13
- brief resolved unexplained event (BRUE) R68.13

Eversion
- cervix (uteri) N86
  - with cervicitis N72

Evisceration
- birth injury P15.8

Examination (for) (following) (general) (of) (routine) Z00.00
- with abnormal findings Z00.01
- abuse, physical (alleged), ruled out
  - child Z04.72
- adolescent (development state) Z00.3
- alleged rape or sexual assault (victim), ruled out
  - child Z04.42
- annual (adult) (periodic) (physical) Z00.00
  - with abnormal findings Z00.01
  - gynecological Z01.419
    - with abnormal findings Z01.411
- blood—*see* Examination, laboratory
- blood pressure Z01.30
  - with abnormal findings Z01.31
- cervical Papanicolaou smear Z12.4
  - as part of routine gynecological examination Z01.419
    - with abnormal findings Z01.411
- child (over 28 days old) Z00.129
  - with abnormal findings Z00.121
  - under 28 days old—*see* Newborn, examination
- contraceptive (drug) maintenance (routine) Z30.8
  - device (intrauterine) Z30.431
- developmental—*see* Examination, child
- ear Z01.10
  - with abnormal findings NEC Z01.118
- eye Z01.00
  - with abnormal findings Z01.01
  - after failed exam Z01.02
- following
  - accident NEC Z04.3
    - transport Z04.1
    - work Z04.2
  - assault, alleged, ruled out
    - child Z04.72
  - motor vehicle accident Z04.1
  - treatment (for) Z09
    - combined NEC Z09
      ~ fracture Z09
      ~ malignant neoplasm Z08
    - malignant neoplasm Z08
    - mental disorder Z09
    - specified condition NEC Z09
- follow-up (routine) (following) Z09
  - chemotherapy NEC Z09
    - malignant neoplasm Z08
  - fracture Z09
  - malignant neoplasm Z08
  - radiotherapy NEC Z09
    - malignant neoplasm Z08
  - surgery NEC Z09
    - malignant neoplasm Z08

Examination, *continued*
- forced labor exploitation Z04.82
- forced sexual exploitation Z04.81
- gynecological Z01.419
  - with abnormal findings Z01.411
  - for contraceptive maintenance Z30.8
- health—*see* Examination, medical
- hearing Z01.10
  - with abnormal findings NEC Z01.118
  - following failed hearing screening Z01.110
  - infant or child (28 days and older) Z00.129
    - with abnormal findings Z00.121
- immunity status testing Z01.84
- laboratory (as part of a general medical examination) Z00.00
  - with abnormal findings Z00.01
  - preprocedural Z01.812
- lactating mother Z39.1
- medical (adult) (for) (of) Z00.00
  - with abnormal findings Z00.01
  - administrative purpose only Z02.9
    - specified NEC Z02.89
  - admission to
    - school Z02.0
      ~ following illness or medical treatment Z02.0
    - summer camp Z02.89
  - adoption Z02.82
  - blood alcohol or drug level Z02.83
  - camp (summer) Z02.89
  - general (adult) Z00.00
    - with abnormal findings Z00.01
  - medicolegal reasons NEC Z04.89
  - participation in sport Z02.5
  - pre-operative—*see* Examination, pre-procedural
  - pre-procedural
    - cardiovascular Z01.810
    - respiratory Z01.811
    - specified NEC Z01.818
  - preschool children
    - for admission to school Z02.0
  - sport competition Z02.5
- medicolegal reason NEC Z04.89
  - following
    - forced labor exploitation Z04.82
    - forced sexual exploitation Z04.81
- newborn—*see* Newborn, examination
- pelvic (annual) (periodic) Z01.419
  - with abnormal findings Z01.411
- period of rapid growth in childhood Z00.2
- periodic (adult) (annual) (routine) Z00.00
  - with abnormal findings Z00.01
- physical (adult)—*see also* Examination, medical Z00.00
  - sports Z02.5
- pre-chemotherapy (antineoplastic) Z01.818
- pre-procedural (pre-operative)
  - cardiovascular Z01.810
  - laboratory Z01.812
  - respiratory Z01.811
  - specified NEC Z01.818
- prior to chemotherapy (antineoplastic) Z01.818
- radiological (as part of a general medical examination) Z00.00
  - with abnormal findings Z00.01
- repeat cervical smear to confirm findings of recent normal smear following initial abnormal smear Z01.42
- skin (hypersensitivity) Z01.82
- special (*see also* Examination) Z01.89
  - specified type NEC Z01.89
- specified type or reason NEC Z04.89
- urine—*see* Examination, laboratory
- vision Z01.00
  - following failed vision screening Z01.020
    - with abnormal findings Z01.021
  - infant or child (over 28 days old) Z00.129
    - with abnormal findings Z00.121
  - with abnormal findings Z01.01

Exanthem, exanthema—*see also* Rash
- with enteroviral vesicular stomatitis B08.4
- subitum B08.20
  - due to human herpesvirus 6 B08.21
  - due to human herpesvirus 7 B08.22
- viral, virus B09
  - specified type NEC B08.8

Excess, excessive, excessively
- alcohol level in blood R78.0
- crying
  - in child, adolescent, or adult R45.83
  - in infant R68.11
- development, breast N62
- drinking (alcohol) NEC (without dependence) F10.10
  - habitual (continual) (without remission) F10.20
- eating R63.2
- foreskin N47.8
- gas R14.0
- large
  - colon K59.39
    - congenital Q43.8
    - toxic K59.31
  - infant P08.0
  - organ or site, congenital NEC—*see* Anomaly, by site
- long
  - organ or site, congenital NEC—*see* Anomaly, by site
- menstruation (with regular cycle) N92.0
  - with irregular cycle N92.1
- napping Z72.821
- natrium E87.0
- secretion—*see also* Hypersecretion
  - sweat R61
- skin and subcutaneous tissue L98.7
  - eyelid (acquired)—*see* Blepharochalasis
    - congenital Q10.3
- sodium (Na) E87.0
- sweating R61
- thirst R63.1
  - due to deprivation of water T73.1
- weight
  - gain R63.5
  - loss R63.4

Excitability, abnormal, under minor stress (personality disorder) F60.3

Excitation
- anomalous atrioventricular I45.6

Excoriation (traumatic)—*see also* Abrasion
- neurotic L98.1
- skin picking disorder F42.4

Exhaustion, exhaustive (physical NEC) R53.83
- battle F43.0
- cardiac—*see* Failure, heart
- delirium F43.0
- heat (*see also* Heat, exhaustion) T67.5
  - due to
    - salt depletion T67.4
    - water depletion T67.3
- psychosis F43.0

Exomphalos Q79.2
- meaning hernia—*see* Hernia, umbilicus

Exotropia—*see* Strabismus, divergent concomitant

Explanation of
- investigation finding Z71.2
- medication Z71.89

Exposure (to) (*see also* Contact) T75.89
- AIDS virus Z20.6
- anthrax Z20.810
- aromatic amines Z77.020
- aromatic (hazardous) compounds NEC Z77.028
- aromatic dyes NOS Z77.028
- arsenic Z77.010
- asbestos Z77.090
- bacterial disease NEC Z20.818
- benzene Z77.021
- body fluids (potentially hazardous) Z77.21
- chemicals (chiefly nonmedicinal) (hazardous) NEC Z77.098
- chromium compounds Z77.018
- communicable disease Z20.9
  - bacterial NEC Z20.818
  - specified NEC Z20.89
  - viral NEC Z20.828
- dyes Z77.098
- environmental tobacco smoke (acute) (chronic) Z77.22
- Escherichia coli (E. coli) Z20.01
- German measles Z20.4
- gonorrhea Z20.2
- hazardous metals NEC Z77.018

Exposure, *continued*
- hazardous substances NEC Z77.29
- hazards in the physical environment NEC Z77.128
- hazards to health NEC Z77.9
- human immunodeficiency virus (HIV) Z20.6
- human T-lymphotropic virus type-1 (HTLV-1) Z20.89
- infestation (parasitic) NEC Z20.7
- intestinal infectious disease NEC Z20.09
  - Escherichia coli (E. coli) Z20.01
- lead Z77.011
- meningococcus Z20.811
- mold (toxic) Z77.120
- nickel dust Z77.018
- poliomyelitis Z20.89
- polycyclic aromatic hydrocarbons Z77.028
- prenatal (drugs) (toxic chemicals)—*see* Newborn, noxious substances transmitted via placenta or breast milk
- rabies Z20.3
- rubella Z20.4
- second hand tobacco smoke (acute) (chronic) Z77.22
  - in the perinatal period P96.81
- sexually-transmitted disease Z20.2
- smallpox (laboratory) Z20.89
- syphilis Z20.2
- tuberculosis Z20.1
- varicella Z20.820
- venereal disease Z20.2
- viral disease NEC Z20.828
- Zika virus Z20.821

Exstrophy
- abdominal contents Q45.8
- bladder Q64.10
  - cloacal Q64.12
  - specified type NEC Q64.19
  - supravesical fissure Q64.11

Extrasystoles (supraventricular) I49.49
- atrial I49.1
- auricular I49.1

Extravasation
- pelvicalyceal N13.8
- pyelosinus N13.8
- vesicant agent
  - antineoplastic chemotherapy T80.810
  - other agent NEC T80.818

F

Failure, failed
- aortic (valve) I35.8
  - rheumatic I06.8
- biventricular I50.82
- cardiorenal (chronic) I50.9
- cardiorespiratory (*see also* Failure, heart) R09.2
- circulation, circulatory (peripheral) R57.9
  - newborn P29.89
- compensation—*see* Disease, heart
- compliance with medical treatment or regimen—*see* Noncompliance
- expansion terminal respiratory units (newborn) (primary) P28.0
- gain weight (child over 28 days old) R62.51
  - newborn P92.6
- heart (acute) (senile) (sudden) I50.9
  - biventricular I50.82
  - combined left-right sided I50.82
  - compensated I50.9
  - congestive (compensated) (decompensated) I50.9
    - with rheumatic fever (conditions in I00)
      - ~ active I01.8
      - ~ inactive or quiescent (with chorea) I09.81
    - newborn P29.0
    - rheumatic (chronic) (inactive) (with chorea) I09.81
      - ~ active or acute I01.8
        - ◊ with chorea I02.0
  - decompensated I50.9
    - newborn P29.0
  - diastolic (congestive) (left ventricular) I50.3-
    - combined with systolic (congestive) I50.40
      - ~ acute (congestive) I50.41
        - ◊ and (on) chronic (congestive) I50.43

Failure, failed, *continued*
- ~ chronic (congestive) I50.42
  - ◊ and (on) acute (congestive) I50.43
- due to presence of cardiac prosthesis I97.13-
- following cardiac surgery I97.13-
- high output NOS I50.83
- low output (syndrome) NOS I50.9
- postprocedural I97.13-
- specified NEC I50.89
- Note: heart failure stages A, B, C, and D are based on the American College of Cardiology and American Heart Association stages of heart failure, which complement and should not be confused with the New York Heart Association Classification of Heart Failure, into Class I, Class II, Class III, and Class IV
- stage A Z91.89
- stage B—*see also* Failure, heart, by type as diastolic or systolic I50.9
- stage C—*see also* Failure, heart, by type as diastolic or systolic I50.9
- stage D—*see also* Failure, heart, by type as diastolic or systolic, chronic I50.84
- systolic (congestive) (left ventricular) I50.2-
  - combined with diastolic (congestive) I50.40
    - ~ acute (congestive) I50.41
    - ~ chronic (congestive) I50.42
      - ◊ and (on) acute (congestive) I50.43
- kidney (*see also* Disease, kidney, chronic) N19
  - acute (*see also* Failure, renal, acute) N17.9-
  - diabetic—*see* E08-E13 with .22
- lactation (complete) O92.3
  - partial O92.4
- mitral I05.8
- myocardial, myocardium (*see also* Failure, heart) I50.9
  - chronic (*see also* Failure, heart, congestive) I50.9
  - congestive (*see also* Failure, heart, congestive) I50.9
- ovulation causing infertility N97.0
- renal N19
  - with
    - tubular necrosis (acute) N17.0
  - acute N17.9
    - with
      - ~ cortical necrosis N17.1
      - ~ medullary necrosis N17.2
      - ~ tubular necrosis N17.0
    - specified NEC N17.8
  - chronic N18.9
  - congenital P96.0
  - end stage N18.6
    - due to hypertension I12.0
- respiration, respiratory J96.90
  - with
    - hypercapnia J96.92
    - hypercarbia J96.92
    - hypoxia J96.91
  - acute J96.00
    - with
      - ~ hypercapnia J96.02
      - ~ hypercarbia J96.02
      - ~ hypoxia J96.01
  - center G93.89
  - chronic J96.10
    - with
      - ~ hypercapnia J96.12
      - ~ hypercarbia J96.12
      - ~ hypoxia J96.11
  - newborn P28.5
  - postprocedural (acute) J95.821
    - acute and chronic J95.822
- to thrive (child over 28 days old) R62.51
  - newborn P92.6
- transplant T86.-
  - bone
    - marrow T86.02
  - heart T86.22
    - with lung(s) T86.32
  - kidney T86.12
  - liver T86.42
  - lung(s) T86.811
    - with heart T86.32
  - stem cell (peripheral blood) (umbilical cord) T86.5
- ventricular (*see also* Failure, heart) I50.9

Failure, failed, *continued*
- left I50.1
  - with rheumatic fever (conditions in I00)
    - ~ active I01.8
      - ◊ with chorea I02.0
    - ~ inactive or quiescent (with chorea) I09.81
  - rheumatic (chronic) (inactive) (with chorea) I09.81
    - ~ active or acute I01.8
      - ◊ with chorea I02.0
- right (*see also* Failure, heart, congestive) I50.9
- vital centers, newborn P91.88

Fainting (fit) R55

Fallot's
- tetrad or tetralogy Q21.3

Family, familial—*see also* Disease, diseased
- disruption Z63.8
  - involving divorce or separation Z63.5
- planning advice Z30.09
- problem Z63.9
  - specified NEC Z63.8
- retinoblastoma C69.2-

Fanconi's anemia (congenital pancytopenia) D61.09

Fasciitis M72.9
- infective M72.8
  - necrotizing M72.6
- necrotizing M72.6

Fascioscapulohumeral myopathy G71.02

Fast pulse R00.0

Fat
- in stool R19.5

Fatigue R53.83
- auditory deafness—*see* Deafness
- chronic R53.82
- combat F43.0
- general R53.83
- muscle M62.89

Fatty—*see also* Disease, diseased
- liver NEC K76.0
  - nonalcoholic K76.0

Faucitis J02.9

Favism (anemia) D55.0

Favus—*see* Dermatophytosis

Fear complex or reaction F40.9

Fear of—*see* Phobia

Febris, febrile—*see also* Fever
- rubra A38.9

Fecal
- incontinence R15.9
- smearing R15.1
- soiling R15.1
- urgency R15.2

Fecalith (impaction) K56.41

Fede's disease K14.0

Feeble rapid pulse due to shock following injury T79.4

Feeble-minded F70

Feeding
- difficulties R63.3
- problem R63.3
  - newborn P92.9
    - specified NEC P92.8
  - nonorganic (adult)—*see* Disorder, eating

Feeling (of)
- foreign body in throat R09.89

Feet—*see* Disease, diseased

Feigned illness Z76.5

Fetid
- breath R19.6

Fetus, fetal—*see also* Disease, diseased
- alcohol syndrome (dysmorphic) Q86.0
- lung tissue P28.0

Fever (inanition) (of unknown origin) (persistent) (with chills) (with rigor) R50.9
- African tick bite A77.8
- American
  - mountain (tick) A93.2
  - spotted A77.0

Fever, *continued*
- Bullis A77.0
- catarrhal (acute) J00
  - chronic J31.0
- cerebrospinal meningococcal A39.0
- Colorado tick (virus) A93.2
- due to
  - conditions classified elsewhere R50.81
  - heat T67.0-
- ephemeral (of unknown origin) R50.9
- epidemic hemorrhagic A98.5
- erysipelatous—*see* Erysipelas
- glandular—*see* Mononucleosis, infectious
- Haverhill A25.1
- hay (allergic) J30.1
  - with asthma (bronchial) J45.909
    - with
      - ~ exacerbation (acute) J45.901
      - ~ status asthmaticus J45.902
  - due to
    - allergen other than pollen J30.89
    - pollen, any plant or tree J30.1
- heat (effects) T67.0-
- hemorrhagic (arthropod-borne) NOS A94
  - arenaviral A96.9
- intermittent (bilious)—*see also* Malaria
  - of unknown origin R50.9
- Lone Star A77.0
- mountain
  - meaning Rocky Mountain spotted fever A77.0
  - tick (American) (Colorado) (viral) A93.2
- newborn P81.9
  - environmental P81.0
- non-exanthematous tick A93.2
- persistent (of unknown origin) R50.9
- petechial A39.0
- postimmunization R50.83
- postoperative R50.82
  - due to infection T81.40
- posttransfusion R50.84
- postvaccination R50.83
- presenting with conditions classified elsewhere R50.81
- rat-bite A25.9
  - due to
    - Spirillum A25.0
      - ~ Streptobacillus moniliformis A25.1
- relapsing (Borrelia) A68.9
  - louse borne A68.0
  - Novy's
    - louse-borne A68.0
    - tick-bourne A68.1
  - tick borne A68.1
- rheumatic (active) (acute) (chronic) (subacute) I00
  - with central nervous system involvement I02.9
  - active with heart involvement (*see* category) I01
  - inactive or quiescent with
    - cardiac hypertrophy I09.89
    - carditis I09.9
    - endocarditis I09.1
      - ~ aortic (valve) I06.9
        - ◊ with mitral (valve) disease I08.0
      - ~ mitral (valve) I05.9
        - ◊ with aortic (valve) disease I08.0
      - ~ pulmonary (valve) I09.89
      - ~ tricuspid (valve) I07.8
    - heart disease NEC I09.89
    - heart failure (congestive) (conditions in I50) I09.81
    - left ventricular failure (conditions in I50.1–I50.4-) I09.81
    - myocarditis, myocardial degeneration (conditions in I51.4) I09.0
    - pancarditis I09.9
    - pericarditis I09.2
- Rocky Mountain spotted A77.0
- rose J30.1
- Sao Paulo A77.0
- scarlet A38.9
- specified NEC A96.8
  - viral A99
    - specified NEC A98.8
- spirillary A25.0
- spotted A77.9
  - American A77.0

Fever, *continued*
- Brazilian A77.0
- cerebrospinal meningitis A39.0
- Columbian A77.0
- due to Rickettsia
  - rickettsii A77.0
- Ehrlichiosis A77.40
- Rocky Mountain spotted A77.0
- streptobacillary A25.1
- swine A02.8
- thermic T67.0-
- unknown origin R50.9
- uveoparotid D86.69
- West Nile (viral) A92.30
  - with
    - complications NEC A92.39
    - cranial nerve disorders A92.32
    - encephalitis A92.31
    - encephalomyelitis A92.31
    - neurologic manifestation NEC A92.32
    - optic neuritis A92.32
    - polyradiculitis A92.32
- yellow A95.9
  - jungle A95.0
  - sylvatic A95.0
  - urban A95.1
- Zika virus A92.5

Fibrillation
- atrial or auricular (established) I48.91
  - cardiac I49.8
  - chronic I48.20
    - persistent I48.19
  - paroxysmal I48.0
  - permanent I48.21
  - persistent (chronic) (NOS) (other) I48.19
    - longstanding I48.11
- heart I49.8
  - muscular M62.89
  - ventricular I49.01

Fibrinogenopenia D68.8
- acquired D65
- congenital D68.2

Fibrinolysis (hemorrhagic) (acquired) D65
- newborn, transient P60

Fibrocystic
- disease—*see also* Fibrosis, cystic
  - pancreas E84.9

Fibromatosis M72.9
- gingival K06.1

Fibromyxolipoma D17.9

Fibroplasia, retrolental H35.17-

Fibrosis, fibrotic
- anal papillae K62.89
- cystic (of pancreas) E84.9
  - with
    - distal intestinal obstruction syndrome E84.19
    - fecal impaction E84.19
    - intestinal manifestations NEC E84.19
    - pulmonary manifestations E84.0
    - specified manifestations NEC E84.8
- meninges G96.198
- pericardium I31.0
- rectal sphincter K62.89
- skin L90.5

Fiedler's
- myocarditis (acute) I40.1

Fifth disease B08.3

Filatov's disease—*see* Mononucleosis, infectious

Fimbrial cyst Q50.4

Findings, abnormal, inconclusive, without diagnosis—*see also* Abnormal
- alcohol in blood R78.0
- antenatal screening of mother O28.9
  - biochemical O28.1
  - chromosomal O28.5
  - cytological O28.2
  - genetic O28.5
  - hematological O28.0
  - radiological O28.4

Findings, abnormal, inconclusive, without diagnosis, *continued*
  - specified NEC O28.8
  - ultrasonic O28.3
- bacteriuria R82.71
- bicarbonate E87.8
- blood sugar R73.09
  - high R73.9
  - low (transient) E16.2
- casts or cells, urine R82.998
- chloride E87.8
- cholesterol E78.9
  - high E78.00
    - with high triglycerides E78.2
- creatinine clearance R94.4
- crystals, urine R82.998
- culture
  - blood R78.81
  - positive—*see* Positive, culture
- echocardiogram R93.1
- electrolyte level, urinary R82.998
- function study NEC R94.8
  - bladder R94.8
  - endocrine NEC R94.7
    - kidney R94.4
    - liver R94.5
    - pancreas R94.8
    - placenta R94.8
    - pulmonary R94.2
    - spleen R94.8
    - thyroid R94.6
- glycosuria R81
- heart
  - shadow R93.1
  - sounds R01.2
- hematinuria R82.3
- hemoglobinuria R82.3
- in blood (of substance not normally found in blood) R78.9
  - alcohol (excessive level) R78.0
  - lead R78.71
- lactic acid dehydrogenase (LDH) R74.02
- neonatal screening P09
- PPD R76.11
- radiologic (X-ray) R93.89
  - abdomen R93.5
  - intrathoracic organs NEC R93.1
  - musculoskeletal
    - limbs R93.6
    - other than limb R93.7
  - retroperitoneum R93.5
  - testis R93.81-
- scan NEC R94.8
  - bladder R94.8
  - bone R94.8
  - kidney R94.4
  - liver R93.2
  - lung R94.2
  - pancreas R94.8
  - placental R94.8
  - spleen R94.8
  - thyroid R94.6
- sedimentation rate, elevated R70.0
- SGOT R74.01
- SGPT R74.01
- sodium (deficiency) E87.1
  - excess E87.0
- stress test R94.39
- thyroid (function) (metabolic rate) (scan) (uptake) R94.6
- transaminase (level) R74.01
- triglycerides E78.9
  - high E78.1
    - with high cholesterol E78.2
- tuberculin skin test (without active tuberculosis) R76.11
- urine
  - bacteriuria R82.71
  - casts or cells R82.998
  - culture positive R82.79
  - glucose R81
  - hemoglobin R82.3
  - sugar R81
- vectorcardiogram (VCG) R94.39

Fire, Saint Anthony's—*see* Erysipelas

Foreign body, *continued*

- ~ puncture—*see* Puncture, eyelid, with foreign body
- ~ superficial injury—*see* Foreign body, superficial, eyelid
  - – gastrointestinal tract T18.9
    - ▪ multiple parts T18.8
    - ▪ specified part NEC T18.8
  - – genitourinary tract T19.9
    - ▪ multiple parts T19.8
    - ▪ specified part NEC T19.8
  - – Highmore's antrum T17.0
  - – hypopharynx—*see* Foreign body, pharynx
  - – lacrimal apparatus (punctum) T15.-
  - – larynx—*see* Foreign body, larynx
  - – lung—*see* Foreign body, respiratory tract
  - – maxillary sinus T17.0
  - – mouth T18.0
  - – nasal sinus T17.0
  - – nasopharynx—*see* Foreign body, pharynx
  - – nose (passage) T17.1
  - – nostril T17.1
  - – pharynx—*see* Foreign body, pharynx
  - – piriform sinus—*see* Foreign body, pharynx
  - – respiratory tract—*see* Foreign body, respiratory tract
  - – sinus (accessory) (frontal) (maxillary) (nasal) T17.0
    - ▪ piriform—*see* Foreign body, pharynx
  - – suffocation by—*see* Foreign body, by site
  - – tear ducts or glands—*see* Foreign body, entering through orifice, eye, specified part NEC
  - – throat—*see* Foreign body, pharynx
  - – tongue T18.0
  - – tonsil, tonsillar (fossa)—*see* Foreign body, pharynx
  - – trachea—*see* Foreign body, trachea
  - – vagina T19.2
  - – vulva T19.2
- • esophagus T18.108
  - – causing
    - ▪ injury NEC T18.108
      - ~ food (bone) (seed) T18.128
      - ~ gastric contents (vomitus) T18.118
      - ~ specified type NEC T18.19-
    - ▪ tracheal compression T18.100
      - ~ food (bone) (seed) T18.120
      - ~ gastric contents (vomitus) T18.110
      - ~ specified type NEC T18.190
- • feeling of, in throat R09.89
- • fragment—*see* Retained, foreign body fragments (type of)
- • genitourinary tract T19.9
  - – vagina T19.2
  - – vulva T19.2
- • granuloma (old) (soft tissue)—*see also* Granuloma, foreign body
  - – skin L92.3
- • in
  - – laceration—*see* Laceration, by site, with foreign body
  - – puncture wound—*see* Puncture, by site, with foreign body
  - – soft tissue (residual) M79.5
- • ingestion, ingested NOS T18.9
- • inhalation or inspiration—*see* Foreign body, by site
- • larynx T17.308
  - – causing
    - ▪ asphyxiation T17.300
      - ~ food (bone) (seed) T17.320
      - ~ gastric contents (vomitus) T17.310
      - ~ specified type NEC T17.390
    - ▪ injury NEC T17.308
      - ~ food (bone) (seed) T17.328
      - ~ gastric contents (vomitus) T17.318
      - ~ specified type NEC T17.398
- • old or residual
  - – soft tissue (residual) M79.5
- • pharynx T17.208
  - – causing
    - ▪ asphyxiation T17.200
      - ~ food (bone) (seed) T17.220
      - ~ gastric contents (vomitus) T17.210
      - ~ specified type NEC T17.290

Foreign body, *continued*

- ▪ injury NEC T17.208
  - ~ food (bone) (seed) T17.228
  - ~ gastric contents (vomitus) T17.218
  - ~ specified type NEC T17.298
- • respiratory tract T17.908
  - – bronchioles—*see* Foreign body, respiratory tract, specified site NEC
  - – bronchus—*see* Foreign body, bronchus
  - – causing
    - ▪ asphyxiation T17.900
      - ~ food (bone) (seed) T17.920
      - ~ gastric contents (vomitus) T17.910
      - ~ specified type NEC T17.990
    - ▪ injury NEC T17.908
      - ~ food (bone) (seed) T17.928
      - ~ gastric contents (vomitus) T17.918
      - ~ specified type NEC T17.998
  - – larynx—*see* Foreign body, larynx
  - – multiple parts—*see* Foreign body, respiratory tract
  - – nasal sinus T17.0
  - – nasopharynx—*see* Foreign body, pharynx
  - – nose T17.1
  - – nostril T17.1
  - – pharynx—*see* Foreign body, pharynx
- • specified site NEC T17.80- (See complete *ICD-10-CM* Manual for codes)
  - – fragments—*see* Retained, foreign body fragments (type of)
  - – soft tissue M79.5
  - – throat—*see* Foreign body, pharynx
  - – trachea—*see* Foreign body, trachea
- • superficial, without open wound
  - – abdomen, abdominal (wall) S30.851
  - – alveolar process S00.552
  - – ankle S90.55-
  - – antecubital space S40.85-
  - – anus S30.857
  - – arm (upper) S40.85-
  - – auditory canal S00.45-
  - – axilla S40.85-
  - – back, lower S30.850
  - – breast S20.15-
  - – brow S00.85
  - – buttock S30.850
  - – calf S80.85-
  - – canthus S00.25-
  - – cheek S00.85
    - ▪ internal S00.552
  - – chest wall S20.95
  - – chin S00.85
  - – clitoris S30.854
  - – costal region S20.95
  - – digit(s)
    - ▪ hand—*see* Foreign body, superficial, without open wound, finger
    - ▪ foot—*see* Foreign body, superficial, without open wound, toe
  - – ear S00.45-
  - – elbow S50.35-
  - – epididymis S30.853
  - – epigastric region S30.851
  - – epiglottis S10.15
  - – esophagus, cervical S10.15
  - – eyebrow S00.25-
  - – eyelid S00.25-
  - – face S00.85
  - – finger(s) S60.45-
    - ▪ index S60.45-
    - ▪ little S60.45-
    - ▪ middle S60.45-
    - ▪ ring S60.45-
  - – flank S30.851
  - – foot (except toe(s) alone) S90.85-
    - ▪ toe—*see* Foreign body, superficial, without open wound, toe
  - – forearm S50.85-
    - ▪ elbow only S50.35-
  - – forehead S00.85
  - – genital organs, external
    - ▪ female S30.856
    - ▪ male S30.855

Foreign body, *continued*

- – groin S30.851
- – gum S00.552
- – hand S60.55-
- – head S00.95
  - ▪ ear S00.45-
  - ▪ eyelid S00.25-
  - ▪ lip S00.551
  - ▪ nose S00.35
  - ▪ oral cavity S00.552
  - ▪ scalp S00.05
  - ▪ specified site NEC S00.85
- – heel—*see* Foreign body, superficial, without open wound, foot
- – hip S70.25-
- – inguinal region S30.851
- – interscapular region S20.459
- – jaw S00.85
- – knee S80.25-
- – labium (majus) (minus) S30.854
- – larynx S10.15
- – leg (lower) S80.85-
  - ▪ knee S80.25-
  - ▪ upper—*see* Foreign body, superficial, without open wound, thigh
- – lip S00.551
- – lower back S30.850
- – lumbar region S30.850
- – malar region S00.85
- – mammary—*see* Foreign body, superficial, without open wound, breast
- – mastoid region S00.85
- – mouth S00.552
- – nail
  - ▪ finger—*see* Foreign body, superficial, without open wound, finger
  - ▪ toe—*see* Foreign body, superficial, without open wound, toe
- – nape S10.85
- – nasal S00.35
- – neck S10.95
  - ▪ specified site NEC S10.85
  - ▪ throat S10.15
- – nose S00.35
- – occipital region S00.05
- – oral cavity S00.552
- – orbital region—*see* Foreign body, superficial, without open wound, eyelid
- – palate S00.552
- – palm—*see* Foreign body, superficial, without open wound, hand
- – parietal region S00.05
- – pelvis S30.850
- – penis S30.852
- – perineum
  - ▪ female S30.854
  - ▪ male S30.850
- – periocular area S00.25-
- – phalanges
  - ▪ finger—*see* Foreign body, superficial, without open wound, finger
  - ▪ toe—*see* Foreign body, superficial, without open wound, toe
- – pharynx S10.15
- – pinna S00.45-
- – popliteal space S80.25-
- – prepuce S30.852
- – pubic region S30.850
- – pudendum
  - ▪ female S30.856
  - ▪ male S30.855
- – sacral region S30.850
- – scalp S00.05
- – scapular region S40.25-
- – scrotum S30.853
- – shin S80.85-
- – shoulder S40.25-
- – sternal region S20.359
- – submaxillary region S00.85
- – submental region S00.85
- – subungual
  - ▪ finger(s)—*see* Foreign body, superficial, without open wound, finger

Foreign body, *continued*
- ■ toe(s)—*see* Foreign body, superficial, without open wound, toe
- – supraclavicular fossa S10.85
- – supraorbital S00.85
- – temple S00.85
- – temporal region S00.85
- – testis S30.853
- – thigh S70.35-
- – thorax, thoracic (wall) S20.95
  - ■ back S20.45-
  - ■ front S20.35-
- – throat S10.15
- – thumb S60.35-
- – toe(s) (lesser) S90.45-
  - ■ great S90.45-
- – tongue S00.552
- – trachea S10.15
- – tunica vaginalis S30.853
- – tympanum, tympanic membrane S00.45-
- – uvula S00.552
- – vagina S30.854
- – vocal cords S10.15
- – vulva S30.854
- – wrist S60.85-
- • swallowed T18.9
- • trachea T17.40- (See complete *ICD-10-CM* Manual for codes)
- • type of fragment—*see* Retained, foreign body fragments (type of)

Fothergill's
- • disease (trigeminal neuralgia)—*see also* Neuralgia
  - – scarlatina anginosa A38.9

Foul breath R19.6

Foundling Z76.1

FPIES (food protein-induced enterocolitis syndrome) K52.21

Fracture (abduction) (adduction) (separation) T14.8
- • acetabulum S32.40-
  - – column
    - ■ anterior (displaced) (iliopubic) S32.43-
      - ~ nondisplaced S32.43-
    - ■ posterior (displaced) (ilioischial) S32.44-
      - ~ nondisplaced S32.44-
  - – dome (displaced) S32.48-
    - ■ nondisplaced S32.48
  - – specified NEC S32.49-
  - – transverse (displaced) S32.45-
    - ■ with associated posterior wall fracture (displaced) S32.46-
      - ~ nondisplaced S32.46-
    - ■ nondisplaced S32.45-
  - – wall
    - ■ anterior (displaced) S32.41-
      - ~ nondisplaced S32.41-
    - ■ medial (displaced) S32.47-
      - ~ nondisplaced S32.47-
    - ■ posterior (displaced) S32.42-
      - ~ with associated transverse fracture (displaced) S32.46-
        - ◊ nondisplaced S32.46-
      - ~ nondisplaced S32.42-
- • ankle S82.89-
  - – bimalleolar (displaced) S82.84-
    - ■ nondisplaced S82.84-
  - – lateral malleolus only (displaced) S82.6-
    - ■ nondisplaced S82.6-
  - – medial malleolus (displaced) S82.5-
    - ■ associated with Maisonneuve's fracture—*see* Fracture, Maisonneuve's
    - ■ nondisplaced S82.5-
  - – talus—*see* Fracture
  - – trimalleolar (displaced) S82.85-
    - ■ nondisplaced S82.85-
- • arm (upper)—*see also* Fracture, humerus, shaft
  - – humerus—*see* Fracture, humerus
  - – radius—*see* Fracture, radius
  - – ulna—*see* Fracture, ulna
- • astragalus—*see* Fracture
- • Barton's—*see* Barton's fracture
- • base of skull—*see* Fracture, skull, base

Fracture, *continued*
- • basicervical (basal) (femoral) S72.0
- • Bennett's—*see* Bennett's fracture
- • bimalleolar—*see* Fracture, ankle, bimalleolar
- • blowout S02.3-
- • bone NEC T14.8
  - – birth injury P13.9
  - – following insertion of orthopedic implant, joint prosthesis or bone plate—*see* Fracture
- • burst—*see* Fracture, traumatic, by site
- • calcaneus—*see* Fracture, tarsal, calcaneus
- • carpal bone(s) S62.10-
  - – capitate (displaced) S62.13-
    - ■ nondisplaced S62.13-
  - – cuneiform—*see* Fracture, carpal bone, triquetrum
  - – hamate (body) (displaced) S62.14-
    - ■ hook process (displaced) S62.15-
      - ~ nondisplaced S62.15-
    - ■ nondisplaced S62.14-
  - – larger multangular—*see* Fracture, carpal bones, trapezium
  - – lunate (displaced) S62.12-
    - ■ nondisplaced S62.12-
  - – navicular S62.00-
    - ■ distal pole (displaced) S62.01-
      - ~ nondisplaced S62.01-
    - ■ middle third (displaced) S62.02-
      - ~ nondisplaced S62.02-
    - ■ proximal third (displaced) S62.03-
      - ~ nondisplaced S62.03-
    - ■ volar tuberosity—*see* Fracture, carpal bones, navicular, distal pole
  - – os magnum—*see* Fracture, carpal bones, capitate
  - – pisiform (displaced) S62.16-
    - ■ nondisplaced S62.16-
  - – semilunar—*see* Fracture, carpal bones, lunate
  - – smaller multangular—*see* Fracture, carpal bones, trapezoid
  - – trapezium (displaced) S62.17-
    - ■ nondisplaced S62.17-
  - – trapezoid (displaced) S62.18-
    - ■ nondisplaced S62.18-
  - – triquetrum (displaced) S62.11-
    - ■ nondisplaced S62.11-
  - – unciform—*see* Fracture, carpal bones, hamate
- • clavicle S42.00-
  - – acromial end (displaced) S42.03-
    - ■ nondisplaced S42.03-
  - – birth injury P13.4
  - – lateral end—*see* Fracture, clavicle, acromial end
  - – shaft (displaced) S42.02-
    - ■ nondisplaced S42.02-
  - – sternal end (anterior) (displaced) S42.01-
    - ■ nondisplaced S42.01-
    - ■ posterior S42.01-
- • coccyx S32.2
- • collar bone—*see* Fracture, clavicle
- • Colles'—*see* Colles' fracture
- • coronoid process—*see* Fracture, ulna, upper end, coronoid process
- • costochondral, costosternal junction—*see* Fracture, rib
- • cranium—*see* Fracture, skull
- • cricoid cartilage S12.8
- • cuboid (ankle)—*see* Fracture, tarsal, cuboid
- • cuneiform
  - – foot—*see* Fracture, tarsal, cuneiform
  - – wrist—*see* Fracture, carpal, triquetrum
- • delayed union—*see* Delay
- • due to
  - – birth injury—*see* Birth, injury, fracture
- • Dupuytren's—*see* Fracture, ankle, lateral malleolus only
- • elbow S42.40-
- • ethmoid (bone) (sinus)—*see* Fracture, skull, base
- • face bone S02.92-
- • fatigue—*see also* Fracture, stress
- • femur, femoral S72.9-
  - – basicervical (basal) S72.0
  - – birth injury P13.2
  - – capital epiphyseal S79.01-
  - – condyles, epicondyles—*see* Fracture, femur, lower end
  - – distal end—*see* Fracture, femur, lower end

Fracture, *continued*
- – epiphysis
  - ■ head—*see* Fracture, femur, upper end, epiphysis
  - ■ lower—*see* Fracture, femur, lower end, epiphysis
  - ■ upper—*see* Fracture, femur, upper end, epiphysis
- – head—*see* Fracture, femur, upper end, head
- – intertrochanteric—*see* Fracture, femur
- – intratrochanteric—*see* Fracture, femur
- – lower end S72.40-
  - ■ condyle (displaced) S72.41-
    - ~ lateral (displaced) S72.42-
      - ◊ nondisplaced S72.42-
    - ~ medial (displaced) S72.43-
      - ◊ nondisplaced S72.43-
    - ~ nondisplaced S72.41-
  - ■ epiphysis (displaced) S72.44-
    - ~ nondisplaced S72.44-
  - ■ physeal S79.10-
    - ~ Salter-Harris
      - ◊ Type I S79.11-
      - ◊ Type II S79.12-
      - ◊ Type III S79.13-
      - ◊ Type IV S79.14-
    - ~ specified NEC S79.19-
  - ■ specified NEC S72.49-
  - ■ supracondylar (displaced) S72.45-
    - ~ with intracondylar extension (displaced) S72.46-
      - ◊ nondisplaced S72.46-
    - ~ nondisplaced S72.45-
  - ■ torus S72.47-
- – neck—*see* Fracture, femur, upper end, neck
- – pertrochanteric—*see* Fracture, femur
- – shaft (lower third) (middle third) (upper third) S72.30-
  - ■ comminuted (displaced) S72.35-
    - ~ nondisplaced S72.35-
  - ■ oblique (displaced) S72.33-
    - ~ nondisplaced S72.33-
  - ■ segmental (displaced) S72.36-
    - ~ nondisplaced S72.36-
  - ■ specified NEC S72.39-
  - ■ spiral (displaced) S72.34-
    - ~ nondisplaced S72.34-
  - ■ transverse (displaced) S72.32-
    - ~ nondisplaced S72.32-
- – specified site NEC—*see* subcategory S72.8
- – transcervical—*see* Fracture, femur, upper end, neck
- – transtrochanteric—*see* Fracture, femur, trochanteric
- – upper end S72.00-
  - ■ cervicotrochanteric—*see* Fracture, femur, upper end, neck, base
  - ■ epiphysis (displaced) S72.02-
    - ~ nondisplaced S72.02-
  - ■ midcervical (displaced) S72.03-
    - ~ nondisplaced S72.03-
  - ■ neck S72.00-
    - ~ base (displaced) S72.04-
      - ◊ nondisplaced S72.04-
  - ■ pertrochanteric—*see* Fracture, femur, upper end
  - ■ physeal S79.00-
    - ~ Salter-Harris type I S79.01-
    - ~ specified NEC S79.09-
  - ■ transcervical—*see* Fracture, femur, upper end, midcervical
- • fibula (shaft) (styloid) S82.40-
  - – comminuted (displaced or nondisplaced) S82.45- (See complete *ICD-10-CM* Manual for codes)
    - ■ involving ankle or malleolus—*see* Fracture, fibula
    - ■ lateral malleolus (displaced) S82.6-
      - ~ nondisplaced S82.6-
    - ■ lower end
      - ~ physeal S89.30-
        - ◊ Salter-Harris
          - » Type I S89.31-
          - » Type II S89.32-
        - ◊ specified NEC S89.39-
      - ~ specified NEC S82.83-
      - ~ torus S82.82-
  - – oblique (displaced or nondisplaced) S82.43- (See complete *ICD-10-CM* Manual for codes)
  - – segmental (displaced or nondisplaced) S82.46- (See complete *ICD-10-CM* Manual for codes)

Fracture, *continued*
- spiral (displaced or nondisplaced) S82.44- (See complete *ICD-10-CM* Manual for codes)
- transverse (displaced or nondisplaced) S82.42- (See complete *ICD-10-CM* Manual for codes)
  - upper end
    - ~ physeal S89.20-
      - ◊ Salter-Harris
        - » Type I S89.21-
        - » Type II S89.22-
      - ◊ specified NEC S89.29-
    - ~ specified NEC S82.83-
    - ~ torus S82.81-
- finger (except thumb) S62.6-
  - distal phalanx (displaced) S62.63-
    - nondisplaced S62.66-
  - index S62.6-
    - distal phalanx (displaced) S62.63-
      - ~ nondisplaced S62.66-
    - medial phalanx (displaced) S62.62-
      - ~ nondisplaced S62.65-
    - proximal phalanx (displaced) S62.61-
      - ~ nondisplaced S62.64-
  - little S62.6-
    - distal phalanx (displaced) S62.63-
      - ~ nondisplaced S62.66-
    - medial phalanx (displaced) S62.62-
      - ~ nondisplaced S62.65-
    - proximal phalanx (displaced) S62.61-
      - ~ nondisplaced S62.64-
  - medial phalanx (displaced) S62.62-
    - nondisplaced S62.65-
  - middle S62.6-
    - distal phalanx (displaced) S62.63-
      - ~ nondisplaced S62.66-
    - medial phalanx (displaced) S62.62-
      - ~ nondisplaced S62.65-
    - proximal phalanx (displaced) S62.61-
      - ~ nondisplaced S62.64-
  - proximal phalanx (displaced) S62.61-
    - nondisplaced S62.64-
  - ring S62.6-
    - distal phalanx (displaced) S62.63-
      - ~ nondisplaced S62.66-
    - medial phalanx (displaced) S62.62-
      - ~ nondisplaced S62.65-
    - proximal phalanx (displaced) S62.61-
      - ~ nondisplaced S62.64-
  - thumb—*see* Fracture, thumb
- foot S92.90-
  - astragalus—*see* Fracture, tarsal, talus
  - calcaneus—*see* Fracture, tarsal, calcaneus
  - cuboid—*see* Fracture, tarsal, cuboid
  - cuneiform—*see* Fracture, tarsal, cuneiform
  - metatarsal—*see* Fracture, metatarsal bone
  - navicular—*see* Fracture, tarsal, navicular
  - sesamoid S92.81-
  - talus—*see* Fracture, tarsal, talus
  - tarsal—*see* Fracture, tarsal
  - toe—*see* Fracture, toe
- forearm S52.9-
  - radius—*see* Fracture, radius
  - ulna—*see* Fracture, ulna
- fossa (anterior) (middle) (posterior) S02.19-
- frontal (bone) (skull) S02.0-
  - sinus S02.19-
- greenstick—*see* Fracture, by site
- hallux—*see* Fracture, toe, great
- hand
  - carpal—*see* Fracture, carpal bone
  - finger (except thumb)—*see* Fracture, finger
  - metacarpal—*see* Fracture, metacarpal
  - navicular (scaphoid) (hand)—*see* Fracture, carpal bone, navicular
  - thumb—*see* Fracture, thumb
- healed or old
  - with complications—*code by* Nature of the complication
- heel bone—*see* Fracture, tarsal, calcaneus
- Hill-Sachs S42.29-
- hip—*see* Fracture, femur, neck

Fracture, *continued*
- humerus S42.30-
  - anatomical neck—*see* Fracture, humerus, upper end
  - articular process—*see* Fracture, humerus, lower end
  - capitellum—*see* Fracture, humerus, lower end, condyle, lateral
  - distal end—*see* Fracture, humerus, lower end
  - epiphysis
    - lower—*see* Fracture, humerus, lower end, physeal
    - upper—*see* Fracture, humerus, upper end, physeal
  - external condyle—*see* Fracture, humerus, lower end, condyle, lateral
  - great tuberosity—*see* Fracture, humerus, upper end, greater tuberosity
  - intercondylar—*see* Fracture, humerus, lower end
  - internal epicondyle—*see* Fracture, humerus, lower end, epicondyle, medial
  - lesser tuberosity—*see* Fracture, humerus, upper end, lesser tuberosity
  - lower end S42.40-
    - condyle
      - ~ lateral (displaced) S42.45-
        - ◊ nondisplaced S42.45-
      - ~ medial (displaced) S42.46-
        - ◊ nondisplaced S42.46-
    - epicondyle
      - ~ lateral (displaced) S42.43-
        - ◊ nondisplaced S42.43-
      - ~ medial (displaced) S42.44-
        - ◊ incarcerated S42.44-
        - ◊ nondisplaced S42.44-
    - physeal S49.10-
      - ~ Salter-Harris
        - ◊ Type I S49.11-
        - ◊ Type II S49.12-
        - ◊ Type III S49.13-
        - ◊ Type IV S49.14-
      - ~ specified NEC S49.19-
    - specified NEC (displaced) S42.49-
      - ~ nondisplaced S42.49-
    - supracondylar (simple) (displaced) S42.41-
      - ~ comminuted (displaced) S42.42-
        - ◊ nondisplaced S42.42-
      - ~ nondisplaced S42.41-
    - torus S42.48-
    - transcondylar (displaced) S42.47-
      - ~ nondisplaced S42.47-
  - proximal end—*see* Fracture, humerus, upper end
  - shaft S42.30-
    - comminuted (displaced) S42.35-
      - ~ nondisplaced S42.35-
    - greenstick S42.31-
    - oblique (displaced) S42.33
      - ~ nondisplaced S42.33-
    - segmental (displaced) S42.36-
      - ~ nondisplaced S42.36-
    - specified NEC S42.39-
    - spiral (displaced) S42.34-
      - ~ nondisplaced S42.34-
    - transverse (displaced) S42.32-
      - ~ nondisplaced S42.32-
  - supracondylar—*see* Fracture, humerus, lower end
  - surgical neck—*see* Fracture, humerus, upper end, surgical neck
  - trochlea—*see* Fracture, humerus, lower end, condyle, medial
  - tuberosity—*see* Fracture, humerus, upper end
  - upper end S42.20-
    - anatomical neck—*see* Fracture, humerus, upper end, specified NEC
    - articular head—*see* Fracture, humerus, upper end, specified NEC
    - epiphysis—*see* Fracture, humerus, upper end, physeal
    - greater tuberosity (displaced) S42.25-
      - ~ nondisplaced S42.25-
    - lesser tuberosity (displaced) S42.26-
      - ~ nondisplaced S42.26-
    - physeal S49.00-
      - ~ Salter-Harris
        - ◊ Type I S49.01-

Fracture, *continued*
- ◊ Type II S49.02-
- ◊ Type III S49.03-
- ◊ Type IV S49.04-
- ~ specified NEC S49.09-
  - specified NEC (displaced) S42.29-
    - ~ nondisplaced S42.29-
  - surgical neck (displaced) S42.21-
    - ~ four-part S42.24-
    - ~ nondisplaced S42.21-
    - ~ three-part S42.23-
    - ~ two-part (displaced) S42.22-
      - ◊ nondisplaced S42.22-
  - torus S42.27-
  - transepiphyseal—*see* Fracture, humerus, upper end, physeal
- hyoid bone S12.8
- ilium S32.30-
  - avulsion (displaced) S32.31-
    - nondisplaced S32.31-
  - specified NEC S32.39-
- impaction, impacted—*code as* Fracture, by site
- innominate bone—*see* Fracture, ilium
- instep—*see* Fracture, foot
- ischium S32.60-
  - avulsion (displaced) S32.61-
    - nondisplaced S32.61-
  - specified NEC S32.69-
- jaw (bone) (lower)—*see* Fracture, mandible
- knee cap—*see* Fracture, patella
- larynx S12.8
- late effects—*see* Sequelae
- leg (lower)
  - ankle—*see* Fracture, ankle
  - femur—*see* Fracture, femur
  - fibula—*see* Fracture, fibula
  - malleolus—*see* Fracture, ankle
  - patella—*see* Fracture, patella
  - specified site NEC S82.89-
  - tibia—*see* Fracture, tibia
- lumbosacral spine S32.9
- Maisonneuve's (displaced) S82.86-
  - nondisplaced S82.86-
- malar bone (*see also* Fracture) S02.40-
- malleolus—*see* Fracture, ankle
- malunion—*see* Fracture, by site
- mandible (lower jaw (bone)) S02.609-
  - alveolus S02.67-
  - angle (of jaw) S02.65-
  - body, unspecified S02.60-
  - condylar process S02.61-
  - coronoid process S02.63-
  - ramus, unspecified S02.64-
  - specified site NEC S02.69-
  - subcondylar process S02.62-
  - symphysis S02.66-
- march—*see* Fracture
- metacarpal S62.30-
  - base (displaced) S62.31-
    - nondisplaced S62.34-
  - fifth S62.30-
    - base (displaced) S62.31-
      - ~ nondisplaced S62.34-
    - neck (displaced) S62.33-
      - ~ nondisplaced S62.36-
    - shaft (displaced) S62.32-
      - ~ nondisplaced S62.35-
    - specified NEC S62.39-
  - first S62.20-
    - base NEC (displaced) S62.23-
      - ~ nondisplaced S62.23-
    - Bennett's—*see* Bennett's fracture
    - neck (displaced) S62.25-
      - ~ nondisplaced S62.25-
    - shaft (displaced) S62.24-
      - ~ nondisplaced S62.24-
    - specified NEC S62.29-
  - fourth S62.30-
    - base (displaced) S62.31-
      - ~ nondisplaced S62.34-
    - neck (displaced) S62.33-
      - ~ nondisplaced S62.36-

Fracture, *continued*

- shaft (displaced) S62.32-
  - ~ nondisplaced S62.35-
  - specified NEC S62.39-
- neck (displaced) S62.33-
  - nondisplaced S62.36-
- Rolando's—*see* Rolando's fracture
- second S62.30-
  - base (displaced) S62.31-
    - ~ nondisplaced S62.34-
  - neck (displaced) S62.33-
    - ~ nondisplaced S62.36-
  - shaft (displaced) S62.32-
    - ~ nondisplaced S62.35-
  - specified NEC S62.39-
- shaft (displaced) S62.32-
  - nondisplaced S62.35-
- third S62.30-
  - base (displaced) S62.31-
    - ~ nondisplaced S62.34-
  - neck (displaced) S62.33-
    - ~ nondisplaced S62.36-
  - shaft (displaced) S62.32-
    - ~ nondisplaced S62.35-
  - specified NEC S62.39-
- specified NEC S62.39-
- metatarsal bone S92.30-
  - fifth (displaced) S92.35-
    - nondisplaced S92.35-
  - first (displaced) S92.31-
    - nondisplaced S92.31-
  - fourth (displaced) S92.34-
    - nondisplaced S92.34-
  - physeal S99.10-
    - Salter-Harris
      - ~ Type I S99.11-
      - ~ Type II S99.12-
      - ~ Type III S99.13-
      - ~ Type IV S99.14-
  - second (displaced) S92.32-
    - nondisplaced S92.32-
  - third (displaced) S92.33-
    - nondisplaced S92.33-
    - specified NEC S99.19-
- Monteggia's—*see* Monteggia's fracture
- multiple
  - hand (and wrist) NEC—*see* Fracture, by site
  - ribs—*see* Fracture, rib, multiple
- nasal (bone(s)) S02.2-
- navicular (scaphoid) (foot)—*see also* Fracture, tarsal bone(s), navicular
  - hand—*see* Fracture, carpal bone(s), navicular
- neck S12.9
  - cervical vertebra S12.9
    - fifth (displaced) S12.400
      - ~ nondisplaced S12.401
    - first (displaced) S12.000
      - ~ burst (stable) S12.0-
        - ◊ unstable S12.0-
      - ~ nondisplaced S12.001
      - ~ posterior arch (displaced) S12.030
        - ◊ nondisplaced S12.031
    - fourth (displaced) S12.300
      - ~ nondisplaced S12.301
    - second (displaced) S12.100
      - ~ nondisplaced S12.101
    - seventh (displaced) S12.600
      - ~ nondisplaced S12.601~
    - sixth (displaced) S12.500
      - ~ nondisplaced S12.501
    - third (displaced) S12.200
      - ~ nondisplaced S12.201
  - hyoid bone S12.8
  - larynx S12.8
  - specified site NEC S12.8
  - thyroid cartilage S12.8
  - trachea S12.8
- newborn—*see* Birth, injury, fracture
- nonunion—*see* Nonunion, fracture
- nose, nasal (bone) (septum) S02.2-
- occiput—*see* Fracture, skull, base, occiput
- olecranon (process) (ulna)—*see* Fracture, ulna, upper end, olecranon process

Fracture, *continued*

- orbit, orbital (bone) (region) S02.85
  - calcis—*see* Fracture, tarsal bone(s), calcaneus
  - floor (blow-out) S02.3-
  - magnum—*see* Fracture, carpal bone(s), capitate
  - pubis—*see* Fracture, pubis
  - roof S02.12-
  - wall
    - lateral S02.83-
    - medial S02.84-
- palate S02.8-
- parietal bone (skull) S02.0-
- patella S82.00-
  - comminuted (displaced or nondisplaced) S82.04- (See complete *ICD-10-CM* Manual for codes)
  - longitudinal (displaced or nondisplaced) S82.02- (See complete *ICD-10-CM* Manual for codes)
  - osteochondral (displaced or nondisplaced) S82.01- (See complete *ICD-10-CM* Manual)
  - transverse (displaced or nondisplaced) S82.03- (See complete *ICD-10-CM* Manual for codes)
- pedicle (of vertebral arch)—*see* Fracture, vertebra
- pelvis, pelvic (bone) S32.9
  - acetabulum—*see* Fracture, acetabulum
  - ilium—*see* Fracture, ilium
  - ischium—*see* Fracture, ischium
  - multiple
    - without disruption of pelvic ring (circle) S32.82
  - pubis—*see* Fracture, pubis
  - specified site NEC S32.89
  - sacrum—*see* Fracture, sacrum
- phalanx
  - foot—*see* Fracture, toe
  - hand—*see* Fracture, finger
- pisiform—*see* Fracture, carpal bone(s), pisiform
- pond—*see* Fracture, skull
- prosthetic device, internal—*see* Complications, prosthetic device, by site, mechanical
- pubis S32.50-
  - with disruption of pelvic ring—*see* Disruption
  - specified site NEC S32.59-
  - superior rim S32.51-
- radius S52.9-
  - distal end—*see* Fracture, radius, lower end
  - head—*see* Fracture, radius, upper end, head
  - lower end S52.50-
    - Barton's—*see* Barton's fracture
    - Colles'—*see* Colles' fracture
    - extraarticular NEC S52.55-
    - intraarticular NEC S52.57-
    - physeal S59.20-
      - ~ Salter-Harris
        - ◊ Type I S59.21-
        - ◊ Type II S59.22-
        - ◊ Type III S59.23-
        - ◊ Type IV S59.24-
      - ~ specified NEC S59.29-
    - Smith's—*see* Smith's fracture
    - specified NEC S52.59-
    - styloid process (displaced) S52.51-
      - ~ nondisplaced S52.51-
    - torus S52.52-
  - neck—*see* Fracture, radius, upper end
  - proximal end—*see* Fracture, radius, upper end
  - shaft S52.30-
    - bent bone S52.38-
    - comminuted (displaced) S52.35-
      - ~ nondisplaced S52.35-
    - Galeazzi's—*see* Galeazzi's fracture
    - greenstick S52.31-
    - oblique (displaced) S52.33-
      - ~ nondisplaced S52.33-
    - segmental (displaced) S52.36-
      - ~ nondisplaced S52.36-
    - specified NEC S52.39-
    - spiral (displaced) S52.34-
      - ~ nondisplaced S52.34-
    - transverse (displaced) S52.32-
      - ~ nondisplaced S52.32-
  - upper end S52.10-
    - head (displaced) S52.12-
      - ~ nondisplaced S52.12-

Fracture, *continued*

- neck (displaced) S52.13-
  - ~ nondisplaced S52.13-
- specified NEC S52.18-
- physeal S59.10-
  - ~ Salter-Harris
    - ◊ Type I S59.11-
    - ◊ Type II S59.12-
    - ◊ Type III S59.13-
    - ◊ Type IV S59.14-
  - ~ specified NEC S59.19-
- torus S52.11-
- ramus
  - inferior or superior, pubis—*see* Fracture, pubis
  - mandible—*see* Fracture, mandible
- rib S22.3-
  - with flail chest—*see* Flail, chest
  - multiple S22.4-
    - with flail chest—*see* Flail, chest
- root, tooth—*see* Fracture, tooth
- sacrum S32.10
  - specified NEC S32.19
  - Type
    - 1 S32.14
    - 2 S32.15
    - 3 S32.16
    - 4 S32.17
  - Zone
    - I S32.119
      - ~ displaced (minimally) S32.111
        - ◊ severely S32.112
      - ~ nondisplaced S32.110
    - II S32.129
      - ~ displaced (minimally) S32.121
        - ◊ severely S32.122
      - ~ nondisplaced S32.120
    - III S32.139
      - ~ displaced (minimally) S32.131
        - ◊ severely S32.132
      - ~ nondisplaced S32.130
- scaphoid (hand)—*see also* Fracture, carpal bone(s), navicular
  - foot—*see* Fracture, tarsal, navicular
- semilunar bone, wrist—*see* Fracture, carpal, lunate
- sequela—*see* Sequelae
- sequelae—*see* Sequelae
- sesamoid bone
  - foot S92.81-
  - hand—*see* Fracture, carpal bone(s)
  - other—*code by* site under Fracture
- shepherd's—*see* Fracture, tarsal bone(s), talus
- shoulder (girdle) S42.9-
- sinus (ethmoid) (frontal) S02.19-
- skull S02.91-
  - base S02.10-
    - occiput S02.119
      - ~ condyle S02.11-
        - ◊ type I S02.11-
        - ◊ type II S02.11-
        - ◊ type III S02.11
      - ~ specified NEC S02.118-
    - specified NEC S02.19-
  - birth injury P13.0
  - frontal bone S02.0-
  - parietal bone S02.0-
  - specified site NEC S02.8-
  - temporal bone S02.19-
  - vault S02.0-
- Smith's—*see* Smith's fracture
- sphenoid (bone) (sinus) S02.19-
- stave (of thumb)—*see* Fracture, metacarpal, first
- sternum S22.20
  - with flail chest—*see* Flail, chest
  - body S22.22
  - manubrium S22.21
  - xiphoid (process) S22.24
- stress M84.30-
  - ankle M84.37-
  - carpus M84.34-
  - clavicle M84.31-
  - femoral neck M84.359
  - femur M84.35-
  - fibula M84.36-
  - finger M84.34-

Fracture, *continued*
- hip M84.359
- humerus M84.32-
- ilium M84.350
- ischium M84.350
- metacarpus M84.34-
- metatarsus M84.37-
- pelvis M84.350
- radius M84.33-
- rib M84.38
- scapula M84.31-
- skull M84.38
- tarsus M84.37-
- tibia M84.36-
- toe M84.37-
- ulna M84.33-
- supracondylar, elbow—*see* Fracture, humerus, lower end, supracondylar
- symphysis pubis—*see* Fracture, pubis
- talus (ankle bone)—*see* Fracture, tarsal bone(s), talus
- tarsal bone(s) S92.20-
  - astragalus—*see* Fracture, tarsal bone(s), talus
  - calcaneus S92.00-
    - anterior process (displaced) S92.02-
      - ~ nondisplaced S92.02-
    - body (displaced) S92.01-
      - ~ nondisplaced S92.01-
    - extraarticular NEC (displaced) S92.05-
      - ~ nondisplaced S92.05-
    - intraarticular (displaced) S92.06-
      - ~ nondisplaced S92.06-
    - physeal S99.00-
      - ~ Salter-Harris
        - ◊ Type I S99.01-
        - ◊ Type II S99.02-
        - ◊ Type III S99.03-
        - ◊ Type IV S99.04-
      - ~ specified NEC S99.09-
    - tuberosity (displaced) S92.04-
      - ~ avulsion (displaced) S92.03-
        - ◊ nondisplaced S92.03-
      - ~ nondisplaced S92.04-
  - cuboid (displaced) S92.21-
    - nondisplaced S92.21-
  - cuneiform
    - intermediate (displaced) S92.23-
      - ~ nondisplaced S92.23-
    - lateral (displaced) S92.22-
      - ~ nondisplaced S92.22-
    - medial (displaced) S92.24-
      - ~ nondisplaced S92.24-
  - navicular (displaced) S92.25-
    - nondisplaced S92.25-
  - scaphoid—*see* Fracture, tarsal bone(s), navicular
  - talus S92.10-
    - avulsion (displaced) S92.15-
      - ~ nondisplaced S92.15-
    - body (displaced) S92.12-
      - ~ nondisplaced S92.12-
    - dome (displaced) S92.14-
      - ~ nondisplaced S92.14-
    - head (displaced) S92.12-
      - ~ nondisplaced S92.12-
    - lateral process (displaced) S92.14-
      - ~ nondisplaced S92.14-
    - neck (displaced) S92.11-
      - ~ nondisplaced S92.11-
    - posterior process (displaced) S92.13-
      - ~ nondisplaced S92.13-
    - specified NEC S92.19-
- temporal bone (styloid) S02.19-
- thorax (bony) S22.9
  - with flail chest—*see* Flail, chest
  - rib S22.3-
    - multiple S22.4-
      - ~ with flail chest—*see* Flail, chest
- thumb S62.50-
  - distal phalanx (displaced) S62.52-
    - nondisplaced S62.52-
  - proximal phalanx (displaced) S62.51-
    - nondisplaced S62.51-
- thyroid cartilage S12.8

Fracture, *continued*
- tibia (shaft) S82.20-
  - comminuted (displaced or nondisplaced) S82.25- (See complete *ICD-10-CM* Manual)
  - condyles—*see* Fracture, tibia
  - distal end—*see* Fracture, tibia
  - epiphysis
    - lower—*see* Fracture, tibia
    - upper—*see* Fracture, tibia
  - head (involving knee joint)—*see* Fracture, tibia
  - intercondyloid eminence—*see* Fracture, tibia
  - involving ankle or malleolus—*see* Fracture, ankle, medial malleolus
  - lower end S82.30-
    - physeal S89.10-
      - ~ Salter-Harris
        - ◊ Type I S89.11-
        - ◊ Type II S89.12-
        - ◊ Type III S89.13-
        - ◊ Type IV S89.14-
      - ~ specified NEC S89.19-
    - pilon (displaced) S82.87-
      - ~ nondisplaced S82.87-
    - specified NEC S82.39-
    - torus S82.31-
  - malleolus—*see* Fracture, ankle, medial malleolus
  - oblique (displaced or nondisplaced) S82.23- - (See complete *ICD-10-CM* Manual)
  - pilon—*see* Fracture, tibia
  - proximal end—*see* Fracture, tibia
  - segmental (displaced or nondisplaced) S82.26- - (See complete *ICD-10-CM* Manual)
  - spiral (displaced) S82.24-
    - nondisplaced S82.24-
  - transverse (displaced or nondisplaced) S82.22- - (See complete *ICD-10-CM* Manual)
  - tuberosity—*see* Fracture, tibia
  - upper end S82.10-
    - bicondylar (displaced) or nondisplaced) S82.14— (See complete *ICD-10-CM* Manual)
    - lateral condyle (displaced) or nondisplaced) S82.12—(See complete *ICD-10-CM* Manual)
    - medial condyle (displaced) or nondisplaced) S82.13—(See complete *ICD-10-CM* Manual)
    - physeal S89.00-
      - ~ Salter-Harris
        - ◊ Type I S89.01-
        - ◊ Type II S89.02-
        - ◊ Type III S89.03-
        - ◊ Type IV S89.04-
      - ~ specified NEC S89.09-
    - plateau—*see* Fracture, tibiar
    - spine (displaced or nondisplaced) S82.11- (See complete *ICD-10-CM* Manual)
    - torus S82.16-
    - specified NEC S82.19-
    - tuberosity (displacedor nondisplaced) S82.15- (See complete *ICD-10-CM* Manual)
- toe S92.91-
  - great (displaced) S92.4-
    - distal phalanx (displaced) S92.42-
      - ~ nondisplaced S92.42-
    - nondisplaced S92.4-
    - proximal phalanx (displaced) S92.41-
      - ~ nondisplaced S92.41-
    - specified NEC S92.49-
  - lesser (displaced) S92.5-
    - distal phalanx (displaced) S92.53-
      - ~ nondisplaced S92.53-
    - middle phalanx (displaced) S92.52-
      - ~ nondisplaced S92.52-
    - nondisplaced S92.5-
    - proximal phalanx (displaced) S92.51-
      - ~ nondisplaced S92.51-
    - specified NEC S92.59-
- tooth (root) S02.5-
- trachea (cartilage) S12.8
- trapezium or trapezoid bone—*see* Fracture, carpal bone(s)
- trimalleolar—*see* Fracture, ankle, trimalleolar
- triquetrum (cuneiform of carpus)—*see* Fracture, carpal bone(s), triquetrum
- trochanter—*see* Fracture, femur

Fracture, *continued*
- tuberosity (external)—*code by* site under Fracture
- ulna (shaft) S52.20-
  - bent bone S52.28-
  - coronoid process—*see* Fracture, ulna, upper end, coronoid process
  - distal end—*see* Fracture, ulna, lower end
  - head S52.60-
  - lower end S52.60-
    - physeal S59.00-
      - ~ Salter-Harris
        - ◊ Type I S59.01-
        - ◊ Type II S59.02-
        - ◊ Type III S59.03-
        - ◊ Type IV S59.04-
      - ~ specified NEC S59.09-
    - specified NEC S52.69-
    - styloid process (displaced) S52.61-
      - ~ nondisplaced S52.61-
    - torus S52.62-
  - proximal end—*see* Fracture, ulna, upper end
  - shaft S52.20-
    - comminuted (displaced) S52.25-
      - ~ nondisplaced S52.25-
    - greenstick S52.21-
    - Monteggia's—*see* Monteggia's fracture
    - oblique (displaced) S52.23-
      - ~ nondisplaced S52.23-
    - segmental (displaced) S52.26-
      - ~ nondisplaced S52.26-
    - specified NEC S52.29-
    - spiral (displaced) S52.24-
      - ~ nondisplaced S52.24-
    - transverse (displaced) S52.22-
      - ~ nondisplaced S52.22-
  - upper end S52.00-
    - coronoid process (displaced) S52.04-
      - ~ nondisplaced S52.04-
    - olecranon process (displaced) S52.02-
      - ~ with intraarticular extension S52.03-
      - ~ nondisplaced S52.02-
        - ◊ with intraarticular extension S52.03-
    - specified NEC S52.09-
    - torus S52.01-
- unciform—*see* Fracture, carpal bone(s), hamate
- vault of skull S02.0-
- vertebra, vertebral (arch) (body) (column) (neural arch) (pedicle) (spinous process) (transverse process)
  - atlas—*see* Fracture, neck, cervical vertebra, first
  - axis—*see* Fracture, neck, cervical vertebra, second
  - cervical (teardrop) S12.9
    - axis—*see* Fracture, neck, cervical vertebra, second
    - first (atlas)—*see* Fracture, neck, cervical vertebra, first
    - second (axis)—*see* Fracture, neck, cervical vertebra, second
- vertex S02.0-
- vomer (bone) S02.2-
- wrist S62.10-
  - carpal—*see* Fracture, carpal bone
  - navicular (scaphoid) (hand)—*see* Fracture, carpal bone(s), navicular
- zygoma S02.402
  - left side S02.40F
  - right side S02.40E

Fragile, fragility
- bone, congenital (with blue sclera) Q78.0
- X chromosome Q99.2

Fragilitas
- ossium (with blue sclerae) (hereditary) Q78.0

Frank's essential thrombocytopenia D69.3

Fraser's syndrome Q87.0

Freckle(s) L81.2

Frederickson's hyperlipoproteinemia, type
- IIA E78.0
- IIB and III E78.2

Freeman Sheldon syndrome Q87.0

Frenum, frenulum
- tongue (shortening) (congenital) Q38.1

Frequency micturition (nocturnal) R35.0
- psychogenic F45.8

Friction
- burn—*see* Burn, by site
- sounds, chest R09.89

Friedreich's
- ataxia G11.11
- combined systemic disease G11.11
- facial hemihypertrophy Q67.4
- sclerosis (cerebellum) (spinal cord) G11.11

Fröhlich's syndrome E23.6

Fucosidosis E77.1

Fugue R68.89
- reaction to exceptional stress (transient) F43.0

Fulminant, fulminating—*see* Disease, diseased

Functional—*see also* Disease, diseased
- bleeding (uterus) N93.8

Fungus, fungous
- cerebral G93.89
- disease NOS B49
- infection—*see* Infection, fungus

Funnel
- breast (acquired) M95.4
  - congenital Q67.6
- chest (acquired) M95.4
  - congenital Q67.6
- pelvis (acquired) M95.5
  - congenital Q74.2

FUO (fever of unknown origin) R50.9

Furfur L21.0
- microsporon B36.0

Furuncle L02.92
- abdominal wall L02.221
- ankle L02.42-
- anus K61.0
- axilla (region) L02.42-
- back (any part) L02.222
- breast N61.1
- buttock L02.32
- cheek (external) L02.02
- chest wall L02.223
- chin L02.02
- face L02.02
- flank L02.221
- foot L02.62-
- forehead L02.02
- gluteal (region) L02.32
- groin L02.224
- hand L02.52-
- head L02.821
  - face L02.02
- hip L02.42-
- knee L02.42-
- leg (any part) L02.42-
- lower limb L02.42-
- malignant A22.0
- mouth K12.2
- navel L02.226
- neck L02.12
- nose J34.0
- partes posteriores L02.32
- pectoral region L02.223
- perineum L02.225
- scalp L02.821
- specified site NEC L02.828
- submandibular K12.2
- temple (region) L02.02
- thumb L02.52-
- toe L02.62-
- trunk L02.229
  - abdominal wall L02.221
  - back L02.222
  - chest wall L02.223
  - groin L02.224
  - perineum L02.225
  - umbilicus L02.226
- umbilicus L02.226
- upper limb L02.42-
- vulva N76.4

Fusion, fused (congenital)
- astragaloscaphoid Q74.2
- atria Q21.1

Fusion, fused, *continued*
- auricles, heart Q21.1
- choanal Q30.0
- cusps, heart valve NEC Q24.8
  - pulmonary Q22.1
- fingers Q70.0-
- hymen Q52.3
- limb, congenital Q74.8
  - lower Q74.2
  - upper Q74.0
- nares, nose, nasal, nostril(s) Q30.0
- ossicles Q79.9
  - auditory Q16.3
- pulmonic cusps Q22.1
- sacroiliac (joint) (acquired) M43.28
  - congenital Q74.2
- toes Q70.2
- ventricles, heart Q21.0

Fussy baby R68.12

G

Gain in weight (abnormal) (excessive)—*see also* Weight, gain

Gaisböck's disease (polycythemia hypertonica) D75.1

Gait abnormality R26.9
- ataxic R26.0
- hysterical (ataxic) (staggering) F44.4
- paralytic R26.1
- spastic R26.1
- specified type NEC R26.89
- staggering R26.0
- unsteadiness R26.81
- walking difficulty NEC R26.2

Galactocele (breast)
- puerperal, postpartum O92.79

Galactophoritis N61.0

Galactorrhea O92.6
- not associated with childbirth N64.3

GALD (gestational alloimmune liver disease) P78.84

Galeazzi's fracture S52.37-

Gallbladder—*see also* Disease, diseased
- acute K81.0

Gambling Z72.6

Ganglion (compound) (diffuse) (joint) (tendon (sheath)) M67.40
- ankle M67.47-
- foot M67.47-
- forearm M67.43-
- hand M67.44-
- lower leg M67.46-
- multiple sites M67.49
- pelvic region M67.45-
- shoulder region M67.41-
- specified site NEC M67.48
- thigh region M67.45-
- upper arm M67.42-
- wrist M67.43-

Ganglionitis
- newborn (birth injury) P11.3

Gangliosidosis E75.10
- GM2 E75.00
  - Sandhoff disease E75.01
  - Tay-Sachs disease E75.02

Gangrene, gangrenous (connective tissue) (dropsical) (dry) (moist) (skin) (ulcer) (*see also* Necrosis)
- appendix K35.80
  - with
    - peritonitis, localized (*see also* Appendicitis) K35.31
- epididymis (infectional) N45.1
- erysipelas—*see* Erysipelas
- glossitis K14.0
- laryngitis J04.0
- pancreas
  - idiopathic
    - infected K85.02
    - uninfected K85.01
  - infected K85.82
  - uninfected K85.81

Gangrene, gangrenous, *continued*
- quinsy J36
- testis (infectional) N45.2
  - noninfective N44.8
- uvulitis K12.2

Gardner-Diamond syndrome (autoerythrocyte sensitization) D69.2

Gargoylism E76.01

Gartner's duct
- cyst Q52.4
- persistent Q50.6

Gas R14.3
- excessive R14.0
- on stomach R14.0
- pains R14.1

Gastrectasis K31.0
- psychogenic F45.8

Gastric—*see* Disease, diseased

Gastritis (simple) K29.70
- with bleeding K29.71
- acute (erosive) K29.00
  - with bleeding K29.01
- dietary counseling and surveillance Z71.3
- eosinophilic K52.81
- viral NEC A08.4

Gastroduodenitis K29.90
- with bleeding K29.91
- virus, viral A08.4
  - specified type NEC A08.39

Gastroenteritis (acute) (chronic) (noninfectious) (*see also* Enteritis) K52.9
- allergic K52.29
  - with
    - eosinophilic gastritis or gastroenteritis K52.81
    - food protein-induced enterocolitis syndrome K52.21
    - food protein-induced enteropathy K52.22
- dietetic K52.29
- eosinophilic K52.81
- epidemic (infectious) A09
- food hypersensitivity K52.29
- infectious—*see* Enteritis, infectious
- noninfectious K52.9
  - specified NEC K52.89
- rotaviral A08.0
- Salmonella A02.0
- viral NEC A08.4
  - acute infectious A08.39
  - infantile (acute) A08.39
  - rotaviral A08.0
  - severe of infants A08.39
  - specified type NEC A08.39

Gastroenteropathy (*see also* Gastroenteritis) K52.9
- infectious A09

Gastrojejunitis (*see also* Enteritis) K52.9

Gastropathy K31.9
- erythematous K29.70
- exudative K90.89

Gastrorrhagia K92.2
- psychogenic F45.8

Gastroschisis (congenital) Q79.3

Gastrospasm (neurogenic) (reflex) K31.89
- neurotic F45.8
- psychogenic F45.8

Gastrostomy
- attention to Z43.1
- status Z93.1

Gee (-Herter) (-Thaysen) disease (nontropical sprue) K90.0

Gemistocytoma
- specified site—*see* Neoplasm, malignant, by site in Table of Neoplasms in the complete *ICD-10-CM* manual
- unspecified site C71.9

General, generalized—*see* Disease, diseased

Genetic
- carrier (status)
  - cystic fibrosis Z14.1
  - hemophilia A (asymptomatic) Z14.01
    - symptomatic Z14.02
  - specified NEC Z14.8

Genu
- congenital Q74.1
- extrorsum (acquired) M21.16-
  - congenital Q74.1
- introrsum (acquired) M21.06-
  - congenital Q74.1
- recurvatum (acquired) M21.86-
  - congenital Q68.2
- valgum (acquired) (knock-knee) M21.06-
  - congenital Q74.1
- varum (acquired) (bowleg) M21.16-
  - congenital Q74.1

Geographic tongue K14.1

Geophagia—*see* Pica

Gerbode defect Q21.0

GERD (gastroesophageal reflux disease) K21.9

Gerhardt's
- syndrome (vocal cord paralysis) J38.00
  - bilateral J38.02
  - unilateral J38.01

German measles—*see also* Rubella
- exposure to Z20.4

Germinoblastoma (diffuse) C85.9-

Gerstmann's syndrome R48.8
- developmental F81.2

Gianotti-Crosti disease L44.4

Giant
- urticaria T78.3

Giardiasis A07.1

Gibert's disease or pityriasis L42

Giddiness R42
- hysterical F44.89
- psychogenic F45.8

Gigantism (cerebral) (hypophyseal) (pituitary) E22.0
- constitutional E34.4

Gilbert's disease or syndrome E80.4

Gilles de la Tourette's disease or syndrome (motor-verbal tic) F95.2

Gingivitis
- acute (catarrhal) K05.00
  - plaque induced K05.00

Gingivoglossitis K14.0

Gingivostomatitis
- herpesviral B00.2

Glaucoma
- childhood Q15.0
- congenital Q15.0
- in (due to)
  - endocrine disease NOS E34.9 [H42]
  - Lowe's syndrome E72.03 [H42]
  - metabolic disease NOS E88.9 [H42]
- infantile Q15.0
- newborn Q15.0
- secondary (to)
  - trauma H40.3-
- traumatic—*see also* Glaucoma, secondary, trauma
  - newborn (birth injury) P15.3

Gleet (gonococcal) A54.01

Glioblastoma (multiforme)
- with sarcomatous component
  - specified site—*see* Neoplasm, malignant, by site in Table of Neoplasms in the complete *ICD-10-CM* manual
  - unspecified site C71.9
- giant cell
  - specified site—*see* Neoplasm, malignant, by site in Table of Neoplasms in the complete *ICD-10-CM* manual
  - unspecified site C71.9
- specified site—*see* Neoplasm, malignant, by site in Table of Neoplasms in the complete *ICD-10-CM* manual
- unspecified site C71.9

Glioma (malignant)
- astrocytic
  - specified site—*see* Neoplasm, malignant, by site in Table of Neoplasms in the complete *ICD-10-CM* manual

Glioma, *continued*
- unspecified site C71.9
- mixed
  - specified site—*see* Neoplasm, malignant, by site in Table of Neoplasms in the complete *ICD-10-CM* manual
  - unspecified site C71.9
- nose Q30.8
- specified site NEC—*see* Neoplasm, malignant, by site in Table of Neoplasms in the complete *ICD-10-CM* manual
  - specified site—*see* Neoplasm, uncertain behavior, by site in Table of Neoplasms in the complete *ICD-10-CM* manual
- unspecified site C71.9

Gliosarcoma
- specified site—*see* Neoplasm, malignant, by site in Table of Neoplasms in the complete *ICD-10-CM* manual
- unspecified site C71.9

Gliosis (cerebral) G93.89

Globinuria R82.3

Globus (hystericus) F45.8

Glomangioma D18.00
- skin D18.01
- specified site NEC D18.09

Glomangiomyoma D18.00
- intra-abdominal D18.03
- intracranial D18.02
- skin D18.01
- specified site NEC D18.09

Glomerulonephritis (*see also* Nephritis) N05.9
- with
  - C3
    - glomerulonephritis N05.A
    - glomerulopathy N05.A
      ~ with dense deposit disease N05.6
  - edema—*see* Nephrosis
  - minimal change N05.0
  - minor glomerular abnormality N05.0
- acute N00.9
- chronic N03.9
- in (due to)
  - defibrination syndrome D65 [N08]
  - disseminated intravascular coagulation D65 [N08]
  - hemolytic-uremic syndrome D59.3
  - Henoch (-Schönlein) purpura D69.0 [N08]
  - sepsis A41.9 [N08]
    - streptococcal A40- [N08]
  - subacute bacterial endocarditis I33.0 [N08]
  - systemic lupus erythematosus M32.14
- poststreptococcal NEC N05.9
  - acute N00.9
  - chronic N03.9
- proliferative NEC (*see also* N00-N07 with fourth character .8) N05.8
  - diffuse (lupus) M32.14

Glossitis (chronic superficial) (gangrenous) (Moeller's) K14.0
- areata exfoliativa K14.1
- benign migratory K14.1
- cortical superficial, sclerotic K14.0
- interstitial, sclerous K14.0
- superficial, chronic K14.0

Glottitis (*see also* Laryngitis) J04.0

Glue
- ear H65.3-
- sniffing (airplane)—*see* Abuse, drug
  - dependence—*see* Dependence, drug
- GLUT1 deficiency syndrome 1, infantile onset E74.810
- GLUT1 deficiency syndrome 2, childhood onset E74.810

Glycogenosis (diffuse) (generalized)
- pulmonary interstitial J84.842

Glycopenia E16.2

Glycosuria R81
- renal E74.818

Goiter (plunging) (substernal) E04.9
- with
  - hyperthyroidism (recurrent)—*see* Hyperthyroidism, with, goiter
  - thyrotoxicosis—*see* Hyperthyroidism, with, goiter

Goiter, *continued*
- adenomatous—*see* Goiter, nodular
- congenital
  - transitory, with normal functioning P72.0
- due to
  - iodine-deficiency (endemic) E01.2
- endemic (iodine-deficiency) E01.2
  - diffuse E01.0
  - multinodular E01.1
- iodine-deficiency (endemic) E01.2
  - diffuse E01.0
  - multinodular E01.1
  - nodular E01.1
- lingual Q89.2
- lymphadenoid E06.3
- neonatal NEC P72.0
- nodular (nontoxic) (due to) E04.9
  - endemic E01.1
  - iodine-deficiency E01.1
  - sporadic E04.9
- nontoxic E04.9
  - diffuse (colloid) E04.0
  - multinodular E04.2
  - simple E04.0
  - specified NEC E04.8
  - uninodular E04.1
- simple E04.0

Goldberg syndrome Q89.8

Goldberg-Maxwell syndrome E34.51

Goldenhar (-Gorlin) syndrome Q87.0

Goldflam-Erb disease or syndrome G70.00
- with exacerbation (acute) G70.01
- in crisis G70.01

Goldscheider's disease Q81.8

Goldstein's disease (familial hemorrhagic telangiectasia) I78.0

Gonococcus, gonococcal (disease) (infection) (*see also* Disease, diseased) A54.9
- conjunctiva, conjunctivitis (neonatorum) A54.31
- eye A54.30
  - conjunctivitis A54.31
  - newborn A54.31
- fallopian tubes (acute) (chronic) A54.24
- genitourinary (organ) (system) (tract) (acute)
  - lower A54.00
- pelviperitonitis A54.24
- pelvis (acute) (chronic) A54.24
- pyosalpinx (acute) (chronic) A54.24
- urethra (acute) (chronic) A54.01
  - with abscess (accessory gland) (periurethral) A54.1
- vulva (acute) (chronic) A54.02

Gonorrhea (acute) (chronic) A54.9
- Bartholin's gland (acute) (chronic) (purulent) A54.02
  - with abscess (accessory gland) (periurethral) A54.1
- bladder A54.01
- cervix A54.03
- conjunctiva, conjunctivitis (neonatorum) A54.31
- contact Z20.2
- exposure to Z20.2
- fallopian tube A54.24
- lower genitourinary tract A54.00
- ovary (acute) (chronic) A54.24
- pelvis (acute) (chronic) A54.24
  - female pelvic inflammatory disease A54.24
- urethra A54.01
- vagina A54.02
- vulva A54.02

Gorlin-Chaudry-Moss syndrome Q87.0

Gougerot-Carteaud disease or syndrome (confluent reticulate papillomatosis) L83

Gouley's syndrome (constrictive pericarditis) I31.1

Gout, gouty (acute) (attack) (flare)—*see also* Gout M10.9
- idiopathic M10.0-
  - ankle M10.07-
  - elbow M10.02-
  - foot joint M10.07-
  - hand joint M10.04-
  - hip M10.05-
  - knee M10.06-
  - multiple site M10.09

Gout, gouty (acute) (attack) (flare), *continued*
- – shoulder M10.01-
- – vertebrae M10.08

Gower's
- muscular dystrophy G71.01
- syndrome (vasovagal attack) R55

Graft-versus-host disease D89.813
- acute D89.810
- acute on chronic D89.812
- chronic D89.811

Grain mite (itch) B88.0

Granular—*see also* Disease, diseased
- inflammation, pharynx J31.2

Granuloma L92.9
- abdomen
  - – from residual foreign body L92.3
  - – pyogenicum L98.0
- annulare (perforating) L92.0
- beryllium (skin) L92.3
- brain (any site) G06.0
- candidal (cutaneous) B37.2
- cerebral (any site) G06.0
- foreign body (in soft tissue) NEC M60.2-
  - – ankle M60.27-
  - – foot M60.27-
  - – forearm M60.23-
  - – hand M60.24-
  - – lower leg M60.26-
  - – pelvic region M60.25-
  - – shoulder region M60.21-
  - – skin L92.3
  - – specified site NEC M60.28
  - – subcutaneous tissue L92.3
  - – thigh M60.25-
  - – upper arm M60.22-
- gland (lymph) I88.8
- hepatic NEC K75.3
  - – in (due to)
    - ■ sarcoidosis D86.89
- Hodgkin C81.9-
- intracranial (any site) G06.0
- monilial (cutaneous) B37.2
- operation wound T81.89
  - – foreign body—*see* Foreign body
  - – stitch T81.89
- orbit, orbital H05.11-
- pyogenic, pyogenicum (of) (skin) L98.0
- rectum K62.89
- reticulohistiocytic D76.3
- septic (skin) L98.0
- silica (skin) L92.3
- skin L92.9
  - – from residual foreign body L92.3
  - – pyogenicum L98.0
- stitch (postoperative) T81.89
- suppurative (skin) L98.0
- telangiectaticum (skin) L98.0
- umbilical (umbilicus) P83.81

Granulomatosis L92.9
- with polyangiitis M31.3
- eosinophilic, with polyangiitis [EGPA] M30.1
- progressive septic D71

Grawitz tumor C64.-

Green sickness D50.8

Grief F43.21
- prolonged F43.29
- reaction (*see also* Disorder, adjustment) F43.20

Grinding, teeth
- psychogenic F45.8
- sleep related G47.63

Grisel's disease M43.6

Growing pains, children R29.898

Growth (fungoid) (neoplastic) (new)—*see also* Table of Neoplasms in the complete *ICD-10-CM* manual
- adenoid (vegetative) J35.8
- benign—*see* Neoplasm, benign, by site in Table of Neoplasms in the complete *ICD-10-CM* manual
- malignant—*see* Neoplasm, malignant, by site in Table of Neoplasms in the complete *ICD-10-CM* manual

Growth, *continued*
- rapid, childhood Z00.2
- secondary—*see* Neoplasm, secondary, by site in Table of Neoplasms in the complete *ICD-10-CM* manual

Gruby's disease B35.0

Guerin-Stern syndrome Q74.3

Guinon's disease (motor-verbal tic) F95.2

Gumboil K04.7

Gynecological examination (periodic) (routine) Z01.419
- with abnormal findings Z01.411

Gynecomastia N62

Gyrate scalp Q82.8

H

Haemophilus (H.) influenzae, as cause of disease classified elsewhere B96.3

Hailey-Hailey disease Q82.8

Hair—*see also* Disease, diseased
- plucking F63.3
  - – in stereotyped movement disorder F98.4
- tourniquet syndrome—*see also* Constriction, external, by site
  - – finger S60.44-
  - – penis S30.842
  - – thumb S60.34-
  - – toe S90.44-

Hairball in stomach T18.2

Hair-pulling, pathological (compulsive) F63.3

Halitosis R19.6

Hallerman-Streiff syndrome Q87.0

Hallucination R44.3
- auditory R44.0
- gustatory R44.2
- olfactory R44.2
- specified NEC R44.2
- tactile R44.2
- visual R44.1

Hallux
- deformity (acquired) NEC M20.5X-
- limitus M20.5X-
- rigidus congenital Q74.2
- valgus (acquired) M20.1-
  - – congenital Q66.6
- varus congenital Q66.3-

Hamartoma, hamartoblastoma Q85.9

Hamartosis Q85.9

Hammer toe (acquired) NEC—*see also* Deformity, toe, hammer toe
- congenital Q66.89

Hand-foot syndrome L27.1

Handicap, handicapped
- educational Z55.9
  - – specified NEC Z55.8

Hangover (alcohol) F10.129

Hanhart's syndrome Q87.0

Hardening
- brain G93.89

Harelip (complete) (incomplete)—*see* Cleft, lip

Harlequin (newborn) Q80.4

Harmful use (of)
- alcohol F10.10
- cannabinoids—*see* Abuse, drug, cannabis
- cocaine—*see* Abuse, drug, cocaine
- drug—*see* Abuse, drug
- hallucinogens—*see* Abuse, drug
- PCP (phencyclidine)—*see* Abuse, drug

Hashimoto's (struma lymphomatosa) E06.3

Hashitoxicosis (transient) E06.3

Haverhill fever A25.1

Hay fever (*see also* Fever, hay) J30.1

Hb (abnormal)
- Bart's disease D56.0
- disease—*see* Disease, hemoglobin
- trait—*see* Trait

Head—*see* Disease, diseased

Headache R51.9
- with
  - – orthostatic component NEC R51.0
  - – positional component NEC R51.0
- chronic daily R51.9
- cluster G44.009
  - – intractable G44.001
  - – not intractable G44.009
- daily chronic R51.9
- histamine G44.009
  - – intractable G44.001
  - – not intractable G44.009
- migraine (type)—*see also* Migraine G43.909
- nasal septum R51.9
- periodic syndromes in adults and children G43.C0
  - – with refractory migraine G43.C1
  - – intractable G43.C1
  - – not intractable G43.C0
  - – without refractory migraine G43.C0
- tension (-type) G44.209
  - – chronic G44.229
    - ■ intractable G44.221
    - ■ not intractable G44.229
  - – episodic G44.219
    - ■ intractable G44.211
    - ■ not intractable G44.219
  - – intractable G44.201
  - – not intractable G44.209

Hearing examination Z01.10
- abnormal findings NEC Z01.118
- following failed hearing screening Z01.110
- for hearing conservation and treatment Z01.12
- infant or child (over 28 days old) Z00.12-

Heart—*see* condition

Heart beat
- abnormality R00.9
  - – specified NEC R00.8
- awareness R00.2
- rapid R00.0
- slow R00.1

Heartburn R12
- psychogenic F45.8

Heat (effects) T67.9
- apoplexy T67.01
- burn (*see also* Burn) L55.9
- cramps T67.2
- exertional T67.02
- exhaustion T67.5
  - – anhydrotic T67.3
  - – due to
    - ■ salt (and water) depletion T67.4
    - ■ water depletion T67.3
      - ~ with salt depletion T67.4
- fatigue (transient) T67.6
- fever T67.01
- hyperpyrexia T67.01
- prickly L74.0
- pyrexia T67.01
- rash L74.0
- stroke T67.01
  - – exertional T67.02
  - – specified NEC T67.09
- syncope T67.1

Heavy-for-dates NEC (infant) (4000g to 4499g) P08.1
- exceptionally (4500g or more) P08.0

Heerfordt's disease D86.89

Hegglin's anomaly or syndrome D72.0

Heinz body anemia, congenital D58.2

Heloma L84

Hemangioendothelioma—*see also* Neoplasm, uncertain behavior, by site in Table of Neoplasms in the complete *ICD-10-CM* manual
- benign D18.00
  - – skin D18.01
  - – specified site NEC D18.09
- bone (diffuse)—*see* Neoplasm, bone, malignant in Table of Neoplasms in the complete *ICD-10-CM* manual

Hemangioendothelioma, *continued*
- epithelioid—*see also* Neoplasm, uncertain behavior, by site in Table of Neoplasms in the complete *ICD-10-CM* manual
  - malignant—*see* Neoplasm, malignant, by site in Table of Neoplasms in the complete *ICD-10-CM* manual
- malignant—*see* Neoplasm, connective tissue, malignant in Table of Neoplasms in the complete *ICD-10-CM* manual

Hemangiofibroma—*see* Neoplasm, benign, by site in Table of Neoplasms in the complete *ICD-10-CM* manual

Hemangiolipoma—*see* Lipoma

Hemangioma D18.00
- arteriovenous D18.00
  - skin D18.01
  - specified site NEC D18.09
- capillary I78.1
  - skin D18.01
  - specified site NEC D18.09
- cavernous D18.00
  - skin D18.01
  - specified site NEC D18.09
- epithelioid D18.00
  - skin D18.01
  - specified site NEC D18.09
- histiocytoid D18.00
  - skin D18.01
  - specified site NEC D18.09
- infantile D18.00
  - skin D18.01
  - specified site NEC D18.09
- intramuscular D18.00
  - skin D18.01
  - specified site NEC D18.09
- juvenile D18.00
- malignant—*see* Neoplasm, connective tissue, malignant in Table of Neoplasms in the complete *ICD-10-CM* manual
- plexiform D18.00
  - skin D18.01
  - specified site NEC D18.09
- racemose D18.00
  - skin D18.01
  - specified site NEC D18.09
- sclerosing—*see* Neoplasm, skin, benign in Table of Neoplasms in the complete *ICD-10-CM* manual
- simplex D18.00
  - skin D18.01
  - specified site NEC D18.09
- skin D18.01
- specified site NEC D18.09
- venous D18.00
  - skin D18.01
  - specified site NEC D18.09
- verrucous keratotic D18.00
  - skin D18.01
  - specified site NEC D18.09

Hemangiomatosis (systemic) I78.8
- involving single site—*see* Hemangioma

Hemarthrosis (nontraumatic) M25.00
- ankle M25.07-
- elbow M25.02-
- foot joint M25.07-
- hand joint M25.04-
- hip M25.05-
- in hemophilic arthropathy—*see* Arthropathy, hemophilic
- knee M25.06-
- shoulder M25.01-
- specified joint NEC M25.08
- traumatic—*see* Sprain, by site
- vertebrae M25.08
- wrist M25.03

Hematemesis K92.0
- with ulcer—*code by* site under Ulcer, with hemorrhage K27.4
- newborn, neonatal P54.0
  - due to swallowed maternal blood P78.2

Hematocele
- female NEC N94.89
  - with ectopic pregnancy O00.90
    - with uterine pregnancy O00.91

Hematochezia (*see also* Melena) K92.1

Hematoma (traumatic) (skin surface intact)—*see also* Contusion
- with
  - injury of internal organs—*see* Injury, by site
  - open wound—*see* Wound, open
- auricle—*see* Contusion, ear
  - nontraumatic—*see* Disorder
- birth injury NEC P15.8
- brain (traumatic)
  - with
    - cerebral laceration or contusion (diffuse)—*see* Injury, intracranial, diffuse
  - cerebellar, traumatic S06.37-
  - newborn NEC P52.4
    - birth injury P10.1
  - intracerebral, traumatic—*see* Injury, intracranial, intracerebral hemorrhage
  - nontraumatic—*see* Hemorrhage, intracranial
  - subarachnoid, arachnoid, traumatic—*see* Injury, intracranial, subarachnoid hemorrhage
  - subdural, traumatic—*see* Injury, intracranial, subdural hemorrhage
- breast (nontraumatic) N64.89
- cerebral—*see* Hematoma, brain
- cerebrum
  - left S06.35-
  - right S06.34-
- face, birth injury P15.4
- genital organ NEC (nontraumatic)
  - female (nonobstetric) N94.89
    - traumatic S30.202
- internal organs—*see* Injury, by site
- intracerebral, traumatic—*see* Injury, intracranial, intracerebral hemorrhage
- intraoperative—*see* Complications
- labia (nontraumatic) (nonobstetric) N90.89
- pelvis (female) (nontraumatic) (nonobstetric) N94.89
  - traumatic—*see* Injury, by site
- perianal (nontraumatic) K64.5
- pinna H61.12-
- superficial, newborn P54.5
- vagina (ruptured) (nontraumatic) N89.8

Hematomyelitis G04.90

Hematopneumothorax (*see* Hemothorax)

Hematopoiesis, cyclic D70.4

Hematuria R31.9
- benign (familial) (of childhood)
  - essential microscopic R31.1
- gross R31.0
- microscopic NEC (with symptoms) R31.29
  - asymptomatic R31.21
  - benign essential R31.1

Hemiatrophy R68.89
- face, facial, progressive (Romberg) G51.8

Hemichorea G25.5

Hemiplegia G81.9-
- ascending NEC G81.9-
  - spinal G95.89
- flaccid G81.0-
- hysterical F44.4
- newborn NEC P91.88
  - birth injury P11.9
- spastic G81.1-
  - congenital G80.2

Hemispasm (facial) R25.2

Hemitremor R25.1

Hemochromatosis E83.119
- due to repeated red blood cell transfusion E83.111
- hereditary (primary) E83.110
- neonatal P78.84
- primary E83.110
- specified NEC E83.118

Hemoglobin—*see also* Disease, diseased
- abnormal (disease)—*see* Disease, hemoglobin
- AS genotype D57.3

Hemoglobin, *continued*
- Constant Spring D58.2
- E-beta thalassemia D56.5
- fetal, hereditary persistence (HPFH) D56.4
- H Constant Spring D56.0
- low NOS D64.9
- S (Hb S), heterozygous D57.3

Hemoglobinemia D59.9
- paroxysmal D59.6
  - nocturnal D59.5

Hemoglobinopathy (mixed) D58.2
- with thalassemia D56.8
- sickle-cell D57.1
  - with thalassemia D57.40
    - with
      - ~ acute chest syndrome D57.411
      - ~ cerebral vascular involvement D57.413
      - ~ crisis (painful) D57.419
      - ~ with specified complication NEC D57.418
        - ◊ splenic sequestration D57.412
        - ◊ vasoocclusive pain D57.419
    - without crisis D57.40

Hemoglobinuria R82.3
- with anemia, hemolytic, acquired (chronic) NEC D59.6
- cold (paroxysmal) (with Raynaud's syndrome) D59.6
  - agglutinin D59.12
- due to exertion or hemolysis NEC D59.6
- intermittent D59.6
- march D59.6
- nocturnal (paroxysmal) D59.5
- paroxysmal (cold) D59.6
  - nocturnal D59.5

Hemopericardium I31.2
- newborn P54.8

Hemophilia (classical) (familial) (hereditary) D66
- A D66
- B D67
- C D68.1
- acquired D68.311
- autoimmune D68.311
- secondary D68.311
- vascular D68.0

Hemoptysis R04.2
- newborn P26.9

Hemorrhage, hemorrhagic (concealed) R58
- acute idiopathic pulmonary, in infants R04.81
- adenoid J35.8
- adrenal (capsule) (gland) E27.49
  - medulla E27.8
  - newborn P54.4
- alveolar
  - lung, newborn P26.8
- anemia (chronic) D50.0
  - acute D62
- antepartum (with)
  - before 20 weeks gestation O20.9
    - specified type NEC O20.8
    - threatened abortion O20.0
- anus K62.5
- basilar (ganglion) I61.0
- bowel K92.2
  - newborn P54.3
- brain (miliary) (nontraumatic)—*see* Hemorrhage, intracranial, intracerebral
  - due to
    - birth injury P10.1
  - newborn P52.4
    - birth injury P10.1
- brainstem (nontraumatic) I61.3
  - traumatic S06.38-
- breast N64.59
- bulbar I61.5
- cecum K92.2
- cerebellar, cerebellum (nontraumatic) I61.4
  - newborn P52.6
  - traumatic S06.37-
- cerebral, cerebrum—*see also* Hemorrhage, intracranial, intracerebral
  - newborn (anoxic) P52.4
    - birth injury P10.1
  - lobe I61.1

Hemorrhage, hemorrhagic, *continued*
- cerebromeningeal I61.8
- cerebrospinal—*see* Hemorrhage, intracranial, intracerebral
- colon K92.2
- conjunctiva H11.3-
  - newborn P54.8
- corpus luteum (ruptured) cyst N83.1-
- cortical (brain) I61.1
- cranial—*see* Hemorrhage, intracranial
- cutaneous R23.3
  - due to autosensitivity, erythrocyte D69.2
  - newborn P54.5
- disease D69.9
  - newborn P53
- duodenum, duodenal K92.2
  - ulcer—*see* Ulcer, duodenum, with, hemorrhage
- epicranial subaponeurotic (massive), birth injury P12.2
- epidural (traumatic)—*see also* Injury, intracranial
  - nontraumatic I62.1
- esophagus K22.8
  - varix I85.01
- extradural (traumatic)—*see* Injury, intracranial, epidural hemorrhage
  - birth injury P10.8
  - newborn (anoxic) (nontraumatic) P52.8
  - nontraumatic I62.1
- gastric—*see* Hemorrhage, stomach
- gastroenteric K92.2
  - newborn P54.3
- gastrointestinal (tract) K92.2
  - newborn P54.3
- genitourinary (tract) NOS R31.9
- graafian follicle cyst (ruptured) N83.0-
- intermenstrual (regular) N92.3
  - irregular N92.1
- internal (organs) EC R58
  - capsule I61.0
  - newborn P54.8
- intestine K92.2
  - newborn P54.3
- intra-alveolar (lung), newborn P26.8
- intracerebral (nontraumatic)—*see* Hemorrhage, intracranial, intracerebral
- intracranial (nontraumatic) I62.9
  - birth injury P10.9
  - epidural, nontraumatic I62.1
  - extradural, nontraumatic I62.1
  - intracerebral (nontraumatic) (in) I61.9
    - brain stem I61.3
    - cerebellum I61.4
    - hemisphere I61.2
      - ~ cortical (superficial) I61.1
      - ~ subcortical (deep) I61.0
    - intraventricular I61.5
    - multiple localized I61.6
    - newborn P52.4
      - ~ birth injury P10.1
    - specified NEC I61.8
    - superficial I61.1
  - subarachnoid (nontraumatic) (from) I60.9
    - intracranial (cerebral) artery I60.7
      - ~ anterior communicating I60.2-
      - ~ basilar I60.4
      - ~ carotid siphon and bifurcation I60.0-
      - ~ communicating I60.7
        - ◊ anterior I60.2-
        - ◊ posterior I60.3-
      - ~ middle cerebral I60.1-
      - ~ posterior communicating I60.3-
      - ~ specified artery NEC I60.6
      - ~ vertebral I60.5-
    - newborn P52.5
      - ~ birth injury P10.3
    - specified NEC I60.8-
    - traumatic S06.6X-
  - subdural (nontraumatic) I62.00
    - acute I62.01
    - birth injury P10.0
    - chronic I62.03
    - newborn (anoxic) (hypoxic) P52.8
      - ~ birth injury P10.0
    - spinal G95.19

Hemorrhage, hemorrhagic, *continued*
    - subacute I62.02
    - traumatic—*see* Injury, intracranial, subdural hemorrhage
- intrapontine I61.3
- intraventricular I61.5
  - newborn (nontraumatic) (*see also* Newborn, affected by, hemorrhage) P52.3
    - due to birth injury P10.2
    - grade
      - ~ 1 P52.0
      - ~ 2 P52.1
      - ~ 3 P52.21
      - ~ 4 P52.22
- lenticular striate artery I61.0
- lung R04.89
  - newborn P26.9
    - massive P26.1
    - specified NEC P26.8
- medulla I61.3
- membrane (brain) I60.8-
- meninges, meningeal (brain) (middle) I60.8-
- mouth K13.79
- mucous membrane NEC R58
  - newborn P54.8
- nail (subungual) L60.8
- nasal turbinate R04.0
  - newborn P54.8
- newborn P54.9
  - specified NEC P54.8
- nipple N64.59
- nose R04.0
  - newborn P54.8
- ovary NEC N83.8
- pericardium, pericarditis I31.2
- peritonsillar tissue J35.8
  - due to infection J36
- pituitary (gland) E23.6
- petechial R23.3
  - due to autosensitivity, erythrocyte D69.2
- pons, pontine I61.3
- posterior fossa (nontraumatic) I61.8
  - newborn P52.6
- postnasal R04.0
- pulmonary R04.89
  - newborn P26.9
    - massive P26.1
    - specified NEC P26.8
- purpura (primary) D69.3
- rectum (sphincter) K62.5
  - newborn P54.2
- skin R23.3
  - newborn P54.5
- slipped umbilical ligature P51.8
- stomach K92.2
  - newborn P54.3
  - ulcer—*see* Ulcer, stomach, with, hemorrhage
- subconjunctival—*see also* Hemorrhage, conjunctiva
  - birth injury P15.3
- subcortical (brain) I61.0
- subcutaneous R23.3
- subependymal
  - newborn P52.0
    - with intraventricular extension P52.1
    - and intracerebral extension P52.22
- subungual L60.8
- suprarenal (capsule) (gland) E27.49
  - newborn P54.4
- tonsil J35.8
- ulcer—*code by* site under Ulcer, with hemorrhage K27.4
- umbilicus, umbilical
  - cord
    - after birth, newborn P51.9
  - newborn P51.9
    - massive P51.0
    - slipped ligature P51.8
  - stump P51.9
- uterus, uterine (abnormal) N93.9
  - dysfunctional or functional N93.8
  - intermenstrual (regular) N92.3
    - irregular N92.1
  - pubertal N92.2

Hemorrhage, hemorrhagic, *continued*
- vagina (abnormal) N93.9
  - newborn P54.6
- ventricular I61.5
- viscera NEC R58
  - newborn P54.8

Hemorrhoids (bleeding) (without mention of degree) K64.9
- 1st degree (grade/stage I) (without prolapse outside of anal canal) K64.0
- 2nd degree (grade/stage II) (that prolapse with straining but retract spontaneously) K64.1
- 3rd degree (grade/stage III) (that prolapse with straining and require manual replacement back inside anal canal) K64.2
- 4th degree (grade/stage IV) (with prolapsed tissue that cannot be manually replaced) K64.3
- external K64.4
  - with
    - thrombosis K64.5
- internal (without mention of degree) K64.8
- prolapsed K64.8
- skin tags
  - anus K64.4
  - residual K64.4
- specified NEC K64.8
- strangulated (*see also* Hemorrhoids, by degree) K64.8
- thrombosed (*see also* Hemorrhoids, by degree) K64.5
- ulcerated (*see also* Hemorrhoids, by degree) K64.8

Hemothorax
- newborn P54.8

Henoch (-Schönlein) disease or syndrome (purpura) D69.0

Hepatitis K75.9
- acute (infectious) (viral) B17.9
- B B19.10
  - acute B16.9
- C (viral) B19.20
  - acute B17.10
  - chronic B18.2
- catarrhal (acute) B15.9
- chronic K73.9
  - active NEC K73.2
- epidemic B15.9
- fulminant NEC K75.3
  - neonatal giant cell P59.29
- history of
  - B Z86.19
  - C Z86.19
- homologous serum—*see* Hepatitis, viral, type B
- in (due to)
  - congenital (active) P37.1 *[K77]*
- infectious, infective (acute) (chronic) (subacute) B15.9
- neonatal (idiopathic) (toxic) P59.29
- newborn P59.29
- viral, virus B19.9
  - acute B17.9
    - C B18.2
  - in remission, any type—*code to* Hepatitis, chronic, by type
  - type
    - A B15.9
    - B 19.10
      - ~ acute B16.9
    - C B19.20
      - ~ acute B17.10
      - ~ chronic B18.2

Hepatomegaly—*see also* Hypertrophy, liver
- in mononucleosis
  - gammaherpesviral B27.09
  - infectious specified NEC B27.89

Herlitz' syndrome Q81.1

Hernia, hernial (acquired) (recurrent) K46.9
- with
  - gangrene—*see* Hernia, by site, with, gangrene
  - incarceration—*see* Hernia, by site, with, obstruction
  - irreducible—*see* Hernia, by site, with, obstruction
  - obstruction—*see* Hernia, by site, with, obstruction
  - strangulation—*see* Hernia, by site, with, obstruction
- abdomen, abdominal K46.-
- bladder (mucosa) (sphincter)
  - congenital (female) (male) Q79.51
- diaphragm, diaphragmatic K44.9

Hernia, hernial, *continued*
- – with
  - gangrene (and obstruction) K44.1
  - obstruction K44.0
  - – congenital Q79.0
- direct (inguinal)—*see* Hernia, inguinal
- diverticulum, intestine—*see* Hernia
- double (inguinal)—*see* Hernia, inguinal, bilateral
- epigastric (*see also* Hernia, ventral) K43.9
- esophageal hiatus—*see* Hernia, hiatal
- external (inguinal)—*see* Hernia, inguinal
- foramen magnum G93.5
  - – congenital Q01.8
- hiatal (esophageal) (sliding) K44.9
  - – with
    - gangrene (and obstruction) K44.1
    - obstruction K44.0
  - – congenital Q40.1
- indirect (inguinal)—*see* Hernia, inguinal
- incisional K43.2
  - – with
    - gangrene (and obstruction) K43.1
    - obstruction K43.0
- inguinal (direct) (external) (funicular) (indirect) (internal) (oblique) (scrotal) (sliding) K40.90
  - – with
    - gangrene (and obstruction) K40.40
      - ~ not specified as recurrent K40.40
      - ~ recurrent K40.41
    - obstruction K40.30
      - ~ not specified as recurrent K40.30
      - ~ recurrent K40.31
  - – bilateral K40.20
    - with
      - ~ gangrene (and obstruction) K40.10
        - ◊ not specified as recurrent K40.10
        - ◊ recurrent K40.11
      - ~ obstruction K40.00
        - ◊ not specified as recurrent K40.00
        - ◊ recurrent K40.01
    - not specified as recurrent K40.20
    - recurrent K40.21
  - – not specified as recurrent K40.90
  - – recurrent K40.91
  - – unilateral K40.90
    - with
      - ~ gangrene (and obstruction) K40.40
        - ◊ not specified as recurrent K40.40
        - ◊ recurrent K40.41
      - ~ obstruction K40.30
        - ◊ not specified as recurrent K40.30
        - ◊ recurrent K40.31
    - not specified as recurrent K40.90
    - recurrent K40.91
- irreducible—*see also* Hernia, by site, with obstruction
  - – with gangrene—*see* Hernia, by site, with gangrene
- linea (alba) (semilunaris)—*see* Hernia, ventral
- midline—*see* Hernia, ventral
- oblique (inguinal)—*see* Hernia, inguinal
- obstructive—*see also* Hernia, by site, with obstruction
  - – with gangrene—*see* Hernia, by site, with gangrene
- scrotum, scrotal—*see* Hernia, inguinal
- sliding (inguinal)—*see also* Hernia, inguinal
  - – hiatus—*see* Hernia, hiatal
- spigelian—*see* Hernia, ventral
- spinal—*see* Spina bifida
- strangulated—*see also* Hernia, by site, with obstruction
  - – with gangrene—*see* Hernia, by site, with gangrene
- subxiphoid—*see* Hernia, ventral
- supra-umbilicus—*see* Hernia, ventral
- tunica vaginalis Q55.29
- umbilicus, umbilical K42.9
  - – with
    - gangrene (and obstruction) K42.1
    - obstruction K42.0
- ventral K43.9
  - – recurrent—*see* Hernia, incisional
  - – incisional K43.2
    - with
      - ~ gangrene (and obstruction) K43.1
      - ~ obstruction K43.0
  - – specified NEC K43.9

Herpangina B08.5

Herpes, herpesvirus, herpetic B00.9
- anogenital A60.9
  - – urogenital tract A60.00
    - cervix A60.03
    - male genital organ NEC A60.02
    - penis A60.01
    - specified site NEC A60.09
    - vagina A60.04
    - vulva A60.04
- circinatus B35.4
- encephalitis B00.4
  - – due to herpesvirus 7 B10.09
  - – specified NEC B10.09
- genital, genitalis A60.00
  - – female A60.09
  - – male A60.02
- gingivostomatitis B00.2
- human B00.9
  - – 1—*see* Herpes, simplex
  - – 2—*see* Herpes, simplex
  - – 4—*see* Mononucleosis, Epstein-Barr (virus)
  - – 7
    - encephalitis B10.09
- meningitis (simplex) B00.3
- pharyngitis, pharyngotonsillitis B00.2
- simplex B00.9
  - – complicated NEC B00.89
  - – congenital P35.2
  - – specified complication NEC B00.89
  - – visceral B00.89
- stomatitis B00.2
- tonsurans B35.0 visceral B00.89
- whitlow B00.89

Herter-Gee Syndrome K90.0

Hesitancy
- of micturition R39.11
- urinary R39.11

Heubner-Herter disease K90.0

Hiccup, hiccough R06.6
- psychogenic F45.8

Hidden penis (congenital) Q55.64

Hidradenitis (axillaris) (suppurative) L73.2

High
- altitude effects T70.20
  - – anoxia T70.29
  - – on
    - ears T70.0
    - sinuses T70.1
  - – polycythemia D75.1
- arch
  - – foot Q66.7-
  - – palate, congenital Q38.5
- basal metabolic rate R94.8
- blood pressure—*see also* Hypertension
  - – borderline R03.0
  - – reading (incidental) (isolated) (nonspecific), without diagnosis of hypertension R03.0
- cholesterol E78.00
  - – with high triglycerides E78.2
- expressed emotional level within family Z63.8
- palate, congenital Q38.5
- risk
  - – infant NEC Z76.2
  - – sexual behavior (heterosexual) Z72.51
    - bisexual Z72.53
    - homosexual Z72.52
- scrotal testis, testes
  - – bilateral Q53.23
  - – unilateral Q53.13
- temperature (of unknown origin) R50.9
- triglycerides E78.1
  - – with high cholesterol E78.2

Hippel's disease Q85.8

Hirschsprung's disease or megacolon Q43.1

Hirsutism, hirsuties L68.0

Hirudiniasis
- external B88.3

Histiocytosis D76.3
- lipid, lipoid D76.3
- mononuclear phagocytes NEC D76.1

Histiocytosis, *continued*
- non-Langerhans cell D76.3
- polyostotic sclerosing D76.3
- sinus, with massive lymphadenopathy D76.3
- syndrome NEC D76.3

Histoplasmosis B39.9
- with pneumonia NEC B39.2
  - – capsulati B39.4
- disseminated B39.3
- generalized B39.3
- pulmonary B39.2
  - – acute B39.0
  - – chronic B39.1

History
- family (of)—*see also* History, personal (of)
  - – alcohol abuse Z81.1
  - – allergy NEC Z84.89
  - – anemia Z83.2
  - – arthritis Z82.61
  - – asthma Z82.5
  - – blindness Z82.1
  - – cardiac death (sudden) Z82.41
  - – carrier of genetic disease Z84.81
  - – chromosomal anomaly Z82.79
  - – chronic
    - disabling disease NEC Z82.8
    - lower respiratory disease Z82.5
  - – colonic polyps Z83.71
  - – congenital malformations and deformations Z82.79
    - polycystic kidney Z82.71
  - – consanguinity Z84.3
  - – deafness Z82.2
  - – diabetes mellitus Z83.3
  - – disability NEC Z82.8
  - – disease or disorder (of)
    - allergic NEC Z84.89
    - behavioral NEC Z81.8
    - blood and blood-forming organs Z83.2
    - cardiovascular NEC Z82.49
    - chronic disabling NEC Z82.8
    - digestive Z83.79
    - ear NEC Z83.52
    - elevated lipoprotein(a) (Lp(a)) Z83.430
    - endocrine NEC Z83.49
    - eye NEC Z83.518
      - ~ glaucoma Z83.511
    - familial hypercholesterolemia Z83.42
    - genitourinary NEC Z84.2
    - glaucoma Z83.511
    - hematological Z83.2
    - immune mechanism Z83.2
    - infectious NEC Z83.1
    - ischemic heart Z82.49
    - kidney Z84.1
    - lipoprotein metabolism Z83.438
    - mental NEC Z81.8
    - metabolic Z83.49
    - musculoskeletal NEC Z82.69
    - neurological NEC Z82.0
    - nutritional Z83.49
    - parasitic NEC Z83.1
    - psychiatric NEC Z81.8
    - respiratory NEC Z83.6
    - skin and subcutaneous tissue NEC Z84.0
    - specified NEC Z84.89
  - – drug abuse NEC Z81.3
  - – elevated lipoprotein (a) (LP(a)) Z83.430
  - – epilepsy Z82.0
  - – familial hypercholesterolemia Z83.42
  - – genetic disease carrier Z84.81
  - – glaucoma Z83.511
  - – hearing loss Z82.2
  - – human immunodeficiency virus (HIV) infection Z83.0
  - – Huntington's chorea Z82.0
  - – hypercholesterolemia (familial) Z83.42
  - – hyperlipidemia, familial combined Z83.438
  - – intellectual disability Z81.0
  - – leukemia Z80.6
  - – lipidemia NEC Z83.438
  - – malignant neoplasm (of) NOS Z80.9
    - bladder Z80.52
    - breast Z80.3

History, *continued*
- bronchus Z80.1
- digestive organ Z80.0
- gastrointestinal tract Z80.0
- genital organ Z80.49
  - ~ ovary Z80.41
  - ~ prostate Z80.42
  - ~ specified organ NEC Z80.49
  - ~ testis Z80.43
- hematopoietic NEC Z80.7
- intrathoracic organ NEC Z80.2
- kidney Z80.51
- lung Z80.1
- lymphatic NEC Z80.7
- ovary Z80.41
- prostate Z80.42
- respiratory organ NEC Z80.2
- specified site NEC Z80.8
- testis Z80.43
- trachea Z80.1
- urinary organ or tract Z80.59
  - ~ bladder Z80.52
  - ~ kidney Z80.51
- mental
  - disorder NEC Z81.8
- multiple endocrine neoplasia (MEN) syndrome Z83.41
- osteoporosis Z82.62
- polycystic kidney Z82.71
- polyps (colon) Z83.71
- psychiatric disorder Z81.8
- psychoactive substance abuse NEC Z81.3
- respiratory condition NEC Z83.6
  - asthma and other lower respiratory conditions Z82.5
- self-harmful behavior Z81.8
- SIDS (sudden infant death syndrome) Z84.82
- skin condition Z84.0
- specified condition NEC Z84.89
- stroke (cerebrovascular) Z82.3
- substance abuse NEC Z81.4
  - alcohol Z81.1
  - drug NEC Z81.3
  - psychoactive NEC Z81.3
  - tobacco Z81.2
- sudden cardiac death Z82.41
- sudden infant death syndrome Z84.82
- tobacco abuse Z81.2
- violence, violent behavior Z81.8
- visual loss Z82.1
- personal (of)—*see also* History, family (of)
  - abuse
    - childhood Z62.819
      - ~ forced labor or sexual exploitation in childhood Z62.813
      - ~ physical Z62.810
      - ~ psychological Z62.811
      - ~ sexual Z62.810
  - alcohol dependence F10.21
  - allergy (to) Z88.9
    - antibiotic agent NEC Z88.1
    - drugs, medicaments and biological substances Z88.9
      - ~ specified NEC Z88.8
    - food Z91.018
      - ~ additives Z91.02
      - ~ eggs Z91.012
      - ~ milk products Z91.011
      - ~ peanuts Z91.010
      - ~ seafood Z91.013
      - ~ specified food NEC Z91.018
    - insect Z91.038
      - ~ bee Z91.030
    - latex Z91.040
    - medicinal agents Z88.9
      - ~ specified NEC Z88.8
    - narcotic agent Z88.5
    - nonmedicinal agents Z91.048
    - penicillin Z88.0
    - serum Z88.7
    - sulfonamides Z88.2
    - vaccine Z88.7
  - anaphylactic shock Z87.892
  - anaphylaxis Z87.892

History, *continued*
- behavioral disorders Z86.59
- brain injury (traumatic) Z87.820
- cancer—*see* History, personal (of), malignant neoplasm (of)
- cardiac arrest (death), successfully resuscitated Z86.74
- cerebral infarction without residual deficit Z86.73
- chemotherapy for neoplastic condition Z92.21
- cleft lip (corrected) Z87.730
- cleft palate (corrected) Z87.730
- congenital malformation (corrected) Z87.798
  - circulatory system (corrected) Z87.74
  - digestive system (corrected) NEC Z87.738
  - ear (corrected) Z87.721
  - eye (corrected) Z87.720
  - face and neck (corrected) Z87.790
  - genitourinary system (corrected) NEC Z87.718
  - heart (corrected) Z87.74
  - integument (corrected) Z87.76
  - limb(s) (corrected) Z87.76
  - musculoskeletal system (corrected) Z87.76
  - neck (corrected) Z87.790
  - nervous system (corrected) NEC Z87.728
  - respiratory system (corrected) Z87.75
  - sense organs (corrected) NEC Z87.728
  - specified NEC Z87.798
- disease or disorder (of) Z87.898
  - blood and blood-forming organs Z86.2
  - connective tissue NEC Z87.39
  - ear Z86.69
  - endocrine Z86.39
    - ~ specified type NEC Z86.39
  - eye Z86.69
  - hematological Z86.2
  - Hodgkin Z85.71
  - immune mechanism Z86.2
  - infectious Z86.19
    - ~ Methicillin resistant Staphylococcus aureus (MRSA) Z86.14
    - ~ tuberculosis Z86.11
  - mental NEC Z86.59
  - metabolic Z86.39
    - ~ specified type NEC Z86.39
  - musculoskeletal NEC Z87.39
  - nervous system Z86.69
  - nutritional Z86.39
  - respiratory system NEC Z87.09
  - sense organs Z86.69
  - specified site or type NEC Z87.898
  - urinary system NEC Z87.448
- drug therapy
  - antineoplastic chemotherapy Z92.21
  - immunosupression Z92.25
  - inhaled steroids Z92.240
  - monoclonal drug Z92.22
  - specified NEC Z92.29
  - steroid Z92.241
  - systemic steroids Z92.241
- encephalitis Z86.61
- extracorporeal membrane oxygenation (ECMO) Z92.81
- fall, falling Z91.81
- forced labor or sexual exploitation in childhood Z62.813
- hepatitis
  - B Z86.19
  - C Z86.19
- Hodgkin disease Z85.71
- hypospadias (corrected) Z87.710
- immunosupression therapy Z92.25
- infection NEC Z86.19
  - central nervous system Z86.61
  - latent tuberculosis Z86.15
  - Methicillin resistant Staphylococcus aureus (MRSA) Z86.14
- in situ neoplasm
  - breast Z86.000
  - cervix uteri Z86.001
  - digestive organs, specified NEC Z86.004
  - esophagus Z86.003
  - genital organs, specified NEC Z86.002
  - melanoma Z86.006

History, *continued*
- middle ear Z86.005
- oral cavity Z86.003
- respiratory system Z86.005
- skin Z86.007
- specified NEC Z86.008
- stomach Z86.003
- in utero procedure while a fetus Z98.871
- latent tuberculosis Z86.15
- leukemia Z85.6
- lymphoma (non-Hodgkin) Z85.72
- malignant melanoma (skin) Z85.820
- malignant neoplasm (of) Z85.9
  - bone Z85.830
  - brain Z85.841
  - carcinoid—*see* History, personal (of), malignant neoplasm, by site, carcinoid
  - endocrine gland NEC Z85.858
  - eye Z85.840
  - hematopoietic NEC Z85.79
  - kidney NEC Z85.528
    - ~ carcinoid Z85.520
- maltreatment Z91.89
- melanoma Z85.820
- meningitis Z86.61
- mental disorder Z86.59
- Methicillin resistant Staphylococcus aureus (MRSA) Z86.14
- neglect (in)
  - childhood Z62.812
- neoplasm
  - in situ—*see* Table of Neoplasms in the complete *ICD-10-CM* manual
  - malignant—*see* Table of Neoplasms in the complete *ICD-10-CM* manual
  - uncertain behavior Z86.03
- nephrotic syndrome Z87.441
- nicotine dependence Z87.891
- noncompliance with medical treatment or regimen—*see* Noncompliance
- nutritional deficiency Z86.39
- parasuicide (attempt) Z91.5
- physical trauma NEC Z87.828
  - self-harm or suicide attempt Z91.5
- pneumonia (recurrent) Z87.01
- poisoning NEC Z91.89
  - self-harm or suicide attempt Z91.5
- procedure while a fetus Z98.871
- prolonged reversible ischemic neurologic deficit (PRIND) Z86.73
- psychological
  - abuse
    - ~ child Z62.811
  - trauma, specified NEC Z91.49
- respiratory condition NEC Z87.09
- retained foreign body fully removed Z87.821
- risk factors NEC Z91.89
- self-harm Z91.5
- self-poisoning attempt Z91.5
- specified NEC Z87.898
- steroid therapy (systemic) Z92.241
  - inhaled Z92.240
- stroke without residual deficits Z86.73
- substance abuse NEC F10-F19
- sudden cardiac arrest Z86.74
- sudden cardiac death successfully resuscitated Z86.74
- suicide attempt Z91.5
- surgery NEC Z98.890
- tobacco dependence Z87.891
- transient ischemic attack (TIA) without residual deficits Z86.73
- trauma (physical) NEC Z87.828
  - psychological NEC Z91.49
  - self-harm Z91.5
- traumatic brain injury Z87.820

HIV (*see also* Human, immunodeficiency virus) B20
- laboratory evidence (nonconclusive) R75
- positive, seropositive Z21
- nonconclusive test (in infants) R75

Hives (bold)—*see* Urticaria

Hoarseness R49.0

Hoffmann's syndrome E03.9 *[G73.7]*

Homelessness Z59.0

Hooded
- clitoris Q52.6
- penis Q55.69

Hordeolum (eyelid) (externum) (recurrent) H00.01-
- internum H00.02-
  - left H00.026
    - lower H00.025
    - upper H00.024
  - right H00.023
    - lower H00.022
    - upper H00.021
- left H00.016
  - lower H00.015
  - upper H00.014
- right H00.013
  - lower H00.012
  - upper H00.011

Horseshoe kidney (congenital) Q63.1

Hospitalism in children—*see* Disorder, adjustment

Human
- bite (open wound)—*see also* Bite
  - intact skin surface—*see* Bite
- herpesvirus—*see* Herpes
- immunodeficiency virus (HIV) disease (infection) B20
  - asymptomatic status Z21
  - contact Z20.6
  - counseling Z71.7
  - exposure to Z20.6
  - laboratory evidence R75
- papillomavirus (HPV)
  - screening for Z11.51

Hunger T73.0
- air, psychogenic F45.8

Hunter's
- syndrome E76.1

Hunt's
- dyssynergia cerebellaris myoclonica G11.19

Hutchinson's
- disease, meaning
  - pompholyx (cheiropompholyx) L30.1

Hyaline membrane (disease) (lung) (pulmonary) (newborn) P22.0

Hydatid
- Morgagni
  - female Q50.5
  - male (epididymal) Q55.4
    - testicular Q55.29

Hydradenitis (axillaris) (suppurative) L73.2

Hydramnios O40.-

Hydrarthrosis—*see also* Effusion, joint
- intermittent M12.4-
  - ankle M12.47-
  - elbow M12.42-
  - foot joint M12.47-
  - hand joint M12.44-
  - hip M12.45-
  - knee M12.46-
  - multiple site M12.49
  - shoulder M12.41-
  - specified joint NEC M12.48
  - wrist M12.43-

Hydroadenitis (axillaris) (suppurative) L73.2

Hydrocele (spermatic cord) (testis) (tunica vaginalis) N43.3
- communicating N43.2
  - congenital P83.5
- congenital P83.5
- encysted N43.0
- female NEC N94.89
- infected N43.1
- newborn P83.5
- round ligament N94.89
- specified NEC N43.2
- spinalis—*see* Spina bifida
- vulva N90.89

Hydrocephalus (acquired) (external) (internal) (malignant) (recurrent) G91.9
- aqueduct Sylvius stricture Q03.0
- communicating G91.0
- congenital (external) (internal) Q03.9
  - with spina bifida Q05.4
    - cervical Q05.0
    - dorsal Q05.1
    - lumbar Q05.2
    - lumbosacral Q05.2
    - sacral Q05.3
    - thoracic Q05.1
    - thoracolumbar Q05.1
  - specified NEC Q03.8
- due to toxoplasmosis (congenital) P37.1
- foramen Magendie block (acquired) G91.1
  - congenital (*see also* Hydrocephalus, congenital) Q03.1
- in (due to)
  - infectious disease NEC B89 [G91.4]
  - neoplastic disease NEC (*see also* Table of Neoplasms in the complete *ICD-10-CM* manual) G91.4
  - parasitic disease B89 [G91.4]
- newborn Q03.9
  - with spina bifida—*see* Spina bifida, with hydrocephalus
- noncommunicating G91.1
- normal pressure G91.2
  - secondary G91.0
- obstructive G91.1
- otitic G93.2
- post-traumatic NEC G91.3
- secondary G91.4
  - post-traumatic G91.3
- specified NEC G91.8

Hydromicrocephaly Q02

Hydromphalos (since birth) Q45.8

Hydronephrosis (atrophic) (early) (functionless) (intermittent) (primary) (secondary) NEC N13.30
- with
  - obstruction (by) (of)
    - renal calculus N13.2
    - ureteral NEC N13.1
      - calculus N13.2
    - ureteropelvic junction N13.0
      - congenital Q62.11
      - with infection N13.6
  - ureteral stricture NEC N13.1
- congenital Q62.0
- specified type NEC N13.39

Hydroperitoneum R18.8

Hydrophthalmos Q15.0

Hydrops R60.9
- abdominis R18.8
- endolymphatic H81.0-
- fetalis P83.2
  - due to
    - ABO isoimmunization P56.0
    - alpha thalassemia D56.0
    - hemolytic disease P56.90
      - specified NEC P56.99
    - isoimmunization (ABO) (Rh) P56.0
    - other specified nonhemolytic disease NEC P83.2
    - Rh incompatibility P56.0
- newborn (idiopathic) P83.2
  - due to
    - ABO isoimmunization P56.0
    - alpha thalassemia D56.0
    - hemolytic disease P56.90
      - specified NEC P56.99
    - isoimmunization (ABO) (Rh) P56.0
    - Rh incompatibility P56.0
- pericardium—*see* Pericarditis
- spermatic cord—*see* Hydrocele

Hydropyonephrosis N13.6

Hydrorrhea (nasal) J34.89

Hydrosadenitis (axillaris) (suppurative) L73.2

Hydroxykynureninuria E70.89

Hyperacidity (gastric) K31.89
- psychogenic F45.8

Hyperactive, hyperactivity F90.9
- bowel sounds R19.12
- child F90.9
  - attention deficit—*see* Disorder, attention-deficit hyperactivity
- detrusor muscle N32.81
- gastrointestinal K31.89
  - psychogenic F45.8
- nasal mucous membrane J34.3

Hyperadrenocorticism E24.9
- congenital E25.0
- iatrogenic E24.2
  - correct substance properly administered—*see* Table of Drugs and Chemicals, by drug, adverse effect
  - overdose or wrong substance given or taken—*see* Table of Drugs and Chemicals, by drug, poisoning
- not associated with Cushing's syndrome E27.0
- pituitary-dependent E24.0

Hyperalimentation R63.2

Hyperbetalipoproteinemia (familial) E78.0
- with prebetalipoproteinemia E78.2

Hyperbicarbonatemia P74.41

Hyperbilirubinemia
- constitutional E80.6
- familial conjugated E80.6
- neonatal (transient)—*see* Jaundice, newborn

Hypercalcemia, hypocalciuric, familial E83.52

Hypercalciuria, idiopathic R82.994

Hypercapnia R06.89
- newborn P84

Hyperchloremia E87.8

Hyperchlorhydria K31.89
- neurotic F45.8
- psychogenic F45.8

Hypercholesterolemia (essential) (primary) (pure) E78.00
- with hyperglyceridemia, endogenous E78.2
- dietary counseling and surveillance Z71.3
- familial E78.01
- family history of Z83.42
- hereditary E78.01

Hyperchylia gastrica, psychogenic F45.8

Hypercorticalism, pituitary-dependent E24.0

Hypercorticosolism—*see* Cushing's, syndrome

Hypercorticosteronism E24.2
- correct substance properly administered—*see* Table of Drugs and Chemicals, by drug, adverse effect
- overdose or wrong substance given or taken—*see* Table of Drugs and Chemicals, by drug, poisoning

Hypercortisonism E24.2
- correct substance properly administered—*see* Table of Drugs and Chemicals, by drug, adverse effect
- overdose or wrong substance given or taken—*see* Table of Drugs and Chemicals, by drug, poisoning

Hyperekplexia Q89.8

Hyperelectrolytemia E87.8

Hyperemesis R11.10
- with nausea R11.2
- projectile R11.12
- psychogenic F45.8

Hyperemia (acute) (passive) R68.89
- anal mucosa K62.89
- ear internal, acute—*see* subcategory H83.0
- labyrinth—*see* subcategory H83.0

Hyperexplexia Q89.8

Hyperfunction
- adrenal cortex, not associated with Cushing's syndrome E27.0
  - virilism E25.9
    - congenital E25.0

Hyperglycemia, hyperglycemic (transient) R73.9
- coma—*see* Diabetes, by type, with coma
- postpancreatectomy E89.1

Hyperheparinemia D68.32

Hyperhidrosis, hyperidrosis R61
- generalized R61
- psychogenic F45.8
- secondary R61
  - focal L74.52

Hyperinsulinism (functional) E16.1
- therapeutic misadventure (from administration of insulin)—see subcategory T38.3

Hyperkeratosis (see also Keratosis) L85.9
- follicularis Q82.8
- universalis congenita Q80.8

Hyperlipemia, hyperlipidemia E78.5
- combined E78.2
  - familial E78.49
- group
  - A E78.00
  - C E78.2
- mixed E78.2
  - specified NEC E78.49

Hyperlipoproteinemia E78.5
- Fredrickson's type
  - IIa E78.00
  - IIb E78.2
  - III E78.2
- low-density-lipoprotein-type (LDL) E78.00
- very-low-density-lipoprotein-type (VLDL) E78.1

Hypermagnesemia E83.41
- neonatal P71.8

Hypermenorrhea N92.0

Hypermetropia (congenital) H52.0-

Hypermobility, hypermotility
- colon—see Syndrome, irritable bowel
  - psychogenic F45.8
- intestine (see also Syndrome, irritable bowel) K58.9
  - psychogenic F45.8
- stomach K31.89
  - psychogenic F45.8
- syndrome M35.7

Hypernatremia E87.0

Hypernephroma C64.-

Hyperopia—see Hypermetropia

Hyperorexia nervosa F50.2

Hyperosmolality E87.0

Hyperostosis (monomelic)—see also Disorder
- skull M85.2
  - congenital Q75.8

Hyperperistalsis R19.2
- psychogenic F45.8

Hyperpigmentation—see also Pigmentation
- melanin NEC L81.4

Hyperplasia, hyperplastic
- adenoids J35.2
- adrenal (capsule) (cortex) (gland) E27.8
  - with
    - sexual precocity (male) E25.9
      - congenital E25.0
    - virilism, adrenal E25.9
      - congenital E25.0
    - virilization (female) E25.9
      - congenital E25.0
  - congenital E25.0
    - salt-losing E25.0
- angiolymphoid, eosinophilia (ALHE) D18.01
- bone NOS Q79.9
  - face Q75.8
  - skull—see Hypoplasia, skull
- cervix (uteri) (basal cell) (endometrium) (polypoid)
  - congenital Q51.828
- endocervicitis N72
- epithelial L85.9
  - nipple N62
  - skin L85.9
- face Q18.8
  - bone(s) Q75.8
- genital
  - female NEC N94.89
  - male N50.89
- gingiva K06.1

Hyperplasia, hyperplastic, continued
- gum K06.1
- nose
  - lymphoid J34.89
  - polypoid J33.9
- tonsils (faucial) (infective) (lingual) (lymphoid) J35.1
  - with adenoids J35.3

Hyperpnea—see Hyperventilation

Hyperproteinemia E88.09

Hyperpyrexia R50.9
- heat (effects) T67.01
  - rheumatic—see Fever, rheumatic
- unknown origin R50.9

Hypersecretion
- ACTH (not associated with Cushing's syndrome) E27.0
  - pituitary E24.0
- corticoadrenal E24.9
- cortisol E24.9
- gastric K31.89
  - psychogenic F45.8
- hormone(s)
  - ACTH (not associated with Cushing's syndrome) E27.0
    - pituitary E24.0
  - antidiuretic E22.2
  - growth E22.0

Hypersegmentation, leukocytic, hereditary D72.0

Hypersensitive, hypersensitiveness, hypersensitivity—see also Allergy
- gastrointestinal K52.29
  - psychogenic F45.8
- reaction T78.40

Hypertension, hypertensive (accelerated) (benign) (essential) (idiopathic) (malignant) (systemic) I10
- benign, intracranial G93.2
- borderline R03.0
- complicating
  - pregnancy
    - gestational (pregnancy induced) (transient) (without proteinuria)
      - with proteinuria O14.9
        ◊ mild pre-eclampsia O14.0-
        ◊ moderate pre-eclampsia O14.0-
        ◊ severe pre-eclampsia O14.1-
          » with hemolysis, elevated liver enzymes and low platelet count (HELLP) O14.2-
    - pre-existing
      ~ with
        ◊ pre-eclampsia O11.-
      ~ essential O10.01-
      ~ secondary O10.41-
- crisis I16.9
- emergency I16.1
- encephalopathy I67.4
- kidney I12.9
  - with
    - stage 5 chronic kidney disease (CKD) or end stage renal disease (ESRD) I12.0
- lesser circulation I27.0
- newborn P29.2
  - pulmonary (persistent) P29.30
- psychogenic F45.8
- pulmonary I27.20
  - with
    - cor pulmonale (chronic) I27.29
      ~
    - right heart ventricular strain/failure I27.29
  - due to
    - hematologic disorders I27.29
    - left heart disease I27.22
    - lung diseases and hypoxia I27.23
    - metabolic disorders I27.29
    - specified systemic disorders NEC I27.29
  - group 1 (associated) (drug-induced) (toxin-induced) I27.21
  - group 2 I27.22
  - group 3 I27.23
  - group 4 I27.24
  - group 5 I27.29
  - of newborn (persistent) P29.3

Hypertension, hypertensive, continued
- primary (idiopathic) I27.0
  - secondary
    ~ arterial I27.21
    ~ specified NEC I27.29
- urgency I16.0

Hyperthermia (of unknown origin)—see also Hyperpyrexia
- newborn P81.9
  - environmental P81.0

Hyperthyroidism (latent) (pre-adult) (recurrent) E05.90
- with
  - goiter (diffuse) E05.00
    - with thyroid storm E05.01
  - storm E05.91
- intracranial (benign) G93.2
- neonatal, transitory P72.1

Hypertony, hypertonia, hypertonicity
- stomach K31.89
  - psychogenic F45.8

Hypertrophy, hypertrophic
- adenoids (infective) J35.2
  - with tonsils J35.3
- anal papillae K62.89
- bladder (sphincter) (trigone) N32.89
- brain G93.89
- breast N62
  - newborn P83.4
  - pubertal, massive N62
- cardiac (chronic) (idiopathic) I51.7
  - with rheumatic fever (conditions in I00)
    - active I01.8
    - inactive or quiescent (with chorea) I09.89
  - congenital NEC Q24.8
  - rheumatic (with chorea) I09.89
    - active or acute I01.8
      ~ with chorea I02.0
- foot (congenital) Q74.2
- frenulum, frenum (tongue) K14.8
  - lip K13.0
- gland, glandular R59.9
  - generalized R59.1
  - localized R59.0
- gum (mucous membrane) K06.1
- hemifacial 67.4
- lingual tonsil (infective) J35.1
  - with adenoids J35.3
- lip K13.0
  - congenital Q18.6
- liver R16.0
- lymph, lymphatic gland R59.9
  - generalized R59.1
  - localized R59.0
- Meckel's diverticulum (congenital) Q43.0
- mucous membrane
  - gum K06.1
  - nose (turbinate) J34.3
- myocardium—see also Hypertrophy, cardiac
  - idiopathic I42.2
- nasal J34.89
  - alae J34.89
  - bone J34.89
  - cartilage J34.89
  - mucous membrane (septum) J34.3
  - sinus J34.89
  - turbinate J34.3
- nasopharynx, lymphoid (infectional) (tissue) (wall) J35.2
- nipple N62
- palate (hard) M27.8
  - soft K13.79
- pharyngeal tonsil J35.2
- pharynx J39.2
  - lymphoid (infectional) (tissue) (wall) J35.2
- pituitary (anterior) (fossa) (gland) E23.6
- prepuce (congenital) N47.8
  - female N90.89
- pseudomuscular G71.09
- pylorus (adult) (muscle) (sphincter) K31.1
  - congenital or infantile Q40.0
- rectal, rectum (sphincter) K62.89
- rhinitis (turbinate) J31.0
- scar L91.0
  - specified NEC L91.8

Hypertrophy, hypertrophic, *continued*
- skin L91.9
- testis N44.8
  - congenital Q55.29
- toe (congenital) Q74.2
  - acquired—*see also* Deformity, toe
- tonsils (faucial) (infective) (lingual) (lymphoid) J35.1
  - with adenoids J35.3
- uvula K13.79
- ventricle, ventricular (heart)—*see also* Hypertrophy, cardiac
  - congenital Q24.8
  - in tetralogy of Fallot Q21.3
- vulva N90.60
  - childhood asymmetric labium majus enlargement (CALME) N90.61
  - other specified N90.69

Hyperuricemia (asymptomatic) E79.0

Hyperuricosuria R82.993

Hyperventilation (tetany) R06.4
- hysterical F45.8
- psychogenic F45.8
- syndrome F45.8

Hypoacidity, gastric K31.89
- psychogenic F45.8

Hypoadrenalism, hypoadrenia E27.40
- primary E27.1

Hypoadrenocorticism E27.40
- pituitary E23.0
- primary E27.1

Hypoalbuminemia E88.09

Hypoaldosteronism E27.40

Hypocalcemia E83.51
- dietary E58
- neonatal P71.1
  - due to cow's milk P71.0
- phosphate-loading (newborn) P71.1

Hypochloremia E87.8

Hypochlorhydria K31.89
- neurotic F45.8
- psychogenic F45.8

Hypochondria, hypochondriac, hypochondriasis (reaction) F45.21
- sleep F51.03

Hypochondrogenesis Q77.0

Hypochondroplasia Q77.4

Hypochromasia, blood cells D50.8

Hypocitraturia R82.991

Hypoeosinophilia D72.89

Hypofibrinogenemia D68.8
- acquired D65
- congenital (hereditary) D68.2

Hypofunction
- adrenocortical E27.40
  - primary E27.1
- corticoadrenal NEC E27.40
- pituitary (gland) (anterior) E23.0

Hypogalactia O92.4

Hypogammaglobulinemia (*see also* Agammaglobulinemia) D80.1
- hereditary D80.0
- nonfamilial D80.1
- transient, of infancy D80.7

Hypoglycemia (spontaneous) E16.2
- coma E15
  - diabetic—*see* Diabetes
- diabetic—*see* Diabetes
- dietary counseling and surveillance Z71.3
- due to insulin E16.0
  - therapeutic misadventure—*see* subcategory T38.3
- neonatal (transitory) P70.4
- transitory neonatal P70.4

Hypogonadism
- female E28.39
- hypogonadotropic E23.0
- ovarian (primary) E28.39
- pituitary E23.0

Hypometabolism R63.8

Hypomotility
- gastrointestinal (tract) K31.89
  - psychogenic F45.8
- intestine K59.89
  - psychogenic F45.8
- stomach K31.89
  - psychogenic F45.8

Hyponatremia E87.1

Hypo-osmolality E87.1

Hypoparathyroidism E20.9
- familial E20.8
- idiopathic E20.0
- neonatal, transitory P71.4
- postprocedural E89.2
- specified NEC E20.8

Hypoperfusion (in)
- newborn P96.89

Hypophyseal, hypophysis—*see also* Disease, diseased
- gigantism E22.0

Hypopituitarism (juvenile) E23.0
- drug-induced E23.1
- iatrogenic NEC E23.1

Hypoplasia, hypoplastic
- alimentary tract, congenital Q45.8
  - upper Q40.8
- anus, anal (canal) Q42.3
  - with fistula Q42.2
- aorta, aortic Q25.42
  - ascending, in hypoplastic left heart syndrome Q23.4
  - valve Q23.1
    - in hypoplastic left heart syndrome Q23.4
- artery (peripheral) Q27.8
  - pulmonary Q25.79
  - umbilical Q27.0
- biliary duct or passage Q44.5
- bone NOS Q79.9
  - marrow D61.9
    - megakaryocytic D69.49
  - skull—*see* Hypoplasia, skull
- brain Q02
- cecum Q42.8
- cephalic Q02
- clavicle (congenital) Q74.0
- colon Q42.9
  - specified NEC Q42.8
- corpus callosum Q04.0
- digestive organ(s) or tract NEC Q45.8
  - upper (congenital) Q40.8
- ear (auricle) (lobe) Q17.2
  - middle Q16.4
- endocrine (gland) NEC Q89.2
- erythroid, congenital D61.01
- eye Q11.2
- eyelid (congenital) Q10.3
- focal dermal Q82.8
- gallbladder Q44.0
- genitalia, genital organ(s)
  - female, congenital Q52.8
    - external Q52.79
    - internal NEC Q52.8
  - in adiposogenital dystrophy E23.6
- intestine (small) Q41.9
  - large Q42.9
    - specified NEC Q42.8
- jaw M26.09
  - lower M26.04
- kidney(s)
  - bilateral Q60.4
  - unilateral Q60.3
- left heart syndrome Q23.4
- lung (lobe) (not associated with short gestation) Q33.6
  - associated with immaturity, low birth weight, prematurity, or short gestation P28.0
- mandible, mandibular M26.04
- medullary D61.9
- megakaryocytic D69.49
- metacarpus—*see* Defect, reduction, limb, upper, specified type NEC
- metatarsus—*see* Defect, reduction, limb, lower, specified type NEC

Hypoplasia, hypoplastic, *continued*
- optic nerve H47.03-
- ovary, congenital Q50.39
- parathyroid (gland) Q89.2
- pelvis, pelvic girdle Q74.2
- penis (congenital) Q55.62
- pituitary (gland) (congenital) Q89.2
- pulmonary (not associated with short gestation) Q33.6
  - associated with short gestation P28.0
- rectum Q42.1
  - with fistula Q42.0
- scapula Q74.0
- shoulder girdle Q74.0
- skin Q82.8
- skull (bone) Q75.8
  - with
    - anencephaly Q00.0
    - encephalocele—*see* Encephalocele
    - hydrocephalus Q03.9
      ~ with spina bifida—*see* Spina bifida, by site, with hydrocephalus
    - microcephaly Q02
- thymic, with immunodeficiency D82.1
- thymus (gland) Q89.2
  - with immunodeficiency D82.1
- thyroid (gland) E03.1
  - cartilage Q31.2
- umbilical artery Q27.0
- zonule (ciliary) Q12.8

Hypoplasminogenemia E88.02

Hypopnea, obstructive sleep apnea G47.33

Hypoproteinemia E77.8

Hypopyrexia R68.0

Hyposecretion
- ACTH E23.0
- antidiuretic hormone E23.2
- ovary E28.39
- vasopressin E23.2

Hyposegmentation, leukocytic, hereditary D72.0

Hypospadias Q54.9
- balanic Q54.0
- coronal Q54.0
- glandular Q54.0
- penile Q54.1
- penoscrotal Q54.2
- perineal Q54.3
- specified NEC Q54.8

Hypotension (arterial) (constitutional) I95.9
- intracranial G96.810
  - following
    - lumbar cerebrospinal fluid shunting G97.83
    - specified procedure NEC G97.84
    - ventricular shunting (ventriculostomy) G97.2
  - specified NEC G96.819
  - spontaneous G96.811
- orthostatic (chronic) I95.1
- postural I95.1

Hypothermia (accidental) T68
- low environmental temperature T68
- neonatal P80.9
  - environmental (mild) NEC P80.8
  - mild P80.8
  - severe (chronic) (cold injury syndrome) P80.0
  - specified NEC P80.8
- not associated with low environmental temperature R68.0

Hypothyroidism (acquired) E03.9
- congenital (without goiter) E03.1
  - with goiter (diffuse) E03.0
- due to
  - iodine-deficiency, acquired E01.8
    - subclinical E02
  - iodine-deficiency (acquired) E01.8
  - congenital—*see* Syndrome
  - subclinical E02
- neonatal, transitory P72.2
- specified NEC E03.8

Hypotonia, hypotonicity, hypotony
- congenital (benign) P94.2

Hypoventilation R06.89

Hypovolemia E86.1
- surgical shock T81.19
- traumatic (shock) T79.4

Hypoxemia R09.02
- newborn P84

Hypoxia (*see also* Anoxia) R09.02
- intrauterine P84
- newborn P84

Hysteria, hysterical (conversion) (dissociative state) F44.9
- anxiety F41.8
- psychosis, acute F44.9

I

Ichthyoparasitism due to Vandellia cirrhosa B88.8

Ichthyosis (congenital) Q80.9
- fetalis Q80.4
- hystrix Q80.8
- lamellar Q80.2
- palmaris and plantaris Q82.8
- simplex Q80.0
- vera Q80.8
- vulgaris Q80.0
- X-linked Q80.1

Icterus—*see also* Jaundice
- conjunctiva R17
  - newborn P59.9
- hemorrhagic (acute) (leptospiral) (spirochetal) A27.0
  - newborn P53
- infectious B15.9

Ictus solaris, solis T67.01

Ideation
- homicidal R45.850
- suicidal R45.851

Identity disorder (child) F64.9
- gender role F64.2
- psychosexual F64.2

Idioglossia F80.0

Idiopathic—*see* Disease, diseased

Idiot, idiocy (congenital) F73
- microcephalic Q02

IgE asthma J45.909

IIAC (idiopathic infantile arterial calcification) Q28.8

Ileitis (chronic) (noninfectious) (*see also* Enteritis) K52.9
- infectious A09
- regional (ulcerative)—*see* Enteritis, regional, small intestine
- segmental—*see* Enteritis, regional
- terminal (ulcerative)—*see* Enteritis, regional, small intestine

Ileocolitis (*see also* Enteritis) K52.9
- regional—*see* Enteritis, regional
- infectious A09
- ulcerative K51.0-

Ileus (bowel) (colon) (inhibitory) (intestine) K56.7
- adynamic K56.0
- meconium P76.0
  - in cystic fibrosis E84.11
  - meaning meconium plug (without cystic fibrosis) P76.0
- neurogenic K56.0
  - Hirschsprung's disease or megacolon Q43.1
- newborn
  - due to meconium P76.0
    - in cystic fibrosis E84.11
    - meaning meconium plug (without cystic fibrosis) P76.0
  - transitory P76.1
- obstructive K56.69
- paralytic K56.0

Illness (*see also* Disease) R69

Imbalance R26.89
- constituents of food intake E63.1
- electrolyte E87.8
  - neonatal, transitory NEC P74.49
    - potassium
      - ~ hyperkalemia P74.31
      - ~ hypokalemia P74.32

Imbalance, *continued*
- sodium
  - ~ hypernatremia P74.21
  - ~ hyponatremia P74.22
- endocrine E34.9
- eye muscle NOS H50.9
- hysterical F44.4
- posture R29.3
- protein-energy—*see* Malnutrition

Immaturity (less than 37 completed weeks)—*see also* Preterm, newborn
- extreme of newborn (less than 28 completed weeks of gestation) (less than 196 completed days of gestation) (unspecified weeks of gestation) P07.20
  - gestational age
    - 23 completed weeks (23 weeks, 0 days through 23 weeks, 6 days) P07.22
    - 24 completed weeks (24 weeks, 0 days through 24 weeks, 6 days) P07.23
    - 25 completed weeks (25 weeks, 0 days through 25 weeks, 6 days) P07.24
    - 26 completed weeks (26 weeks, 0 days through 26 weeks, 6 days) P07.25
    - 27 completed weeks (27 weeks, 0 days through 27 weeks, 6 days) P07.26
    - less than 23 completed weeks P07.21
- fetus or infant light-for-dates—*see* Light-for-dates
- lung, newborn P28.0
- organ or site NEC—*see* Hypoplasia
- pulmonary, newborn P28.0
- sexual (female) (male), after puberty E30.0

Immersion T75.1

Immunization—*see also* Vaccination
- ABO—*see* Incompatibility, ABO
  - in newborn P55.1
- complication—*see* Complications, vaccination
- encounter for Z23
- not done (not carried out) Z28.9
  - because (of)
    - acute illness of patient Z28.01
    - allergy to vaccine (or component) Z28.04
    - caregiver refusal Z28.82
    - chronic illness of patient Z28.02
    - contraindication NEC Z28.09
    - delay in delivery of vaccine Z28.83
    - group pressure Z28.1
    - guardian refusal Z28.82
    - immune compromised state of patient Z28.03
    - lack of availability of vaccine Z28.83
    - manufacturer delay of vaccine Z28.83
    - parent refusal Z28.82
    - patient's belief Z28.1
    - patient had disease being vaccinated against Z28.81
    - patient refusal Z28.21
    - religious beliefs of patient Z28.1
    - specified reason NEC Z28.89
      - ~ of patient Z28.29
    - unavailability of vaccine Z28.83
    - unspecified patient reason Z28.20
- Rh factor
  - affecting management of pregnancy NEC O36.09-
    - anti-D antibody O36.01-

Immunocompromised NOS D84.9

Immunodeficiency D84.9
- with
  - adenosine-deaminase deficiency D81.30
    - adenosine deaminase 2 D81.32
    - other adenosine deaminase D81.39
    - severe combined immunodeficiency due to adenosine deaminase deficiency D81.31
  - antibody defects D80.9
    - specified type NEC D80.8
  - thrombocytopenia and eczema D82.0
- common variable D83.9
  - with
    - abnormalities of B-cell numbers and function D83.0
    - autoantibodies to B- or T-cells D83.2
    - immunoregulatory T-cell disorders D83.1
    - specified type NEC D83.8

Immunodeficiency, *continued*
- due to
  - conditions classified elsewhere D84.81
  - drugs D84.821
  - external causes D84.822
  - medication (current or past) D84.821
- combined D81.9
  - severe D81.9
    - due to adenosine deaminase deficiency D81.31
- following hereditary defective response to Epstein-Barr virus (EBV) D82.3
- severe combined (SCID) D81.9
  - due to adenosine deaminase deficiency D81.31
- specified type NEC D84.89

Immunodeficient NOS D84.9

Immunosuppressed NOS D84.9

Impaction, impacted
- bowel, colon, rectum (*see also* Impaction, fecal) K56.49
- cerumen (ear) (external) H61.2-
- fecal, feces K56.41
- intestine (calculous) NEC (*see also* Impaction, fecal) K56.49
- turbinate J34.89

Impaired, impairment (function)
- auditory discrimination—*see* Abnormal, auditory perception
- dual sensory Z73.82
- fasting glucose R73.01
- glucose tolerance (oral) R73.02
- hearing—*see* Deafness
- heart—*see* Disease, heart
- rectal sphincter R19.8
- vision NEC H54.7
  - both eyes H54.3

Impediment, speech R47.9
- psychogenic (childhood) F98.8
- slurring R47.81
- specified NEC R47.89

Imperception auditory (acquired)—*see also* Deafness
- congenital H93.25

Imperfect
- aeration, lung (newborn) NEC—*see* Atelectasis
- closure (congenital)
  - alimentary tract NEC Q45.8
    - lower Q43.8
    - upper Q40.8
  - atrioventricular ostium Q21.2
  - atrium (secundum) Q21.1
  - branchial cleft NOS Q18.2
    - cyst Q18.0
    - fistula Q18.0
    - sinus Q18.0
  - choroid Q14.3
  - ductus
    - arteriosus Q25.0
    - Botalli Q25.0
  - ear drum (causing impairment of hearing) Q16.4
  - esophagus with communication to bronchus or trachea Q39.1
  - eyelid Q10.3
  - foramen
    - botalli Q21.1
    - ovale Q21.1
  - genitalia, genital organ(s)or system
    - female Q52.8
      - ~ external Q52.79
      - ~ internal NEC Q52.8
    - male Q55.8
  - interatrial ostium or septum Q21.1
  - interauricular ostium or septum Q21.1
  - interventricular ostium or septum Q21.0
  - omphalomesenteric duct Q43.0
  - ostium
    - interatrial Q21.1
    - interauricular Q21.1
    - interventricular Q21.0
  - roof of orbit Q75.8
  - septum
    - atrial (secundum) Q21.1
    - interatrial (secundum) Q21.1
    - interauricular (secundum) Q21.1

Imperfect, *continued*
- ■ interventricular Q21.0
  - ~ in tetralogy of Fallot Q21.3
- ■ ventricular Q21.0
  - ~ with pulmonary stenosis or atresia, dextraposition of aorta, and hypertrophy of right ventricle Q21.3
  - ~ in tetralogy of Fallot Q21.3
- – skull Q75.0
  - ■ with
    - ~ anencephaly Q00.0
    - ~ encephalocele—*see* Encephalocele
    - ~ hydrocephalus Q03.9
      - ◊ with spina bifida—*see* Spina bifida, by site, with hydrocephalus
    - ~ microcephaly Q02
- – spine (with meningocele)—*see* Spina bifida
- – vitelline duct Q43.0
- • posture R29.3
- • rotation, intestine Q43.3
- • septum, ventricular Q21.0

Imperfectly descended testis—*see* Cryptorchid

Imperforate (congenital)—*see also* Atresia
- • anus Q42.3
  - – with fistula Q42.2
- • esophagus Q39.0
  - – with tracheoesophageal fistula Q39.1
- • hymen Q52.3
- • jejunum Q41.1
- • rectum Q42.1
  - – with fistula Q42.0

Impervious (congenital)—*see also* Atresia
- • anus Q42.3
  - – with fistula Q42.2
- • bile duct Q44.2
- • esophagus Q39.0
  - – with tracheoesophageal fistula Q39.1
- • intestine (small) Q41.9
  - – large Q42.9
    - ■ specified NEC Q42.8
- • rectum Q42.1
  - – with fistula Q42.0

Impetigo (any organism) (any site) (circinate) (contagiosa) (simplex) (vulgaris) L01.00
- • external ear L01.00 [H62.4-]
- • furfuracea L30.5

Implantation
- • cyst
  - – vagina N89.8

Impression, basilar Q75.8

Improper care (child) (newborn)—*see* Maltreatment

Improperly tied umbilical cord (causing hemorrhage) P51.8

Impulsiveness (impulsive) R45.87

Inability to swallow—*see* Aphagia

Inadequate, inadequacy
- • development
  - – child R62.50
  - – genitalia
    - ■ after puberty NEC E30.0
    - ■ congenital
      - ~ female Q52.8
        - ◊ external Q52.79
        - ◊ internal Q52.8
      - ~ male Q55.8
  - – lungs Q33.6
    - ■ associated with short gestation P28.0
  - – organ or site not listed—*see* Anomaly, by site
- • eating habits Z72.4
- • environment, household Z59.1
- • family support Z63.8
- • food (supply) NEC Z59.4
  - – hunger effects T73.0
- • household care, due to
  - – family member
    - ■ handicapped or ill Z74.2
    - ■ temporarily away from home Z74.2
- • housing (heating) (space) Z59.1
- • intrafamilial communication Z63.8
- • mental—*see* Disability, intellectual

Inadequate, inadequacy, *continued*
- • pulmonary
  - – function R06.89
    - ■ newborn P28.5
  - – ventilation, newborn P28.5
- • social
  - – insurance Z59.7
  - – skills NEC Z73.4

Inanition R64
- • fever R50.9

Inappropriate
- • diet or eating habits Z72.4
- • secretion
  - – antidiuretic hormone (ADH) (excessive) E22.2
  - – pituitary (posterior) E22.2

Inattention at or after birth—*see* Neglect

Incarceration, incarcerated
- • exomphalos K42.0
  - – gangrenous K42.1
- • hernia—*see also* Hernia, by site, with obstruction
  - – with gangrene—*see* Hernia, by site, with gangrene
- • omphalocele K42.0
- • rupture—*see* Hernia, by site
- • sarcoepiplomphalocele K42.0
  - – with gangrene K42.1

Incision, incisional
- • hernia K43.2
  - – with
    - ■ gangrene (and obstruction) K43.1
    - ■ obstruction K43.0

Inclusion
- • azurophilic leukocytic D72.0
- • blennorrhea (neonatal) (newborn) P39.1
- • gallbladder in liver (congenital) Q44.1

Incompatibility
- • ABO
  - – affecting management of pregnancy O36.11-
    - ■ anti-A sensitization O36.11-
    - ■ anti-B sensitization O36.19-
    - ■ specified NEC O36.19-
  - – infusion or transfusion reaction T80.30-
  - – newborn P55.1
- • blood (group) (Duffy) (K(ell)) (Kidd) (Lewis) (M) (S) NEC
  - – affecting management of pregnancy O36.11-
    - ■ anti-A sensitization O36.11-
    - ■ anti-B sensitization O36.19-
  - – infusion or transfusion reaction T80.89
  - – newborn P55.8
- • Rh (blood group) (factor)
  - – affecting management of pregnancy NEC O36.09-
    - ■ anti-D antibody O36.01-
  - – infusion or transfusion reaction—*see* Complication(s), transfusion, incompatibility reaction, Rh (factor)
  - – newborn P55.0
- • rhesus—*see* Incompatibility, Rh

Incompetency, incompetent, incompetence
- • annular
  - – aortic (valve)—*see* Insufficiency, aortic
  - – mitral (valve) I34.0
  - – pulmonary valve (heart) I37.1
- • aortic (valve)—*see* Insufficiency, aortic
- • cardiac valve—*see* Endocarditis
- • pulmonary valve (heart) I37.1
  - – congenital Q22.3

Incomplete—*see also* Disease, diseased
- • bladder, emptying R33.9
- • defecation R15.0
- • expansion lungs (newborn) NEC—*see* Atelectasis
- • rotation, intestine Q43.3

Incontinence R32
- • anal sphincter R15.9
- • feces R15.9
  - – nonorganic origin F98.1
- • psychogenic F45.8
- • rectal R15.9
- • urethral sphincter R32
- • urine (urinary) R32
  - – nocturnal N39.44
  - – nonorganic origin F98.0

Increase, increased
- • abnormal, in development R63.8
- • function
  - – adrenal
    - ■ cortex—*see* Cushing's, syndrome
    - ■ pituitary (gland) (anterior) (lobe) E22.9
    - ■ posterior E22.2
- • intracranial pressure (benign) G93.2
- • pressure, intracranial G93.2
- • sphericity, lens Q12.4

Indeterminate sex Q56.4

India rubber skin Q82.8

Indigestion (acid) (bilious) (functional) K30
- • due to decomposed food NOS A05.9
- • nervous F45.8
- • psychogenic F45.8

Induration
- • brain G93.89
- • breast (fibrous) N64.51
- • chancre
  - – congenital A50.07
  - – extragenital NEC A51.2

Inertia
- • stomach K31.89
  - – psychogenic F45.8

Infancy, infantile, infantilism—*see also* Disease, diseased
- • celiac K90.0
- • genitalia, genitals (after puberty) E30.0
- • Herter's (nontropical sprue) K90.0
- • intestinal K90.0
- • Lorain E23.0
- • pituitary E23.0
- • uterus—*see* Infantile, genitalia

Infant(s)—*see also* Infancy
- • excessive crying R68.11
- • irritable child R68.12
- • lack of care—*see* Neglect
- • liveborn (singleton) Z38.2
  - – born in hospital Z38.00
    - ■ by cesarean Z38.01
  - – born outside hospital Z38.1
  - – multiple NEC Z38.8
    - ■ born in hospital Z38.68
      - ~ by cesarean Z38.69
    - ■ born outside hospital Z38.7
  - – quadruplet Z38.8
    - ■ born in hospital Z38.63
      - ~ by cesarean Z38.64
    - ■ born outside hospital Z38.7
  - – quintuplet Z38.8
    - ■ born in hospital Z38.65
      - ~ by cesarean Z38.66
    - ■ born outside hospital Z38.7
  - – triplet Z38.8
    - ■ born in hospital Z38.61
      - ~ by cesarean Z38.62
    - ■ born outside hospital Z38.7
  - – twin Z38.5
    - ■ born in hospital Z38.30
      - ~ by cesarean Z38.31
    - ■ born outside hospital Z38.4
- • of diabetic mother (syndrome of) P70.1
  - – gestational diabetes P70.0

Infantile—*see also* Disease, diseased
- • genitalia, genitals E30.0
- • os, uterine E30.0
- • penis E30.0
- • uterus E30.0

Infantilism—*see* Infancy

Infarct, infarction
- • adrenal (capsule) (gland) E27.49
- • cerebral (acute) (chronic) (*see also* Occlusion, artery) I63.9-
  - – neonatal P91.82-
  - – perinatal (arterial ischemic) P91.82-
- • hypophysis (anterior lobe) E23.6
  - – diffuse acute K55.062
  - – focal (segmental) K55.061
  - – intestine, part unspecified
  - – unspecified extent K55.069

Infarct, infarction, *continued*
- large intestine
  - diffuse acute K55.042
  - focal (segmental) K55.041
  - unspecified extent K55.049
- myocardium, myocardial (acute) (with stated duration of 4 weeks or less)
  - postprocedural
    - following cardiac surgery I97.190
    - following other surgery I97.191
- pituitary (gland) E23.6
- small intestine
  - diffuse acute K55.022
  - focal (segmental) K55.021
  - unspecified extent K55.029
- suprarenal (capsule) (gland) E27.49

Infection
- with
  - drug resistant organism—*see* Resistance, organism(s), to, drug—*see also* specific organism
  - organ dysfunction (acute) R65.20
    - with septic shock R65.21
- acromioclavicular M00.9
- adenoid (and tonsil) J03.90
  - chronic J35.02
- adenovirus NEC
  - as cause of disease classified elsewhere B97.0
  - unspecified nature or site B34.0
- alveolus, alveolar (process) K04.7
- antrum (chronic)—*see* Sinusitis, acute, maxillary
- anus, anal (papillae) (sphincter) K62.89
- axillary gland (lymph) L04.2
- bacterial NOS A49.9
  - as cause of disease classified elsewhere B96.89
    - Enterococcus B95.2
    - Escherichia coli [E. coli] (*see also* Escherichia coli) B96.20
    - Helicobacter pylori [H. pylori] B96.81
    - Hemophilus influenzae [H. influenzae] B96.3
    - Mycoplasma pneumoniae [M. pneumoniae] B96.0
    - Proteus (mirabilis) (morganii) B96.4
    - Pseudomonas (aeruginosa) (mallei) (pseudomallei) B96.5
    - Staphylococcus B95.8
      - ~ aureus (methicillin susceptible) (MSSA) B95.61
        - ◊ methicillin resistant (MRSA) B95.62
      - ~ specified NEC B95.7
    - Streptococcus B95.5
      - ~ group A B95.0
      - ~ group B B95.1
      - ~ pneumoniae B95.3
      - ~ specified NEC B95.4
  - specified NEC A48.8
- Blastomyces, blastomycotic—*see also* Blastomycosis
  - North American B40.9
- Borrelia burgdorferi A69.20
- brain (*see also* Encephalitis) G04.90
  - membranes—*see* Meningitis
  - septic G06.0
    - meninges—*see* Meningitis, bacterial
- buttocks (skin) L08.9
- Campylobacter, intestinal A04.5
  - as cause of disease classified elsewhere B96.81
- Candida (albicans) (tropicalis)—*see* Candidiasis
- candiru B88.8
- central line-associated T80.219
  - bloodstream (CLABSI) T80.211
  - specified NEC T80.218
- cervical gland (lymph) L04.0
- Chlamydia, chlamydial A74.9
  - anus A56.3
  - genitourinary tract A56.2
    - lower A56.00
    - specified NEC A56.19
  - pharynx A56.4
  - rectum A56.3
  - sexually transmitted NEC A56.8
- Clostridium NEC
  - botulinum (food poisoning) A05.1
    - infant A48.51
    - wound A48.52

Infection, *continued*
- difficile
  - foodborne (disease) A04.7-
  - necrotizing enterocolitis A04.7-
  - sepsis A41.4
- perfringens
  - due to food A05.2
  - foodborne (disease) A05.2
  - necrotizing enterocolitis A05.2
  - sepsis A41.4
- welchii
  - foodborne (disease) A05.2
  - sepsis A41.4
- congenital P39.9
  - Candida (albicans) P37.5
  - cytomegalovirus P35.1
  - herpes simplex P35.2
  - infectious or parasitic disease P37.9
    - specified NEC P37.8
  - listeriosis (disseminated) P37.2
  - rubella P35.0
  - toxoplasmosis (acute) (subacute) (chronic) P37.1
  - urinary (tract) P39.3
- coronavirus-2019 U07.1
- coronavirus NEC B34.2
  - as cause of disease classified elsewhere B97.29
  - severe acute respiratory syndrome (SARS associated) B97.21
- COVID-19 U07.1
- cytomegalovirus, cytomegaloviral B25.9
  - congenital P35.1
  - maternal, maternal care for (suspected) damage to fetus O35.3
  - mononucleosis B27.10
    - with
      - ~ complication NEC B27.19
      - ~ meningitis B27.12
      - ~ polyneuropathy B27.11
- dental (pulpal origin) K04.7
- due to or resulting from
  - central venous catheter T80.219
    - bloodstream T80.211
    - exit or insertion site T80.212
    - localized T80.212
    - port or reservoir T80.212
    - specified NEC T80.218
    - tunnel T80.212
  - device, implant or graft (*see also* Complications, by site and type, infection or inflammation) T85.79
    - arterial graft NEC T82.7
    - catheter NEC T85.79
      - ~ dialysis (renal) T82.7
      - ~ infusion NEC T82.7
      - ~ urinary T83.518
        - ◊ cystostomy T83.510
        - ◊ Hopkins T83.518
        - ◊ ileostomy T83.518
        - ◊ nephrostomy T83.512
        - ◊ specified NEC T83.518
        - ◊ urethral indwelling T83.511
        - ◊ urostomy T83.518
  - Hickman catheter T80.219
    - bloodstream T80.211
    - localized T80.212
    - specified NEC T80.218
  - immunization or vaccination T88.0
  - infusion, injection or transfusion NEC T80.29
    - acute T80.22
  - peripherally inserted central catheter (PICC) T80.219
    - bloodstream T80.211
    - localized T80.212
    - specified NEC T80.218
  - portacath (port-a-cath) T80.219
    - bloodstream T80.211
    - localized T80.212
    - specified NEC T80.218
  - postoperative (postprocedural) T81.4
    - sepsis T81.49
    - specified surgical site NEC T81.4-
    - superficial incisional surgical site T81.41
  - surgery T81.40

Infection, *continued*
- triple lumen catheter T80.219
  - bloodstream T80.211
  - localized T80.212
  - specified NEC T80.218
- umbilical venous catheter T80.219
  - bloodstream T80.211
  - localized T80.212
  - specified NEC T80.218
- ear (middle)—*see also* Otitis, media
  - external—*see* Otitis, externa, infective
  - inner—*see* subcategory H83.0
- echovirus
  - as cause of disease classified elsewhere B97.12
  - unspecified nature or site B34.1
- endocardium I33.0
- Enterobius vermicularis B80
- enterovirus B34.1
  - as cause of disease classified elsewhere B97.10
    - coxsackievirus B97.11
    - echovirus B97.12
    - specified NEC B97.19
- erythema infectiosum B08.3
- Escherichia (E.) coli NEC A49.8
  - as cause of disease classified elsewhere (*see also* Escherichia coli) B96.20
  - congenital P39.8
    - sepsis P36.4
  - generalized A41.51
  - intestinal—*see* Enteritis, infectious, due to, Escherichia coli
- eyelid H01.-
  - abscess—*see* Abscess, eyelid
  - blepharitis—*see* Blepharitis
  - chalazion—*see* Chalazion
  - dermatosis (noninfectious)—*see* Dermatitis, eyelid
  - hordeolum—*see* Hordeolum
  - specified NEC H01.8
- finger (skin) L08.9
  - nail L03.01-
    - fungus B35.1
- focal
  - teeth (pulpal origin) K04.7
  - tonsils J35.01
- foot (skin) L08.9
  - dermatophytic fungus B35.3
- fungus NOS B49
  - beard B35.0
  - dermatophytic—*see* Dermatophytosis
  - foot B35.3
  - groin B35.6
  - hand B35.2
  - nail B35.1
  - perianal (area) B35.6
  - scalp B35.0
  - skin B36.9
    - foot B35.3
    - hand B35.2
    - toenails B35.1
- Giardia lamblia A07.1
- gingiva (chronic)
  - acute K05.00
    - plaque induced K05.00
- gram-negative bacilli NOS A49.9
- gum (chronic)
  - acute K05.00
    - plaque induced K05.00
- Helicobacter pylori A04.8
  - as the cause of disease classified elsewhere B96.81
- Hemophilus
  - influenzae NEC A49.2
    - as cause of disease classified elsewhere B96.3
  - generalized A41.3
- herpes (simplex)—*see also* Herpes
  - congenital P35.2
  - disseminated B00.7
  - herpesvirus, herpesviral—*see* Herpes
- hip (joint) NEC M00.9
  - skin NEC L08.9
- human
  - papilloma virus A63.0
- hydrocele N43.0
- inguinal (lymph) glands L04.1

Infection, *continued*
- joint NEC M00.9
- knee (joint) NEC M00.9
  - joint M00.9
  - skin L08.9
- leg (skin) NOS L08.9
- listeria monocytogenes—*see also* Listeriosis
  - congenital P37.2
- local, skin (staphylococcal) (streptococcal) L08.9
  - abscess—*code by* site under Abscess
  - cellulitis—*code by* site under Cellulitis
  - ulcer—*see* Ulcer
- lung (*see also* Pneumonia) J18.9
  - virus—*see* Pneumonia, viral
- lymph gland—*see also* Lymphadenitis, acute
  - mesenteric I88.0
- lymphoid tissue, base of tongue or posterior pharynx, NEC (chronic) J35.03
- Malassezia furfur B36.0
- mammary gland N61.0
- meningococcal (*see also* Disease, diseased) A39.9
  - cerebrospinal A39.0
  - meninges A39.0
  - meningococcemia A39.4
    - acute A39.2
    - chronic A39.3
- mesenteric lymph nodes or glands NEC I88.0
- metatarsophalangeal M00.9
- mouth, parasitic B37.0
- Mycoplasma NEC A49.3
  - pneumoniae, as cause of disease classified elsewhere B96.0
- myocardium NEC I40.0
- nail (chronic)
  - with lymphangitis—*see* Lymphangitis, acute
  - finger L03.01-
    - fungus B35.1
  - ingrowing L60.0
  - toe L03.03-
    - fungus B35.1
- newborn P39.9
  - intra-amniotic NEC P39.2
  - skin P39.4
  - specified type NEC P39.8
- nipple N61.0
- Oidium albicans B37.9
- operative wound T81.49
- Oxyuris vermicularis B80
- pancreas (acute) K85.92
  - abscess—*see* Pancreatitis, acute
  - specified NEC K85.82
- parameningococcus A39.9
- paraurethral ducts N34.2
- parvovirus NEC B34.3
  - as the cause of disease classified elsewhere B97.6
- Pasteurella NEC A28.0
  - multocida A28.0
  - pseudotuberculosis A28.0
  - septica (cat bite) (dog bite) A28.0
- perinatal period P39.9
  - specified type NEC P39.8
- perirectal K62.89
- perirenal—*see* Infection, kidney
- peritoneal—*see* Peritonitis
- pharynx—*see also* Pharyngitis
  - coxsackievirus B08.5
  - posterior, lymphoid (chronic) J35.03
- pinworm B80
- pityrosporum furfur B36.0
- pleuro-pneumonia-like organism (PPLO) NEC A49.3
  - as cause of disease classified elsewhere B96.0
- pneumococcus, pneumococcal NEC A49.1
  - as cause of disease classified elsewhere B95.3
  - generalized (purulent) A40.3
    - with pneumonia J13
- port or reservoir T80.212
- postoperative T81.40
  - surgical site
    - deep incisional T81.42
    - organ and space T81.43
    - specified NEC T81.49
    - superficial incisional T81.41
- postprocedural T81.40

Infection, *continued*
- prepuce NEC N47.7
  - with penile inflammation N47.6
- Proteus (mirabilis) (morganii) (vulgaris) NEC A49.8
  - as cause of disease classified elsewhere B96.4
- Pseudomonas NEC A49.8
  - as cause of disease classified elsewhere B96.5
  - pneumonia J15.1
- rectum (sphincter) K62.89
- renal
  - pelvis and ureter (cystic) N28.85
- respiratory (tract) NEC J98.8
  - acute J22
  - chronic J98.8
  - influenzal (upper) (acute)—*see* Influenza, with, respiratory manifestations NEC
  - lower (acute) J22
    - chronic—*see* Bronchitis
  - rhinovirus J00
  - syncytial virus (RSV) J06.9 [B97.4]
  - upper (acute) NOS J06.9
    - streptococcal J06.9
    - viral NOS J06.9
- rhinovirus
  - as cause of disease classified elsewhere B97.89
  - unspecified nature or site B34.8
- rickettsial NOS A79.9
- roundworm (large) NEC B82.0
  - Ascariasis (*see also* Ascariasis) B77.9
- Salmonella (aertrycke) (arizonae) (callinarum) (choleraesuis) (enteritidis) (suipestifer) (typhimurium)
  - with
    - (gastro) enteritis A02.0
    - specified manifestation NEC A02.8
  - due to food (poisoning) A02.9
- scabies B86
- Shigella A03.9
  - boydii A03.2
  - dysenteriae A03.0
  - flexneri A03.1
  - group
    - A A03.0
    - B A03.1
    - C A03.2
    - D A03.3
- shoulder (joint) NEC M00.9
  - skin NEC L08.9
- skin (local) (staphylococcal) (streptococcal) L08.9
  - abscess—*code by* site under Abscess
  - cellulitis—*code by* site under Cellulitis
- spinal cord NOS (*see also* Myelitis) G04.91
  - abscess G06.1
  - meninges—*see* Meningitis
  - streptococcal G04.89
- staphylococcal, unspecified site
  - aureus (methicillin susceptible) (MSSA) A49.01
    - methicillin resistant (MRSA) A49.02
  - as cause of disease classified elsewhere B95.8
    - aureus (methicillin susceptible) (MSSA) B95.61
      - methicillin resistant (MRSA) B95.62
    - specified NEC B95.7
  - food poisoning A05.0
  - generalized (purulent) A41.2
  - pneumonia—*see* Pneumonia, staphylococcal
- streptobacillus moniliformis A25.1
- streptococcal NEC A49.1
  - as the cause of disease classified elsewhere B95.5
  - congenital
    - sepsis P36.10
      - group B P36.0
      - specified NEC P36.19
  - generalized (purulent) A40.9
- subcutaneous tissue, local L08.9
- threadworm B80
- toe (skin) L08.9
  - cellulitis L03.03-
    - fungus B35.1
  - nail L03.03-
    - fungus B35.1
- tongue NEC K14.0
  - parasitic B37.0
- tooth, teeth K04.7
  - periapical K04.7

Infection, *continued*
- TORCH—*see* Infection, congenital
  - without active infection P00.2
- Trichomonas A59.9
  - cervix A59.09
  - specified site NEC A59.8
  - urethra A59.03
  - urogenitalis A59.00
  - vagina A59.01
  - vulva A59.01
- Trombicula (irritans) B88.0
- tuberculous
  - latent (LTBI) Z22.7
  - NEC—*see* Tuberculosis
- tunnel T80.212
- urinary (tract) N39.0
  - bladder—*see* Cystitis
  - newborn P39.3
  - urethra—*see* Urethritis
- varicella B01.9
- Vibrio
  - parahaemolyticus (food poisoning) A05.3
  - vulnificus
    - foodborne intoxication A05.5
- virus, viral NOS B34.9
  - adenovirus
    - as the cause of disease classified elsewhere B97.0
    - unspecified nature or site B34.0
  - as the cause of disease classified elsewhere B97.89
    - adenovirus B97.0
    - coxsackievirus B97.11
    - echovirus B97.12
    - enterovirus B97.10
      - ~ coxsackievirus B97.11
      - ~ echovirus B97.12
      - ~ specified NEC B97.19
    - parvovirus B97.6
    - specified NEC B97.89
  - central nervous system A89
    - enterovirus NEC A88.8
      - ~ meningitis A87.0
  - coxsackie B34.1
    - as cause of disease classified elsewhere B97.11
  - ECHO
    - as cause of disease classified elsewhere B97.12
    - unspecified nature or site B34.1
  - enterovirus, as cause of disease classified elsewhere B97.10
    - coxsackievirus B97.11
    - echovirus B97.12
    - specified NEC B97.19
  - exanthem NOS B09
  - respiratory syncytial (RSV)
    - as cause of disease classified elsewhere B97.4
    - bronchiolitis J21.0
    - bronchitis J20.5
    - bronchopneumonia J12.1
    - otitis media H65.- [B97.4]
    - pneumonia J12.1
    - upper respiratory infection J06.9 [B97.4]
  - rhinovirus
    - as the cause of disease specified elsewhere B97.89
  - specified type NEC B33.8
    - as the cause of disease specified elsewhere B97.89
- yeast (*see also* Candidiasis) B37.9
- Zika virus A92.5
  - congenital P35.4

Infertility
- female N97.9
  - associated with
    - anovulation N97.0
    - Stein-Leventhal syndrome E28.2
  - due to
    - Stein-Leventhal syndrome E28.2

Infestation B88.9
- Acariasis B88.0
  - demodex folliculorum B88.0
  - sarcoptes scabiei B86
  - trombiculae B88.0
- arthropod NEC B88.2

Infestation, *continued*
- Ascaris lumbricoides—*see* Ascariasis
- candiru B88.8
- cestodes B71.9
- chigger B88.0
- chigo, chigoe B88.1
- crab-lice B85.3
- Demodex (folliculorum) B88.0
- Dermanyssus gallinae B88.0
- Enterobius vermicularis B80
- eyelid
  - in (due to)
    ■ phthiriasis B85.3
- fluke B66.9
  - specified type NEC B66.8
- Giardia lamblia A07.1
- helminth
  - intestinal B82.0
    ■ enterobiasis B80
- intestinal NEC B82.9
- Linguatula B88.8
- Lyponyssoides sanguineus B88.0
- mites B88.9
  - scabic B86
- Monilia (albicans)—*see* Candidiasis
- mouth B37.0
- nematode NEC (intestinal) B82.0
  - Enterobius vermicularis B80
  - physaloptera B80
- Oxyuris vermicularis B80
- parasite, parasitic B89
  - eyelid B89
  - intestinal NOS B82.9
  - mouth B37.0
  - skin B88.9
  - tongue B37.0
- Pediculus B85.2
  - body B85.1
  - capitis (humanus) (any site) B85.0
  - corporis (humanus) (any site) B85.1
  - mixed (classifiable to more than one of the titles B85.0–B85.3) B85.4
  - pubis (any site) B85.3
- Pentastoma B88.8
- Phthirus (pubis) (any site) B85.3
  - with any infestation classifiable to B85.0-B85.2 B85.4
- pinworm B80
- pubic louse B85.3
- red bug B88.0
- sand flea B88.1
- Sarcoptes scabiei B86
- scabies B86
- Schistosoma B65.9
  - cercariae B65.3
- skin NOS B88.9
- specified type NEC B88.8
- tapeworm B71.9
- Tetranychus molestissimus B88.0
- threadworm B80
- tongue B37.0
- Trombicula (irritans) B88.0
- Tunga penetrans B88.1
- Vandella cirrhosa B88.8

Infiltrate, infiltration
- leukemic—*see* Leukemia
- lung R91.8
- lymphatic (*see also* Leukemia) C91.9-
  - gland I88.9
- on chest x-ray R91.8
- pulmonary R91.8
- vesicant agent
  - antineoplastic chemotherapy T80.810
  - other agent NEC T80.818

Inflammation, inflamed, inflammatory (with exudation)
- anal canal, anus K62.89
- areola N61.0
- areolar tissue NOS L08.9
- breast N61.0
- bronchi—*see* Bronchitis
- catarrhal J00

Inflammation, inflamed, inflammatory, *continued*
- cerebrospinal
  - meningococcal A39.0
- due to device, implant or graft—*see also* Complications, by site and type, infection or inflammation
  - arterial graft T82.7
  - catheter T85.79
    ■ cardiac T82.7
    ■ dialysis (renal) T82.7
    ■ infusion T82.7
    ■ urinary T83.518
      ~ cystostomy T83.510
      ~ Hopkins T83.518
      ~ ileostomy T83.518
      ~ nephrostomy T83.512
      ~ specified NEC T83.518
      ~ urethral indwelling T83.511
      ~ urostomy T83.518
  - electronic (electrode) (pulse generator) (stimulator)
  - vascular NEC T82.7
- duodenum K29.80
  - with bleeding K29.81
- esophagus K20.9-
- follicular, pharynx J31.2
- gland (lymph)—*see* Lymphadenitis
- glottis—*see* Laryngitis
- granular, pharynx J31.2
- leg NOS L08.9
- lip K13.0
- mouth K12.1
- nipple N61.0
- orbit (chronic) H05.10-
  - acute H05.00
    ■ abscess—*see* Abscess
  - granuloma—*see* Granuloma, orbit
- parotid region L08.9
- perianal K62.89
- pericardium—*see* Pericarditis
- perineum (female) (male) L08.9
- perirectal K62.89
- peritoneum—*see* Peritonitis
- polyp, colon (*see also* Polyp, colon, inflammatory) K51.40
- rectum (*see also* Proctitis) K62.89
- respiratory, upper (*see also* Infection, respiratory, upper) J06.9
- skin L08.9
- subcutaneous tissue L08.9
- tongue K14.0
- tonsil—*see* Tonsillitis
- vein—*see also* Phlebitis
  - intracranial or intraspinal (septic) G08
  - thrombotic I80.9
    ■ leg—*see* Phlebitis, leg
    ■ lower extremity—*see* Phlebitis, leg

Influenza (bronchial) (epidemic) (respiratory (upper)) (unidentified influenza virus) J11.1
- with
  - digestive manifestations J11.2
  - encephalopathy J11.81
  - enteritis J11.2
  - gastroenteritis J11.2
  - gastrointestinal manifestations J11.2
  - laryngitis J11.1
  - myocarditis J11.82
  - otitis media J11.83
  - pharyngitis J11.1
  - pneumonia J11.00
    ■ specified type J11.08
  - respiratory manifestations NEC J11.1
  - specified manifestation NEC J11.89
- A (non-novel) J10-
- A/H5N1 (*see also* Influenza, due to, identified novel influenza A virus) J09.X2
- avian (*see also* Influenza, due to, identified novel influenza A virus) J09.X2
- B J10-
- bird (*see also* Influenza, due to, identified novel influenza A virus) J09.X2
- C J10-
- novel (2009) H1N1 influenza (*see also* Influenza, due to, identified influenza virus NEC) J10.1

Influenza, *continued*
- novel influenza A/H1N1 (*see also* Influenza, due to, identified influenza virus NEC) J10.1
- due to
  - avian (*see also* Influenza, due to, identified novel influenza A virus) J09.X2
  - identified influenza virus NEC J10.1
    ■ with
      ~ digestive manifestations J10.2
      ~ encephalopathy J10.81
      ~ enteritis J10.2
      ~ gastroenteritis J10.2
      ~ gastrointestinal manifestations J10.2
      ~ laryngitis J10.1
      ~ myocarditis J10.82
      ~ otitis media J10.83
      ~ pharyngitis J10.1
      ~ pneumonia (unspecified type) J10.00
        ◊ with same identified influenza virus J10.01
        ◊ specified type NEC J10.08
      ~ respiratory manifestations NEC J10.1
      ~ specified manifestation NEC J10.89
  - identified novel influenza A virus J09.X2
    ■ with
      ~ digestive manifestations J09.X3
      ~ encephalopathy J09.X9
      ~ enteritis J09.X3
      ~ gastroenteritis J09.X3
      ~ gastrointestinal manifestations J09.X3
      ~ laryngitis J09.X2
      ~ myocarditis J09.X9
      ~ otitis media J09.X9
      ~ pharyngitis J09.X2
      ~ pneumonia J09.X1
      ~ respiratory manifestations NEC J09.X2
      ~ specified manifestation NEC J09.X9
      ~ upper respiratory symptoms J09.X2
- of other animal origin, not bird or swine (*see also* Influenza, due to, identified novel influenza A virus) J09.X2
- swine (viruses that normally cause infections in pigs) (*see also* Influenza, due to, identified novel influenza A virus) J09.X2

Influenza-like disease—*see* Influenza

Influenzal—*see* Influenza

Ingestion
- chemical—*see* Table of Drugs and Chemicals, by substance, poisoning
- drug or medicament
  - correct substance properly administered—*see* Table of Drugs and Chemicals, by drug, adverse effect
  - overdose or wrong substance given or taken—*see* Table of Drugs and Chemicals, by drug, poisoning
- foreign body—*see* Foreign body, alimentary tract

Ingrowing
- hair (beard) L73.1
- nail (finger) (toe) L60.0

Inguinal—*see also* Disease, diseased
- testicle Q53.9
  - bilateral Q53.212
  - unilateral Q53.112

Inhalation
- anthrax A22.1
- gases, fumes, or vapors
  - specified agent—*see* Table of Drugs and Chemicals, by substance T59.89-
- liquid or vomitus—*see* Asphyxia
- meconium (newborn) P24.00
  - with
    ■ pneumonia (pneumonitis) P24.01
    ■ with respiratory symptoms P24.01
- mucus—*see* Asphyxia
- oil or gasoline (causing suffocation)—*see* Foreign body, by site
- smoke T59.81-
  - with respiratory conditions J70.5

See also the *ICD-10-CM* External Cause of Injuries Table for codes describing accident details.

Injury (*see also* specified type of injury) T14.90
- ankle S99.91-
  - specified type NEC S99.81-
- blood vessel NEC T14.8
  - hand (level) S65.9-
    - laceration S65.91-
    - specified
      - type NEC S65.99-
  - neck S15.9
    - specified site NEC S15.8
  - palmar arch (superficial) S65.2-
    - deep S65.30-
      - laceration S65.31-
      - specified type NEC S65.39-
    - laceration S65.21-
    - specified type NEC S65.29-
- brachial plexus S14.3
  - newborn P14.3
- cord
  - spermatic (pelvic region)
    - scrotal region S39.848
- eye S05.9-
  - conjunctiva S05.0-
  - cornea
    - abrasion S05.0-
- foot S99.92-
  - specified type NEC S99.82-
- genital organ(s)
  - external S39.94
    - specified NEC S39.848
- head S09.90
  - with loss of consciousness S06.9-
  - specified NEC S09.8
- internal T14.8
  - pelvis, pelvic (organ) S39.9-
  - specified NEC S39.83
- intra-abdominal S36.90
- intracranial (traumatic) S06.9-
  - intracerebral hemorrhage, traumatic
    - intracranial (trauma)
      - epidural, hemorrhage (traumatic) S06.4X
    - left side S06.35-
    - right side S06.34-
  - subarachnoid hemorrhage, traumatic S06.6X-
  - subdural hemorrhage, traumatic S06.5X-
- intrathoracic
  - lung S27.30-
    - aspiration J69.0
    - bilateral S27.302
    - contusion S27.329
      - bilateral S27.322
      - unilateral S27.321
    - unilateral S27.301
  - pneumothorax S27.0-
- kidney S37.0-
  - acute (nontraumatic) N17.9
  - contusion—*see* Contusion, kidney
- lung—*see also* Injury, intrathoracic, lung
  - aspiration J69.0
  - dabbing (related) U07.0
  - electronic cigarette (related) U07.0
  - EVALI- [e-cigarette, or vaping, product use associated] U07.0
  - transfusion-related (TRALI) J95.84
  - - vaping (device) (product) (use) (associated) U07.0
- multiple NOS T07
- muscle
  - finger
    - extensor S56.4-
      - hand level S66.3-
        - strain S66.31-
      - laceration S56.42-
      - strain S56.41-
    - flexor (forearm level) S56.1-
      - hand level S66.1-
        - laceration S66.12- (See complete *ICD-10-CM* Manual)
        - strain S66.11-
      - laceration S56.12-
      - strain S56.11-
    - intrinsic S66.5-
      - strain S66.51-

Injury, *continued*
- foot S96.9-
  - intrinsic S96.2-
    - laceration S96.22-
    - strain S96.21-
  - laceration S96.92-
  - specified
    - site NEC S96.8-
      - strain S96.81-
  - strain S96.91-
- forearm (level) S56.90-
  - extensor S56.5-
    - laceration S56.52-
    - strain S56.51-
  - flexor
    - laceration S56.22-
    - strain S56.21-
  - laceration S56.92-
  - specified
    - site NEC S56.8-
      - laceration S56.82-
      - strain S56.81-
  - strain S56.91-
- hand (level) S66.9-
  - strain S66.91-
- thumb
  - abductor (forearm level) S56.3-
    - laceration S56.32-
    - strain S56.31-
  - extensor (forearm level) S56.3-
    - hand level S66.2-
      - strain S66.21-
    - laceration S56.32-
    - specified type NEC S56.39-
    - strain S56.31-
  - flexor (forearm level) S56.0 -
    - hand level S66.0-
      - laceration S66.02-
      - strain S66.01-
    - laceration S56.02-
    - strain S56.01-
  - intrinsic S66.4-
    - strain S66.41-
- toe—*see also* Injury, muscle, foot
  - extensor, long S96.1-
    - laceration S96.12-
    - strain S96.11-
  - flexor, long S96.0-
    - laceration S96.02-
    - strain S96.01-
- neck (level) S16.9
  - laceration S16.2
  - specified type NEC S16.8
  - strain S16.1
- nerve NEC T14.8
  - facial S04.5-
    - newborn P11.3
- pelvis, pelvic (floor) S39.93
  - specified NEC S39.83
- postcardiac surgery (syndrome) I97.0
- rectovaginal septum NEC S39.83
- scalp S09.90
  - newborn (birth injury) P12.9
    - due to monitoring (electrode) (sampling incision) P12.4
    - specified NEC P12.89
      - caput succedaneum P12.81
- spermatic cord (pelvic region)
  - scrotal region S39.848
- spinal (cord)
  - cervical (neck) S14.109
    - C1 level S14.101
    - C2 level S14.102
    - C3 level S14.103
    - C4 level S14.104
    - C5 level S14.105
    - C6 level S14.106
    - C7 level S14.107
    - C8 level S14.108
  - lumbar S34.109
    - complete lesion S34.11- (See complete *ICD-10-CM* Manual)

Injury, *continued*
- incomplete lesion S34.129
  - L1 level S34.121
  - L2 level S34.122
  - L3 level S34.123
  - L4 level S34.124
  - L5 level S34.125
- L1 level S34.101
- L2 level S34.102
- L3 level S34.103
- L4 level S34.104
- L5 level S34.105
- sacral S34.139
  - complete lesion S34.131
  - incomplete lesion S34.132
- thoracic S24.109
  - T1 level S24.101
  - T2-T6 level S24.102
  - T7-T10 level S24.103
  - T11-T12 level S24.104
- spleen S36.0-
  - laceration S36.03-
    - superficial (capsular) (minor) S36.030
- toe S99.92-
  - specified type NEC S99.82-
- transfusion-related acute lung (TRALI) J95.84
- vagina S39.93
  - abrasion S30.814
  - bite S31.45
    - insect S30.864
    - superficial NEC S30.874
  - contusion S30.23
  - external constriction S30.844
  - insect bite S30.864
  - laceration S31.41
    - with foreign body S31.42
  - open wound S31.4-
  - puncture S31.43
    - with foreign body S31.44
  - superficial S30.95
    - foreign body S30.854
- vulva S39.94
  - abrasion S30.814
  - bite S31.45
    - insect S30.864
    - superficial NEC S30.874
  - contusion S30.23
  - external constriction S30.844
  - insect bite S30.864
  - laceration S31.41
    - with foreign body S31.42
  - open wound S31.4-
  - puncture S31.43
    - with foreign body S31.44
  - superficial S30.95
    - foreign body S30.854
- whiplash (cervical spine) S13.4

Insensitivity
- adrenocorticotropin hormone (ACTH) E27.49
- androgen E34.50
  - complete E34.51
  - partial E34.52

Insolation (sunstroke) T67.01

Insomnia (organic) G47.00
- adjustment F51.02
  - adjustment disorder F51.02
- behavioral, of childhood Z73.819
  - combined type Z73.812
  - limit setting type Z73.811
  - sleep-onset association type Z73.810
- childhood Z73.819
- chronic F51.04
  - somatized tension F51.04
- conditioned F51.04
- due to
  - anxiety disorder F51.05
  - depression F51.05
  - medical condition G47.01
  - mental disorder NEC F51.05
- idiopathic F51.01
- learned F51.3
- nonorganic origin F51.01

Insomnia, *continued*
- not due to a substance or known physiological condition F51.01
  - specified NEC F51.09
- paradoxical F51.03
- primary F51.01
- psychiatric F51.05
- psychophysiologic F51.04
- related to psychopathology F51.05
- short-term F51.02
- specified NEC G47.09
- stress-related F51.02
- transient F51.02
- without objective findings F51.02

Inspissated bile syndrome (newborn) P59.1

Instability
- emotional (excessive) F60.3
- joint (post-traumatic) M25.30
  - specified site NEC M25.39
- personality (emotional) F60.3
- vasomotor R55

Insufficiency, insufficient
- adrenal (gland) E27.40
  - primary E27.1
- adrenocortical E27.40
  - primary E27.1
- anus K62.89
- aortic (valve) I35.1
  - with
    - mitral (valve) disease I08.0
      ~ with tricuspid (valve) disease I08.3
    - stenosis I35.2
    - tricuspid (valve) disease I08.2
      ~ with mitral (valve) disease I08.3
  - congenital Q23.1
  - rheumatic I06.1
    - with
      ~ mitral (valve) disease I08.0
        ◊ with tricuspid (valve) disease I08.3
      ~ stenosis I06.2
        ◊ with mitral (valve) disease I08.0
          » with tricuspid (valve) disease I08.3
      ~ tricuspid (valve) disease I08.2
        ◊ with mitral (valve) disease I08.3
  - specified cause NEC I35.1
- cardiac—*see also* Insufficiency, myocardial
  - due to presence of (cardiac) prosthesis I97.11-
  - postprocedural I97.11-
- corticoadrenal E27.40
  - primary E27.1
- kidney N28.9
  - acute N28.9
  - chronic N18.9
- mitral (valve) I34.0
  - with
    - aortic valve disease I08.0
      ~ with tricuspid (valve) disease I08.3
    - obstruction or stenosis I05.2
      ~ with aortic valve disease I08.0
    - tricuspid (valve) disease I08.1
      ~ with aortic (valve) disease I08.3
  - congenital Q23.3
  - rheumatic I05.1
    - with
      ~ aortic valve disease I08.0
        ◊ with tricuspid (valve) disease I08.3
      ~ obstruction or stenosis I05.2
        ◊ with aortic valve disease I08.0
          » with tricuspid (valve) disease I08.3
      ~ tricuspid (valve) disease I08.1
        ◊ with aortic (valve) disease I08.3
    - active or acute I01.1
      ~ with chorea, rheumatic (Sydenham's) I02.0
  - specified cause, except rheumatic I34.0
- muscle—*see also* Disease, muscle
  - heart—*see* Insufficiency, myocardium, myocardial
  - ocular NEC H50.9
- myocardial, myocardium (with arteriosclerosis) I50.9
  - with
    - rheumatic fever (conditions in I00) I09.0
      ~ active, acute or subacute I01.2
        ◊ with chorea I02.0

Insufficiency, insufficient, *continued*
  ~ inactive or quiescent (with chorea) I09.0
  - congenital Q24.8
  - newborn P29.0
  - rheumatic I09.0
    - active, acute, or subacute I01.2
- placental (mother) O36.51
- pulmonary J98.4
  - newborn P28.89
  - valve I37.1
    - with stenosis I37.2
    - congenital Q22.2
    - rheumatic I09.89
      ~ with aortic, mitral or tricuspid (valve) disease I08.8
- renal (acute) N28.9
  - chronic N18.9
- respiratory R06.89
  - newborn P28.5
- rotation—*see* Malrotation
- suprarenal E27.40
  - primary E27.1
- tarso-orbital fascia, congenital Q10.3
- thyroid (gland) (acquired) E03.9
  - congenital E03.1
- tricuspid (valve) (rheumatic) I07.1
  - with
    - aortic (valve) disease I08.2
      ~ with mitral (valve) disease I08.3
    - mitral (valve) disease I08.1
      ~ with aortic (valve) disease I08.3
    - obstruction or stenosis I07.2
      ~ with aortic (valve) disease I08.2
        ◊ with mitral (valve) disease I08.3
  - congenital Q22.8
  - nonrheumatic I36.1
    - with stenosis I36.2
- urethral sphincter R32
- velopharyngeal
  - acquired K13.79
  - congenital Q38.8

Intertrigo L30.4
- labialis K13.0

Intolerance
- carbohydrate K90.49
- disaccharide, hereditary E73.0
- fat NEC K90.49
  - pancreatic K90.3
- food K90.49
  - dietary counseling and surveillance Z71.3
- gluten
  - celiac K90.0
  - non-celiac K90.41
- lactose E73.9
  - specified NEC E73.8
- milk NEC K90.49
  - lactose E73.9
- protein K90.49
- starch NEC K90.49

Intoxication
- drug
  - acute (without dependence)—*see* Abuse, drug, by type, with intoxication
    - with dependence—*see* Dependence, drug, by type with intoxication
  - addictive
    - via placenta or breast milk—*see* Absorption, drug
  - newborn P93.8
    - gray baby syndrome P93.0
  - overdose or wrong substance given or taken—*see* Table of Drugs and Chemicals, by drug, poisoning
- foodborne A05.9
  - bacterial A05.9
  - classical (Clostridium botulinum) A05.1
  - due to
    - Bacillus cereus A05.4
    - bacterium A05.9
      ~ specified NEC A05.8
    - Clostridium
      ~ botulinum A05.1
      ~ perfringens A05.2
      ~ welchii A05.2

Intoxication, *continued*
    - Salmonella A02.9
      ~ with
        ◊ (gastro) enteritis A02.0
        ◊ specified manifestation NEC A02.8
    - Staphylococcus A05.0
    - Vibrio
      ~ parahaemolyticus A05.3
      ~ vulnificus A05.5
  - enterotoxin, staphylococcal A05.0
  - noxious—*see* Poisoning, food, noxious
- meaning
  - inebriation—*see* category F10
  - poisoning—*see* Table of Drugs and Chemicals
- serum (*see also* Reaction, serum) T80.69

Intraabdominal testis, testes
- bilateral Q53.211
- unilateral Q53.111

Intrahepatic gallbladder Q44.1

Intrauterine contraceptive device
- checking Z30.431
- insertion Z30.430
  - immediately following removal Z30.433
- in situ Z97.5
- management Z30.431
- reinsertion Z30.433
- removal Z30.432
- replacement Z30.433

Intussusception (bowel) (colon) (enteric) (ileocecal) (ileocolic) (intestine) (rectum) K56.1

Invagination (bowel, colon, intestine or rectum) K56.1

Inversion
- albumin-globulin (A-G) ratio E88.09
- nipple N64.59
- testis (congenital) Q55.29

Investigation (*see also* Examination) Z04.9

I. Q.
- under 20 F73
- 20–34 F72
- 35–49 F71
- 50–69 F70

IRDS (type I) P22.0
- type II P22.1

Iritis
- diabetic—*see* E08 –E13 with .39

Irradiated enamel (tooth, teeth) K03.89

Irradiation effects, adverse T66

Irregular, irregularity
- action, heart I49.9
- bleeding N92.6
- breathing R06.89
- menstruation (cause unknown) N92.6
- periods N92.6
- respiratory R06.89
- septum (nasal) J34.2
- sleep-wake pattern (rhythm) G47.23

Irritable, irritability R45.4
- bladder N32.89
- bowel (syndrome) K58.9
  - with constipation K58.1
  - with diarrhea K58.0
  - mixed K58.2
  - other K58.8
  - psychogenic F45.8
- cerebral, in newborn P91.3
- colon K58.9
  - with constipation K58.1
  - with diarrhea K58.0
  - mixed K58.2
  - other K58.8
  - psychogenic F45.8
- heart (psychogenic) F45.8
- infant R68.12 stomach K31.89
  - psychogenic F45.8

Irritation
- anus K62.89
- bladder N32.89
- gastric K31.89
  - psychogenic F45.8

Irritation, *continued*
- nervous R45.0
- perineum NEC L29.3
- stomach K31.89
  - psychogenic F45.8
- vaginal N89.8

Ischemia, ischemic I99.8
- brain—*see* Ischemia, cerebral
- cerebral (chronic) (generalized) I67.82
  - intermittent G45.9
  - newborn P91.0
  - recurrent focal G45.8
  - transient G45.9
- intestine, unspecified part
  - diffuse acute (reversible) K55.052
  - focal (segmental) acute (reversible) K55.051
  - unspecified extent K55.059
- large intestine
  - diffuse acute (reversible) K55.032
  - focal (segmental) acute (reversible) K55.031
  - unspecified extent K55.039
- small intestine
  - diffuse acute (reversible) K55.012
  - focal (segmental) acute (reversible) K55.011
  - unspecified extent K55.019

Ischuria R34

Isoimmunization NEC—*see also* Incompatibility
- affecting management of pregnancy (ABO) (with hydrops fetalis) O36.11-
  - anti-A sensitization O36.11-
  - anti-B sensitization O36.19-
  - anti-c sensitization O36.09-
  - anti-C sensitization O36.09-
  - anti-e sensitization O36.09-
  - anti-E sensitization O36.09-
  - Rh NEC O36.09-
    - anti-D antibody O36.01-
  - specified NEC O36.19-
- newborn P55.9
  - with
    - hydrops fetalis P56.0
    - kernicterus P57.0
  - ABO (blood groups) P55.1
  - Rhesus (Rh) factor P55.0
  - specified type NEC P55.8

Isolation, isolated
- family Z63.79

Issue of
- medical certificate Z02.79
  - for disability determination Z02.71
- repeat prescription (appliance) (glasses) (medicinal substance, medicament, medicine) Z76.0
  - contraception—*see* Contraception

Itch, itching—*see also* Pruritus
- baker's L23.6
- barber's B35.0
- cheese B88.0
- clam digger's B65.3
- copra B88.0
- dhobi B35.6
- grain B88.0
- grocer's B88.0
- harvest B88.0
- jock B35.6
- Malabar B35.5
  - beard B35.0
  - foot B35.3
  - scalp B35.0
- meaning scabies B86
- Norwegian B86
- perianal L29.0
- poultrymen's B88.0
- sarcoptic B86
- scabies B86
- scrub B88.0
- straw B88.0
- swimmer's B65.3
- winter L29.8

Ixodiasis NEC B88.8

J

Jacquet's dermatitis (diaper dermatitis) L22

Jamaican
- neuropathy G92
- paraplegic tropical ataxic-spastic syndrome G92

Jaundice (yellow) R17
- breast-milk (inhibitor) P59.3
- catarrhal (acute) B15.9
- cholestatic (benign) R17
- due to or associated with
  - delayed conjugation P59.8
    - associated with (due to) preterm delivery P59.0
  - preterm delivery P59.0
- epidemic (catarrhal) B15.9
- familial nonhemolytic (congenital) (Gilbert) E80.4
  - Crigler-Najjar E80.5
- febrile (acute) B15.9
- infectious (acute) (subacute) B15.9
- neonatal—*see* Jaundice, newborn
- newborn P59.9
  - due to or associated with
    - ABO
      - ~ antibodies P55.1
      - ~ incompatibility, maternal/fetal P55.1
      - ~ isoimmunization P55.1
    - breast milk inhibitors to conjugation P59.3
      - ~ associated with preterm delivery P59.0
    - Crigler-Najjar syndrome E80.5
    - delayed conjugation P59.8
      - ~ associated with preterm delivery P59.0
    - Gilbert syndrome E80.4
    - hemolytic disease P55.9
      - ~ ABO isoimmunization P55.1
    - hepatocellular damage P59.20
      - ~ specified NEC P59.29
    - hypothyroidism, congenital E03.1
    - inspissated bile syndrome P59.1
    - mucoviscidosis E84.9
    - preterm delivery P59.0
  - spherocytosis (congenital) D58.0
- nonhemolytic congenital familial (Gilbert) E80.4
- symptomatic R17
  - newborn P59.9

Jealousy
- childhood F93.8
- sibling F93.8

Jejunitis—*see* Enteritis

Jejunostomy status Z93.4

Jejunum, jejunal—*see* Disease, diseased

Jerks, myoclonic G25.3

Jervell-Lange-Nielsen syndrome I45.81

Jeune's disease Q77.2

Jigger disease B88.1

Job's syndrome (chronic granulomatous disease) D71

Joseph-Diamond-Blackfan anemia (congenital hypoplastic) D61.01

K

Kallmann's syndrome E23.0

Kaposi's
- vaccinia T88.1

Kartagener's syndrome or triad (sinusitis, bronchiectasis, situs inversus) Q89.3

Karyotype
- 46,XX Q98.3
  - with streak gonads Q50.32
  - hermaphrodite (true) Q99.1
  - male Q98.3
- 47,XXX Q97.0
- 47,XYY Q98.5

Kawasaki's syndrome M30.3

Kaznelson's syndrome (congenital hypoplastic anemia) D61.01

Kelis L91.0

Keloid, cheloid L91.0
- Hawkin's L91.0
- scar L91.0

Keloma L91.0

Keratitis (nodular) (nonulcerative) (simple) (zonular) H16.9
- dendritic (a) (herpes simplex) B00.52
- disciform (is) (herpes simplex) B00.52
  - varicella B01.81
- gonococcal (congenital or prenatal) A54.33
- herpes, herpetic (simplex) B00.52
- in (due to)
  - exanthema (*see also* Exanthem) B09
  - herpes (simplex) virus B00.52
  - measles B05.81
- postmeasles B05.81

Keratoconjunctivitis H16.20-
- herpes, herpetic (simplex) B00.52
- in exanthema (*see also* Exanthem) B09
- postmeasles B05.81

Keratoderma, keratodermia (congenital) (palmaris et plantaris) (symmetrical) Q82.8

Keratoglobus H18.79
- congenital Q15.8
  - with glaucoma Q15.0

Keratoma
- palmaris and plantaris hereditarium Q82.8

Keratosis
- congenital, specified NEC Q80.8
- female genital NEC N94.89
- follicularis Q82.8
  - congenita Q82.8
  - spinulosa (decalvans) Q82.8
- gonococcal A54.89
- nigricans L83
- palmaris et plantaris (inherited) (symmetrical) Q82.8
  - acquired L85.1
- tonsillaris J35.8
- vegetans Q82.8

Kerion (celsi) B35.0

Kink, kinking
- ureter (pelvic junction) N13.5
  - with
    - hydronephrosis N13.1

Klinefelter's syndrome Q98.4

Klumpke (-Déjerine) palsy, paralysis (birth) (newborn) P14.1

Knee—*see* Disease, diseased

Knock knee (acquired) M21.06-
- congenital Q74.1

Knot(s)
- intestinal, syndrome (volvulus) K56.2

Knotting (of)
- intestine K56.2

Köebner's syndrome Q81.8

Koplik's spots B05.9

Kraft-Weber-Dimitri disease Q85.8

Kraurosis
- ani K62.89

Kreotoxism A05.9

Kwashiokor E40

Kyphoscoliosis, kyphoscoliotic (acquired) (*see also* Scoliosis) M41.9
- congenital Q67.5
- heart (disease) I27.1

Kyphosis, kyphotic (acquired) M40.209
- Morquio-Brailsford type (spinal) E76.219

L

Labile
- blood pressure R09.89

Labium leporinum—*see* Cleft, lip

Labyrinthitis (circumscribed) (destructive) (diffuse) (inner ear) (latent) (purulent) (suppurative) H83.0

Laceration
- abdomen, abdominal
  - wall S31.119
    - with
      - ~ foreign body S31.129

Laceration, *continued*
- epigastric region S31.112
  - ~ with
    - ◊ foreign body S31.122
  - left
    - ~ lower quadrant S31.114
      - ◊ with
        - » foreign body S31.124
    - ~ upper quadrant S31.111
      - ◊ with
        - » foreign body S31.121
  - periumbilic region S31.115
    - ~ with
      - ◊ foreign body S31.125
  - right
    - ~ lower quadrant S31.113
      - ◊ with
        - » foreign body S31.123
    - ~ upper quadrant S31.110
      - ◊ with
        - » foreign body S31.120
- Achilles tendon S86.02-
- ankle S91.01-
  - with
    - foreign body S91.02-
- antecubital space—*see* Laceration
- anus (sphincter) S31.831
  - with
    - foreign body S31.832
  - nontraumatic, nonpuerperal—*see* Fissure, anus
- arm (upper) S41.11-
  - with foreign body S41.12-
  - lower—*see* Laceration, forearm
- auditory canal (external) (meatus)—*see* Laceration, ear
- auricle, ear—*see* Laceration, ear
- axilla—*see* Laceration, arm
- back—*see also* Laceration, thorax, back
  - lower S31.010
    - with
      - ~ foreign body S31.020
- buttock S31.8-
  - with foreign body S31.8-
  - left S31.821
    - with foreign body S31.822
  - right S31.811
    - with foreign body S31.812
- calf—*see* Laceration, leg
- canaliculus lacrimalis—*see* Laceration, eyelid
- canthus, eye—*see* Laceration, eyelid
- capsule, joint—*see* Sprain
- cerebral
  - left side S06.32-
  - during birth P10.8
    - with hemorrhage P10.1
  - right side S06.31-
- cheek (external) S01.41-
  - with foreign body S01.42-
  - internal—*see* Laceration, oral cavity
- chest wall—*see* Laceration, thorax
- chin—*see* Laceration, head, specified site NEC
- digit(s)
  - hand—*see* Laceration, finger
  - foot—*see* Laceration, toe
- ear (canal) (external) S01.31-
  - with foreign body S01.32-
  - drum S09.2-
- elbow S51.01-
  - with foreign body S51.02-
- epididymis—*see* Laceration, testis
- epigastric region—*see* Laceration, abdomen, wall, epigastric region
- eyebrow—*see* Laceration, eyelid
- eyelid S01.11-
  - with foreign body S01.12-
- face NEC—*see* Laceration, head, specified site NEC
- finger(s) S61.21-
  - with
    - damage to nail S61.31-
      - ~ with
        - ◊ foreign body S61.32-

Laceration, *continued*
- foreign body S61.22-
- index S61.21-
  - with
    - ~ damage to nail S61.31-
      - ◊ with
        - » foreign body S61.32-
    - ~ foreign body S61.22-
  - left S61.211
    - ~ with
      - ◊ damage to nail S61.311
        - » with
          - ◊ foreign body S61.221
  - right S61.210
    - ~ with
      - ◊ damage to nail S61.310
        - » with
          - ❖ foreign body S61.320
      - ◊ foreign body S61.220
- little S61.218
  - with
    - ~ damage to nail S61.31-
      - ◊ with
        - » foreign body S61.32-
    - ~ foreign body S61.22-
  - left S61.217
    - ~ with
      - ◊ damage to nail S61.317
        - » with
          - ❖ foreign body S61.327
      - ◊ foreign body S61.227
  - right S61.216
    - ~ with
      - ◊ damage to nail S61.316
        - » with
          - ❖ foreign body S61.326
      - ◊ foreign body S61.226
- middle S61.218
  - with
    - ~ damage to nail S61.31-
      - ◊ with
        - » foreign body S61.32-
    - ~ foreign body S61.22-
  - left S61.213
    - ~ with
      - ◊ damage to nail S61.313
        - » with
          - ❖ foreign body S61.323
      - ◊ foreign body S61.223
  - right S61.212
    - ~ with
      - ◊ damage to nail S61.312
        - » with
          - ❖ foreign body S61.322
      - ◊ foreign body S61.222
- ring S61.218
  - with
    - ~ damage to nail S61.31-
      - ◊ with
        - » foreign body S61.32-
    - ~ foreign body S61.22-
  - left S61.215
    - ~ with
      - ◊ damage to nail S61.315
        - » with
          - ❖ foreign body S61.325
      - ◊ foreign body S61.225
  - right S61.214
    - ~ with
      - ◊ damage to nail S61.314
        - » with
          - ❖ foreign body S61.324
      - ◊ foreign body S61.224
- flank S31.119
  - with foreign body S31.129
- foot (except toe(s) alone) S91.31-
  - with foreign body S91.32-
  - left S91.312
    - with foreign body S91.322
  - right S91.311
    - with foreign body S91.321
  - toe—*see* Laceration, toe

Laceration, *continued*
- forearm S51.81-
  - with
    - foreign body S51.82-
  - elbow only—*see* Laceration
  - left S51.812
    - with
      - ~ foreign body S51.822
  - right S51.811
    - with
      - ~ foreign body S51.821
- forehead S01.81
  - with foreign body S01.82
- gum—*see* Laceration, oral cavity
- hand S61.41-
  - with
    - foreign body S61.42-
  - finger—*see* Laceration, finger
  - left S61.412
    - with
      - ~ foreign body S61.422
  - right S61.411
    - with
      - ~ foreign body S61.421
  - thumb—*see* Laceration, thumb
- head S01.91
  - with foreign body S01.92
  - cheek—*see* Laceration, cheek
  - ear—*see* Laceration, ear
  - eyelid—*see* Laceration, eyelid
  - lip—*see* Laceration, lip
  - nose—*see* Laceration, nose
  - oral cavity—*see* Laceration, oral cavity
  - scalp S01.01
    - with foreign body S01.02
  - specified site NEC S01.81
    - with foreign body S01.82
  - temporomandibular area—*see* Laceration, cheek
- heel—*see* Laceration, foot
- hip S71.01-
  - with foreign body S71.02-
  - left S71.012
    - with foreign body S71.022
  - right S71.011
    - with foreign body S71.021
- hypochondrium—*see* Laceration, abdomen, wall
- hypogastric region—*see* Laceration, abdomen, wall
- inguinal region—*see* Laceration, abdomen, wall
- instep—*see* Laceration, foot
- interscapular region—*see* Laceration, thorax, back
- jaw—*see* Laceration, head, specified site NEC
- joint capsule—*see* Sprain, by site
- knee S81.01-
  - with foreign body S81.02-
- labium (majus) (minus)—*see* Laceration, vulva
- lacrimal duct—*see* Laceration, eyelid
- leg (lower) S81.81-
  - with foreign body S81.82-
  - foot—*see* Laceration, foot
  - knee—*see* Laceration, knee
  - left S81.812
    - with foreign body S81.822
  - right S81.811
    - with foreign body S81.821
  - upper—*see* Laceration, thigh
- ligament—*see* Sprain
- lip S01.511
  - with foreign body S01.521
- loin—*see* Laceration, abdomen, wall
- lower back—*see* Laceration, back, lower
- lumbar region—*see* Laceration, back, lower
- malar region—*see* Laceration, head, specified site NEC
- mammary—*see* Laceration
- mastoid region—*see* Laceration, head, specified site NEC
- mouth—*see* Laceration, oral cavity
- muscle—*see* Injury, muscle, by site, laceration
- nail
  - finger—*see* Laceration, finger, with, damage to nail
  - toe—*see* Laceration, toe, with, damage to nail
- nasal (septum) (sinus)—*see* Laceration, nose
- nasopharynx—*see* Laceration, head, specified site NEC

Laceration, *continued*
- neck S11.91
  - with foreign body S11.92
- nerve—*see* Injury, nerve
- nose (septum) (sinus) S01.21
  - with foreign body S01.22
- ocular NOS
  - adnexa NOS S01.11-
- oral cavity S01.512
  - with foreign body S01.522
- palate—*see* Laceration, oral cavity
- palm—*see* Laceration, hand
- pelvic S31.010
  - with
    - foreign body S31.020
- penis S31.21
- perineum
  - female S31.41
    - with
      - foreign body S31.42
  - male S31.119
    - with foreign body S31.129
- periocular area (with or without lacrimal passages)— *see* Laceration, eyelid
- periumbilic region—*see* Laceration, abdomen, wall, periumbilic
- phalanges
  - finger—*see* Laceration, finger
  - toe—*see* Laceration, toe
- pinna—*see* Laceration, ear
- popliteal space—*see* Laceration, knee
- prepuce—*see* Laceration, penis
- pubic region S31.119
  - with foreign body S31.129
- pudendum—*see* Laceration
- rectovaginal septum—*see* Laceration, vagina
- rectum S36.63
- sacral region—*see* Laceration, back, lower
- sacroiliac region—*see* Laceration, back, lower
- salivary gland—*see* Laceration, oral cavity
- scalp S01.01
  - with foreign body S01.02
- scapular region—*see* Laceration, shoulder
- scrotum S31.31
- shin—*see* Laceration, leg
- shoulder S41.01-
  - with foreign body S41.02-
  - left S41.012
    - with foreign body S41.022
  - right S41.011
    - with foreign body S41.021
- spleen S36.03-
  - superficial (minor) S36.030
- submaxillary region—*see* Laceration, head, specified site NEC
- submental region—*see* Laceration, head, specified site NEC
- subungual
  - finger(s)—*see* Laceration, finger, with, damage to nail
  - toe(s)—*see* Laceration, toe, with, damage to nail
- temple, temporal region—*see* Laceration, head, specified site NEC
- temporomandibular area—*see* Laceration, cheek
- tendon—*see* Injury, muscle, by site, laceration
  - Achilles S86.02-
- testis S31.31
- thigh S71.11-
  - with foreign body S71.12-
- thorax, thoracic (wall) S21.91
  - with foreign body S21.92
    - back S21.22-
    - front S21.12-
  - back S21.21-
    - with
      - foreign body S21.22-
  - front S21.11-
    - with
      - foreign body S21.12-
- thumb S61.01-
  - with
    - damage to nail S61.11-

Laceration, *continued*
- ~ with
  - ◊ foreign body S61.12-
- foreign body S61.02-
- left S61.012
  - with
    - ~ damage to nail S61.112
      - ◊ with
        - » foreign body S61.122
    - ~ foreign body S61.022
- right S61.011
  - with
    - ~ damage to nail S61.111
      - ◊ with
        - » foreign body S61.121
    - ~ foreign body S61.021
- toe(s) S91.11-
  - with
    - damage to nail S91.21-
      - ~ with
        - ◊ foreign body S91.22-
    - foreign body S91.12-
  - great S91.11-
    - with
      - ~ damage to nail S91.21-
        - ◊ with
          - » foreign body S91.22-
      - ~ foreign body S91.12-
    - left S91.112
      - ~ with
        - ◊ damage to nail S91.212
          - » with
            - ❖ foreign body S91.222
        - ◊ foreign body S91.122
    - right S91.111
      - ~ with
        - ◊ damage to nail S91.211
          - » with
            - ❖ foreign body S91.221
        - ◊ foreign body S91.121
  - lesser S91.11-
    - with
      - ~ damage to nail S91.21-
        - ◊ with
          - » foreign body S91.22-
      - ~ foreign body S91.12-
    - left S91.115
      - ~ with
        - ◊ damage to nail S91.215
          - » with
            - ❖ foreign body S91.225
        - ◊ foreign body S91.125
    - right S91.114
      - ~ with
        - ◊ damage to nail S91.214
          - » with
            - ❖ foreign body S91.224
        - ◊ foreign body S91.124
- tongue—*see* Laceration, oral cavity
- tunica vaginalis—*see* Laceration, testis
- tympanum, tympanic membrane—*see* Laceration, ear, drum
- umbilical region S31.115
  - with foreign body S31.125
- uvula—*see* Laceration, oral cavity
- vagina S31.41
  - with
    - foreign body S31.42
  - nonpuerperal, nontraumatic N89.8
  - old (postpartal) N89.8
- vulva S31.41
  - with
    - foreign body S31.42
- wrist S61.51-
  - with
    - foreign body S61.52-
  - left S61.512
    - with
      - ~ foreign body S61.522
  - right S61.511
    - with
      - ~ foreign body S61.521

Lack of
- adequate
  - food Z59.4
  - sleep Z72.820
- appetite (*see* Anorexia) R63.0
- care
  - in home Z74.2
  - of infant (at or after birth) T76.02
    - confirmed T74.02
- coordination R27.9
  - ataxia R27.0
  - specified type NEC R27.8
- development (physiological) R62.50
  - failure to thrive (child over 28 days old) R62.51
    - newborn P92.6
  - short stature R62.52
  - specified type NEC R62.59
- energy R53.83
- growth R62.52
- heating Z59.1
- housing (permanent) (temporary) Z59.0
  - adequate Z59.1
- ovulation N97.0
- person able to render necessary care Z74.2
- physical exercise Z72.3
- shelter Z59.0

Lactation, lactating (breast) (puerperal, postpartum)
- associated
  - cracked nipple O92.13
  - retracted nipple O92.03
- defective O92.4
- disorder NEC O92.79
- excessive O92.6
- failed (complete) O92.3
  - partial O92.4
- mastitis NEC N61.1
- mother (care and/or examination) Z39.1
- nonpuerperal N64.3

Lacunar skull Q75.8

Lalling F80.0

Lambliasis, lambliosis A07.1

Landouzy-Déjérine dystrophy or facioscapulohumeral atrophy G71.02

Lapsed immunization schedule status Z28.3

Large
- baby (regardless of gestational age) (4000g-4499g) P08.1

Large-for-dates (infant) (4000g to 4499g) P08.1
- affecting management of pregnancy O36.6-
- exceptionally (4500g or more) P08.0

Larsen-Johansson disease or osteochondrosis—*see* Osteochondrosis, juvenile, patella

Laryngismus (stridulus) J38.5
- congenital P28.89

Laryngitis (acute) (edematous) (fibrinous) (infective) (infiltrative) (malignant) (membranous) (phlegmonous) (pneumococcal) (pseudomembranous) (septic) (subglottic) (suppurative) (ulcerative) J04.0
- with
  - influenza, flu, or grippe—*see* Influenza, laryngitis
  - tracheitis (acute)—*see* Laryngotracheitis
- atrophic J37.0
- catarrhal J37.0
- chronic J37.0
  - with tracheitis (chronic) J37.1
- Hemophilus influenzae J04.0
- H. influenzae J04.0
- hypertrophic J37.0
- influenzal—*see* Influenza, respiratory manifestations NEC
- obstructive J05.0
- sicca J37.0
- spasmodic J05.0
  - acute J04.0
- streptococcal J04.0
- stridulous J05.0

Laryngomalacia (congenital) Q31.5

Laryngopharyngitis (acute) J06.0
- chronic J37.0

Laryngoplegia J38.00
- bilateral J38.02
- unilateral J38.01

Laryngotracheitis (acute) (Infectional) (infective) (viral) J04.2
- atrophic J37.1
- catarrhal J37.1
- chronic J37.1
- Hemophilus influenzae J04.2
- hypertrophic J37.1
- influenzal—*see* Influenza, respiratory manifestations NEC
- sicca J37.1
- spasmodic J38.5
  - acute J05.0
- streptococcal J04.2

Laryngotracheobronchitis—*see* Bronchitis

Late
- talker R62.0
- walker R62.0

Late effects—*see* Sequela

Latent tuberculosis (LTBI) Z22.7

Launois' syndrome (pituitary gigantism) E22.0

Lax, laxity—*see also* Relaxation
- ligament(ous)—*see also* Disorder
  - familial M35.7
- skin congenital Q82.8

Lazy leukocyte syndrome D70.8

Leak, leakage
- air NEC J93.82
  - postprocedural J95.812
- cerebrospinal fluid G96.00
  - cranial
  - postoperative G96.08
    - specified NEC G96.08
    - spontaneous G96.01
    - traumatic G96.08
  - spinal
    - postoperative G96.09
    - post-traumatic G96.09
    - specified NEC G96.09
    - spontaneous G96.02
  - spontaneous
    - from
      ~ skull base G96.01
      ~ spine G96.02
- device, implant or graft—*see also* Complications, by site and type, mechanical
  - persistent air J93.82

Leaky heart—*see* Endocarditis

Learning defect (specific) F81.9

Leber's
- congenital amaurosis H35.50

Lederer's anemia D59.19

Legg (-Calvé)-Perthes disease, syndrome or osteochondrosis M91.1-

Leiner's disease L21.1

Lenegre's disease I44.2

Lengthening, leg—*see* Deformity, limb

Lennox-Gastaut syndrome G40.812
- intractable G40.814
  - with status epilepticus G40.813
  - without status epilepticus G40.814
- not intractable G40.812
  - with status epilepticus G40.811
  - without status epilepticus G40.812

Lenticonus (anterior) (posterior) (congenital) Q12.8

Lentiglobus (posterior) (congenital) Q12.8

Lentigo (congenital) L81.4

Leptocytosis, hereditary D56.9

Leptomeningitis (chronic) (circumscribed) (hemorrhagic) (nonsuppurative)—*see* Meningitis

Leptomeningopathy G96.198

Leptus dermatitis B88.0

Leri-Weill syndrome Q77.8

Lesch-Nyhan syndrome E79.1

Lesion(s) (nontraumatic)
- angiocentric immunoproliferative D47.Z9
- anorectal K62.9
- aortic (valve) I35.9
- basal ganglion G25.9
- brain G93.9
  - congenital Q04.9
    - hypertensive I67.4
- buccal cavity K13.79
- cardiac (*see also* Disease, heart) I51.9
  - congenital Q24.9
- cerebrovascular I67.9
  - degenerative I67.9
  - hypertensive I67.4
- chorda tympani G51.8
- hypothalamic E23.7
- joint—*see* Disorder, joint
  - sacroiliac (old) M53.3
- lip K13.0
- maxillary sinus J32.0
- mitral I05.9
- motor cortex NEC G93.89
- mouth K13.79
- nervous system, congenital Q07.9
- nose (internal) J34.89
- oral mucosa K13.70
- peptic K27.9
- primary (*see also* Syphilis, primary) A51.0
- pulmonary J98.4
  - valve I37.9
- sacroiliac (joint) (old) M53.3
- sinus (accessory) (nasal) J34.89
- skin L98.9
  - suppurative L08.0
- tonsillar fossa J35.9
- tricuspid (valve) I07.9
  - nonrheumatic I36.9
- vascular I99.9
- vagina N89.8
- vulva N90.89

Lethargy R53.83

Leukemia, leukemic C95.9-
- acute lymphoblastic C91.0-
- acute myeloblastic (minimal differentiation) (with maturation) C92.0-
- AML (1/ETO) (M0) (M1) (M2) (without a FAB classification) NOS C92.0-
- chronic myelomonocytic C93.1-
- CMML (-1) (-2) (with eosinophilia) C93.1-
- juvenile myelomonocytic C93.3-
- lymphoid C91.9-
- monocytic (subacute) C93.9-
- myelogenous (*see also* Category C92) C92.9-
- myeloid C92.9-
- subacute lymphocytic C91.9-

Leukemoid reaction (*see also* Reaction, leukemoid) D72.823-

Leukocytopenia D72.819

Leukocytosis D72.829
- eosinophilic D72.19

Leukoencephalitis G04.81
- acute (subacute) hemorrhagic G36.1
  - postimmunization or postvaccinal G04.02
- postinfectious G04.01

Leukoencephalopathy (Encephalopathy) G93.49
- postimmunization and postvaccinal G04.02
- reversible, posterior G93.6

Leukomalacia, cerebral, newborn P91.2

Leukomelanopathy, hereditary D72.0
- periventricular P91.2

Leukonychia (punctata) (striata) L60.8
- congenital Q84.4

Leukopathia unguium L60.8
- congenital Q84.4

Leukopenia D72.819
- basophilic D72.818
- chemotherapy (cancer) induced D70.1
- congenital D70.0
- cyclic D70.0
- drug induced NEC D70.2

Leukopenia, *continued*
  - due to cytoreductive cancer chemotherapy D70.1
- eosinophilic D72.818
- familial D70.0
- infantile genetic D70.0
- malignant D70.9
- periodic D70.0
- transitory neonatal P61.5

Leukoplakia
- anus K62.89
- rectum K62.89

Leukorrhea N89.8
- due to Trichomonas (vaginalis) A59.00
- trichomonal A59.00

Leukosarcoma C85.9-

Levocardia (isolated) Q24.1
- with situs inversus Q89.3

Lev's disease or syndrome (acquired complete heart block) I44.2

Leyden-Moebius dystrophy G71.09

Liar, pathologic F60.2

Libman-Sacks disease M32.11

Lice (infestation) B85.2
- body (Pediculus corporis) B85.1
- crab B85.3
- head (Pediculus corporis) B85.0
- mixed (classifiable to more than one of the titles B85.0–B85.3) B85.4
- pubic (Phthirus pubis) B85.3

Lichen L28.0
- congenital Q82.8
- pilaris Q82.8
  - acquired L85.8

Light
- for gestational age—*see* Light for dates
- headedness R42

Light-for-dates (infant) P05.00
- with weight of
  - 499 grams or less P05.01
  - 500–749 grams P05.02
  - 750–999 grams P05.03
  - 1000–1249 grams P05.04
  - 1250–1499 grams P05.05
  - 1500–1749 grams P05.06
  - 1750–1999 grams P05.07
  - 2000–2499 grams P05.08
  - 2500 g and over P05.09
- and small-for-dates—*see* Small for dates
- affecting management of pregnancy O36.59-

Ligneous thyroiditis E06.5

Lindau (-von Hippel) disease Q85.8

Line(s)
- Harris'—*see* Arrest, epiphyseal

Lingua
- geographica K14.1

Linguatulosis B88.8

Lipochondrodystrophy E76.01

Lipochrome histiocytosis (familial) D71

Lipodystrophy (progressive) E88.1
- intestinal K90.81

Lipoid—*see also* Disease, diseased
- histiocytosis D76.3
- nephrosis N04.9

Lipoma D17.9
- infiltrating D17.9
- intramuscular D17.9
- pleomorphic D17.9
- site classification
  - arms (skin) (subcutaneous) D17.2-
  - connective tissue D17.30
    - intra-abdominal D17.5
    - intrathoracic D17.4
    - peritoneum D17.79
    - retroperitoneum D17.79
    - specified site NEC D17.39
    - spermatic cord D17.6

Lipoma, *continued*
- face (skin) (subcutaneous) D17.0
- genitourinary organ NEC D17.72
- head (skin) (subcutaneous) D17.0
- intra-abdominal D17.5
- intrathoracic D17.4
- kidney D17.71
- legs (skin) (subcutaneous) D17.2-
- neck (skin) (subcutaneous) D17.0
- peritoneum D17.79
- retroperitoneum D17.79
- skin D17.30
  - specified site NEC D17.39
- specified site NEC D17.79
- spermatic cord D17.6
- subcutaneous D17.30
  - specified site NEC D17.39
- trunk (skin) (subcutaneous) D17.1
- unspecified D17.9
- spindle cell D17.9

Lipoproteinemia E78.5
- broad-beta E78.2
- floating-beta E78.2

Lisping F80.0

Listeriosis, Listerellosis A32.9
- congenital (disseminated) P37.2
- cutaneous A32.0
- neonatal, newborn (disseminated) P37.2
- oculoglandular A32.81
- specified NEC A32.89

Lithemia E79.0

Little leaguer's elbow—*see* Epicondylitis, medial

Little's disease G80.9

Livedo (annularis) (racemosa) (reticularis) R23.1

Living alone (problems with) Z60.2
- with handicapped person Z74.2

Lobstein (-Ekman) disease or syndrome Q78.0

Lone Star fever A77.0

Long
- QT syndrome I45.81

Long-term (current) (prophylactic) drug therapy (use of)
- antibiotics Z79.2
  - short-term use—omit code
- anti-inflammatory, non-steroidal (NSAID) Z79.1
- aspirin Z79.82
- drug, specified NEC Z79.899
- hypoglycemic, oral, drugs Z79.84
- insulin Z79.4
- non-steroidal anti-inflammatories (NSAID) Z79.1
- steroids
  - inhaled Z79.51
  - systemic Z79.52

Longitudinal stripes or grooves, nails L60.8
- congenital Q84.6

Lorain (-Levi) short stature syndrome E23.0

Lordosis M40.50
- acquired—*see* Lordosis, specified type NEC
- congenital Q76.429
  - lumbar region Q76.426
  - lumbosacral region Q76.427
  - sacral region Q76.428
  - sacrococcygeal region Q76.428
  - thoracolumbar region Q76.425
- lumbar region M40.56
- lumbosacral region M40.57
- postural—*see* Lordosis, specified type NEC
- specified type NEC M40.40
  - lumbar region M40.46
  - lumbosacral region M40.47
  - thoracolumbar region M40.45
- thoracolumbar region M40.55

Loss (of)
- appetite (*see* Anorexia) R63.0
  - hysterical F50.89
  - nonorganic origin F50.89
  - psychogenic F50.89
- blood—*see* Hemorrhage
- consciousness, transient R55
  - traumatic—*see* Injury, intracranial

Loss, *continued*
- control, sphincter, rectum R15.9
  - nonorganic origin F98.1
- fluid (acute) E86.9
  - with
    - hypernatremia E87.0
    - hyponatremia E87.1
- hearing—*see also* Deafness
  - central NOS H90.5
  - conductive H90.2
    - bilateral H90.0
    - unilateral
      - ~ with
        - ◊ restricted hearing on the contralateral side H90.A1-
        - ◊ unrestricted hearing on the contralateral side H90.1-
  - mixed conductive and sensorineural hearing loss H90.8
    - bilateral H90.6
    - unilateral
      - ~ with
        - ◊ restricted hearing on the contralateral side H90.A3-
        - ◊ unrestricted hearing on the contralateral side H90.7-
  - neural NOS H90.5
  - perceptive NOS H90.5
  - sensorineural NOS H90.5
    - bilateral H90.3
    - unilateral
      - ~ with
        - ◊ restricted hearing on the contralateral side H90.A2-
        - ◊ unrestricted hearing on the contralateral side H90.4-
  - sensory NOS H90.5
- parent in childhood Z63.4
- self-esteem, in childhood Z62.898
- sense of
  - smell—*see* Disturbance, sensation
  - taste—*see* Disturbance, sensation
  - touch R20.8
- sensory R44.9
  - dissociative F44.6
- vision, visual H54.7
- weight (abnormal) (cause unknown) R63.4

Louis-Bar syndrome (ataxia-telangiectasia) G11.3

Louping ill (encephalitis) A84.89

Louse, lousiness—*see* Lice

Low
- achiever, school Z55.3
- back syndrome M54.5
- basal metabolic rate R94.8
- birthweight (2499 grams or less) P07.10
  - with weight of
    - 1000–1249 grams P07.14
    - 1250–1499 grams P07.15
    - 1500–1749 grams P07.16
    - 1750–1999 grams P07.17
    - 2000–2499 grams P07.18
  - extreme (999 grams or less) P07.00
    - with weight of
      - ~ 499 grams or less P07.01
      - ~ 500–749 grams P07.02
      - ~ 750–999 grams P07.03
  - for gestational age—*see* Light for dates
- blood pressure—*see also* Hypotension
  - reading (incidental) (isolated) (nonspecific) R03.1
- cardiac reserve—*see* Disease, heart
- hematocrit D64.9
- hemoglobin D64.9
- salt syndrome E87.1
- self-esteem R45.81
- vision H54.2X-
  - one eye (other eye normal) H54.5-
    - left (normal vision on right) H54.52A-
    - other eye blind—*see* Blindness
    - right (normal vision on left) H54.511-

Low-density-lipoprotein-type (LDL) hyperlipoproteinemia E78.00

Lowe's syndrome E72.03

Lown-Ganong-Levine syndrome I45.6

Ludwig's angina or disease K12.2

Luetscher's syndrome E86.0

Lumbago, lumbalgia M54.5
- with sciatica M54.4-

Lumbermen's itch B88.0

Lump—*see also* Mass
- breast N63.0
  - axillary tail N63.3-
  - left N63.2-
  - right N63.1-
  - subareolar N63.4-

Lupoid (miliary) **of Boeck** D86.3

Lupus
- anticoagulant D68.62
  - with
    - hemorrhagic disorder D68.312
- erythematosus (discoid) (local)
  - disseminated M32.9
  - systemic M32.9
    - with organ or system involvement M32.10
      - ~ endocarditis M32.11
      - ~ lung M32.13
      - ~ pericarditis M32.12
      - ~ renal (glomerular) M32.14
        - ◊ tubulo-interstitial M32.15
      - ~ specified organ or system NEC M32.19
    - drug-induced M32.0
    - inhibitor (presence of) D68.62
      - with
        - ◊ hemorrhagic disorder D68.312
- nephritis (chronic) M32.14

Lutembacher's disease or syndrome (atrial septal defect with mitral stenosis) Q21.1

Luxation—*see also* Dislocation
- eyeball (nontraumatic)
  - birth injury P15.3
- lens (old) (partial) (spontaneous)
  - congenital Q12.1

Lyell's syndrome L51.2
- due to drug L51.2
  - correct substance properly administered—*see* Table of Drugs and Chemicals, by drug, adverse effect
  - overdose or wrong substance given or taken—*see* Table of Drugs and Chemicals, by drug, poisoning

Lyme disease A69.20

Lymphadenitis I88.9
- acute L04.9
  - axilla L04.2
  - face L04.0
  - head L04.0
  - hip L04.3
  - limb
    - lower L04.3
    - upper L04.2
  - neck L04.0
  - shoulder L04.2
  - specified site NEC L04.8
  - trunk L04.1
- any site, except mesenteric I88.9
  - chronic I88.1
  - subacute I88.1
- chronic I88.1
  - mesenteric I88.0
- gonorrheal A54.89
- infective—*see* Lymphadenitis, acute
- mesenteric (acute) (chronic) (nonspecific) (subacute) I88.0
  - tuberculous A18.39
- mycobacterial A31.8
- purulent—*see* Lymphadenitis, acute
- pyogenic—*see* Lymphadenitis, acute
- regional, nonbacterial I88.8
- septic—*see* Lymphadenitis, acute
- subacute, unspecified site I88.1
- suppurative—*see* Lymphadenitis, acute
- syphilitic
  - late A52.79

Lymphadenoid goiter E06.3

Lymphadenopathy (generalized) R59.1
- due to toxoplasmosis (acquired) B58.89
  - congenital (acute) (subacute) (chronic) P37.1

Lymphadenosis R59.1

Lymphangitis I89.1
- with
  - abscess—*code by* site under Abscess
  - cellulitis—*code by* site under Cellulitis
- acute L03.91
  - abdominal wall L03.321
  - auricle (ear)—*see* Lymphangitis, acute
  - axilla L03.12-
  - back (any part) L03.322
  - buttock L03.327
  - cervical (meaning neck) L03.222
  - cheek (external) L03.212
  - chest wall L03.323
- digit
  - finger—*see* Cellulitis, finger
  - toe—*see* Cellulitis, toe
- ear (external) H60.1-
- eyelid—*see* Abscess, eyelid
- face NEC L03.212
- finger (intrathecal) (periosteal) (subcutaneous) (subcuticular) L03.02-
- gluteal (region) L03.327
- groin L03.324
- head NEC L03.891
  - face (any part, except ear, eye and nose) L03.212
- jaw (region) L03.212
- lower limb L03.12-
- navel L03.326
- neck (region) L03.222
- orbit, orbital—*see* Cellulitis, orbit
- pectoral (region) L03.323
- perineal, perineum L03.325
- scalp (any part) L03.891
- specified site NEC L03.898
- strumous tuberculous A18.2
- subacute (any site) I89.1
- toe (intrathecal) (periosteal) (subcutaneous) (subcuticular) L03.04-
- trunk L03.329
  - abdominal wall L03.321
  - back (any part) L03.322
  - buttock L03.327
  - chest wall L03.323
  - groin L03.324
  - perineal, perineum L03.325
  - umbilicus L03.326
- umbilicus L03.326
- upper limb L03.12-

Lymphocytoma, benign cutis L98.8

Lymphocytopenia D72.810

Lymphocytosis (symptomatic) D72.820
- infectious (acute) B33.8

Lymphogranulomatosis (malignant)—*see also* Lymphoma, Hodgkin
- benign (Boeck's sarcoid) (Schaumann's) D86.1

Lymphohistiocytosis, hemophagocytic (familial) D76.1

Lymphoma (of) (malignant) C85.90
- diffuse large cell C83.3-
  - anaplastic C83.3-
  - B-cell C83.3-
  - CD30-positive C83.3-
  - centroblastic C83.3-
  - immunoblastic C83.3-
  - plasmablastic C83.3-
  - subtype not specified C83.3-
  - T-cell rich C83.3-
- histiocytic C85.9-
  - true C96.A
- Hodgkin C81.-
  - mixed cellularity classical C81.2-
    - nodular lymphocyte predominant C81.0-
- Lennert's C84.4-
- lymphoepithelioid C84.4-
- mature T-cell NEC C84.4-
- non-Hodgkin (*see also* Lymphoma, by type) C85.9-
- peripheral T-cell, not classified C84.4-

Lymphopenia D72.810

Lymphoproliferation, X-linked disease D82.3

Lymphosarcoma (diffuse) (*see also* Lymphoma) C85.9-

M

Macrocolon (*see also* Megacolon) Q43.1

Macrocornea Q15.8
- with glaucoma Q15.0

Macrocytosis D75.89

Macrodactylia, macrodactylism (fingers) (thumbs) Q74.0
- toes Q74.2

Macrogenitosomia (adrenal) (male) (praecox) E25.9
- congenital E25.0

Macrophthalmos Q11.3
- in congenital glaucoma Q15.0

Macrosigmoid K59.39
- congenital Q43.2
- toxic K59.31

Macrospondylitis, acromegalic E22.0

Maculae ceruleae B85.1

Madelung's
- deformity (radius) Q74.0
- disease
  - radial deformity Q74.0

Main en griffe (acquired)
- congenital Q74.0

Maintenance (encounter for)
- antineoplastic chemotherapy Z51.11
- antineoplastic radiation therapy Z51.0

Malabsorption K90.9
- calcium K90.89
- carbohydrate K90.49
- disaccharide E73.9
- fat K90.49
- intestinal K90.9
  - specified NEC K90.89
- lactose E73.9
- postgastrectomy K91.2
- postsurgical K91.2
- protein K90.49
- starch K90.49
- syndrome K90.9
  - postsurgical K91.2

Maladaptation—*see* Maladjustment

Maladie de Roger Q21.0

Maladjustment
- educational Z55.4
- family Z63.9
- social Z60.9
  - due to
    - acculturation difficulty Z60.3

Malaise R53.81

Malaria, malarial (fever) B54
- clinically diagnosed (without parasitological confirmation) B54
- congenital NEC P37.4
  - falciparum P37.3
- congestion, congestive B54
- hemorrhagic B54
- recurrent B54
- remittent B54
- specified type NEC (parasitologically confirmed) B53.8
- spleen B54
- typhoid B54

Malassimilation K90.9

Mal de mer T75.3

Maldescent, testis Q53.9
- bilateral Q53.20
  - abdominal Q53.211
  - perineal Q53.22
- unilateral Q53.10
  - abdominal Q53.111
  - perineal Q53.12

Maldevelopment—*see also* Anomaly
- brain Q07.9
- hip Q74.2
  - congenital dislocation Q65.2
    - bilateral Q65.1
    - unilateral Q65.0-
- mastoid process Q75.8
- toe Q74.2

Male type pelvis Q74.2

Malformation (congenital)—*see also* Anomaly
- alimentary tract Q45.9
  - specified type NEC Q45.8
  - upper Q40.9
    - specified type NEC Q40.8
- aorta Q25.40
  - absence Q25.41
  - aneurysm, congenital Q25.43
  - aplasia Q25.41
  - atresia Q25.29
    - aortic arch Q25.21
  - coarctation (preductal) (postductal) Q25.1
  - dilatation, congenital Q25.44
  - hypoplasia Q25.42
  - patent ductus arteriosus Q25.0
  - specified type NEC Q25.49
  - stenosis Q25.1
    - supravalvular Q25.3
- arteriovenous, aneurysmatic (congenital) Q27.3-
  - brain Q28.2
    - ruptured I60.8-
      - ~ intracerebral I61.8
      - ~ intraparenchymal I61.8
      - ~ intraventricular I61.5
      - ~ subarachnoid I60.8-
  - cerebral—*see also* Malformation, arteriovenous, brain Q28.2
  - peripheral Q27.3-
- bile duct Q44.5
- bone Q79.9
  - face Q75.9
    - specified type NEC Q75.8
  - skull Q75.9
    - specified type NEC Q75.8
- broad ligament Q50.6
- bursa Q79.9
- corpus callosum (congenital) Q04.0
- digestive system NEC, specified type NEC Q45.8
- dura Q07.9
  - brain Q04.9
  - spinal Q06.9
- ear Q17.9
  - causing impairment of hearing Q16.9
  - external Q17.9
    - accessory auricle Q17.0
      - ~ absence of
        - ◊ auditory canal Q16.1
        - ◊ auricle Q16.0
    - macrotia Q17.1
    - microtia Q17.2
    - misplacement Q17.4
    - misshapen NEC Q17.3
    - prominence Q17.5
    - specified type NEC Q17.8
  - inner Q16.5
  - middle Q16.4
    - absence of eustachian tube Q16.2
    - ossicles (fusion) Q16.3
  - ossicles Q16.3
    - external Q17.9
- eye Q15.9
  - lid Q10.3
  - specified NEC Q15.8
- fallopian tube Q50.6
- great
  - vein Q26.9
    - anomalous
      - ~ pulmonary venous connection Q26.4
        - ◊ partial Q26.3
        - ◊ total Q26.2
- heart Q24.9
  - specified type NEC Q24.8
- integument Q84.9

Malformation, *continued*
- joint Q74.9
  - ankle Q74.2
  - sacroiliac Q74.2
- kidney Q63.9
  - accessory Q63.0
  - giant Q63.3
  - horseshoe Q63.1
  - hydronephrosis (congenital) Q62.0
  - malposition Q63.2
  - specified type NEC Q63.8
- lacrimal apparatus Q10.6
- meninges or membrane (congenital) Q07.9
  - cerebral Q04.8
  - spinal (cord) Q06.9
- multiple types NEC Q89.7
- musculoskeletal system Q79.9
- nervous system (central) Q07.9
- ovary Q50.39
- parathyroid gland Q89.2
- penis Q55.69
  - aplasia Q55.5
  - curvature (lateral) Q55.61
  - hypoplasia Q55.62
- pulmonary
  - arteriovenous Q25.72
  - artery Q25.9
    - atresia Q25.5
    - specified type NEC Q25.79
- respiratory system Q34.9
- scrotum—*see* Malformation, testis and scrotal transposition
- sense organs NEC Q07.9
- specified NEC Q89.8
- tendon Q79.9
- testis and scrotum Q55.20
  - aplasia Q55.0
  - hypoplasia Q55.1
  - polyorchism Q55.21
  - retractile testis Q55.22
  - scrotal transposition Q55.23
  - specified NEC Q55.29
- thyroid gland Q89.2
- tongue (congenital) Q38.3
  - hypertrophy Q38.2
  - tie Q38.1
- urinary system Q64.9

Malibu disease L98.8

Malignancy—*see also* Neoplasm
- unspecified site (primary) C80.1

Malignant—*see* Disease, diseased

Malingerer, malingering Z76.5

Mallet finger (acquired) M20.01-
- congenital Q74.0

Malnutrition E46
- degree
  - first E44.1
  - mild (protein) E44.1
  - moderate (protein) E44.0
  - second E44.0
- following gastrointestinal surgery K91.2
- lack of care, or neglect (child) (infant) T76.02
  - confirmed T74.02
- protein E46
  - calorie E46
    - mild E44.1
    - moderate E44.0
  - energy E46
    - mild E44.1
    - moderate E44.0

Malocclusion (teeth) M26.4
- temporomandibular (joint) M26.69

Malposition
- arterial trunk Q20.0
- cervix—*see* Malposition
- congenital
  - alimentary tract Q45.8
    - lower Q43.8
    - upper Q40.8
  - aorta Q25.4

Malposition, *continued*
- artery (peripheral) Q27.8
  - pulmonary Q25.79
- biliary duct or passage Q44.5
- clavicle Q74.0
- digestive organ or tract NEC Q45.8
  - lower Q43.8
  - upper Q40.8
- endocrine (gland) NEC Q89.2
- fallopian tube Q50.6
- finger(s) Q68.1
  - supernumerary Q69.0
- gallbladder Q44.1
- gastrointestinal tract Q45.8
- genitalia, genital organ(s) or tract
  - female Q52.8
    - ~ external Q52.79
    - ~ internal NEC Q52.8
  - male Q55.8
- heart Q24.8
  - dextrocardia Q24.0
    - ~ with complete transposition of viscera Q89.3
- hepatic duct Q44.5
- hip (joint) Q65.89
- ovary Q50.39
- parathyroid (gland) Q89.2
- pituitary (gland) Q89.2
- scapula Q74.0
- shoulder Q74.0
- symphysis pubis Q74.2
- thymus (gland) Q89.2
- thyroid (gland) (tissue) Q89.2
  - cartilage Q31.8
- toe(s) Q66.9-
  - supernumerary Q69.2
- gastrointestinal tract, congenital Q45.8

Malposture R29.3

Malrotation
- cecum Q43.3
- colon Q43.3
- intestine Q43.3
- kidney Q63.2

Maltreatment
- child
  - abandonment
    - confirmed T74.02
    - suspected T76.02
  - bullying
    - confirmed T74.32
    - suspected T76.32
  - confirmed T74.92
  - history of—*see* History, personal (of), abuse
  - intimidation (through social media)
    - confirmed T74.32
    - suspected T76.32
  - neglect
    - confirmed T74.02
    - history of—*see* History, personal (of), abuse
    - suspected T76.02
  - physical abuse
    - confirmed T74.12
    - history of—*see* History, personal (of), abuse
    - suspected T76.12
  - psychological abuse
    - confirmed T74.32
    - history of—*see* History, personal (of), abuse
    - suspected T76.32
  - sexual abuse
    - confirmed T74.22
    - history of—*see* History, personal (of), abuse
    - suspected T76.22
  - suspected T76.92
- personal history of Z91.89

Mammillitis N61.0

Mammitis—*see* Mastitis

Mammogram (examination) Z12.39
- routine Z12.31

Mammoplasia N62

Manic depression F31.9

Mannosidosis E77.1

Maple-syrup-urine disease E71.0

Marchesani (-Weill) syndrome Q87.0

Marie's
- cerebellar ataxia (late-onset) G11.2
- disease or syndrome (acromegaly) E22.0

Marion's disease (bladder neck obstruction) N32.0

Mark
- port wine Q82.5
- raspberry Q82.5
- strawberry Q82.5
- tattoo L81.8

Maroteaux-Lamy syndrome (mild) (severe) E76.29

Marrow (bone)
- arrest D61.9

Masculinization (female) with adrenal hyperplasia E25.9
- congenital E25.0

Mass
- abdominal R19.00
  - epigastric R19.06
  - generalized R19.07
  - left lower quadrant R19.04
  - left upper quadrant R19.02
  - periumbilic R19.05
  - right lower quadrant R19.03
  - right upper quadrant R19.01
  - specified site NEC R19.09
- breast (*see also* Lump, breast) N63.0
- chest R22.2
- cystic—*see* Cyst
- ear H93.8-
- head R22.0
- intra-abdominal (diffuse) (generalized)—*see* Mass, abdominal
- kidney N28.89
- liver R16.0
- localized (skin) R22.9
  - chest R22.2
  - head R22.0
  - limb
    - lower R22.4-
    - upper R22.3-
  - neck R22.1
  - trunk R22.2
- lung R91.8
- malignant—*see* Neoplasm, malignant, by site in Table of Neoplasms in the complete *ICD-10-CM* manual
- neck R22.1
- pelvic (diffuse) (generalized)—*see* Mass, abdominal
- specified organ NEC—*see* Disease, by site
- splenic R16.1
- substernal thyroid—*see* Goiter
- superficial (localized) R22.9
- umbilical (diffuse) (generalized) R19.09

Mast cell
- disease, systemic tissue D47.02
- leukemia C94.3-
- neoplasm
  - malignant C96.20
    - specified type NEC C96.29
  - of uncertain behavior NEC D47.09
- sarcoma C96.22
- tumor D47.09

Mastalgia N64.4

Mastitis (acute) (diffuse) (nonpuerperal) (subacute) N61.0
- infective N61.0
  - newborn P39.0
- neonatal (noninfective) P83.4
  - infective P39.0

Mastocytosis D47.09
- aggressive systemic C96.21
- cutaneous (diffuse) (maculopapular) D47.01
  - congenital Q82.2
  - of neonatal onset Q82.2
  - of newborn onset Q82.2
- indolent systemic D47.02
- isolated bone marrow D47.02
- malignant C96.29
- systemic (indolent) (smoldering)
  - with an associated hematological non-mast cell lineage disease (SM-AHNMD) D47.02

Mastodynia N64.4

Mastoidalgia—*see* subcategory H92.0

Mastoplasia, mastoplastia N62

Masturbation (excessive) F98.8

May (-Hegglin) anomaly or syndrome D72.0

McQuarrie's syndrome (idiopathic familial hypoglycemia) E16.2

Measles (black) (hemorrhagic) (suppressed) B05.9
- with
  - complications NEC B05.89
  - encephalitis B05.0
  - intestinal complications B05.4
  - keratitis (keratoconjunctivitis) B05.81
  - meningitis B05.1
  - otitis media B05.3
  - pneumonia B05.2
- French—*see* Rubella
- German—*see* Rubella
- Liberty—*see* Rubella

Meckel-Gruber syndrome Q61.9

Meckel's diverticulitis, diverticulum (displaced) (hypertrophic) Q43.0

Meconium
- ileus, newborn P76.0
  - in cystic fibrosis E84.11
  - meaning meconium plug (without cystic fibrosis) P76.0
- obstruction, newborn P76.0
  - due to fecaliths P76.0
  - in mucoviscidosis E84.11
- plug syndrome (newborn) NEC P76.0

Mediastinopericarditis—*see also* Pericarditis
- acute I30.9
- adhesive I31.0
- chronic I31.8
  - rheumatic I09.2

Medulloblastoma
- desmoplastic C71.6
- specified site—*see* Neoplasm, malignant, by site in Table of Neoplasms in the complete *ICD-10-CM* manual
- unspecified site C71.6

Medullomyoblastoma
- specified site—*see* Neoplasm, malignant, by site in Table of Neoplasms in the complete *ICD-10-CM* manual
- unspecified site C71.6

Meekeren-Ehlers-Danlos syndrome Q79.69
- classical Ehlers-Danlos syndrome Q79.61
- hypermobile Ehlers-Danlos syndrome Q79.62
- other Ehlers-Danlos syndromes Q79.69
- vascular Ehlers-Danlos syndrome Q79.63

Megacolon (acquired) (functional) (not Hirschsprung's disease) (in) K59.39
- congenital, congenitum (aganglionic) Q43.1
- Hirschsprung's (disease) Q43.1
- toxic K59.31

Megalerythema (epidemic) B08.3

Megalocornea Q15.8
- with glaucoma Q15.0

Megalodactylia (fingers) (thumbs) (congenital) Q74.0
- toes Q74.2

Megarectum K62.89

Megasigmoid K59.39
- congenital Q43.2
- toxic K59.31

Melancholia F32.9
- hypochondriac F45.29
- intermittent (single episode) F32.89
  - recurrent episode F33.9

Melanocytosis, neurocutaneous Q82.8

Melanoderma, melanodermia L81.4

Melanodontia, infantile K03.89

Melanodontoclasia K03.89

Melanoma (malignant) C43.9
- benign—*see* Nevus
- skin C43.-

Melanosis L81.4
- Riehl's L81.4
- tar L81.4
- toxic L81.4

MELAS syndrome E88.41

Melena K92.1
- with ulcer—*code by* site under Ulcer, with hemorrhage K27.4
- due to swallowed maternal blood P78.2
- newborn, neonatal P54.1
  - due to swallowed maternal blood P78.2

Membrane(s), membranous—*see also* Disease, diseased
- over face of newborn P28.9

Menarche
- delayed E30.0
- precocious E30.1

Meningism—*see* Meningismus

Meningismus (infectional) (pneumococcal) R29.1
- due to serum or vaccine R29.1
- influenzal—*see* Influenza

Meningitis (basal) (basic) (brain) (cerebral) (cervical) (congestive) (diffuse) (hemorrhagic) (infantile) (membranous) (metastatic) (nonspecific) (pontine) (progressive) (simple) (spinal) (subacute) (sympathetic) (toxic) G03.9
- abacterial G03.0
- arbovirus A87.8
- aseptic G03.0
- bacterial G00.9
  - Escherichia Coli (E. coli) G00.8
  - gram-negative G00.9
  - H. influenzae G00.0
  - pneumococcal G00.1
  - specified organism NEC G00.8
  - streptococcal (acute) G00.2
- candidal B37.5
- caseous (tuberculous) A17.0
- cerebrospinal A39.0
- clear cerebrospinal fluid NEC G03.0
- coxsackievirus A87.0
- diplococcal (gram positive) A39.0
- echovirus A87.0
- enteroviral A87.0
- epidemic NEC A39.0
- Escherichia Coli (E. coli) G00.8
- fibrinopurulent G00.9
  - specified organism NEC G00.8
- gram-negative cocci G00.9
- gram-positive cocci G00.9
- Haemophilus (influenzae) G00.0
- H. influenzae G00.0
- in (due to)
  - bacterial disease NEC A48.8 *[G01]*
  - chickenpox B01.0
  - Diplococcus pneumoniae G00.1
  - enterovirus A87.0
  - herpes (simplex) virus B00.3
  - infectious mononucleosis B27.92
  - Lyme disease A69.21
  - measles B05.1
  - parasitic disease NEC B89 [G02}
  - Streptococcal pneumoniae G00.1
  - varicella B01.0
  - viral disease NEC A87.8
  - whooping cough A37.90
- infectious G00.9
- influenzal (H. influenzae) G00.0
- meningococcal A39.0
- monilial B37.5
- mycotic NEC B49 [G02]
- Neisseria A39.0
- nonbacterial G03.0
- nonpyogenic G03.0
- ossificans G96.198
- pneumococcal streptococcus pneumoniae G00.1
- postmeasles B05.1
- purulent G00.9
  - specified organism NEC G00.8
- pyogenic G00.9
  - specified organism NEC G00.8
- septic G00.9
  - specified organism NEC G00.8

Meningitis, *continued*
- serosa circumscripta NEC G03.0
- serous NEC G93.2
- specified organism NEC G00.8
- sterile G03.0
- streptococcal (acute) G00.2
- suppurative G00.9
  - specified organism NEC G00.8
- tuberculous A17.0
- viral NEC A87.9

Meningocele (spinal) — *see also* Spina bifida
- acquired (traumatic) G96.198

Meningococcemia A39.4
- acute A39.2
- chronic A39.3

Meningococcus, meningococcal (*see also* Disease, diseased) A39.9
- carrier (suspected) of Z22.31
- meningitis (cerebrospinal) A39.0

Meningoencephalitis (*see also* Encephalitis) G04.90
- acute NEC (*see also* Encephalitis, viral) A86
  - disseminated G04.00
    - postimmunization or postvaccination G04.02
- California A83.5
- herpesviral, herpetic B00.4
  - due to herpesvirus 7 B10.09
  - specified NEC B10.09
- in (due to)
  - diseases classified elsewhere G05.3
  - Haemophilus influenzae (H. Influenzae) G00.0
  - herpes B00.4
    - due to herpesvirus 7 B10.09
    - specified NEC B10.09
  - H. influenzae G00.0
  - Lyme disease A69.22
  - toxoplasmosis (acquired) B58.2
    - congenital P37.1
- infectious (acute) (viral) A86
- parasitic NEC B89 *[G05.3]*
- pneumococcal G04.2
- toxic NEC G92
- virus NEC A86

Meningoencephalomyelitis—*see also* Encephalitis
- acute NEC (viral) A86
  - disseminated G04.00
    - postimmunization or postvaccination G04.02
    - postinfectious G04.01
- due to
  - Toxoplasma or toxoplasmosis (acquired) B58.2
    - congenital P37.1
- postimmunization or postvaccination G04.02

Meningomyelitis—*see also* Meningoencephalitis
- in diseases classified elsewhere G05.4

Menkes' disease or syndrome E83.09
- meaning maple-syrup-urine disease E71.0

Menometrorrhagia N92.1

Menorrhagia (primary) N92.0
- pubertal (menses retained) N92.2

Menostaxis N92.0

Menses, retention N94.89

Menstrual—*see* Menstruation

Menstruation
- absent—*see* Amenorrhea
- anovulatory N97.0
- cycle, irregular N92.6
- during pregnancy O20.8
- excessive (with regular cycle) N92.0
  - with irregular cycle N92.1
  - at puberty N92.2
- frequent N92.0
- irregular N92.6
  - specified NEC N92.5
- latent N92.5
- membranous N92.5
  - painful (*see also* Dysmenorrhea) N94.6 primary N94.4
  - psychogenic F45.8
  - secondary N94.5
- passage of clots N92.0
- precocious E30.1

Morbilli—*see* Measles

Morbus—*see also* Disease
- angelicus, anglorum E55.0
- celiacus K90.0
- hemorrhagicus neonatorum P53
- maculosus neonatorum P54.5

Morgagni's
- cyst, organ, hydatid, or appendage
  - female Q50.5
  - male (epididymal) Q55.4
    - testicular Q55.29

Morgagni-Stokes-Adams syndrome I45.9

Morgagni-Turner (-Albright) syndrome Q96.9

Moron (I.Q.50-69) F70

Morvan's disease or syndrome G60.8

Mosaicism, mosaic (autosomal) (chromosomal)
- 45,X/other cell lines NEC with abnormal sex chromosome Q96.4
- 45,X/46,XX Q96.3
- sex chromosome
  - female Q97.8
  - lines with various numbers of X chromosomes Q97.2
  - male Q98.7
- XY Q96.3

Motion sickness (from travel, any vehicle) (from roundabouts or swings) T75.3

Mountain
- sickness T70.29
  - with polycythemia, acquired (acute) D75.1
- tick fever A93.2

MRSA (Methicillin resistant Staphylococcus aureus)
- infection A49.02
  - as the cause of disease classified elsewhere B95.62
- sepsis A41.02

MSD (multiple sulfatase deficiency) E75.26

MSSA (Methicillin susceptible Staphylococcus aureus)
- infection A49.02
  - as the cause of disease classified elsewhere B95.61
- sepsis A41.01

Mucinosis (cutaneous) (focal) (papular) (reticular erythematous) (skin) L98.5
- oral K13.79

Mucocele
- buccal cavity K13.79
- nasal sinus J34.1
- nose J34.1
- sinus (accessory) (nasal) J34.1
- turbinate (bone) (middle) (nasal) J34.1

Mucolipidosis
- I E77.1
- II, III E77.0

Mucopolysaccharidosis E76.3
- beta-gluduronidase deficiency E76.29
- cardiopathy E76.3 *[I52]*
- Hunter's syndrome E76.1
- Hurler's syndrome E76.01
- Maroteaux-Lamy syndrome E76.29
- Morquio syndrome E76.219
  - A E76.210
  - B E76.211
  - classic E76.210
- Sanfilippo syndrome E76.22
- specified NEC E76.29
- type
  - I
    - Hurler's syndrome E76.01
    - Hurler-Scheie syndrome E76.02
    - Scheie's syndrome E76.03
  - II E76.1
  - III E76.22
  - IV E76.219
  - IVA E76.210
  - IVB E76.211
  - VI E76.29
  - VII E76.29

Mucositis (ulcerative) K12.30
- nasal J34.81

Mucoviscidosis E84.9
- with meconium obstruction E84.11

Mucus
- asphyxiation or suffocation—*see* Asphyxia
- in stool R19.5
- plug—*see* Asphyxia

Muguet B37.0

Multicystic kidney (development) Q61.4

Mumps B26.9

Murmur (cardiac) (heart) (organic) R01.1
- aortic (valve)—*see* Endocarditis, aortic
- benign R01.0
- diastolic—*see* Endocarditis
- Flint I35.1
- functional R01.0
- Graham Steell I37.1
- innocent R01.0
- mitral (valve)—*see* Insufficiency, mitral
- nonorganic R01.0
- presystolic, mitral—*see* Insufficiency, mitral
- pulmonic (valve) I37.8
- systolic R01.1
- tricuspid (valve) I07.9
- valvular—*see* Endocarditis

Muscle, muscular—*see also* Disease, diseased
- carnitine (palmityltransferase) deficiency E71.314

Mutation(s)
- surfactant, of lung J84.83

Mutism—*see also* Aphasia
- deaf (acquired) (congenital) NEC H91.3
- elective (adjustment reaction) (childhood) F94.0
- hysterical F44.4
- selective (childhood) F94.0

Myalgia M79.1-
- traumatic NEC T14.8

Myasthenia G70.9
- congenital G70.2
- cordis—*see* Failure, heart
- developmental G70.2
- gravis G70.00
  - with exacerbation (acute) G70.01
  - in crisis G70.01
  - neonatal, transient P94.0
  - pseudoparalytica G70.00
    - with exacerbation (acute) G70.01
    - in crisis G70.01
- stomach, psychogenic F45.8
- syndrome
  - in
    - diabetes mellitus—*see* E08-E13 with .44
    - neoplastic disease (*see also* Table of Neoplasms in the complete *ICD-10-CM* manual) D49.9 *[G73.3]*
    - thyrotoxicosis E05.90 *[G73.3]*
      ~ with thyroid storm E05.91 *[G73.3]*

Myasthenic M62.81

Mycoplasma (M.) pneumoniae, as cause of disease classified elsewhere B96.0

Mycosis, mycotic B49
- mouth B37.0
- nails B35.1
- stomatitis B37.0
- vagina, vaginitis (candidal) B37.3

Myelitis (acute) (ascending) (childhood) (chronic) (descending) (diffuse) (disseminated) (idiopathic) (pressure) (progressive) (spinal cord) (subacute) (*see also* Encephalitis) G04.91
- flaccid G04.89
- in diseases classified elsewhere G05.4
- post–chicken pox B01.12
- postimmunization G04.02
- postinfectious G04.89
- postvaccinal G04.02
- specified NEC G04.89
- toxic G92
- varicella B01.12

Myelogenous—*see* Disease, diseased

Myeloid—*see* Disease, diseased

Myelokathexis D70.9

Myelopathy (spinal cord) G95.9
- in (due to)
  - infection—*see* Encephalitis
  - mercury—*see* subcategory T56.1
  - neoplastic disease (*see also* Table of Neoplasms in the complete *ICD-10-CM* manual) D49.9 *[G99.2]*

Myelophthisis D61.82

Myelosclerosis D75.89
- disseminated, of nervous system G35

Myelosis
- acute C92.0-
- aleukemic C92.9-
- nonleukemic D72.828
- subacute C92.9-

Myocardiopathy (congestive) (constrictive) (familial) (hypertrophic nonobstructive) (idiopathic) (infiltrative) (obstructive) (primary) (restrictive) (sporadic) (*see also* Cardiomyopathy) I42.9
- hypertrophic obstructive I42.1
- in (due to)
  - Friedreich's ataxia G11.11 [I43]
  - progressive muscular dystrophy G71.09 [I43]
- secondary I42.9
- thyrotoxic E05.90 [I43]
  - with storm E05.91 [I43]

Myocarditis (with arteriosclerosis) (chronic) (fibroid) (interstitial) (old) (progressive) (senile) I51.4
- with
  - rheumatic fever (conditions in I00) I09.0
    - active—*see* Myocarditis, acute, rheumatic
    - inactive or quiescent (with chorea) I09.0
- active I40.9
  - rheumatic I01.2
    - with chorea (acute) (rheumatic) (Sydenham's) I02.0
- acute or subacute (interstitial) I40.9
  - due to
    - streptococcus (beta-hemolytic) I01.2
  - idiopathic I40.1
  - rheumatic I01.2
    - with chorea (acute) (rheumatic) (Sydenham's) I02.0
  - specified NEC I40.8
- bacterial (acute) I40.0
- eosinophilic I40.1
- epidemic of newborn (Coxsackie) B33.22
- Fiedler's (acute) (isolated) I40.1
- giant cell (acute) (subacute) I40.1
- granulomatous (idiopathic) (isolated) (nonspecific) I40.1
- idiopathic (granulomatous) I40.1
- in (due to)
  - Lyme disease A69.29
  - sarcoidosis D86.85
- infective I40.0
- influenzal—*see* Influenza, myocarditis
- isolated (acute) I40.1
- nonrheumatic, active I40.9
- parenchymatous I40.9
- pneumococcal I40.0
- rheumatic (chronic) (inactive) (with chorea) I09.0
  - active or acute I01.2
    - with chorea (acute) (rheumatic) (Sydenham's) I02.0
- septic I40.0
- staphylococcal I40.0
- suppurative I40.0
- toxic I40.8
- virus, viral I40.0
  - of newborn (Coxsackie) B33.22

Myoclonus, myoclonic, myoclonia (familial) (essential) (multifocal) (simplex) G25.3
- drug-induced G25.3
- epilepsy (*see also* Epilepsy, generalized, specified NEC) G40.4-
  - familial (progressive) G25.3
- familial progressive G25.3
- Friedreich's G25.3
- jerks G25.3
- massive G25.3
- palatal G25.3
- pharyngeal G25.3

Myofibromatosis
- infantile Q89.8

Myopathy G72.9
- autosomal (dominant) (recessive) G71.228
  - other specified NEC G71.228
- benign congenital G71.20
- central core G71.29
- centronuclear G71.228
- congenital (benign) G71.20
- distal G71.09
- facioscapulohumeral G71.02hyaline body G71.29
- in (due to)
  - Cushing's syndrome E24.9 [G73.7]
  - hyperadrenocorticism E24.9 [G73.7]
  - *hypopituitarism E23.0 [G73.7]*
  - hypothyroidism E03.9 [G73.7]
  - myxedema E03.9 [G73.7]
  - sarcoidosis D86.87
  - scarlet fever A38.1
  - systemic lupus erythematosus M32.19
  - thyrotoxicosis (hyperthyroidism) E05.90 *[G73.7]*
    - with thyroid storm E05.91 *[G73.7]*
- limb-girdle G71.09
- myosin storage G71.29
  - myotubular (centronuclear) G71.220
    - X-linked G71.220
- nemaline G71.21
- ocular G71.09
- oculopharyngeal G71.09
- rod (body) G71.21
- scapulohumeral G71.02

Myopia (axial) (congenital) H52.1-

Myositis M60.9
- in (due to)
  - sarcoidosis D86.87
- infective M60.009
  - arm
    - left M60.001
    - right M60.000
  - leg
    - left M60.004
    - right M60.003
  - lower limb
    - ankle M60.07-
    - foot M60.07-
    - lower leg M60.06-
    - thigh M60.05-
    - toe M60.07-
  - multiple sites M60.09
  - specified site NEC M60.08
  - upper limb
    - finger M60.04-
    - forearm M60.03-
    - hand M60.04-
    - shoulder region M60.01-
    - upper arm M60.02-

Myospasia impulsiva F95.2

Myotonia (acquisita) (intermittens) M62.89
- congenita (acetazolamide responsive) (dominant) (recessive) G71.12
- levior G71.12

Myriapodiasis B88.2

Myringitis H73.2-
- with otitis media—*see* Otitis, media
- acute H73.00-
  - bullous H73.01-
- bullous—*see* Myringitis, acute, bullous
- chronic H73.1-

Myxadenitis labialis K13.0

Myxedema (adult) (idiocy) (infantile) (juvenile) (*see also* Hypothyroidism) E03.9
- circumscribed E05.90
  - with storm E05.91
- congenital E00.1
- cutis L98.5
- localized (pretibial) E05.90
  - with storm E05.91

Myxolipoma D17.9

N

Naegeli's
- disease Q82.8

Nail—*see also* Disease, diseased
- biting F98.8

Nanism, nanosomia—*see* Dwarfism

Napkin rash L22

Narcosis R06.89

Narcotism—*see* Dependence

NARP (Neuropathy, Ataxia and Retinitis pigmentosa) syndrome E88.49

Narrowness, abnormal, eyelid Q10.3

Nasopharyngeal—*see also* Disease, diseased
- pituitary gland Q89.2
- torticollis M43.6

Nasopharyngitis (acute) (infective) (streptococcal) (subacute) J00
- chronic (suppurative) (ulcerative) J31.1

Nasopharynx, nasopharyngeal—*see* Disease, diseased

Natal tooth, teeth K00.6

Nausea (without vomiting) R11.0
- with vomiting R11.2
- marina T75.3
- navalis T75.3

Near drowning T75.1

Nearsightedness—*see* Myopia

Near-syncope R55

Necrolysis, toxic epidermal L51.2
- due to drug
  - correct substance properly administered—*see* Table of Drugs and Chemicals, by drug, adverse effect
  - overdose or wrong substance given or taken—*see* Table of Drugs and Chemicals, by drug, poisoning

Necrosis, necrotic (ischemic)—*see also* Gangrene
- adrenal (capsule) (gland) E27.49
- antrum J32.0
- cortical (acute) (renal) N17.1
- ethmoid (bone) J32.2
- fat, fatty (generalized)—*see also* Disorder, specified type NEC
  - skin (subcutaneous), newborn P83.0
  - subcutaneous due to birth injury P15.6
- kidney (bilateral) N28.0
  - acute N17.9
  - cortical (acute) (bilateral) N17.1
  - medullary (bilateral) (in acute renal failure) (papillary) N17.2
  - papillary (bilateral) (in acute renal failure) N17.2
  - tubular N17.0
    - medullary (acute) (renal) N17.2
- papillary (acute) (renal) N17.2
- pharynx J02.9
  - in granulocytopenia—*see* Neutropenia
- phosphorus—*see* subcategory T54.2
- pituitary (gland) E23.0
- subcutaneous fat, newborn P83.88
- suprarenal (capsule) (gland) E27.49
- tonsil J35.8
- tubular (acute) (anoxic) (renal) (toxic) N17.0
  - postprocedural N99.0

Need (for)
- care provider because (of)
  - assistance with personal care Z74.1
  - continuous supervision required Z74.3
  - impaired mobility Z74.09
  - no other household member able to render care Z74.2
  - specified reason NEC Z74.8
- immunization—*see* Vaccination
- vaccination—*see* Vaccination

Neglect
- child (childhood)
  - confirmed T74.02
  - history of Z62.812
  - suspected T76.02
- emotional, in childhood Z62.898

Nelaton's syndrome G60.8

Neonatal—*see also* Newborn
- acne L70.4
- bradycardia P29.12
- screening, abnormal findings on P09
- tachycardia P29.11
- tooth, teeth K00.6

Neonatorum—*see* Disease, diseased

Neoplasia
- intraepithelial (histologically confirmed)
  - anal (AIN) (histologically confirmed) K62.82
    - grade I K62.82
    - grade II K62.82

Neoplasm, neoplastic—*see also* Table of Neoplasms in the complete *ICD-10-CM* manual.
- lipomatous, benign—*see* Lipoma

Nephralgia N23

Nephritis, nephritic (albuminuric) (azotemic) (congenital) (disseminated) (epithelial) (familial) (focal) (granulomatous) (hemorrhagic) (infantile) (nonsuppurative, excretory) (uremic) N05.9
- with
  - C3
    - glomerulonephritis N05.A
    - glomerulopathy N05.A
      - with dense deposit disease N05.6
- acute N00.9
  - with
    - C3
      - glomerulonephritis N00.A
      - glomerulopathy N00.A
        - with dense deposit disease N00.6
        - dense deposit disease N00.6
    - diffuse
      - crescentic glomerulonephritis N00.7
      - endocapillary proliferative glomerulonephritis N00.4
      - membranous glomerulonephritis N00.2
      - mesangial proliferative glomerulonephritis N00.3
      - mesangiocapillary glomerulonephritis N00.5
    - focal and segmental glomerular lesions N00.1
    - minor glomerular abnormality N00.0
    - specified morphological changes NEC N00.8
- chronic N03.9
  - with
    - C3
      - glomerulonephritis N03.A
      - glomerulopathy N03.A
        - with dense deposit disease N03.6
- croupous N00.9
- due to
  - diabetes mellitus—*see* E08-E13 with .21
  - subacute bacterial endocarditis I33.0
  - systemic lupus erythematosus (chronic) M32.14
- in
  - diabetes mellitus—*see* E08–E13 with.21
- polycystic Q61.3
  - autosomal
    - dominant Q61.2
    - recessive NEC Q61.19
  - childhood type NEC Q61.19
  - infantile type NEC Q61.19
- poststreptococcal N05.9
  - acute N00.9
  - chronic N03.9
- rapidly progressive N01.-
  - with
    - C3
      - glomerulonephritis N01.A
      - glomerulopathy N01.A
        - with dense deposit disease N01.6
- tubulo-interstitial (in) N12
  - acute (infectious) N10
- war N00.9

Nephroblastoma (epithelial) (mesenchymal) C64.-

Nephrocystitis, pustular—*see* Nephritis, tubulo-interstitial

Nephroma C64-

Nephronephritis—*see* Nephrosis

Nephronophthisis Q61.5

Nephropathy (*see also* Nephritis) N28.9
- analgesic N14.0
  - with medullary necrosis, acute N17.2
- diabetic—*see* E08–E13 with .21
- hereditary NEC N07.9
  - with
    - C3
      ~ glomerulonephritis N07.A
      ~ glomerulopathy N07.A
        ◊ with dense deposit disease N07.6
- obstructive N13.8
- phenacetin N17.2
- vasomotor N17.0

Nephrosis, nephrotic (Epstein's) (syndrome) (congenital) N04.9
- with
  - glomerular lesion N04.1
  - hypocomplementemic N04.5
- acute N04.9
- anoxic—*see* Nephrosis, tubular
- chemical—*see* Nephrosis, tubular
- Finnish type (congenital) Q89.8
- hemoglobin N10
- hemoglobinuric—*see* Nephrosis, tubular
- in
  - diabetes mellitus—*see* E08–E13 with .21
- lipoid N04.9
- minimal change N04.0
- myoglobin N10
- radiation N04.9
- toxic—*see* Nephrosis, tubular
- tubular (acute) N17.0
  - postprocedural N99.0
  - radiation N04.9

Nerves R45.0

Nervous (*see also* Disease, diseased) R45.0
- heart F45.8
- stomach F45.8
- tension R45.0

Nervousness R45.0

Nettleship's syndrome—*see* Urticaria pigmentosa

Neuralgia, neuralgic (acute) M79.2
- ciliary G44.009
  - intractable G44.001
  - not intractable G44.009
- ear—*see* subcategory H92.0
- migrainous G44.009
  - intractable G44.001
  - not intractable G44.009
- perineum R10.2
- pubic region R10.2
- scrotum R10.2
- spermatic cord R10.2

Neurasthenia F48.8
- cardiac F45.8
- gastric F45.8
- heart F45.8

Neuritis (rheumatoid) M79.2
- cranial nerve
  - due to Lyme disease A69.22
  - fifth or trigeminal G51.0
  - seventh or facial G51.8
    - newborn (birth injury) P11.3
  - sixth or abducent—*see* Strabismus, paralytic, sixth nerve
- facial G51.8
  - newborn (birth injury) P11.3
- serum (*see also* Reaction, serum) T80.69

Neuroblastoma
- specified site—*see* Neoplasm, malignant, by site in Table of Neoplasms in the complete *ICD-10-CM* manual
- unspecified site C74.90

Neurocirculatory asthenia F45.8

Neurodermatitis (circumscribed) (circumscripta) (local) L28.0
- atopic L20.81
- diffuse (Brocq) L20.81
- disseminated L20.81

Neurofibromatosis (multiple) (nonmalignant) Q85.00
- acoustic Q85.02
- malignant—*see* Neoplasm, nerve, malignant in Table of Neoplasms in the complete *ICD-10-CM* manual
- specified NEC Q85.09
- type 1 (von Recklinghausen) Q85.01
- type 2 Q85.02

Neurogenic—*see also* Disease, diseased
- bladder (*see also* Dysfunction) N31.9
  - cauda equina syndrome G83.4
- bowel NEC K59.2
- heart F45.8

Neuromyopathy G70.9
- paraneoplastic D49.9 *[G13.0]*

Neuropathy, neuropathic G62.9
- hereditary G60.9
  - motor and sensory (types I-IV) G60.0
  - sensory G60.8
  - specified NEC G60.8
- idiopathic G60.9
  - progressive G60.3
  - specified NEC G60.8
- peripheral (nerve) (*see also* Polyneuropathy) G62.9
  - autonomic G90.9
    - in (due to)
      ~ hyperthyroidism E05.90 [G99.0]
        ◊ with thyroid storm E05.91 [G99.0]

Neurosis, neurotic F48.9
- anankastic F42.8
- anxiety (state) F41.1
  - panic type F41.0
- bladder F45.8
- cardiac (reflex) F45.8
- cardiovascular F45.8
- character F60.9
- colon F45.8
- compulsive, compulsion F42.9
- conversion F44.9
- cutaneous F45.8
- excoriation F42.4
- gastric F45.8
- gastrointestinal F45.8
- heart F45.8
- hysterical F44.9
- incoordination F45.8
  - larynx F45.8
  - vocal cord F45.8
- intestine F45.8
- larynx (sensory) F45.8
  - hysterical F44.4
- mixed NEC F48.8
- musculoskeletal F45.8
- obsessional F42.9
- obsessive-compulsive F42.9
- ocular NEC F45.8
- pharynx F45.8
- phobic F40.9
- posttraumatic (situational) F43.10
  - acute F43.11
  - chronic F43.12
- rectum F45.8
- respiratory F45.8
- rumination F45.8
- state F48.9
- stomach F45.8
- traumatic F43.10
  - acute F43.11
  - chronic F43.12
- vasomotor F45.8
- visceral F45.8

Neurospongioblastosis diffusa Q85.1

Neutropenia, neutropenic (chronic) (genetic) (idiopathic) (immune) (infantile) (malignant) (pernicious) (splenic) D70.9
- congenital (primary) D70.0
- cyclic D70.4
- cytoreductive cancer chemotherapy sequela D70.1
- drug-induced D70.2
  - due to cytoreductive cancer chemotherapy D70.1
- due to infection D70.3
- fever D70.9

Neutropenia, neutropenic, *continued*
- neonatal, transitory (isoimmune) (maternal transfer) P61.5
- periodic D70.4
- secondary (cyclic) (periodic) (splenic) D70.4
  - drug-induced D70.2
    - due to cytoreductive cancer chemotherapy D70.1
- toxic D70.8

Neutrophilia, hereditary giant D72.0

Nevus D22-
- achromic—*see* Neoplasm, skin, benign in Table of Neoplasms in the complete *ICD-10-CM* manual
- amelanotic—*see* Neoplasm, skin, benign in Table of Neoplasms in the complete *ICD-10-CM* manual
- angiomatous D18.00
  - skin D18.01
  - specified site NEC D18.09
- araneus I78.1
- blue—(*see* Neoplasm, skin, benign for blue, cellular, giant, or Jadassohn's or other than malignant in Table of Neoplasms in the complete *ICD-10-CM* manual)
  - malignant—*see* Melanoma
- capillary D18.00
  - skin D18.01
  - specified site NEC D18.09
- cavernous D18.00
  - skin D18.01
  - specified site NEC D18.09
- cellular—*see* Neoplasm, skin, benign in Table of Neoplasms in the complete *ICD-10-CM* manual
  - blue—*see* Neoplasm, skin, benign in Table of Neoplasms in the complete *ICD-10-CM* manual
- comedonicus Q82.5
- dermal—*see* Neoplasm, skin, benign in Table of Neoplasms in the complete *ICD-10-CM* manual
  - with epidermal nevus—*see* Neoplasm, skin, benign in Table of Neoplasms in the complete *ICD-10-CM* manual
- dysplastic—*see* Neoplasm, skin, benign in Table of Neoplasms in the complete *ICD-10-CM* manual
- flammeus Q82.5
- hemangiomatous D18.00
  - skin D18.01
  - specified site NEC D18.09
- lymphatic D18.1
- meaning hemangioma D18.00
  - skin D18.01
  - specified site NEC D18.09
- multiplex Q85.1
- non-neoplastic I78.1
- portwine Q82.5
- sanguineous Q82.5
- skin D22.9
  - abdominal wall D22.5
  - ala nasi D22.39
  - ankle D22.7-
  - anus, anal D22.5
  - arm D22.6-
  - auditory canal (external) D22.2-
  - auricle (ear) D22.2-
  - auricular canal (external) D22.2-
  - axilla, axillary fold D22.5
  - back D22.5
  - breast D22.5
  - brow D22.39
  - buttock D22.5
  - canthus (eye) D22.1-
  - cheek (external) D22.39
  - chest wall D22.5
  - chin D22.39
  - ear (external) D22.2-
    - external meatus (ear) D22.2-
  - eyebrow D22.39
  - eyelid (lower) (upper) D22.1-
  - face D22.3-
  - finger D22.6-
  - flank D22.5
  - foot D22.7-
  - forearm D22.6-
  - forehead D22.39
  - foreskin D29.0

Nevus, *continued*
- genital organ (external) NEC
  - female D28.0
  - male D29.9
- gluteal region D22.5
- groin D22.5
- hand D22.6-
- heel D22.7-
- helix D22.2-
- hip D22.7-
- interscapular region D22.5
- jaw D22.39
- knee D22.7-
- leg D22.7-
- lip (lower) (upper) D22.0
- lower limb D22.7-
- nail D22.9
  - finger D22.6-
  - toe D22.7-
- nasolabial groove D22.39
- nates D22.5
- neck D22.4
- nose (external) D22.39
- palpebra D22.1-
- penis D29.0
- perianal skin D22.5
- perineum D22.5
- pinna D22.2-
- popliteal fossa or space D22.7-
- scalp D22.4
- shoulder D22.6-
- submammary fold D22.5
- temple D22.39
- thigh D22.7-
- toe D22.7-
- trunk NEC D22.5
- umbilicus D22.5
- upper limb D22.6-
- vulva D28.0
- specified site NEC -see Neoplasm, by site, benign in Table of Neoplasms in the complete *ICD-10-CM* manual
- Sutton's benign D22.9
  - spider I78.1
  - stellar I78.1
  - strawberry Q82.5
  - unius lateris Q82.5
  - Unna's Q82.5
  - vascular Q82.5
  - verrucous Q82.5

Newborn (infant) (liveborn) (singleton) Z38.2
- abstinence syndrome P96.1
- acne L70.4
- affected by
  - abruptio placenta P02.1
  - amniocentesis (while in utero) P00.6
  - amnionitis P02.78
  - apparent life threatening event (ALTE) R68.13
  - bleeding (into)
    - cerebral cortex P52.22
    - germinal matrix P52.0
    - ventricles P52.1
  - breech delivery P03.0
  - cardiac arrest P29.81
  - cerebral ischemia P91.0
  - Cesarean delivery P03.4
  - chemotherapy agents P04.1
  - chorioamnionitis P02.78
  - cocaine (crack) P04.41
  - complications of labor and delivery P03.9
    - specified NEC P03.89
  - compression of umbilical cord NEC P02.5
  - contracted pelvis P03.1
  - cyanosis P28.2
  - delivery P03.9
    - Cesarean P03.4
    - forceps P03.2
    - vacuum extractor P03.3
  - drugs of addiction P04.40
    - cocaine P04.41
    - hallucinogens P04.42
    - specified drug NEC P04.49

Newborn, *continued*
- entanglement (knot) in umbilical cord P02.5
- fetal (intrauterine)
  - growth retardation P05.9
  - inflammatory response syndrome (FIRS) P02.70
- FIRS (fetal inflammatory response syndrome) P02.70
- forceps delivery P03.2
- heart rate abnormalities
  - bradycardia P29.12
  - intrauterine P03.819
    - ~ before onset of labor P03.810
    - ~ during labor P03.811
  - tachycardia P29.11
- hemorrhage (antepartum) P02.1
  - intraventricular (nontraumatic) P52.3
    - ~ grade 1 P52.0
    - ~ grade 2 P52.1
    - ~ grade 3 P52.21
    - ~ grade 4 P52.22
  - subependymal P52.0
    - ~ with intracerebral extension P52.22
    - ~ with intraventricular extension P52.1
      - ◊ with enlargement of ventricles P52.21
    - ~ without intraventricular extension P52.0
- hypoxic ischemic encephalopathy [HIE] P91.60
  - mild P91.61
  - moderate P91.62
  - severe P91.63
- induction of labor P03.89
- intrauterine (fetal) blood loss P50.9
- intrauterine (fetal) hemorrhage P50.9
- malpresentation (malposition) NEC P03.1
- maternal (complication of) (use of)
  - alcohol P04.3
  - amphetamines P04.16
  - analgesia (maternal) P04.0
  - anesthesia (maternal) P04.0
  - anticonvulsants P04.13
  - antidepressants P04.15
  - antineoplastic chemotherapy P04.11
  - anxiolytics P04.1A
  - blood loss P02.1
  - cannabis P04.81
  - circulatory disease P00.3
  - condition P00.9
    - ~ specified NEC P00.89
  - cytotoxic drugs P04.12
  - delivery P03.9
    - ~ Cesarean P03.4
    - ~ forceps P03.2
    - ~ vacuum extractor P03.3
  - diabetes mellitus (pre-existing) P70.1
  - disorder P00.9
    - ~ specified NEC P00.89
  - drugs (addictive) (illegal) NEC P04.49
  - hemorrhage P02.1
  - incompetent cervix P01.0
  - infectious disease P00.2
  - malpresentation before labor P01.7
  - medical procedure P00.7
  - medication (legal) (maternal use) (prescribed) P04.19
  - opiates P04.14
    - ~ administered for procedures during pregnancy or labor and delivery P04.0
  - parasitic disease P00.2
  - placenta previa P02.0
  - premature rupture of membranes P01.1
  - respiratory disease P00.3
  - sedative-hypnotics P04.17
    - ~ tranquilizers administered for procedures during pregnancy or labor and delivery P04.0
  - surgical procedure P00.6
  - medication (legal) (maternal use) (prescribed) P04.19
  - specified type NEC P04.18
- membranitis P02.78
- methamphetamine(s) P04.49
- mixed metabolic and respiratory acidosis P84
- neonatal abstinence syndrome P96.1

Newborn, *continued*
- noxious substances transmitted via placenta or breast milk P04.9
  - cannabis P04.81
  - specified NEC P04.89
- placenta previa P02.0
- placental
  - abnormality (functional) (morphological) P02.20
    - ~ specified NEC P02.29
  - dysfunction P02.29
  - infarction P02.29
  - insufficiency P02.29
  - separation NEC P02.1
  - transfusion syndromes P02.3
- placentitis P02.78
- prolapsed cord P02.4
- respiratory arrest P28.81
- slow intrauterine growth P05.9
- tobacco P04.2
- twin to twin transplacental transfusion P02.3
- umbilical cord (tightly) around neck P02.5
- umbilical cord condition P02.60
  - short cord P02.69
  - specified NEC P02.69
- uterine contractions (abnormal) P03.6
- vasa previa P02.69
  - from intrauterine blood loss P50.0
- apnea P28.4
  - primary P28.3
  - obstructive P28.4
  - sleep (central) (obstructive) (primary) P28.3
- born in hospital Z38.00
  - by cesarean Z38.01
- born outside hospital Z38.1
- breast buds P96.89
- breast engorgement P83.4
- check-up—*see* Newborn, examination
- convulsion P90
- dehydration P74.1
- examination
  - 8 to 28 days old Z00.111
  - under 8 days old Z00.110
- fever P81.9
  - environmentally-induced P81.0
- hyperbilirubinemia P59.9
  - of prematurity P59.0
- hypernatremia P74.21
- hyponatremia P74.22
- infection P39.9
  - candidal P37.5
  - specified NEC P39.8
  - urinary tract P39.3
- jaundice P59.9
  - due to
    - breast milk inhibitor P59.3
    - hepatocellular damage P59.20
      - ~ specified NEC P59.29
    - preterm delivery P59.0
  - of prematurity P59.0
  - specified NEC P59.8
- mastitis P39.0
  - infective P39.0
  - noninfective P83.4
- multiple born NEC Z38.8
  - born in hospital Z38.68
    - by cesarean Z38.69
  - born outside hospital Z38.7
- omphalitis P38.9
  - with mild hemorrhage P38.1
  - without hemorrhage P38.9
- post-term P08.21
- prolonged gestation (over 42 completed weeks) P08.22
- quadruplet Z38.8
  - born in hospital Z38.63
    - by cesarean Z38.64
  - born outside hospital Z38.7
- quintuplet Z38.8
  - born in hospital Z38.65
    - by cesarean Z38.66
  - born outside hospital Z38.7
- seizure P90
- sepsis (congenital) P36.9
  - due to

Newborn, *continued*
- ■ anaerobes NEC P36.5
- ■ Escherichia coli P36.4
- ■ Staphylococcus P36.30
  - ~ aureus P36.2
  - ~ specified NEC P36.39
- ■ Streptococcus P36.10
  - ~ group B P36.0
  - ~ specified NEC P36.19
- − specified NEC P36.8
- • triplet Z38.8
  - − born in hospital Z38.61
    - ■ by cesarean Z38.62
  - − born outside hospital Z38.7
- • twin Z38.5
  - − born in hospital Z38.30
    - ■ by cesarean Z38.31
  - − born outside hospital Z38.4
- • vomiting P92.09
  - − bilious P92.01
- • weight check Z00.111

Night
- • sweats R61
- • terrors (child) F51.4

Nightmares (REM sleep type) F51.5

Nipple—*see* Disease, diseased

Nitrosohemoglobinemia D74.8

Nocturia R35.1
- • psychogenic F45.8

Nocturnal—*see* Disease, diseased

Node(s)—*see also* Nodule
- • Osler's I33.0

Nodule(s), **nodular**
- • breast NEC N63.0
- • cutaneous—*see* Swelling, localized
- • inflammatory—*see* Inflammation
- • lung, solitary (subsegmental branch of the bronchial tree) R91.1
  - − multiple R91.8
- • retrocardiac R09.89
- • solitary, lung (subsegmental branch of the bronchial tree) R91.1
  - − multiple R91.8
- • subcutaneous—*see* Swelling, localized

Nonclosure—*see also* Imperfect, closure
- • ductus arteriosus (Botallo's) Q25.0
- • foramen
  - − botalli Q21.1
  - − ovale Q21.1

Noncompliance Z91.19
- • with
  - − dietary regimen Z91.11
  - − medical treatment Z91.19
  - − medication regimen NEC Z91.14
    - ■ underdosing (*see also* Table of Drugs and Chemicals, categories T36 − T50, with final character 6) Z91.14
      - ~ intentional NEC Z91.128
        - ◊ due to financial hardship of patient Z91.120
      - ~ unintentional NEC Z91.138

Nondescent (congenital)—*see also* Malposition, congenital
- • testicle Q53.9
  - − bilateral Q53.20
    - ■ abdominal Q53.211
    - ■ perineal Q53.22
  - − unilateral Q53.10
    - ■ abdominal Q53.111
    - ■ perineal Q53.12

Nondevelopment
- • brain Q02
  - − part of Q04.3
- • heart Q24.8
- • organ or site, congenital NEC—*see* Hypoplasia

Nonexpansion, lung (newborn) P28.0

Nonovulation N97.0

Non-palpable testicle(s)
- • bilateral R39.84
- • unilateral R39.83

Nonpneumatization, lung NEC P28.0

Nonunion
- • fracture—*see* Fracture, by site
- • organ or site, congenital NEC—*see* Imperfect, closure
- • symphysis pubis, congenital Q74.2

Noonan's syndrome Q87.19

Norcardiosis, nocardiasis A43.9
- • cutaneous A43.1
- • lung A43.0
- • pneumonia A43.0
- • pulmonary A43.0
- • specified site NEC A43.8

Normocytic anemia (infectional) due to blood loss (chronic) D50.0
- • acute D62

Norwegian itch B86

Nose, nasal—*see* Disease, diseased

Nosebleed R04.0

Nose-picking F98.8

Nosophobia F45.22

Nostalgia F43.20

Nothnagel's
- • syndrome—*see* Strabismus, paralytic, third nerve
- • vasomotor acroparesthesia I73.89

Novy's relapsing fever A68.9
- • louse-borne A68.0
- • tick-borne A68.1

Noxious
- • foodstuffs, poisoning by—*see* Poisoning, food, noxious, plants NEC
- • substances transmitted through placenta or breast milk P04.9

Nursemaid's elbow S53.03-

Nutrition deficient or insufficient (*see also* Malnutrition) E46
- • due to
  - − insufficient food T73.0
  - − lack of
    - ■ care (child) T76.02
    - ■ food T73.0

Nycturia R35.1
- • psychogenic F45.8

Nystagmus H55.00
- • benign paroxysmal—*see* Vertigo, benign paroxysmal
- • central positional H81.4
- • congenital H55.01
- • dissociated H55.04
- • latent H55.02
- • miners' H55.09
- • positional
  - − benign paroxysmal H81.4
    - ■ central H81.4
- • specified form NEC H55.09
- • visual deprivation H55.03

O

Obesity E66.9
- • with alveolar hypoventilation E66.2
- • constitutional E66.8
- • dietary counseling and surveillance Z71.3
- • drug-induced E66.1
- • due to
  - − drug E66.1
  - − excess calories E66.09
    - ■ morbid E66.01
    - ■ severe E66.01
- • endocrine E66.8
- • endogenous E66.8
- • familial E66.8
- • glandular E66.8
- • hypothyroid—*see* Hypothyroidism
- • morbid E66.01
  - − with alveolar hypoventilation E66.2
  - − due to excess calories E66.01
  - − with obesity hypoventilation syndrome (OHS) E66.2
- • nutritional E66.09
- • pituitary E23.6
- • severe E66.01
- • specified type NEC E66.8

Observation (following) (for) (without need for further medical care) Z04.9
- • accident NEC Z04.3
  - − at work Z04.2
  - − transport Z04.1
- • adverse effect of drug Z03.6
- • alleged rape or sexual assault (victim), ruled out
  - − child Z04.42
- • criminal assault Z04.89
- • development state
  - − adolescent Z00.3
  - − period of rapid growth in childhood Z00.2
  - − puberty Z00.3
- • disease, specified NEC Z03.89
- • following work accident Z04.2
- • forced labor exploitation Z04.82
- • forced sexual exploitation Z04.81
- • newborn (for suspected condition, ruled out)—*see* Newborn, affected by (suspected to be), maternal (complication of) (use of)
- • suicide attempt, alleged NEC Z03.89
  - − self-poisoning Z03.6
- • suspected, ruled out—*see also* Suspected condition
  - − abuse, physical
    - ■ child Z04.72
  - − accident at work Z04.2
  - − child battering victim Z04.72
  - − condition NEC Z03.89
  - − drug poisoning or adverse effect Z03.6
  - − exposure (to)
    - ■ anthrax Z03.810
    - ■ biological agent NEC Z03.818
  - − foreign body
    - ■ aspirated (inhaled) Z03.822
    - ■ ingested Z03.821
    - ■ inserted (injected), in (eye) (orifice) (skin) Z03.823
  - − inflicted injury NEC Z04.89
  - − newborn, ruled-out
    - ■ cardiac condition Z05.0
    - ■ connective tissue condition Z05.73
    - ■ gastrointestinal condition Z05.5
    - ■ genetic condition Z05.41
    - ■ genitourinary condition Z05.6
    - ■ immunologic condition Z05.43
    - ■ infectious condition Z05.1
    - ■ metabolic condition Z05.42
    - ■ musculoskeletal condition Z05.72
    - ■ neurological condition Z05.2
    - ■ other condition Z05.8
    - ■ respiratory condition Z05.3
    - ■ skin and subcutaneous tissue condition Z05.71
    - ■ unspecified suspected condition Z05.9
  - − suicide attempt, alleged Z03.89
    - ■ self-poisoning Z03.6
  - − toxic effects from ingested substance (drug) (poison) Z03.6
- • toxic effects from ingested substance (drug) (poison) Z03.6

Obsession, obsessional state F42

Obsessive-compulsive neurosis or reaction F42.8
- • mixed thoughts and acts F42.2

Obstruction, obstructed, obstructive
- • airway J98.8
  - − with
    - ■ asthma J45.909
      - ~ with
        - ◊ exacerbation (acute) J45.901
        - ◊ status asthmaticus J45.902
- • aqueduct of Sylvius G91.1
  - − congenital Q03.0
    - ■ with spina bifida—*see* Spina bifida, by site, with hydrocephalus
- • artery (*see also* Embolism, artery) I74.9
- • bile duct or passage (common) (hepatic) (noncalculous) K83.1
  - − with calculus K80.51
  - − congenital (causing jaundice) Q44.3
- • bladder-neck (acquired) N32.0
  - − congenital Q64.31
- • cystic duct—*see also* Obstruction, gallbladder
  - − with calculus K80.21

Obstruction, obstructed, obstructive, *continued*
- device, implant or graft (*see also* Complications, by site and type, mechanical) T85.698
  - catheter NEC T85.628
    - cystostomy T83.090
    - Hopkins T83.098
    - ileostomy T83.098
    - nephrostomy T83.092
    - urethral indwelling T83.091
    - urinary T83.098
    - urostomy T83.098
  - ventricular intracranial shunt T85.09
- fecal K56.41
  - with hernia—*see* Hernia, by site, with obstruction
- foramen of Monro (congenital) Q03.8
  - with spina bifida—*see* Spina bifida, by site, with hydrocephalus
- foreign body—*see* Foreign body
- gallbladder K82.0
  - with calculus, stones K80.21
  - congenital Q44.1
- intestine K56.609
  - adynamic K56.0
  - complete K56.601
  - congenital (small) Q41.9
    - large Q42.9
      ~ specified part NEC Q42.8
  - incomplete K56.600
  - neurogenic K56.0
    - Hirschsprung's disease or megacolon Q43.1
  - newborn P76.9
    - due to
      ~ fecaliths P76.8
      ~ inspissated milk P76.2
      ~ meconium (plug) P76.0
        ◊ in mucoviscidosis E84.11
    - specified NEC P76.8
  - partial K56.600
  - reflex K56.0
  - specified NEC K56.699
    - complete K56.691
    - incomplete K56.690
    - partial K56.690
  - volvulus K56.2
- lacrimal (passages) (duct)
  - by
    - stenosis—*see* Stenosis, lacrimal
  - congenital Q10.5
  - neonatal H04.53-
- lacrimonasal duct—*see* Obstruction, lacrimal
- meconium (plug)
  - newborn P76.0
    - due to fecaliths P76.0
    - in mucoviscidosis E84.11
- nasal J34.89
- nasolacrimal duct—*see also* Obstruction, lacrimal
  - congenital Q10.5
- nose J34.89
- portal (circulation) (vein) I81
- pulmonary valve (heart) I37.0
- pylorus
  - congenital or infantile Q40.0
- rectum K62.4
- renal N28.89
  - outflow N13.8
  - pelvis, congenital Q62.39
- sinus (accessory) (nasal) J34.89
- stomach NEC K31.89
  - congenital Q40.2
  - due to pylorospasm K31.3
- ureter (functional) (pelvic junction) NEC N13.5
  - with
    - hydronephrosis N13.0
- urinary (moderate) N13.9
  - organ or tract (lower) N13.9
  - specified NEC N13.8
- uropathy N13.9
- vagina N89.5
- vesical NEC N32.0
- vesicourethral orifice N32.0
  - congenital Q64.31

Occlusion, occluded
- anus K62.4
  - congenital Q42.3
    - with fistula Q42.2
- aqueduct of Sylvius G91.1
  - congenital Q03.0
    - with spina bifida—*see* Spina bifida, by site, with hydrocephalus
- artery (*see also* Embolism, artery) I70.9
- choanal Q30.0
- fallopian tube N97.1
  - congenital Q50.6
- gallbladder—*see also* Obstruction, gallbladder
  - congenital (causing jaundice) Q44.1
- hymen N89.6
  - congenital Q52.3
- nose J34.89
  - congenital Q30.0
- oviduct N97.1
  - congenital Q50.6
- posterior lingual, of mandibular teeth M26.29
- teeth (mandibular) (posterior lingual) M26.29
- ureter (complete) (partial) N13.5
  - congenital Q62.10
- ureteropelvic junction N13.5
  - congenital Q62.11
- ureterovesical orifice N13.5
  - congenital Q62.12
- vagina N89.5
- ventricle (brain) NEC G91.1

Occult
- blood in feces (stools) R19.5

Oculogyric crisis or disturbance H51.8
- psychogenic F45.8

Odontoclasia K03.89

Oligoastrocytoma
- specified site—*see* Neoplasm, malignant, by site in Table of Neoplasms in the complete *ICD-10-CM* manual
- unspecified site C71.9

Oligocythemia D64.9

Oligodendroblastoma
- specified site—*see* Neoplasm, malignant in Table of Neoplasms in the complete *ICD-10-CM* manual
- unspecified site C71.9

Oligodendroglioma
- anaplastic type
  - specified site—*see* Neoplasm, malignant, by site in Table of Neoplasms in the complete *ICD-10-CM* manual
  - unspecified site C71.9
- specified site—*see* Neoplasm, malignant, by site in Table of Neoplasms in the complete *ICD-10-CM* manual
- unspecified site C71.9

Oligodontia—*see* Anodontia

Oligoencephalon Q02

Oligohydramnios O41.0-

Oligophrenia—*see also* Disability, intellectual
- phenylpyruvic E70.0

Oliguria R34
- postprocedural N99.0

Omphalitis (congenital) (newborn) P38.9
- with mild hemorrhage P38.1
- without hemorrhage P38.9

Omphalocele Q79.2

Omphalomesenteric duct, persistent Q43.0

Omphalorrhagia, newborn P51.9

Onanism (excessive) F98.8

Onychia—*see also* Cellulitis
- with lymphangitis—*see* Lymphangitis, acute
- candidal B37.2
- dermatophytic B35.1

Onychocryptosis L60.0

Onycholysis L60.1

Onychomadesis L60.8

Onychomycosis (finger) (toe) B35.1

Onychophagia F98.8

Onychophosis L60.8

Onychoptosis L60.8

Onyxis (finger) (toe) L60.0

Oophoritis (cystic) (infectional) (interstitial) N70.92
- with salpingitis N70.93

Ophthalmia (*see also* Conjunctivitis) H10.9
- blennorrhagic (gonococcal) (neonatorum) A54.31
- gonococcal (neonatorum) A54.31
- neonatorum, newborn P39.1
  - gonococcal A54.31

Orchitis (gangrenous) (nonspecific) (septic) (suppurative) N45.2
- blennorrhagic (gonococcal) (acute) (chronic) A54.23
- chlamydial A56.19
- gonococcal (acute) (chronic) A54.23
- mumps B26.0
- syphilitic A52.76

Orotaciduria, oroticaciduria (congenital) (hereditary) (pyrimidine deficiency) E79.8
- anemia D53.0

Orthopnea R06.01

Osgood-Schlatter disease or osteochondrosis M92.52-

Osler (-Weber)-Rendu disease I78.0

Osler's nodes I33.0

Ossification
- diaphragm J98.6
- falx cerebri G96.198
- meninges (cerebral) (spinal) G96.198

Osteitis—*see also* Osteomyelitis
- deformans M88.9
- fragilitans Q78.0
  - in (due to)
    - malignant neoplasm of bone C41.9
    - neoplastic disease (*see also* Table of Neoplasms in the complete *ICD-10-CM* manual) D49.9
      ~ carpus D49.9
      ~ clavicle D49.9
      ~ femur D49.9
      ~ fibula D49.9
      ~ finger D49.9
      ~ humerus D49.9
      ~ ilium D49.9
      ~ ischium D49.9
      ~ metacarpus D49.9
      ~ metatarsus D49.9
      ~ multiple sites D49.9
      ~ neck D49.9
      ~ radius D49.9
      ~ rib D49.9
      ~ scapula D49.9
      ~ skull D49.9
      ~ tarsus D49.9
      ~ tibia D49.9
      ~ toe D49.9
      ~ ulna D49.9
      ~ vertebra D49.9
  - skull M88.0
  - specified NEC—*see* Paget's disease, bone, by site
  - vertebra M88.1
- tuberculosa A18.09
  - cystica D86.89
  - multiplex cystoides D86.89

Osteochondritis—*see also* Osteochondropathy
- juvenile M92.9
  - patellar M92.4-

Osteochondrodysplasia Q78.9
- with defects of growth of tubular bones and spine Q77.9
- specified NEC Q78.8

Osteochondropathy M93.9-
- slipped upper femoral epiphysis—*see* Slipped, epiphysis, upper femoral

Osteochondrosis—*see also* Osteochondropathy
- acetabulum (juvenile) M91.0
- astragalus (juvenile) M92.6-
- Blount's M92.51-
- Buchanan's M91.0
- Burns' M92.1-
- calcaneus (juvenile) M92.6-
- capitular epiphysis (femur) (juvenile) M91.1-
- carpal (juvenile) (lunate) (scaphoid) M92.21-

Osteochondrosis, *continued*
- coxae juvenilis M91.1-
- deformans juvenilis, coxae M91.1-
- Diaz's M92.6-
- femoral capital epiphysis (juvenile) M91.1-
- femur (head), juvenile M91.1-
- fibula (juvenile) M92.5-
- foot NEC (juvenile) M92.8
- Freiberg's M92.7-
- Haas' (juvenile) M92.0-
- Haglund's M92.6-
- hip (juvenile) M91.1-
- humerus (capitulum) (head) (juvenile) M92.0-
- ilium, iliac crest (juvenile) M91.0
- ischiopubic synchondrosis M91.0
- Iselin's M92.7-
- juvenile, juvenilis M92.9
  - after congenital dislocation of hip reduction M91.8-
  - arm M92.3-
  - capitular epiphysis (femur) M91.1-
  - clavicle, sternal epiphysis M92.3-
  - coxae M91.1-
  - deformans M92.9
  - fibula M92.50-
  - foot NEC M92.8
  - hand M92.20-
    - carpal lunate M92.21-
    - metacarpal head M92.22-
    - specified site NEC M92.29-
  - head of femur M91.1-
  - hip and pelvis M91.9-
    - femoral head M91.1-
    - pelvis M91.0
    - specified NEC M91.8-
  - humerus M92.0-
  - limb
    - lower NEC M92.8
    - upper NEC M92.3-
  - medial cuneiform bone M92.6-
  - metatarsus M92.7-
  - patella M92.4-
  - radius M92.1-
  - specified site NEC M92.8
  - tarsus M92.6-
  - tibia M92.50-
  - proximal M92.51-
  - tubercle M92.52
  - ulna M92.1-
  - upper limb NEC M92.3-
- Kienböck's M92.21-
- Köhler's
  - patellar M92.4-
  - tarsal navicular M92.6-
- Legg-Perthes (-Calvé) (-Waldenström) M91.1-
- limb
  - lower NEC (juvenile) M92.8
  - tibia and fibula M92.59-
  - upper NEC (juvenile) M92.3-
- lunate bone (carpal) (juvenile) M92.21-
- Mauclaire's M92.22-
- metacarpal (head) (juvenile) M92.22-
- metatarsus (fifth) (head) (juvenile) (second) M92.7-
- navicular (juvenile) M92.6-
- os
  - calcis (juvenile) M92.6-
  - tibiale externum (juvenile) M92.6-
- Osgood-Schlatter M92.52-
- Panner's M92.0-
- patellar center (juvenile) (primary) (secondary) M92.4-
- pelvis (juvenile) M91.0
- Pierson's M91.0
- radius (head) (juvenile) M92.1-
- Sever's M92.6-
- Sinding-Larsen M92.4-
- symphysis pubis (juvenile) M91.0
- talus (juvenile) M92.6-
- tarsus (navicular) (juvenile) M92.6-
- tibia (proximal) (tubercle) (juvenile) M92.5-
- ulna (lower) (juvenile) M92.1-
- van Neck's M91.0

Osteogenesis imperfecta Q78.0

Osteomyelitis (general) (infective) (localized) (neonatal) (purulent) (septic) (staphylococcal) (streptococcal) (suppurative) (with periostitis) M86.9
- acute M86.10
  - carpus M86.14-
  - clavicle M86.11-
  - femur M86.15-
  - fibula M86.16-
  - finger M86.14-
  - humerus M86.12-
  - ilium M86.18
  - ischium M86.18
  - metacarpus M86.14-
  - metatarsus M86.17-
  - multiple sites M86.19
  - neck M86.18
  - radius M86.13-
  - rib M86.18
  - scapula M86.11-
  - skull M86.18
  - tarsus M86.17-
  - tibia M86.16-
  - toe M86.17-
  - ulna M86.13-

Osteonecrosis M87.9
- secondary
  - due to
    - hemoglobinopathy NEC D58.2 [M90.50]
      ~ carpus D58.2 [M90.54-]
      ~ clavicle D58.2 [M90.51-]
      ~ femur D58.2 [M90.55-]
      ~ fibula D58.2 [M90.56-]
      ~ finger D58.2 [M90.54-]
      ~ humerus D58.2 [M90.52-]
      ~ ilium D58.2 [M90.55-]
      ~ ischium D58.2 [M90.55-]
      ~ metacarpus D58.2 [M90.54-]
      ~ metatarsus D58.2 [M90.57-]
      ~ multiple sites D58.2 [M90.58]
      ~ neck D58.2 [M90.58]
      ~ radius D58.2 [M90.53-]
      ~ rib D58.2 [M90.58]
      ~ scapula D58.2 [M90.51-]
      ~ skull D58.2 [M90.58]
      ~ tarsus D58.2 [M90.57-]
      ~ tibia D58.2 [M90.56-]
      ~ toe D58.2 [M90.57-]
      ~ ulna D58.2 [M90.53-]
      ~ vertebra D58.2 [M90.58]

Osteophyte M25.70
- ankle M25.77-
- elbow M25.72-
- foot joint M25.77-
- hand joint M25.74-
- hip M25.75-
- knee M25.76-
- shoulder M25.71-
- spine M25.78
- vertebrae M25.78
- wrist M25.73-

Osteopsathyrosis (idiopathica) Q78.0

Osteosclerosis Q78.2
- acquired M85.8-
- congenita Q77.4
- fragilitas (generalisata) Q78.2
- myelofibrosis D75.81

Osteosis
- cutis L94.2

Ostium
- atrioventriculare commune Q21.2
- primum (arteriosum) (defect) (persistent) Q21.2
- secundum (arteriosum) (defect) (patent) (persistent) Q21.1

Ostrum-Furst syndrome Q75.8

Otalgia—*see* subcategory H92.0

Otitis (acute) H66.9-
- with effusion—*see also* Otitis, media, nonsuppurative
  - purulent—*see* Otitis, media
- chronic—*see also* Otitis, media, chronic
  - with effusion—*see also* Otitis, media, nonsuppurative

Otitis, *continued*
- externa H60.9-
  - abscess—*see also* Abscess, ear, external
  - acute (noninfective) H60.50-
    - infective—*see* Otitis, externa, infective
  - cellulitis—*see* Cellulitis, ear
  - in (due to)
    - aspergillosis B44.89
    - candidiasis B37.84
    - erysipelas A46 [H62.4-]
    - herpes (simplex) virus infection B00.1
    - impetigo L01.00 [H62.4-]
    - infectious disease NEC B99 [H62.4-]
    - mycosis NEC B36.9 [H62.4-]
    - parasitic disease NEC B89 [H62.4-]
    - viral disease NEC B34.9 [H62.4-]
  - infective NEC H60.39-
    - abscess—*see* Abscess, ear, external
    - cellulitis—*see* Cellulitis, ear
    - swimmer's ear H60.33-
  - mycotic NEC B36.9 [H62.4-]
    - in
      ~ aspergillosis B44.89
      ~ candidiasis B37.84
      ~ moniliasis B37.84
  - specified NEC—*see* subcategory H60.8-
  - tropical NEC B36.8
    - in
      ~ aspergillosis B44.89
      ~ candidiasis B37.84
      ~ moniliasis B37.84
- interna—*see* subcategory H83.0
- media (hemorrhagic) (staphylococcal) (streptococcal) H66.9-
  - with effusion (nonpurulent)—*see* Otitis, media, nonsuppurative
  - acute, subacute H66.9-
    - allergic—*see* Otitis, media, nonsuppurative, acute or subacute NEC allergic
    - exudative—*see* Otitis, media, nonsuppurative, acute or subacute NEC allergic
    - mucoid—*see* Otitis, media, nonsuppurative, acute or subacute NEC allergic
    - necrotizing—*see also* Otitis, media, suppurative, acute
      ~ in
        ◊ measles B05.3
        ◊ scarlet fever A38.0
    - nonsuppurative NEC—*see* Otitis, media, nonsuppurative, acute or subacute NEC allergic
    - purulent—*see* Otitis, media, suppurative, acute
    - sanguinous—*see* Otitis, media, nonsuppurative, acute or subacute NEC allergic
    - secretory—*see* Otitis, media, nonsuppurative, acute or subacute NEC allergic, serous
    - seromucinous—*see* Otitis, media, nonsuppurative, acute or subacute NEC allergic
    - serous—*see* Otitis, media, nonsuppurative, acute or subacute NEC allergic, serous
    - suppurative—*see* Otitis, media, suppurative, acute
  - allergic—*see* Otitis, media, nonsuppurative
  - catarrhal—*see* Otitis, media, nonsuppurative
  - chronic H66.9-
    - with effusion (nonpurulent)—*see* Otitis, media, nonsuppurative, chronic
    - allergic—*see* Otitis, media, nonsuppurative, chronic, allergic
    - benign suppurative—*see* Otitis, media, suppurative, chronic
    - catarrhal—*see* Otitis, media, nonsuppurative, chronic, serous
    - exudative—*see* Otitis, media, suppurative, chronic
    - mucinous—*see* Otitis, media, nonsuppurative, chronic, mucoid
    - mucoid—*see* Otitis, media, nonsuppurative, chronic, mucoid
    - nonsuppurative NEC—*see* Otitis, media, nonsuppurative, chronic
    - purulent—*see* Otitis, media, suppurative, chronic
    - secretory—*see* Otitis, media, nonsuppurative, chronic, mucoid
    - seromucinous—*see* Otitis, media, nonsuppurative, chronic

Otitis, *continued*
- ■ serous—*see* Otitis, media, nonsuppurative, chronic, serous
- ■ suppurative—*see* Otitis, media, suppurative, chronic
- ■ transudative—*see* Otitis, media, nonsuppurative, chronic, mucoid
- – exudative—*see* Otitis, media, suppurative
- – in (due to) (with)
  - ■ influenza—*see* Influenza, with, otitis media
  - ■ measles B05.3
  - ■ scarlet fever A38.0
  - ■ tuberculosis A18.6
  - ■ viral disease NEC B34.- *[H67.-]*
- – mucoid—*see* Otitis, media, nonsuppurative
- – nonsuppurative H65.9-
  - ■ acute or subacute NEC allergic H65.11- (6th characters 1—3, 9)
    - ~ recurrent H65.11- (6th characters 4—7)
    - ~ secretory—*see* Otitis, media, nonsuppurative, serous
    - ~ serous H65.0- (6th characters 0—3)
      - ◊ recurrent H65.0- (6th characters 4—7)
  - ■ chronic H65.49-
    - ~ allergic H65.41-
    - ~ mucoid H65.3-
    - ~ serous H65.2-
- – postmeasles B05.3
- – purulent—*see* Otitis, media, suppurative
- – secretory—*see* Otitis, media, nonsuppurative
- – seromucinous—*see* Otitis, media, nonsuppurative
- – serous—*see* Otitis, media, nonsuppurative
- – suppurative H66.4-
  - ■ acute H66.00- (6th characters 1 – 3, 9)
    - ~ with rupture of ear drum H66.01- (6th characters 1 – 3, 9)
    - ~ recurrent H66.00- (6th characters 4 – 7)
      - ◊ with rupture of ear drum H66.01- (6th characters 4 – 7)
  - ■ chronic (*see also* subcategory) H66.3
    - ~ atticoantral H66.2-
    - ~ tubotympanic (benign) H66.1-
- – transudative—*see* Otitis, media, nonsuppurative
- – tuberculous A18.6

Otomycosis (diffuse) NEC B36.9 [H62.4-]
- ● in
  - – aspergillosis B44.89
  - – candidiasis B37.84
  - – moniliasis B37.84

Otorrhea H92.1-
- ● cerebrospinal (fluid) G96.01
  - – postoperative G96.08
  - – specified NEC G96.08
  - – spontaneous G96.01
  - – traumatic G96.08

Ovary, ovarian—*see also* Disease, diseased
- ● vein syndrome N13.8

Overactive—*see also* Hyperfunction
- ● bladder N32.81
- ● hypothalamus E23.3

Overactivity R46.3
- ● child—*see* Disorder, attention-deficit hyperactivity

Overbite (deep) (excessive) (horizontal) (vertical) M26.29

Overconscientious personality F60.5

Overeating R63.2
- ● nonorganic origin F50.89
- ● psychogenic F50.89

Overlapping toe (acquired)—*see also* Deformity, toe
- ● congenital (fifth toe) Q66.89

Overload
- ● circulatory, due to transfusion (blood) (blood components) (TACO) E87.71
- ● fluid E87.70
  - – due to transfusion (blood) (blood components) E87.71
  - – specified NEC E87.79
- ● iron, due to repeated red blood cell transfusions E83.111
- ● potassium (K) E87.5
- ● sodium (Na) E87.0

Overnutrition—*see* Hyperalimentation

Overproduction—*see also* Hypersecretion
- ● growth hormone E22.0

Overriding
- ● toe (acquired)—*see also* Deformity, toe
  - – congenital Q66.89

Overstrained R53.83

Overweight E66.3

Overworked R53.83

Ovulation (cycle)
- ● failure or lack of N97.0
- ● pain N94.0

Oxyuriasis B80

Oxyuris vermicularis (infestation) B80

Ozena J31.0

P

Pachydermatocele (congenital) Q82.8

Paget's disease
- ● bone M88.9
  - – carpus M88.84-
  - – clavicle M88.81-
  - – femur M88.85-
  - – fibula M88.86-
  - – finger M88.84-
  - – humerus M88.82-
  - – ilium M88.85-
  - – in neoplastic disease D49.9 *[M90.6-]*
  - – ischium M88.85-
  - – metacarpus M88.84-
  - – metatarsus M88.87-
  - – multiple sites M88.89
  - – neck M88.88
  - – radius M88.83-
  - – rib M88.88
  - – scapula M88.81-
  - – skull M88.0
  - – specified NEC M88.88
  - – tarsus M88.87-
  - – tibia M88.86-
  - – toe M88.87-
  - – ulna M88.83-
  - – vertebra M88.1
- ● osteitis deformans—*see* Paget's disease, bone

Pain(s) (*see also* Painful) R52
- ● abdominal R10.9
  - – colic R10.83
  - – generalized R10.84
    - ■ with acute abdomen R10.0
  - – lower R10.30
    - ■ left quadrant R10.32
    - ■ pelvic or perineal R10.2
    - ■ periumbilical R10.33
    - ■ right quadrant R10.31
  - – rebound—*see* Tenderness, abdominal, rebound
  - – severe with abdominal rigidity R10.0
  - – tenderness—*see* Tenderness, abdominal
  - – upper R10.10
    - ■ epigastric R10.13
    - ■ left quadrant R10.12
    - ■ right quadrant R10.11
- ● acute R52
  - – due to trauma G89.11
  - – neoplasm related G89.3
  - – postprocedural NEC G89.18
- ● adnexa (uteri) R10.2
- ● anus K62.89
- ● axillary (axilla) M79.62-
- ● back (postural) M54.9
- ● bladder R39.89
  - – associated with micturition—*see* Micturition, painful
  - – chronic R39.82
- ● breast N64.4
- ● broad ligament R10.2
- ● cancer associated (acute) (chronic) G89.3
- ● chest (central) R07.9
- ● chronic G89.29
  - – neoplasm related G89.3
- ● coccyx M53.3
- ● due to cancer G89.3
- ● due to malignancy (primary) (secondary) G89.3

Pain, *continued*
- ● ear—*see* subcategory H92.0
- ● epigastric, epigastrium R10.13
- ● face, facial R51.9
- ● female genital organs NEC N94.89
- ● gastric—*see* Pain, abdominal
- ● generalized NOS R52
- ● genital organ
  - – female N94.89
  - – male
    - ■ scrotal N50.82
    - ■ testicular N50.81-
- ● groin—*see* Pain, abdominal, lower
- ● hand M79.64-
  - – joints M25.54-
- ● head—*see* Headache
- ● intermenstrual N94.0
- ● jaw R68.84
- ● joint M25.50
  - – ankle M25.57-
  - – elbow M25.52-
  - – finger M25.54-
  - – foot M25.57-
  - – hand M79.64-
  - – hip M25.55-
  - – knee M25.56-
  - – shoulder M25.51-
  - – specified site NEC M25.59
  - – toe M25.57-
  - – wrist M25.53-
- ● kidney N23
- ● laryngeal R07.0
- ● limb M79.60-
  - – lower M79.60-
    - ■ foot M79.67-
    - ■ lower leg M79.66-
    - ■ thigh M79.65-
    - ■ toe M79.67-
  - – upper M79.60-
    - ■ axilla M79.62-
    - ■ finger M79.64-
    - ■ forearm M79.63-
    - ■ hand M79.64-
    - ■ upper arm M79.62-
- ● mandibular R68.84
- ● mastoid—*see* subcategory H92.0
- ● maxilla R68.84
- ● menstrual (*see also* Dysmenorrhea) N94.6
- ● mouth K13.79
- ● muscle—*see* Myalgia
- ● musculoskeletal (*see also* Pain, by site) M79.18
- ● myofascial M79.18
- ● nasal J34.89
- ● nasopharynx J39.2
- ● neck NEC M54.2
- ● nose J34.89
- ● ocular H57.1-
- ● ophthalmic H57.1-
- ● orbital region H57.1-
- ● ovary N94.89
- ● ovulation N94.0
- ● pelvic (female) R10.2
- ● perineal, perineum R10.2
- ● postoperative NOS G89.18
- ● postprocedural NOS G89.18
- ● premenstrual F32.81
- ● psychogenic (persistent) (any site) F45.41
- ● rectum K62.89
- ● round ligament (stretch) R10.2
- ● sacroiliac M53.3
- ● scrotal N50.82
- ● shoulder M25.51-
- ● spine M54.9
  - – cervical M54.2
  - – low back M54.5
    - ■ with sciatica M54.4-
- ● temporomandibular (joint) M26.62-
- ● testicular N50.81-
- ● throat R07.0
- ● tibia M79.66-
- ● toe M79.67-
- ● tumor associated G89.3
- ● ureter N23

Pain, *continued*
- urinary (organ) (system) N23
- uterus NEC N94.89
- vagina R10.2
- vesical R39.89
  - associated with micturition—*see* Micturition, painful
- vulva R10.2

Painful—*see also* Pain
- menstruation—*see* Dysmenorrhea
  - psychogenic F45.8
- micturition—*see* Micturition, painful
- scar NEC L90.5
- wire sutures T81.89

Painter's colic—*see* subcategory T56.0

Palate—*see* Disease, diseased

Palatoplegia K13.79

Palatoschisis—*see* Cleft, palate

Palliative care Z51.5

Pallor R23.1

Palpitations (heart) R00.2
- psychogenic F45.8

Palsy (*see also* Paralysis) G83.9
- Bell's—*see also* Palsy, facial
  - newborn P11.3
- brachial plexus NEC G54.0
  - newborn (birth injury) P14.3
- cerebral (congenital) G80.9
- cranial nerve—*see also* Disorder, nerve, cranial
  - multiple G52.7
    - in
      - ~ neoplastic disease (*see also* Table of Neoplasms in the complete *ICD-10-CM* manual) D49.9 [G53]
      - ~ sarcoidosis D86.82
- Erb's P14.0
- facial G51.0
  - newborn (birth injury) P11.3
- Klumpke (-Déjérine) P14.1
- lead—*see* subcategory T56.0
- seventh nerve—*see also* Palsy, facial
  - newborn P11.3

Pancake heart R93.1
- with cor pulmonale (chronic) I27.81

Pancarditis (acute) (chronic) I51.89
- rheumatic I09.89
  - active or acute I01.8

Pancolitis, ulcerative (chronic) K51.00
- with
  - abscess K51.014
  - complication K51.019
  - fistula K51.013
  - obstruction K51.012
  - rectal bleeding K51.011
  - specified complication NEC K51.018

Pancreatitis (annular) (apoplectic) (calcareous) (edematous) (hemorrhagic) (malignant) (subacute) (suppurative) K85.90
- acute K85.90
- idiopathic K85.00
  - with infected necrosis K85.02
  - with uninfected necrosis K85.01
  - with infected necrosis K85.92
  - with uninfected necrosis K85.91

Pancytopenia (acquired) D61.818
- with
  - malformations D61.09
  - myelodysplastic syndrome—*see* Syndrome, myelodysplastic
- antineoplastic chemotherapy induced D61.810
- congenital D61.09
- drug-induced NEC D61.811

PANDAS (pediatric autoimmune neuropsychiatric disorders associated with streptococcal infections syndrome) D89.89

Panhematopenia D61.9
- congenital D61.09
- constitutional D61.09

Panhemocytopenia D61.9
- congenital D61.09
- constitutional D61.09

Panhypopituitarism E23.0
- prepubertal E23.0

Panic (attack) (state) F41.0
- reaction to exceptional stress (transient) F43.0

Panmyelopathy, familial, constitutional D61.09

Panmyelophthisis D61.82
- congenital D61.09

Pansinusitis (chronic) (hyperplastic) (nonpurulent) (purulent) J32.4
- acute J01.40
  - recurrent J01.41

Papanicolaou smear, cervix Z12.4
- as part of routine gynecological examination Z01.419
  - with abnormal findings Z01.411
- for suspected neoplasm Z12.4
- routine Z01.419
  - with abnormal findings Z01.411

Papilledema (choked disc) H47.10
- associated with
  - decreased ocular pressure H47.12
  - increased intracranial pressure H47.11
  - retinal disorder H47.13

Papillitis
- anus K62.89
- necrotizing, kidney N17.2
- renal, necrotizing N17.2
- tongue K14.0

Papilloma—*see also* Neoplasm, benign, by site in Table of Neoplasms in the complete *ICD-10-CM* manual
- acuminatum (female) (male) (anogenital) A63.0
- choroid plexus (lateral ventricle) (third ventricle)
  - anaplastic C71.5
  - malignant C71.5
- rectum K62.89

Papillomatosis—*see also* Neoplasm, benign, by site in Table of Neoplasms in the complete *ICD-10-CM* manual
- confluent and reticulated L83

Papillon-Léage and Psaume syndrome Q87.0

Para-albuminemia E88.09

Paracephalus Q89.7

Parageusia R43.2
- psychogenic F45.8

Paralysis, paralytic (complete) (incomplete) G83.9
- anus (sphincter) K62.89
- asthenic bulbar G70.00
  - with exacerbation (acute) G70.01
  - in crisis G70.01
- Bell's G51.0
  - newborn P11.3
- bowel, colon or intestine K56.0
- brachial plexus G54.0
  - birth injury P14.3
  - newborn (birth injury) P14.3
- brain G83.9
- bulbospinal G70.00
  - with exacerbation (acute) G70.01
  - in crisis G70.01
- cardiac (*see also* Failure, heart) I50.9
- Clark's G80.9
- colon K56.0
- conjugate movement (gaze) (of eye) H51.0
  - cortical (nuclear) (supranuclear) H51.0
- deglutition R13.0
  - hysterical F44.4
- diaphragm (flaccid) J98.6
  - due to accidental dissection of phrenic nerve during procedure—*see* Puncture
- Duchenne's
  - birth injury P14.0
  - due to or associated with
    - muscular dystrophy G71.01
- due to intracranial or spinal birth injury—*see* Palsy, cerebral
- Erb (-Duchenne) (birth) (newborn) P14.0
- facial (nerve) G51.0
  - birth injury P11.3
  - congenital P11.3
  - following operation NEC—*see* Puncture, accidental complicating surgery

Paralysis, paralytic, *continued*
- newborn (birth injury) P11.3
- gait R26.1
- glottis J38.00
  - bilateral J38.02
  - unilateral J38.01
- Hoppe-Goldflam G70.00
  - with exacerbation (acute) G70.01
  - in crisis G70.01
- hysterical F44.4
- ileus K56.0
- infantile A80.30
- infective A80.-
- inferior nuclear G83.9
- intestine K56.0
- Klumpke (-Déjérine) (birth) (newborn) P14.1
- laryngeal nerve (recurrent) (superior) (unilateral) J38.00
  - bilateral J38.02
  - unilateral J38.01
- larynx J38.00
  - bilateral J38.02
  - unilateral J38.01
- lead—*see* subcategory T56.0
- left side—*see* Hemiplegia
- leg G83.1-
  - both—*see* Paraplegia
  - hysterical F44.4
  - psychogenic F44.4
- lip K13.0
- monoplegic—*see* Monoplegia
- motor G83.9
- muscle, muscular NEC G72.89
- nerve—*see also* Disorder, nerve
  - facial G51.0
    - birth injury P11.3
    - congenital P11.3
    - newborn (birth injury) P11.3
  - seventh or facial G51.0
    - newborn (birth injury) P11.3
- oculofacial, congenital (Moebius) Q87.0
- palate (soft) K13.79
- progressive, spinal G12.25
- pseudohypertrophic (muscle) G71.09
- psychogenic F44.4
- radicular NEC
  - upper limbs, newborn (birth injury) P14.3
- recurrent isolated sleep G47.53
- respiratory (muscle) (system) (tract) R06.81
  - center NEC G93.89
  - congenital P28.89
  - newborn P28.89
- right side—*see* Hemiplegia
- saturnine—*see* subcategory T56.0
- sleep, recurrent isolated G47.53
- spastic G83.9
  - cerebral G80.-
  - congenital (cerebral) G80.-
- spinal (cord) G83.9
- spinal progressive G12.25
  - pseudohypertrophic G71.02
- syndrome G83.9
- uveoparotitic D86.89
- uvula K13.79
- velum palate K13.79
- vocal cords J38.00
  - bilateral J38.02
  - unilateral J38.01

Paramenia N92.6

Paramyoclonus multiplex G25.3

Paranoid
- personality F60.0
- traits F60.0
- trends F60.0
- type, psychopathic personality F60.0

Paraphimosis (congenital) N47.2

Paraplegia (lower) G82.20
- complete G82.21
- functional (hysterical) F44.4
- hysterical F44.4
- incomplete G82.22
- psychogenic F44.4

Parasitic—*see also* Disease, diseased
- disease NEC B89
- stomatitis B37.0
- sycosis (beard) (scalp) B35.0

Parasitism B89
- intestinal B82.9
- skin B88.9
- specified—*see* Infestation

Parasomnia G47.50
- in conditions classified elsewhere G47.54
- nonorganic origin F51.8
- organic G47.50
- specified NEC G47.59

Paraspadias Q54.9

Paraspasmus facialis G51.8

Parasuicide (attempt)
- history of (personal) Z91.5
  - in family Z81.8

Paratrachoma A74.0

Parencephalitis—*see also* Encephalitis
- sequelae G09

Parent-child conflict—*see* Conflict, parent-child
- estrangement NEC Z62.890

Paresis—*see also* Paralysis
- bowel, colon or intestine K56.0
- pseudohypertrophic G71.09

Paronychia—*see also* Cellulitis
- with lymphangitis—*see* Lymphangitis, digit
- candidal (chronic) B37.2

Parorexia (psychogenic) F50.89

Parosmia R43.1
- psychogenic F45.8

Parry-Romberg syndrome G51.8

Particolored infant Q82.8

Parulis K04.7

Parvovirus, as the cause of disease classified elsewhere B97.6

Passage
- meconium (newborn) during delivery P03.82
- of sounds or bougies—*see* Attention to, artificial, opening

Passive—*see* Disease, diseased
- smoking Z77.22

Pasteurella septica A28.0

PAT (paroxysmal atrial tachycardia) I47.1

Patent—*see also* Imperfect, closure
- ductus arteriosus or Botallo's Q25.0
- foramen
  - botalli Q21.1
  - ovale Q21.1
- interauricular septum Q21.1
- interventricular septum Q21.0
- omphalomesenteric duct Q43.0
- ostium secundum Q21.1
- vitelline duct Q43.0

Pathologic, pathological—*see also* Disease, diseased
- asphyxia R09.01

Pattern, sleep-wake, irregular G47.23

Patulous—*see also* Imperfect, closure (congenital)
- alimentary tract Q45.8
  - lower Q43.8
  - upper Q40.8

Pause, sinoatrial I49.5

Pectenosis K62.4

Pectus
- carinatum (congenital) Q67.7
- excavatum (congenital) Q67.6
- recurvatum (congenital) Q67.6

Pediculosis (infestation) B85.2
- capitis (head-louse) (any site) B85.0
- corporis (body-louse) (any site) B85.1
- eyelid B85.0
- mixed (classifiable to more than one of the titles B85.0–B85.3) B85.4
- pubis (pubic louse) (any site) B85.3
- vestimenti B85.1
- vulvae B85.3

Pediculus (infestation)—*see* Pediculosis

Pelger-Huët anomaly or syndrome D72.0

Pelvic—*see also* Disease, diseased
- examination (periodic) (routine) Z01.419
  - with abnormal findings Z01.411
- kidney, congenital Q63.2

Pelviperitonitis—*see also* Peritonitis, pelvic
- gonococcal A54.24

Pemphigus
- benign familial (chronic) Q82.8

Pentosuria (essential) E74.89

Perforation, perforated (nontraumatic) (of)
- accidental during procedure (blood vessel) (nerve) (organ)— *see* Complication
- antrum—*see* Sinusitis, maxillary
- appendix K35.32
- atrial septum, multiple Q21.1
- by
  - device, implant or graft (*see also* Complications, by site and type, mechanical) T85.628
    - catheter NEC T85.698
      - ~ cystostomy T83.090
      - ~ urinary—*see also* Complications, catheter, urinary T83.098
    - ventricular intracranial shunt T85.09
  - instrument (any) during a procedure, accidental—*see* Puncture
- cecum K35.32
- ear drum—*see* Perforation, tympanum
- nasal
  - septum J34.89
    - congenital Q30.3
  - sinus J34.89
    - congenital Q30.8
    - due to sinusitis—*see* Sinusitis
- palate (*see also* Cleft, palate) Q35.9
- palatine vault (*see also* Cleft, palate, hard) Q35.1
- sinus (accessory) (chronic) (nasal) J34.89
- sphenoidal sinus—*see* Sinusitis, sphenoidal
- tympanum, tympanic (membrane) (persistent post-traumatic) (postinflammatory) H72.9-
  - attic H72.1-
    - multiple H72.81-
    - total H72.82-
  - central H72.0-
    - multiple H72.81-
    - total H72.82-
  - marginal NEC—*see* subcategory H72.2
  - multiple H72.81-
  - pars flaccida—*see* Perforation, tympanum, attic
  - total H72.82-
  - traumatic, current episode S09.2-
- uvula K13.79

Periadenitis mucosa necrotica recurrens K12.0

Pericarditis (with decompensation) (with effusion) I31.9
- with rheumatic fever (conditions in I00)
  - active—*see* Pericarditis, rheumatic
  - inactive or quiescent I09.2
- acute (hemorrhagic) (nonrheumatic) (Sicca) I30.9
  - with chorea (acute) (rheumatic) (Sydenham's) I02.0
  - benign I30.8
  - nonspecific I30.0
  - rheumatic I01.0
    - with chorea (acute) (Sydenham's) I02.0
- adhesive or adherent (chronic) (external) (internal) I31.0
  - acute—*see* Pericarditis, acute
  - rheumatic I09.2
- bacterial (acute) (subacute) (with serous or seropurulent effusion) I30.1
- calcareous I31.1
- cholesterol (chronic) I31.8
  - acute I30.9
- chronic (nonrheumatic) I31.9
  - rheumatic I09.2
- constrictive (chronic) I31.1
- coxsackie B33.23
- fibrinopurulent I30.1
- fibrinous I30.8
- fibrous I31.0
- idiopathic I30.0
- in systemic lupus erythematosus M32.12

Pericarditis, *continued*
- infective I30.1
- meningococcal A39.53
- neoplastic (chronic) I31.8
  - acute I30.9
- obliterans, obliterating I31.0
- plastic I31.0
- pneumococcal I30.1
- purulent I30.1
- rheumatic (active) (acute) (with effusion) (with pneumonia) I01.0
  - with chorea (acute) (rheumatic) (Sydenham's) I02.0
  - chronic or inactive (with chorea) I09.2
- septic I30.1
- serofibrinous I30.8
- staphylococcal I30.1
- streptococcal I30.1
- suppurative I30.1
- syphilitic A52.06
- tuberculous A18.84
- viral I30.1

Perichondritis
- auricle—*see* Perichondritis, ear
- bronchus J98.09
- ear (external) H61.00-
  - acute H61.01-
  - chronic H61.02-
- nose J34.89

Periepididymitis N45.1

Perilabyrinthitis (acute)—*see* subcategory H83.0

Periods—*see also* Menstruation
- heavy N92.0
- irregular N92.6
- shortened intervals (irregular) N92.1

Periorchitis N45.2

Periproctitis K62.89

Peritonitis (adhesive) (bacterial) (fibrinous) (hemorrhagic) (idiopathic) (localized) (perforative) (primary) (with adhesions) (with effusion) K65.9
- with or following
  - abscess K65.1
  - appendicitis
    - with perforation or rupture K35.32
    - generalized K35.20
    - localized K35.30
- acute (generalized) K65.0
- chlamydial A74.81
- diaphragmatic K65.0
- diffuse K65.0
- disseminated K65.0
- eosinophilic K65.8
  - acute K65.0
- fibropurulent K65.0
- general (ized) K65.0
- meconium (newborn) P78.0
- neonatal P78.1
  - meconium P78.0
- pancreatic K65.0
- pelvic
  - female N73.5
    - acute N73.3
    - chronic N73.4
      - ~ with adhesions N73.6
  - male K65.0
- purulent K65.0
- septic K65.0
- specified NEC K65.8
- spontaneous bacterial K65.2
- subdiaphragmatic K65.0
- subphrenic K65.0
- suppurative K65.0

Peritonsillitis J36

Perlèche NEC K13.0
- due to
  - candidiasis B37.83
  - moniliasis B37.83

Persistence, persistent (congenital)
- anal membrane Q42.3
  - with fistula Q42.2
- atrioventricular canal Q21.2

Persistence, persistent, *continued*
- branchial cleft NOS Q18.2
  - cyst Q18.0
  - fistula Q18.0
  - sinus Q18.0
- canal of Cloquet Q14.0
- capsule (opaque) Q12.8
- cilioretinal artery or vein Q14.8
- convolutions
  - aortic arch Q25.46
  - fallopian tube Q50.6
  - oviduct Q50.6
  - uterine tube Q50.6
- fetal
  - circulation P29.38
  - hemoglobin, hereditary (HPFH) D56.4
- foramen
  - Botalli Q21.1
  - ovale Q21.1
- hemoglobin, fetal (hereditary) (HPFH) D56.4
- Meckel's diverticulum Q43.0
- omphalomesenteric duct Q43.0
- ostium
  - atrioventriculare commune Q21.2
  - primum Q21.2
  - secundum Q21.1
- ovarian rests in fallopian tube Q50.6
- primary (deciduous)
  - teeth K00.6
- sinus
  - urogenitalis
    - female Q52.8
    - male Q55.8
- thyroglossal duct Q89.2
- thyrolingual duct Q89.2
- truncus arteriosus or communis Q20.0
- tunica vasculosa lentis Q12.2
- vitelline duct Q43.0

Person (with)
- concern (normal) about sick person in family Z63.6
- consulting on behalf of another Z71.0
- feigning illness Z76.5
- living (in)
  - without
    - adequate housing (heating) (space) Z59.1
    - housing (permanent) (temporary) Z59.0
    - person able to render necessary care Z74.2
    - shelter Z59.0

Personality (disorder) F60.9
- affective F34.0
- aggressive F60.3
- amoral F60.2
- anacastic, anankastic F60.5
- antisocial F60.2
- anxious F60.6
- asocial F60.2
- asthenic F60.7
- avoidant F60.6
- borderline F60.3
- compulsive F60.5
- cycloid F34.0
- cyclothymic F34.0
- depressive F34.1
- dissocial F60.2
- emotionally unstable F60.3
- expansive paranoid F60.0
- explosive F60.3
- fanatic F60.0
- histrionic F60.4
- hyperthymic F34.0
- hypothymic F34.1
- hysterical F60.4
- obsessional F60.5
- obsessive (-compulsive) F60.5
- organic F07.0
- overconscientious F60.5
- paranoid F60.0
- pathologic F60.9
- pattern defect or disturbance F60.9
- psychoinfantile F60.4
- psychopathic F60.2
- querulant F60.0

Personality, *continued*
- schizoid F60.1
- sensitive paranoid F60.0
- sociopathic (amoral) (antisocial) (asocial) (dissocial) F60.2
- specified NEC F60.89

Perthes' disease M91.1-

Pertussis (*see also* Whooping cough) A37.90

Perversion, perverted
- appetite F50.89
  - psychogenic F50.89
- function
  - pituitary gland E23.2
    - posterior lobe E22.2
- sense of smell and taste R43.8
  - psychogenic F45.8
- sexual—*see* Deviation, sexual transvestism

Pervious, congenital—*see also* Imperfect, closure
- ductus arteriosus Q25.0

Pes (congenital)—*see also* Talipes
- adductus Q66.89
- cavus Q66.7-
- valgus Q66.6

Petechia, petechiae R23.3
- newborn P54.5

Petit mal seizure—*see* Epilepsy, generalized, specified NEC

Petit's hernia—*see* Hernia
- Peutz-Jeghers disease or syndrome Q85.8

Pfeiffer's disease—*see* Mononucleosis, infectious

Phagedena (dry) (moist) (sloughing)—*see also* Gangrene
- geometric L88

Phakomatosis Q85.9
- Bourneville's Q85.1
- specified NEC Q85.8

Pharyngeal pouch syndrome D82.1

Pharyngitis (acute) (catarrhal) (gangrenous) (infective) (malignant) (membranous) (phlegmonous) (pseudomembranous) (simple) (subacute) (suppurative) (ulcerative) (viral) J02.9
- aphthous B08.5
- atrophic J31.2
- chlamydial A56.4
- chronic (atrophic) (granular) (hypertrophic) J31.2
- coxsackievirus B08.5
- enteroviral vesicular B08.5
- follicular (chronic) J31.2
- granular (chronic) J31.2
- herpesviral B00.2
- hypertrophic J31.2
- infectional, chronic J31.2
- influenzal—*see* Influenza, with, respiratory manifestations NEC
- pneumococcal J02.8
- purulent J02.9
- putrid J02.9
- septic J02.0
- sicca J31.2
- specified organism NEC J02.8
- staphylococcal J02.8
- streptococcal J02.0
- vesicular, enteroviral B08.5
- viral NEC J02.8

Pharyngolaryngitis (acute) J06.0
- chronic J37.0

Pharyngotonsillitis, herpesviral B00.2

Phenomenon
- vasomotor R55
- vasovagal R55
- Wenckebach's I44.1

Phenylketonuria E70.1
- classical E70.0

Phimosis (congenital) (due to infection) N47.1

Phlebitis (infective) (pyemic) (septic) (suppurative) I80.9
- calf muscular vein (NOS) I80.25-
- femoral vein (superficial) I80.1-
- femoropopliteal vein I80.0-
- gastrocnemial vein I80.25-
- hepatic veins I80.8
- iliac vein (common) (external) (internal) I80.21-
- iliofemoral—*see* Phlebitis, femoral vein

Phlebitis, *continued*
- leg I80.3
  - deep (vessels) NEC I80.20-
    - iliac I80.21-
    - popliteal vein I80.22-
    - specified vessel NEC I80.29-
    - tibial vein I80.23-
  - femoral vein (superficial) I80.1-
  - superficial (vessels) I80.0-
- lower limb—*see* Phlebitis, leg
- peroneal vein I80.24-
- popliteal vein—*see* Phlebitis, leg
- saphenous (accessory) (great) (long) (small)—*see* Phlebitis, leg
- soleal vein I80.25-
- specified site NEC I80.8
- tibial vein—*see* Phlebitis, leg
- ulcerative I80.9
  - leg—*see* Phlebitis, leg
- umbilicus I80.8

Phobia, phobic F40.9
- reaction F40.9
- state F40.9

Photodermatitis (sun) L56.8
- chronic L57.8
- due to drug L56.8

Photosensitivity, photosensitization (sun) skin L56.8

Phthiriasis (pubis) B85.3
- with any infestation classifiable to B85.0–B85.2 B85.4

Physical restraint status Z78.1

Pica F50.89
- in adults F50.89
- infant or child F98.3

Picking, nose F98.8

Pickwickian syndrome E66.2

Pierre Robin deformity or syndrome Q87.0

Pig-bel A05.2

Pigeon
- breast or chest (acquired) M95.4
  - congenital Q67.7

Pigmentation (abnormal) (anomaly) L81.9
- iron L81.8
- lids, congenital Q82.8
- metals L81.8
- optic papilla, congenital Q14.2
- retina, congenital (grouped) (nevoid) Q14.1
- scrotum, congenital Q82.8
- tattoo L81.8

Piles (*see also* Hemorrhoids) K64.9

Pinhole meatus (*see also* Stricture, urethra) N35.919

Pink
- eye—*see* Conjunctivitis, acute, mucopurulent

Pinworm (disease) (infection) (infestation) B80

Pithecoid pelvis Q74.2

Pitting (*see also* Edema) R60.9
- lip R60.0
- nail L60.8

Pityriasis (capitis) L21.0
- alba L30.5
- circinata (et maculata) L42
- furfuracea L21.0
- maculata (et circinata) L30.5
- rosea L42
- simplex L30.5
- specified type NEC L30.5
- streptogenes L30.5
- versicolor (scrotal) B36.0

Plagiocephaly
- aquired M95.2
- congenital Q67.3

Plaque(s)
- epicardial I31.8

Planning, family
- contraception Z30.9
- procreation Z31.69

Plasmacytopenia D72.818

Plasmacytosis D72.822

Platybasia Q75.8

Platyonychia (congenital) Q84.6
- acquired L60.8

Platypelloid pelvis M95.5
- congenital Q74.2

Plethora R23.2
- newborn P61.1

Pleurisy (acute) (adhesive) (chronic) (costal) (diaphragmatic) (double) (dry) (fibrinous) (fibrous) (interlobar) (latent) (plastic) (primary) (residual) (sicca) (sterile) (subacute) (unresolved) R09.1
- with
  - adherent pleura J86.0
  - effusion J90
- pneumococcal J90
- purulent—*see* Pyothorax
- septic—*see* Pyothorax
- serofibrinous—*see* Pleurisy, with effusion
- seropurulent—*see* Pyothorax
- serous—*see* Pleurisy, with effusion
- staphylococcal J86.9
- streptococcal J90
- suppurative—*see* Pyothorax

Pleuropericarditis—*see also* Pericarditis
- acute I30.9

Pleuro-pneumonia-like organism (PPLO), as the cause of disease classified elsewhere B96.0

Plica
- polonica B85.0
- tonsil J35.8

Plug
- meconium (newborn) NEC syndrome P76.0
- mucus—*see* Asphyxia

Plumbism—*see* subcategory T56.0

PMEI (polymorphic epilepsy in infancy) G40.83-

Pneumatocele (lung) J98.4
- intracranial G93.89

Pneumaturia R39.89

Pneumocephalus G93.89

Pneumococcemia A40.3

Pneumococcus, pneumococcal—*see* Disease, diseased

Pneumohemopericardium I31.2

Pneumomediastinum J98.2
- congenital or perinatal P25.2

Pneumonia (acute) (double) (migratory) (purulent) (septic) (unresolved) J18.9
- with
  - due to specified organism—*see* Pneumonia, in (due to)
  - influenza—*see* Influenza, with, pneumonia
- anaerobes J15.8
- anthrax A22.1
- Ascaris B77.81
- aspiration J69.0
  - due to
    - aspiration of microorganisms
      - ~ bacterial J15.9
      - ~ viral J12.9
    - food (regurgitated) J69.0
    - gastric secretions J69.0
    - milk (regurgitated) J69.0
    - oils, essences J69.1
    - solids, liquids NEC J69.8
    - vomitus J69.0
  - newborn P24.81
    - amniotic fluid (clear) P24.11
    - blood P24.21
    - food (regurgitated) P24.31
    - liquor (amnii) P24.11
    - meconium P24.01
    - milk P24.31
    - mucus P24.11
    - specified NEC P24.81
    - stomach contents P24.31
- atypical NEC J18.9
- bacillus J15.9
  - specified NEC J15.8

Pneumonia, *continued*
- bacterial J15.9
  - specified NEC J15.8
- Bacteroides (fragilis) (oralis) (melaninogenicus) J15.8
- broncho-, bronchial (confluent) (croupous) (diffuse) (disseminated) (hemorrhagic) (involving lobes) (lobar) (terminal) J18.0
  - aspiration—*see* Pneumonia, aspiration
  - bacterial J15.9
    - specified NEC J15.8
  - diplococcal J13
  - Eaton's agent J15.7
  - Escherichia coli (E. coli) J15.5
  - Friedländer's bacillus J15.0
  - Hemophilus influenzae J14
  - inhalation—*see also* Pneumonia, aspiration
    - of oils or essences J69.1
  - Klebsiella (pneumoniae) J15.0
  - lipid, lipoid J69.1
  - Mycoplasma (pneumoniae) J15.7
  - pleuro-pneumonia-like-organisms (PPLO) J15.7
  - pneumococcal J13
  - Proteus J15.6
  - Pseudomonas J15.1
  - Serratia marcescens J15.6
  - specified organism NEC J16.8
  - streptococcal NEC J15.4
    - group B J15.3
    - pneumoniae J13
- Butyrivibrio (fibriosolvens) J15.8
- Candida B37.1
- chlamydial J16.0
  - congenital P23.1
- Clostridium (haemolyticum) (novyi) J15.8
- confluent—*see* Pneumonia, broncho
- congenital (infective) P23.9
  - due to
    - bacterium NEC P23.6
    - Chlamydia P23.1
    - Escherichia coli P23.4
    - Haemophilus influenzae P23.6
    - infective organism NEC P23.8
    - Klebsiella pneumoniae P23.6
    - Mycoplasma P23.6
    - Pseudomonas P23.5
    - Staphylococcus P23.2
    - Streptococcus (except group B) P23.6
      - ~ group B P23.3
    - viral agent P23.0
  - specified NEC P23.8
- croupous—*see* Pneumonia, lobar
- cytomegalovirus (CMV) B25.0
- diplococcal, diplococcus (broncho-) (lobar) J13
- Eaton's agent J15.7
- Enterobacter J15.6
- Escherichia coli (E. coli) J15.5
- Eubacterium J15.8
- Friedländer's bacillus J15.0
- Fusobacterium (nucleatum) J15.8
- giant cell (measles) B05.2
- gram-negative bacteria NEC J15.6
  - anaerobic J15.8
- Hemophilus influenzae (broncho-) (lobar) J14
- human metapneumovirus (hMPV) J12.3
- in (due to)
  - actinomycosis A42.0
  - adenovirus J12.0
  - anthrax A22.1
  - ascariasis B77.81
  - aspergillosis B44.9
  - Bacillus anthracis A22.1
  - Bacterium anitratum J15.6
  - candidiasis B37.1
  - chickenpox B01.2
  - Chlamydia J16.0
    - neonatal P23.1
  - cytomegalovirus disease B25.0
  - Diplococcus (pneumoniae) J13
  - Eaton's agent J15.7
  - Enterobacter J15.6
  - Escherichia coli (E. coli) J15.5
  - Friedländer's bacillus J15.0
  - gonorrhea A54.84

Pneumonia, *continued*
- Hemophilus influenzae (H. influenzae) J14
- Herellea J15.6
- human metapneumovirus (hMPV) J12.3
- Klebsiella (pneumoniae) J15.0
- measles B05.2
- Mycoplasma (pneumoniae) J15.7
- nocardiosis, nocardiasis A43.0
- parainfluenza virus J12.2
- pleuro-pneumonia-like-organism (PPLO) J15.7
- pneumococcus J13
- Proteus J15.6
- Pseudomonas NEC J15.1
- rheumatic fever I00 *[J17]*
- Serratia marcescens J15.6
- specified
  - bacterium NEC J15.8
  - organism NEC J16.8
- Staphylococcus J15.20
  - aureus (methicillin susceptible) (MSSA) J15.211
    - ~ methicillin resistant (MRSA) J15.212
  - specified NEC J15.29
- Streptococcus J15.4
  - group B J15.3
  - pneumoniae J13
  - specified NEC J15.4
- varicella B01.2
- whooping cough A37.91
  - due to
    - ~ Bordetella parapertussis A37.11
    - ~ Bordetella pertussis A37.01
    - ~ specified NEC A37.81
- inhalation of food or vomit—*see* Pneumonia, aspiration
- interstitial J84.9
  - pseudomonas J15.1
- Klebsiella (pneumoniae) J15.0
- lipid, lipoid (exogenous) J69.1
- lobar (disseminated) (double) (interstitial) J18.1
  - bacterial J15.9
    - specified NEC J15.8
  - Escherichia coli (E. coli) J15.5
  - Friedländer's bacillus J15.0
  - Hemophilus influenzae J14
  - Klebsiella (pneumoniae) J15.0
  - pneumococcal J13
  - Proteus J15.6
  - Pseudomonas J15.1
  - specified organism NEC J16.8
  - staphylococcal—*see* Pneumonia, staphylococcal
  - streptococcal NEC J15.4
  - Streptococcus pneumoniae J13
  - viral, virus—*see* Pneumonia, viral
- lobular—*see* Pneumonia, broncho
- massive—*see* Pneumonia, lobar
- meconium P24.01
- MRSA (methicillin resistant Staphylococcus aureus) J15.212
- MSSA (methicillin susceptible Staphylococcus aureus) J15.211
- multilobar—*see* Pneumonia, by type
- Mycoplasma (pneumoniae) J15.7
- neonatal P23.9
  - aspiration—*see* Aspiration, by substance, with pneumonia
- parainfluenza virus J12.2
- Peptococcus J15.8
- Peptostreptococcus J15.8
- pleuro-pneumonia-like organism (PPLO) J15.7
- pneumococcal (broncho-) (lobar) J13
- postinfectional NEC B99 *[J17]*
- postmeasles B05.2
- Proteus J15.6
- Pseudomonas J15.1
- respiratory syncytial virus (RSV) J12.1
- resulting from a procedure J95.89
- rheumatic I00 *[J17]*
- SARS-associated coronavirus J12.81
- Serratia marcescens J15.6
- specified NEC J18.8
  - bacterium NEC J15.8
  - organism NEC J16.8
  - virus NEC J12.89

Pneumonia, *continued*
- staphylococcal (broncho) (lobar) J15.20
  - aureus (methicillin susceptible) (MSSA) J15.211
    - methicillin resistant (MRSA) J15.212
  - specified NEC J15.29
- streptococcal NEC (broncho) (lobar) J15.4
  - group
    - A J15.4
    - B J15.3
    - specified NEC J15.4
- Streptococcus pneumoniae J13
- varicella B01.2
- Veillonella J15.8
- ventilator associated J95.851
- viral, virus (broncho) (interstitial) (lobar) J12.9
  - congenital P23.0
  - human metapneumovirus (hMPV) J12.3
  - parainfluenza J12.2
  - respiratory syncytial (RSV) J12.1
  - SARS-associated coronavirus J12.81
  - specified NEC J12.89

Pneumonitis (acute) (primary)—*see also* Pneumonia
- aspiration J69.0
- congenital rubella P35.0
- due to
  - detergent J69.8
  - food, vomit (aspiration) J69.0
  - inhalation
    - blood J69.8
    - essences J69.1
    - food (regurgitated), milk, vomit J69.0
    - oils, essences J69.1
    - saliva J69.0
    - solids, liquids NEC J69.8
  - oils, essences J69.1
  - solids, liquids NEC J69.8
  - toxoplasmosis (acquired) B58.3
    - congenital P37.1
  - ventilator J95.851
- meconium P24.01
- rubella, congenital P35.0
- ventilator associated J95.851

Pneumopathy NEC J98.4
- alveolar J84.09
- parietoalveolar J84.09

Pneumopericarditis—*see also* Pericarditis
- acute I30.9

Pneumopericardium—*see also* Pericarditis
- congenital P25.3
- newborn P25.3

Pneumophagia (psychogenic) F45.8

Pneumopyopericardium I30.1

Pneumopyothorax—*see* Pyopneumothorax
- with fistula J86.0

Pneumothorax NOS J93.9
- acute J93.83
- chronic J93.81
- congenital P25.1
- perinatal period P25.1
- postprocedural J95.811
- specified NEC J93.83
- spontaneous NOS J93.83
  - newborn P25.1
  - primary J93.11
  - secondary J93.12
  - tension J93.0
- tense valvular, infectional J93.0
- tension (spontaneous) J93.0
- traumatic S27.0

Podencephalus Q01.9

Poikiloderma L81.6
- congenital Q82.8

Pointed ear (congenital) Q17.3

Poison ivy, oak, sumac or other plant dermatitis (allergic) (contact) L23.7

Poisoning (acute)—*see also* Table of Drugs and Chemicals
- algae and toxins T65.82-
- Bacillus B (aertrycke) (cholerae (suis)) (paratyphosus) (suipestifer) A02.9
  - botulinus A05.1

Poisoning, *continued*
- bacterial toxins A05.9
- berries, noxious—*see* Poisoning, food, noxious, berries
- botulism A05.1
- Clostridium botulinum A05.1
- drug—*see* Table of Drugs and Chemicals, by drug, poisoning
- epidemic, fish (noxious)—*see* Poisoning, food, noxious or naturally toxic, seafood
  - bacterial A05.9
- fava bean D55.0
- food (acute) (diseased) (infected) (noxious) NEC A05.9
  - bacterial—*see* Intoxication, foodborne, by agent
  - due to
    - Bacillus (aertrycke) (choleraesuis) (paratyphosus) (suipestifer) A02.9
      - ~ botulinus A05.1
    - Clostridium (perfringens) (Welchii) A05.2
    - salmonella (aertrycke) (callinarum) (choleraesuis) (enteritidis) (paratyphi) (suipestifer) A02.9
      - ~ with
        - ◊ gastroenteritis A02.0
        - ◊ sepsis A02.1
    - staphylococcus A05.0
    - Vibrio
      - ~ parahaemolyticus A05.3
      - ~ vulnificus A05.5
  - noxious or naturally toxic
    - berries—*see* subcategory T62.1-
    - fish—*see* Poisoning, food, noxious or naturally toxic, seafood
    - mushrooms—*see* subcategory T62.0X-
    - plants NEC—*see* subcategory T62.2X-
    - seafood—*see* Poisoning, food, noxious or naturally toxic, seafood
    - specified NEC—*see* subcategory T62.8X-
- kreotoxism, food A05.9
- lead T56.0-
- mushroom—*see* Poisoning, food, noxious, mushroom
- mussels—*see also* Poisoning
  - bacterial—*see* Intoxication, foodborne, by agent
- shellfish (amnesic) (azaspiracid) (diarrheic) (neurotoxic) (noxious) (paralytic) T61.78-
- Staphylococcus, food A05.0

Poliomyelitis (acute) (anterior) (epidemic) A80.9
- congenital P35.8 (if included in tabular list)
- imported A80.1
- indigenous A80.2
  - spinal, acute A80.9
- nonepidemic A80.9
- paralytic
  - specified NEC A80.39
  - wild virus

Pollakiuria R35.0
- psychogenic F45.8

Pollinosis J30.1

Pollitzer's disease L73.2

Polycystic (disease)
- degeneration, kidney Q61.3
  - autosomal recessive (infantile type) NEC Q61.19
- kidney Q61.3
  - autosomal
    - recessive NEC Q61.19
  - autosomal recessive (childhood type) NEC Q61.19
  - infantile type NEC Q61.19
- ovary, ovaries E28.2

Polycythemia (secondary) D75.1
- acquired D75.1
- benign (familial) D75.0
- due to
  - donor twin P61.1
  - erythropoietin D75.1
  - fall in plasma volume D75.1
  - high altitude D75.1
  - maternal-fetal transfusion P61.1
  - stress D75.1
- emotional D75.1
- erythropoietin D75.1
- familial (benign) D75.0
- Gaisböck's (hypertonica) D75.1
- high altitude D75.1

Polycythemia, *continued*
- hypertonica D75.1
- hypoxemic D75.1
- neonatorum P61.1
- nephrogenous D75.1
- relative D75.1
- secondary D75.1
- spurious D75.1
- stress D75.1

Polycytosis cryptogenica D75.1

Polydactylism, polydactyly Q69.9
- toes Q69.2

Polydipsia R63.1

Polydystrophy, pseudo-Hurler E77.0

Polyhydramnios O40.-

Polymenorrhea N92.0

Polyneuritis, polyneuritic—*see also* Polyneuropathy
- cranialis G52.7
- inflammatory G61.9

Polyneuropathy (peripheral) G62.9
- hereditary G60.9
  - specified NEC G60.8
- in (due to)
  - hypoglycemia E16.2 *[G63]*
  - infectious
    - disease NEC B99 *[G63]*
    - mononucleosis B27.91
  - Lyme disease A69.22
  - neoplastic disease (*see also* Table of Neoplasms in the complete *ICD-10-CM* manual) D49.9 *[G63]*
  - sarcoidosis D86.89
  - systemic
    - lupus erythematosus M32.19
- sensory (hereditary) (idiopathic) G60.8

Polyopia H53.8

Polyorchism, polyorchidism Q55.21

Polyp, polypus
- accessory sinus J33.8
- adenoid tissue J33.0
- antrum J33.8
- anus, anal (canal) K62.0
- choanal J33.0
- colon K63.5
  - adenomatous D12.6
  - ascending D12.2
  - cecum D12.0
  - descending D12.4
  - inflammatory K51.40
    - with
      - ~ abscess K51.414
      - ~ complication K51.419
        - ◊ specified NEC K51.418
      - ~ fistula K51.413
      - ~ intestinal obstruction K51.412
      - ~ rectal bleeding K51.411
  - sigmoid D12.5
  - transverse D12.3
- ethmoidal (sinus) J33.8
- frontal (sinus) J33.8
- maxillary (sinus) J33.8
- nares
  - anterior J33.9
  - posterior J33.0
- nasal (mucous) J33.9
  - cavity J33.0
  - septum J33.0
- nasopharyngeal J33.0
- nose (mucous) J33.9
- rectum (nonadenomatous) K62.1
- septum (nasal) J33.0
- sinus (accessory) (ethmoidal) (frontal) (maxillary) (sphenoidal) J33.8
- sphenoidal (sinus) J33.8
- turbinate, mucous membrane J33.8
- umbilical, newborn P83.6

Polyposis—*see also* Polyp
- coli (adenomatous) D12.6
- colon (adenomatous) D12.6
- familial D12.6
- intestinal (adenomatous) D12.6

Polyserositis
- due to pericarditis I31.1
- pericardial I31.1

Polysyndactyly (*see also* Syndactylism) Q70.4

Polyuria R35.8
- nocturnal R35.1
- psychogenic F45.8

Pomphylox L30.1

Poor
- urinary stream R39.12
- vision NEC H54.7

Porencephaly (congenital) (developmental) (true) Q04.6
- acquired G93.0
- nondevelopmental G93.0
- traumatic (post) F07.89

Porocephaliasis B88.8

Porokeratosis Q82.8

Port wine nevus, mark, or stain Q82.5

Positive
- culture (nonspecific)
  - blood R78.81
  - bronchial washings R84.5
  - cerebrospinal fluid R83.5
  - nose R84.5
    - staphylococcus (Methicillin susceptible) Z22.321
      - Methicillin resistant Z22.322
  - urine R82.79
- PPD (skin test) R76.11
- serology for syphilis A53.0
  - false R76.8
  - with signs or symptoms—*code as* Syphilis, by site and stage
- skin test, tuberculin (without active tuberculosis) R76.11
- test, human immunodeficiency virus (HIV) R75
- VDRL A53.0
  - with signs and symptoms—*code by* site and stage under Syphilis A53.9
- Wassermann reaction A53.0

Postcardiotomy syndrome I97.0

Postcommissurotomy syndrome I97.0

Postconcussional syndrome F07.81

Postcontusional syndrome F07.81

Posthemorrhagic anemia (chronic) D50.0
- acute D62
- newborn P61.3

Postmaturity, postmature (over 42 weeks)
- newborn P08.22

Postmeasles complication NEC (*see also* Disease, diseased) B05.89

Postnasal drip R09.82
- due to
  - allergic rhinitis—*see* Rhinitis, allergic
  - common cold J00
  - gastroesophageal reflux—*see* Reflux, gastroesophageal
  - nasopharyngitis—*see* Nasopharyngitis
  - other known condition—*code to* condition
  - sinusitis—*see* Sinusitis

Postoperative (postprocedural)—*see* Complication, postprocedural
- state NEC Z98.890

Post-term (40-42 weeks) (pregnancy) (mother)
- infant P08.21

Post-traumatic brain syndrome, nonpsychotic F07.81

Postvaccinal reaction or complication—*see* Complications, vaccination

Postvalvulotomy syndrome I97.0

Potter's
- facies Q60.6
- syndrome (with renal agenesis) Q60.6

Poultrymen's itch B88.0

Poverty NEC Z59.6
- extreme Z59.5

Prader-Willi syndrome Q87.11

Precocious
- adrenarche E30.1
- menarche E30.1
- menstruation E30.1
- pubarche E30.1
- puberty E30.1
  - central E22.8
- sexual development NEC E30.1

Precocity, sexual (constitutional) (female) (idiopathic) (male) E30.1
- with adrenal hyperplasia E25.9
  - congenital E25.0

Prediabetes, prediabetic R73.03

Pre-eclampsia O14.9
- with pre-existing hypertension—*see* Hypertension, complicating, pregnancy, pre-existing, with, pre-eclampsia
- mild O14.0-
- moderate O14.0-
- severe O14.1
  - with hemolysis, elevated liver enzymes and low platelet count (HELLP) O14.2-

Pre-excitation atrioventricular conduction I45.6

Pregnancy (single) (uterine)—*see also* Delivery

Note: The Tabular must be reviewed for assignment of the appropriate character indicating the trimester of the pregnancy

Note: The Tabular must be reviewed for assignment of appropriate seventh character for multiple gestation codes in Chapter 15
- abdominal (ectopic) O00.00
  - with uterine pregnancy O00.01
  - with viable fetus O36.7-
- ampullar O00.10-
- broad ligament O00.80
- cervical O00.80
- complicated by (care of) (management affected by)
  - abnormal, abnormality
    - findings on antenatal screening of mother O28.9
      - biochemical O28.1
      - chromosomal O28.5
      - cytological O28.2
      - genetic O28.5
      - hematological O28.0
      - radiological O28.4
      - specified NEC O28.8
      - ultrasonic O28.3
  - conjoined twins O30.02-
  - death of fetus (near term) O36.4
    - early pregnancy O02.1
  - decreased fetal movement O36.81-
  - diabetes (mellitus)
    - gestational (pregnancy induced—*see* Diabetes, gestational
      - type 1 O24.01-
      - type 2 O24.11-
  - edema
    - with
      - gestational hypertension, mild (*see also* Pre-eclampsia) O14.0-
  - fetal (maternal care for)
    - abnormality or damage O35.9
      - specified type NEC O35.8
    - anemia and thrombocytopenia O36.82-
    - anencephaly O35.0
    - bradycardia O36.83-
    - chromosomal abnormality (conditions in Q90 – Q99) O35.1
    - conjoined twins O30.02-
    - damage from
      - amniocentesis O35.7
      - biopsy procedures O35.7
      - drug addiction O35.5
      - hematological investigation O35.7
      - intrauterine contraceptive device O35.7
      - maternal
        - alcohol addiction O35.4
        - cytomegalovirus infection O35.3
        - disease NEC O35.8
        - drug addiction O35.5
        - listeriosis O35.8

Pregnancy, *continued*
- rubella O35.3
- toxoplasmosis O35.8
- viral infection O35.3
  - medical procedure NEC O35.7
  - radiation O35.6
  - death (near term) O36.4
    - early pregnancy O02.1
  - decreased movement O36.81-
  - depressed heart rate tones O36.83-
  - excessive growth (large for dates) O36.6-
  - fetal heart rate or rhythm O36.83-
  - growth retardation O36.59-
    - light for dates O36.59-
    - small for dates O36.59-
  - heart rate irregularity (abnormal variability) (bradycardia) (decelerations) (tachycardia) O36.83-
  - hereditary disease O35.2
  - hydrocephalus O35.0
  - intrauterine death O36.4
  - non-reassuring heart rate or rhythm O36.83-
  - poor growth O36.59-
    - light for dates O36.59-
    - small for dates O36.59-
  - problem O36.9-
    - specified NEC O36.89-
  - spina bifida O35.0
  - thrombocytopenia O36.82-
  - HELLP syndrome (hemolysis, elevated liver enzymes and low platelet count) O14.2-
  - hemorrhage
    - before 20 completed weeks gestation O20.9
      - specified NEC O20.8
    - early O20.9
      - specified NEC O20.8
    - threatened abortion O20.0
  - hydramnios O40.-
  - hydrops
    - amnii O40.-
    - fetalis O36.2-
      - associated with isoimmunization (*see also* Pregnancy, complicated by, isoimmunization) O36.11-
  - hydrorrhea O42.90
  - inconclusive fetal viability O36.80
  - intrauterine fetal death (near term) O36.4
    - early pregnancy O02.1
  - isoimmunization O36.11-
    - anti-A sensitization O36.11-
    - anti-B sensitization O36.19-
    - Rh O36.09-
      - anti-D antibody O36.01-
    - specified NEC O36.19-
  - missed
    - abortion O02.1
    - delivery O36.4
  - multiple gestations
    - conjoined twins O30.02-
    - specified number of multiples NEC—*see* Pregnancy, multiple (gestation), specified NEC
    - quadruplet—*see* Pregnancy, quadruplet
    - specified complication NEC O31.8X-
    - triplet—*see* Pregnancy, triplet
    - twin—*see* Pregnancy, twin
  - oligohydramnios O41.0-
    - with premature rupture of membranes (*see also* Pregnancy, complicated by, premature rupture of membranes) O42.-
  - placental insufficiency O36.51-
  - polyhydramnios O40.-
  - pre-eclampsia O14.9-
    - mild O14.0-
    - moderate O14.0-
    - severe O14.1-
      - with hemolysis, elevated liver enzymes and low platelet count (HELLP) O14.2-
  - premature rupture of membranes O42.90
    - after 37 weeks gestation O42.92
    - full-term, unspec as to length of time between rupture and onset of labor O42.92
    - with onset of labor

Pregnancy, *continued*
- ~ within 24 hours O42.00
  - ◊ at or after 37 weeks gestation O42.02
  - ◊ pre-term (before 37 completed weeks of gestation) O42.01-
- ~ after 24 hours O42.10
  - ◊ at or after 37 weeks gestation O42.12
  - ◊ pre-term (before 37 completed weeks of gestation) O42.11-
  - ■ pre-term (before 37 completed weeks of gestation) O42.91-
- – preterm labor
  - ■ second trimester
    - ~ without delivery O60.02
  - ■ third trimester
    - ~ without delivery O60.03
  - ■ without delivery
    - ~ second trimester O60.02
    - ~ third trimester O60.03
- – Rh immunization, incompatibility or sensitization NEC O36.09-
  - ■ anti-D antibody O36.01-
- – threatened
  - ■ abortion O20.0
- – young mother
  - ■ multigravida O09.62-
  - ■ primigravida O09.61-
- • cornual O00.8-
- • ectopic (ruptured) O00.9-
  - – abdominal O00.00
    - ■ with uterine pregnancy O00.01
    - ■ with viable fetus O36.7-
  - – cervical O00.8-
  - – cornual O00.8-
  - – intraligamentous O00.8-
  - – mural O00.8-
  - – ovarian O00.20-
  - – specified site NEC O00.8-
  - – tubal (ruptured) O00.10-
    - ■ with intrauterine pregnancy O00.11
- • fallopian O00.10-
  - – with intrauterine pregnancy O00.11
- • incidental finding Z33.1
- • interstitial O00.8-
- • intraligamentous O00.8-
- • intramural O00.8-
- • intraperitoneal O00.00
  - – with intrauterine pregnancy O00.01
- • isthmian O00.10-
- • mesometric (mural) O00.8-
- • multiple (gestation)
  - – greater than quadruplets—*see* Pregnancy, multiple (gestation), specified NEC
  - – specified NEC O30.80-
    - ■ number of chorions and amnions are both equal to the number of fetuses O30.83-
    - ■ two or more monoamniotic fetuses O30.82-
    - ■ two or more monochorionic fetuses O30.81-
    - ■ unable to determine number of placenta and number of amniotic sacs O30.89-
    - ■ unspecified number of placenta and unspecified number of amniotic sacs O30.80-
- • mural O00.8-
- • ovarian O00.2-
- • quadruplet O30.20-
  - – with
    - ■ two or more monoamniotic fetuses O30.22-
    - ■ two or more monochorionic fetuses O30.21-
  - – quadrachorionic/quadra-amniotic O30.23-
  - – two or more monoamniotic fetuses O30.22-
  - – two or more monochorionic fetuses O30.21-
  - – unable to determine number of placenta and number of amniotic sacs O30.29-
  - – unspecified number of placenta and unspecified number of amniotic sacs O30.20-
- • quintuplet—*see* Pregnancy, multiple (gestation), specified NEC
- • sextuplet—*see* Pregnancy, multiple (gestation), specified NEC
- • supervision of
  - – young mother
    - ■ multigravida O09.62-
    - ■ primigravida O09.61-

Pregnancy, *continued*
- • triplet O30.10-
  - – with
    - ■ two or more monoamniotic fetuses O30.12-
    - ■ two or more monochrorionic fetuses O30.11-
  - – trichorionic/triamniotic O30.13-
  - – two or more monoamniotic fetuses O30.12-
  - – two or more monochrorionic fetuses O30.11-
  - – unable to determine number of placenta and number of amniotic sacs O30.19-
  - – unspecified number of placenta and unspecified number of amniotic sacs O30.10-
- • tubal (with abortion) (with rupture) O00.10-
  - – with intrauterine pregnancy O00.11
- • twin O30.00-
  - – conjoined O30.02-
  - – dichorionic/diamniotic (two placentae, two amniotic sacs) O30.04-
  - – monochorionic/diamniotic (one placenta, two amniotic sacs) O30.03-
  - – monochorionic/monoamniotic (one placenta, one amniotic sac) O30.01-
  - – unable to determine number of placenta and number of amniotic sacs O30.09-
  - – unspecified number of placenta and unspecified number of amniotic sacs O30.00-
- • unwanted Z64.0
- • weeks of gestation
  - – 8 weeks Z3A.08
  - – 9 weeks Z3A.09
  - – 10 weeks Z3A.10
  - – 11 weeks Z3A.11
  - – 12 weeks Z3A.12
  - – 13 weeks Z3A.13
  - – 14 weeks Z3A.14
  - – 15 weeks Z3A.15
  - – 16 weeks Z3A.16
  - – 17 weeks Z3A.17
  - – 18 weeks Z3A.18
  - – 19 weeks Z3A.19
  - – 20 weeks Z3A.20
  - – 21 weeks Z3A.21
  - – 22 weeks Z3A.22
  - – 23 weeks Z3A.23
  - – 24 weeks Z3A.24
  - – 25 weeks Z3A.25
  - – 26 weeks Z3A.26
  - – 27 weeks Z3A.27
  - – 28 weeks Z3A.28
  - – 29 weeks Z3A.29
  - – 30 weeks Z3A.30
  - – 31 weeks Z3A.31
  - – 32 weeks Z3A.32
  - – 33 weeks Z3A.33
  - – 34 weeks Z3A.34
  - – 35 weeks Z3A.35
  - – 36 weeks Z3A.36
  - – 37 weeks Z3A.37
  - – 38 weeks Z3A.38
  - – 39 weeks Z3A.39
  - – 40 weeks Z3A.40
  - – 41 weeks Z3A.41
  - – 42 weeks Z3A.42
  - – greater than 42 weeks Z3A.49
  - – less than 8 weeks Z3A.01
  - – not specified Z3A.00

Premature—*see also* Disease, diseased
- • beats I49.40
  - – atrial I49.1
  - – auricular I49.1
  - – supraventricular I49.1
- • birth NEC—*see* Preterm, newborn
- • closure, foramen ovale Q21.8
- • contraction
  - – atrial I49.1
  - – auricular I49.1
  - – auriculoventricular I49.49
  - – heart (extrasystole) I49.49
- • lungs P28.0
- • newborn
  - – extreme (less than 28 completed weeks)—*see* Immaturity, extreme

Pregnancy, *continued*
- – less than 37 completed weeks—*see* Preterm, newborn
- • puberty E30.1

Premenstrual
- • dysphoric disorder (PMDD) F32.81
- • tension N94.3

Prenatal
- • teeth K00.6

Preponderance, left or right ventricular I51.7

Prescription of contraceptives (initial) Z30.019
- • barrier Z30.018
- • diaphragm Z30.018
- • emergency (postcoital) Z30.012
- • implantable subdermal Z30.017
- • injectable Z30.013
- • intrauterine contraceptive device Z30.014
- • pills Z30.011
- • postcoital (emergency) Z30.012
- • repeat Z30.40
  - – barrier Z30.49
  - – diaphragm Z30.49
  - – implantable subdermal Z30.46
  - – injectable Z30.42
  - – pills Z30.41
  - – specified type NEC Z30.49
  - – transdermal patch Z30.45
  - – vaginal ring Z30.44
- • specified type NEC Z30.018
- • transdermal patch Z30.016
- • vaginal ring Z30.015

Presence (of)
- • arterial-venous shunt (dialysis) Z99.2
- • artificial
  - – heart (fully implantable) (mechanical) Z95.812
    - ■ valve Z95.2
- • bladder implant (functional) Z96.0
- • cardiac
  - – pacemaker Z95.0
- • cerebrospinal fluid drainage device Z98.2
- • contact lens(es) Z97.3
- • CSF shunt Z98.2
- • endocrine implant (functional) NEC Z96.49
- • external hearing-aid or device Z97.4
- • functional implant Z96.9
  - – specified NEC Z96.89
- • heart valve implant (functional) Z95.2
  - – prosthetic Z95.2
  - – specified type NEC Z95.4
  - – xenogenic Z95.3
- • implanted device (artificial) (functional) (prosthetic) Z96.9
  - – cardiac pacemaker Z95.0
  - – heart valve Z95.2
    - ■ prosthetic Z95.2
    - ■ specified NEC Z95.4
    - ■ xenogenic Z95.3
  - – neurostimulator Z96.82
  - – skin Z96.81

Prespondylolisthesis (congenital) Q76.2

Pressure
- • area, skin—*see* Ulcer, pressure, by site
- • increased
  - – intracranial (benign) G93.2
    - ■ injury at birth P11.0

Pre-syncope R55

Preterm
- • newborn (infant) P07.30
  - – gestational age
    - ■ 28 completed weeks (28 weeks, 0 days through 28 weeks, 6 days) P07.31
    - ■ 29 completed weeks (29 weeks, 0 days through 29 weeks, 6 days) P07.32
    - ■ 30 completed weeks (30 weeks, 0 days through 30 weeks, 6 days) P07.33
    - ■ 31 completed weeks (31 weeks, 0 days through 31 weeks, 6 days) P07.34
    - ■ 32 completed weeks (32 weeks, 0 days through 32 weeks, 6 days) P07.35
    - ■ 33 completed weeks (33 weeks, 0 days through 33 weeks, 6 days) P07.36

Preterm, *continued*
- 34 completed weeks (34 weeks, 0 days through 34 weeks, 6 days) P07.37
- 35 completed weeks (35 weeks, 0 days through 35 weeks, 6 days) P07.38
- 36 completed weeks (36 weeks, 0 days through 36 weeks, 6 days) P07.39

Priapism N48.30
- due to
  - disease classified elsewhere N48.32
  - drug N48.33
  - specified cause NEC N48.39
  - trauma N48.31

Prickly heat L74.0

Primus varus (bilateral) Q66.21-

Pringle's disease (tuberous sclerosis) Q85.1

Problem (with) (related to)
- academic Z55.8
- acculturation Z60.3
- adopted child Z62.821
- alcoholism in family Z63.72
- atypical parenting situation Z62.9
- behavioral (adult)
  - drug seeking Z76.5
- birth of sibling affecting child Z62.898
- care (of)
- child
  - abuse (affecting the child)—*see* Maltreatment, child
  - custody or support proceedings Z65.3
  - in care of non-parental family member Z62.21
  - in foster care Z62.21
  - in welfare custody Z62.21
  - living in orphanage or group home Z62.22
- conflict or discord (with)
  - classmates Z55.4
  - counselor Z64.4
  - family Z63.9
    - specified NEC Z63.8
  - probation officer Z64.4
  - social worker Z64.4
  - teachers Z55.4
- drug addict in family Z63.72
- education Z55.9
  - specified NEC Z55.8
- enuresis, child F98.0
- failed examinations (school) Z55.2
- falling Z91.81
- family (*see also* Disruption, family) Z63.9-
  - specified NEC Z63.8
- feeding (elderly) (infant) R63.3
  - newborn P92.9
    - breast P92.5
    - overfeeding P92.4
    - slow P92.2
    - specified NEC P92.8
    - underfeeding P92.3
  - nonorganic F50.89
- foster child Z62.822
- genital NEC
  - female N94.9
  - male N50.9
- homelessness Z59.0
- housing Z59.9
  - inadequate Z59.1
- identity (of childhood) F93.8
- intrafamilial communication Z63.8
- jealousy, child F93.8
- language (developmental) F80.9
- learning (developmental) F81.9
- lifestyle Z72.9
  - gambling Z72.6
  - high-risk sexual behavior (heterosexual) Z72.51
    - bisexual Z72.53
    - homosexual Z72.5
  - inappropriate eating habits Z72.4
  - self-damaging behavior NEC Z72.89
  - specified NEC Z72.89
  - tobacco use Z72.0
- literacy Z55.9
  - low level Z55.0
  - specified NEC Z55.8

Problem (with) (related to), *continued*
- mental F48.9
- presence of sick or disabled person in family or household Z63.79
  - needing care Z63.6
- primary support group (family) Z63.9
  - specified NEC Z63.8
- psychosocial Z65.9
  - specified NEC Z65.8
- relationship Z63.9
  - childhood F93.8
- seeking and accepting known hazardous and harmful
  - behavioral or psychological interventions Z65.8
  - chemical, nutritional or physical interventions Z65.8
- sight H54.7
- speech R47.9
  - developmental F80.9
  - specified NEC R47.89
- swallowing—*see* Dysphagia
- taste—*see* Disturbance, sensation
- tic, child F95.0
- underachievement in school Z55.3
- voice production R47.89

Procedure (surgical)
- for purpose other than remedying health state Z41.9
  - specified NEC Z41.8
- not done Z53.9
  - because of
    - administrative reasons Z53.8
    - contraindication Z53.09
      - smoking Z53.01
    - patient's decision Z53.20
      - for reasons of belief or group pressure Z53.1
      - left against medical advice (AMA) Z53.21
      - specified reason NEC Z53.29
    - specified reason NEC Z53.8

Proctalgia K62.89

Proctitis K62.89
- amebic (acute) A06.0
- chlamydial A56.3
- gonococcal A54.6
- granulomatous—*see* Enteritis, regional, large intestine
- herpetic A60
- ulcerative (chronic) K51.20
  - with
    - complication K51.219
      - abscess K51.214
      - fistula K51.213
      - obstruction K51.212
      - rectal bleeding K51.211
      - specified NEC K51.218

Proctocele
- male K62.3

Proctoptosis K62.3

Proctorrhagia K62.5

Proctospasm K59.4
- psychogenic F45.8

Prolapse, prolapsed
- anus, anal (canal) (sphincter) K62.2
- bladder (mucosa) (sphincter) (acquired)
  - congenital Q79.4
- rectum (mucosa) (sphincter) K62.3

Prolonged, prolongation (of)
- bleeding (time) (idiopathic) R79.1
- coagulation (time) R79.1
- gestation (over 42 completed weeks)
  - newborn P08.22
- interval I44.0
- partial thromboplastin time (PTT) R79.1
- prothrombin time R79.1
- QT interval R94.31

Pronation
- ankle—*see* Deformity, limb, foot, specified NEC
- foot—*see also* Deformity, limb, foot, specified NEC
  - congenital Q74.2

Prophylactic
- administration of
  - antibiotics, long-term Z79.2
  - antivenin Z29.12
    - short-term use—omit code

Prophylactic, *continued*
- drug (*see also* Long-term (current) (prophylactic) drug therapy (use of)) Z79.899-
- fluoride varnish application Z29.3
- other specified Z29.8
- rabies immune therapry Z29.14
- respiratory syncytial virus (RSV) immune globulin Z29.11
- Rho (D) immune globulin Z29.13
- unspecified Z29.9
- medication Z79.899
- vaccination Z23

Prostatitis (congestive) (suppurative) (with cystitis) N41.9
- acute N41.0

Prostration R53.83
- heat—*see also* Heat, exhaustion
  - anhydrotic T67.3
  - due to
    - salt (and water) depletion T67.4
    - water depletion T67.3

Protein
- sickness (*see also* Reaction, serum) T80.69

Proteinuria R80.9
- Bence Jones R80.3
- isolated R80.0
- orthostatic R80.2
  - with glomerular lesion—*see* Proteinuria, isolated, with glomerular lesion
- postural R80.2
  - with glomerular lesion—*see* Proteinuria, isolated, with glomerular lesion
- specified type NEC R80.8

Proteolysis, pathologic D65

Proteus (mirabilis) (morganii), **as the cause of disease classified elsewhere** B96.4

Protrusion, protrusio
- device, implant or graft (*see also* Complications, by site and type, mechanical) T85.698
  - catheter NEC T85.698
    - cystostomy T83.090
    - urinary—*see also* Complications, catheter, urinary T83.098
  - ventricular intracranial shunt T85.09

Prune belly (syndrome) Q79.4

Prurigo (ferox) (gravis) (Hebrae) (Hebra's) (mitis) (simplex) L28.2
- Besnier's L20.0
- psychogenic F45.8

Pruritus, pruritic (essential) L29.9
- ani, anus L29.0
  - psychogenic F45.8
- anogenital L29.3
  - psychogenic F45.8
- hiemalis L29.8
- neurogenic (any site) F45.8
- perianal L29.0
- psychogenic (any site) F45.8
- scroti, scrotum L29.1
  - psychogenic F45.8
- specified NEC L29.8
  - psychogenic F45.8
- Trichomonas A59.9
- vulva, vulvae L29.2
  - psychogenic F45.8

Pseudo-Hurler's polydystrophy E77.0

Pseudoangioma I81

Pseudarthrosis, pseudoarthrosis (bone)
- clavicle, congenital Q74.0

Pseudocirrhosis, liver, pericardial I31.1

Pseudocyesis F45.8

Pseudohemophilia (Bernuth's) (hereditary) (type B) D68.0

Pseudohermaphroditism Q56.3
- adrenal E25.8
- female Q56.2
  - with adrenocortical disorder E25.8
  - without adrenocortical disorder Q56.2
  - adrenal, congenital E25.0

Pseudohermaphroditism, *continued*
- male Q56.1
  - with
    - androgen resistance E34.51
    - feminizing testis E34.51

Pseudohydrocephalus G93.2

Pseudohypertrophic muscular dystrophy (Erb's) G71.02

Pseudohypertrophy, muscle G71.09

Pseudoinsomnia F51.03

Pseudomeningocele (cerebral) (infective) (post-traumatic) G96.198

Pseudomonas
- aeruginosa, as cause of disease classified elsewhere B96.5
- mallei infection
  - as cause of disease classified elsewhere B96.5
- pseudomallei, as cause of disease classified elsewhere B96.5

Pseudoparalysis
- atonic, congenital P94.2

Pseudopolycythemia D75.1

Pseudopuberty, precocious
- female heterosexual E25.8
- male isosexual E25.8

Pseudorubella B08.20

Pseudosclerema, newborn P83.88

Pseudotuberculosis A28.2
- enterocolitis A04.8
- pasteurella (infection) A28.0

Pseudotumor G93.2

Pseudoxanthoma elasticum Q82.8

Psilosis (sprue) (tropical) K90.1
- nontropical K90.0

Psoriasis L40.9
- flexural L40.8
- specified NEC L40.8

Psychological and behavioral factors affecting medical condition F59

Psychoneurosis, psychoneurotic—*see also* Neurosis
- hysteria F44.9

Psychopathy, psychopathic
- autistic F84.5
- constitution, post-traumatic F07.81
- personality—*see* Disorder, personality

Psychosexual identity disorder of childhood F64.2

Psychosis, psychotic
- acute (transient)
  - hysterical F44.9
- affective—*see* Disorder, mood
- childhood F84.0
  - atypical F84.8
- exhaustive F43.0
- hysterical (acute) F44.9
- infantile F84.0
  - atypical F84.8

Ptosis—*see also* Blepharoptosis
- brow or eyebrow H57.81-
- eyelid—*see* Blepharoptosis
  - congenital Q10.0

PTP D69.51

Ptyalism (periodic) K11.7
- hysterical F45.8

Pubarche, precocious E30.1

Pubertas praecox E30.1

Puberty (development state) Z00.3
- bleeding (excessive) N92.2
- delayed E30.0
- precocious (constitutional) (cryptogenic) (idiopathic) E30.1
  - central E22.8
  - due to
    - ovarian hyperfunction E28.1
      - estrogen E28.0

Puberty, *continued*
- premature E30.1
  - due to
    - adrenal cortical hyperfunction E25.8
    - pineal tumor E34.8
    - pituitary (anterior) hyperfunction E22.8

Puente's disease (simple glandular cheilitis) K13.0

Pulse
- alternating R00.8
- bigeminal R00.8
- fast R00.0
- feeble, rapid due to shock following injury T79.4
- rapid R00.0
- weak R09.89

Punch drunk F07.81

Punctum lacrimale occlusion—*see* Obstruction, lacrimal

Puncture
- abdomen, abdominal
  - wall S31.139
    - with
      - ~ foreign body S31.149
    - epigastric region S31.132
      - ~ with
        - ◊ foreign body S31.142
    - left
      - ~ lower quadrant S31.134
        - ◊ with
          - » foreign body S31.144
      - ~ upper quadrant S31.131
        - ◊ with
          - » foreign body S31.141
    - periumbilic region S31.135
      - ~ with
        - ◊ foreign body S31.145
    - right
      - ~ lower quadrant S31.133
        - ◊ with
          - » foreign body S31.143
      - ~ upper quadrant S31.130
        - ◊ with
          - » foreign body S31.140
- accidental, complicating surgery—*see* Complication
- alveolar (process)—*see* Puncture, oral cavity
- ankle S91.03-
  - with
    - foreign body S91.04-
  - left S91.032
    - with
      - ~ foreign body S91.042
  - right S91.031
    - with
      - ~ foreign body S91.041
- anus S31.833
  - with foreign body S31.834
- arm (upper) S41.13-
  - with foreign body S41.14-
  - left S41.132
    - with foreign body S41.142
  - lower—*see* Puncture, forearm
  - right S41.131
    - with foreign body S41.141
- auditory canal (external) (meatus)—*see* Puncture, ear
- auricle, ear—*see* Puncture, ear
- axilla—*see* Puncture, arm
- back—*see also* Puncture, thorax, back
  - lower S31.030
    - with
      - ~ foreign body S31.040
- bladder (traumatic)
  - nontraumatic N32.89
- buttock S31.8-
  - with foreign body S31.8-
  - left S31.823
    - with foreign body S31.824
  - right S31.813
    - with foreign body S31.814
- by
  - device, implant or graft—*see* Complications, by site and type, mechanical
  - instrument (any) during a procedure, accidental—*see* Puncture, accidental complicating surgery

Puncture, *continued*
- calf—*see* Puncture, leg
- canaliculus lacrimalis—*see* Puncture, eyelid
- canthus, eye—*see* Puncture, eyelid
- cheek (external) S01.43-
  - with foreign body S01.44
  - internal—*see* Puncture, oral cavity
  - left S01.432
    - with foreign body S01.442
  - right S01.431
    - with foreign body S01.441
- chest wall—*see* Puncture, thorax
- chin—*see* Puncture, head, specified site NEC
- clitoris—*see* Puncture, vulva
- costal region—*see* Puncture, thorax
- digit(s)
  - hand—*see* Puncture, finger
  - foot—*see* Puncture, toe
- ear (canal) (external) S01.33-
  - drum S09.2-
  - with foreign body S01.34-
  - left S01.332
    - with foreign body S01.342
  - right S01.331
    - with foreign body S01.341
- elbow S51.03-
  - with
    - foreign body S51.04-
  - left S51.032
    - with
      - ~ foreign body S51.042
  - right S51.031
    - with
      - ~ foreign body S51.041
- epididymis—*see* Puncture
- epigastric region—*see* Puncture, abdomen, wall, epigastric region
- epiglottis S11.83
  - with foreign body S11.84
  - eyebrow—*see* Puncture, eyelid
- eyelid S01.13-
  - with foreign body S01.14-
  - left S01.132
    - with foreign body S01.142
  - right S01.131
    - with foreign body S01.141
- face NEC—*see* Puncture, head, specified site NEC
- finger(s) S61.23-
  - with
    - damage to nail S61.33-
      - ~ with
        - ◊ foreign body S61.34-
    - foreign body S61.24-
  - index S61.23-
    - with
      - ~ damage to nail S61.33-
        - ◊ with
          - » foreign body S61.34-
      - ~ foreign body S61.24-
    - left S61.231
      - ~ with
        - ◊ damage to nail S61.331
          - » with
            - ❖ foreign body S61.341
        - ◊ foreign body S61.241
    - right S61.230
      - ~ with
        - ◊ damage to nail S61.330
          - » with
            - ❖ foreign body S61.340
        - ◊ foreign body S61.240
  - little S61.23-
    - with
      - ~ damage to nail S61.33-
        - ◊ with
          - » foreign body S61.34-
      - ~ foreign body S61.24-
    - left S61.237
      - ~ with
        - ◊ damage to nail S61.337
          - » with
            - ❖ foreign body S61.347
        - ◊ foreign body S61.247

Puncture, *continued*
- ■ right S61.236
  - ~ with
    - ◊ damage to nail S61.336
      - » with
        - ❖ foreign body S61.346
    - ◊ foreign body S61.246
- − middle S61.23-
  - ■ with
    - ~ damage to nail S61.33-
      - ◊ with
        - » foreign body S61.34-
    - ~ foreign body S61.24-
  - ■ left S61.233
    - ~ with
      - ◊ damage to nail S61.333
        - » with
          - ❖ foreign body S61.343
      - ◊ foreign body S61.243
  - ■ right S61.232
    - ~ with
      - ◊ damage to nail S61.332
        - » with
          - ❖ foreign body S61.342
      - ◊ foreign body S61.242
- − ring S61.238
  - ■ with
    - ~ damage to nail S61.33-
      - ◊ with
        - » foreign body S61.34-
    - ~ foreign body S61.24-
  - ■ left S61.235
    - ~ with
      - ◊ damage to nail S61.335
        - » with
          - ❖ foreign body S61.345
      - ◊ foreign body S61.245
  - ■ right S61.234
    - ~ with
      - ◊ damage to nail S61.334
        - » with
          - ❖ foreign body S61.344
      - ◊ foreign body S61.244
- • flank S31.139
  - − with foreign body S31.149
- • foot (except toe(s) alone) S91.33-
  - − with foreign body S91.34-
  - − left S91.332
    - ■ with foreign body S91.342
  - − right S91.331
    - ■ with foreign body S91.341
  - − toe—*see* Puncture, toe
- • forearm S51.83-
  - − with
    - ■ foreign body S51.84-
  - − elbow only—*see* Puncture, elbow
  - − left S51.832
    - ■ with
      - ~ foreign body S51.842
  - − right S51.831
    - ■ with
      - ~ foreign body S51.841
- • forehead—*see* Puncture, head, specified site NEC
- • genital organs, external
  - − female (*code to* Puncture by specific site for vagina or vulva)
  - − male (*code to* Puncture by specific site for penis, scrotum, or testis)
- • groin—*see* Puncture, abdomen, wall
- • gum—*see* Puncture, oral cavity
- • hand (*code to* Puncture by specific site for finger or thumb) S61.43-
  - − with
    - ■ foreign body S61.44-
  - − left S61.432
    - ■ with
      - ~ foreign body S61.442
  - − right S61.431
    - ■ with
      - ~ foreign body S61.441

Puncture, *continued*
- • head (*code to* Puncture by specific site for cheek/temporomandibular area, ear, eyelid, nose, or oral cavity) S01.93
  - − with foreign body S01.94
  - − scalp S01.03
    - ■ with foreign body S01.04
  - − specified site NEC S01.83
    - ■ with foreign body S01.84
- • heel—*see* Puncture, foot
- • hip S71.03-
  - − with foreign body S71.04-
  - − left S71.032
    - ■ with foreign body S71.042
  - − right S71.031
    - ■ with foreign body S71.041
- • hypochondrium—*see* Puncture, abdomen, wall
- • hypogastric region—*see* Puncture, abdomen, wall
- • inguinal region—*see* Puncture, abdomen, wall
- • instep—*see* Puncture, foot
- • interscapular region—*see* Puncture, thorax, back
- • jaw—*see* Puncture, head, specified site NEC
- • knee S81.03-
  - − with foreign body S81.04-
  - − left S81.032
    - ■ with foreign body S81.042
  - − right S81.031
    - ■ with foreign body S81.041
- • leg (lower) (*code to* Puncture by specified site for foot, knee, or upper leg/thigh) S81.83-
  - − with foreign body S81.84-
  - − left S81.832
    - ■ with foreign body S81.842
  - − right S81.831
    - ■ with foreign body S81.841
- • lip S01.531
  - − with foreign body S01.541
- • loin—*see* Puncture, abdomen, wall
- • lower back—*see* Puncture, back, lower
- • lumbar region—*see* Puncture, back, lower
- • malar region—*see* Puncture, head, specified site NEC
- • mastoid region—*see* Puncture, head, specified site NEC
- • mouth—*see* Puncture, oral cavity
- • nail
  - − finger—*see* Puncture, finger, with, damage to nail
  - − toe—*see* Puncture, toe, with, damage to nail
- • nasal (septum) (sinus)—*see* Puncture, nose
- • nasopharynx—*see* Puncture, head, specified site NEC
- • neck S11.93
  - − with foreign body S11.94
- • nose (septum) (sinus) S01.23
  - − with foreign body S01.24
- • oral cavity S01.532
  - − with foreign body S01.542
- • palate—*see* Puncture, oral cavity
- • palm—*see* Puncture, hand
- • penis S31.23
  - − with foreign body S31.24
- • perineum
  - − female S31.43
    - ■ with foreign body S31.44
  - − male S31.139
    - ■ with foreign body S31.149
- • phalanges
  - − finger—*see* Puncture, finger
  - − toe—*see* Puncture, toe
- • pinna—*see* Puncture, ear
- • popliteal space—*see* Puncture, knee
- • scalp S01.03
  - − with foreign body S01.04
- • scapular region—*see* Puncture, shoulder
- • scrotum S31.33
  - − with foreign body S31.34
- • shin—*see* Puncture, leg
- • shoulder S41.03-
  - − with foreign body S41.04-
  - − left S41.032
    - ■ with foreign body S41.042
  - − right S41.031
    - ■ with foreign body S41.041
- • subungual
  - − finger(s)—*see* Puncture, finger, with, damage to nail
  - − toe—*see* Puncture, toe, with, damage to nail

Puncture, *continued*
- • testis S31.33
- • thigh S71.13-
  - − with foreign body S71.14-
  - − left S71.132
    - ■ with foreign body S71.142
  - − right S71.131
    - ■ with foreign body S71.141
- • thorax, thoracic (wall) S21.93
  - − with foreign body S21.94
  - − back S21.23-
    - ■ with
      - ~ foreign body S21.24-
  - − front S21.13-
    - ■ with
      - ~ foreign body S21.14-
- • throat—*see* Puncture, neck
- • thumb S61.03-
  - − with
    - ■ damage to nail S61.13-
      - ~ with
        - ◊ foreign body S61.14-
    - ■ foreign body S61.04-
  - − left S61.032
    - ■ with
      - ~ damage to nail S61.132
        - ◊ with
          - » foreign body S61.142
      - ~ foreign body S61.042
  - − right S61.031
    - ■ with
      - ~ damage to nail S61.131
        - ◊ with
          - » foreign body S61.141
      - ~ foreign body S61.041
- • toe(s) S91.13-
  - − with
    - ■ damage to nail S91.23-
      - ~ with
        - ◊ foreign body S91.24-
    - ■ foreign body S91.14-
  - − great S91.13-
    - ■ with
      - ~ damage to nail S91.23-with
        - » foreign body S91.24-
      - ~ foreign body S91.14-
    - ■ left S91.132
      - ~ with
        - ◊ damage to nail S91.232
          - » with
            - ❖ foreign body S91.242
        - ◊ foreign body S91.142
    - ■ right S91.131
      - ~ with
        - ◊ damage to nail S91.231
          - » with
            - ❖ foreign body S91.241
        - ◊ foreign body S91.141
  - − lesser S91.13-
    - ■ with
      - ~ damage to nail S91.23-
        - ◊ with
          - » foreign body S91.24-
      - ~ foreign body S91.14-
    - ■ left S91.135
      - ~ with
        - ◊ damage to nail S91.235
          - » with
            - ❖ foreign body S91.245
        - ◊ foreign body S91.145
    - ■ right S91.134
      - ~ with
        - ◊ damage to nail S91.234
          - » with
            - ❖ foreign body S91.244
        - ◊ foreign body S91.144
- • tympanum, tympanic membrane S09.2-
- • umbilical region S31.135
  - − with foreign body S31.145
- • vagina S31.43
  - − with foreign body S31.44

Puncture, *continued*
- vulva S31.43
  - with foreign body S31.44
- wrist S61.53-
  - with
    - foreign body S61.54-
  - left S61.532
    - with
      ~ foreign body S61.542
  - right S61.531
    - with
      ~ foreign body S61.541

PUO (pyrexia of unknown origin) R50.9

Purpura D69.2
- abdominal D69.0
- allergic D69.0
- anaphylactoid D69.0
- arthritic D69.0
- autoerythrocyte sensitization D69.2
- autoimmune D69.0
- bacterial D69.0
- Bateman's (senile) D69.2
- capillary fragility (hereditary) (idiopathic) D69.8
- Devil's pinches D69.2
- fibrinolytic—*see* Fibrinolysis
- fulminans, fulminous D65
- gangrenous D65
- hemorrhagic, hemorrhagica D69.3
  - not due to thrombocytopenia D69.0
- Henoch (-Schönlein) (allergic) D69.0
- idiopathic (thrombocytopenic) D69.3
  - nonthrombocytopenic D69.0
- immune thrombocytopenic D69.3
- infectious D69.0
- malignant D69.0
- neonatorum P54.5
- nervosa D69.0
- newborn P54.5
- nonthrombocytopenic D69.2
  - hemorrhagic D69.0
  - idiopathic D69.0
- nonthrombopenic D69.2
- peliosis rheumatica D69.0
- posttransfusion (post-transfusion) (from (fresh) whole blood or blood products) D69.51
- primary D69.49
- red cell membrane sensitivity D69.2
- rheumatica D69.0
- Schönlein (-Henoch) (allergic) D69.0
- senile D69.2
- simplex D69.2
- symptomatica D69.0
- telangiectasia annularis L81.7
- thrombocytopenic D69.49
  - congenital D69.42
  - hemorrhagic D69.3
  - hereditary D69.42
  - idiopathic D69.3
  - immune D69.3
  - neonatal, transitory P61.0
  - thrombotic M31.1
- thrombohemolytic—*see* Fibrinolysis
- thrombolytic—*see* Fibrinolysis
- thrombopenic D69.49
- thrombotic, thrombocytopenic M31.1
- toxic D69.0
- vascular D69.0
- visceral symptoms D69.0

Purpuric spots R23.3

Purulent—*see* Disease, diseased

Pus
- in
  - stool R19.5
  - urine N39.0
- tube (rupture)—*see* Salpingo-oophoritis

Pustular rash L08.0

Pustule (nonmalignant) L08.9
- malignant A22.0

Pyelectasis—*see* Hydronephrosis

Pyelitis (congenital) (uremic)—*see also* Pyelonephritis
- with
  - calculus—*see* category N20
    - with hydronephrosis N13.6
- acute N10
- chronic N11.9
  - with calculus—*see* category N20
    - with hydronephrosis N13.6

Pyelonephritis—*see also* Nephritis, tubulo-interstitial
- with
  - calculus—*see* category N20
    - with hydronephrosis N13.6
- acute N10
- calculous—*see* category N20
  - with hydronephrosis N13.6
- chronic N11.9
  - with calculus—*see* category N20
    - with hydronephrosis N13.6
- in (due to)
  - lymphoma NEC C85.90 *[N16]*
  - sarcoidosis D86.84
  - sepsis A41.9 *[N16]*
  - transplant rejection T86.- *[N16]*

Pyelophlebitis I80.8

Pyemia, pyemic (fever) (infection) (purulent)—*see also* Sepsis
- pneumococcal
- specified organism NEC A41.89

Pyloritis K29.90
- with bleeding K29.91

Pylorospasm (reflex) NEC K31.3
- congenital or infantile Q40.0
- newborn Q40.0
- neurotic F45.8
- psychogenic F45.8

Pylorus, pyloric—*see* Disease, diseased

Pyoarthrosis—*see* Arthritis, pyogenic or pyemic

Pyocele
- sinus (accessory)—*see* Sinusitis
- turbinate (bone) J32.9

Pyoderma, pyodermia L08.0
- gangrenosum L88
- newborn P39.4
- phagedenic L88

Pyodermatitis L08.0

Pyopericarditis, pyopericardium I30.1

Pyopneumopericardium I30.1

Pyopneumothorax (infective) J86.9
- with fistula J86.0

Pyothorax J86.9
- with fistula J86.0

Pyrexia (of unknown origin) R50.9
- atmospheric T67.01
- heat T67.01
- newborn P81.9
  - environmentally-induced P81.0
- persistent R50.9

Pyroglobulinemia NEC E88.09

Pyrosis R12

Pyuria R82.81
- abnormal laboratory finding R82.81
- bacterial N39.0

Pityriasis (capitis) L21.0
- furfuracea L21.0

Q

Quadriparesis—*see* Quadriplegia
- meaning muscle weakness M62.81

Quadriplegia G82.50
- complete
  - C1–C4 level G82.51
  - C5–C7 level G82.53
- incomplete
  - C1–C4 level G82.52
  - C5–C7 level G82.54
- traumatic *code to* injury with seventh character S
  - current episode—*see* Injury, spinal (cord), cervical

Quervain's disease M65.4
- thyroid E06.1

Quincke's disease or edema T78.3

Quinsy (gangrenous) J36

R

Rabies A82.9
- contact Z20.3
- exposure to Z20.3
- inoculation reaction—*see* Complications, vaccination

Radiation
- therapy, encounter for Z51.0

Radiotherapy session Z51.0

Rag picker's disease A22.1

Rag sorter's disease A22.1

Rales R09.89

Ramsay-Hunt disease or syndrome (*see also* Hunt's)
- meaning dyssynergia cerebellaris myoclonica G11.19

Rape
- alleged, observation or examination, ruled out
  - child Z04.42
- child
  - confirmed T74.22
  - suspected T76.22

Rapid
- feeble pulse, due to shock, following injury T79.4
- heart (beat) R00.0
  - psychogenic F45.8

Rash (toxic) R21
- canker A38.9
- diaper L22
- drug (internal use) L27.0
  - contact (*see also* Dermatitis, due to, drugs and medicaments) L25.1
- following immunization T88.1-
- food—*see* Dermatitis, due to, food
- heat L74.0
- napkin (psoriasiform) L22
- nettle—*see* Urticaria
- pustular L08.0
- rose R21
  - epidemic B06.9
- scarlet A38.9
- serum (*see also* Reaction, serum) T80.69
- wandering tongue K14.1

Rat-bite fever A25.9
- due to Streptobacillus moniliformis A25.1
- spirochetal (morsus muris) A25.0

RDS (newborn) (type I) P22.0
- type II P22.1

Reaction—*see also* Disorder
- adverse
  - food (any) (ingested) NEC T78.1
    - anaphylactic—*see* Shock, anaphylactic, due to food
- allergic—*see* Allergy
- anaphylactic—*see* Shock, anaphylactic
- anaphylactoid—*see* Shock, anaphylactic
- antitoxin (prophylactic) (therapeutic)—*see* Complications, vaccination
- combat and operational stress F43.0
- compulsive F42.8
- conversion F44.9
- crisis, acute F43.0
- deoxyribonuclease (DNA) (DNase) hypersensitivity D69.2
- depressive (single episode) F32.9
  - psychotic F32.3
  - recurrent—*see* Disorder, depressive, recurrent
- dissociative F44.9
- drug NEC T88.7
  - allergic—*see* Allergy, drug
  - newborn P93.8
    - gray baby syndrome P93.0
  - overdose or poisoning (by accident)—*see* Table of Drugs and Chemicals, by drug, poisoning
  - photoallergic L56.1
  - phototoxic L56.0
  - withdrawal—*see* Dependence, by drug, with, withdrawal

Reaction, *continued*
- ▪ infant of dependent mother P96.1
- ▪ newborn P96.1
- – wrong substance given or taken (by accident)—*see* Table of Drugs and Chemicals, by drug, poisoning
- • fear F40.9
  - – child (abnormal) F93.8
- • febrile nonhemolytic transfusion (FNHTR) R50.84
- • hypoglycemic, due to insulin E16.0
  - – therapeutic misadventure—*see* subcategory T38.3
- • hysterical F44.9
- • immunization—*see* Complications, vaccination
- • insulin T38.3-
- • leukemoid D72.823
  - – basophilic D72.823
  - – lymphocytic D72.823
  - – monocytic D72.823
  - – myelocytic D72.823
  - – neutrophilic D72.823
- • neurogenic—*see* Neurosis
- • neurotic F48.9
- • nonspecific
  - – to
    - ▪ cell mediated immunity measurement of gamma interferon antigen response without active tuberculosis R76.12
    - ▪ QuantiFERON-TB test (QFT) without active tuberculosis R76.12
    - ▪ tuberculin test (*see also* Reaction) R76.11
- • obsessive-compulsive F42.8
- • phobic F40.9
- • psychoneurotic—*see also* Neurosis
  - – compulsive F42
  - – obsessive F42
- • psychophysiologic—*see* Disorder, somatoform
- • psychosomatic—*see* Disorder, somatoform
- • psychotic—*see* Psychosis
- • scarlet fever toxin—*see* Complications, vaccination
- • serum T80.69-
  - – anaphylactic (immediate) (*see also* Shock, anaphylactic) T80.59-
  - – specified reaction NEC
    - ▪ due to
      - ~ administration of blood and blood products T80.61-
      - ~ immunization T80.62-
      - ~ serum specified NEC T80.69-
      - ~ vaccination T80.62-
- • spinal puncture G97.1
  - – dural G97.1
- • stress (severe) F43.9
  - – acute (agitation) ("daze") (disorientation) (disturbance of consciousness) (flight reaction) (fugue) F43.0
  - – specified NEC F43.8
- • surgical procedure—*see* Complications, surgical procedure
- • tetanus antitoxin—*see* Complications, vaccination
- • toxic, to local anesthesia T81.89
- • toxin-antitoxin—*see* Complications, vaccination
- • tuberculin skin test, abnormal R76.11
- • withdrawing, child or adolescent F93.8

Reactive airway disease—*see* Asthma

Reactive depression—*see* Reaction, depressive

Recklinghausen disease Q85.01

Rectalgia K62.89

Rectitis K62.89

Rectocele
- • male K62.3

Rectosigmoiditis K63.89
- • ulcerative (chronic) K51.30
  - – with
    - ▪ complication K51.319
      - ~ abscess K51.314
      - ~ fistula K51.313
      - ~ obstruction K51.312
      - ~ rectal bleeding K51.311
      - ~ specified NEC K51.318

Red bugs B88.0

Reduced
- • mobility Z74.09
- • ventilatory or vital capacity R94.2

Redundant, redundancy
- • foreskin (congenital) N47.8
- • prepuce (congenital) N47.8

Reflex R29.2
- • vasovagal R55

Reflux K21.9
- • acid K21.9
- • esophageal K21.9
  - – with esophagitis K21.0-
  - – newborn P78.83
- • gastroesophageal K21.9
  - – with esophagitis K21.0-
- • vesicoureteral (with scarring) N13.70
  - – without nephropathy N13.71

Refusal of
- • food, psychogenic F50.89

Regurgitation R11.10
- • aortic (valve)—*see* Insufficiency, aortic
- • food—*see also* Vomiting
  - – with reswallowing—*see* Rumination
  - – newborn P92.1
- • gastric contents—*see* Vomiting
- • heart—*see* Endocarditis
- • mitral (valve)—*see* Insufficiency, mitral
  - – congenital Q23.3
- • myocardial—*see* Endocarditis
- • pulmonary (valve) (heart) I37.1
  - – congenital Q22.2
  - – syphilitic A52.03
- • tricuspid—*see* Insufficiency, tricuspid
- • valve, valvular—*see* Endocarditis
  - – congenital Q24.8

Reifenstein syndrome E34.52

Reinsertion
- • implantable subdermal contraceptive Z30.46
- • intrauterine contraceptive device Z30.433

Rejection
- • food, psychogenic F50.89
- • transplant
  - – bone
    - ▪ marrow T86.01
  - – heart T86.21
    - ▪ with lung(s) T86.31
  - – kidney T86.11
  - – liver T86.41
  - – lung(s) T86.810
    - ▪ with heart T86.31
  - – organ (immune or nonimmune cause) T86.-
  - – stem cell (peripheral blood) (umbilical cord) T86.5

Relapsing fever A68.9
- • louse-borne (epidemic) A68.0
- • Novy's (American) A68.1
- • tick borne (endemic) A68.1

Relaxation
- • anus (sphincter) K62.89
  - – psychogenic F45.8
- • cardioesophageal K21.9
- • diaphragm J98.6
- • posture R29.3
- • rectum (sphincter) K62.89

Remittent fever (malarial) B54

Remnant
- • fingernail L60.8
  - – congenital Q84.6
- • thyroglossal duct Q89.2
- • tonsil J35.8
  - – infected (chronic) J35.01

Removal (from) (of)
- • device
  - – contraceptive Z30.432
    - ▪ implantable subdermal Z30.46
  - – dressing (nonsurgical) Z48.00
    - – surgical Z48.01
- • home in childhood (to foster home or institution) Z62.29
- • staples Z48.02
- • suture Z48.02

Rendu-Osler-Weber disease or syndrome I78.0

Renon-Delille syndrome E23.3

Replacement by artificial or mechanical device or prosthesis of
- • heart Z95.812
  - – valve Z95.2
    - ▪ prosthetic Z95.2
    - ▪ specified NEC Z95.4
    - ▪ xenogenic Z95.3
- • organ replacement
  - – by artificial or mechanical device or prosthesis of
    - ▪ heart Z95.812
      - ~ valve Z95.2

Request for expert evidence Z04.89

Residual—*see also* Disease, diseased
- • urine R39.198

Resistance, resistant (to)
- • insulin E88.81
- • organism(s)
  - – to
    - ▪ drug Z16.30
      - ~ aminoglycosides Z16.29
      - ~ amoxicillin Z16.11
      - ~ ampicillin Z16.11
      - ~ antibiotic(s) Z16.20
        - ◊ multiple Z16.24
        - ◊ specified NEC Z16.29
      - ~ antimicrobial (single) Z16.30
        - ◊ multiple Z16.35
        - ◊ specified NEC Z16.39
      - ~ beta lactam antibiotics Z16.10
        - ◊ specified NEC Z16.19
      - ~ cephalosporins Z16.19
      - ~ extended beta lactamase (ESBL) Z16.12
      - ~ macrolides Z16.29
      - ~ methicillin—*see* MRSA
      - ~ multiple drugs (MDRO)
        - ◊ antibiotics Z16.24
        - ◊ antimycobacterial (single) Z16.341
      - ~ penicillins Z16.11
      - ~ sulfonamides Z16.29
      - ~ tetracyclines Z16.29
      - ~ vancomycin Z16.21
        - ◊ related antibiotics Z16.22

Respiration
- • Cheyne-Stokes R06.3
- • decreased due to shock, following injury T79.4
- • disorder of, psychogenic F45.8
- • insufficient, or poor R06.89
  - – newborn P28.5
- • painful R07.1
- • sighing, psychogenic F45.8

Respiratory—*see also* Disease, diseased
- • distress syndrome (newborn) (type I) P22.0
  - – type II P22.1
- • syncytial virus (RSV), as cause of disease classified elsewhere B97

Restless legs (syndrome) G25.81

Rests, ovarian, in fallopian tube Q50.6

Retained—*see also* Retention
- • foreign body fragments (type of) Z18.9
  - – acrylics Z18.2
  - – animal quill(s) or spines Z18.31
  - – cement Z18.83
  - – concrete Z18.83
  - – crystalline Z18.83
  - – diethylhexylphthalates Z18.2
  - – glass Z18.81
  - – isocyanate Z18.2
  - – magnetic metal Z18.11
  - – metal Z18.10
  - – nonmagnetic metal Z18.12
  - – organic NEC Z18.39
  - – plastic Z18.2
  - – quill(s) (animal) Z18.31
  - – specified NEC Z18.89
  - – spine(s) (animal) Z18.31
  - – stone Z18.83
  - – tooth (teeth) Z18.32
  - – wood Z18.33

Retained, *continued*
- fragments (type of) Z18.9
  - acrylics Z18.2
  - animal quill(s) or spines Z18.31
  - cement Z18.83
  - concrete Z18.83
  - crystalline Z18.83
  - diethylhexylphthalates Z18.2
  - glass Z18.81
  - isocyanate Z18.2
  - magnetic metal Z18.11
  - metal Z18.10
  - nonmagnetic metal Z18.12
  - organic NEC Z18.39
  - plastic Z18.2
  - quill(s) (animal) Z18.31
  - specified NEC Z18.89
  - spine(s) (animal) Z18.31
  - stone Z18.83
  - tooth (teeth) Z18.32
  - wood Z18.33

Retardation
- development, developmental, specific—*see* Disorder, developmental
- growth R62.50
  - due to malnutrition E45
- mental—*see* Disability, intellectual
- motor function, specific F82
- physical (child) R62.52
  - due to malnutrition E45
- reading (specific) F81.0
- spelling (specific) (without reading disorder) F81.81

Retching—*see* Vomiting

Retention—*see also* Retained
- cyst—*see* Cyst
- dead
  - fetus (at or near term) (mother) O36.4
- deciduous tooth K00.6
- fetus
  - dead O36.4
- fluid R60.9
- foreign body
  - current trauma—*code as* Foreign body, by site or type
- menses N94.89
- urine R33.9
  - psychogenic F45.8

Reticulocytosis R70.1

Reticulohistiocytoma (giant-cell) D76.3

Reticulosis (skin)
- hemophagocytic, familial D76.1

Retina, retinal—*see also* Disease, diseased

Retinoblastoma C69.2-
- differentiated C69.2-
- undifferentiated C69.2-

Retinopathy (background) H35.00
- of prematurity H35.10-
  - stage 0 H35.11-
  - stage 1 H35.12-
  - stage 2 H35.13-
  - stage 3 H35.14-
  - stage 4 H35.15-
  - stage 5 H35.16-

Retractile testis Q55.22

Retraction
- nipple N64.53
  - associated with
  - congenital Q83.8

Retrograde menstruation N92.5

Retrosternal thyroid (congenital) Q89.2

Retroversion, retroverted
- testis (congenital) Q55.29

Rett's disease or syndrome F84.2

Rh (factor)
- hemolytic disease (newborn) P55.0
- incompatibility, immunization or sensitization
  - affecting management of pregnancy NEC O36.09-
    - anti-D antibody O36.01-

Rh, *continued*
  - newborn P55.0
  - transfusion reaction—*see* Complication(s), transfusion, incompatibility reaction
- negative mother affecting newborn P55.0
- titer elevated—*see* Complication(s), transfusion, incompatibility reaction
- transfusion reaction—*see* Complication(s), transfusion, incompatibility reaction

Rhabdomyolysis (idiopathic) NEC M62.82

Rheumatic (acute) (subacute)
- chronic I09.89
- coronary arteritis I01.8
- fever (acute)—*see* Fever, rheumatic
- heart—*see* Disease, heart, rheumatic
- myocardial degeneration—*see* Degeneration, myocardium
- myocarditis (chronic) (inactive) (with chorea) I09.0
  - active or acute I01.2
  - with chorea (acute) (rheumatic) (Sydenham's) I02.0
- pancarditis, acute I01.8
  - with chorea (acute) (rheumatic) Sydenham's) I02.0
- pericarditis (active) (acute) (with effusion) (with pneumonia) I01.0
  - with chorea (acute) (rheumatic) (Sydenham's) I02.0
  - chronic or inactive I09.2
- pneumonia I00 *[J17]*
- torticollis M43.6

Rheumatism (articular) (neuralgic) (nonarticular) M79.0
- intercostal, meaning Tietze's disease M94.0
- sciatic M54.4-

Rhinitis (atrophic) (catarrhal) (chronic) (croupous) (fibrinous) (granulomatous) (hyperplastic) (hypertrophic) (membranous) (obstructive) (purulent) (suppurative) (ulcerative) J31.0
- with
  - sore throat—*see* Nasopharyngitis
- acute J00
- allergic J30.9
  - with asthma J45.909
    - with
      - ~ exacerbation (acute) J45.901
      - ~ status asthmaticus J45.902
  - due to
    - food J30.5
    - pollen J30.1
  - nonseasonal J30.89
  - perennial J30.89
  - seasonal NEC J30.2
  - specified NEC J30.89
- infective J00
- pneumococcal J00
- vasomotor J30.0

Rhinoantritis (chronic)—*see* Sinusitis, maxillary

Rhinolith (nasal sinus) J34.89

Rhinomegaly J34.89

Rhinopharyngitis (acute) (subacute)—*see also* Nasopharyngitis

Rhinorrhea J34.89
- cerebrospinal (fluid) G96.01
  - postoperative G96.08
  - specified NEC G96.08
  - spontaneous G96.01
  - traumatic G96.08
- paroxysmal—*see* Rhinitis, allergic
- spasmodic—*see* Rhinitis, allergic

Rhinovirus infection NEC B34.8

Rhizomelic chondrodysplasia punctata E71.540

Rhythm
- disorder I49.9
- escape I49.9
- heart, abnormal I49.9
- idioventricular I44.2
- sleep, inversion G47.2-

Rhytidosis facialis L98.8

Rickets (active) (acute) (adolescent) (chest wall) (congenital) (current) (infantile) (intestinal) E55.0
- celiac K90.0
- hypophosphatemic with nephrotic-glycosuric dwarfism E72.09

Rickettsial disease A79.9
- specified type NEC A79.89

Rickettsialpox (rickettsia akari) A79.1

Rickettsiosis A79.9
- due to
  - Rickettsia akari (rickettsialpox) A79.1
- specified type NEC A79.89
- tick-borne A77.9
- vesicular A79.1

Riedel's
- struma, thyroiditis or disease E06.5

Riehl's melanosis L81.4

Rietti-Greppi-Micheli anemia D56.9

Rieux's hernia—*see* Hernia

Riga (-Fede) **disease** K14.0

Right middle lobe syndrome J98.11

Rigid, rigidity—*see also* Disease, diseased
- abdominal R19.30
  - with severe abdominal pain R10.0
- nuchal R29.1

Rigors R68.89
- with fever R50.9

Ringworm B35.9
- beard B35.0
- black dot B35.0
- body B35.4
- corporeal B35.4
- foot B35.3
- groin B35.6
- hand B35.2
- honeycomb B35.0
- nails B35.1
- perianal (area) B35.6
- scalp B35.0
- specified NEC B35.8

Risk
- for
  - dental caries Z91.849
    - high Z91.843
    - low Z91.841
    - moderate Z91.842
  - suicidal
    - meaning personal history of attempted suicide Z91.5
    - meaning suicidal ideation—*see* Ideation, suicidal

Ritter's disease L00

Robert's pelvis Q74.2

Robin (-Pierre) syndrome Q87.0

Robinow-Silvermann-Smith syndrome Q87.19

Rocky Mountain (spotted) **fever** A77.0

Roger's disease Q21.0

Rolando's fracture (displaced) S62.22-
- nondisplaced S62.22-

Romano-Ward (prolonged QT interval) **syndrome** I45.81

Romberg's disease or syndrome G51.8

Roof, mouth—*see* Disease, diseased

Rosary, rachitic E55.0

Rose
- cold J30.1
- fever J30.1
- rash R21
  - epidemic B06.9

Rosenthal's disease or syndrome D68.1

Roseola B09
- infantum B08.20
  - due to human herpesvirus 6 B08.21
  - due to human herpesvirus 7 B08.22

Rossbach's disease K31.89
- psychogenic F45.8

Rothmund (-Thomson) syndrome Q82.8

Rotor's disease or syndrome E80.6

Round
- worms (large) (infestation) NEC B82.0
  - Ascariasis (*see also* Ascariasis) B77.9

Rubella (German measles) B06.9
- complication NEC B06.09
  - neurological B06.00
- congenital P35.0
- contact Z20.4
- exposure to Z20.4
- maternal
  - care for (suspected) damage to fetus O35.3
  - manifest rubella in infant P35.0
  - suspected damage to fetus affecting management of pregnancy O35.3
- specified complications NEC B06.89

Rubeola (meaning measles)—*see* Measles
- meaning rubella—*see* Rubella

Rudimentary (congenital)—*see also* Agenesis
- bone Q79.9

Ruled out condition—*see* Observation, suspected

Rumination R11.10
- with nausea R11.2
- disorder of infancy F98.21
- neurotic F42.8
- newborn P92.1
- obsessional F42.8
- psychogenic F42.8

Runny nose R09.89

Rupture, ruptured
- abscess (spontaneous)—*code by* site under Abscess
- aorta, aortic I71.8
  - valve or cusp (*see also* Endocarditis, aortic) I35.8
- appendix (with peritonitis) K35.32
  - with localized peritonitis K35.32
- arteriovenous fistula, brain I60.8-
- cardiac (auricle) (ventricle) (wall) I23.3
  - with hemopericardium I23.0
  - infectional I40.9
- cecum (with peritonitis) K65.0
  - with peritoneal abscess K35.33
- cerebral aneurysm (congenital) (*see* Hemorrhage, intracranial, subarachnoid)
- circle of Willis I60.6
- corpus luteum (infected) (ovary) N83.1-
- cyst—*see* Cyst
- ear drum (nontraumatic)—*see also* Perforation, tympanum
  - traumatic S09.2-
- fallopian tube NEC (nonobstetric) (nontraumatic) N83.8
  - due to pregnancy O00.10
- gastric
  - vessel K92.2
- graafian follicle (hematoma) N83.0-
- hymen (nontraumatic) (nonintentional) N89.8
- kidney (traumatic) birth injury P15.8
- meningeal artery I60.8-
- ovary, ovarian N83.8
  - corpus luteum cyst N83.1-
  - follicle (graafian) N83.0-
- oviduct (nonobstetric) (nontraumatic) N83.8
  - due to pregnancy O00.10
- pulmonary
  - valve (heart) I37.8
- rotator cuff (nontraumatic) M75.10-
  - complete M75.12-
  - incomplete M75.11-
- spleen (traumatic) S36.03-
  - birth injury P15.1
- tonsil J35.8
- traumatic
  - spleen S36.03-
- tricuspid (heart) (valve) I07.8
- tube, tubal (nonobstetric) (nontraumatic) N83.8
  - abscess—*see* Salpingitis
  - due to pregnancy O00.10
- tympanum, tympanic (membrane) (nontraumatic) (*see also* Perforation, tympanic membrane) H72.9-
  - traumatic—*see* Rupture, ear drum, traumatic
- viscus R19.8

Russell-Silver syndrome Q87.19

Ruvalcaba-Myhre-Smith syndrome E71.440

Rytand-Lipsitch syndrome I44.2

S

Saccharomyces infection B37.9

Sachs' amaurotic familial idiocy or disease E75.02

Sachs-Tay disease E75.02

Sacks-Libman disease M32.11

Sacralgia M53.3

Sacrodynia M53.3

Saint
- Anthony's fire—*see* Erysipelas

Salmonella—*see* Infection, Salmonella

Salmonellosis A02.0

Salpingitis (catarrhal) (fallopian tube) (nodular) (pseudofollicular) (purulent) (septic) N70.91
- with oophoritis N70.93
- acute N70.01
  - with oophoritis N70.03
- chlamydial A56.11
- chronic N70.11
  - with oophoritis N70.13
- gonococcal (acute) (chronic) A54.24
- specific (gonococcal) (acute) (chronic) A54.24
- venereal (gonococcal) (acute) (chronic) A54.24

Salpingo-oophoritis (catarrhal) (purulent) (ruptured) (septic) (suppurative) N70.93
- acute N70.03
  - gonococcal A54.24
- chronic N70.13
- gonococcal (acute) (chronic) A54.24
- specific (gonococcal) (acute) (chronic) A54.24
- venereal (gonococcal) (acute) (chronic) A54.24

Sandhoff's disease E75.01

Sanfilippo (Type B) (Type C) (Type D) syndrome E76.22

Sanger-Brown ataxia G11.2

Sao Paulo fever or typhus A77.0

Sarcoepiplocele—*see* Hernia

Sarcoepiplomphalocele Q79.2

Sarcoid—*see also* Sarcoidosis
- arthropathy D86.86
- Boeck's D86.9
- Darier-Roussy D86.3
- iridocyclitis D86.83
- meningitis D86.81
- myocarditis D86.85
- myositis D86.87
- pyelonephritis D86.84

Sarcoidosis D86.9
- with
  - cranial nerve palsies D86.82
  - hepatic granuloma D86.89
  - polyarthritis D86.86
  - tubulo-interstitial nephropathy D86.84
- combined sites NEC D86.89
- lung D86.0
  - and lymph nodes D86.2
- lymph nodes D86.1
  - and lung D86.2
- meninges D86.81
- skin D86.3
- specified type NEC D86.89

Sarcoma (of)—*see also* Neoplasm, connective tissue, malignant in Table of Neoplasms in the complete *ICD-10-CM* manual
- cerebellar C71.6
  - circumscribed (arachnoidal) C71.6
- circumscribed (arachnoidal) cerebellar C71.6
- clear cell—*see also* Neoplasm, connective tissue, malignant in Table of Neoplasms in the complete *ICD-10-CM* manual
  - kidney C64.-
- monstrocellular
  - specified site—*see* Neoplasm, malignant, by site in Table of Neoplasms in the complete *ICD-10-CM* manual
  - unspecified site C71.9

SBE (subacute bacterial endocarditis) I33.0

Scabies (any site) B86

Scaglietti-Dagnini syndrome E22.0

Scald—*see* Burn

Scapulohumeral myopathy G71.02

Scar, scarring (*see also* Cicatrix) L90.5
- adherent L90.5
- atrophic L90.5
- cheloid L91.0
- hypertrophic L91.0
- keloid L91.0
- painful L90.5
- vagina N89.8
  - postoperative N99.2
- vulva N90.89

Scarabiasis B88.2

Scarlatina (anginosa) (maligna) A38.9
- myocarditis (acute) A38.1
  - old—*see* Myocarditis
- otitis media A38.0
- ulcerosa A38.8

Scarlet fever (albuminuria) (angina) A38.9

Schaumann's
- benign lymphogranulomatosis D86.1
- disease or syndrome—*see* Sarcoidosis

Schistosomiasis B65.9
- cutaneous B65.3

Schizencephaly Q04.6

Schizophrenia, schizophrenic
- childhood type F84.5
- syndrome of childhood F84.5

Schlatter-Osgood disease or osteochondrosis M92.52-

Schlatter's tibia M92.52-

Schmorl's disease or nodes
- sacrococcygeal region M53.3

Schönlein (-Henoch) disease or purpura (primary) (rheumatic) D69.0

Schultze's type acroparesthesia, simple I73.89

Schwannomatosis Q85.03

Schwartz-Bartter syndrome E22.2

Sciatica (infective)
- with lumbago M54.4-

Scleredema
- newborn P83.0

Sclerema (adiposum) (edematosum) (neonatorum) (newborn) P83.0

Sclerocystic ovary syndrome E28.2

Scleroderma, sclerodermia (acrosclerotic) (diffuse) (generalized) (progressive) (pulmonary) (*see also* Sclerosis)
- newborn P83.88

Sclérose en plaques G35

Sclerosis, sclerotic
- ascending multiple G35
- brain (generalized) (lobular) G37.9
  - disseminated G35
  - insular G35
  - miliary G35
  - multiple G35
  - stem, multiple G35
  - tuberous Q85.1
- bulbar, multiple G35
- cerebrospinal (disseminated) (multiple) G35
- disseminated G35
- dorsal G35
- extrapyramidal G25.9
- Friedreich's (spinal cord) G11.11
- hereditary
  - spinal (Friedreich's ataxia) G11.11
- hippocampal G93.81
- insular G35
- mesial temporal G93.81
- mitral I05.8
- multiple (brain stem) (cerebral) (generalized) (spinal cord) G35
- plaques G35
- pulmonary
  - artery I27.0
- spinal (cord) (progressive) G95.89
  - hereditary (Friedreich's) (mixed form) G11.11
- temporal (mesial) G93.81

Sclerosis, sclerotic, *continued*
- tricuspid (heart) (valve) I07.8
- tuberous (brain) Q85.1

Scoliosis (acquired) (postural) M41.9
- adolescent (idiopathic)—*see* Scoliosis, idiopathic, juvenile
- congenital Q67.5
  - due to bony malformation Q76.3
- idiopathic M41.20
  - adolescent M41.129
    - cervical region M41.122
    - cervicothoracic region M41.123
    - lumbar region M41.126
    - lumbosacral region M41.127
    - thoracic region M41.124
    - thoracolumbar region M41.125
  - cervical region M41.22
  - cervicothoracic region M41.23
  - infantile M41.00
    - cervical region M41.02
    - cervicothoracic region M41.03
    - lumbar region M41.06
    - lumbosacral region M41.07
    - sacrococcygeal region M41.08
    - thoracic region M41.04
    - thoracolumbar region M41.05
  - juvenile M41.119
    - cervical region M41.112
    - cervicothoracic region M41.113
    - lumbar region M41.116
    - lumbosacral region M41.117
    - thoracic region M41.114
    - thoracolumbar region M41.115
  - lumbar M41.26
    - lumbosacral M41.27
    - thoracic M41.24
    - thoracolumbar M41.25
- sciatic M54.4-

Scratch—*see* Abrasion

Scratchy throat R09.89

Screening (for) Z13.9
- alcoholism Z13.89
- anemia Z13.0
- autism Z13.41
- behavioral disorders Z13.30
- cardiovascular disorder Z13.6
- chlamydial diseases Z11.8
- chromosomal abnormalities (nonprocreative) NEC Z13.79
- congenital
  - dislocation of hip Z13.89
  - eye disorder Z13.5
  - malformation or deformation Z13.89
- cystic fibrosis Z13.228
- depression (adult) (adolescent) (child) Z13.31
  - maternal or perinatal Z13.32
- developmental
  - delays Z13.40
    - global (milestones) Z13.42
    - specified NEC Z13.49
  - handicap Z13.42
    - in early childhood Z13.42
- diabetes mellitus Z13.1
- disability, intellectual Z13.39
  - infant Z13.41
- disease or disorder Z13.9
  - bacterial NEC Z11.2
    - intestinal infectious Z11.0
    - respiratory tuberculosis Z11.1
  - behavioral Z13.30
    - specified NEC Z13.49
  - blood or blood-forming organ Z13.0
  - cardiovascular Z13.6
  - chlamydial Z11.8
  - dental Z13.89
  - developmental delays Z13.40
    - global (milestones) Z13.42
    - specified NEC Z13.49
  - endocrine Z13.29
  - heart Z13.6
  - human immunodeficiency virus (HIV) infection Z11.4
  - immunity Z13.0
  - infectious Z11.9

Screening, *continued*
- mental health and behavioral Z13.30
- metabolic Z13.228
- neurological Z13.89
- nutritional Z13.21
  - metabolic Z13.228
    - lipid disorders Z13.220
- respiratory Z13.83
- rheumatic Z13.828
- rickettsial Z11.8
- sexually-transmitted NEC Z11.3
  - human immunodeficiency virus (HIV) Z11.4
- sickle cell trait Z13.0
- spirochetal Z11.8
- thyroid Z13.29
- venereal Z11.3
- viral NEC Z11.59
  - human immunodeficiency virus (HIV) Z11.4
- elevated titer Z13.89
- galactosemia Z13.228
- gonorrhea Z11.3
- hematopoietic malignancy Z12.89
- hemoglobinopathies Z13.0
- Hodgkin disease Z12.89
- human immunodeficiency virus (HIV) Z11.4
- human papillomavirus (HPV) Z11.51
- hypertension Z13.6
- immunity disorders Z13.0
- infant or child (over 28 days old) Z00.12-
- infection
  - mycotic Z11.8
  - parasitic Z11.8
- intellectual disability Z13.39
- leukemia Z12.89
- lymphoma Z12.89
- malaria Z11.6
- measles Z11.59
- mental health disorder Z13.30
- metabolic errors, inborn Z13.228
- musculoskeletal disorder Z13.828
- mycoses Z11.8
- neoplasm (malignant) (of) Z12.9
  - blood Z12.89
  - breast Z12.39
    - routine mammogram Z12.31
  - cervix Z12.4
  - hematopoietic system Z12.89
  - lymph (glands) Z12.89
  - nervous system Z12.82
- nephropathy Z13.89
- nervous system disorders NEC Z13.858
- neurological condition Z13.89
- parasitic infestation Z11.9
  - specified NEC Z11.8
- phenylketonuria Z13.228
- poisoning (chemical) (heavy metal) Z13.88
- postnatal, chromosomal abnormalities Z13.89
- rheumatoid arthritis Z13.828
- sexually-transmitted disease NEC Z11.3
  - human immunodeficiency virus (HIV) Z11.4
- sickle-cell disease or trait Z13.0
- special Z13.9
  - specified NEC Z13.89
- syphilis Z11.3
- traumatic brain injury Z13.850
- tuberculosis, respiratory
  - active Z11.1
  - latent Z11.7
- venereal disease Z11.3
- viral encephalitis (mosquito- or tick-borne) Z11.59
- whooping cough Z11.2

Scrofula, scrofulosis (tuberculosis of cervical lymph glands) A18.2

Scurvy, scorbutic
- anemia D53.2
- rickets E55.0 /M90.80/

Seasickness T75.3

Seatworm (infection) (infestation) B80

Seborrhea, seborrheic L21.9
- capillitii R23.8
- capitis L21.0

Seborrhea, seborrheic, *continued*
- dermatitis L21.9
  - infantile L21.1
- eczema L21.9
  - infantile L21.1
- sicca L21.0

Seckel's syndrome Q87.19

Second hand tobacco smoke exposure (acute) (chronic) Z77.22
- in the perinatal period P96.81

Secretion
- antidiuretic hormone, inappropriate E22.2
- hormone
  - antidiuretic, inappropriate (syndrome) E22.2
- urinary
  - excessive R35.8
  - suppression R34

Seitelberger's syndrome (infantile neuraxonal dystrophy) G31.89

Seizure(s) (*see also* Convulsions) R56.9
- akinetic—*see* Epilepsy, generalized, specified NEC
- atonic—*see* Epilepsy, generalized, specified NEC
- convulsive—*see* Convulsions
- disorder (*see also* Epilepsy) G40.909
- epileptic—*see* Epilepsy
- febrile (simple) R56.00
  - with status epilepticus G40.901
  - complex (atypical) (complicated) R56.01
    - with status epilepticus G40.901
- newborn P90
- nonspecific epileptic
  - atonic—*see* Epilepsy, generalized, specified NEC
  - clonic—*see* Epilepsy, generalized, specified NEC
  - myoclonic—*see* Epilepsy, generalized, specified NEC
  - tonic—*see* Epilepsy, generalized, specified NEC
  - tonic-clonic—*see* Epilepsy, generalized, specified NEC
- partial, developing into secondarily generalized seizures
  - complex—*see* Epilepsy, localization-related, symptomatic, with complex partial seizures
  - simple—*see* Epilepsy, localization-related, symptomatic
- post traumatic R56.1
- recurrent G40.909
- specified NEC G40.89

Self-damaging behavior (life-style) Z72.89

Self-harm (attempted)
- history (personal) Z91.5
  - in family Z81.8

Self-mutilation (attempted)
- history (personal) Z91.5
  - in family Z81.8

Self-poisoning
- history (personal) Z91.5
  - in family Z81.8
- observation following (alleged) attempt Z03.6

Semicoma R40.1

Sensitive, sensitivity—*see also* Allergy
- child (excessive) F93.8
- cold, autoimmune D59.12
- dentin K03.89
- gluten (non-celiac) K90.41
- methemoglobin D74.8
- tuberculin, without clinical or radiological symptoms R76.11

Sensitization, auto-erythrocytic D69.2

Separation
- anxiety, abnormal (of childhood) F93.0
- apophysis, traumatic—*code as* Fracture, by site
- epiphysis, epiphyseal
  - nontraumatic—*see also* Osteochondropathy
    - upper femoral—*see* Slipped, epiphysis, upper femoral
  - traumatic—*code as* Fracture, by site

Sepsis (generalize) (unspecified organism) A41.9
- with
  - organ dysfunction (acute) (multiple) R65.20
    - with septic shock R65.21
- anaerobic A41.4

Sepsis, *continued*
- candidal B37.7
- cryptogenic A41.9
- due to device, implant or graft T85.79
  - catheter NEC T85.79
    - dialysis (renal) T82.7
    - infusion NEC T82.7
    - urethral indwelling T83.511
    - urinary T83.518
  - vascular T82.7
- Enterococcus A41.81
- Escherichia coli (E. coli) A41.51
- following
  - immunization T88.0
  - infusion, therapeutic injection or transfusion NEC T80.29
- gangrenous A41.9
- Gram-negative (organism) A41.5-
  - anaerobic A41.4
- Haemophilus influenzae A41.3
- localized—code to specific localized infection
  - in operation wound T81.49
  - postprocedural T81.44
- meningeal—*see* Meningitis
- meningococcal A39.4
  - acute A39.2
  - chronic A39.3
- MSSA (Methicillin susceptible Staphylococcus aureus) A41.01
- newborn P36.9
  - due to
    - anaerobes NEC P36.5
    - Escherichia coli P36.4
    - Staphylococcus P36.30
      - aureus P36.2
      - specified NEC P36.39
    - Streptococcus P36.10
      - group B P36.0
      - specified NEC P36.19
  - specified NEC P36.8
- Pasteurella multocida A28.0
- pneumococcal A40.3
- severe R65.20
  - with septic shock R65.21
- Shigella (*see also* Dysentery, bacillary) A03.9
- skin, localized—*see* Abscess
- specified organism NEC A41.89
- Staphylococcus, staphylococcal A41.2
  - aureus (methicillin susceptible) (MSSA) A41.01
    - methicillin resistant (MRSA) A41.02
  - coagulase-negative A41.1
  - specified NEC A41.1
- Streptococcus, streptococcal A40.9
  - group
    - D A41.81
  - neonatal P36.10
    - group B P36.0
    - specified NEC P36.19
  - pneumoniae A40.3

Septic—*see* Disease, diseased
- gallbladder (acute) K81.0
- sore—*see also* Abscess
  - throat J02.0
    - streptococcal J02.0
- tonsils, chronic J35.01
  - with adenoiditis J35.03

Septicemia A41.9
- meaning sepsis—*see* Sepsis

Septum, septate (congenital)—*see also* Anomaly, by site
- anal Q42.3
  - with fistula Q42.2
- aqueduct of Sylvius Q03.0
  - with spina bifida—*see* Spina bifida, by site, with hydrocephalus
- uterus Q51.2-
- vaginal, longitudinal Q52.129
  - microperforate
    - left side Q52.124
    - right side Q52.123
  - nonobstructing Q52.120
  - obstructing

Septum, septate, *continued*
    - left side Q52.122
    - right side Q52.121

Sequelae (of)—*see also* Disease, diseased
- encephalitis or encephalomyelitis (conditions in G04) G09
  - in infectious disease NEC B94.8
  - viral B94.1
- hepatitis, viral B94.2
- infectious disease B94.9
  - specified NEC B94.8
- parasitic disease B94.9
- viral
  - encephalitis B94.1
  - hepatitis B94.2

Serology for syphilis
- doubtful
  - with signs or symptoms—*code by* site and stage under Syphilis
- reactivated A53.0
- positive A53.0

Serositis, multiple K65.8
- pericardial I31.1

Serum
- allergy, allergic reaction (*see also* Reaction, serum) T80.69
  - shock (*see also* Shock, anaphylactic) T80.59
- arthritis (*see also* Reaction, serum) T80.69
- complication or reaction NEC (*see also* Reaction, serum) T80.69
- disease NEC (*see also* Reaction, serum) T80.69
- hepatitis—*see also* Hepatitis, viral, type B
  - carrier (suspected) of B18.1
- intoxication (*see also* Reaction, serum) T80.69
- neuritis (*see also* Reaction, serum) T80.69
- poisoning NEC (*see also* Reaction, serum) T80.69
- rash NEC (*see also* Reaction, serum) T80.69
- reaction NEC (*see also* Reaction, serum) T80.69
- sickness NEC (*see also* Reaction, serum) T80.69
- urticaria (*see also* Reaction, serum) T80.69

Severe sepsis R65.20
- with septic shock R65.21

Sexual
- immaturity (female) (male) E30.0
- precocity (constitutional) (cryptogenic) (female) (idiopathic) (male) E30.1

Shadow lung R91.8

Shedding
- nail L60.8
- premature, primary (deciduous) teeth K00.6

Sheehan's disease or syndrome E23.0

Shelf, rectal K62.89

Shellshock (current) F43.0
- lasting state—*see* Disorder, post-traumatic stress

Shigellosis A03.9
- Group A A03.0
- Group B A03.1
- Group C A03.2
- Group D A03.3

Shock R57.9
- adverse food reaction (anaphylactic)—*see* Shock, anaphylactic, due to food
- allergic—*see* Shock, anaphylactic
- anaphylactic T78.2
  - chemical—*see* Table of Drugs and Chemicals
  - due to drug or medicinal substance
    - correct substance properly administered T88.6-
    - overdose or wrong substance given or taken (by accident)—*see* Table of Drugs and Chemicals, by drug, poisoning
  - due to food (nonpoisonous) T78.00
    - additives T78.06
    - dairy products T78.07
    - eggs T78.08
    - fish T78.03
      - shellfish T78.02
    - fruit T78.04
    - milk T78.07

Shock, *continued*
    - nuts T78.05
      - peanuts T78.01
    - peanuts T78.01
    - seeds T78.05
    - specified type NEC T78.09
    - vegetable T78.04
  - following sting(s)—*see* Table of Drugs and Chemicals, by animal or substance, poisoning
  - immunization T80.52-
  - serum T80.59-
    - blood and blood products T80.51-
    - immunization T80.52-
    - specified NEC T80.59-
    - vaccination T80.52-
- anaphylactoid—*see* Shock, anaphylactic
- cardiogenic R57.0
- chemical substance—*see* Table of Drugs and Chemicals
- culture—*see* Disorder, adjustment
- drug
  - due to correct substance properly administered T88.6
  - overdose or wrong substance given or taken (by accident)—*see* Table of Drugs and Chemicals, by drug, poisoning
- electric T75.4
  - (taser) T75.4
- endotoxic R65.21
  - postprocedural (during or resulting from a procedure, not elsewhere classified) T81.12-
- following
  - injury (immediate) (delayed) T79.4
- food (anaphylactic)—*see* Shock, anaphylactic, due to food
- from electroshock gun (taser) T75.4
- gram-negative R65.21
  - postprocedural (during or resulting from a procedure, NEC) T81.12
- hematologic R57.8
- hemorrhagic R57.8
  - surgery (intraoperative) (postoperative) T81.19
  - trauma T79.4
- hypovolemic R57.1
  - surgical T81.19
  - traumatic T79.4
- insulin E15
  - therapeutic misadventure—*see* subcategory T38.3
- kidney N17.0
- lung J80
- pleural (surgical) T81.19
  - due to trauma T79.4
- postprocedural (postoperative) T81.10
  - cardiogenic T81.11
  - endotoxic T81.12-
  - gram-negative T81.12-
  - hypovolemic T81.19
  - septic T81.12-
  - specified type NEC T81.19
- psychic F43.0
- septic (due to severe sepsis) R65.21
- specified NEC R57.8
- surgical T81.10
- taser gun (taser) T75.4
- therapeutic misadventure NEC T81.10
- toxic, syndrome A48.3
- transfusion—*see* Complications, transfusion
- traumatic (immediate) (delayed) T79.4

Short, shortening, shortness
- arm (acquired)—*see also* Deformity, limb length
  - congenital Q71.81-
- breath R06.02
- bowel syndrome K91.2
- common bile duct, congenital Q44.5
- cystic duct, congenital Q44.5
- frenum, frenulum, linguae (congenital) Q38.1
- hip (acquired)—*see also* Deformity, limb
  - congenital Q65.89
- leg (acquired)—*see also* Deformity, limb
  - congenital Q72.81-
- lower limb (acquired)—*see also* Deformity, limb
  - congenital Q72.81-
- rib syndrome Q77.2

Short, shortening, shortness, *continued*
- stature (child) (hereditary) (idiopathic) NEC R62.52
  - constitutional E34.3
  - due to endocrine disorder E34.3
  - Laron-type E34.3
- tendon—*see also* Contraction
  - with contracture of joint—*see* Contraction, joint
  - Achilles (acquired) M67.0-
    - congenital Q66.89
  - congenital Q79.8

Shunt
- arterial-venous (dialysis) Z99.2
- arteriovenous, pulmonary (acquired) I28.0
  - congenital Q25.72
- cerebral ventricle (communicating) in situ Z98.2

Sialitis, silitis (any gland) (chronic) (suppurative)—*see* Sialoadenitis

Sialoadenitis (any gland) (periodic) (suppurative) K11.20
- acute K11.21
  - recurrent K11.22
- chronic K11.23

Sialidosis E77.1

Sibling rivalry Z62.891

Sicard's syndrome G52.7

Sick R69
- or handicapped person in family Z63.79
  - needing care at home Z63.6
- sinus (syndrome) I49.5

Sickle-cell
- anemia—*see* Disease, sickle-cell
- beta plus—*see* Disease, sickle-cell, thalassemia, beta plus
- beta zero—*see* Disease, sickle-cell, thalassemia, beta zero
- trait D57.3

Sicklemia—*see also* Disease, sickle-cell
- trait D57.3

Sickness
- air (travel) T75.3
- airplane T75.3
- car T75.3
- green D50.8
- milk—*see* Poisoning, food, noxious
- motion T75.3
- mountain T70.29
  - acute D75.1
- protein (*see also* Reaction, serum) T80.69
- roundabout (motion) T75.3
- sea T75.3
- serum NEC (*see also* Reaction, serum) T80.69
- swing (motion) T75.3
- train (railway) (travel) T75.3
- travel (any vehicle) T75.3

Siemens' syndrome (ectodermal dysplasia) Q82.8

Sighing R06.89
- psychogenic F45.8

Sigmoiditis (*see also* Enteritis) K52.9
- infectious A09
- noninfectious K52.9

Silver's syndrome Q87.19

Simple, simplex—*see* Disease, diseased

Simulation, conscious (of illness) Z76.5

Single
- atrium Q21.2
- umbilical artery Q27.0

Sinus—*see also* Fistula
- bradycardia R00.1
- dermal (congenital) Q06.8
  - with abscess Q06.8
- pilonidal (infected) (rectum) L05.92
  - with abscess L05.02
- preauricular Q18.1
- tachycardia R00.0
  - paroxysmal I47.1
- tarsi syndrome—M25.57-

Sinusitis (accessory) (chronic) (hyperplastic) (nasal) (nonpurulent) (purulent) J32.9
- acute J01.90
  - ethmoidal J01.20
    - recurrent J01.21
  - frontal J01.10
    - recurrent J01.11
  - involving more than one sinus, other than pansinusitis J01.80
    - recurrent J01.81
  - maxillary J01.00
    - recurrent J01.01
  - pansinusitis J01.40
    - recurrent J01.41
  - recurrent J01.91
  - specified NEC J01.80
    - recurrent J01.81
  - sphenoidal J01.30
    - recurrent J01.31
- allergic—*see* Rhinitis, allergic
- ethmoidal J32.2
  - acute J01.20
    - recurrent J01.21
- frontal J32.1
  - acute J01.10
    - recurrent J01.11
- influenzal—*see* Influenza, with, respiratory manifestations NEC
- involving more than one sinus but not pansinusitis J32.8
  - acute J01.80
    - recurrent J01.81
- maxillary J32.0
  - acute J01.00
    - recurrent J01.01
- sphenoidal J32.3
  - acute J01.30
    - recurrent J01.31

Sinusitis-bronchiectasis-situs inversus (syndrome) (triad) Q89.3

Siriasis T67.01

Situation, psychiatric F99

Situational
- disturbance (transient)—*see* Disorder, adjustment
  - acute F43.0
- maladjustment—*see* Disorder, adjustment
- reaction—*see* Disorder, adjustment
  - acute F43.0

Situs inversus or transversus (abdominalis) (thoracis) Q89.3

Sixth disease B08.20
- due to human herpesvirus 6 B08.21
- due to human herpesvirus 7 B08.22

Sjögren-Larsson syndrome Q87.19

Skin—*see also* Disease, diseased
- clammy R23.1

Sleep
- disorder or disturbance G47.9
  - child F51.9
  - nonorganic origin F51.9
  - specified NEC G47.8
- disturbance G47.9
  - nonorganic origin F51.9
- drunkenness F51.9
- rhythm inversion G47.2-
- terrors F51.4
- walking F51.3
  - hysterical F44.89

Sleep-wake schedule disorder G47.20

Slim disease (in HIV infection) B20

Slipped, slipping
- epiphysis (traumatic)—*see also* Osteochondropathy
  - capital femoral (traumatic)
    - acute (on chronic) S79.01-
  - current traumatic—*code as* Fracture, by site
  - upper femoral (nontraumatic) M93.00-
    - acute M93.01-
      - on chronic M93.03-
    - chronic M93.02-
- ligature, umbilical P51.8

Slow
- feeding, newborn P92.2
- heart (beat) R00.1

Slowing, urinary stream R39.198

Small(ness)
- for gestational age—*see* Small for dates
- introitus, vagina N89.6
- kidney (unknown cause)
  - bilateral N27.1
  - unilateral N27.0
- ovary (congenital) Q50.39
- uterus N85.8
- white kidney N03.9

Small-and-light-for-dates—*see* Small for dates

Small-for-dates (infant) P05.10
- with weight of
  - 499 grams or less P05.11
  - 500–749 grams P05.12
  - 750–999 grams P05.13
  - 1000–1249 grams P05.14
  - 1250–1499 grams P05.15
  - 1500–1749 grams P05.16
  - 1750–1999 grams P05.17
  - 2000–2499 grams P05.18
  - 2500 grams and over P05.19

Smearing, fecal R15.1

SMEI (severe myoclonic epilepsy in infancy) G40.83-

Smith's fracture S52.54-

Smoker—*see* Dependence, drug, nicotine

Smoking
- passive Z77.22

Smothering spells R06.81

Sneezing (intractable) R06.7

Sniffing
- cocaine
  - abuse—*see* Abuse, drug, cocaine
  - dependence—*see* Dependence, drug, cocaine
- gasoline
  - abuse—*see* Abuse, drug, inhalant
  - dependence—*see* Dependence, drug, inhalant
- glue (airplane)
  - abuse—*see* Abuse, drug, inhalant
  - drug dependence—*see* Dependence, drug, inhalant

Sniffles
- newborn P28.89

Snoring R06.83

Snuffles (non-syphilitic) R06.5
- newborn P28.89

Social
- exclusion Z60.4
- migrant Z59.0
  - acculturation difficulty Z60.3
- skills inadequacy NEC Z73.4
- transplantation Z60.3

Sodoku A25.0

Softening
- brain (necrotic) (progressive) G93.89
  - congenital Q04.8
- cartilage M94.2-
  - patella M22.4-

Soldier's
- heart F45.8
- patches I31.0

Solitary
- cyst, kidney N28.1
- kidney, congenital Q60.0

Soor B37.0

Sore
- mouth K13.79
  - canker K12.0
- muscle M79.10
- skin L98.9
- throat (acute)—*see also* Pharyngitis
  - with influenza, flu, or grippe—*see* Influenza, with, respiratory manifestations NEC
  - chronic J31.2
  - coxsackie (virus) B08.5

Sore, *continued*
- herpesviral B00.2
- influenzal—*see* Influenza, with, respiratory manifestations NEC
- septic J02.0
- streptococcal (ulcerative) J02.0
- viral NEC J02.8
  - coxsackie B08.5

Soto's syndrome (cerebral gigantism) Q87.3

Spading nail L60.8
- congenital Q84.6

Spanish collar N47.1

Spasm(s), spastic, spasticity (*see also* Disease, diseased) R25.2
- artery I73.9
  - cerebral G45.9
- anus, ani (sphincter) (reflex) K59.4
  - psychogenic F45.8
- bladder (sphincter, external or internal) N32.89
  - psychogenic F45.8
- bronchus, bronchiole J98.01
- cerebral (arteries) (vascular) G45.9
- colon K58.9
  - with constipation K58.1
  - with diarrhea K58.0
  - mixed K58.2
  - other K58.8
  - psychogenic F45.8
- diaphragm (reflex) R06.6
  - psychogenic F45.8
- esophagus (diffuse) K22.4
  - psychogenic F45.8
- gastrointestinal (tract) K31.89
  - psychogenic F45.8
- glottis J38.5
  - hysterical F44.4
  - psychogenic F45.8
    - conversion reaction F44.4
  - reflex through recurrent laryngeal nerve J38.5
- habit—*see* Tic
- hysterical F44.4
- intestinal (*see also* Syndrome, irritable, bowel) K58.9
  - psychogenic F45.8
- larynx, laryngeal J38.5
  - hysterical F44.4
  - psychogenic F45.8
    - conversion reaction F44.4
- muscle NEC M62.838
  - back M62.830
- nerve, trigeminal G51.0
- nervous F45.8
- nodding F98.4
- oculogyric H51.8
  - psychogenic F45.8
- perineal, female N94.89
- pharynx (reflex) J39.2
  - hysterical F45.8
  - psychogenic F45.8
- psychogenic F45.8
- pylorus NEC K31.3
  - congenital or infantile Q40.0
  - psychogenic F45.8
- rectum (sphincter) K59.4
  - psychogenic F45.8
- sigmoid (*see also* Syndrome, irritable, bowel) K58.9
  - psychogenic F45.8
- stomach K31.89
  - neurotic F45.8
- throat J39.2
  - hysterical F45.8
  - psychogenic F45.8
- tic F95.9
  - chronic F95.1
  - transient of childhood F95.0
- urethra (sphincter) N35.919

Spasmodic—*see* Disease, diseased

Spasmus nutans F98.4

Spastic, spasticity—*see also* Spasm
- child (cerebral) (congenital) (paralysis) G80.1

Specific, specified—*see* Disease, diseased

Speech
- defect, disorder, disturbance, impediment R47.9
  - psychogenic, in childhood and adolescence F98.8
  - slurring R47.81
  - specified NEC R47.89

Spens' syndrome (syncope with heart block) I45.9

Spermatocele N43.40
- congenital Q55.4
- multiple N43.42
- single N43.41

Sphericity, increased, lens (congenital) Q12.4

Spherocytosis (congenital) (familial) (hereditary) D58.0
- hemoglobin disease D58.0
- sickle-cell (disease) D57.8-

Spherophakia Q12.4

Spider
- bite—*see* Table of Drugs and Chemicals, by animal or substance, poisoning
- fingers—*see* Syndrome, Marfan's
- nevus I78.1
- toes—*see* Syndrome, Marfan's
- vascular I78.1

Spiegler-Fendt
- benign lymphocytoma L98.8

Spina bifida (aperta) Q05.9
- with hydrocephalus NEC Q05.4
- cervical Q05.5
  - with hydrocephalus Q05.0
- dorsal Q05.6
  - with hydrocephalus Q05.1
- lumbar Q05.7
  - with hydrocephalus Q05.2
- lumbosacral Q05.7
  - with hydrocephalus Q05.2
- occulta Q76.0
- sacral Q05.8
  - with hydrocephalus Q05.3
- thoracic Q05.6
  - with hydrocephalus Q05.1
- thoracolumbar Q05.6
  - with hydrocephalus Q05.1

Spirillosis A25.0

Splenitis (interstitial) (malignant) (nonspecific) D73.89
- malarial (*see also* Malaria) B54 *[D77]*
- tuberculous A18.85

Splenomegaly, splenomegalia (Bengal) (cryptogenic) (idiopathic) (tropical) R16.1
- with hepatomegaly R16.2
- malarial (*see also* Malaria) B54 *[D77]*
- neutropenic D73.81

Spondylolisthesis (acquired) (degenerative) M43.1-
- congenital Q76.2

Spondylolysis (acquired) M43.0-
- congenital Q76.2

Spongioblastoma (any type)—*see* Neoplasm, malignant, by site in Table of Neoplasms in the complete *ICD-10-CM* manual
- specified site—*see* Neoplasm, malignant, by site in Table of Neoplasms in the complete *ICD-10-CM* manual
- unspecified site C71.9

Spongioneuroblastoma—*see* Neoplasm, malignant, by site in Table of Neoplasms in the complete *ICD-10-CM* manual

Sporadic—*see* Disease, diseased

Spots, spotting (in) (of)
- café au lait L81.3
- Cayenne pepper I78.1
- de Morgan's (senile angiomas) I78.1
- intermenstrual (regular) N92.0
  - irregular N92.1
- liver L81.4
- purpuric R23.3
- ruby I78.1

Sprain (joint) (ligament)
- ankle S93.40-
  - calcaneofibular ligament S93.41-
  - deltoid ligament S93.42-
  - internal collateral ligament S93.49-
  - specified ligament NEC S93.49-

Sprain (joint) (ligament), *continued*
- talofibular ligament S93.49-
- tibiofibular ligament S93.43-
- anterior longitudinal, cervical S13.4
- atlas, atlanto-axial, atlanto-occipital S13.4
- cervical, cervicodorsal, cervicothoracic S13.4
- elbow S53.40-
  - radial collateral ligament S53.43-
  - radiohumeral S53.41-
  - specified type NEC S53.49-
  - ulnar collateral ligament S53.44-
  - ulnohumeral S53.42-
- finger(s) S63.61-
  - index S63.61-
  - interphalangeal (joint) S63.63-
    - index S63.63-
    - little S63.63-
    - middle S63.63-
    - ring S63.63-
  - little S63.61-
  - middle S63.61-
  - ring S63.61-
  - metacarpophalangeal (joint) S63.65-
  - specified site NEC S63.69-
    - index S63.69-
    - little S63.69-
    - middle S63.69-
    - ring S63.69-
- foot S93.60-
  - specified ligament NEC S93.69-
  - tarsal ligament S93.61-
  - tarsometatarsal ligament S93.62-
- hand S63.9-
  - specified site NEC—*see* subcategory S63.8
- innominate
  - sacral junction S33.6
- jaw (articular disc) (cartilage) (meniscus) S03.4-
  - old M26.69
- knee S83.9-
  - collateral ligament S83.40-
    - lateral (fibular) S83.42-
    - medial (tibial) S83.41-
  - cruciate ligament S83.50-
    - anterior S83.51-
    - posterior S83.52-
- lumbar (spine) S33.5
- lumbosacral S33.9
- mandible (articular disc) S03.4-
  - old M26.69
- meniscus
  - jaw S03.4-
    - old M26.69
  - mandible S03.4
    - old M26.69
- neck S13.9
  - anterior longitudinal cervical ligament S13.4
  - atlanto-axial joint S13.4
  - atlanto-occipital joint S13.4
  - cervical spine S13.4
- pelvis NEC S33.8
- rotator cuff (capsule) S43.42-
- sacroiliac (region)
  - joint S33.6
- spine
  - cervical S13.4
  - lumbar S33.5
- symphysis
  - jaw S03.4-
    - old M26.69
  - mandibular S03.4-
    - old M26.69
- talofibular S93.49-
- tarsal—*see* Sprain, foot, specified site NEC
- tarsometatarsal—*see* Sprain, foot, specified site NEC
- temporomandibular S03.4-
  - old M26.69
- thumb S63.60-
  - interphalangeal (joint) S63.62-
  - metacarpophalangeal (joint) S63.64-
  - specified site NEC S63.68-
- toe(s) S93.50-
  - great S93.50-

Sprain (joint) (ligament), *continued*
- – interphalangeal joint S93.51-
  - ■ great S93.51-
  - ■ lesser S93.51-
  - – lesser S93.50-
  - – metatarsophalangeal joint S93.52-
    - ■ great S93.52-
    - ■ lesser S93.52-
- • wrist S63.50-
  - – carpal S63.51-
  - – radiocarpal S63.52-
  - – specified site NEC S63.59-

Sprengel's deformity (congenital) Q74.0

Sprue (tropical) K90.1
- • celiac K90.0
- • idiopathic K90.49
- • meaning thrush B37.0
- • nontropical K90.0

Spur, bone—*see also* Enthesopathy
- • iliac crest M76.2-
- • nose (septum) J34.89

Spurway's syndrome Q78.0

Sputum
- • abnormal (amount) (color) (odor) (purulent) R09.3
- • blood-stained R04.2
- • excessive (cause unknown) R09.3

Squashed nose M95.0
- • congenital Q67.4

SSADHD (succinic semialdehyde dehydrogenase deficiency) E72.81

St. Hubert's disease A82.9

Staggering gait R26.0
- • hysterical F44.4

Stain, staining
- • meconium (newborn) P96.83
- • port wine Q82.5

Stammering (*see also* Disorder, fluency) F80.81

Staphylitis (acute) (catarrhal) (chronic) (gangrenous) (membranous) (suppurative) (ulcerative) K12.2

Staphylococcal scalded skin syndrome L00

Staphylococcemia A41.2

Staphylococcus, staphylococcal—*see also* Disease, diseased
- • as cause of disease classified elsewhere B95.8
  - – aureus (methicillin susceptible) (MSSA) B95.61
    - ■ methicillin resistant (MRSA) B95.62
- • specified NEC, as the cause of disease classified elsewhere B95.7

Stasis
- • renal N19
  - – tubular N17.0

State (of)
- • agitated R45.1
  - – acute reaction to stress F43.0
- • compulsive F42.8
  - – mixed with obsessional thoughts F42.2
- • crisis F43.0
- • depressive F32.9
- • dissociative F44.9
- • neurotic F48.9
- • obsessional F42.8
- • panic F41.0
- • persistent vegetative R40.3
- • phobic F40.9
- • pregnant, incidental Z33.1
- • tension (mental) F48.9
  - – specified NEC F48.8
- • vegetative, persistent R40.3
- • withdrawal—*see* Withdrawal state

Status (post)—*see also* Presence (of)
- • absence, epileptic—*see* Epilepsy, by type, with status epilepticus
- • asthmaticus—*see* Asthma, by type, with, status asthmaticus
- • awaiting organ transplant Z76.82
- • colectomy (complete) (partial) Z90.49
- • colonization—*see* Carrier (suspected) of
- • delinquent immunization Z28.3

Status (post), *continued*
- • dialysis (hemodialysis) (peritoneal) Z99.2
- • do not resuscitate (DNR) Z66
- • epileptic, epilepticus (*see also* Epilepsy, by type, with status epilepticus) G40.901
- • gastrostomy Z93.1
- • human immunodeficiency virus (HIV) infection, asymptomatic Z21
- • lapsed immunization schedule Z28.3
- • nephrectomy (unilateral) (bilateral) Z90.5
- • pacemaker
  - – cardiac Z95.0
- • physical restraint Z78.1
- • postcommotio cerebri F07.81
- • postoperative (postprocedural) NEC Z98.890
- • postsurgical (postprocedural) NEC Z98.890
- • pregnant, incidental Z33.1
- • renal dialysis (hemodialysis) (peritoneal) Z99.2
- • retained foreign body—*see* Retained, foreign body fragments (type of)
- • shunt
  - – arteriovenous (for dialysis) Z99.2
  - – cerebrospinal fluid Z98.2
- • transplant—*see* Transplant
  - – organ removed Z98.85
- • underimmunization Z28.3
  - – ventricular (communicating) (for drainage) Z98.2

Stealing
- • child problem F91.8
  - – in company with others Z72.810

Steam burn—*see* Burn

Steatoma L72.3
- • eyelid (cystic)—*see* Dermatitis
  - – infected—*see* Hordeolum

Steatorrhea (chronic) K90.49
- • idiopathic (adult) (infantile) K90.9
- • primary K90.0

Stein-Leventhal syndrome E28.2

Stein's syndrome E28.2

Stenocephaly Q75.8

Stenosis, stenotic (cicatricial)—*see also* Stricture
- • anus, anal (canal) (sphincter) K62.4
  - – and rectum K62.4
  - – congenital Q42.3
    - ■ with fistula Q42.2
- • aorta (ascending) (supraventricular) (congenital) Q25.1
- • aortic (valve) I35.0
  - – with insufficiency I35.2
  - – congenital Q23.0
  - – rheumatic I06.0
    - ■ with
      - ~ incompetency, insufficiency or regurgitation I06.2
        - ◊ with mitral (valve) disease I08.0
          - » with tricuspid (valve) disease I08.3
      - ~ mitral (valve) disease I08.0
        - ◊ with tricuspid (valve) disease I08.3
      - ~ tricuspid (valve) disease I08.2
        - ◊ with mitral (valve) disease I08.3
  - – specified cause NEC I35.0
- • aqueduct of Sylvius (congenital) Q03.0
  - – with spina bifida—*see* Spina bifida, by site, with hydrocephalus
  - – acquired G91.1
- • bile duct (common) (hepatic) K83.1
  - – congenital Q44.3
- • brain G93.89
- • colon—*see also* Obstruction, intestine
  - – congenital Q42.9
    - ■ specified NEC Q42.8
- • common (bile) duct K83.1
  - – congenital Q44.3
- • heart valve (congenital) Q24.8
  - – aortic Q23.0
  - – pulmonary Q22.1
- • hypertrophic subaortic (idiopathic) I42.1
- • intestine—*see also* Obstruction, intestine
  - – congenital (small) Q41.9
    - ■ large Q42.9
      - ~ specified NEC Q42.8
    - ■ specified NEC Q41.8

Stenosis, stenotic, *continued*
- • lacrimal (passage)
  - – congenital Q10.5
  - – duct H04.55-
  - – sac H04.57-
- • lacrimonasal duct—*see* Stenosis, lacrimal, duct
  - – congenital Q10.5
- • mitral (chronic) (inactive) (valve) I05.0
  - – with
    - ■ aortic valve disease I08.0
    - ■ incompetency, insufficiency or regurgitation I05.2
  - – active or acute I01.1
    - ■ with rheumatic or Sydenham's chorea I02.0
  - – congenital Q23.2
  - – specified cause, except rheumatic I34.2
- • myocardium, myocardial—*see also* Degeneration, myocardial
  - – hypertrophic subaortic (idiopathic) I42.1
- • nares (anterior) (posterior) J34.89
  - – congenital Q30.0
- • nasal duct—*see also* Stenosis, lacrimal, duct
  - – congenital Q10.5
- • nasolacrimal duct—*see also* Stenosis, lacrimal, duct
  - – congenital Q10.5
- • pulmonary (artery) (congenital) Q25.6
  - – with ventricular septal defect, transposition of aorta, and hypertrophy of right ventricle Q21.3
  - – in tetralogy of Fallot Q21.3
  - – infundibular Q24.3
  - – subvalvular Q24.3
  - – supravalvular Q25.6
  - – valve I37.0
    - ■ with insufficiency I37.2
    - ■ congenital Q22.1
    - ■ rheumatic I09.89
      - ~ with aortic, mitral or tricuspid (valve) disease I08.8
- • pulmonic (congenital) Q22.1
- • pylorus (hypertrophic) (acquired) K31.1
  - – congenital Q40.0
  - – infantile Q40.0
- • spinal M48.0-
- • subaortic (congenital) Q24.4
  - – hypertrophic (idiopathic) I42.1
- • tricuspid (valve) I07.0
  - – with
    - ■ aortic (valve) disease I08.2
    - ■ incompetency, insufficiency or regurgitation I07.2
      - ~ with aortic (valve) disease I08.2
        - ◊ with mitral (valve) disease I08.3
    - ■ mitral (valve) disease I08.1
      - ~ with aortic (valve) disease I08.3
  - – congenital Q22.4
  - – nonrheumatic I36.0
    - ■ with insufficiency I36.2
- • ureteropelvic junction, congenital Q62.11
- • ureterovesical orifice, congenital Q62.12
- • vagina N89.5
  - – congenital Q52.4
- • valve (cardiac) (heart) (*see also* Endocarditis) I38
  - – congenital Q24.8
    - ■ aortic Q23.0
    - ■ pulmonary Q22.1

Stercolith (impaction) K56.41

Stercoraceous, stercoral ulcer K63.3
- • anus or rectum K62.6

Stereotypies NEC F98.4

Steroid
- • effects (adverse) (adrenocortical) (iatrogenic)
  - – cushingoid E24.2
    - ■ correct substance properly administered—*see* Table of Drugs and Chemicals, by drug, adverse effect
    - ■ overdose or wrong substance given or taken—*see* Table of Drugs and Chemicals, by drug, poisoning

Stevens-Johnson disease or syndrome L51.1
- • toxic epidermal necrolysis overlap L51.3

Sticker's disease B08.3

Stiffness, joint NEC M25.60-
- • ankle M25.67-
- • contracture—*see* Contraction, joint

Stiffness, joint NEC, *continued*
- elbow M25.62-
- foot M25.67-
- hand M25.64-
- hip M25.65-
- knee M25.66-
- shoulder M25.61-
- wrist M25.63-

Stillbirth P95

Still's disease or syndrome (juvenile) M08.20
- specified site NEC M08.2A

Stitch
- abscess T81.41

Stokes-Adams disease or syndrome I45.9

Stomatitis (denture) (ulcerative) K12.1
- angular K13.0
- aphthous K12.0
- candidal B37.0
- catarrhal K12.1
- due to
  - thrush B37.0
- follicular K12.1
- herpesviral, herpetic B00.2
- herpetiformis K12.0
- malignant K12.1
- membranous acute K12.1
- monilial B37.0
- mycotic B37.0
- parasitic B37.0
- septic K12.1
- suppurative (acute) K12.2
- vesicular K12.1
  - with exanthem (enteroviral) B08.4

Stomatocytosis D58.8

Stomatomycosis B37.0

Stomatorrhagia K13.79

Stovkis (-Talma) **disease** D74.8

Strabismus (congenital) (nonparalytic) H50.9
- concomitant H50.40
  - convergent—*see* Strabismus, convergent concomitant
  - divergent—*see* Strabismus, divergent concomitant
- convergent concomitant H50.00
  - accommodative component H50.43
  - alternating H50.05
    - with
      - ~ A pattern H50.06
      - ~ specified nonconcomitances NEC H50.08
      - ~ V pattern H50.07
    - monocular H50.01-
      - with
        - ~ A pattern H50.02-
        - ~ specified nonconcomitances NEC H50.04-
        - ~ V pattern H50.03-
      - intermittent H50.31-
        - ~ alternating H50.32
- cyclotropia H50.41
- divergent concomitant H50.10
  - alternating H50.15
    - with
      - ~ A pattern H50.16
      - ~ specified nonconcomitances NEC H50.18
      - ~ V pattern H50.17
    - monocular H50.11-
      - with
        - ~ A pattern H50.12-
        - ~ specified nonconcomitances NEC H50.14-
        - ~ V pattern H50.13-
      - intermittent H50.33
        - ~ alternating H50.34
- Duane's syndrome H50.81-
- due to adhesions, scars H50.69
- heterophoria H50.50
  - alternating H50.55
  - cyclophoria H50.54
  - esophoria H50.51
  - exophoria H50.52
  - vertical H50.53
- heterotropia H50.40
  - intermittent H50.30

Strabismus, *continued*
- hypertropia H50.2-
- hypotropia—*see* Strabismus, Hypertropia
- latent H50.50
- mechanical H50.60
  - Brown's sheath syndrome H50.61-
  - specified type NEC H50.69
- monofixation syndrome H50.42
- paralytic H49.9
  - abducens nerve H49.2-
  - fourth nerve H49.1-
  - Kearns-Sayre syndrome H49.81-
  - ophthalmoplegia (external)
    - progressive H49.4-
      - ~ with pigmentary retinopathy H49.81-
    - total H49.3-
  - sixth nerve H49.2-
  - specified type NEC H49.88-
  - third nerve H49.0-
  - trochlear nerve H49.1-
- specified type NEC H50.89
- vertical H50.2-

Strain
- cervical S16.1
- neck S16.1

Strangulation, strangulated—*see also* Asphyxia, traumatic
- bladder-neck N32.0
- bowel or colon K56.2
- intestine (large) (small) K56.2
  - with hernia—*see also* Hernia, by site, with, obstruction
    - with gangrene—*see* Hernia, by site, with, gangrene
- mesentery K56.2
- omentum K56.2
- organ or site, congenital NEC—*see* Atresia, by site
- vesicourethral orifice N32.0

Strangury R30.0

Strawberry
- mark Q82.5

Straw itch B88.0

Strephosymbolia F81.0
- secondary to organic lesion R48.8

Streptobacillary fever A25.1

Streptococcus, streptococcal—*see also* Disease, diseased
- as cause of disease classified elsewhere B95.5
- group
  - A, as cause of disease classified elsewhere B95.0
  - B, as cause of disease classified elsewhere B95.1
  - D, as cause of disease classified elsewhere B95.2
- pneumoniae, as cause of disease classified elsewhere B95.3
- specified NEC, as cause of disease classified elsewhere B95.4

Stress F43.9
- family—*see* Disruption, family
- fetal P84
- polycythemia D75.1
- reaction (*see also* Reaction, stress) F43.9

Stricture—*see also* Stenosis
- anus (sphincter) K62.4
  - congenital Q42.3
    - with fistula Q42.2
  - infantile Q42.3
    - with fistula Q42.3
- aorta (ascending) (congenital) Q25.1
- aortic (valve)—*see* Stenosis, aortic
- aqueduct of Sylvius (congenital) Q03.0
  - with spina bifida—*see* Spina bifida, by site, with hydrocephalus
  - acquired G91.1
- artery I77.1
  - congenital (peripheral) Q27.8
    - umbilical Q27.0
- bile duct (common) (hepatic) K83.1
  - congenital Q44.3
- bladder N32.89
  - neck N32.0
- brain G93.89

Stricture, *continued*
- colon—*see also* Obstruction, intestine
  - congenital Q42.9
    - specified NEC Q42.8
- digestive organs NEC, congenital Q45.8
- fallopian tube N97.1
  - gonococcal A54.24
- heart—*see also* Disease, heart
  - valve (*see also* Endocarditis) I38
    - aortic Q23.0
    - mitral Q23.4
    - pulmonary Q22.1
- intestine—*see also* Obstruction, intestine
  - congenital (small) Q41.9
    - large Q42.9
      - ~ specified NEC Q42.8
    - specified NEC Q41.8
  - ischemic K55.1
- myocardium, myocardial I51.5
  - hypertrophic subaortic (idiopathic) I42.1
- nares (anterior) (posterior) J34.89
  - congenital Q30.0
- nose J34.89
  - congenital Q30.0
- nostril (anterior) (posterior) J34.89
  - congenital Q30.0
- pelviureteric junction (congenital) Q62.11
- pulmonary, pulmonic
  - artery (congenital) Q25.6
  - infundibulum (congenital) Q24.3
  - valve I37.0
    - congenital Q22.1
- punctum lacrimale
  - congenital Q10.5
- pylorus (hypertrophic) K31.1
  - congenital Q40.0
  - infantile Q40.0
- rectum (sphincter) K62.4
  - congenital Q42.1
    - with fistula Q42.0
  - gonococcal A54.6
- subaortic Q24.4
  - hypertrophic (acquired) (idiopathic) I42.1
- ureter (postoperative) N13.5
  - with
    - hydronephrosis N13.1
- ureteropelvic junction N13.0
  - congenital Q62.11
- urethra (organic) (spasmodic) N35.9-
  - congenital Q64.39
    - valvular (posterior) Q64.2
  - female N35.92
  - gonococcal, gonorrheal A54.01
  - male N35.919
    - anterior urethra N35.914
    - bulbous urethra N35.912
    - meatal N35.911
    - membranous urethra N35.913
    - overlapping sites N35.116
  - postinfective NEC
    - female N35.12
    - male N35.119
      - ~ anterior urethra N35.114
      - ~ bulbous urethra N35.112
      - ~ meatal N35.111
      - ~ membranous urethra N35.113
      - ~ overlapping sites N35.116
  - post-traumatic
    - female N35.028
    - male N35.014
      - ~ anterior urethra N35.013
      - ~ bulbous urethra N35.011
      - ~ meatal N35.010
      - ~ membranous urethra N35.012
      - ~ overlapping sites N35.016
  - specified cause NEC
    - female N35.82
    - male N35.819
      - ~ anterior urethra N35.814
      - ~ bulbous urethra N35.812
      - ~ meatal N35.811
      - ~ membranous urethra N35.813
      - ~ overlapping sites N35.816

Stricture, *continued*
- valve (cardiac) (heart)—*see also* Endocarditis
  - congenital
    - aortic Q23.0
    - pulmonary Q22.1
- vesicourethral orifice N32.0
  - congenital Q64.31

Stridor R06.1
- congenital (larynx) P28.89

Stroke (apoplectic) (brain) (embolic) (ischemic) (paralytic) (thrombotic)
- cerebral, perinatal P91.82-
- epileptic—*see* Epilepsy
- heat T67.01
  - exertional T67.02
  - specified NEC T67.09
- ischemic, perinatal arterial P91.82-
- neonatal P91.82-
- sun T67.01
  - specified NEC T67.09

Struma—*see also* Goiter
- Hashimoto E06.3
- lymphomatosa E06.3
- nodosa (simplex) E04.9
  - endemic E01.2
    - multinodular E01.1
- Riedel's E06.5

Stupor (catatonic) R40.1
- reaction to exceptional stress (transient) F43.0

Sturge (-Weber) (-Dimitri) (-Kalischer) **disease or syndrome** Q85.8

Stuttering F80.81
- childhood onset F80.81
- in conditions classified elsewhere R47.82

Sty, stye (external) (internal) (meibomian) (zeisian)—*see* Hordeolum

Subacidity, gastric K31.89
- psychogenic F45.8

Subacute—*see* Disease, diseased

Subarachnoid—*see* Disease, diseased

Subcortical—*see* Disease, diseased

Subglossitis—*see* Glossitis

Subhemophilia D66

Subluxation—*see also* Dislocation
- finger S63.20-
  - index S63.20-
  - interphalangeal S63.2-
    - distal S63.24-
      - ~ index S63.24-
      - ~ little S63.24-
      - ~ middle S63.24-
      - ~ ring S63.24-
    - index S63.2-
    - little S63.2-
    - middle S63.2-
    - proximal S63.23-
      - ~ index S63.23-
      - ~ little S63.23-
      - ~ middle S63.23-
      - ~ ring S63.23-
    - ring S63.2-
  - little S63.20-
  - metacarpophalangeal (joint) S63.21-
    - index S63.26-
    - little S63.26-
    - middle S63.26-
    - ring S63.26-
  - middle S63.20-
  - ring S63.20
- hip S73.0-
  - anterior S73.03-
    - obturator S73.02-
  - central S73.04-
  - posterior S73.01-
- interphalangeal (joint)
  - finger S63.2-
    - distal joint S63.24-
      - ~ index S63.24-
      - ~ little S63.24-

Subluxation, *continued*
  - ~ middle S63.24-
  - ~ ring S63.24-
    - index S63.2-
    - little S63.2-
    - middle S63.2-
    - proximal joint S63.23-
      - ~ index S63.23-
      - ~ little S63.23-
      - ~ middle S63.23-
      - ~ ring S63.23-
    - ring S63.2-
  - thumb S63.12-
- knee S83.10-
  - cap—*see* Subluxation, patella
  - patella—*see* Subluxation, patella
  - proximal tibia
    - anteriorly S83.11-
    - laterally S83.14-
    - medially S83.13-
    - posteriorly S83.12-
  - specified type NEC S83.19-
- metacarpal (bone)
  - proximal end S63.06-
- metacarpophalangeal (joint)
  - finger S63.21-
    - index S63.21-
    - little S63.21-
    - middle S63.21-
    - ring S63.21-
  - thumb S63.11-
- patella S83.00-
  - lateral S83.01-
  - recurrent (nontraumatic) M22.1-
  - specified type NEC S83.09-
- radial head S53.00-
  - nursemaid's elbow S53.03-
  - specified type NEC S53.09-
- thumb S63.10-
  - interphalangeal joint—*see* Subluxation, interphalangeal (joint), thumb
  - metacarpophalangeal joint S63.11-

Submersion (fatal) (nonfatal) T75.1

Substernal thyroid E04.9
- congenital Q89.2

Substitution disorder F44.9

Subthyroidism (acquired)—*see also* Hypothyroidism
- congenital E03.1

Sucking thumb, child (excessive) F98.8

Sudamen, sudamina L74.1

Sugar
- blood
  - high (transient) R73.9
  - low (transient) E16.2
- in urine R81

Suicide, suicidal (attempted) T14.91
- by poisoning—*see* Table of Drugs and Chemicals
- history of (personal) Z91.5
  - in family Z81.8
- ideation—*see* Ideation, suicidal
- risk
  - meaning personal history of attempted suicide Z91.5
  - meaning suicidal ideation—*see* Ideation, suicidal
- tendencies
  - meaning personal history of attempted suicide Z91.5
  - meaning suicidal ideation—*see* Ideation, suicidal
- trauma—*see* nature of injury by site

Sulfhemoglobinemia, sulphemoglobinemia (acquired) (with methemoglobinemia) D74.8

Sunburn L55.9
- due to
  - tanning bed (acute) L56.8
- first degree L55.0
- second degree L55.1
- third degree L55.2

Sunstroke T67.01

Supernumerary (congenital)
- carpal bones Q74.0
- fallopian tube Q50.6
- finger Q69.0

Supernumerary, *continued*
- lacrimonasal duct Q10.6
- lobule (ear) Q17.0
- nipple(s) Q83.3
- ovary Q50.31
- oviduct Q50.6.
- ossicles, auditory Q16.3
- tarsal bones Q74.2
- testis Q55.29
- thumb Q69.1
- toe Q69.2
- uterus Q51.28

Supervision (of)
- contraceptive—*see* Prescription of contraceptives
- dietary (for) Z71.3
  - allergy (food) Z71.3
  - colitis Z71.3
  - diabetes mellitus Z71.3
  - food allergy or intolerance Z71.3
  - gastritis Z71.3
  - hypercholesterolemia Z71.3
  - hypoglycemia Z71.3
  - intolerance (food) Z71.3
  - obesity Z71.3
  - specified NEC Z71.3
- healthy infant or child Z76.2
  - foundling Z76.1
- lactation Z39.1

Suppression
- menstruation N94.89
- urine, urinary secretion R34

Suppuration, suppurative—*see also* Disease, diseased
- accessory sinus (chronic)—*see* Sinusitis
- antrum (chronic)—*see* Sinusitis, maxillary
- bladder—*see* Cystitis
- brain G06.0
  - sequelae G09
- breast N61.1
- ear (middle)—*see also* Otitis, media
  - external NEC—*see* Otitis, externa, infective
  - internal—*see* subcategory H83.0
- ethmoidal (chronic) (sinus)—*see* Sinusitis, ethmoidal
- frontal (chronic) (sinus)—*see* Sinusitis, frontal
- gallbladder (acute) K81.0
- intracranial G06.0
- joint—*see* Arthritis, pyogenic or pyemic
- labyrinthine—*see* subcategory H83.0
- mammary gland N61.1
- maxilla, maxillary M27.2
  - sinus (chronic)—*see* Sinusitis, maxillary
- muscle—*see* Myositis, infective
- nasal sinus (chronic)—*see* Sinusitis
- pelvis, pelvic
  - female—*see* Disease, pelvis, inflammatory
  - male K65.0
- sinus (accessory) (chronic) (nasal)—*see* Sinusitis
- sphenoidal sinus (chronic)—*see* Sinusitis, sphenoidal
- thyroid (gland) E06.0
- tonsil—*see* Tonsillitis
- uterus—*see* Endometritis

Supraglottitis J04.30
- with obstruction J04.31

Surgical
- shock T81.10

Surveillance (of) (for)—*see also* Observation
- alcohol abuse Z71.41
- contraceptive—*see* Prescription of contraceptives
- dietary Z71.3
- drug abuse Z71.51

Suspected condition, ruled out—*see also* Observation, suspected
- fetal anomaly Z03.73
- fetal growth Z03.74
- newborn—*see* Observation, newborn (for suspected condition, ruled out) Z05-

Suture
- burst (in operation wound) T81.31
  - external operation wound T81.31
- removal Z48.02

Swearing, compulsive F42.8
- in Gilles de la Tourette's syndrome F95.2

Sweat, sweats
- night R61

Sweating, excessive R61

Swelling (of) R60.9
- abdomen, abdominal (not referable to any particular organ)—*see* Mass, abdominal
- ankle—*see* Effusion, joint, ankle
- arm M79.89
  - forearm M79.89
- breast (*see also*, Lump, breast) N63.0
- chest, localized R22.2
- extremity (lower) (upper)—*see* Disorder
- finger M79.89
- foot M79.89
- glands R59.9
  - generalized R59.1
  - localized R59.0
- hand M79.89
- head (localized) R22.0
- inflammatory—*see* Inflammation
- intra-abdominal—*see* Mass, abdominal
- joint—*see* Effusion, joint
- leg M79.89
  - lower M79.89
- limb—*see* Disorder
- localized (skin) R22.9
  - chest R22.2
  - head R22.0
  - limb
    - lower—*see* Mass, localized, limb, lower
    - upper—*see* Mass, localized, limb, upper
  - neck R22.1
  - trunk R22.2
- neck (localized) R22.1
- pelvic—*see* Mass, abdominal
- scrotum N50.89
- splenic—*see* Splenomegaly
- testis N50.89
- toe M79.89
- umbilical R19.09

Swimmer's
- cramp T75.1
- ear H60.33-
- itch B65.3

Swimming in the head R42

Swollen—*see* Swelling

Sycocis L73.8
- barbae (not parasitic) L73.8
- contagiosa (mycotic) B35.0
- lupoides L73.8
- mycotic B35.0
- parasitic B35.0
- vulgaris L73.8

Symblepharon
- congenital Q10.3

Symond's syndrome G93.2

Sympathetic—*see* Disease, diseased

Sympathicoblastoma
- specified site—*see* Neoplasm, malignant, by site in Table of Neoplasms in the complete *ICD-10-CM* manual
- unspecified site C74.90

Sympathogonioma—*see* Sympathicoblastoma

Symphalangy (fingers) (toes) Q70.9

Symptoms NEC R68.89
- breast NEC N64.59
- cold J00
- development NEC R63.8
- genital organs, female R10.2
- involving
  - abdomen NEC R19.8
  - awareness R41.9
    - altered mental status R41.82
  - cardiovascular system NEC R09.89
  - chest NEC R09.89
  - circulatory system NEC R09.89
  - cognitive functions R41.9
    - altered mental status R41.82
  - development NEC R62.50
  - digestive system R19.8
  - food and fluid intake R63.8

Symptoms NEC, *continued*
- general perceptions and sensations R44.9
  - specified NEC R44.8
- musculoskeletal system R29.91
  - specified NEC R29.898
- nervous system R29.90
  - specified NEC R29.818
- pelvis R19.8
- respiratory system NEC R09.89
- metabolism NEC R63.8
- of infancy R68.19
- pelvis NEC, female R10.2
- viral syndrome J00

Sympus Q74.2

Syncope (near) (pre-) R55
- bradycardia R00.1
- cardiac R55
- heart R55
- heat T67.1
- laryngeal R05
- psychogenic F48.8
- tussive R05
- vasoconstriction R55
- vasodepressor R55
- vasomotor R55
- vasovagal R55

Syndactylism, syndactyly Q70.9
- complex (with synostosis)
  - fingers Q70.0-
  - toes Q70.2-
- simple (without synostosis)
  - fingers Q70.1-
  - toes Q70.3-

Syndrome—*see also* Disease
- abdominal
  - acute R10.0
  - muscle deficiency Q79.4
- abstinence, neonatal P96.1
- acquired immunodeficiency—*see* Human, immuno-deficiency virus (HIV) disease
- acute abdominal R10.0
- acute respiratory distress (adult) (child) J80
- Adair-Dighton Q78.0
- Adams-Stokes (-Morgagni) I45.9
- adrenocortical—*see* Cushing's, syndrome
- adrenogenital E25.9
  - congenital, associated with enzyme deficiency E25.0
- Alder's D72.0
- Aldrich (-Wiskott) D82.0
- Alport Q87.81
- alveolar hypoventilation E66.2
- androgen insensitivity E34.50
  - complete E34.51
  - partial E34.52
- androgen resistance (*see also* Syndrome, androgen insensitivity) E34.50
- Angelman Q93.51
- ankyloglossia superior Q38.1
- antibody deficiency D80.9
  - agammaglobulinemic D80.1
    - hereditary D80.0
  - congenital D80.0
  - hypogammaglobulinemic D80.1
    - hereditary D80.0
- Arnold-Chiari—*see* Arnold-Chiari disease
- Arrillaga-Ayerza I27.0
- arterial tortuosity Q87.82
- aspiration, of newborn—*see* Aspiration, by substance, with, pneumonia
  - meconium P24.01
- ataxia-telangiectasia G11.3
- autoerythrocyte sensitization (Gardner-Diamond) D69.2
- autoimmune lymphoproliferative *[ALPS]* D89.82
- Ayerza (-Arrillaga) I27.0
- Beals Q87.40
- bilateral polycystic ovarian E28.2
- black
  - widow spider bite—*see* Table of Drugs and Chemicals, by animal or substance, poisoning
- Blackfan-Diamond D61.01

Syndrome, *continued*
- blind loop K90.2
  - congenital Q43.8
  - postsurgical K91.2
- blue sclera Q78.0
- Boder-Sedgwick G11.3
- Borjeson Forssman Lehmann Q89.8
- Bouillaud's I01.9
- Bourneville (-Pringle) Q85.1
- bradycardia-tachycardia I49.5
- brain (nonpsychotic) F09
  - with psychosis, psychotic reaction F09
  - acute or subacute—*see* Delirium
  - congenital—*see* Disability, intellectual
  - organic F09
    - post-traumatic (nonpsychotic) F07.81
  - postcontusional F07.81
  - post-traumatic, nonpsychotic F07.81
- Brock's J98.11
- bronze baby P83.88
- Burnett's (milk-alkali) E83.52
- carbohydrate-deficient glycoprotein (CDGS) E77.8
- cardiacos negros I27.0
- cardiopulmonary-obesity E66.2
- cardiorespiratory distress (idiopathic), newborn P22.0
- cat cry Q93.4
- celiac K90.0
- cerebral
  - gigantism E22.0
- CHARGE Q89.8
- child maltreatment—*see* Maltreatment, child
- chondrocostal junction M94.0
- chondroectodermal dysplasia Q77.6
- chromosome 5 short arm deletion Q93.4
- Clerambault's automatism G93.89
- clumsiness, clumsy child F82
- cluster headache G44.009
  - intractable G44.001
  - not intractable G44.009
- Coffin-Lowry Q89.8
- combined immunity deficiency D81.9
- concussion F07.81
- congenital
  - facial diplegia Q87.0
  - oculo-auriculovertebral Q87.0
  - oculofacial diplegia (Moebius) Q87.0
  - rubella (manifest) P35.0
- congestive dysmenorrhea N94.6
- Costen's (complex) M26.69
- costochondral junction M94.0
- costovertebral E22.0
- Cowden Q85.8
- cri-du-chat Q93.4
- crib death R99
- croup J05.0
- Cushing's E24.9
  - due to
    - drugs E24.2
    - overproduction of pituitary ACTH E24.0
  - drug-induced E24.2
  - overdose or wrong substance given or taken—*see* Table of Drugs and Chemicals, by drug, poisoning
  - pituitary-dependent E24.0
  - specified type NEC E24.8
- cryptophthalmos Q87.0
- cytokine release D89.839
  - grade 1 D89.831
  - grade 2 D89.832
  - grade 3 D89.833
  - grade 4 D89.834
  - grade 5 D89.835
- Dandy-Walker Q03.1
  - with spina bifida Q07.01
- defibrination—*see also* Fibrinolysis
  - newborn P60
- dependence—*see* F10-F19 with fourth character .2
- De Quervain E34.51
- de Vivo syndrome E74.810
- diabetes mellitus in newborn infant P70.2
- Diamond-Blackfan D61.01
- Diamond-Gardner D69.2
- DIC (diffuse or disseminated intravascular coagulopathy) D65

Syndrome, *continued*

- di George's D82.1
- Dighton's Q78.0
- disequilibrium E87.8
- Döhle body-panmyelopathic D72.0
- Down (*see also* Down syndrome) Q90.9
- Dravet (intractable) G40.834
  - with status epilepticus G40.833
  - without status epilepticus G40.834
- DRESS (drug rash with eosinophilia and systemic symptoms) D72.12
- Dressler's (postmyocardial infarction) I24.1
  - postcardiotomy I97.0
- drug rash with eosinophilia and systemic symptoms (DRESS) D72.12
- drug withdrawal, infant of dependent mother P96.1
- dry eye H04.12-
- due to abnormality
  - chromosomal Q99.9
    - sex
      - ~ female phenotype Q97.9
      - ~ male phenotype Q98.9
    - specified NEC Q99.8
- Dupré's (meningism) R29.1
- dysmetabolic X E88.81
- dyspraxia, developmental F82
- Eagle-Barrett Q79.4
- eczema-thrombocytopenia D82.0
- Eddowes' Q78.0
- effort (psychogenic) F45.8
- Ehlers-Danlos Q79.60
  - classical Ehlers-Danlos syndrome Q79.61
  - hypermobile Ehlers-Danlos syndrome Q79.62
  - other Ehlers-Danlos syndromes Q79.69
  - vascular Ehlers-Danlos syndrome Q79.63
- Eisenmenger's I27.83
- Ekman's Q78.0
- Ellis-van Creveld Q77.6
- eosinophilia-myalgia M35.8
- epileptic—*see* Epilepsy, by type
- Erdheim's E22.0
- Evans D69.41
- eye retraction—*see* Strabismus
- eyelid-malar-mandible Q87.0
- facet M47.89-
- Fallot's Q21.3
- familial eczema-thrombocytopenia (Wiskott-Aldrich) D82.0
- Fanconi's (anemia) (congenital pancytopenia) D61.09
- fatigue
  - chronic R53.82
- faulty bowel habit K59.39
- fetal
  - alcohol (dysmorphic) Q86.0
- Fiedler's I40.1
- first arch Q87.0
- fish odor E72.89
- floppy
  - baby P94.2
- food protein-induced enterocolitis (FPIES) K52.21
- fragile X Q99.2
- Fukuhara E88.49
- functional
  - bowel K59.9
- Gaisböck's D75.1
- Gardener-Diamond D69.2
- Gee-Herter-Heubner K90.0
- Gianotti-Crosti L44.4
- Gilles de la Tourette's F95.2
- Gleich's D72.118
- Goldberg Q89.8
- Goldberg-Maxwell E34.51
- Good's D83.8
- Gouley's I31.1
- Gower's R55
- hand-foot L27.1
- Hegglin's D72.0
- hemolytic-uremic D59.3
- hemophagocytic, infection-associated D76.2
- Henoch-Schönlein D69.0
- hepatopulmonary K76.81
- Herter (-Gee) (nontropical sprue) K90.0
- Heubner-Herter K90.0

Syndrome, *continued*

- histamine-like (fish poisoning)—*see* Poisoning, food, noxious or naturally toxic, fish
- histiocytic D76.3
- histiocytosis NEC D76.3
- HIV infection, acute B20
- Hoffmann-Werdnig G12.0
- hypereosinophilic (HES) D72.119
  - idiopathic (IHES) D72.110
  - lymphocytic variant (LHES) D72.111
  - specified NEC D72.118
- hyperkinetic—*see* Hyperkinesia
- hypermobility M35.7
- hypernatremia E87.0
- hyperosmolarity E87.0
- hypertransfusion, newborn P61.1
- hyperventilation F45.8
- hyperviscosity (of serum)
  - polycythemic D75.1
- hypoglycemic (familial) (neonatal) E16.2
- hyponatremic E87.1
- hypoplastic left-heart Q23.4
- hyposmolality E87.1
- hypothenar hammer I73.89
- ICF (intravascular coagulation-fibrinolysis) D65
- idiopathic
  - cardiorespiratory distress, newborn P22.0
  - nephrotic (infantile) N04.9
- immunity deficiency, combined D81.9
- immunodeficiency
  - acquired—*see* Human, immunodeficiency virus (HIV) disease
  - combined D81.9
- inappropriate secretion of antidiuretic hormone E22.2
- inspissated bile (newborn) P59.1
- intestinal
  - knot K56.2
- intravascular coagulation-fibrinolysis (ICF) D65
- iodine-deficiency, congenital E00.-
- IRDS (idiopathic respiratory distress, newborn) P22.0
- irritable
  - bowel K58.9
    - with constipation K58.1
    - with diarrhea K58.0
    - mixed K58.2
    - other K58.8
    - psychogenic F45.8
  - heart (psychogenic) F45.8
- IVC (intravascular coagulopathy) D65
- Jervell-Lange-Nielsen I45.81
- Job's D71
- Joseph-Diamond-Blackfan D61.01
- jugular foramen G52.7
- Kabuki Q89.8
- Kanner's (autism) F84.0
- Kartagener's Q89.3
- Kostmann's D70.0
- Lambert-E
  - in neoplastic disease G73.1
- Launois' E22.0
- lazy
  - leukocyte D70.8
- Lemiere I80.8
- Lennox-Gastaut G40.812
  - intractable G40.814
    - with status epilepticus G40.813
    - without status epilepticus G40.814
  - not intractable G40.812
    - with status epilepticus G40.811
    - without status epilepticus G40.812
- Leopold-Levi's E05.90
- Lev's I44.2
- long arm 18 or 21 deletion Q93.89
- long QT I45.81
- Louis-Barré G11.3
- low
  - output (cardiac) I50.9
- Luetscher's (dehydration) E86.0
- Lutembacher's Q21.1
- macrophage activation D76.1
  - due to infection D76.2
- Mal de Debarquement R42

Syndrome, *continued*

- malabsorption K90.9
  - postsurgical K91.2
- malformation, congenital, due to
  - alcohol Q86.0
- maple-syrup-urine E71.0
- Marfan's Q87.40
  - with
    - cardiovascular manifestations Q87.418
      - ~ aortic dilation Q87.410
    - ocular manifestations Q87.42
    - skeletal manifestations Q87.43
- Marie's E22.0
- mast cell activation D89.40
  - idiopathic D89.42
  - monoclonal D89.41
  - other D89.49
  - secondary D89.43
- May (-Hegglin) D72.0
- McQuarrie's E16.2
- meconium plug (newborn) P76.0
- Meekeren-Ehlers-Danlos Q79.6-
- MELAS E88.41
- MERRF (myoclonic epilepsy associated with ragged-red fibers) E88.42
- metabolic E88.81
- micrognathia-glossoptosis Q87.0
- midbrain NEC G93.89
- migraine—*see also* Migraine G43.909
- milk-alkali E83.52
- Miller-Dieker Q93.88
- Minkowski-Chauffard D58.0
- MNGIE (Mitochondrial Neurogastrointestinal Encephalopathy) E88.49
- Morgagni-Adams-Stokes I45.9
- mucocutaneous lymph node (acute febrile) (MCLS) M30.3
- myasthenic G70.9
  - in
    - diabetes mellitus—*see* Diabetes, type 1, with, amyotrophy
    - endocrine disease NEC E34.9 [G73.3]
    - neoplastic disease (*see also* Table of Neoplasms in the complete *ICD-10-CM* manual) D49.9 [G73.3]
    - thyrotoxicosis (hyperthyroidism) E05.90 [G73.3]
      - ~ with thyroid storm E05.91 [G73.3]
- myelodysplastic D46.9
  - with
    - multilineage dysplasia D46.A
      - ~ with ringed sideroblasts D46.B
  - myeloid hypereosinophilic D72.118
- myofascial pain M79.18
- NARP (Neuropathy, Ataxia and Retinitis pigmentosa) E88.49
- neonatal abstinence P96.1
- nephritic—*see also* Nephritis
  - with edema—*see* Nephrosis
  - acute N00.9
  - chronic N03.9
- nephrotic (congenital) (*see also* Nephrosis) N04.9
  - with
    - C3
      - ~ glomerulonephritis N04.A
      - ~ glomerulopathy N04.A
        - ◊ with dense deposit disease N04.6
    - dense deposit disease N04.6
    - diffuse
      - ~ crescentic glomerulonephritis N04.7
      - ~ endocapillary proliferative glomerulonephritis N04.4
      - ~ membranous glomerulonephritis N04.2
      - ~ mesangial proliferative glomerulonephritis N04.3
      - ~ mesangiocapillary glomerulonephritis N04.5
    - focal and segmental glomerular lesions N04.1
    - minor glomerular abnormality N04.0
    - specified morphological changes NEC N04.8
- Nothnagel's vasomotor acroparesthesia I73.89
- Ogilvie K59.81
- ophthalmoplegia-cerebellar ataxia—*see* Strabismus, paralytic, third nerve
- oral-facial-digital Q87.0
- oro-facial-digital Q87.0

Syndrome, *continued*
- Osler-Weber-Rendu I78.0
- oto-palatal-digital Q87.0
- ovary
  - polycystic E28.2
  - sclerocystic E28.2
- pain—*see also* Pain
  - complex regional I G90.5-
    - lower limb G90.52-
    - specified site NEC G90.59
    - upper limb G90.51-
- painful
  - bruising D69.2
- paralytic G83.9
- pediatric autoimmune neuropsychiatric disorders associated with streptococcal infections (PANDAS) D89.89
- pharyngeal pouch D82.1
- Pick's (heart) (liver) I31.1
- Pickwickian E66.2
- pituitary E22.0
- pontine NEC G93.89
- postcardiac injury
  - postcardiotomy I97.0
- postcommissurotomy I97.0
- postconcussional F07.81
- postcontusional F07.81
- postvalvulotomy I97.0
- prune belly Q79.4
- pseudoparalytica G70.00
  - with exacerbation (acute) G70.01
  - in crisis G70.01
- pseudo-Turner's Q87.19
- pulmonary
  - arteriosclerosis I27.0
  - dysmaturity (Wilson-Mikity) P27.0
  - hypoperfusion (idiopathic) P22.0
- QT interval prolongation I45.81
- RDS (respiratory distress syndrome, newborn) P22.0
- Reifenstein E34.52
- Rendu-Osler-Weber I78.0
- respiratory
  - distress
    - acute J80
      - ~ child J80
    - newborn (idiopathic) (type I) P22.0
      - ~ type II P22.1
- retinoblastoma (familial) C69.2
- retroviral seroconversion (acute) Z21
- Romano-Ward (prolonged QT interval) I45.81
- rubella (congenital) P35.0
- Ruvalcaba-Myhre-Smith E71.440
- Rytand-Lipsitch I44.2
- salt
  - depletion E87.1
    - due to heat NEC T67.8
      - ~ causing heat exhaustion or prostration T67.4
  - low E87.1
- Scaglietti-Dagnini E22.0
- scapuloperoneal G71.09
- schizophrenic, of childhood NEC F84.5
- Schwartz-Bartter E22.2
- sclerocystic ovary E28.2
- Seitelberger's G31.89
- seroconversion, retroviral (acute) Z21
- serous meningitis G93.2
- severe acute respiratory (SARS) J12.81
- shaken infant T74.4
- shock (traumatic) T79.4
  - kidney N17.0
  - toxic A48.3
- shock-lung J80
- short
  - bowel K91.2
  - rib Q77.2
- Shwachman's D70.4
- sick
  - cell E87.1
  - sinus I49.5
- sinus tarsi M25.57-
- sinusitis-bronchiectasis-situs inversus Q89.3
- Smith-Magenis Q93.88
- Soto's Q87.3

Syndrome, *continued*
- Spen's I45.9
- splenic
  - neutropenia D73.81
- Spurway's Q78.0
- staphylococcal scalded skin L00
- Stein-Leventhal E28.2
- Stein's E28.2
- Stevens-Johnson syndrome L51.1
  - toxic epidermal necrolysis overlap L51.3
- Stickler Q89.8
- stiff baby Q89.8
- Stokes (-Adams) I45.9
- swallowed blood P78.2
- sweat retention L74.0
- Symond's G93.2
- systemic inflammatory response (SIRS), of non-infectious origin (without organ dysfunction) R65.10
  - with acute organ dysfunction R65.11
- tachycardia-bradycardia I49.5
- teething K00.7
- tegmental G93.89
- telangiectasia-pigmentation-cataract Q82.8
- temporal pyramidal apex—*see* Otitis, media, suppurative, acute
- temporomandibular joint-pain-dysfunction M26.62-
- testicular feminization (*see also* Syndrome, androgen insensitivity) E34.51
- Tietze's M94.0
- toxic shock A48.3
- triple X, female Q97.0
- trisomy Q92.9
  - 13 Q91.7
    - meiotic nondisjunction Q91.4
  - 18 Q91.3
    - meiotic nondisjunction Q91.0
  - 21 Q90.9
- tumor lysis (following antineoplastic chemotherapy) (spontaneous) NEC E88.3
- uremia, chronic (*see also* Disease, kidney, chronic) N18.9
- vago-hypoglossal G52.7
- van der Hoeve's Q78.0
- vasovagal R55
- velo-cardio-facial Q93.81
- visual disorientation H53.8
- von Willebrand (-Jürgens) D68.0
- Werdnig-Hoffman G12.0
- wet
  - lung, newborn P22.1
- whiplash S13.4
- whistling face Q87.0
- Willebrand (-Jürgens) D68.0
- Williams Q93.82
- Wiskott-Aldrich D82.0
- withdrawal—*see* Withdrawal state
  - drug
    - infant of dependent mother P96.1
    - therapeutic use, newborn P96.2
- Yao M04.8
- Zahorsky's B08.5
- Zellweger syndrome E71.510
- Zellweger-like syndrome E71.541

Synostosis (congenital) Q78.8
- astragalo-scaphoid Q74.2
- radioulnar Q74.0

Syphilis, syphilitic (acquired) A52.79
- age under 2 years NOS—*see also* Syphilis, congenital, early
  - acquired A51.9
- anemia (late) A52.79 *[D63.8]*
- asymptomatic—*see* Syphilis, latent
- bubo (primary) A51.0
- chancre (multiple) A51.0
  - extragenital A51.2
  - Rollet's A51.0
- congenital A50.9
  - early, or less than 2 years after birth NEC A50.2
    - with manifestations—*see* Syphilis, congenital, early
- contact Z20.2
- cutaneous A51.39

Syndrome, *continued*
- early A51.9
  - symptomatic A51.9
    - extragenital chancre A51.2
    - primary, except extragenital chancre A51.0
- exposure to Z20.2
- genital (primary) A51.0
- inactive—*see* Syphilis, latent
- infantum—*see* Syphilis, congenital
- inherited—*see* Syphilis, congenital
- latent A53.0
  - with signs or symptoms—*code by* site and stage under Syphilis
  - date of infection unspecified A53.0
  - early, or less than 2 years after infection A51.5
  - follow-up of latent syphilis A53.0
    - date of infection unspecified A53.0
    - late, or 2 years or more after infection A52.8
  - late, or 2 years or more after infection A52.8
  - positive serology (only finding) A53.0
    - date of infection unspecified A53.0
    - early, or less than 2 years after infection A51.5
    - late, or 2 years or more after infection A52.8
- lip A51.39
  - chancre (primary) A51.2
  - late A52.79
- penis (chancre) A51.0
- primary A51.0
  - extragenital chancre NEC A51.2
  - fingers A51.2
  - genital A51.0
  - lip A51.2
  - specified site NEC A51.2
  - tonsils A51.2
- skin (with ulceration) (early) (secondary) A51.39
- tonsil (lingual) (late) A52.76
  - primary A51.2
- vagina A51.0
  - late A52.76
- vulva A51.0
  - late A52.76
  - secondary A51.39

System, systemic—*see also* Disease, diseased
- inflammatory response syndrome (SIRS) of non-infectious origin (without organ dysfunction) R65.10
  - with acute organ dysfunction R65.11
- lupus erythematosus M32.9

T

Tachyalimentation K91.2

Tachyarrhythmia, tachyrhythmia—*see* Tachycardia

Tachycardia R00.0
- atrial (paroxysmal) I47.1
- auricular I47.1
- AV nodal re-entry (re-entrant) I47.1
- junctional (paroxysmal) I47.1
- newborn P29.11
- nodal (paroxysmal) I47.1
- paroxysmal (sustained) (nonsustained) I47.9
  - with sinus bradycardia I49.5
  - atrial (PAT) I47.1
  - atrioventricular (AV) (re-entrant) I47.1
    - psychogenic F54
  - junctional I47.1
    - ectopic I47.1
  - nodal I47.1
  - supraventricular (sustained) I47.1
- psychogenic F45.8
- sick sinus I49.5
- sinoauricular NOS R00.0
  - paroxysmal I47.1
- sinus [sinusal] NOS R00.0
  - paroxysmal I47.1
- supraventricular I47.1
- ventricular (paroxysmal) (sustained) I47.2

Tachypnea R06.82
- hysterical F45.8
- newborn (idiopathic) (transitory) P22.1
- psychogenic F45.8
- transitory, of newborn P22.1

TACO (transfusion associated circulatory overload) E87.71

Tag (hypertrophied skin) (infected) L91.8
- adenoid J35.8
- anus K64.4
- hemorrhoidal K64.4
- sentinel K64.4
- skin L91.8
  - accessory (congenital) Q82.8
  - anus K64.4
  - congenital Q82.8
  - preauricular Q17.0
- tonsil J35.8

Talipes (congenital) Q66.89
- acquired, planus—*see* Deformity, limb, flat foot
- asymmetric Q66.89
- calcaneovalgus Q66.4-
- calcaneovarus Q66.1-
- calcaneus Q66.89
- cavus Q66.7-
- equinovalgus Q66.6
- equinovarus Q66.0-
- equinus Q66.89
- percavus Q66.7-
- planovalgus Q66.6
- planus (acquired) (any degree)—*see also* Deformity, limb, flat foot
  - congenital Q66.5-
- valgus Q66.6
- varus Q66.3-

Tall stature, constitutional E34.4

Tamponade, heart I31.4

Tantrum, child problem F91.8

Tapeworm (infection) (infestation)—*see* Infestation, tapeworm

Tapia's syndrome G52.7

Tattoo (mark) L81.8

Tay-Sachs amaurotic familial idiocy or disease E75.02

TBI (traumatic brain injury) S06.9

Tear, torn (traumatic)—*see also* Laceration
- anus, anal (sphincter) S31.831
  - nontraumatic (healed) (old) K62.81
- rotator cuff (nontraumatic) M75.10-
  - complete M75.12-
  - incomplete M75.11-
  - traumatic S46.01-
    - capsule S43.42-
- vagina—*see* Laceration, vagina

Teeth—*see also* Disease, diseased
- grinding
  - psychogenic F45.8
  - sleep related G47.63

Teething (syndrome) K00.7

Telangiectasia, telangiectasis (verrucous) I78.1
- ataxic (cerebellar) (Louis-Bar) G11.3
- familial I78.0
- hemorrhagic, hereditary (congenital) (senile) I78.0
- hereditary, hemorrhagic (congenital) (senile) I78.0
- spider I78.1

Telescoped bowel or intestine K56.1
- congenital Q43.8

Temperature
- body, high (of unknown origin) R50.9
- cold, trauma from
  - newborn P80.0

Temporomandibular joint pain-dysfunction syndrome M26.62-

Tendency
- bleeding—*see* Defect, coagulation
- suicide
  - meaning personal history of attempted suicide Z91.5
  - meaning suicidal ideation—*see* Ideation, suicidal

Tenderness, abdominal R10.819
- epigastric R10.816
- generalized R10.817
- left lower quadrant R10.814
- left upper quadrant R10.812
- periumbilic R10.815
- right lower quadrant R10.813
- right upper quadrant R10.811

Tenderness, abdominal, *continued*
- rebound R10.829
  - epigastric R10.826
  - generalized R10.827
  - left lower quadrant R10.824
  - left upper quadrant R10.822
  - periumbilic R10.825
  - right lower quadrant R10.823
  - right upper quadrant R10.821

Tendinitis, tendonitis—*see also* Enthesopathy
- Achilles M76.6-

Tenesmus (rectal) R19.8

Tennis elbow—*see* Epicondylitis, lateral

Tenosynovitis M65.9
- adhesive—*see* Tenosynovitis, specified type NEC
- shoulder region M65.81-
  - adhesive—*see* Capsulitis, adhesive
- specified type NEC M65.88
  - ankle M65.87-
  - foot M65.87-
  - forearm M65.83-
  - hand M65.84-
  - lower leg M65.86-
  - multiple sites M65.89
  - pelvic region M65.85-
  - shoulder region M65.81-
  - specified site NEC M65.88
  - thigh M65.85-
  - upper arm M65.82-

Tension
- arterial, high—*see also* Hypertension
  - without diagnosis of hypertension R03.0
- headache G44.209
  - intractable G44.201
  - not intractable G44.209
- nervous R45.0
- pneumothorax J93.0
- state (mental) F48.9

Tentorium—*see* Disease, diseased

Teratencephalus Q89.8

Teratism Q89.7

Terror(s) night (child) F51.4

Test, tests, testing (for)
- blood-alcohol Z04.89
  - positive—*see* Findings
- blood-drug Z04.89
  - positive—*see* Findings
- hearing Z01.10
  - with abnormal findings NEC Z01.118
  - infant or child (over 28 days old) Z00.129
    - with abnormal findings Z00.121
- HIV (human immunodeficiency virus)
  - nonconclusive (in infants) R75
  - positive Z21
  - seropositive Z21
- immunity status Z01.84
- laboratory (as part of a general medical examination) Z00.00
  - with abnormal finding Z00.01
  - for medicolegal reason NEC Z04.89
- Mantoux (for tuberculosis) Z11.1
  - abnormal result R76.11
- skin, diagnostic
  - allergy Z01.82
    - special screening examination—*see* Screening, by name of disease
  - Mantoux Z11.1
  - tuberculin Z11.1
- specified NEC Z01.89
- tuberculin Z11.1
  - abnormal result R76.11
- vision Z01.00
  - with abnormal findings Z01.01
  - after failed exam Z01.02-
  - infant or child (over 28 days old) Z00.129
    - with abnormal findings Z00.121
- Wassermann Z11.3
  - positive—*see* Serology for syphilis

Testicle, testicular, testes—*see also* Disease, diseased
- feminization syndrome (*see also* Syndrome, androgen insensitivity) E34.51
- migrans Q55.29

Tetanus, tetanic (cephalic) (convulsions) A35

Tetany (due to) R29.0
- associated with rickets E55.0
- hyperpnea R06.4
  - hysterical F44.5
  - psychogenic F45.8
- hyperventilation (*see also* Hyperventilation) R06.4
  - hysterical F44.5
- neonatal (without calcium or magnesium deficiency) P71.3
- psychogenic (conversion reaction) F44.5

Tetralogy of Fallot Q21.3

Tetraplegia (chronic) (*see also* Quadriplegia) G82.50

Thalassemia (anemia) (disease) D56.9
- with other hemoglobinopathy D56.8
- alpha (major) (severe) (triple gene defect) D56.0
  - minor D56.3
  - silent carrier D56.3
  - trait D56.3
- beta (severe) D56.1
  - homozygous D56.1
  - major D56.1
  - minor D56.3
  - trait D56.3
- delta-beta (homozygous) D56.2
  - minor D56.3
  - trait D56.3
- dominant D56.8
- hemoglobin
  - C D56.8
  - E-beta D56.5
- intermedia D56.1
- major D56.1
- minor D56.3
- mixed D56.8
- sickle-cell—*see* Disease, sickle-cell, thalassemia
- specified type NEC D56.8
- trait D56.3
- variants D56.8

Thanatophoric dwarfism or short stature Q77.1

Thaysen-Gee disease (nontropical sprue) K90.0

Thaysen's disease K90.0

Thelitis N61.0

Therapy
- drug, long-term (current) (prophylactic)
  - antibiotics Z79.2
  - anti-inflammatory Z79.1
  - aspirin Z79.82
  - drug, specified NEC Z79.899
  - hypoglycemic drugs, oral Z79.84
  - insulin Z79.4
  - steroids
    - inhaled Z79.51
    - systemic Z79.52

Thermoplegia T67.0

Thickening
- breast N64.59

Thirst, excessive R63.1
- due to deprivation of water T73.1

Thomsen disease G71.12

Threadworm (infection) (infestation) B80

Threatened
- abortion O20.0
  - with subsequent abortion O03.9
- miscarriage O20.0

Thrombocythemia (essential) (hemorrhagic) (idiopathic) (primary) D47.3

Thrombocytopenia, thrombocytopenic D69.6
- with absent radius (TAR) Q87.2
- congenital D69.42
- dilutional D69.59
- due to
  - drugs D69.59
    - heparin induced (HIT) D75.82

Thrombocytopenia, thrombocytopenic, *continued*
- – extracorporeal circulation of blood D69.59
- – (massive) blood transfusion D69.59
- – platelet alloimmunization D69.59
- • essential D69.3
- • heparin induced (HIT) D75.82
- • hereditary D69.42
- • idiopathic D69.3
- • neonatal, transitory P61.0
  - – due to
    - ■ exchange transfusion P61.0
    - ■ idiopathic maternal thrombocytopenia P61.0
    - ■ isoimmunization P61.0
- • primary NEC D69.49
  - – idiopathic D69.3
- • secondary D69.59
- • transient neonatal P61.0

Thrombocytosis, essential D47.3
- • primary D47.3

Thromboembolism—*see* Embolism

Thrombopathy (Bernard-Soulier) D69.1
- • constitutional D68.0
- • Willebrand-Jürgens D68.0

Thrombophlebitis I80.9
- • calf muscular vein (NOS) I80.25-
- • femoral vein (superficial) I80.1-
- • femoropopliteal vein I80.0-
- • gastrocnemial vein I80.25-
- • hepatic (vein) I80.8
- • iliac vein (common) (external) (internal) I80.21-
- • iliofemoral I80.1-
- • leg I80.3
  - – superficial I80.0-
- • lower extremity I80.299
- • peroneal vein I80.24-
- • popliteal vein—*see* Phlebitis, leg
- • saphenous (greater) (lesser) I80.0-
- • soleal vein I80.25-
- • specified site NEC I80.8
- • tibial vein (anterior) (posterior) I80.23-

Thrombosis, thrombotic (bland) (multiple) (progressive) (silent) (vessel) I82.90
- • anus K64.5
- • artery, arteries (postinfectional) I74.9
- • genital organ
  - – female NEC N94.89
- • liver (venous) I82.0
  - – artery I74.8
  - – portal vein I81
- • mesenteric (artery) (with gangrene) K55.0
  - – vein (inferior) (superior) I81
- • perianal venous K64.5
- • portal I81
- • renal (artery) N28.0
  - – vein I82.3
- • tricuspid I07.8
- • vein (acute) I82.90
  - – perianal K64.5
  - – renal I82.3
- • venous, perianal K64.5

Thrombus—*see* Thrombosis

Thrush—*see also* Candidiasis
- • oral B37.0
- • newborn P37.5
- • vagina B37.3

Thumb—*see also* Disease, diseased
- • sucking (child problem) F98.8

Thyroglossal—*see also* Disease, diseased
- • cyst Q89.2
- • duct, persistent Q89.2

Thyroid (gland) (body)—*see also* Disease, diseased
- • lingual Q89.2

Thyroiditis E06.9
- • acute (nonsuppurative) (pyogenic) (suppurative) E06.0
- • autoimmune E06.3
- • chronic (nonspecific) (sclerosing) E06.5
  - – with thyrotoxicosis, transient E06.2
  - – fibrous E06.5
  - – lymphadenoid E06.3

Thyroiditis, *continued*
- – lymphocytic E06.3
- – lymphoid E06.3
- • de Quervain's E06.1
- • drug-induced E06.4
- • fibrous (chronic) E06.5
- • giant-cell (follicular) E06.1
- • granulomatous (de Quervain) (subacute) E06.1
- • Hashimoto's (struma lymphomatosa) E06.3
- • iatrogenic E06.4
- • ligneous E06.5
- • lymphocytic (chronic) E06.3
- • lymphoid E06.3
- • lymphomatous E06.3
- • nonsuppurative E06.1
- • pseudotuberculous E06.1
- • pyogenic E06.0
- • radiation E06.4
- • Riedel's E06.5
- • subacute (granulomatous) E06.1
- • suppurative E06.0
- • viral E06.1
- • woody E06.5

Thyrolyngual duct, persistent Q89.2

Thyrotoxic
- • crisis—*see* Thyrotoxicosis
- • heart disease or failure (*see also* Thyrotoxicosis) E05.90 *[I43]*
  - – with thyroid storm E05.91 *[I43]*
- • storm—*see* Thyrotoxicosis

Thyrotoxicosis (recurrent) E05.90
- • with
  - – goiter (diffuse) E05.00
    - ■ with thyroid storm E05.01
  - – heart E05.90 *[I43]*
    - – with thyroid storm E05.91 *[I43]*
    - – failure E05.90 *[I43]*
- • neonatal (transient) P72.1
- • transient with chronic thyroiditis E06.2

Tibia vara M92.51-

Tic (disorder) F95.9
- • child problem F95.0
- • compulsive F95.1
- • de la Tourette F95.2
- • disorder
  - – chronic
    - ■ motor F95.1
    - ■ vocal F95.1
  - – combined vocal and multiple motor F95.2
  - – transient F95.0
- • habit F95.9
  - – transient of childhood F95.0
- • lid, transient of childhood F95.0
- • motor-verbal F95.2
- • orbicularis F95.8
  - – transient of childhood F95.0
- • provisional F95.0
- • spasm (motor or vocal) F95.9
  - – chronic F95.1
  - – transient of childhood F95.0

Tick-borne—*see* Disease, diseased

Tietze's disease or syndrome M94.0

Tight, tightness
- • anus K62.89
- • foreskin (congenital) N47.1
- • rectal sphincter K62.89
- • urethral sphincter N35.919

Timidity, child F93.8

Tinea (intersecta) (tarsi) B35.9
- • asbestina B35.0
- • barbae B35.0
- • beard B35.0
- • black dot B35.0
- • capitis B35.0
- • corporis B35.4
- • cruris B35.6
- • flava B36.0
- • foot B35.3
- • furfuracea B36.0
- • imbricata (Tokelau) B35.5

Tinea, *continued*
- • kerion B35.0
- • microsporic—*see* Dermatophytosis
- • nodosa B36.-
- • pedis B35.3
- • scalp B35.0
- • specified NEC B35.8
- • sycosis B35.0
- • tonsurans B35.0
- • trichophytic—*see* Dermatophytosis
- • unguium B35.1
- • versicolor B36.0

Tinnitus NOS H93.1-
- • audible H93.1-
- • aurium H93.1-
- • pulsatile H93.A-
- • subjective H93.1-

Tiredness R53.83

Tobacco (nicotine)
- • abuse—*see* Tobacco, use
- • dependence—*see* Dependence, drug, nicotine
- • harmful use Z72.0
- • heart—*see* Tobacco, toxic effect
- • maternal use, affecting newborn P04.2
- • toxic effect—*see* Table of Drugs and Chemicals, by substance, poisoning
  - – chewing tobacco—*see* Table of Drugs and Chemicals, by substance, poisoning
  - – cigarettes—*see* Table of Drugs and Chemicals, by substance, poisoning
- • use Z72.0
  - – counseling and surveillance Z71.6
  - – history Z87.891
- • withdrawal state—*see* Dependence, drug, nicotine F17.203

Tongue—*see also* Disease, diseased
- • tie Q38.1

Tonsillitis (acute) (catarrhal) (croupous) (follicular) (gangrenous) (infective) (lacunar) (lingual) (malignant) (membranous) (parenchymatous) (phlegmonous) (pseudomembranous) (purulent) (septic) (subacute) (suppurative) (toxic) (ulcerative) (vesicular) (viral) J03.90
- • chronic J35.01
  - – with adenoiditis J35.03
- • hypertrophic J35.01
  - – with adenoiditis J35.03
- • recurrent J03.91
- • specified organism NEC J03.80
  - – recurrent J03.81
- • staphylococcal J03.80
  - – recurrent J03.81
- • streptococcal J03.00
  - – recurrent J03.01

Tooth, teeth—*see* Disease, diseased

TORCH infection—*see* Infection, congenital
- • without active infection P00.2

Torsion
- • appendix epididymis N44.04
- • appendix testis N44.03
- • bile duct (common) (hepatic) K83.8
  - – congenital Q44.5
- • bowel, colon or intestine K56.2
- • epididymis (appendix) N44.04
- • gallbladder K82.8
  - – congenital Q44.1
- • hydatid of Morgagni
  - – male N44.03
- • Meckel's diverticulum (congenital) Q43.0
- • mesentery K56.2
- • omentum K56.2
- • organ or site, congenital NEC—*see* Anomaly, by site
- • ovary (pedicle) N83.51-
  - – with fallopian tube N83.53
  - – congenital Q50.2
- • penis (acquired) N48.82
  - – congenital Q55.63
- • spermatic cord N44.02
  - – extravaginal N44.01
  - – intravaginal N44.02
- • testis, testicle N44.00
  - – appendix N44.03

Torsion, *continued*
- tibia—*see* Deformity, limb, specified type NEC, lower leg

Torticollis (intermittent) (spastic) M43.6
- congenital (sternomastoid) Q68.0
- due to birth injury P15.8
- hysterical F44.4
- ocular R29.891
- psychogenic F45.8
  - conversion reaction F44.4
- rheumatic M43.6
- traumatic, current S13.4

Tortuous
- ureter N13.8

Tourette's syndrome F95.2

Tourniquet syndrome—*see* Constriction, external, by site

Tower skull Q75.0
- with exophthalmos Q87.0

Toxemia
- erysipelatous—*see* Erysipelas
- food—*see* Poisoning, food
- staphylococcal, due to food A05.0

Toxic (poisoning) (*see also* Disease, diseased) T65.91
- effect—*see* Table of Drugs and Chemicals, by substance, poisoning
- shock syndrome A48.3

Toxicity—*see* Table of Drugs and Chemicals, by substance, poisoning
- fava bean D55.0
- food, noxious—*see* Poisoning, food
- from drug or nonmedicinal substance—*see* Table of Drugs and Chemicals, by drug

Toxicosis—*see also* Toxemia
- capillary, hemorrhagic D69.0

Toxoplasma, toxoplasmosis (acquired) B58.9
- with
  - meningoencephalitis B58.2
  - ocular involvement B58.00
  - other organ involvement B58.89
  - pneumonia, pneumonitis B58.3
- congenital (acute) (subacute) (chronic) P37.1
- maternal, manifest toxoplasmosis in infant (acute) (subacute) (chronic) P37.1

Tracheitis (catarrhal) (infantile) (membranous) (plastic) (septal) (suppurative) (viral) J04.10
- with
  - bronchitis (15 years of age and above) J40
    - acute or subacute—*see* Bronchitis, acute
    - under 15 years of age J20.9
  - laryngitis (acute) J04.2
    - chronic J37.1
- acute J04.10
  - with obstruction J04.11
- chronic J42
  - with
    - laryngitis (chronic) J37.1

Tracheomalacia J39.8
- congenital Q32.0

Tracheopharyngitis (acute) J06.9
- chronic J42

Trachoma, trachomatous A71.9
- Türck's J37.0

Train sickness T75.3

Trait
- Hb-S D57.3
- hemoglobin
  - abnormal NEC D58.2
    - with thalassemia D56.3
  - C—*see* Disease, hemoglobin or Hb
  - S (Hb-S) D57.3
- Lepore D56.3
- sickle-cell D57.3
  - with elliptocytosis or spherocytosis D57.3

Transaminasemia R74.01

Transfusion
- associated (red blood cell) hemochromatosis E83.111
- reaction (adverse)—*see* Complications, transfusion
- related acute lung injury (TRALI) J95.84

Transient (meaning homeless) (*see also* Disease, diseased) Z59.0

Translocation
- balanced autosomal Q95.9
  - in normal individual Q95.0
- chromosomes NEC Q99.8
  - balanced and insertion in normal individual Q95.0
- Down syndrome Q90.2
- trisomy
  - 13 Q91.6
  - 18 Q91.2
  - 21 Q90.2

Transplant (ed) (status) Z94.9
- awaiting organ Z76.82
- bone Z94.6
  - marrow Z94.81
- candidate Z76.82
- heart Z94.1
  - valve Z95.2
    - prosthetic Z95.2
    - specified NEC Z95.4
    - xenogenic Z95.3
- intestine Z94.82
- kidney Z94.0
- liver Z94.4
- lung(s) Z94.2
  - and heart Z94.3
- organ (failure) (infection) (rejection) Z94.9
  - removal status Z98.85
- pancreas Z94.83
- skin Z94.5
- social Z60.3
- specified organ or tissue NEC Z94.89
- stem cells Z94.84
- tissue Z94.9

Transposition (congenital)—*see also* Malposition, congenital
- abdominal viscera Q89.3
- aorta (dextra) Q20.3
- great vessels (complete) (partial) Q20.3
- heart Q24.0
  - with complete transposition of viscera Q89.3
- scrotum Q55.23
- stomach Q40.2
  - with general transposition of viscera Q89.3
- vessels, great (complete) (partial) Q20.3
- viscera (abdominal) (thoracic) Q89.3

Transsexualism F64.0

Transvestism, transvestitism (dual-role) F64.1

Trauma, traumatism—*see also* Injury
- acoustic—*see* subcategory H83.3
- occlusal
  - primary K08.81
  - secondary K08.82

Tremor(s) R25.1
- hysterical F44.4
- psychogenic (conversion reaction) F44.4

Triad
- Kartagener's Q89.3

Trichocephaliasis, trichocephalosis B79

Trichocephalus infestation B79

Trichomoniasis A59.9
- bladder A59.03
- cervix A59.09
- seminal vesicles A59.09
- specified site NEC A59.8
- urethra A59.03
- urogenitalis A59.00
- vagina A59.01
- vulva A59.01

Trigger finger (acquired)
- congenital Q74.0

Triphalangeal thumb Q74.0

Triple—*see also* Anomaly
- X, female Q97.0

Trismus R25.2

Trisomy (syndrome) Q92.9
- 13 (partial) Q91.7
  - meiotic nondisjunction Q91.4
- 18 (partial) Q91.3
  - meiotic nondisjunction Q91.0
- 21 (partial) Q90.9

Trombiculosis, trombiculiasis, trombidiosis B88.0

Trophoneurosis NEC G96.89

Trouble—*see also* Disease
- nervous R45.0

Truancy, childhood
- from school Z72.810

Truncus
- arteriosus (persistent) Q20.0
- communis Q20.0

Trunk—*see* Disease, diseased

Tuberculoma—*see also* Tuberculosis
- brain A17.81
- meninges (cerebral) (spinal) A17.1
- spinal cord A17.81

Tuberculosis, tubercular, tuberculous (calcification) (calcified) (caseous) (chromogenic acid-fast bacilli) (degeneration) (fibrocaseous) (fistula) (interstitial) (isolated circumscribed lesions) (necrosis) (parenchymatous) (ulcerative) A15.9
- abscess (respiratory) A15.9
  - latent Z22.7
  - meninges (cerebral) (spinal) A17.0
  - scrofulous A18.2
- arachnoid A17.0
- axilla, axillary (gland) A18.2
- cachexia A15.9
- cerebrospinal A17.81
  - meninges A17.0
- cervical (lymph gland or node) A18.2
- contact Z20.1
- dura (mater) (cerebral) (spinal) A17.0
  - abscess (cerebral) (spinal) A17.81
- exposure (to) Z20.1
- glandular, general A18.2
- immunological findings only A15.7
- infection A15.9
  - without clinical manifestation A15.7
- infraclavicular gland A18.2
- inguinal gland A18.2
- inguinalis A18.2
- latent Z22.7
- leptomeninges, leptomeningitis (cerebral) (spinal) A17.0
- lymph gland or node (peripheral) A18.2
  - cervical A18.2
- marasmus A15.9
- neck gland A18.2
- meninges, meningitis (basilar) (cerebral) (cerebrospinal) (spinal) A17.0
- pachymeningitis A17.0
- respiratory A15.9
  - primary A15.7
  - specified site NEC A15.8
- scrofulous A18.2
- senile A15.9
- spine, spinal (column) A18.01
  - cord A17.81
  - medulla A17.81
  - membrane A17.0
  - meninges A17.0
- supraclavicular gland A18.2
- unspecified site A15.9

Tuberous sclerosis (brain) Q85.1

Tumefaction—*see also* Swelling
- liver—*see* Hypertrophy, liver

Tumor—*see also* Neoplasm, unspecified behavior, by site in Table of Neoplasms in the complete *ICD-10-CM* manual
- Cock's peculiar L72.3
- glomus D18.00
  - skin D18.00
  - specified site NEC D18.09
- Grawitz's C64.-
- neuroectodermal (peripheral)—*see* Neoplasm, malignant, by site in Table of Neoplasms in the complete *ICD-10-CM* manual

Tumor, *continued*
- – primitive
  - ▪ specified site—*see* Neoplasm, malignant, by site in Table of Neoplasms in the complete *ICD-10-CM* manual
  - ▪ unspecified site C71.9
- • phantom F45.8
- • sternomastoid (congenital) Q68.0
- • turban D23.4
- • Wilms' C64.-

Tumor lysis syndrome (following antineoplastic chemotherapy) (spontaneous) NEC E88.3

Tungiasis B88.1

Tunica vasculosa lentis Q12.2

Turban tumor D23.4

Türck's trachoma J37.0

Turner-like syndrome Q87.19

Turner's syndrome Q96.9

Turner-Ullrich syndrome Q96.9

Twist, twisted
- • bowel, colon or intestine K56.2
- • mesentery K56.2
- • omentum K56.2
- • organ or site, congenital NEC—*see* Anomaly, by site

Tylosis (acquired) L84
- • palmaris et plantaris (congenital) (inherited) Q82.8
  - – acquired L85.1

Tympanism R14.0

Tympanites (abdominal) (intestinal) R14.0

Tympanitis—*see* Myringitis

Tympany
- • abdomen R14.0
- • chest R09.89

Typhus (fever)
- • Sao Paulo A77.0

U

Ulcer, ulcerated, ulcerating, ulceration, ulcerative
- • anorectal K62.6
- • anus (sphincter) (solitary) K62.6
- • aphthous (oral) (recurrent) K12.0
- • bleeding K27.4
- • breast N61.1
- • buccal (cavity) (traumatic) K12.1
- • cervix (uteri) (decubitus) (trophic) N86
  - – with cervicitis N72
- • Dieulafoy's K25.0
- • duodenum, duodenal (eroded) (peptic) K26.9
  - – with
    - ▪ hemorrhage K26.4
      - ~ and perforation K26.6
    - ▪ perforation K26.5
  - – acute K26.3
    - ▪ with
      - ~ hemorrhage K26.0
        - ◊ and perforation K26.2
      - ~ perforation K26.1
  - – chronic K26.7
    - ▪ with
      - ~ hemorrhage K26.4
        - ◊ and perforation K26.6
      - ~ perforation K26.5
- • dysenteric A09
- • esophagus (peptic) K22.10
  - – due to
    - ▪ gastrointestinal reflux disease K21.0-
- • frenum (tongue) K14.0
- • hemorrhoid (*see also* Hemorrhoids, by degree) K64.8
- • intestine, intestinal K63.3
  - – rectum K62.6
- • lip K13.0
- • meatus (urinarius) N34.2
- • Meckel's diverticulum Q43.0
- • oral mucosa (traumatic) K12.1
- • palate (soft) K12.1
- • peptic (site unspecified) K27.9
  - – with

Ulcer, ulcerated, ulcerating, ulceration, ulcerative, *continued*
- - ▪ hemorrhage K27.4
    - ~ and perforation K27.6
  - ▪ perforation K27.5
- – acute K27.3
  - ▪ with
    - ~ hemorrhage K27.0
      - ◊ and perforation K27.2
    - ~ perforation K27.1
- – chronic K27.7
  - ▪ with
    - ~ hemorrhage K27.4
      - ◊ and perforation K27.6
    - ~ perforation K27.5
- – esophagus K22.10
  - ▪ with bleeding K22.11
- – newborn P78.82
- • perforating K27.5
- • peritonsillar J35.8
- • pressure (pressure area) L89.9-
  - – ankle L89.5-
  - – back L89.1-
  - – buttock L89.3-
  - – coccyx L89.15-
  - – contiguous site of back, buttock, hip L89.4-
  - – elbow L89.0-
  - – face L89.81-
  - – head L89.81-
  - – heel L89.6-
  - – hip L89.2-
  - – sacral region (tailbone) L89.15-
  - – specified site NEC L89.89-
  - – stage 1 (healing) (pre-ulcer skin changes limited to persistent focal edema)
    - ▪ ankle L89.5-
    - ▪ back L89.1-
    - ▪ buttock L89.3-
    - ▪ coccyx L89.15-
    - ▪ contiguous site of back, buttock, hip L89.4-
    - ▪ elbow L89.0-
    - ▪ face L89.81-
    - ▪ head L89.81-
    - ▪ heel L89.6-
    - ▪ hip L89.2-
    - ▪ sacral region (tailbone) L89.15-
    - ▪ specified site NEC L89.89-
  - – stage 2 (healing) (abrasion, blister, partial thickness skin loss involving epidermis and/or dermis)
    - ▪ ankle L89.5-
    - ▪ back L89.1-
    - ▪ buttock L89.3-
    - ▪ coccyx L89.15-
    - ▪ contiguous site of back, buttock, hip L89.4-
    - ▪ elbow L89.0-
    - ▪ face L89.81-
    - ▪ head L89.81-
    - ▪ heel L89.6-
    - ▪ hip L89.2-
    - ▪ sacral region (tailbone) L89.15-
    - ▪ specified site NEC L89.89-
  - – stage 3 (healing) (full thickness skin loss involving damage or necrosis of subcutaneous tissue)
    - ▪ ankle L89.5-
    - ▪ back L89.1-
    - ▪ buttock L89.3-
    - ▪ coccyx L89.15-
    - ▪ contiguous site of back, buttock, hip L89.4-
    - ▪ elbow L89.0-
    - ▪ face L89.81-
    - ▪ head L89.81-
    - ▪ heel L89.6-
    - ▪ hip L89.2-
    - ▪ sacral region (tailbone) L89.15-
    - ▪ specified site NEC L89.89-
  - – stage 4 (healing) (necrosis of soft tissues through to underlying muscle, tendon, or bone)
    - ▪ ankle L89.5-
    - ▪ back L89.1-
    - ▪ buttock L89.3-
    - ▪ coccyx L89.15-
    - ▪ contiguous site of back, buttock, hip L89.4-
    - ▪ elbow L89.0-

Ulcer, ulcerated, ulcerating, ulceration, ulcerative, *continued*
- - ▪ face L89.81-
  - ▪ head L89.81-
  - ▪ heel L89.6-
  - ▪ hip L89.2-
  - ▪ sacral region (tailbone) L89.15-
  - ▪ specified site NEC L89.89-
- • rectum (sphincter) (solitary) K62.6
  - – stercoraceous, stercoral K62.6
- • scrofulous (tuberculous) A18.2
- • scrotum N50.89
  - – varicose I86.1
- • solitary, anus or rectum (sphincter) K62.6
- • sore throat J02.9
  - – streptococcal J02.0
- • stercoraceous, stercoral K63.3
  - – anus or rectum K62.6
- • stomach (eroded) (peptic) (round) K25.9
  - – with
    - ▪ hemorrhage K25.4
      - ~ and perforation K25.6
    - ▪ perforation K25.5
  - – acute K25.3
    - ▪ with
      - ~ hemorrhage K25.0
        - ◊ and perforation K25.2
      - ~ perforation K25.1
  - – chronic K25.7
    - ▪ with
      - ~ hemorrhage K25.4
        - ◊ and perforation K25.6
      - ~ perforation K25.5
- • stomatitis K12.1
- • strumous (tuberculous) A18.2
- • tongue (traumatic) K14.0
- • tonsil J35.8
- • turbinate J34.89
- • uterus N85.8
  - – cervix N86
    - ▪ with cervicitis N72
  - – neck N86
    - ▪ with cervicitis N72
- • valve, heart I33.0
- • varicose (lower limb, any part)—*see also* Varix
  - – scrotum I86.1

Ulcerosa scarlatina A38.8

Ulcus—*see also* Ulcer
- • durum (syphilitic) A51.0
  - – extragenital A51.2

Ulerythema
- • ophryogenes, congenital Q84.2
- • sycosiforme L73.8

Ullrich (-Bonnevie) (-Turner) syndrome Q87.19

Ullrich-Feichtiger syndrome Q87.0

Unavailability (of)
- • medical facilities (at) Z75.3
  - – due to
    - ▪ lack of services at home Z75.0
  - – home Z75.0

Underdevelopment—*see also* Undeveloped
- • sexual E30.0

Underdosing (*see also* Table of Drugs and Chemicals, categories T36–T50, with final character 6) Z91.14
- • intentional NEC Z91.128
  - – due to financial hardship of patient Z91.120
- • unintentional NEC Z91.138

Underimmunization status Z28.3

Underweight R63.6
- • for gestational age—*see* Light for dates

Underwood's disease P83.0

Undeveloped, undevelopment—*see also* Hypoplasia
- • brain (congenital) Q02
- • cerebral (congenital) Q02
- • heart Q24.8
- • lung Q33.6
- • uterus E30.0

Undiagnosed (disease) R69

Unguis incarnatus L60.0

Unstable
- hip (congenital) Q65.6

Unsteadiness on feet R26.81

Untruthfulness, child problem F91.8

Upbringing, institutional Z62.22
- away from parents NEC Z62.29
- in care of non-parental family member Z62.21
- in foster care Z62.21
- in orphanage or group home Z62.22
- in welfare custody Z62.21

Upper respiratory—*see* Disease, diseased

Upset
- gastric K30
- gastrointestinal K30
  - psychogenic F45.8
- intestinal (large) (small) K59.9
  - psychogenic F45.8
- mental F48.9
- stomach K30
  - psychogenic F45.8

Uremia, uremic N19
- chronic NOS (*see also* Disease, kidney, chronic) N18.9
  - due to hypertension—*see* Hypertensive, kidney
- congenital P96.0

Ureteralgia N23

Ureteritis N28.89
- due to calculus N20.1
  - with calculus, kidney N20.2
    - with hydronephrosis N13.2
- nonspecific N28.89

Ureterocele N28.89
- congenital (orthotopic) Q62.31

Urethralgia R39.89

Urethritis (anterior) (posterior) N34.2
- candidal B37.41
- chlamydial A56.01
- diplococcal (gonococcal) A54.01
  - with abscess (accessory gland) (periurethral) A54.1
- gonococcal A54.01
  - with abscess (accessory gland) (periurethral) A54.1
- nongonococcal N34.1
- nonspecific N34.1
- nonvenereal N34.1
- specified NEC N34.2
- trichomonal or due to Trichomonas (vaginalis) A59.03

Urethrorrhea R36.9

Urgency
- fecal R15.2
- urinary R39.15

Uric acid in blood (increased) E79.0

Uricacidemia (asymptomatic) E79.0

Uricemia (asymptomatic) E79.0

Uricosuria R82.998

Urination
- frequent R35.0

Urine
- blood in—*see* Hematuria
- discharge, excessive R35.8
- enuresis, nonorganic origin F98.0
- frequency R35.0
- incontinence R32
  - nonorganic origin F98.0
- intermittent stream R39.198
- pus in N39.0
- retention or stasis R33.9
  - psychogenic F45.8
- secretion
  - deficient R34
  - excessive R35.8
  - frequency R35.0
- stream
  - intermittent R39.198
  - slowing R39.198
  - weak R39.12

Urodialysis R34

Uropathy N39.9
- obstructive N13.9
  - specified NEC N13.8
- reflux N13.9
  - specified NEC N13.8

Urticaria L50.9
- with angioneurotic edema T78.3
- allergic L50.0
- cholinergic L50.5
- chronic L50.8
- due to
  - cold or heat L50.2
  - drugs L50.0
  - food L50.0
  - inhalants L50.0
  - plants L50.6
  - serum (*see also* Reaction, serum) T80.69
- factitial L50.3
- giant T78.3
- gigantea T78.3
- idiopathic L50.1
- larynx T78.3
- neonatorum P83.88
- pigmentosa D47.01
  - congenital Q82.2
  - of neonatal onset Q82.2
- nonallergic L50.1
- pigmentosa D47.01
  - congenital Q82.2
  - of neonatal onset Q82.2
- recurrent periodic L50.8
- serum (*see also* Reaction, serum) T80.69
- specified type NEC L50.8
- thermal (cold) (heat) L50.2
- vibratory L50.4

Use (of)
- alcohol Z72.89
  - harmful—*see* Abuse, alcohol
- caffeine—*see* Use, stimulant NEC
- cannabis F12.90
  - withdrawal F12.93
- inhalants F18.9-
- stimulant NEC F15.90
  - with
    - withdrawal F15.93
  - harmful—*see* Abuse, drug, stimulant NEC
- tobacco Z72.0
  - with dependence—*see* Dependence, drug, nicotine
- volatile solvents (*see also* Use, inhalant) F18.90
  - harmful—*see* Abuse, drug, inhalant

Uveitis (anterior)
- due to toxoplasmosis (acquired) B58.09
  - congenital P37.1

Uveoparotitis D86.89

Uvulitis (acute) (catarrhal) (chronic) (membranous) (suppurative) (ulcerative) K12.2

V

Vaccination (prophylactic)
- complication or reaction—*see* Complications, vaccination
- delayed Z28.9
- encounter for Z23
- not done—*see* Immunization, not done, because (of)

Vaccinia (generalized) (localized) T88.1
- congenital P35.8

Vacuum, in sinus (accessory) (nasal) J34.89

Vagabond's disease B85.1

Vaginitis (acute) (circumscribed) (diffuse) (emphysematous) (nonvenereal) (ulcerative) N76.0
- with abscess (accessory gland) (periurethral) A54.1
- bacterial N76.0
- blennorrhagic (gonococcal) A54.02
- candidal B37.3
- chlamydial A56.02
- chronic N76.1
- due to Trichomonas (vaginalis) A59.01
- gonococcal A54.02

Vaginitis, *continued*
- in (due to)
  - candidiasis B37.3
  - herpesviral (herpes simplex) infection A60.04
  - pinworm infection B80 [N77.1]
- monilial B37.3
- mycotic (candidal) B37.3
- syphilitic (early) A51.0
  - late A52.76
- trichomonal A59.01

Vaginosis—*see* Vaginitis

Valve, valvular (formation)—*see also* Disease, diseased
- cerebral ventricle (communicating) in situ Z98.2

Van der Hoeve (-de Kleyn) **syndrome** Q78.0

Vapor asphyxia or suffocation
- specified agent—*see* Table of Drugs and Chemicals

Variants, thalassemic D56.8

Varicella B01.9
- with
  - complications NEC B01.89
  - encephalitis B01.11
  - encephalomyelitis B01.11
  - meningitis B01.0
  - myelitis B01.12
  - pneumonia B01.2
- congenital P35.8

Varices—*see* Varix

Varicocele (scrotum) (thrombosed) I86.1
- spermatic cord (ulcerated) I86.1

Varicose
- ulcer
  - anus (*see also* Hemorrhoids) K64.8
  - scrotum I86.1

Varix (lower limb) I83.9-
- esophagus (idiopathic) (primary) (ulcerated) I85.00
  - bleeding I85.01
  - congenital Q27.8
- scrotum (ulcerated) I86.1

Vascular—*see also* Disease, diseased
- spider I78.1

Vasculitis I77.6
- allergic D69.0
- systemic M31.8

Vasovagal attack (paroxysmal) R55
- psychogenic F45.8

Vegetation, vegetative
- adenoid (nasal fossa) J35.8
- endocarditis (acute) (any valve) (subacute) I33.0
- heart (mycotic) (valve) I33.0

Venereal
- disease A64

Venom, venomous—*see* Table of Drugs and Chemicals, by animal or substance, poisoning

Ventriculitis (cerebral) (*see also* Encephalitis) G04.90

Ventriculostomy status Z98.2

Vernet's syndrome G52.7

Verruca (due to HPV) (filiformis) (simplex) (viral) (vulgaris) B07.9
- acuminata A63.0
- plana B07.8
- plantaris B07.0
- venereal A63.0

Vertigo R42
- aural H81.31-
- benign paroxysmal (positional) H81.1-
- central (origin) H81.4
- cerebral H81.4
- laryngeal R05
- peripheral NEC H81.39-
  - malignant H81.4

Vesiculitis (seminal) N49.0
- trichomonal A59.09

Vestibulitis (ear) (*see also* subcategory) H83.0
- nose (external) J34.89
- vulvar N94.810

Villaret's syndrome G52.7

Virilism (adrenal) E25.9
- congenital E25.0

Virilization (female) (suprarenal) E25.9
- congenital E25.0
- isosexual E28.2

Virus, viral—*see also* Disease, diseased
- as cause of disease classified elsewhere B97.89
- cytomegalovirus B25.9
- human immunodeficiency (HIV)—*see* Human, immunodeficiency virus (HIV) disease
- infection—*see* Infection, virus
- respiratory syncytial (RSV)
  - as cause of disease classified elsewhere B97.4
  - bronchiolitis J21.0
  - bronchitis J20.5
  - bronchopneumonia J12.1
  - otitis media H65.- [B97.4]
  - pneumonia J12.1
  - upper respiratory infection J06.9 [B97.4]
- specified NEC B34.8
- swine influenza (viruses that normally cause infections in pigs) (*see also* Influenza, due to, identified novel influenza A virus) J09.X2
- West Nile (fever) A92.30
  - with
    - complications NEC A92.39
    - cranial nerve disorders A92.32
    - encephalitis A92.31
    - encephalomyelitis A92.31
    - neurologic manifestation NEC A92.32
    - optic neuritis A92.32
    - polyradiculitis A92.32
- Zika virus disease A92.5

Vision, visual
- blurred, blurring H53.8
  - hysterical F44.6
- defect, defective NEC H54.7
- disorientation (syndrome) H53.8
- disturbance H53.9
  - hysterical F44.6
- double H53.2
- examination Z01.00
  - with abnormal findings Z01.01
  - after failed exam Z01.02-
- hallucinations R44.1

Vitality, lack or want of R53.83
- newborn P96.89

Vitamin deficiency—*see* Deficiency, vitamin

Vitelline duct, persistent Q43.0

Vitiligo L80

Volvulus (bowel) (colon) (intestine) K56.2
- with perforation K56.2
- congenital Q43.8
- duodenum K31.5
  - without refractory migraine G43.A0

Vomiting R11.10
- with nausea R11.2
- bilious (cause unknown) R11.14
  - in newborn P92.01
- cyclical, in migraine G43.A0
  - with refractory migraine G43.A1
  - intractable G43.A1
  - not intractable G43.A0
  - psychogenic F50.89
  - without refractory migraine G43.A0
- cyclical syndrome NOS (unrelated to migraine) R11.1
- fecal matter R11.13
- following gastrointestinal surgery K91.0
  - psychogenic F50.89
- functional K31.89
- hysterical F50.89
- nervous F50.89
- neurotic F50.89
- newborn NEC P92.09
  - bilious P92.01
- periodic R11.10
  - psychogenic F50.89
- projectile R11.12
- psychogenic F50.89
- without nausea R11.11

Von Hippel (-Lindau) **disease or syndrome** Q85.8

Von Recklinghausen
- disease (neurofibromatosis) Q85.01

Vrolik's disease Q78.0

Vulvitis (acute) (allergic) (atrophic) (hypertrophic) (intertriginous) (senile) N76.2
- adhesive, congenital Q52.79
- blennorrhagic (gonococcal) A54.02
- candidal B37.3
- chlamydial A56.02
- gonococcal A54.02
  - with abscess (accessory gland) (periurethral) A54.1
- monilial B37.3
- syphilitic (early) A51.0
  - late A52.76
- trichomonal A59.01

Vulvodynia N94.819
- specified NEC N94.818

Vulvorectal—*see* Disease, diseased

Vulvovaginitis (acute)—*see* Vaginitis

W

Waiting list
- for organ transplant Z76.82

Walking
- difficulty R26.2
  - psychogenic F44.4
- sleep F51.3
  - hysterical F44.89

Wall, abdominal—*see* Disease, diseased

Wandering
- gallbladder, congenital Q44.1
- in diseases classified elsewhere Z91.83

Wart (due to HPV) (filiform) (infectious) (viral) B07.9
- anogenital region (venereal) A63.0
- common B07.8
- external genital organs (venereal) A63.0
- flat B07.8
- plantar B07.0
- venereal A63.0

Waterbrash R12

Weak, weakening, weakness (generalized) R53.1
- bladder (sphincter) R32
- mind F70
- muscle M62.81
- newborn P96.89
- urinary stream R39.12

Weaver's syndrome Q87.3

Web, webbed (congenital)
- fingers Q70.1-
- toes Q70.3-

Weber-Cockayne syndrome (epidermolysis bullosa) Q81.8

Weber-Osler syndrome I78.0

Weight
- 1000–2499 grams at birth (low)—*see* Low, birthweight
- 999 grams or less at birth (extremely low)—*see* Low, birthweight, extreme
- and length below 10th percentile for gestational age P05.1-
- below 10th percentile but length above 10th percentile P05.0-
- gain (abnormal) (excessive) R63.5
- loss (abnormal) (cause unknown) R63.4

Weil (l)-Marchesani syndrome Q87.19

Wen—*see* Cyst, sebaceous

Wenckebach's block or phenomenon I44.1

Werdnig-Hoffmann syndrome (muscular atrophy) G12.0

Werlhof's disease D69.3

Wernicke's
- developmental aphasia F80.2

West's syndrome—*see* Epilepsy, spasms

Wet
- lung (syndrome), newborn P22.1

Wheal—*see* Urticaria

Wheezing R06.2

Whiplash injury S13.4

Whipple's disease (*see also* subcategory M14.8-) K90.81

Whistling face Q87.0

White—*see also* Disease, diseased
- kidney, small N03.9
- mouth B37.0

Whitehead L70.0

Whitlow—*see also* Cellulitis
- with lymphangitis—*see* Lymphangitis, digit
- herpesviral B00.89

Whooping cough A37.90
- with pneumonia A37.91

Williams syndrome Q93.82

Wilms' tumor C64.-

Wiskott-Aldrich syndrome D82.0

Withdrawal state—*see also* Dependence, drug by type, with withdrawal
- newborn
  - correct therapeutic substance properly administered P96.2
  - infant of dependent mother P96.1
- therapeutic substance, neonatal P96.2

Witts' anemia D50.8

Wolff-Parkinson-White syndrome I45.6

Wool sorter's disease A22.1

Word
- blindness (congenital) (developmental) F81.0
- deafness (congenital) (developmental) H93.25

Worries R45.82

Wound, open T14.8

See Bite, Laceration, or Puncture by site for types of wounds not referenced here.
- abdomen, abdominal
  - wall S31.109
- ankle S91.0-
- antecubital space S51.0-
- anterior chamber, eye—*see* Wound, open, ocular
- anus S31.83-
  - bite S31.835
- arm (upper) S41.1-
  - forearm S51.8-
- axilla S41.10-
- back—*see also* Wound, open, thorax, back
  - lower S31.000
- buttock S31.8-
  - left S31.82-
  - right S31.81-
- calf S81.8-
- canaliculus lacrimalis S01.10-
- canthus, eye S01.10-
- cheek (external) S01.4-
- chest wall—*see* Wound, open, thorax
- chin S01.8-
- choroid—*see* Wound, open, ocular
- ciliary body (eye)—*see* Wound, open, ocular
- clitoris S31.4-
  - bite S31.45
- conjunctiva—*see* Wound, open, ocular
- cornea—*see* Wound, open, ocular
- costal region—*see* Wound, open, thorax
- Descemet's membrane—*see* Wound, open, ocular
- digit(s)
  - foot—*see* Wound, open, toe
  - hand—*see* Wound, open, finger
- ear (canal) (external)
  - with amputation—*see* Amputation, traumatic, ear
  - drum S09.2-
- elbow S51.0-
- epididymis—*see* Wound, open, testis
- epiglottis S11.80
- eye—*see* Wound, open, ocular
- eyeball—*see* Wound, open, ocular
- eyebrow S01.10-
- eyelid S01.10-
- face NEC—*see* Wound, open, head, specified site NEC
- finger(s) S61.2-
  - with
    - amputation—*see* Amputation, traumatic, finger
    - damage to nail S61.3-

Chapter 1. Certain infectious and parasitic diseases (A00–B99)

GUIDELINES

HIV Infections
See category B20.

Coding of Sepsis and Severe Sepsis

SEPSIS
For a diagnosis of sepsis, assign the appropriate code for the underlying systemic infection. If the type of infection or causal organism is not further specified, assign code A41.9, Sepsis, unspecified organism. A code from subcategory R65.2, Severe sepsis, should not be assigned unless severe sepsis or an associated acute organ dysfunction is documented.

Negative or inconclusive blood cultures and sepsis
Negative or inconclusive blood cultures do not preclude a diagnosis of sepsis in patients with clinical evidence of the condition, however, the provider should be queried.

Urosepsis
The term urosepsis is a nonspecific term. It is not to be considered synonymous with sepsis. It has no default code in the Alphabetic Index. Should a provider use this term they should be queried.

Sepsis with organ dysfunction
If a patient has sepsis and associated acute organ dysfunction or multiple organ dysfunction (MOD), follow the instructions for coding severe sepsis.

Acute organ dysfunction that is not clearly associated with the sepsis
If a patient has sepsis and an acute organ dysfunction, but the medical record documentation indicates that the acute organ dysfunction is related to a medical condition other than the sepsis, do not assign a code from subcategory R65.2, Severe sepsis. An acute organ dysfunction must be associated with the sepsis in order to assign the severe sepsis code. If the documentation is not clear as to whether an acute organ dysfunction is related to the sepsis or another medical condition, query the provider.

SEVERE SEPSIS
The coding of severe sepsis requires a minimum of 2 codes: first a code for the underlying systemic infection, followed by a code from subcategory R65.2, Severe sepsis. If the causal organism is not documented, assign code A41.9, Sepsis, unspecified organism, for the infection. Additional code(s) for the associated acute organ dysfunction are also required.

Due to the complex nature of severe sepsis, some cases may require querying the provider prior to assignment of the codes.

Septic shock
Septic shock generally refers to circulatory failure associated with severe sepsis, and therefore, it represents a type of acute organ dysfunction. For cases of septic shock, the code for the systemic infection should be sequenced first, followed by code R65.21, Severe sepsis with septic shock or code T81.12, Postprocedural septic shock. Any additional codes for the other acute organ dysfunctions should also be assigned. As noted in the sequencing instructions in the Tabular List, the code for septic shock cannot be assigned as a principal diagnosis.

Sequencing of severe sepsis
If severe sepsis is present on admission, and meets the definition of principal diagnosis, the underlying systemic infection should be assigned as principal diagnosis followed by the appropriate code from subcategory R65.2 as required by the sequencing rules in the Tabular List. A code from subcategory R65.2 can never be assigned as a principal diagnosis. When severe sepsis develops during an encounter (it was not present on admission) the underlying systemic infection and the appropriate code from subcategory R65.2 should be assigned as secondary diagnoses. Severe sepsis may be present on admission but the diagnosis may not be confirmed until sometime after admission. If the documentation is not clear whether severe sepsis was present on admission, the provider should be queried.

Sepsis *or* severe sepsis with a localized infection
If the reason for admission is both sepsis or severe sepsis and a localized infection, such as pneumonia or cellulitis, a code(s) for the underlying systemic infection should be assigned first and the code for the localized infection should be assigned as a secondary diagnosis. If the patient has severe sepsis, a code from subcategory R65.2 should also be assigned as a secondary diagnosis. If the patient is admitted with a localized infection, such as pneumonia, and sepsis/severe sepsis doesn't develop until after admission, the localized infection should be assigned first, followed by the appropriate sepsis/severe sepsis codes.

SEPSIS DUE TO A POSTPROCEDURAL INFECTION

Documentation of causal relationship
As with all postprocedural complications, code assignment is based on the provider's documentation of the relationship between the infection and the procedure.

Sepsis due to a postprocedural infection
For infections following a procedure, a code from T81.40, to T81.43 Infection following a procedure, or a code from O86.00 to O86.03, Infection of obstetric surgical wound, that identifies the site of the infection should be coded first, if known. Assign an additional code for sepsis following a procedure (T81.44) or sepsis following an obstetrical procedure (O86.04). Use an additional code to identify the infectious agent. If the patient has severe sepsis, the appropriate code from subcategory R65.2 should also be assigned with the additional code(s) for any acute organ dysfunction.

For infections following infusion, transfusion, therapeutic injection, or immunization, a code from subcategory T80.2, Infections following infusion, transfusion, and therapeutic injection, or code T88.0-, Infection following immunization, should be coded first, followed by the code for the specific infection. If the patient has severe sepsis, the appropriate code from subcategory R65.2 should also be assigned, with the additional codes(s) for any acute organ dysfunction.

Postprocedural infection and postprocedural septic shock
If a postprocedural infection has resulted in postprocedural septic shock, assign the codes indicated above for sepsis due to a postprocedural infection, followed by code T81.12-, Postprocedural septic shock. Do not assign code R65.21, Severe sepsis with septic shock. Additional code(s) should be assigned for any acute organ dysfunction.

SEPSIS AND SEVERE SEPSIS ASSOCIATED WITH A NONINFECTIOUS PROCESS (CONDITION)
In some cases a noninfectious process (condition), such as trauma, may lead to an infection which can result in sepsis or severe sepsis. If sepsis or severe sepsis is documented as associated with a noninfectious condition, such as a burn or serious injury, and this condition meets the definition for principal diagnosis, the code for the noninfectious condition should be sequenced first, followed by the code for the resulting infection. If severe sepsis, is present a code from subcategory R65.2 should also be assigned with any associated organ dysfunction(s) codes. It is not necessary to assign a code from subcategory R65.1, SIRS of non-infectious origin, for these cases.

If the infection meets the definition of principal diagnosis it should be sequenced before the non-infectious condition. When both the associated non-infectious condition and the infection meet the definition of principal diagnosis either may be assigned as principal diagnosis.

Only one code from category R65, Symptoms and signs specifically associated with systemic inflammation and infection, should be assigned. Therefore, when a non-infectious condition leads to an infection resulting in severe sepsis, assign the appropriate code from subcategory R65.2, Severe sepsis. Do not additionally assign a code from subcategory R65.1, SIRS of non-infectious origin.

Includes: diseases generally recognized as communicable or transmissible
Use additional code to identify resistance to antimicrobial drugs (Z16.-)
Excludes1: certain localized infections — see body system-related chapters
Excludes2: carrier or suspected carrier of infectious disease (Z22.-)
    infectious and parasitic diseases specific to the perinatal period (P35–P39)
    influenza and other acute respiratory infections (J00–J22)

(A00–A09) INTESTINAL INFECTIOUS DISEASES

A02 **OTHER SALMONELLA INFECTIONS**
[4th]   ***Includes:*** infection or foodborne intoxication due to any Salmonella species other than S. typhi and S. paratyphi
  A02.0 **Salmonella enteritis**
    Salmonellosis
  A02.1 **Salmonella sepsis**
  A02.2 **Localized salmonella infections**
    [5th] **A02.20** **Localized salmonella infection, unspecified**
      A02.21 **Salmonella meningitis**
      A02.22 **Salmonella pneumonia**
      A02.23 **Salmonella arthritis**
      A02.24 **Salmonella osteomyelitis**

 [4th] [5th] [6th] [7th] Additional Character Required   ✔ 3-character code

 •=New Code   ***Excludes1***—Not coded here, do not use together
▲=Revised Code   ***Excludes2***—Not included here

A02.25   **Salmonella pyelonephritis**
Salmonella tubulointerstitial nephropathy
A02.29   **Salmonella with other localized infection**
A02.8   **Other specified salmonella infections**
A02.9   **Salmonella infection, unspecified**

A03   SHIGELLOSIS
4th
A03.0   **Shigellosis due to Shigella dysenteriae**
Group A shigellosis [Shiga-Kruse dysentery]
A03.1   **Shigellosis due to Shigella flexneri**
Group B shigellosis
A03.2   **Shigellosis due to Shigella boydii**
Group C shigellosis
A03.3   **Shigellosis due to Shigella sonnei**
Group D shigellosis
A03.8   **Other shigellosis**
A03.9   **Shigellosis, unspecified**
Bacillary dysentery NOS

A04   OTHER BACTERIAL INTESTINAL INFECTIONS
4th
Excludes1: bacterial foodborne intoxications, NEC (A05.-)
     tuberculous enteritis (A18.32)
A04.0   **Enteropathogenic E. coli infection**
A04.1   **Enterotoxigenic E. coli infection**
A04.2   **Enteroinvasive E. coli infection**
A04.3   **Enterohemorrhagic E. coli infection**
A04.4   **Other intestinal E. coli infections**
E. coli enteritis NOS
A04.5   **Campylobacter enteritis**
A04.6   **Enteritis due to Yersinia enterocolitica**
Excludes1: extraintestinal yersiniosis (A28.2)
A04.7   **Enterocolitis due to Clostridium difficile**
5th
Foodborne intoxication by Clostridium difficile
Pseudomembraneous colitis
     A04.71   **Enterocolitis due to Clostridium difficile, recurrent**
     A04.72   **Enterocolitis due to Clostridium difficile, not specified as recurrent**
A04.8   **Other specified bacterial intestinal infections**
H. pylori
A04.9   **Bacterial intestinal infection, unspecified**
Bacterial enteritis NOS

A05   OTHER BACTERIAL FOODBORNE INTOXICATIONS, NOT ELSEWHERE CLASSIFIED
4th
Excludes1: Clostridium difficile foodborne intoxication and infection (A04.7-)
     E. coli infection (A04.0–A04.4)
     listeriosis (A32.-)
     salmonella foodborne intoxication and infection (A02.-)
     toxic effect of noxious foodstuffs (T61–T62)
A05.0   **Foodborne staphylococcal intoxication**
A05.1   **Botulism food poisoning**
Botulism NOS
Classical foodborne intoxication due to Clostridium botulinum
Excludes1: infant botulism (A48.51)
       wound botulism (A48.52)
A05.2   **Foodborne Clostridium perfringens [Clostridium welchii] intoxication**
Enteritis necroticans
Pigbel
A05.3   **Foodborne Vibrio parahaemolyticus intoxication**
A05.4   **Foodborne Bacillus cereus intoxication**
A05.5   **Foodborne Vibrio vulnificus intoxication**
A05.8   **Other specified bacterial foodborne intoxications**
A05.9   **Bacterial foodborne intoxication, unspecified**

A06   AMEBIASIS
4th
Includes: infection due to Entamoeba histolytica
Excludes1: other protozoal intestinal diseases (A07.-)
Excludes2: acanthamebiasis (B60.1-)
     Naegleriasis (B60.2)
A06.0   **Acute amebic dysentery**
Acute amebiasis
Intestinal amebiasis NOS

A07   OTHER PROTOZOAL INTESTINAL DISEASES
4th
A07.1   **Giardiasis [lambliasis]**
A07.2   **Cryptosporidiosis**

A08   VIRAL AND OTHER SPECIFIED INTESTINAL INFECTIONS
4th
Excludes1: influenza with involvement of gastrointestinal tract (J09.X3, J10.2, J11.2)
A08.0   **Rotaviral enteritis**
A08.3   **Other viral enteritis**
5th   **A08.39**   **Other viral enteritis**
Coxsackie virus enteritis
Echovirus enteritis
Enterovirus enteritis NEC
Torovirus enteritis
A08.4   **Viral intestinal infection, unspecified**
Viral enteritis NOS
Viral gastroenteritis NOS
Viral gastroenteropathy NOS
A08.8   **Other specified intestinal infections**

A09   INFECTIOUS GASTROENTERITIS AND COLITIS, UNSPECIFIED
✔
Infectious colitis NOS
Infectious enteritis NOS
Infectious gastroenteritis NOS
Excludes1: colitis NOS (K52.9)
     diarrhea NOS (R19.7)
     enteritis NOS (K52.9)
     gastroenteritis NOS (K52.9)
     noninfective gastroenteritis and colitis, unspecified (K52.9)

(A15–A19) TUBERCULOSIS

Includes: infections due to Mycobacterium tuberculosis and Mycobacterium bovis
Excludes1: congenital tuberculosis (P37.0)
     nonspecific reaction to test for tuberculosis without active tuberculosis (R76.1-)
     pneumoconiosis associated with tuberculosis, any type in A15 (J65)
     positive PPD (R76.11)
     positive tuberculin skin test without active tuberculosis (R76.11)
     sequelae of tuberculosis (B90.-)
     silicotuberculosis (J65)

A15   RESPIRATORY TUBERCULOSIS
4th
A15.0   **Tuberculosis of lung**
Tuberculous bronchiectasis
Tuberculous fibrosis of lung
Tuberculous pneumonia
Tuberculous pneumothorax
A15.4   **Tuberculosis of intrathoracic lymph nodes**
Tuberculosis of hilar lymph nodes
Tuberculosis of mediastinal lymph nodes
Tuberculosis of tracheobronchial lymph nodes
Excludes1: tuberculosis specified as primary (A15.7)
A15.5   **Tuberculosis of larynx, trachea and bronchus**
Tuberculosis of bronchus
Tuberculosis of glottis
Tuberculosis of larynx
Tuberculosis of trachea
A15.6   **Tuberculous pleurisy**
Tuberculosis of pleura Tuberculous empyema
Excludes1: primary respiratory tuberculosis (A15.7)
A15.7   **Primary respiratory tuberculosis**
A15.8   **Other respiratory tuberculosis**
Mediastinal tuberculosis
Nasopharyngeal tuberculosis
Tuberculosis of nose
Tuberculosis of sinus [any nasal]
A15.9   **Respiratory tuberculosis unspecified**

A17   TUBERCULOSIS OF NERVOUS SYSTEM
4th
A17.0   **Tuberculous meningitis**
Tuberculosis of meninges (cerebral)(spinal)
Tuberculous leptomeningitis
Excludes1: tuberculous meningoencephalitis (A17.82)

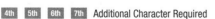

4th **5th** **6th** **7th**   Additional Character Required   ✔   3-character code   •=New Code   *Excludes1*—Not coded here, do not use together
▲=Revised Code   *Excludes2*—Not included here

A17.1 Meningeal tuberculoma
Tuberculoma of meninges (cerebral) (spinal)
Excludes2: tuberculoma of brain and spinal cord (A17.81)

A17.8 Other tuberculosis of nervous system

`5th` **A17.81 Tuberculoma of brain and spinal cord**
Tuberculous abscess of brain and spinal cord

A17.82 Tuberculous meningoencephalitis
Tuberculous myelitis

A17.83 Tuberculous neuritis
Tuberculous mononeuropathy

A17.89 Other tuberculosis of nervous system
Tuberculous polyneuropathy

A17.9 Tuberculosis of nervous system, unspecified

A18 TUBERCULOSIS OF OTHER ORGANS

`4th` **A18.0 Tuberculosis of bones and joints**

`5th` **A18.01 Tuberculosis of spine**
Pott's disease or curvature of spine
Tuberculous arthritis
Tuberculous osteomyelitis of spine
Tuberculous spondylitis

A18.02 Tuberculous arthritis of other joints
Tuberculosis of hip (joint)
Tuberculosis of knee (joint)

A18.03 Tuberculosis of other bones
Tuberculous mastoiditis
Tuberculous osteomyelitis

A18.09 Other musculoskeletal tuberculosis
Tuberculous myositis
Tuberculous synovitis
Tuberculous tenosynovitis

A18.2 Tuberculous peripheral lymphadenopathy
Tuberculous adenitis
Excludes2: tuberculosis of bronchial and mediastinal lymph nodes (A15.4)
tuberculosis of mesenteric and retroperitoneal lymph nodes (A18.39)
tuberculous tracheobronchial adenopathy (A15.4)

A18.3 Tuberculosis of intestines, peritoneum and mesenteric glands

`5th` **A18.31 Tuberculous peritonitis**
Tuberculous ascites

A18.32 Tuberculous enteritis
Tuberculosis of anus and rectum
Tuberculosis of intestine (large) (small)

A18.39 Retroperitoneal tuberculosis
Tuberculosis of mesenteric glands
Tuberculosis of retroperitoneal (lymph glands)

A18.4 Tuberculosis of skin and subcutaneous tissue
Erythema induratum, tuberculous
Lupus excedens
Lupus vulgaris NOS
Lupus vulgaris of eyelid
Scrofuloderma
Tuberculosis of external ear
Excludes2: lupus erythematosus (L93.-)
lupus NOS (M32.9)
systemic lupus erythematosus (M32.-)

A18.6 Tuberculosis of (inner) (middle) ear
Tuberculous otitis media
Excludes2: tuberculosis of external ear (A18.4)
tuberculous mastoiditis (A18.03)

A18.8 Tuberculosis of other specified organs

`5th` **A18.84 Tuberculosis of heart**
Tuberculous cardiomyopathy
Tuberculous endocarditis
Tuberculous myocarditis
Tuberculous pericarditis

A18.85 Tuberculosis of spleen

A18.89 Tuberculosis of other sites
Tuberculosis of muscle
Tuberculous cerebral arteritis

A19 MILIARY TUBERCULOSIS

`4th` *Includes:* disseminated tuberculosis
generalized tuberculosis
tuberculous polyserositis

A19.0 Acute miliary tuberculosis of a single specified site

A19.1 Acute miliary tuberculosis of multiple sites

A19.2 Acute miliary tuberculosis, unspecified

A19.8 Other miliary tuberculosis

A19.9 Miliary tuberculosis, unspecified

(A20–A28) CERTAIN ZOONOTIC BACTERIAL DISEASES

A22 ANTHRAX

`4th` *Includes:* infection due to Bacillus anthracis

A22.0 Cutaneous anthrax
Malignant carbuncle
Malignant pustule

A22.1 Pulmonary anthrax
Inhalation anthrax
Rag picker's disease
Wool sorter's disease

A22.2 Gastrointestinal anthrax

A22.9 Anthrax, unspecified

A25 RAT-BITE FEVERS

`4th` **A25.0 Spirillosis**

A25.1 Streptobacillosis

A25.9 Rat-bite fever, unspecified

A26 ERYSIPELOID

`4th` **A26.0 Cutaneous erysipeloid**

A26.7 Erysipelothrix sepsis

A26.8 Other forms of erysipeloid

A26.9 Erysipeloid, unspecified

A27 LEPTOSPIROSIS

`4th` **A27.0 Leptospirosis icterohemorrhagica**

A27.8 Other forms of leptospirosis

`5th` **A27.81 Aseptic meningitis in leptospirosis**

A27.89 Other forms of leptospirosis

A27.9 Leptospirosis, unspecified

A28 OTHER ZOONOTIC BACTERIAL DISEASES, NEC

`4th` **A28.0 Pasteurellosis**

A28.1 Cat-scratch disease
Cat-scratch fever

A28.2 Extraintestinal yersiniosis
Excludes1: enteritis due to Yersinia enterocolitica (A04.6)

(A30–A49) OTHER BACTERIAL DISEASES

A31 INFECTION DUE TO OTHER MYCOBACTERIA

`4th` *Excludes2:* tuberculosis (A15–A19)

A31.0 Pulmonary mycobacterial infection

A31.1 Cutaneous mycobacterial infection

A31.2 Disseminated mycobacterium avium-intracellulare complex (DMAC)

A31.8 Other mycobacterial infections

A31.9 Mycobacterial infection, unspecified

A32 LISTERIOSIS

`4th` *Includes:* listerial foodborne infection
Excludes1: neonatal (disseminated) listeriosis (P37.2)

A32.0 Cutaneous listeriosis

A32.1 Listerial meningitis and meningoencephalitis

`5th` **A32.11 Listerial meningitis**

A32.12 Listerial meningoencephalitis

A32.7 Listerial sepsis

A32.8 Other forms of listeriosis

`5th` **A32.81 Oculoglandular listeriosis**

A32.82 Listerial endocarditis

A32.89 Other forms of listeriosis
Listerial cerebral arteritis

A32.9 Listeriosis, unspecified

A35 OTHER TETANUS

`✔`

A36 **DIPHTHERIA**
`4th`
- A36.0 Pharyngeal diphtheria
- A36.1 Nasopharyngeal diphtheria
- A36.2 Laryngeal diphtheria
- A36.8 Other diphtheria
  - `5th` A36.89   Other diphtheritic complications
- A36.9 Diphtheria, unspecified

A37 **WHOOPING COUGH**
`4th`
- A37.0 Whooping cough due to Bordetella pertussis;
  - `5th` A37.00   without pneumonia
  - A37.01   with pneumonia
- A37.1 Whooping cough due to Bordetella parapertussis;
  - `5th` A37.10   without pneumonia
  - A37.11   with pneumonia
- A37.8 Whooping cough due to other Bordetella species;
  - `5th` A37.80   without pneumonia
  - A37.81   with pneumonia
- A37.9 Whooping cough, unspecified species;
  - `5th` A37.90   without pneumonia
  - A37.91   with pneumonia

A38 **SCARLET FEVER**
`4th`
Includes: scarlatina
Excludes2: streptococcal sore throat (J02.0)
- A38.0 Scarlet fever with otitis media
- A38.1 Scarlet fever with myocarditis
- A38.8 Scarlet fever with other complications
- A38.9 Scarlet fever, uncomplicated
  - Scarlet fever, NOS

A39 **MENINGOCOCCAL INFECTION**
`4th`
- A39.0 Meningococcal meningitis
- A39.1 Waterhouse-Friderichsen syndrome
  - Meningococcal hemorrhagic adrenalitis
  - Meningococcic adrenal syndrome
- A39.2 Acute meningococcemia
- A39.3 Chronic meningococcemia
- A39.4 Meningococcemia, unspecified
- A39.5 Meningococcal heart disease
  - `5th` A39.50   Meningococcal carditis, unspecified
  - A39.51   Meningococcal endocarditis
  - A39.52   Meningococcal myocarditis
  - A39.53   Meningococcal pericarditis
- A39.8 Other meningococcal infections
  - `5th` A39.89   Other meningococcal infections
    - Meningococcal conjunctivitis
- A39.9 Meningococcal infection, unspecified
  - Meningococcal disease NOS

A40 **STREPTOCOCCAL SEPSIS**
`4th`

GUIDELINES

Refer to Chapter 1 guidelines for sepsis guidelines.
Code first: postprocedural streptococcal sepsis (T81.4-)
streptococcal sepsis following immunization (T88.0)
streptococcal sepsis following infusion, transfusion or therapeutic injection (T80.2-)
Excludes1: neonatal (P36.0–P36.1)
sepsis due to Streptococcus, group D (A41.81)
- A40.0 Sepsis due to streptococcus, group A
- A40.1 Sepsis due to streptococcus, group B
- A40.3 Sepsis due to Streptococcus pneumoniae
  - Pneumococcal sepsis
- A40.8 Other streptococcal sepsis
- A40.9 Streptococcal sepsis, unspecified

A41 **OTHER SEPSIS**
`4th`

GUIDELINES

Refer to Chapter 1 guidelines for sepsis guidelines.
Code first: postprocedural sepsis (T81.4-)
sepsis following immunization (T88.0)
sepsis following infusion, transfusion or therapeutic injection (T80.2-)

Excludes1: bacteremia NOS (R78.81)
neonatal (P36.-)
puerperal sepsis (O85)
streptococcal sepsis (A40.-)
Excludes2: sepsis (due to) (in) actinomycotic (A42.7)
sepsis (due to) (in) anthrax (A22.7)
sepsis (due to) (in) candidal (B37.7)
sepsis (due to) (in) Erysipelothrix (A26.7)
sepsis (due to) (in) extraintestinal yersiniosis (A28.2)
sepsis (due to) (in) gonococcal (A54.86)
sepsis (due to) (in) herpesviral (B00.7)
sepsis (due to) (in) listerial (A32.7)
sepsis (due to) (in) melioidosis (A24.1)
sepsis (due to) (in) meningococcal (A39.2–A39.4)
sepsis (due to) (in) plague (A20.7)
sepsis (due to) (in) tularemia (A21.7)
toxic shock syndrome (A48.3)
- A41.0 Sepsis due to Staphylococcus aureus
  - `5th` A41.01   Sepsis due to MSSA
    - MSSA sepsis
    - Staphylococcus aureus sepsis NOS
  - A41.02   Sepsis due to MRSA
- A41.1 Sepsis due to other specified staphylococcus
  - Coagulase negative staphylococcus sepsis
- A41.2 Sepsis due to unspecified staphylococcus
- A41.3 Sepsis due to H. influenzae
- A41.4 Sepsis due to anaerobes
  - *Excludes1:* gas gangrene (A48.0)
- A41.5 Sepsis due to other Gram-negative organisms
  - `5th` A41.50   Gram-negative sepsis, unspecified
    - Gram-negative sepsis NOS
  - A41.51   Sepsis due to E. coli
  - A41.52   Sepsis due to Pseudomonas
    - Pseudomonas aeroginosa
  - A41.53   Sepsis due to Serratia
  - A41.59   Other Gram-negative sepsis
- A41.8 Other specified sepsis
  - `5th` A41.81   Sepsis due to Enterococcus
  - A41.89   Other specified sepsis
    - If the type of infection or causal organism is not further specified for sepsis, assign code A41.9
- A41.9 Sepsis, unspecified organism
  - Septicemia NOS

A42 **ACTINOMYCOSIS**
`4th`
Excludes1: actinomycetoma (B47.1)
- A42.0 Pulmonary actinomycosis
- A42.1 Abdominal actinomycosis
- A42.2 Cervicofacial actinomycosis
- A42.7 Actinomycotic sepsis
- A42.8 Other forms of actinomycosis
  - `5th` A42.81   Actinomycotic meningitis
  - A42.82   Actinomycotic encephalitis
  - A42.89   Other forms of actinomycosis
- A42.9 Actinomycosis, unspecified

A43 **NOCARDIOSIS**
`4th`
- A43.0 Pulmonary nocardiosis
- A43.1 Cutaneous nocardiosis
- A43.8 Other forms of nocardiosis
- A43.9 Nocardiosis, unspecified

A44 **BARTONELLOSIS**
`4th`
- A44.0 Systemic bartonellosis
- A44.1 Cutaneous and mucocutaneous bartonellosis
- A44.8 Other forms of bartonellosis
- A44.9 Bartonellosis, unspecified

A46 **ERYSIPELAS**
`✔`
Excludes1: postpartum or puerperal erysipelas (O86.89)

A48 **OTHER BACTERIAL DISEASES, NOT ELSEWHERE CLASSIFIED**
`4th`
Excludes1: actinomycetoma (B47.1)
- A48.1 Legionnaires' disease

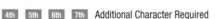

`4th` `5th` `6th` `7th`   Additional Character Required   `✔`   3-character code

●=New Code   *Excludes1*—Not coded here, do not use together
▲=Revised Code   *Excludes2*—Not included here

A48.2   **Nonpneumonic Legionnaires' disease [Pontiac fever]**

A48.3   **Toxic shock syndrome**

     Use additional code to identify the organism (B95, B96)

     Excludes1: endotoxic shock NOS (R57.8)

         sepsis NOS (A41.9)

A48.5   **Other specified botulism**

`5th`   Non-foodborne intoxication due to toxins of Clostridium botulinum [C. botulinum]

     Excludes1: food poisoning due to toxins of Clostridium botulinum (A05.1)

     A48.51   **Infant botulism**

     A48.52   **Wound botulism**

         Non-foodborne botulism NOS

         Use additional code for associated wound

A48.8   **Other specified bacterial diseases**

A49   **BACTERIAL INFECTION OF UNSPECIFIED SITE**

`4th`   *Excludes1:* bacterial agents as the cause of diseases classified elsewhere (B95–B96)

     chlamydial infection NOS (A74.9)

     meningococcal infection NOS (A39.9)

     rickettsial infection NOS (A79.9)

     spirochetal infection NOS (A69.9)

A49.0   **Staphylococcal infection, unspecified site**

`5th`

> **GUIDELINES**
>
> The condition or state of being colonized or carrying MSSA or MRSA is called colonization or carriage, while an individual person is described as being colonized or being a carrier. Colonization means that MSSA or MSRA is present on or in the body without necessarily causing illness. A positive MRSA colonization test might be documented by the provider as "MRSA screen positive" or "MRSA nasal swab positive". Assign code Z22.322, Carrier or suspected carrier of MRSA, for patients documented as having MRSA colonization. Assign code Z22.321, Carrier or suspected carrier of MSSA, for patient documented as having MSSA colonization. Colonization is not necessarily indicative of a disease process or as the cause of a specific condition the patient may have unless documented as such by the provider. If a patient is documented as having both MRSA colonization and infection during a hospital admission, code Z22.322, and a code for the MRSA infection may both be assigned.

     A49.01   **MSSA infection, unspecified site**

         MSSA infection

         Staphylococcus aureus infection NOS

     A49.02   **MRSA infection, unspecified site**

         MRSA infection

A49.1   **Streptococcal infection, unspecified site**

A49.2   **H. influenzae infection, unspecified site**

A49.3   **Mycoplasma infection, unspecified site**

A49.8   **Other bacterial infections of unspecified site**

A49.9   **Bacterial infection, unspecified**

     Excludes1: bacteremia NOS (R78.81)

(A50–A64) INFECTIONS WITH A PREDOMINANTLY SEXUAL MODE OF TRANSMISSION

Excludes1: HIV disease (B20)

     nonspecific and nongonococcal urethritis (N34.1)

     Reiter's disease (M02.3-)

A50   **CONGENITAL SYPHILIS**

`4th`   **A50.0**   **Early congenital syphilis, symptomatic**

`5th`   Any congenital syphilitic condition specified as early or manifest less than two years after birth.

     A50.01   **Early congenital syphilitic; oculopathy**

     A50.02   **osteochondropathy**

     A50.03   **pharyngitis**

         Early congenital syphilitic laryngitis

     A50.04   **pneumonia**

     A50.05   **rhinitis**

     A50.06   **Early cutaneous congenital syphilis**

     A50.07   **Early mucocutaneous congenital syphilis**

     A50.08   **Early visceral congenital syphilis**

     A50.09   **Other early congenital syphilis, symptomatic**

A50.1   **Early congenital syphilis, latent**

     Congenital syphilis without clinical manifestations, with positive serological reaction and negative spinal fluid test, less than two years after birth.

A50.2   **Early congenital syphilis, unspecified**

     Congenital syphilis NOS less than two years after birth.

A50.3   **Late congenital syphilitic oculopathy**

`5th`   *Excludes1:* Hutchinson's triad (A50.53)

     A50.30   **Late congenital syphilitic oculopathy, unspecified**

     A50.31   **Late congenital syphilitic interstitial keratitis**

     A50.32   **Late congenital syphilitic chorioretinitis**

     A50.39   **Other late congenital syphilitic oculopathy**

A50.4   **Late congenital neurosyphilis [juvenile neurosyphilis]**

`5th`   **Use additional code** to identify any associated mental disorder

     Excludes1: Hutchinson's triad (A50.53)

     A50.40   **Late congenital neurosyphilis, unspecified**

         Juvenile neurosyphilis NOS

     A50.41   **Late congenital syphilitic meningitis**

     A50.42   **Late congenital syphilitic encephalitis**

     A50.43   **Late congenital syphilitic polyneuropathy**

     A50.44   **Late congenital syphilitic optic nerve atrophy**

     A50.45   **Juvenile general paresis**

         Dementia paralytica juvenilis

         Juvenile tabetoparetic neurosyphilis

     A50.49   **Other late congenital neurosyphilis**

         Juvenile tabes dorsalis

A50.5   **Other late congenital syphilis, symptomatic**

`5th`   Any congenital syphilitic condition specified as late or manifest two years or more after birth.

     A50.51   **Clutton's joints**

     A50.52   **Hutchinson's teeth**

     A50.53   **Hutchinson's triad**

     A50.54   **Late congenital cardiovascular syphilis**

     A50.55   **Late congenital syphilitic arthropathy**

     A50.56   **Late congenital syphilitic osteochondropathy**

     A50.57   **Syphilitic saddle nose**

     A50.59   **Other late congenital syphilis, symptomatic**

A50.6   **Late congenital syphilis, latent**

     Congenital syphilis without clinical manifestations, with positive serological reaction and negative spinal fluid test, two years or more after birth.

A50.7   **Late congenital syphilis, unspecified**

     Congenital syphilis NOS two years or more after birth.

A50.9   **Congenital syphilis, unspecified**

A51   **EARLY SYPHILIS**

`4th`   **A51.0**   **Primary genital syphilis**

     Syphilitic chancre NOS

A51.1   **Primary anal syphilis**

A51.2   **Primary syphilis of other sites**

A51.3   **Secondary syphilis of skin and mucous membranes**

`5th`   **A51.31**   **Condyloma latum**

     A51.32   **Syphilitic alopecia**

     A51.39   **Other secondary syphilis of skin**

A51.5   **Early syphilis, latent**

     Syphilis (acquired) without clinical manifestations, with positive serological reaction and negative spinal fluid test, less than two years after infection.

A51.9   **Early syphilis, unspecified**

A52   **LATE SYPHILIS**

`4th`   **A52.0**   **Cardiovascular and cerebrovascular syphilis**

`5th`   **A52.00**   **Cardiovascular syphilis, unspecified**

     A52.03   **Syphilitic endocarditis**

         Syphilitic aortic valve incompetence or stenosis

         Syphilitic mitral valve stenosis

         Syphilitic pulmonary valve regurgitation

     A52.06   **Other syphilitic heart involvement**

         Syphilitic coronary artery disease

         Syphilitic myocarditis

         Syphilitic pericarditis

     A52.09   **Other cardiovascular syphilis**

A52.7   **Other symptomatic late syphilis**

`5th`   **A52.76**   **Other genitourinary symptomatic late syphilis**

     A52.79   **Other symptomatic late syphilis**

`4th` `5th` `6th` `7th` Additional Character Required   ✓ 3-character code

•=New Code   *Excludes1*—Not coded here, do not use together

▲=Revised Code   *Excludes2*—Not included here

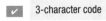

CHAPTER 1. CERTAIN INFECTIOUS AND PARASITIC DISEASES   (A52.8–A68)

A52.8 Late syphilis, latent
Syphilis (acquired) without clinical manifestations, with positive serological reaction and negative spinal fluid test, two years or more after infection

A52.9 Late syphilis, unspecified

A53 OTHER AND UNSPECIFIED SYPHILIS
[4th]

A53.0 Latent syphilis, unspecified as early or late
Latent syphilis NOS
Positive serological reaction for syphilis

A53.9 Syphilis, unspecified
Infection due to Treponema pallidum NOS
Syphilis (acquired) NOS
Excludes1: syphilis NOS under two years of age (A50.2)

A54 GONOCOCCAL INFECTION
[4th]

A54.0 Gonococcal infection of lower genitourinary tract without periurethral or accessory gland abscess
[5th]
Excludes1: gonococcal infection with genitourinary gland abscess (A54.1)
gonococcal infection with periurethral abscess (A54.1)

    A54.00 Gonococcal infection of lower genitourinary tract, unspecified

    A54.01 Gonococcal cystitis and urethritis, unspecified

    A54.02 Gonococcal vulvovaginitis, unspecified

    A54.03 Gonococcal cervicitis, unspecified

    A54.09 Other gonococcal infection of lower genitourinary tract

A54.1 Gonococcal infection of lower genitourinary tract with periurethral and accessory gland abscess
Gonococcal Bartholin's gland abscess

A54.2 Gonococcal pelviperitonitis and other gonococcal genitourinary infection
[5th]
    A54.21 Gonococcal infection of kidney and ureter

    A54.22 Gonococcal prostatitis

    A54.23 Gonococcal infection of other male genital organs
Gonococcal epididymitis
Gonococcal orchitis

    A54.24 Gonococcal female pelvic inflammatory disease
Gonococcal pelviperitonitis
Excludes1: gonococcal peritonitis (A54.85)

    A54.29 Other gonococcal genitourinary infections

A54.3 Gonococcal infection of eye
[5th]
    A54.30 Gonococcal infection of eye, unspecified

    A54.31 Gonococcal conjunctivitis
Ophthalmia neonatorum due to gonococcus

    A54.32 Gonococcal iridocyclitis

    A54.33 Gonococcal keratitis

    A54.39 Other gonococcal eye infection
Gonococcal endophthalmia

A54.4 Gonococcal infection of musculoskeletal system
[5th]
    A54.40 Gonococcal infection of musculoskeletal system, unspecified

    A54.41 Gonococcal spondylopathy
Excludes2: gonococcal infection of spine (A54.41)

    A54.49 Gonococcal infection of other musculoskeletal tissue
Gonococcal bursitis
Gonococcal myositis
Gonococcal synovitis
Gonococcal tenosynovitis

A54.5 Gonococcal pharyngitis

A54.6 Gonococcal infection of anus and rectum

A54.8 Other gonococcal infections
[5th]
    A54.84 Gonococcal pneumonia

    A54.85 Gonococcal peritonitis
Excludes1: gonococcal pelviperitonitis (A54.24)

    A54.86 Gonococcal sepsis

    A54.89 Other gonococcal infections
Gonococcal keratoderma
Gonococcal lymphadenitis

A54.9 Gonococcal infection, unspecified

A56 OTHER SEXUALLY TRANSMITTED CHLAMYDIAL DISEASES
[4th]
Includes: sexually transmitted diseases due to Chlamydia trachomatis
Excludes1: neonatal chlamydial conjunctivitis (P39.1)
neonatal chlamydial pneumonia (P23.1)
Excludes2: chlamydial lymphogranuloma (A55)
conditions classified to A74.-

A56.0 Chlamydial infection of lower genitourinary tract
[5th]
    A56.00 Chlamydial infection of lower genitourinary tract, unspecified

    A56.01 Chlamydial cystitis and urethritis

    A56.02 Chlamydial vulvovaginitis

    A56.09 Other chlamydial infection of lower genitourinary tract
Chlamydial cervicitis

A56.1 Chlamydial infection of pelviperitoneum and other genitourinary organs
[5th]
    A56.11 Chlamydial female pelvic inflammatory disease

    A56.19 Other chlamydial genitourinary infection
Chlamydial epididymitis
Chlamydial orchitis

A56.2 Chlamydial infection of genitourinary tract, unspecified

A56.3 Chlamydial infection of anus and rectum

A56.4 Chlamydial infection of pharynx

A56.8 Sexually transmitted chlamydial infection of other sites

A59 TRICHOMONIASIS
[4th]
Excludes2: intestinal trichomoniasis (A07.8)

A59.0 Urogenital trichomoniasis
[5th]
    A59.00 Urogenital trichomoniasis, unspecified
Fluor (vaginalis) due to Trichomonas
Leukorrhea (vaginalis) due to Trichomonas

    A59.01 Trichomonal vulvovaginitis

    A59.02 Trichomonal prostatitis

    A59.03 Trichomonal cystitis and urethritis

    A59.09 Other urogenital trichomoniasis
Trichomonas cervicitis

A59.8 Trichomoniasis of other sites

A59.9 Trichomoniasis, unspecified

A60 ANOGENITAL HERPESVIRAL [HERPES SIMPLEX] INFECTIONS
[4th]

A60.0 Herpesviral infection of genitalia and urogenital tract
[5th]
    A60.00 Herpesviral infection of urogenital system, unspecified

    A60.01 Herpesviral infection of penis

    A60.02 Herpesviral infection of other male genital organs

    A60.03 Herpesviral cervicitis

    A60.04 Herpesviral vulvovaginitis
Herpesviral [herpes simplex] ulceration
Herpesviral [herpes simplex] vaginitis
Herpesviral [herpes simplex] vulvitis

    A60.09 Herpesviral infection of other urogenital tract

A60.1 Herpesviral infection of perianal skin and rectum

A60.9 Anogenital herpesviral infection, unspecified

A63 OTHER PREDOMINANTLY SEXUALLY TRANSMITTED DISEASES, NEC
[4th]
Excludes2: molluscum contagiosum (B08.1)
papilloma of cervix (D26.0)

A63.0 Anogenital (venereal) warts
Anogenital warts due to (human) papillomavirus [HPV]
Condyloma acuminatum

A63.8 Other specified predominantly sexually transmitted diseases

A64 UNSPECIFIED SEXUALLY TRANSMITTED DISEASE
[✓]
Other spirochetal diseases (A65–A69)
Excludes2: leptospirosis (A27.-)
syphilis (A50–A53)

(A65–A69) OTHER SPIROCHETAL DISEASES

A68 RELAPSING FEVERS
[4th]
Includes: recurrent fever
Excludes2: Lyme disease (A69.2-)

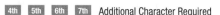 [4th] [5th] [6th] [7th] Additional Character Required   [✓] 3-character code

•=New Code   ***Excludes1***—Not coded here, do not use together
▲=Revised Code   ***Excludes2***—Not included here

A68.0 Louse-borne relapsing fever
Relapsing fever due to Borrelia recurrentis

A68.1 Tick-borne relapsing fever
Relapsing fever due to any Borrelia species other than Borrelia recurrentis

A68.9 Relapsing fever, unspecified

A69 **OTHER SPIROCHETAL INFECTIONS**
[4th] **A69.2 Lyme disease**
[5th] Erythema chronicum migrans due to Borrelia burgdorferi

    A69.20 Lyme disease, unspecified

    A69.21 Meningitis due to Lyme disease

    A69.22 Other neurologic disorders in Lyme disease
        Cranial neuritis
        Meningoencephalitis
        Polyneuropathy

    A69.23 Arthritis due to Lyme disease

    A69.29 Other conditions associated with Lyme disease
        Myopericarditis due to Lyme disease

A69.8 Other specified spirochetal infections

A69.9 Spirochetal infection, unspecified
Other diseases caused by chlamydiae (A70–A74)
Excludes1: sexually transmitted chlamydial diseases (A55–A56)

(A70–A74) OTHER DISEASES CAUSED BY CHLAMYDIAE

A71 **TRACHOMA**
[4th] **A71.0 Initial stage of trachoma**
Trachoma dubium

A71.1 Active stage of trachoma
Granular conjunctivitis (trachomatous)
Trachomatous follicular conjunctivitis
Trachomatous pannus

A71.9 Trachoma, unspecified

A74 **OTHER DISEASES CAUSED BY CHLAMYDIAE**
[4th] *Excludes1:* neonatal chlamydial conjunctivitis (P39.1)
neonatal chlamydial pneumonia (P23.1)
Reiter's disease (M02.3-)
sexually transmitted chlamydial diseases (A55–A56)
Excludes2: chlamydial pneumonia (J16.0)

A74.0 Chlamydial conjunctivitis
Paratrachoma

A74.8 Other chlamydial diseases
[5th]   **A74.81 Chlamydial peritonitis**
    A74.89 Other chlamydial diseases

A74.9 Chlamydial infection, unspecified
Chlamydiosis NOS

(A75–A79) RICKETTSIOSES

A77 **SPOTTED FEVER [TICK-BORNE RICKETTSIOSES]**
[4th] **A77.0 Spotted fever due to Rickettsia rickettsii**
Rocky Mountain spotted fever
Sao Paulo fever

A77.4 Ehrlichiosis
[5th] *Excludes1:* Rickettsiosis due to Ehrlichia sennetsu (A79.81)

    A77.40 Ehrlichiosis, unspecified

    A77.41 Ehrlichiosis chafeensis [E. chafeensis]

    A77.49 Other ehrlichiosis
        Ehrlichiosis due to E. ewingii
        Ehrlichiosis due to E. muris euclairensis

A77.8 Other spotted fevers
Rickettsia 364D/R. philipii (Pacific Coast tick fever)
Spotted fever due to Rickettsia africae (African tick bite fever)
Spotted fever due to Rickettsia parkeri

A77.9 Spotted fever, unspecified
Tick-borne typhus NOS

A79 **OTHER RICKETTSIOSES**
[4th] **A79.1 Rickettsialpox due to Rickettsia akari**
Kew Garden fever
Vesicular rickettsiosis

A79.8 Other specified rickettsioses
[5th]   **A79.89 Other specified rickettsioses**

A79.9 Rickettsiosis, unspecified
Rickettsial infection NOS

(A80–A89) VIRAL AND PRION INFECTIONS OF THE CENTRAL NERVOUS SYSTEM

Excludes1: postpolio syndrome (G14)
sequelae of poliomyelitis (B91)
sequelae of viral encephalitis (B94.1)

A80 **ACUTE POLIOMYELITIS**
[4th] **A80.1 Acute paralytic poliomyelitis, wild virus, imported**

A80.2 Acute paralytic poliomyelitis, wild virus, indigenous

A80.3 Acute paralytic poliomyelitis, other and unspecified
[5th]   **A80.30 Acute paralytic poliomyelitis, unspecified**
    A80.39 Other acute paralytic poliomyelitis

A80.9 Acute poliomyelitis, unspecified

A82 **RABIES**
[4th] **A82.0 Sylvatic rabies**

A82.1 Urban rabies

A82.9 Rabies, unspecified

A83 **MOSQUITO-BORNE VIRAL ENCEPHALITIS**
[4th] *Includes:* mosquito-borne viral meningoencephalitis
Excludes2: Venezuelan equine encephalitis (A92.2)
West Nile fever (A92.3-)
West Nile virus (A92.3-)

A83.2 Eastern equine encephalitis

A83.3 St Louis encephalitis

A83.5 California encephalitis
California meningoencephalitis
La Crosse encephalitis

A83.8 Other mosquito-borne viral encephalitis

A83.9 Mosquito-borne viral encephalitis, unspecified

A84 **TICK-BORNE VIRAL ENCEPHALITIS**
[4th] *Includes:* tick-borne viral meningoencephalitis
▲**A84.8 Other tick-borne viral encephalitis**
[5th]   ●**A84.81 Powassan virus disease**
    ●**A84.89 Other tick-borne viral encephalitis**
        Louping ill
        Code first, if applicable, transfusion related infection (T80.22-)

A84.9 Tick-borne viral encephalitis, unspecified

A85 **OTHER VIRAL ENCEPHALITIS, NEC**
[4th] *Includes:* specified viral encephalomyelitis NEC
specified viral meningoencephalitis NEC
Excludes1: benign myalgic encephalomyelitis (G93.3)
encephalitis due to cytomegalovirus (B25.8)
encephalitis due to herpesvirus NEC (B10.0-)
encephalitis due to herpesvirus [herpes simplex] (B00.4)
encephalitis due to measles virus (B05.0)
encephalitis due to mumps virus (B26.2)
encephalitis due to poliomyelitis virus (A80.-)
encephalitis due to zoster (B02.0)
lymphocytic choriomeningitis (A87.2)

A85.0 Enteroviral encephalitis
Enteroviral encephalomyelitis

A85.1 Adenoviral encephalitis
Adenoviral meningoencephalitis

A85.2 Arthropod-borne viral encephalitis, unspecified
Excludes1: West nile virus with encephalitis (A92.31)

A85.8 Other specified viral encephalitis
Encephalitis lethargica
Von Economo-Cruchet disease

A86 **UNSPECIFIED VIRAL ENCEPHALITIS**
[✔] Viral encephalomyelitis NOS
Viral meningoencephalitis NOS

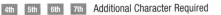 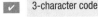

[4th] [5th] [6th] [7th] Additional Character Required   [✔] 3-character code

●=New Code   *Excludes1*—Not coded here, do not use together
▲=Revised Code   *Excludes2*—Not included here

A87 **VIRAL MENINGITIS**
4th
Excludes1: meningitis due to herpesvirus [herpes simplex] (B00.3)
  meningitis due to herpesvirus [herpes simplex] (B00.3)
  meningitis due to measles virus (B05.1)
  meningitis due to mumps virus (B26.1)
  meningitis due to poliomyelitis virus (A80.-)
  meningitis due to zoster (B02.1)

A87.0 **Enteroviral meningitis**
  Coxsackievirus meningitis
  Echovirus meningitis
A87.1 **Adenoviral meningitis**
A87.8 **Other viral meningitis**
A87.9 **Viral meningitis, unspecified**

A88 **OTHER VIRAL INFECTIONS OF CENTRAL NERVOUS**
4th **SYSTEM, NEC**
Excludes1: viral encephalitis NOS (A86)
  viral meningitis NOS (A87.9)
A88.0 **Enteroviral exanthematous fever [Boston exanthem]**
A88.1 **Epidemic vertigo**
A88.8 **Other specified viral infections of central nervous system**

A89 **UNSPECIFIED VIRAL INFECTION OF CENTRAL**
✔ **NERVOUS SYSTEM**

(A90–A99) ARTHROPOD-BORNE VIRAL FEVERS AND VIRAL HEMORRHAGIC FEVERS

A92 **OTHER MOSQUITO-BORNE VIRAL FEVERS**
4th
Excludes1: Ross River disease (B33.1)
A92.3 **West Nile virus infection**
5th   West Nile fever
  A92.30 **West Nile virus infection, unspecified**
    West Nile fever NOS
    West Nile fever without complications
    West Nile virus NOS
  A92.31 **West Nile virus infection with encephalitis**
    West Nile encephalitis
    West Nile encephalomyelitis
  A92.32 **West Nile virus infection with other neurologic manifestation**
    Use additional code to specify the neurologic manifestation
  A92.39 **West Nile virus infection with other complications**
    Use additional code to specify the other conditions
A92.5 **Zika virus disease**

GUIDELINE

1) Code only confirmed cases
Code only a confirmed diagnosis of Zika virus (A92.5, Zika virus disease) as documented by the provider. This is an exception to the hospital inpatient guideline Section II, H. In this context, "confirmation" does not require documentation of the type of test performed; the provider's diagnostic statement that the condition is confirmed is sufficient. This code should be assigned regardless of the stated mode of transmission.

If the provider documents "suspected", "possible" or "probable" Zika, do not assign code A92.5. Assign a code(s) explaining the reason for encounter (such as fever, rash, or joint pain) or Z20.821, Contact with and (suspected) exposure to Zika virus.
Zika virus fever
Zika virus infection
Zika, NOS
Excludes1: congenital Zika virus disease (P35.4)
A92.8 **Other specified mosquito-borne viral fevers**
A92.9 **Mosquito-borne viral fever, unspecified**

A93 **OTHER ARTHROPOD-BORNE VIRAL FEVERS, NOT**
4th **ELSEWHERE CLASSIFIED**
A93.0 **Oropouche virus disease**
  Oropouche fever
A93.1 **Sandfly fever**
  Pappataci fever
  Phlebotomus fever

A93.2 **Colorado tick fever**
A93.8 **Other specified arthropod-borne viral fevers**
  Piry virus disease
  Vesicular stomatitis virus disease [Indiana fever]

A94 **UNSPECIFIED ARTHROPOD-BORNE VIRAL FEVER**
✔ Arboviral fever NOS
  Arbovirus infection NOS

A95 **YELLOW FEVER**
4th
A95.0 **Sylvatic yellow fever**
  Jungle yellow fever
A95.1 **Urban yellow fever**
A95.9 **Yellow fever, unspecified**

A96 **ARENAVIRAL HEMORRHAGIC FEVER**
4th
A96.0 **Junin hemorrhagic fever**
  Argentinian hemorrhagic fever
A96.1 **Machupo hemorrhagic fever**
  Bolivian hemorrhagic fever
A96.2 **Lassa fever**
A96.8 **Other arenaviral hemorrhagic fevers**
A96.9 **Arenaviral hemorrhagic fever, unspecified**

A98 **OTHER VIRAL HEMORRHAGIC FEVERS, NOT ELSEWHERE**
4th **CLASSIFIED**
Excludes1: chikungunya hemorrhagic fever (A92.0)
  dengue hemorrhagic fever (A91)
A98.4 **Ebola virus disease**
A98.5 **Hemorrhagic fever with renal syndrome**
  Epidemic hemorrhagic fever
  Korean hemorrhagic fever
  Russian hemorrhagic fever
  Hantaan virus disease
  Hantavirus disease with renal manifestations
  Nephropathia epidemica
  Songo fever
  Excludes1: hantavirus (cardio)-pulmonary syndrome (B33.4)
A98.8 **Other specified viral hemorrhagic fevers**

A99 **UNSPECIFIED VIRAL HEMORRHAGIC FEVER**
✔

(B00–B09) VIRAL INFECTIONS CHARACTERIZED BY SKIN AND MUCOUS MEMBRANE LESIONS

B00 **HERPESVIRAL [HERPES SIMPLEX] INFECTIONS**
4th
Excludes1: congenital herpesviral infections (P35.2)
Excludes2: anogenital herpesviral infection (A60.-)
  gammaherpesviral mononucleosis (B27.0-)
  herpangina (B08.5)
B00.0 **Eczema herpeticum**
  Kaposi's varicelliform eruption
B00.1 **Herpesviral vesicular dermatitis**
  Herpes simplex facialis
  Herpes simplex labialis
  Herpes simplex otitis externa
  Vesicular dermatitis of ear
  Vesicular dermatitis of lip
B00.2 **Herpesviral gingivostomatitis and pharyngotonsillitis**
  Herpesviral pharyngitis
B00.3 **Herpesviral meningitis**
B00.4 **Herpesviral encephalitis**
  Herpesviral meningoencephalitis
  Simian B disease
  Excludes1: herpesviral encephalitis due to herpesvirus 6 and 7 (B10.01, B10.09)
  non-simplex herpesviral encephalitis (B10.0-)
B00.5 **Herpesviral ocular disease**
5th   **B00.50** **Herpesviral ocular disease, unspecified**
  B00.51 **Herpesviral iridocyclitis**
    Herpesviral iritis
    Herpesviral uveitis, anterior
  B00.52 **Herpesviral keratitis**
    Herpesviral keratoconjunctivitis

4th *5th* *6th* *7th* Additional Character Required   ✔ 3-character code

•=New Code   *Excludes1*—Not coded here, do not use together
▲=Revised Code   *Excludes2*—Not included here

B00.53   **Herpesviral conjunctivitis**
B00.59   **Other herpesviral disease of eye**
         Herpesviral dermatitis of eyelid
B00.7 Disseminated herpesviral disease
     Herpesviral sepsis
B00.8 Other forms of herpesviral infections
5th   B00.81   **Herpesviral hepatitis**
     B00.82   **Herpes simplex myelitis**
     B00.89   **Other herpesviral infection**
         Herpesviral whitlow
B00.9 Herpesviral infection, unspecified
     Herpes simplex infection NOS

B01 VARICELLA [CHICKENPOX]
4th   **B01.0 Varicella meningitis**
     B01.1 Varicella encephalitis, myelitis and encephalomyelitis
     5th   Postchickenpox encephalitis, myelitis and encephalomyelitis
         B01.11   **Varicella encephalitis and encephalomyelitis**
             Postchickenpox encephalitis and encephalomyelitis
         B01.12   **Varicella myelitis**
             Postchickenpox myelitis
     B01.2 Varicella pneumonia
     B01.8 Varicella with other complications
     5th   B01.81   **Varicella keratitis**
         B01.89   **Other varicella complications**
     B01.9 Varicella without complication
         Varicella NOS

B05 MEASLES
4th   *Includes:* morbilli
     Excludes1: subacute sclerosing panencephalitis (A81.1)
     B05.0 Measles complicated by encephalitis
         Postmeasles encephalitis
     B05.1 Measles complicated by meningitis
         Postmeasles meningitis
     B05.2 Measles complicated by pneumonia
         Postmeasles pneumonia
     B05.3 Measles complicated by otitis media
         Postmeasles otitis media
     B05.4 Measles with intestinal complications
     B05.8 Measles with other complications
     5th   B05.81   **Measles keratitis and keratoconjunctivitis**
         B05.89   **Other measles complications**
     B05.9 Measles without complication
         Measles NOS

B06 RUBELLA [GERMAN MEASLES]
4th   *Excludes1:* congenital rubella (P35.0)
     B06.0 Rubella with neurological complications
     5th   B06.00   **Rubella with neurological complication, unspecified**
         B06.09 **Other neurological complications of rubella**
     B06.8 Rubella with other complications
     5th   B06.81   **Rubella pneumonia**
         B06.89   **Other rubella complications**
     B06.9 Rubella without complication
         Rubella NOS

B07 VIRAL WARTS
4th   *Includes:* verruca simplex
         verruca vulgaris
         viral warts due to human papillomavirus
     Excludes2: anogenital (venereal) warts (A63.0)
         papilloma of bladder (D41.4)
         papilloma of cervix (D26.0)
         papilloma larynx (D14.1)
     B07.0 Plantar wart
         Verruca plantaris
     B07.8 Other viral warts
         Common wart
         Flat wart
         Verruca plana
     B07.9 Viral wart, unspecified

B08 OTHER VIRAL INFECTIONS CHARACTERIZED BY SKIN
4th   **AND MUCOUS MEMBRANE LESIONS, NEC**
     Excludes1: vesicular stomatitis virus disease (A93.8)
     B08.1 Molluscum contagiosum
     B08.2 Exanthema subitum [sixth disease]
     5th   Roseola infantum
         B08.20   **Exanthema subitum [sixth disease], unspecified**
             Roseola infantum, unspecified
         B08.21   **Exanthema subitum [sixth disease] due to human herpesvirus 6**
             Roseola infantum due to human herpesvirus 6
         B08.22   **Exanthema subitum [sixth disease] due to human herpesvirus 7**
             Roseola infantum due to human herpesvirus 7
     B08.3 Erythema infectiosum [fifth disease]
     B08.4 Enteroviral vesicular stomatitis with exanthem
         Hand, foot and mouth disease
     B08.5 Enteroviral vesicular pharyngitis
         Herpangina
     B08.8 Other specified viral infections characterized by skin and mucous membrane lesions
         Enteroviral lymphonodular pharyngitis
         Foot-and-mouth disease
         Poxvirus NEC

B09 UNSPECIFIED VIRAL INFECTION CHARACTERIZED BY
✔   **SKIN AND MUCOUS MEMBRANE LESIONS**
     Viral enanthema NOS
     Viral exanthema NOS

(B10) OTHER HUMAN HERPESVIRUSES

B10 OTHER HUMAN HERPESVIRUSES
4th   *Excludes2:* cytomegalovirus (B25.9)
         Epstein-Barr virus (B27.0-)
         herpes NOS (B00.9)
         herpes simplex (B00.-)
         herpes zoster (B02.-)
         human herpesvirus NOS (B00.-)
         human herpesvirus 1 and 2 (B00.-)
         human herpesvirus 3 (B01.-, B02.-)
         human herpesvirus 4 (B27.0-)
         human herpesvirus 5 (B25.-)
         varicella (B01.-)
         zoster (B02.-)
     B10.0 Other human herpesvirus encephalitis
     5th   *Excludes2:* herpes encephalitis NOS (B00.4)
         herpes simplex encephalitis (B00.4)
         human herpesvirus encephalitis (B00.4)
         simian B herpes virus encephalitis (B00.4)
         B10.01   **Human herpesvirus 6 encephalitis**
         B10.09   **Other human herpesvirus encephalitis**
             Human herpesvirus 7 encephalitis
     B10.8 Other human herpesvirus infection
     5th   B10.81   **Human herpesvirus 6 infection**
         B10.82   **Human herpesvirus 7 infection**
         B10.89   **Other human herpesvirus infection**
             Human herpesvirus 8 infection
             Kaposi's sarcoma-associated herpesvirus infection

(B15–B19) VIRAL HEPATITIS

Excludes1: sequelae of viral hepatitis (B94.2)
Excludes2: cytomegaloviral hepatitis (B25.1)
     herpesviral [herpes simplex] hepatitis (B00.81)

B15 ACUTE HEPATITIS A
4th   **B15.9 Hepatitis A without hepatic coma**
         Hepatitis A (acute)(viral) NOS

B16 ACUTE HEPATITIS B
4th   **B16.9 Acute hepatitis B without delta-agent and without hepatic coma**
         Hepatitis B (acute) (viral) NOS

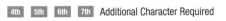 **4th** **5th** **6th** **7th** Additional Character Required   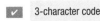 **✔** 3-character code

• =New Code   *Excludes1*—Not coded here, do not use together
▲=Revised Code   *Excludes2*—Not included here

B17 OTHER ACUTE VIRAL HEPATITIS
4th
B17.1 Acute hepatitis C
   5th **B17.10 Acute hepatitis C without hepatic coma**
     Acute hepatitis C NOS
B17.9 Acute viral hepatitis, unspecified
   Acute infectious hepatitis NOS

B18 CHRONIC VIRAL HEPATITIS
4th
Includes: Carrier of viral hepatitis
B18.1 Chronic viral hepatitis B without delta-agent
   Carrier of viral hepatits B
B18.2 Chronic viral hepatitis C
   Carrier of viral hepatitis C
B18.8 Other chronic viral hepatitis
   Carrier of other viral hepatitis
B18.9 Chronic viral hepatitis, unspecified
   Carrier of unspecified viral hepatitis

B19 UNSPECIFIED VIRAL HEPATITIS
4th
B19.1 Unspecified viral hepatitis B
   5th **B19.10 Unspecified viral hepatitis B without hepatic coma**
     Unspecified viral hepatitis B NOS
B19.2 Unspecified viral hepatitis C
   5th **B19.20 Unspecified viral hepatitis C without hepatic coma**
     Viral hepatitis C NOS
B19.9 Unspecified viral hepatitis without hepatic coma
   Viral hepatitis NOS

(B20) HIV DISEASE

GUIDELINES

Code only confirmed cases of HIV infection/illness

In this context, "confirmation" does not require documentation of positive serology or culture for HIV; the provider's diagnostic statement that the patient is HIV positive, or has an HIV-related illness is sufficient.

Asymptomatic HIV

Z21, Asymptomatic HIV infection status, is to be applied when the patient without any documentation of symptoms is listed as being "HIV positive," "known HIV," "HIV test positive," or similar terminology. Do not use this code if the term "AIDS" is used or if the patient is treated for any HIV-related illness or is described as having any condition(s) resulting from his/her HIV positive status; use B20 in these cases.

Patients with inconclusive HIV serology

Patients with inconclusive HIV serology, but no definitive diagnosis or manifestations of the illness, may be assigned code R75, Inconclusive laboratory evidence of HIV.

B20 HIV DISEASE
✔
Includes: acquired immune deficiency syndrome [AIDS]
   AIDS-related complex [ARC]
   HIV infection, symptomatic
Use additional code(s) to identify all manifestations of HIV infection
Excludes1: asymptomatic HIV infection status (Z21)
   exposure to HIV virus (Z20.6)
   inconclusive serologic evidence of HIV (R75)
   Other viral diseases (B25–B34)

(B25–B34) OTHER VIRAL DISEASES

B25 CYTOMEGALOVIRAL DISEASE
4th
Excludes1: congenital cytomegalovirus infection (P35.1)
   cytomegaloviral mononucleosis (B27.1-)
B25.0 Cytomegaloviral pneumonitis
B25.8 Other cytomegaloviral diseases
   Cytomegaloviral encephalitis
B25.9 Cytomegaloviral disease, unspecified

B26 MUMPS
4th
Includes: epidemic parotitis
   infectious parotitis
B26.0 Mumps orchitis
B26.1 Mumps meningitis

B26.2 Mumps encephalitis
B26.8 Mumps with other complications
   5th **B26.89 Other mumps complications**
B26.9 Mumps without complication
   Mumps NOS
   Mumps parotitis NOS

B27 INFECTIOUS MONONUCLEOSIS
4th
Includes: glandular fever
   monocytic angina
   Pfeiffer's disease
B27.0 Gammaherpesviral mononucleosis
   5th Mononucleosis due to Epstein-Barr virus
     B27.00 Gammaherpesviral mononucleosis without complication
     B27.01 Gammaherpesviral mononucleosis with polyneuropathy
     B27.02 Gammaherpesviral mononucleosis with meningitis
     B27.09 Gammaherpesviral mononucleosis with other complications
      Hepatomegaly in gammaherpesviral mononucleosis
B27.1 Cytomegaloviral mononucleosis
   5th **B27.10 Cytomegaloviral mononucleosis without complications**
     B27.11 Cytomegaloviral mononucleosis with polyneuropathy
     B27.12 Cytomegaloviral mononucleosis with meningitis
     B27.19 Cytomegaloviral mononucleosis with other complication
      Hepatomegaly in cytomegaloviral mononucleosis
B27.8 Other infectious mononucleosis
   5th **B27.80 Other infectious mononucleosis without complication**
     B27.81 Other infectious mononucleosis with polyneuropathy
     B27.82 Other infectious mononucleosis with meningitis
     B27.89 Other infectious mononucleosis with other complication
      Hepatomegaly in other infectious mononucleosis
B27.9 Infectious mononucleosis, unspecified
   5th **B27.90 Infectious mononucleosis, unspecified without complication**
     B27.91 Infectious mononucleosis, unspecified with polyneuropathy
     B27.92 Infectious mononucleosis, unspecified with meningitis
     B27.99 Infectious mononucleosis, unspecified with other complication
      Hepatomegaly in unspecified infectious mononucleosis

B30 VIRAL CONJUNCTIVITIS
4th
Excludes1: herpesviral [herpes simplex] ocular disease (B00.5)
   ocular zoster (B02.3)
B30.0 Keratoconjunctivitis due to adenovirus
   Epidemic keratoconjunctivitis
   Shipyard eye
B30.1 Conjunctivitis due to adenovirus
   Acute adenoviral follicular conjunctivitis
   Swimming-pool conjunctivitis
B30.2 Viral pharyngoconjunctivitis
B30.3 Acute epidemic hemorrhagic conjunctivitis (enteroviral)
   Conjunctivitis due to coxsackievirus 24
   Conjunctivitis due to enterovirus 70
   Hemorrhagic conjunctivitis (acute)(epidemic)
B30.8 Other viral conjunctivitis
   Newcastle conjunctivitis
B30.9 Viral conjunctivitis, unspecified

B33 OTHER VIRAL DISEASES, NEC
4th
B33.2 Viral carditis
   5th Coxsackie (virus) carditis
     B33.20 Viral carditis, unspecified
     B33.21 Viral endocarditis
     B33.22 Viral myocarditis
     B33.23 Viral pericarditis
     B33.24 Viral cardiomyopathy
B33.3 Retrovirus infections, NEC
   Retrovirus infection NOS

4th *5th* *6th* *7th* Additional Character Required   ✔ 3-character code

•=New Code   *Excludes1*—Not coded here, do not use together
▲=Revised Code   *Excludes2*—Not included here

B33.8 Other specified viral diseases
> *Excludes1:* anogenital human papillomavirus infection (A63.0)
> viral warts due to human papillomavirus infection (B07)

B34 **VIRAL INFECTION OF UNSPECIFIED SITE**
4th
> *Excludes1:* anogenital human papillomavirus infection (A63.0)
> cytomegaloviral disease NOS (B25.9)
> herpesvirus [herpes simplex] infection NOS (B00.9)
> retrovirus infection NOS (B33.3)
> viral agents as the cause of diseases classified elsewhere (B97.-)
> viral warts due to human papillomavirus infection (B07)

B34.0 Adenovirus infection, unspecified
B34.1 Enterovirus infection, unspecified
> Coxsackievirus infection NOS
> Echovirus infection NOS

B34.2 Coronavirus infection, unspecified
> *Excludes1:* COVID-19 (U07.1)
> pneumonia due to SARS-associated coronavirus (J12.81)

B34.3 Parvovirus infection, unspecified
B34.4 Papovavirus infection, unspecified
B34.8 Other viral infections of unspecified site
B34.9 Viral infection, unspecified
> Viremia NOS

(B35–B49) MYCOSES

Excludes2: hypersensitivity pneumonitis due to organic dust (J67.-)
mycosis fungoides (C84.0-)

B35 **DERMATOPHYTOSIS**
4th
> *Includes:* favus
> infections due to species of Epidermophyton, Micro-sporum and Trichophyton
> tinea, any type except those in B36.-

B35.0 Tinea barbae and tinea capitis
> Beard ringworm
> Kerion
> Scalp ringworm
> Sycosis, mycotic

B35.1 Tinea unguium
> Dermatophytic onychia
> Dermatophytosis of nail
> Onychomycosis
> Ringworm of nails

B35.2 Tinea manuum
> Dermatophytosis of hand
> Hand ringworm

B35.3 Tinea pedis
> Athlete's foot
> Dermatophytosis of foot
> Foot ringworm

B35.4 Tinea corporis
> Ringworm of the body

B35.5 Tinea imbricata
> Tokelau

B35.6 Tinea cruris
> Dhobi itch
> Groin ringworm
> Jock itch

B35.8 Other dermatophytoses
> Disseminated dermatophytosis
> Granulomatous dermatophytosis

B35.9 Dermatophytosis, unspecified
> Ringworm NOS

B36 **OTHER SUPERFICIAL MYCOSES**
4th
B36.0 Pityriasis versicolor
> Tinea flava
> Tinea versicolor

B36.8 Other specified superficial mycoses
B36.9 Superficial mycosis, unspecified

B37 **CANDIDIASIS**
4th
> *Includes:* candidosis
> moniliasis
> *Excludes1:* neonatal candidiasis (P37.5)

B37.0 Candidal stomatitis
> Oral thrush

B37.1 Pulmonary candidiasis
> Candidal bronchitis
> Candidal pneumonia

B37.2 Candidiasis of skin and nail
> Candidal onychia
> Candidal paronychia
> *Excludes2:* diaper dermatitis (L22)

B37.3 Candidiasis of vulva and vagina
> Candidal vulvovaginitis
> Monilial vulvovaginitis
> Vaginal thrush

B37.4 Candidiasis of other urogenital sites
5th **B37.41 Candidal cystitis and urethritis**
> **B37.42 Candidal balanitis**
> **B37.49 Other urogenital candidiasis**
> Candidal pyelonephritis

B37.5 Candidal meningitis
B37.6 Candidal endocarditis
B37.7 Candidal sepsis
> Disseminated candidiasis
> Systemic candidiasis

B37.8 Candidiasis of other sites
5th **B37.81 Candidal esophagitis**
> **B37.82 Candidal enteritis**
> Candidal proctitis
> **B37.83 Candidal cheilitis**
> **B37.84 Candidal otitis externa**
> **B37.89 Other sites of candidiasis**
> Candidal osteomyelitis

B37.9 Candidiasis, unspecified
> Thrush NOS

B39 **HISTOPLASMOSIS**
4th
> **Code first** associated AIDS (B20)
> **Use additional code** for any associated manifestations, such as:
> endocarditis (I39)
> meningitis (G02)
> pericarditis (I32)
> retinitits (H32)

B39.0 Acute pulmonary histoplasmosis capsulati
B39.1 Chronic pulmonary histoplasmosis capsulati
B39.2 Pulmonary histoplasmosis capsulati, unspecified
B39.3 Disseminated histoplasmosis capsulati
> Generalized histoplasmosis capsulati

B39.4 Histoplasmosis capsulati, unspecified
> American histoplasmosis

B39.9 Histoplasmosis, unspecified

B40 **BLASTOMYCOSIS**
4th
> *Excludes1:* Brazilian blastomycosis (B41.-)
> keloidal blastomycosis (B48.0)

B40.0 Acute pulmonary blastomycosis
B40.1 Chronic pulmonary blastomycosis
B40.2 Pulmonary blastomycosis, unspecified
B40.3 Cutaneous blastomycosis
B40.7 Disseminated blastomycosis
> Generalized blastomycosis

B40.8 Other forms of blastomycosis
5th **B40.81 Blastomycotic meningoencephalitis**
> Meningomyelitis due to blastomycosis
> **B40.89 Other forms of blastomycosis**

B40.9 Blastomycosis, unspecified

B44 **ASPERGILLOSIS**
4th
> *Includes:* aspergilloma

B44.8 Other forms of aspergillosis
5th **B44.81 Allergic bronchopulmonary aspergillosis**
> **B44.89 Other forms of aspergillosis**

B44.9 Aspergillosis, unspecified

B49 **UNSPECIFIED MYCOSIS**
✔
Fungemia NOS

4th **5th** **6th** **7th** Additional Character Required   **✔** 3-character code

• =New Code   *Excludes1*—Not coded here, do not use together
▲=Revised Code   *Excludes2*—Not included here

(B50–B64) PROTOZOAL DISEASES

Excludes1: amebiasis (A06.-)
   other protozoal intestinal diseases (A07.-)

B54   **UNSPECIFIED MALARIA**
✔

B58   **TOXOPLASMOSIS**
4th   **Includes:** infection due to Toxoplasma gondii
     Excludes1: congenital toxoplasmosis (P37.1)
     B58.0 Toxoplasma oculopathy
       5th   **B58.00   Toxoplasma oculopathy, unspecified**
           B58.01   Toxoplasma chorioretinitis
           B58.09   Other toxoplasma oculopathy
               Toxoplasma uveitis
     B58.2 Toxoplasma meningoencephalitis
     B58.3 Pulmonary toxoplasmosis
     B58.8 Toxoplasmosis with other organ involvement
       5th   **B58.83   Toxoplasma tubulo-interstitial nephropathy**
               Toxoplasma pyelonephritis
           B58.89   Toxoplasmosis with other organ involvement
     B58.9 Toxoplasmosis, unspecified

B60   **OTHER PROTOZOAL DISEASES, NOT ELSEWHERE**
4th   **CLASSIFIED**
     Excludes1: cryptosporidiosis (A07.2)
       intestinal microsporidiosis (A07.8)
       isosporiasis (A07.3)
     ▲**B60.0 Babesiosis**
       5th   •**B60.00   Babesiosis, unspecified**
               Babesiosis due to unspecified Babesia species
               Piroplasmosis, unspecified
           •**B60.01   Babesiosis due to Babesia microti**
               Infection due to B. microti
           •**B60.02   Babesiosis due to Babesia duncani**
               Infection due to B. duncani and B. duncani-type species
           •**B60.03   Babesiosis due to Babesia divergens**
               Babesiosis due to Babesia MO-1
               Infection due to B. divergens and B. divergens-like strains
           •**B60.09   Other babesiosis**
               Babesiosis due to Babesia KO-1
               Babesiosis due to Babesia venatorum
               Infection due to other Babesia species
               Infection due to other protozoa of the order Piroplasmida
               Other piroplasmosis
     B60.1 Acanthamebiasis
       5th   **B60.10   Acanthamebiasis, unspecified**
           B60.11   Meningoencephalitis due to Acanthamoeba
                (culbertsoni)
           B60.12   Conjunctivitis due to Acanthamoeba
           B60.13   Keratoconjunctivitis due to Acanthamoeba
           B60.19   Other acanthamebic disease

B64   **UNSPECIFIED PROTOZOAL DISEASE**
✔

(B65–B83) HELMINTHIASES

B65   **SCHISTOSOMIASIS [BILHARZIASIS]**
4th   **Includes:** snail fever
     B65.3 Cercarial dermatitis
          Swimmer's itch
     B65.8 Other schistosomiasis
          Infection due to Schistosoma intercalatum
          Infection due to Schistosoma mattheei
          Infection due to Schistosoma mekongi
     B65.9 Schistosomiasis, unspecified

B66   **OTHER FLUKE INFECTIONS**
4th   **B66.8 Other specified fluke infections**
          Echinostomiasis
          Heterophyiasis
          Metagonimiasis
          Nanophyetiasis
          Watsoniasis

     B66.9 Fluke infection, unspecified

B69   **CYSTICERCOSIS**
4th   **Includes:** cysticerciasis infection due to larval form of Taenia solium
     B69.0 Cysticercosis of central nervous system
     B69.8 Cysticercosis of other sites
       5th   **B69.89   Cysticercosis of other sites**
     B69.9 Cysticercosis, unspecified

B71   **OTHER CESTODE INFECTIONS**
4th   **B71.0 Hymenolepiasis**
          Dwarf tapeworm infection
          Rat tapeworm (infection)
     B71.8 Other specified cestode infections
          Coenurosis
     B71.9 Cestode infection, unspecified
          Tapeworm (infection) NOS

B76   **HOOKWORM DISEASES**
4th   **Includes:** uncinariasis
     B76.9 Hookworm disease, unspecified
          Cutaneous larva migrans NOS

B77   **ASCARIASIS**
4th   **Includes:** ascaridiasis
       roundworm infection
     B77.0 Ascariasis with intestinal complications
     B77.8 Ascariasis with other complications
       5th   **B77.81   Ascariasis pneumonia**
           B77.89   Ascariasis with other complications
     B77.9 Ascariasis, unspecified

B79   **TRICHURIASIS**
✔   **Includes:** trichocephaliasis
       whipworm (disease)(infection)

B80   **ENTEROBIASIS**
✔   **Includes:** oxyuriasis
       pinworm infection
       threadworm infection

B82   **UNSPECIFIED INTESTINAL PARASITISM**
4th   **B82.0 Intestinal helminthiasis, unspecified**
     B82.9 Intestinal parasitism, unspecified

(B85–B89) PEDICULOSIS, ACARIASIS AND OTHER INFESTATIONS

B85   **PEDICULOSIS AND PHTHIRIASIS**
4th   **B85.0 Pediculosis due to Pediculus humanus capitis**
          Head-louse infestation
     B85.1 Pediculosis due to Pediculus humanus corporis
          Body-louse infestation
     B85.2 Pediculosis, unspecified
     B85.3 Phthiriasis
          Infestation by crab-louse
          Infestation by Phthirus pubis
     B85.4 Mixed pediculosis and phthiriasis
          Infestation classifiable to more than one of the categories
          B85.0–B85.3

B86   **SCABIES**
✔   Sarcoptic itch

B88   **OTHER INFESTATIONS**
4th   **B88.0 Other acariasis**
          Acarine dermatitis
          Dermatitis due to Demodex species
          Dermatitis due to Dermanyssus gallinae
          Dermatitis due to Liponyssoides sanguineus
          Trombiculosis
          Excludes2: scabies (B86)
     B88.1 Tungiasis [sandflea infestation]
     B88.2 Other arthropod infestations
          Scarabiasis
     B88.3 External hirudiniasis
          Leech infestation NOS
          Excludes2: internal hirudiniasis (B83.4)

4th   5th   6th   7th   Additional Character Required   ✔   3-character code   •=New Code   **Excludes1**—Not coded here, do not use together
                                                                 ▲=Revised Code   **Excludes2**—Not included here

 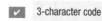

B88.8 Other specified infestations
Ichthyoparasitism due to Vandellia cirrhosa
Linguatulosis
Porocephaliasis

B88.9 Infestation, unspecified
Infestation (skin) NOS
Infestation by mites NOS
Skin parasites NOS

B89   UNSPECIFIED PARASITIC DISEASE
✔

(B90–B94) SEQUELAE OF INFECTIOUS AND PARASITIC DISEASES

Note: Categories B90–B94 are to be used to indicate conditions in categories A00–B89 as the cause of sequelae, which are themselves classified elsewhere. The 'sequelae' include conditions specified as such; they also include residuals of diseases classifiable to the above categories if there is evidence that the disease itself is no longer present. Codes from these categories are not to be used for chronic infections. Code chronic current infections to active infectious disease as appropriate.

     Code first condition resulting from (sequela) the infectious or parasitic disease

B90   SEQUELAE OF TUBERCULOSIS
4th
   B90.0 Sequelae of central nervous system tuberculosis
   B90.1 Sequelae of genitourinary tuberculosis
   B90.2 Sequelae of tuberculosis of bones and joints
   B90.8 Sequelae of tuberculosis of other organs
     Excludes2: sequelae of respiratory tuberculosis (B90.9)
   B90.9 Sequelae of respiratory and unspecified tuberculosis
     Sequelae of tuberculosis NOS

B94   SEQUELAE OF OTHER AND UNSPECIFIED INFECTIOUS AND PARASITIC DISEASES
4th
   B94.1 Sequelae of viral encephalitis
   B94.2 Sequelae of viral hepatitis
   B94.8 Sequelae of other specified infectious and parasitic diseases
   B94.9 Sequelae of unspecified infectious and parasitic disease

(B95–B97) BACTERIAL AND VIRAL INFECTIOUS AGENTS

Note: These categories are provided for use as supplementary or additional codes to identify the infectious agent(s) in diseases classified elsewhere.

B95   STREPTOCOCCUS, STAPHYLOCOCCUS, AND ENTEROCOCCUS AS THE CAUSE OF DISEASES CLASSIFIED ELSEWHERE
4th
   B95.0 Streptococcus, group A, as the cause of diseases classified elsewhere
   B95.1 Streptococcus, group B, as the cause of diseases classified elsewhere
   B95.2 Enterococcus as the cause of diseases classified elsewhere
   B95.3 Streptococcus pneumoniae as the cause of diseases classified elsewhere
   B95.4 Other streptococcus as the cause of diseases classified elsewhere
   B95.5 Unspecified streptococcus as the cause of diseases classified elsewhere
   B95.6 Staphylococcus aureus as the cause of diseases classified elsewhere
5th
     B95.61 MSSA infection as the cause of diseases classified elsewhere
      MSSA infection as the cause of diseases classified elsewhere
      Staphylococcus aureus infection NOS as the cause of diseases classified elsewhere
     B95.62 MRSA infection as the cause of diseases classified elsewhere
      MRSA infection as the cause of diseases classified elsewhere
   B95.7 Other staphylococcus as the cause of diseases classified elsewhere
   B95.8 Unspecified staphylococcus as the cause of diseases classified elsewhere

B96   OTHER BACTERIAL AGENTS AS THE CAUSE OF DISEASES CLASSIFIED ELSEWHERE
4th
   B96.0 M. pneumoniae as the cause of diseases classified elsewhere
     Pleuro-pneumonia-like-organism [PPLO]
   B96.1 K. pneumoniae as the cause of diseases classified elsewhere
   B96.2 E. coli as the cause of diseases classified elsewhere
5th
     B96.20 Unspecified E. coli as the cause of diseases classified elsewhere
      E. coli NOS
     B96.21 STEC O157 as the cause of diseases classified elsewhere
      E. coli O157:H- (nonmotile) with confirmation of Shiga toxin
      E. coli O157 with confirmation of Shiga toxin when H antigen is unknown, or is not H7
      O157:H7 E. coli with or without confirmation of Shiga toxin-production
      STEC O157:H7 with or without confirmation of Shiga toxin-production
      STEC O157:H7 with or without confirmation of Shiga toxin-production
     B96.22 Other specified STEC as the cause of diseases classified elsewhere
      Non-O157 STEC
      Non-O157 STEC with known O group
     B96.23 STEC as the cause of diseases classified elsewhere
      STEC with unspecified O group
      STEC NOS
     B96.29 Other E. coli as the cause of diseases classified elsewhere
      Non-STEC
   B96.3 H. influenzae as the cause of diseases classified elsewhere
   B96.4 Proteus (mirabilis) (morganii) as the cause of diseases classified elsewhere
   B96.5 Pseudomonas (aeruginosa) (mallei) (pseudomallei) as the cause of diseases classified elsewhere
   B96.8 Other specified bacterial agents as the cause of diseases classified elsewhere
5th
     B96.81 H. pylori as the cause of diseases classified elsewhere
     B96.89 Other specified bacterial agents as the cause of diseases classified elsewhere

B97   VIRAL AGENTS AS THE CAUSE OF DISEASES CLASSIFIED ELSEWHERE
4th
   B97.0 Adenovirus as the cause of diseases classified elsewhere
   B97.1 Enterovirus as the cause of diseases classified elsewhere
5th
     B97.10 Unspecified enterovirus as the cause of diseases classified elsewhere
     B97.11 Coxsackievirus as the cause of diseases classified elsewhere
     B97.12 Echovirus as the cause of diseases classified elsewhere
     B97.19 Other enterovirus as the cause of diseases classified elsewhere
   B97.2 Coronavirus as the cause of diseases classified elsewhere
5th
     B97.21 SARS-associated coronavirus as the cause of diseases classified elsewhere
      Excludes1: pneumonia due to SARS-associated coronavirus (J12.81)
     B97.29 Other coronavirus as the cause of diseases classified elsewhere
   B97.4 Respiratory syncytial virus as the cause of diseases classified elsewhere
     RSV as the cause of diseases classified elsewhere
     Code first related disorders, such as:
      otitis media (H65.-)
      upper respiratory infection (J06.9)
     Excludes2: acute bronchiolitis due to respiratory syncytial virus (RSV) (J21.0)
      acute bronchitis due to respiratory syncytial virus (RSV) (J20.5)
      respiratory syncytial virus (RSV) pneumonia (J12.1)
   B97.6 Parvovirus as the cause of diseases classified elsewhere

CHAPTER 1. CERTAIN INFECTIOUS AND PARASITIC DISEASES   (B88.8–B97.6)

4th   5th   6th   7th   Additional Character Required   ✔   3-character code

•=New Code   *Excludes1*—Not coded here, do not use together
▲=Revised Code   *Excludes2*—Not included here

B97.8 Other viral agents as the cause of diseases classified elsewhere
5th

    B97.89 Other viral agents as the cause of diseases classified elsewhere

(B99) OTHER INFECTIOUS DISEASES

B99 OTHER AND UNSPECIFIED INFECTIOUS DISEASES
4th
  B99.8 Other infectious disease
  B99.9 Unspecified infectious disease

  6th 7th Additional Character Required   3-character code   •=New Code   *Excludes1*—Not coded here, do not use together
▲=Revised Code   *Excludes2*—Not included here

Chapter 2. Neoplasms (C00–D49)

GUIDELINES

Chapter 2 of the *ICD-10-CM* contains the codes for most benign and all malignant neoplasms. Certain benign neoplasms, such as prostatic adenomas, may be found in the specific body system chapters. To properly code a neoplasm it is necessary to determine from the record if the neoplasm is benign, in-situ, malignant, or of uncertain histologic behavior. If malignant, any secondary (metastatic) sites should also be determined.

Primary malignant neoplasms overlapping site boundaries

A primary malignant neoplasm that overlaps two or more contiguous (next to each other) sites should be classified to the subcategory/code .8 ('overlapping lesion'), unless the combination is specifically indexed elsewhere. For multiple neoplasms of the same site that are not contiguous such as tumors in different quadrants of the same breast, codes for each site should be assigned.

Malignant neoplasm of ectopic tissue

Malignant neoplasms of ectopic tissue are to be coded to the site of origin mentioned, e.g., ectopic pancreatic malignant neoplasms involving the stomach are coded to malignant neoplasm of pancreas, unspecified (C25.9).

The neoplasm table in the Alphabetic Index should be referenced first. However, if the histological term is documented, that term should be referenced first, rather than going immediately to the Neoplasm Table, in order to determine which column in the Neoplasm Table is appropriate. For example, if the documentation indicates "adenoma," refer to the term in the Alphabetic Index to review the entries under this term and the instructional note to "see also neoplasm, by site, benign." The table provides the proper code based on the type of neoplasm and the site. It is important to select the proper column in the table that corresponds to the type of neoplasm. The Tabular List should then be referenced to verify that the correct code has been selected from the table and that a more specific site code does not exist.

Refer to the *ICD-10-CM* manual for information regarding Z15.0, codes for genetic susceptibility to cancer.

TREATMENT DIRECTED AT THE MALIGNANCY

If the treatment is directed at the malignancy, designate the malignancy as the principal diagnosis.

The only exception to this guideline is if a patient admission/encounter is solely for the administration of chemotherapy, immunotherapy or external beam radiation therapy, assign the appropriate Z51.- code as the first-listed or principal diagnosis, and the diagnosis or problem for which the service is being performed as a secondary diagnosis.

TREATMENT OF SECONDARY SITE

When a patient is admitted because of a primary neoplasm with metastasis and treatment is directed toward the secondary site only, the secondary neoplasm is designated as the principal diagnosis even though the primary malignancy is still present.

CODING AND SEQUENCING OF COMPLICATIONS

Coding and sequencing of complications associated with the malignancies or with the therapy thereof are subject to the following guidelines:

Anemia associated with malignancy

When admission/encounter is for management of an anemia associated with the malignancy, and the treatment is only for anemia, the appropriate code for the malignancy is sequenced as the principal or first-listed diagnosis followed by the appropriate code for the anemia (such as code D63.0, Anemia in neoplastic disease).

Anemia associated with chemotherapy, immunotherapy and radiation therapy

When the admission/encounter is for management of an anemia associated with an adverse effect of the administration of chemotherapy or immunotherapy and the only treatment is for the anemia, the anemia code is sequenced first followed by the appropriate codes for the neoplasm and the adverse effect (T45.1X5, Adverse effect of antineoplastic and immunosuppressive drugs).

When the admission/encounter is for management of an anemia associated with an adverse effect of radiotherapy, the anemia code should be sequenced first, followed by the appropriate neoplasm code and code Y84.2, Radiological procedure and radiotherapy as the cause of abnormal reaction of the patient, or of later complication, without mention of misadventure at the time of the procedure.

Management of dehydration due to the malignancy

When the admission/encounter is for management of dehydration due to the malignancy and only the dehydration is being treated (intravenous rehydration), the dehydration is sequenced first, followed by the code(s) for the malignancy.

Treatment of a complication resulting from a surgical procedure

When the admission/encounter is for treatment of a complication resulting from a surgical procedure, designate the complication as the principal or first-listed diagnosis if treatment is directed at resolving the complication.

PRIMARY MALIGNANCY PREVIOUSLY EXCISED

When a primary malignancy has been previously excised or eradicated from its site and there is no further treatment directed to that site and there is no evidence of any existing primary malignancy at that site, a code from category Z85, Personal history of malignant neoplasm, should be used to indicate the former site of the malignancy. Any mention of extension, invasion, or metastasis to another site is coded as a secondary malignant neoplasm to that site. The secondary site may be the principal or first-listed a diagnosis with the Z85 code used as a secondary code.

ADMISSIONS/ENCOUNTERS INVOLVING CHEMOTHERAPY, IMMUNO-THERAPY AND RADIATION THERAPY

Episode of care involves surgical removal of neoplasm

When an episode of care involves the surgical removal of a neoplasm, primary or secondary site, followed by adjunct chemotherapy or radiation treatment during the same episode of care, the code for the neoplasm should be assigned as principal or first-listed diagnosis.

Patient admission/encounter solely for administration of chemo-therapy, immunotherapy and radiation therapy

If a patient admission/encounter is solely for the administration of chemotherapy, immunotherapy or external beam radiation therapy assign code Z51.0, Encounter for antineoplastic radiation therapy, or Z51.11, Encounter for antineoplastic chemotherapy, or Z51.12, Encounter for antineoplastic immunotherapy as the first-listed or principal diagnosis. If a patient receives more than one of these therapies during the same admission more than one of these codes may be assigned, in any sequence. The malignancy for which the therapy is being administered should be assigned as a secondary diagnosis.

If a patient admission/encounter is for the insertion or implantation of radioactive elements (e.g., brachytherapy) the appropriate code for the malignancy is sequenced as the principal or first-listed diagnosis. Code Z51.0 should not be assigned.

Patient admitted for radiation therapy, chemotherapy or immuno-therapy and develops complications

When a patient is admitted for the purpose of external beam radiotherapy, immunotherapy or chemotherapy and develops complications such as uncontrolled nausea and vomiting or dehydration, the principal or first-listed diagnosis is Z51.0, Encounter for antineoplastic radiation therapy, or Z51.11, Encounter for antineoplastic chemotherapy, or Z51.12, Encounter for antineoplastic immunotherapy followed by any codes for the complications. When a patient is admitted for the purpose of insertion or implantation of radioactive elements (e.g., brachytherapy) and develops complications such as uncontrolled nausea and vomiting or dehydration, the principal or first-listed diagnosis is the appropriate code for the malignancy followed by any codes for the complications.

ADMISSION/ENCOUNTER TO DETERMINE EXTENT OF MALIGNANCY

When the reason for admission/encounter is to determine the extent of the malignancy, or for a procedure such as paracentesis or thoracentesis, the primary malignancy or appropriate metastatic site is designated as the principal or first-listed diagnosis, even though chemotherapy or radiotherapy is administered.

SYMPTOMS, SIGNS, AND ABNORMAL FINDINGS LISTED IN CHAPTER 18 ASSOCIATED WITH NEOPLASMS

Symptoms, signs, and ill-defined conditions listed in Chapter 18 characteristic of, or associated with, an existing primary or secondary site malignancy cannot be used to replace the malignancy as principal or first-listed diagnosis, regardless of the number of admissions or encounters for treatment and care of the neoplasm.

ADMISSION/ENCOUNTER FOR PAIN CONTROL/MANAGEMENT

Refer to category G89 for information on coding admission/encounter for pain control/management.

4th 5th 6th 7th Additional Character Required ✓ 3-character code

Unspecified laterality codes were excluded here.   • =New Code   ▲ =Revised Code   ***Excludes1***—Not coded here, do not use together   ***Excludes2***—Not included here

PEDIATRIC ICD-10-CM 2021: A MANUAL FOR PROVIDER-BASED CODING   139

MALIGNANCY IN TWO OR MORE NONCONTIGUOUS SITES

A patient may have more than one malignant tumor in the same organ. These tumors may represent different primaries or metastatic disease, depending on the site. Should the documentation be unclear, the provider should be queried as to the status of each tumor so that the correct codes can be assigned.

DISSEMINATED MALIGNANT NEOPLASM, UNSPECIFIED

See code C80.0.

MALIGNANT NEOPLASM WITHOUT SPECIFICATION OF SITE

See code C80.1.

SEQUENCING OF NEOPLASM CODES

Encounter for treatment of primary malignancy

If the reason for the encounter is for treatment of a primary malignancy, assign the malignancy as the principal/first-listed diagnosis. The primary site is to be sequenced first, followed by any metastatic sites.

Encounter for treatment of secondary malignancy

When an encounter is for a primary malignancy with metastasis and treatment is directed toward the metastatic (secondary) site(s) only, the metastatic site(s) is designated as the principal/first-listed diagnosis. The primary malignancy is coded as an additional code.

Encounter for complication associated with a neoplasm

When an encounter is for management of a complication associated with a neoplasm, such as dehydration, and the treatment is only for the complication, the complication is coded first, followed by the appropriate code(s) for the neoplasm.

The exception to this guideline is anemia. When the admission/encounter is for management of an anemia associated with the malignancy, and the treatment is only for anemia, the appropriate code for the malignancy is sequenced as the principal or first-listed diagnosis followed by code D63.0, Anemia in neoplastic disease.

Complication from surgical procedure for treatment of a neoplasm

When an encounter is for treatment of a complication resulting from a surgical procedure performed for the treatment of the neoplasm, designate the complication as the principal/first-listed diagnosis. See the guideline regarding the coding of a current malignancy versus personal history to determine if the code for the neoplasm should also be assigned.

Pathologic fracture due to a neoplasm

When an encounter is for a pathological fracture due to a neoplasm, and the focus of treatment is the fracture, a code from subcategory M84.5, should be sequenced first, followed by the code for the neoplasm.

If the focus of treatment is the neoplasm with an associated pathological fracture, the neoplasm code should be sequenced first, followed by a code from M84.5 for the pathological fracture.

CURRENT MALIGNANCY VERSUS PERSONAL HISTORY OF MALIGNANCY

When a primary malignancy has been excised but further treatment, such as additional surgery for the malignancy, radiation therapy or chemotherapy is directed to that site, the primary malignancy code should be used until treatment is completed.

When a primary malignancy has been previously excised or eradicated from its site, there is no further treatment (of the malignancy) directed to that site, and there is no evidence of any existing primary malignancy **at that site,** a code from category Z85, Personal history of malignant neoplasm, should be used to indicate the former site of the malignancy.

Subcategories Z85.0 – Z85.7 should only be assigned for the former site of a primary malignancy, not the site of a secondary malignancy. Codes from subcategory Z85.8-, may be assigned for the former site(s) of either a primary or secondary malignancy included in this subcategory.

Refer to Chapter 21, Factors influencing health status and contact with health services, History (of).

LEUKEMIA, MULTIPLE MYELOMA, AND MALIGNANT PLASMA CELL NEOPLASMS IN REMISSION VERSUS PERSONAL HISTORY

The categories for leukemia, and category C90, have codes indicating whether or not the leukemia has achieved remission. There are also codes Z85.6, Personal history of leukemia, and Z85.79, Personal history of other malignant neoplasms of lymphoid, hematopoietic and related tissues. If the documentation is unclear, as to whether the leukemia has achieved remission, the provider should be queried.

Refer to Chapter 21, Factors influencing health status and contact with health services, History (of)

AFTERCARE FOLLOWING SURGERY FOR NEOPLASM

Refer to Chapter 21, Factors influencing health status and contact with health services, Aftercare

FOLLOW-UP CARE FOR COMPLETED TREATMENT OF A MALIGNANCY

Refer to Chapter 21, Factors influencing health status and contact with health services, Follow-up

PROPHYLACTIC ORGAN REMOVAL FOR PREVENTION OF MALIGNANCY

Refer to Chapter 21, Factors influencing health

MALIGNANT NEOPLASM ASSOCIATED WITH TRANSPLANTED ORGAN

A malignant neoplasm of a transplanted organ should be coded as a transplant complication. Assign first the appropriate code from category T86.-, Complications of transplanted organs and tissue, followed by code C80.2, Malignant neoplasm associated with transplanted organ. Use an additional code for the specific malignancy.

NEOPLASMS (C00–D49)

Note: Functional activity

All neoplasms are classified in this chapter, whether they are functionally active or not. An additional code from Chapter 4 may be used, to identify functional activity associated with any neoplasm.

Morphology [Histology]

Chapter 2 classifies neoplasms primarily by site (topography), with broad groupings for behavior, malignant, in situ, benign, etc. The Table of Neoplasms should be used to identify the correct topography code. In a few cases, such as for malignant melanoma and certain neuroendocrine tumors, the morphology (histologic type) is included in the category and codes.

Primary malignant neoplasms overlapping site boundaries

A primary malignant neoplasm that overlaps two or more contiguous (next to each other) sites should be classified to the subcategory/code .8 ('overlapping lesion'), unless the combination is specifically indexed elsewhere. For multiple neoplasms of the same site that are not contiguous, such as tumors in different quadrants of the same breast, codes for each site should be assigned.

Malignant neoplasm of ectopic tissue

Malignant neoplasms of ectopic tissue are to be coded to the site mentioned, e.g., ectopic pancreatic malignant neoplasms are coded to pancreas, unspecified (C25.9).

(C00–C96) MALIGNANT NEOPLASMS

Includes: Malignant neoplasms, stated or presumed to be primary (of specified sites), and certain specified histologies, except neuroendocrine, and of lymphoid, hematopoietic and related tissue (C00–C75)

(C00–C14) MALIGNANT NEOPLASMS OF LIP, ORAL CAVITY AND PHARYNX

(C15–C26) MALIGNANT NEOPLASMS OF DIGESTIVE ORGANS

Excludes1: Kaposi's sarcoma of gastrointestinal sites (C46.4)

(C30–C39) MALIGNANT NEOPLASMS OF RESPIRATORY AND INTRATHORACIC ORGANS

Includes: malignant neoplasm of middle ear
Excludes1: mesothelioma (C45.-)

(C40–C41) MALIGNANT NEOPLASMS OF BONE AND ARTICULAR CARTILAGE

Includes: malignant neoplasm of cartilage (articular) (joint)
     malignant neoplasm of periosteum
Excludes1: malignant neoplasm of bone marrow NOS (C96.9)
     malignant neoplasm of synovia (C49.-)

C40   **MALIGNANT NEOPLASM OF BONE AND ARTICULAR**
4th   **CARTILAGE OF LIMBS**
     Use additional code to identify major osseous defect, if applicable
     (M89.7-)

4th **5th** **6th** **7th** Additional Character Required   3-character code

Unspecified laterality codes •=New Code   *Excludes1*—Not coded here, do not use together
were excluded here.   ▲=Revised Code   *Excludes2*—Not included here

C40.0 **Malignant neoplasm of scapula and long bones of upper limb**
- `5th` C40.01 **right upper limb**
- C40.02 **left upper limb**

C40.1 **Malignant neoplasm of short bones of; upper limb**
- `5th` C40.11 **right upper limb**
- C40.12 **left upper limb**

C40.2 **Malignant neoplasm of long bones of; lower limb**
- `5th` C40.21 **right lower limb**
- C40.22 **left lower limb**

C40.3 **Malignant neoplasm of short bones of; lower limb**
- `5th` C40.31 **right lower limb**
- C40.32 **left lower limb**

C40.8 **Malignant neoplasm of overlapping sites of bone and articular cartilage of; limb**
- `5th` C40.81 **right limb**
- C40.82 **left limb**

C40.9 **Malignant neoplasm of unspecified bones and articular cartilage of; limb**
- `5th` C40.91 **right limb**
- C40.92 **left limb**

C41 MALIGNANT NEOPLASM OF BONE AND ARTICULAR CARTILAGE OF OTHER AND UNSPECIFIED SITES

Excludes1: malignant neoplasm of bones of limbs (C40.-)
  malignant neoplasm of cartilage of ear (C49.0)
  malignant neoplasm of cartilage of eyelid (C49.0)
  malignant neoplasm of cartilage of larynx (C32.3)
  malignant neoplasm of cartilage of limbs (C40.-)
  malignant neoplasm of cartilage of nose (C30.0)

C41.0 **Malignant neoplasm of bones of skull and face**
Malignant neoplasm of maxilla (superior)
Malignant neoplasm of orbital bone
Excludes2: carcinoma, any type except intraosseous or odontogenic of:
  maxillary sinus (C31.0)
  upper jaw (C03.0)
  malignant neoplasm of jaw bone (lower) (C41.1)

C41.1 **Malignant neoplasm of mandible**
Malignant neoplasm of inferior maxilla
Malignant neoplasm of lower jaw bone
Excludes2: carcinoma, any type except intraosseous or odontogenic of:
  jaw NOS (C03.9)
  lower (C03.1)
  malignant neoplasm of upper jaw bone (C41.0)

C41.2 **Malignant neoplasm of vertebral column**
Excludes1: malignant neoplasm of sacrum and coccyx (C41.4)

C41.3 **Malignant neoplasm of ribs, sternum and clavicle**

C41.4 **Malignant neoplasm of pelvic bones, sacrum and coccyx**

C41.9 **Malignant neoplasm of bone and articular cartilage, unspecified**

(C43–C44) MELANOMA AND OTHER MALIGNANT NEOPLASMS OF SKIN

C43 MALIGNANT MELANOMA OF SKIN
- `4th`
Excludes1: melanoma in situ (D03.-)
Excludes2: malignant melanoma of skin of genital organs (C51-C52, C60.-, C63.-)
  Merkel cell carcinoma (C4A.-)
  sites other than skin-code to malignant neoplasm of the site

C43.0 **Malignant melanoma of lip**
Excludes1: malignant neoplasm of vermilion border of lip (C00.0-C00.2)

C43.1 **Malignant melanoma of eyelid, including canthus**
- `5th` C43.10 **Malignant melanoma of unspecified eyelid, including canthus**
- `6th` C43.11 **Malignant melanoma of right eyelid, including canthus**
  - C43.111 **Malignant melanoma of right upper eyelid, including canthus**
  - C43.112 **Malignant melanoma of right lower eyelid, including canthus**

C43.12 **Malignant melanoma of left eyelid, including canthus**
- `6th` C43.121 **Malignant melanoma of left upper eyelid, including canthus**
  - C43.122 **Malignant melanoma of left lower eyelid, including canthus**

C43.2 **Malignant melanoma of ear and external auricular canal**
- `5th` C43.21 **Malignant melanoma of right ear and external auricular canal**
- C43.22 **Malignant melanoma of left ear and external auricular canal**

C43.3 **Malignant melanoma of other and unspecified parts of face**
- `5th` C43.30 **Malignant melanoma of unspecified part of face**
- C43.31 **Malignant melanoma of nose**
- C43.39 **Malignant melanoma of other parts of face**

C43.4 **Malignant melanoma of scalp and neck**

C43.5 **Malignant melanoma of trunk**
- `5th` *Excludes2:* malignant neoplasm of anus NOS (C21.0)
  malignant neoplasm of scrotum (C63.2)
- C43.51 **Malignant melanoma of anal skin**
  Malignant melanoma of anal margin
  Malignant melanoma of perianal skin
- C43.52 **Malignant melanoma of skin of breast**
- C43.59 **Malignant melanoma of other part of trunk**

C43.6 **Malignant melanoma of upper limb, including shoulder**
- `5th` C43.61 **Malignant melanoma of right upper limb, including shoulder**
- C43.62 **Malignant melanoma of left upper limb, including shoulder**

C43.7 **Malignant melanoma of lower limb, including hip**
- `5th` C43.71 **Malignant melanoma of right lower limb, including hip**
- C43.72 **Malignant melanoma of left lower limb, including hip**

C43.8 **Malignant melanoma of overlapping sites of skin**

C43.9 **Malignant melanoma of skin, unspecified**
Malignant melanoma of unspecified site of skin
Melanoma (malignant) NOS

C4A MERKEL CELL CARCINOMA
- `4th` C4A.0 **Merkel cell carcinoma of lip**
Excludes1: malignant neoplasm of vermilion border of lip (C00.0-C00.2)

C4A.1 **Merkel cell carcinoma of eyelid, including canthus**
- `5th` C4A.10 **Merkel cell carcinoma of unspecified eyelid, including canthus**
- `6th` C4A.11 **Merkel cell carcinoma of right eyelid, including canthus**
  - C4A.111 **Merkel cell carcinoma of right upper eyelid, including canthus**
  - C4A.112 **Merkel cell carcinoma of right lower eyelid, including canthus**
- `6th` C4A.12 **Merkel cell carcinoma of left eyelid, including canthus**
  - C4A.121 **Merkel cell carcinoma of left upper eyelid, including canthus**
  - C4A.122 **Merkel cell carcinoma of left lower eyelid, including canthus**

C4A.2 **Merkel cell carcinoma of ear and external auricular canal**
- `5th` C4A.20 **Merkel cell carcinoma of unspecified ear and external auricular canal**
- C4A.21 **Merkel cell carcinoma of right ear and external auricular canal**
- C4A.22 **Merkel cell carcinoma of left ear and external auricular canal**

C4A.3 **Merkel cell carcinoma of other and unspecified parts of face**
- `5th` C4A.30 **Merkel cell carcinoma of unspecified part of face**
- C4A.31 **Merkel cell carcinoma of nose**
- C4A.39 **Merkel cell carcinoma of other parts of face**

C4A.4 **Merkel cell carcinoma of scalp and neck**

C4A.5 **Merkel cell carcinoma of trunk**
- `5th` *Excludes2:* malignant neoplasm of anus NOS (C21.0)
  malignant neoplasm of scrotum (C63.2)
- C4A.51 **Merkel cell carcinoma of anal skin**
  Merkel cell carcinoma of anal margin
  Merkel cell carcinoma of perianal skin

`4th` `5th` `6th` `7th` Additional Character Required | ✔ 3-character code

Unspecified laterality codes were excluded here. | •=New Code ▲=Revised Code | *Excludes1*—Not coded here, do not use together *Excludes2*—Not included here

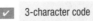

C4A.52 Merkel cell carcinoma of skin of breast

C4A.59 Merkel cell carcinoma of other part of trunk

C4A.6 [5th] Merkel cell carcinoma of upper limb, including shoulder

C4A.61 Merkel cell carcinoma of right upper limb, including shoulder

C4A.62 Merkel cell carcinoma of left upper limb, including shoulder

C4A.7 [5th] Merkel cell carcinoma of lower limb, including hip

C4A.71 Merkel cell carcinoma of right lower limb, including hip

C4A.72 Merkel cell carcinoma of left lower limb, including hip

C4A.8 Merkel cell carcinoma of overlapping sites

C4A.9 Merkel cell carcinoma, unspecified

Merkel cell carcinoma of unspecified site

Merkel cell carcinoma NOS

C44 [4th] **OTHER AND UNSPECIFIED MALIGNANT NEOPLASM OF SKIN**

Includes: malignant neoplasm of sebaceous glands

malignant neoplasm of sweat glands

Excludes1: Kaposi's sarcoma of skin (C46.0)

malignant melanoma of skin (C43.-)

malignant neoplasm of skin of genital organs (C51-C52, C60.-, C63.2)

Merkel cell carcinoma (C4A.-)

C44.0 [5th] Other and unspecified malignant neoplasm of skin of lip

Excludes1: malignant neoplasm of lip (C00.-)

C44.00 Unspecified malignant neoplasm of skin of lip

C44.01 Basal cell carcinoma of skin of lip

C44.02 Squamous cell carcinoma of skin of lip

C44.09 Other specified malignant neoplasm of skin of lip

C44.1 [5th] Other and unspecified malignant neoplasm of skin of eyelid, including canthus

Excludes1: connective tissue of eyelid (C49.0)

C44.10 [6th] Unspecified malignant neoplasm of skin of eyelid, including canthus

C44.101 Unspecified malignant neoplasm of skin of unspecified eyelid, including canthus

C44.102 [7th] Unspecified malignant neoplasm of skin of right eyelid, including canthus

C44.1021 Unspecified malignant neoplasm of skin of right upper eyelid, including canthus

C44.1022 Unspecified malignant neoplasm of skin of right lower eyelid, including canthus

C44.109 [7th] Unspecified malignant neoplasm of skin of left eyelid, including canthus

C44.1091 Unspecified malignant neoplasm of skin of left upper eyelid, including canthus

C44.1092 Unspecified malignant neoplasm of skin of left lower eyelid, including canthus

C44.11 [6th] Basal cell carcinoma of skin of eyelid, including canthus

C44.111 Basal cell carcinoma of skin of unspecified eyelid, including canthus

C44.112 [7th] Basal cell carcinoma of skin of right eyelid, including canthus

C44.1121 Basal cell carcinoma of skin of right upper eyelid, including canthus

C44.1122 Basal cell carcinoma of skin of right lower eyelid, including canthus

C44.119 [7th] Basal cell carcinoma of skin of left eyelid, including canthus

C44.1191 Basal cell carcinoma of skin of left upper eyelid, including canthus

C44.1192 Basal cell carcinoma of skin of left lower eyelid, including canthus

C44.12 [6th] Squamous cell carcinoma of skin of eyelid, including canthus

C44.121 Squamous cell carcinoma of skin of unspecified eyelid, including canthus

C44.122 [7th] Squamous cell carcinoma of skin of right eyelid, including canthus

C44.1221 Squamous cell carcinoma of skin of right upper eyelid, including canthus

C44.1222 Squamous cell carcinoma of skin of right lower eyelid, including canthus

C44.129 [7th] Squamous cell carcinoma of skin of left eyelid, including canthus

C44.1291 Squamous cell carcinoma of skin of left upper eyelid, including canthus

C44.1292 Squamous cell carcinoma of skin of left lower eyelid, including canthus

C44.13 [6th] Sebaceous cell carcinoma of skin of eyelid, including canthus

C44.131 Sebaceous cell carcinoma of skin of unspecified eyelid, including canthus

C44.132 [7th] Sebaceous cell carcinoma of skin of specified lower eyelid

C44.1321 Sebaceous cell carcinoma of skin of right upper eyelid, including canthus

C44.1322 Sebaceous cell carcinoma of skin of right lower eyelid, including canthus

C44.139 [7th] Sebaceous cell carcinoma of skin of specified lower eyelid, including canthus

C44.1391 Sebaceous cell carcinoma of skin of left upper eyelid, including canthus

C44.1392 Sebaceous cell carcinoma of skin of left lower eyelid, including canthus

C44.19 [6th] Other specified malignant neoplasm of skin of eyelid, including canthus

C44.191 Other specified malignant neoplasm of skin of unspecified eyelid, including canthus

C44.192 [7th] Other specified malignant neoplasm of skin of right eyelid, including canthus

C44.1921 Other specified malignant neoplasm of skin of right upper eyelid, including canthus

C44.1922 Other specified malignant neoplasm of skin of right lower eyelid, including canthus

C44.199 [7th] Other specified malignant neoplasm of skin of left eyelid, including canthus

C44.1991 Other specified malignant neoplasm of skin of left upper eyelid, including canthus

C44.1992 Other specified malignant neoplasm of skin of left lower eyelid, including canthus

C44.2 [5th] Other and unspecified malignant neoplasm of skin of ear and external auricular canal

Excludes1: connective tissue of ear (C49.0)

C44.20 [6th] Unspecified malignant neoplasm of skin of ear and external auricular canal

C44.201 Unspecified malignant neoplasm of skin of unspecified ear and external auricular canal

C44.202 Unspecified malignant neoplasm of skin of right ear and external auricular canal

C44.209 Unspecified malignant neoplasm of skin of left ear and external auricular canal

---

[4th] [5th] [6th] [7th] Additional Character Required ✔ 3-character code

Unspecified laterality codes were excluded here.

•=New Code
▲=Revised Code

Excludes1—Not coded here, do not use together
Excludes2—Not included here

 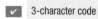

C44.21 **Basal cell carcinoma of skin of ear and external auricular canal** `6th`

C44.212 Basal cell carcinoma of skin of right ear and external auricular canal

C44.219 Basal cell carcinoma of skin of left ear and external auricular canal

C44.22 **Squamous cell carcinoma of skin of ear and external auricular canal** `6th`

C44.222 Squamous cell carcinoma of skin of right ear and external auricular canal

C44.229 Squamous cell carcinoma of skin of left ear and external auricular canal

C44.29 **Other specified malignant neoplasm of skin of ear and external auricular canal** `6th`

C44.292 Other specified malignant neoplasm of skin of right ear and external auricular canal

C44.299 Other specified malignant neoplasm of skin of left ear and external auricular canal

C44.3 **Other and unspecified malignant neoplasm of skin of other and unspecified parts of face** `5th`

C44.30 **Unspecified malignant neoplasm of skin of other and unspecified parts of face** `6th`

C44.300 Unspecified malignant neoplasm of skin of unspecified part of face

C44.301 Unspecified malignant neoplasm of skin of nose

C44.309 Unspecified malignant neoplasm of skin of other parts of face

C44.31 **Basal cell carcinoma of skin of other and unspecified parts of face** `6th`

C44.310 Basal cell carcinoma of skin of unspecified parts of face

C44.311 Basal cell carcinoma of skin of nose

C44.319 Basal cell carcinoma of skin of other parts of face

C44.32 **Squamous cell carcinoma of skin of other and unspecified parts of face** `6th`

C44.320 Squamous cell carcinoma of skin of unspecified parts of face

C44.321 Squamous cell carcinoma of skin of nose

C44.329 Squamous cell carcinoma of skin of other parts of face

C44.39 **Other specified malignant neoplasm of skin of other and unspecified parts of face** `6th`

C44.390 Other specified malignant neoplasm of skin of unspecified parts of face

C44.391 Other specified malignant neoplasm of skin of nose

C44.399 Other specified malignant neoplasm of skin of other parts of face

C44.4 **Other and unspecified malignant neoplasm of skin of scalp and neck** `5th`

C44.40 Unspecified malignant neoplasm of skin of scalp and neck

C44.41 Basal cell carcinoma of skin of scalp and neck

C44.42 Squamous cell carcinoma of skin of scalp and neck

C44.49 Other specified malignant neoplasm of skin of scalp and neck

C44.5 **Other and unspecified malignant neoplasm of skin of trunk** `5th`

Excludes1: anus NOS (C21.0)
scrotum (C63.2)

C44.50 **Unspecified malignant neoplasm of skin of trunk** `6th`

C44.500 Unspecified malignant neoplasm of anal skin

Unspecified malignant neoplasm of anal margin
Unspecified malignant neoplasm of perianal skin

C44.501 Unspecified malignant neoplasm of skin of breast

C44.509 Unspecified malignant neoplasm of skin of other part of trunk

C44.51 **Basal cell carcinoma of skin of trunk** `6th`

C44.510 Basal cell carcinoma of anal skin

Basal cell carcinoma of anal margin
Basal cell carcinoma of perianal skin

C44.511 Basal cell carcinoma of skin of breast

C44.519 Basal cell carcinoma of skin of other part of trunk

C44.52 **Squamous cell carcinoma of skin of trunk** `6th`

C44.520 Squamous cell carcinoma of anal skin

Squamous cell carcinoma of anal margin
Squamous cell carcinoma of perianal skin

C44.521 Squamous cell carcinoma of skin of breast

C44.529 Squamous cell carcinoma of skin of other part of trunk

C44.59 **Other specified malignant neoplasm of skin of trunk** `6th`

C44.590 Other specified malignant neoplasm of anal skin

Other specified malignant neoplasm of anal margin
Other specified malignant neoplasm of perianal skin

C44.591 Other specified malignant neoplasm of skin of breast

C44.599 Other specified malignant neoplasm of skin of other part of trunk

C44.6 **Other and unspecified malignant neoplasm of skin of upper limb, including shoulder** `5th`

C44.60 **Unspecified malignant neoplasm of skin of upper limb, including shoulder** `6th`

C44.602 Unspecified malignant neoplasm of skin of right upper limb, including shoulder

C44.609 Unspecified malignant neoplasm of skin of left upper limb, including shoulder

C44.61 **Basal cell carcinoma of skin of upper limb, including shoulder** `6th`

C44.612 Basal cell carcinoma of skin of right upper limb, including shoulder

C44.619 Basal cell carcinoma of skin of left upper limb, including shoulder

C44.62 **Squamous cell carcinoma of skin of upper limb, including shoulder** `6th`

C44.622 Squamous cell carcinoma of skin of right upper limb, including shoulder

C44.629 Squamous cell carcinoma of skin of left upper limb, including shoulder

C44.69 **Other specified malignant neoplasm of skin of upper limb, including shoulder** `6th`

C44.692 Other specified malignant neoplasm of skin of right upper limb, including shoulder

C44.699 Other specified malignant neoplasm of skin of left upper limb, including shoulder

C44.7 **Other and unspecified malignant neoplasm of skin of lower limb, including hip** `5th`

C44.70 **Unspecified malignant neoplasm of skin of lower limb, including hip** `6th`

C44.702 Unspecified malignant neoplasm of skin of right lower limb, including hip

C44.709 Unspecified malignant neoplasm of skin of left lower limb, including hip

C44.71 **Basal cell carcinoma of skin of lower limb, including hip** `6th`

C44.712 Basal cell carcinoma of skin of right lower limb, including hip

C44.719 Basal cell carcinoma of skin of left lower limb, including hip

C44.72 **Squamous cell carcinoma of skin of lower limb, including hip** `6th`

C44.722 Squamous cell carcinoma of skin of right lower limb, including hip

C44.729 Squamous cell carcinoma of skin of left lower limb, including hip

C44.79 **Other specified malignant neoplasm of skin of lower limb, including hip** `6th`

`4th` `5th` `6th` `7th` Additional Character Required   ✓ 3-character code

Unspecified laterality codes were excluded here.

•=New Code
▲=Revised Code

Excludes1—Not coded here, do not use together
Excludes2—Not included here

C44.792　Other specified malignant neoplasm of skin of right lower limb, including hip
C44.799　Other specified malignant neoplasm of skin of left lower limb, including hip

C44.8 **Other and unspecified malignant neoplasm of overlapping sites of skin** `5th`

　　C44.80　Unspecified malignant neoplasm of overlapping sites of skin
　　C44.81　Basal cell carcinoma of overlapping sites of skin
　　C44.82　Squamous cell carcinoma of overlapping sites of skin
　　C44.89　Other specified malignant neoplasm of overlapping sites of skin

C44.9 **Other and unspecified malignant neoplasm of skin, unspecified** `5th`

　　C44.90　Unspecified malignant neoplasm of skin, unspecified
　　　　　　Malignant neoplasm of unspecified site of skin
　　C44.91　Basal cell carcinoma of skin, unspecified
　　C44.92　Squamous cell carcinoma of skin, unspecified
　　C44.99　Other specified malignant neoplasm of skin, unspecified

(C45–C49) MALIGNANT NEOPLASMS OF MESOTHELIAL AND SOFT TISSUE

(C50) MALIGNANT NEOPLASMS OF BREAST

(C51–C58) MALIGNANT NEOPLASMS OF FEMALE GENITAL ORGANS

Includes: malignant neoplasm of skin of female genital organs

(C60–C63) MALIGNANT NEOPLASMS OF MALE GENITAL ORGANS

Includes: malignant neoplasm of skin of male genital organs

(C64–C68) MALIGNANT NEOPLASMS OF URINARY TRACT

C64 **MALIGNANT NEOPLASM OF KIDNEY, EXCEPT RENAL PELVIS** `4th`

Excludes1: malignant carcinoid tumor of the kidney (C7A.093)
　　malignant neoplasm of renal calyces (C65.-)
　　malignant neoplasm of renal pelvis (C65.-)

　　C64.1　Malignant neoplasm of right kidney, except renal pelvis
　　C64.2　Malignant neoplasm of left kidney, except renal pelvis

(C69–C72) MALIGNANT NEOPLASMS OF EYE, BRAIN AND OTHER PARTS OF CENTRAL NERVOUS SYSTEM

C69 **MALIGNANT NEOPLASM OF EYE AND ADNEXA** `4th`

Excludes1: malignant neoplasm of connective tissue of eyelid (C49.0)
　　malignant neoplasm of eyelid (skin) (C43.1-, C44.1-)
　　malignant neoplasm of optic nerve (C72.3-)

　　C69.2 **Malignant neoplasm of retina** `5th`
　　　Excludes1: dark area on retina (D49.81)
　　　　neoplasm of unspecified behavior of retina and choroid (D49.81)
　　　　retinal freckle (D49.81)
　　　　C69.21　Malignant neoplasm of right retina
　　　　C69.22　Malignant neoplasm of left retina

C71 **MALIGNANT NEOPLASM OF BRAIN** `4th`

Excludes1: malignant neoplasm of cranial nerves (C72.2–C72.5)
　　retrobulbar malignant neoplasm (C69.6-)

　　C71.0　Malignant neoplasm of; cerebrum, except lobes and ventricles
　　　　　　Malignant neoplasm of supratentorial NOS
　　C71.1　frontal lobe
　　C71.2　temporal lobe
　　C71.3　parietal lobe
　　C71.4　occipital lobe
　　C71.5　cerebral ventricle
　　　　Excludes1: malignant neoplasm of fourth cerebral ventricle (C71.7)

C71.6　cerebellum
C71.7　brain stem
　　　　Malignant neoplasm of fourth cerebral ventricle
　　　　Infratentorial malignant neoplasm NOS
C71.8　overlapping sites of brain
C71.9　brain, unspecified

(C73–C75) MALIGNANT NEOPLASMS OF THYROID AND OTHER ENDOCRINE GLANDS

C74 **MALIGNANT NEOPLASM OF ADRENAL GLAND** `4th`

　　C74.0 **Malignant neoplasm of cortex of; adrenal gland**
　　　C74.01　right adrenal gland `5th`
　　　C74.02　left adrenal gland
　　C74.1 **Malignant neoplasm of medulla of; adrenal gland**
　　　C74.11　right adrenal gland `5th`
　　　C74.12　left adrenal gland
　　C74.9 **Malignant neoplasm of unspecified part of; adrenal gland**
　　　C74.91　right adrenal gland `5th`
　　　C74.92　left adrenal gland

(C7A) MALIGNANT NEUROENDOCRINE TUMORS

(C7B) SECONDARY NEUROENDOCRINE TUMORS

(C76–C80) MALIGNANT NEOPLASMS OF ILL-DEFINED, OTHER SECONDARY AND UNSPECIFIED SITES

C80 **MALIGNANT NEOPLASM WITHOUT SPECIFICATION OF SITE** `4th`

Excludes1: malignant carcinoid tumor of unspecified site (C7A.00)
　　malignant neoplasm of specified multiple sites- code to each site

C80.0 **Disseminated malignant neoplasm, unspecified**
　　Use only in those cases where the patient has advanced metastatic disease and no known primary or secondary sites are specified. It should not be used in place of assigning codes for the primary site and all known secondary sites.
　　Carcinomatosis NOS
　　Generalized cancer, unspecified site (primary) (secondary)
　　Generalized malignancy, unspecified site (primary) (secondary)

C80.1 **Malignant (primary) neoplasm, unspecified**
　　Use only be used when no determination can be made as to the primary site of a malignancy.
　　Cancer NOS
　　Cancer unspecified site (primary)
　　Carcinoma unspecified site (primary)
　　Malignancy unspecified site (primary)
　　Excludes1: secondary malignant neoplasm of unspecified site (C79.9)

C80.2 **Malignant neoplasm associated with transplanted organ**
　　Code first complication of transplanted organ (T86.-)
　　Use additional code to identify the specific malignancy

(C81–C96) MALIGNANT NEOPLASMS OF LYMPHOID, HEMATOPOIETIC AND RELATED TISSUE

Excludes2: Kaposi's sarcoma of lymph nodes (C46.3)
　　secondary and unspecified neoplasm of lymph nodes (C77.-)
　　secondary neoplasm of bone marrow (C79.52)
　　secondary neoplasm of spleen (C78.89)

C81 **HODGKIN LYMPHOMA** `4th`

Excludes1: personal history of Hodgkin lymphoma (Z85.71)

　　C81.0 **Nodular lymphocyte predominant Hodgkin lymphoma**
　　　C81.00　Nodular lymphocyte predominant Hodgkin lymphoma, unspecified site `5th`
　　　C81.01　Nodular lymphocyte predominant Hodgkin lymphoma, lymph nodes of head, face, and neck
　　　C81.02　Nodular lymphocyte predominant Hodgkin lymphoma, intrathoracic lymph nodes
　　　C81.03　Nodular lymphocyte predominant Hodgkin lymphoma, intra-abdominal lymph nodes

---

`4th` `5th` `6th` `7th` Additional Character Required　　✔ 3-character code

Unspecified laterality codes were excluded here.　　•=New Code　▲=Revised Code

Excludes1—Not coded here, do not use together
Excludes2—Not included here

C81.04	Nodular lymphocyte predominant Hodgkin lymphoma, lymph nodes of axilla and upper limb
C81.05	Nodular lymphocyte predominant Hodgkin lymphoma, lymph nodes of inguinal region and lower limb
C81.06	Nodular lymphocyte predominant Hodgkin lymphoma, intrapelvic lymph nodes
C81.07	Nodular lymphocyte predominant Hodgkin lymphoma, spleen
C81.08	Nodular lymphocyte predominant Hodgkin lymphoma, lymph nodes of multiple sites
C81.09	Nodular lymphocyte predominant Hodgkin lymphoma, extranodal and solid organ sites

C81.2 Mixed cellularity Hodgkin lymphoma

5th Mixed cellularity classical Hodgkin lymphoma

C81.20	Mixed cellularity Hodgkin lymphoma, unspecified site
C81.21	lymph nodes of head, face, and neck
C81.22	intrathoracic lymph nodes
C81.23	intra-abdominal lymph nodes
C81.24	lymph nodes of axilla and upper limb
C81.25	lymph nodes of inguinal region and lower limb
C81.26	intrapelvic lymph nodes
C81.27	spleen
C81.28	lymph nodes of multiple sites
C81.29	extranodal and solid organ sites

C81.9 Hodgkin lymphoma, unspecified

5th	C81.91	Hodgkin lymphoma, unspecified; lymph nodes of head, face, and neck
	C81.92	intrathoracic lymph nodes
	C81.93	intra-abdominal lymph nodes
	C81.94	lymph nodes of axilla and upper limb
	C81.95	lymph nodes of inguinal region and lower limb
	C81.96	intrapelvic lymph nodes
	C81.97	spleen
	C81.98	lymph nodes of multiple sites
	C81.99	extranodal and solid organ sites

C83 NON-FOLLICULAR LYMPHOMA

4th *Excludes1:* personal history of non-Hodgkin lymphoma (Z85.72)

C83.3 Diffuse large B-cell lymphoma

5th Anaplastic diffuse large B-cell lymphoma
CD30-positive diffuse large B-cell lymphoma
Centroblastic diffuse large B-cell lymphoma
Diffuse large B-cell lymphoma, subtype not specified
Immunoblastic diffuse large B-cell lymphoma
Plasmablastic diffuse large B-cell lymphoma
Diffuse large B-cell lymphoma, subtype not specified
T-cell rich diffuse large B-cell lymphoma

Excludes1: mediastinal (thymic) large B-cell lymphoma (C85.2-)
mature T/NK-cell lymphomas (C84.-)

C83.30	Diffuse large B-cell lymphoma; unspecified site
C83.31	lymph nodes of head, face, and neck
C83.32	intrathoracic lymph nodes
C83.33	intra-abdominal lymph nodes
C83.34	lymph nodes of axilla and upper limb
C83.35	lymph nodes of inguinal region and lower limb
C83.36	intrapelvic lymph nodes
C83.37	spleen
C83.38	lymph nodes of multiple sites
C83.39	extranodal and solid organ sites

C83.7 Burkitt lymphoma

5th Atypical Burkitt lymphoma
Burkitt-like lymphoma

Excludes1: mature B-cell leukemia Burkitt type (C91.A-)

C83.70	Burkitt lymphoma, unspecified site
C83.71	Burkitt lymphoma, lymph nodes of head, face, and neck
C83.72	Burkitt lymphoma, intrathoracic lymph nodes
C83.73	Burkitt lymphoma, intra-abdominal lymph nodes
C83.74	Burkitt lymphoma, lymph nodes of axilla and upper limb
C83.75	Burkitt lymphoma, lymph nodes of inguinal region and lower limb

C83.76	Burkitt lymphoma, intrapelvic lymph nodes
C83.77	Burkitt lymphoma, spleen
C83.78	Burkitt lymphoma, lymph nodes of multiple sites
C83.79	Burkitt lymphoma, extranodal and solid organ sites

C84 MATURE T/NK-CELL LYMPHOMAS

4th *Excludes1:* personal history of non-Hodgkin lymphoma (Z85.72)

C84.4 Peripheral T-cell lymphoma, not classified

5th Lennert's lymphoma
Lymphoepithelioid lymphoma
Mature T-cell lymphoma, not elsewhere classified

C84.41	Peripheral T-cell lymphoma, not classified; lymph nodes of head, face, and neck
C84.42	intrathoracic lymph nodes
C84.43	intra-abdominal lymph nodes
C84.44	lymph nodes of axilla and upper limb
C84.45	lymph nodes of inguinal region and lower limb
C84.46	intrapelvic lymph nodes
C84.47	spleen
C84.48	lymph nodes of multiple sites
C84.49	extranodal and solid organ sites

C85 OTHER SPECIFIED AND UNSPECIFIED TYPES OF NON-HODGKIN LYMPHOMA

4th *Excludes1:* other specified types of T/NK-cell lymphoma (C86.-)
personal history of non-Hodgkin lymphoma (Z85.72)

C85.9 Non-Hodgkin lymphoma, unspecified

5th Lymphoma NOS
Malignant lymphoma NOS
Non-Hodgkin lymphoma NOS

C85.90	Non-Hodgkin lymphoma, unspecified, unspecified site
C85.91	Non-Hodgkin lymphoma, unspecified; lymph nodes of head, face, and neck
C85.92	intrathoracic lymph nodes
C85.93	intra-abdominal lymph nodes
C85.94	lymph nodes of axilla and upper limb
C85.95	lymph nodes of inguinal region and lower limb
C85.96	intrapelvic lymph nodes
C85.97	spleen
C85.98	lymph nodes of multiple sites
C85.99	extranodal and solid organ sites

C91 LYMPHOID LEUKEMIA

4th *Excludes1:* personal history of leukemia (Z85.6)

C91.0 Acute lymphoblastic leukemia [ALL]

5th **Note:** Codes in subcategory C91.0- should only be used for T-cell and B-cell precursor leukemia

C91.00	ALL, not having achieved remission
	ALL with failed remission
	ALL NOS
C91.01	ALL, in remission
C91.02	ALL, in relapse

C91.9 Lymphoid leukemia, unspecified

5th	C91.90	Lymphoid leukemia, unspecified; not having achieved remission
		Lymphoid leukemia with failed remission
		Lymphoid leukemia NOS
	C91.91	in remission
	C91.92	in relapse

C92 MYELOID LEUKEMIA

4th *Includes:* granulocytic leukemia
myelogenous leukemia

Excludes1: personal history of leukemia (Z85.6)

C92.0 Acute myeloblastic leukemia

5th Acute myeloblastic leukemia, minimal differentiation
Acute myeloblastic leukemia (with maturation)
Acute myeloblastic leukemia 1/ETO
Acute myeloblastic leukemia M0 or M1 or M2
Acute myeloblastic leukemia with t(8;21)
Acute myeloblastic leukemia (without a FAB classification) NOS
Refractory anemia with excess blasts in transformation [RAEB T]

Excludes1: acute exacerbation of chronic myeloid leukemia (C92.10)
refractory anemia with excess of blasts not in transformation (D46.2-)

4th	**5th**	**6th**	**7th**	Additional Character Required	✔	3-character code

Unspecified laterality codes were excluded here.   •=New Code   ▲=Revised Code

Excludes1—Not coded here, do not use together
Excludes2—Not included here

C92.00 Acute myeloblastic leukemia; not having achieved remission
Acute myeloblastic leukemia with failed remission
Acute myeloblastic leukemia NOS
C92.01 in remission
C92.02 in relapse
C92.1 Chronic myeloid leukemia, BCR/ABL-positive
`5th`
Chronic myelogenous leukemia, Philadelphia chromosome (Ph1) positive
Chronic myelogenous leukemia, t(9;22) (q34;q11)
Chronic myelogenous leukemia with crisis of blast cells
Excludes1: atypical chronic myeloid leukemia BCR/ABL-negative (C92.2-)
CMML (C93.1-)
chronic myeloproliferative disease (D47.1)
C92.10 Chronic myeloid leukemia, BCR/ABL-positive; not having achieved remission
Chronic myeloid leukemia, BCR/ABL-positive with failed remission
Chronic myeloid leukemia, BCR/ABL-positive NOS
C92.11 in remission
C92.12 in relapse
C92.2 Atypical chronic myeloid leukemia, BCR/ABL-negative
`5th` **C92.20 Atypical chronic myeloid leukemia, BCR/ABL-negative; not having achieved remission**
Atypical chronic myeloid leukemia, BCR/ABL-negative with failed remission
Atypical chronic myeloid leukemia, BCR/ABL-negative NOS
C92.21 in remission
C92.22 in relapse
C92.9 Myeloid leukemia, unspecified
`5th` **C92.90 Myeloid leukemia, unspecified; not having achieved remission**
Myeloid leukemia, unspecified with failed remission
Myeloid leukemia, unspecified NOS
C92.91 in remission
C92.92 unspecified in relapse

C93 `4th` **MONOCYTIC LEUKEMIA**
Includes: monocytoid leukemia
Excludes1: personal history of leukemia (Z85.6)
C93.0 Acute monoblastic/monocytic leukemia
`5th` AML M5 or AML M5a or AML M5b
C93.00 Acute monoblastic/monocytic leukemia; not having achieved remission
Acute monoblastic/monocytic leukemia with failed remission
Acute monoblastic/monocytic leukemia NOS
C93.01 in remission
C93.02 in relapse
C93.1 Chronic myelomonocytic leukemia [CMML]
`5th` Chronic monocytic leukemia
CMML-1 or CMML-2
CMML with eosinophilia
Code also, if applicable, eosinophilia (D72.18)
C93.10 CMML not having achieved remission
CMML with failed remission
CMML NOS
C93.11 CMML, in remission
C93.12 CMML, in relapse
C93.3 Juvenile myelomonocytic leukemia
`5th` **C93.30 Juvenile myelomonocytic leukemia; not having achieved remission**
Juvenile myelomonocytic leukemia with failed remission
Juvenile myelomonocytic leukemia NOS
C93.31 in remission
C93.32 in relapse
C93.Z Other monocytic leukemia
`5th` **C93.Z0 Other monocytic leukemia; not having achieved remission**
Other monocytic leukemia NOS
C93.Z1 in remission
C93.Z2 in relapse

C93.9 Monocytic leukemia, unspecified
`5th` **C93.90 Monocytic leukemia, unspecified; not having achieved remission**
Monocytic leukemia, unspecified with failed remission
leukemia, unspecified NOS
C93.91 in remission
C93.92 in relapse

C94 `4th` **OTHER LEUKEMIAS OF SPECIFIED CELL TYPE**
Excludes1: leukemic reticuloendotheliosis (C91.4-)
myelodysplastic syndromes (D46.-)
personal history of leukemia (Z85.6)
plasma cell leukemia (C90.1-)
C94.0 Acute erythroid leukemia
`5th` Acute myeloid leukemia M6(a)(b)
Erythroleukemia
C94.00 Acute erythroid leukemia, not having achieved remission
Acute erythroid leukemia with failed remission
Acute erythroid leukemia NOS
C94.01 Acute erythroid leukemia, in remission
C94.02 Acute erythroid leukemia, in relapse
C94.3 Mast cell leukemia
`5th` **C94.30 Mast cell leukemia not having achieved remission**
Mast cell leukemia with failed remission
Mast cell leukemia NOS
C94.31 Mast cell leukemia, in remission
C94.32 Mast cell leukemia, in relapse

C95 `4th` **LEUKEMIA OF UNSPECIFIED CELL TYPE**
Excludes1: personal history of leukemia (Z85.6)
C95.9 Leukemia, unspecified
`5th` **C95.90 Leukemia, unspecified not having achieved remission**
Leukemia, unspecified with failed remission
Leukemia NOS
C95.91 Leukemia, unspecified, in remission
C95.92 Leukemia, unspecified, in relapse

C96 `4th` **OTHER AND UNSPECIFIED MALIGNANT NEOPLASMS OF LYMPHOID, HEMATOPOIETIC AND RELATED TISSUE**
Excludes1: personal history of other malignant neoplasms of lymphoid, hematopoietic and related tissues (Z85.79)
C96.2 Malignant mast cell neoplasm
`5th` ***Excludes1:*** indolent mastocytosis (D47.02)
mast cell leukemia (C94.30)
mastocytosis (congenital) (cutaneous) (Q82.2)
C96.20 Malignant mast cell neoplasm, unspecified
C96.21 Aggressive systemic mastocytosis
C96.22 Mast cell sarcoma
C96.29 Other malignant mast cell neoplasm
C96.A Histiocytic sarcoma
Malignant histiocytosis

(D00–D09) IN SITU NEOPLASMS

Includes: Bowen's disease
erythroplasia
grade III intraepithelial neoplasia
Queyrat's erythroplasia

(D10–D36) BENIGN NEOPLASMS, EXCEPT BENIGN NEUROENDOCRINE TUMORS

D12 `4th` **BENIGN NEOPLASM OF COLON, RECTUM, ANUS AND ANAL CANAL**
Excludes1: benign carcinoid tumors of the large intestine, and rectum (D3A.02-)
polyp of colon NOS (K63.5)
D12.0 Benign neoplasm of; cecum
Benign neoplasm of ileocecal valve
D12.1 appendix
Excludes1: benign carcinoid tumor of the appendix (D3A.020)
D12.2 ascending colon

`4th` `5th` `6th` `7th` Additional Character Required ✔ 3-character code

Unspecified laterality codes were excluded here.
•=New Code
▲=Revised Code
Excludes1—Not coded here, do not use together
Excludes2—Not included here

D12.3 transverse colon
Benign neoplasm of hepatic flexure or splenic flexure

D12.4 descending colon

D12.5 sigmoid colon

D12.6 colon, unspecified
Adenomatosis of colon
Benign neoplasm of large intestine NOS
Polyposis (hereditary) of colon
Excludes1: inflammatory polyp of colon (K51.4-)

D12.7 rectosigmoid junction

D12.8 rectum
Excludes1: benign carcinoid tumor of the rectum (D3A.026)

D12.9 Benign neoplasm of anus and anal canal
Benign neoplasm of anus NOS
Excludes1: benign neoplasm of anal margin (D22.5, D23.5)
benign neoplasm of anal skin (D22.5, D23.5)
benign neoplasm of perianal skin (D22.5, D23.5)

D15 | **4th** | **BENIGN NEOPLASM OF OTHER AND UNSPECIFIED INTRATHORACIC ORGANS**
Excludes1: benign neoplasm of mesothelial tissue (D19.-)

D15.1 Benign neoplasm of heart
Excludes1: benign neoplasm of great vessels (D21.3)

D17 | **4th** | **BENIGN LIPOMATOUS NEOPLASM**

D17.0 Benign lipomatous neoplasm of skin and subcutaneous tissue of; head, face and neck

D17.1 trunk

D17.2 | **5th** | **Benign lipomatous neoplasm of skin and subcutaneous tissue of; limb**
    D17.21 right arm
    D17.22 left arm
    D17.23 right leg
    D17.24 left leg

D17.3 | **5th** | **Benign lipomatous neoplasm of skin and subcutaneous tissue of; other and unspecified sites**
    D17.30 unspecified sites
    D17.39 other sites

D17.4 Benign lipomatous neoplasm of intrathoracic organs

D17.5 Benign lipomatous neoplasm of intra-abdominal organs
Excludes1: benign lipomatous neoplasm of peritoneum and retroperitoneum (D17.79)

D17.6 Benign lipomatous neoplasm of spermatic cord

D17.7 Benign lipomatous neoplasm of other sites
  5th **D17.71 Benign lipomatous neoplasm of; kidney**
    D17.72 other genitourinary organ
    D17.79 other sites
      Benign lipomatous neoplasm of peritoneum or retroperitoneum

D17.9 Benign lipomatous neoplasm, unspecified
Lipoma NOS

D18 | **4th** | **HEMANGIOMA AND LYMPHANGIOMA, ANY SITE**
Excludes1: benign neoplasm of glomus jugulare (D35.6)
blue or pigmented nevus (D22.-)
nevus NOS (D22.-)
vascular nevus (Q82.5)

D18.0 | **5th** | **Hemangioma**
Angioma NOS
Cavernous nevus
D18.00 Hemangioma unspecified site
D18.01 Hemangioma of skin and subcutaneous tissue
D18.02 Hemangioma of intracranial structures
D18.03 Hemangioma of intra-abdominal structures
D18.09 Hemangioma of other sites

D18.1 Lymphangioma, any site

D22 | **4th** | **MELANOCYTIC NEVI**
Includes: atypical nevus
blue hairy pigmented nevus
nevus NOS

D22.0 Melanocytic nevi of lip

D22.1 Melanocytic nevi of eyelid, including canthus
  5th **D22.10 Melanocytic nevi of unspecified eyelid, including canthus**

D22.11 Melanocytic nevi of right eyelid, including canthus
  6th **D22.111 Melanocytic nevi of right upper eyelid, including canthus**
    D22.112 Melanocytic nevi of right lower eyelid, including canthus

D22.12 Melanocytic nevi of left eyelid, including canthus
  6th **D22.121 Melanocytic nevi of left upper eyelid, including canthus**
    D22.122 Melanocytic nevi of left lower eyelid, including canthus

D22.2 Melanocytic nevi of ear and external auricular canal
  5th **D22.21 Melanocytic nevi of right ear and external auricular canal**
    D22.22 Melanocytic nevi of left ear and external auricular canal

D22.3 Melanocytic nevi of other and unspecified parts of face
  5th **D22.30 Melanocytic nevi of unspecified part of face**
    D22.39 Melanocytic nevi of other parts of face

D22.4 Melanocytic nevi of scalp and neck

D22.5 Melanocytic nevi of trunk
Melanocytic nevi of anal margin
Melanocytic nevi of anal skin
Melanocytic nevi of perianal skin
Melanocytic nevi of skin of breast

D22.6 Melanocytic nevi of upper limb, including shoulder
  5th **D22.61 Melanocytic nevi of right upper limb, including shoulder**
    D22.62 Melanocytic nevi of left upper limb, including shoulder

D22.7 Melanocytic nevi of lower limb, including hip
  5th **D22.71 Melanocytic nevi of right lower limb, including hip**
    D22.72 Melanocytic nevi of left lower limb, including hip

D22.9 Melanocytic nevi, unspecified

D23 | **4th** | **OTHER BENIGN NEOPLASMS OF SKIN**
Includes: benign neoplasm of hair follicles or sebaceous glands or sweat glands
Excludes1: benign lipomatous neoplasms of skin (D17.0-D17.3)
Excludes 2: melanocytic nevi (D22.-)

D23.0 Other benign neoplasm of skin of lip
Excludes1: benign neoplasm of vermilion border of lip (D10.0)

D23.1 | **5th** | **Other benign neoplasm of skin of; eyelid, including canthus**
  D23.11 right eyelid, including canthus
  6th **D23.111 Other benign neoplasm of skin of right upper eyelid, including canthus**
    D23.112 Other benign neoplasm of skin of right lower eyelid, including canthus
  D23.12 left eyelid, including canthus
  6th **D23.121 Other benign neoplasm of skin of left upper eyelid, including canthus**
    D23.122 Other benign neoplasm of skin of left lower eyelid, including canthus

D23.2 | **5th** | **Other benign neoplasm of skin of; ear and external auricular canal**
  D23.21 right ear and external auricular canal
  D23.22 left ear and external auricular canal

D23.3 | **5th** | **Other benign neoplasm of skin of; other and unspecified parts of face**
  D23.30 unspecified part of face
  D23.39 other parts of face

D23.4 Other benign neoplasm of skin of scalp and neck

D23.5 Other benign neoplasm of skin of trunk
Other benign neoplasm of anal margin or anal skin or perianal skin
Other benign neoplasm of skin of breast
Excludes1: benign neoplasm of anus NOS (D12.9)

D23.6 | **5th** | **Other benign neoplasm of skin of; upper limb, including shoulder**
  D23.61 right upper limb, including shoulder
  D23.62 left upper limb, including shoulder

D23.7 | **5th** | **Other benign neoplasm of skin of; lower limb, including hip**
  D23.71 right lower limb, including hip
  D23.72 left lower limb, including hip

D23.9 Other benign neoplasm of skin, unspecified

4th **5th** **6th** **7th** Additional Character Required   ✓ 3-character code

Unspecified laterality codes were excluded here. •=New Code ▲=Revised Code *Excludes1*—Not coded here, do not use together *Excludes2*—Not included here

CHAPTER 2. NEOPLASMS   (D24–D49.9)

D24   BENIGN NEOPLASM OF BREAST
4th

Includes: benign neoplasm of connective tissue of breast
benign neoplasm of soft parts of breast
fibroadenoma of breast

Excludes2: adenofibrosis of breast (N60.2)
benign cyst of breast (N60.-)
benign mammary dysplasia (N60.-)
benign neoplasm of skin of breast (D22.5, D23.5)
fibrocystic disease of breast (N60.-)

D24.1   Benign neoplasm of right breast
D24.2   Benign neoplasm of left breast

(D3A) BENIGN NEUROENDOCRINE TUMORS

(D37–D48) NEOPLASMS OF UNCERTAIN BEHAVIOR, POLYCYTHEMIA VERA AND MYELODYSPLASTIC SYNDROMES

Note: Categories D37–D44, and D48 classify by site neoplasms of uncertain behavior, i.e., histologic confirmation whether the neoplasm is malignant or benign cannot be made.
Excludes1: neoplasms of unspecified behavior (D49.-)

D47   OTHER NEOPLASMS OF UNCERTAIN BEHAVIOR OF LYMPHOID, HEMATOPOIETIC AND RELATED TISSUE
4th

D47.0   Mast cell neoplasms of uncertain behavior
5th   *Excludes1:*
congenital cutaneous mastocytosis (Q82.2)
histiocytic neoplasms of uncertain behavior (D47.Z9)
malignant mast cell neoplasm (C96.2-)

  D47.01   Cutaneous mastocytosis
Diffuse cutaneous mastocytosis
Maculopapular cutaneous mastocytosis
Solitary mastocytoma
Telangiectasia macularis eruptiva perstans
Urticaria pigmentosa
Excludes1: congenital (diffuse) (maculopapular)
cutaneous mastocytosis (Q82.2)
congenital urticaria pigmentosa (Q82.2)
extracutaneous mastocytoma (D47.09)

  D47.02   Systemic mastocytosis
Indolent systemic mastocytosis
Isolated bone marrow mastocytosis
Smoldering systemic mastocytosis
Systemic mastocytosis, with an associated hematological
non-mast cell lineage disease (SM-AHNMD)
Code also, if applicable, any associated hematological
non-mast cell lineage disease
Excludes1: aggressive systemic mastocytosis (C96.21)
mast cell leukemia (C94.3-)

  D47.09   Other mast cell neoplasms of uncertain behavior
Extracutaneous mastocytoma
Mast cell tumor NOS
Mastocytoma NOS
Mastocytosis NOS
Mastocytosis NOS

D47.3   Essential (hemorrhagic) thrombocythemia
Essential thrombocytosis
Idiopathic hemorrhagic thrombocythemia

D47.Z   Other specified neoplasms of uncertain behavior of lymphoid,
5th   **hematopoietic and related tissue**

  D47.Z1   Post-transplant lymphoproliferative disorder (PTLD)
Code first complications of transplanted organs and
tissue (T86.-)

  D47.Z9   Other specified neoplasms of uncertain behavior of
lymphoid, hematopoietic and related tissue
Histiocytic tumors of uncertain behavior
Use for kaposiform lymphangiomatosis

D47.9   Neoplasm of uncertain behavior of lymphoid, hematopoietic and related tissue, unspecified
Lymphoproliferative disease NOS

(D49) NEOPLASMS OF UNSPECIFIED BEHAVIOR

D49   NEOPLASMS OF UNSPECIFIED BEHAVIOR
4th

Note: Category D49 classifies by site neoplasms of unspecified morphology and behavior. *The term 'mass', unless otherwise stated, is not to be regarded as a neoplastic growth.*
Includes: 'growth' NOS or neoplasm NOS or new growth NOS or tumor NOS
Excludes1: neoplasms of uncertain behavior (D37–D44, D48)

D49.0   Neoplasm of unspecified behavior of; digestive system
Excludes1: neoplasm of unspecified behavior of margin of anus or
perianal skin or skin of anus (D49.2)

D49.1   respiratory system

D49.2   bone, soft tissue, and skin
Excludes1: neoplasm of unspecified behavior of anal canal or anus
NOS (D49.0)
bone marrow (D49.89)
cartilage of larynx or nose (D49.1)
connective tissue of breast (D49.3)
skin of genital organs (D49.59)
vermilion border of lip (D49.0)

D49.3   breast
Excludes1: neoplasm of unspecified behavior of skin of breast
(D49.2)

D49.4   bladder

D49.5   other genitourinary organs
5th   **D49.51   Neoplasm of unspecified behavior of kidney**
6th   **D49.511   right kidney**
   D49.512   left kidney
  D49.59   Neoplasm unspecified behavior of other genitourinary organ

D49.6   brain
Excludes1: neoplasm of unspecified behavior of cerebral meninges
(D49.7)
neoplasm of unspecified behavior of cranial nerves (D49.7)

D49.7   endocrine glands and other parts of nervous system
Excludes1: neoplasm of unspecified behavior of peripheral,
sympathetic, and parasympathetic nerves and ganglia (D49.2)

D49.8   other specified sites
Excludes1: neoplasm of unspecified behavior of eyelid (skin)
(D49.2)

D49.9   unspecified site

4th **5th** **6th** **7th**   Additional Character Required   ✓   3-character code   Unspecified laterality codes were excluded here.   •=New Code   ▲=Revised Code   *Excludes1*—Not coded here, do not use together   *Excludes2*—Not included here

148   PEDIATRIC ICD-10-CM 2021: A MANUAL FOR PROVIDER-BASED CODING

Chapter 3. Diseases of the blood and blood-forming organs and certain disorders involving the immune mechanism (D50–D89)

GUIDELINES

None currently. Reserved for future guideline expansion.

Excludes2: autoimmune disease (systemic) NOS (M35.9)
    certain conditions originating in the perinatal period (P00–P96)
    complications of pregnancy, childbirth and the puerperium (O00–O9A)
    congenital malformations, deformations and chromosomal abnormalities
      (Q00–Q99)
    endocrine, nutritional and metabolic diseases (E00–E88)
    HIV disease (B20)
    injury, poisoning and certain other consequences of external causes (S00–T88)
    neoplasms (C00–D49)
    symptoms, signs and abnormal clinical and laboratory findings, NEC (R00–R94)

(D50–D53) NUTRITIONAL ANEMIAS

D50 IRON DEFICIENCY ANEMIA
`4th`
    Includes: asiderotic anemia
      hypochromic anemia

    D50.0 Iron deficiency anemia secondary to blood loss (chronic)
      Posthemorrhagic anemia (chronic)
      Excludes1: acute posthemorrhagic anemia (D62)
        congenital anemia from fetal blood loss (P61.3)

    D50.1 Sideropenic dysphagia
      Kelly-Paterson syndrome
      Plummer-Vinson syndrome

    D50.8 Other iron deficiency anemias
      Iron deficiency anemia due to inadequate dietary iron intake

    D50.9 Iron deficiency anemia, unspecified

D51 VITAMIN B12 DEFICIENCY ANEMIA
`4th`
    Excludes1: vitamin B12 deficiency (E53.8)

    D51.0 Vitamin B12 deficiency anemia due to intrinsic factor deficiency
      Addison anemia
      Biermer anemia
      Pernicious (congenital) anemia
      Congenital intrinsic factor deficiency

    D51.1 Vitamin B12 deficiency anemia due to selective vitamin B12 malabsorption with proteinuria
      Imerslund (Gräsbeck) syndrome
      Megaloblastic hereditary anemia

    D51.2 Transcobalamin II deficiency

    D51.3 Other dietary vitamin B12 deficiency anemia
      Vegan anemia

    D51.8 Other vitamin B12 deficiency anemias

    D51.9 Vitamin B12 deficiency anemia, unspecified

D52 FOLATE DEFICIENCY ANEMIA
`4th`
    Excludes1: folate deficiency without anemia (E53.8)

    D52.0 Dietary folate deficiency anemia
      Nutritional megaloblastic anemia

    D52.1 Drug-induced folate deficiency anemia
      Use additional code for adverse effect, if applicable, to identify
        drug (T36–T50 with fifth or sixth character 5)

    D52.8 Other folate deficiency anemias

    D52.9 Folate deficiency anemia, unspecified
      Folic acid deficiency anemia NOS

D53 OTHER NUTRITIONAL ANEMIAS
`4th`
    Includes: megaloblastic anemia unresponsive to vitamin B12 or folate
      therapy

    D53.0 Protein deficiency anemia
      Amino-acid deficiency anemia
      Orotaciduric anemia
      Excludes1: Lesch-Nyhan syndrome (E79.1)

    D53.1 Other megaloblastic anemias, NEC
      Megaloblastic anemia NOS
      Excludes1: Di Guglielmo's disease (C94.0)

    D53.2 Scorbutic anemia
      Excludes1: scurvy (E54)

    D53.8 Other specified nutritional anemias
      Anemia associated with deficiency of copper
      Anemia associated with deficiency of molybdenum
      Anemia associated with deficiency of zinc
      Excludes1: nutritional deficiencies without anemia, such as:
        copper deficiency NOS (E61.0)
        molybdenum deficiency NOS (E61.5)
        zinc deficiency NOS (E60)

    D53.9 Nutritional anemia, unspecified
      Simple chronic anemia
      Excludes1: anemia NOS (D64.9)

(D55–D59) HEMOLYTIC ANEMIAS

D55 ANEMIA DUE TO ENZYME DISORDERS
`4th`
    Excludes1: drug-induced enzyme deficiency anemia (D59.2)

    D55.0 Anemia due to glucose-6-phosphate dehydrogenase [G6PD] deficiency
      Excludes1: G6PD deficiency without anemia (D75.A)
      Favism
      G6PD deficiency anemia

    D55.1 Anemia due to other disorders of glutathione metabolism
      Anemia (due to) enzyme deficiencies, except G6PD, related to the
        hexose monophosphate [HMP] shunt pathway
      Anemia (due to) hemolytic nonspherocytic (hereditary), type I

    D55.2 Anemia due to disorders of glycolytic enzymes
      Hemolytic nonspherocytic (hereditary) anemia, type II
      Hexokinase deficiency anemia
      Pyruvate kinase [PK] deficiency anemia
      Triose-phosphate isomerase deficiency anemia
      Excludes1: disorders of glycolysis not associated with anemia
        (E74.81-)

    D55.3 Anemia due to disorders of nucleotide metabolism

    D55.8 Other anemias due to enzyme disorders

    D55.9 Anemia due to enzyme disorder, unspecified

D56 THALASSEMIA
`4th`
    Excludes1: sickle-cell thalassemia (D57.4-)

    D56.0 Alpha thalassemia
      Alpha thalassemia major
      Hemoglobin H Constant Spring
      Hemoglobin H disease
      Hydrops fetalis due to alpha thalassemia
      Severe alpha thalassemia
      Triple gene defect alpha thalassemia
      Use additional code, if applicable, for hydrops fetalis due to alpha
        thalassemia (P56.99)
      Excludes1: alpha thalassemia trait or minor (D56.3)
        asymptomatic alpha thalassemia (D56.3)
        hydrops fetalis due to isoimmunization (P56.0)
        hydrops fetalis not due to immune hemolysis (P83.2)

    D56.1 Beta thalassemia
      Beta thalassemia major
      Cooley's anemia
      Homozygous beta thalassemia
      Severe beta thalassemia
      Thalassemia intermedia
      Thalassemia major
      Excludes1: beta thalassemia minor (D56.3)
        beta thalassemia trait (D56.3)
        delta-beta thalassemia (D56.2)
        hemoglobin E-beta thalassemia (D56.5)
        sickle-cell beta thalassemia (D57.4-)

    D56.2 Delta-beta thalassemia
      Homozygous delta-beta thalassemia
      Excludes1: delta-beta thalassemia minor (D56.3)
        delta-beta thalassemia trait (D56.3)

`4th` `5th` `6th` `7th` Additional Character Required   ✔ 3-character code

•=New Code   *Excludes1*—Not coded here, do not use together
▲=Revised Code   *Excludes2*—Not included here

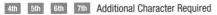

D56.3   Thalassemia minor
Alpha thalassemia minor
Alpha thalassemia silent carrier
Alpha thalassemia trait
Beta thalassemia minor
Beta thalassemia trait
Delta-beta thalassemia minor
Delta-beta thalassemia trait
Thalassemia trait NOS
Excludes1: alpha thalassemia (D56.0)
    beta thalassemia (D56.1)
    delta-beta thalassemia (D56.2)
    hemoglobin E-beta thalassemia (D56.5)
    sickle-cell trait (D57.3)

D56.4   Hereditary persistence of fetal hemoglobin [HPFH]

D56.5   Hemoglobin E-beta thalassemia
Excludes1: beta thalassemia (D56.1)
    beta thalassemia minor (D56.3)
    beta thalassemia trait (D56.3)
    delta-beta thalassemia (D56.2)
    delta-beta thalassemia trait (D56.3)
    hemoglobin E disease (D58.2)
    other hemoglobinopathies (D58.2)
    sickle-cell beta thalassemia (D57.4-)

D56.8   Other thalassemias
Dominant thalassemia
Hemoglobin C thalassemia
Mixed thalassemia
Thalassemia with other hemoglobinopathy
Excludes1: hemoglobin C disease (D58.2)
    hemoglobin E disease (D58.2)
    other hemoglobinopathies (D58.2)
    sickle-cell anemia (D57.-)
    sickle-cell thalassemia (D57.4)

D56.9   Thalassemia, unspecified
Mediterranean anemia (with other hemoglobinopathy)

D57   SICKLE-CELL DISORDERS
[4th] **Use additional code** for any associated fever (R50.81)
Excludes1: other hemoglobinopathies (D58.-)

D57.0   Hb-SS disease with crisis
[5th] Sickle-cell disease with crisis
Hb-SS disease with vaso-occlusive pain
   D57.00   Hb-SS disease with crisis, unspecified
     Hb-SS disease with (painful) crisis NOS
     Hb-SS disease with vasoocclusive pain NOS
   D57.01   Hb-SS disease with acute chest syndrome
   D57.02   Hb-SS disease with splenic sequestration
   •**D57.03   Hb-SS disease with cerebral vascular involvement**
     Code also, if applicable, cerebral infarction (I63.-)
   •**D57.09   Hb-SS disease with crisis with other specified complication**
     Use additional code to identify complications, such as:
      cholelithiasis (K80.-)
      priapism (N48.32)

D57.1   Sickle-cell disease without crisis
Hb-SS disease without crisis
Sickle-cell anemia NOS
Sickle-cell disease NOS
Sickle-cell disorder NOS

D57.2   Sickle-cell/Hb-C disease
[5th] Hb-SC disease
Hb-S/Hb-C disease
   D57.20   Sickle-cell/Hb-C disease without crisis
   D57.21   Sickle-cell/Hb-C disease with crisis
    [6th]   **D57.211   Sickle-cell/Hb-C disease with acute chest syndrome**
      D57.212   Sickle-cell/Hb-C disease with splenic sequestration
     •**D57.213   Sickle-cell/Hb-C disease with cerebral vascular involvement**
      Code also, if applicable, cerebral infarction (I63.-)

     •**D57.218   Sickle-cell/Hb-C disease with crisis with other specified complication**
      Use additional code to identify complications, such as:
       cholelithiasis (K80.-)
       priapism (N48.32)
     D57.219   Sickle-cell/Hb-C disease with crisis, unspecified
      Sickle-cell/Hb-C disease with vasoocclusive pain NOS

D57.3   Sickle-cell trait
Hb-S trait
Heterozygous hemoglobin S

D57.4   Sickle-cell thalassemia
[5th] Sickle-cell beta thalassemia
Thalassemia Hb-S disease
   D57.40   Sickle-cell thalassemia without crisis
     Microdrepanocytosis
     Sickle-cell thalassemia NOS
   D57.41   Sickle-cell thalassemia, unspecified, with crisis
    [6th]   Sickle-cell thalassemia with (painful) crisis NOS
     Sickle-cell thalassemia with vasoocclusive pain NOS
     D57.411   Sickle-cell thalassemia, unspecified, with acute chest syndrome
     D57.412   Sickle-cell thalassemia, unspecified, with splenic sequestration
    •**D57.413   Sickle-cell thalassemia, unspecified, with cerebral vascular involvement**
     Code also, if applicable, cerebral infarction (I63.-)
    •**D57.418   Sickle-cell thalassemia, unspecified, with crisis with other specified complication**
     Use additional code to identify complications, such as:
      cholelithiasis (K80.-)
      priapism (N48.32)
     D57.419   Sickle-cell thalassemia, unspecified, with crisis
     Sickle-cell thalassemia with (painful) crisis NOS
     Sickle-cell thalassemia with vasoocclusive pain

   •**D57.42   Sickle-cell thalassemia beta zero without crisis**
     HbS-beta zero without crisis
     Sickle-cell beta zero without crisis
   •**D57.43   Sickle-cell thalassemia beta zero**
    [6th]   HbS-beta zero with crisis
     Sickle-cell beta zero with crisis
    •**D57.431   Sickle-cell thalassemia beta zero with acute chest syndrome**
     HbS-beta zero with acute chest syndrome
     Sickle-cell beta zero with acute chest syndrome
    •**D57.432   Sickle-cell thalassemia beta zero with splenic sequestration**
     HbS-beta zero with splenic sequestration
     Sickle-cell beta zero with splenic sequestration
    •**D57.433   Sickle-cell thalassemia beta zero with cerebral vascular involvement**
     HbS-beta zero with cerebral vascular involvement
     Sickle-cell beta zero with cerebral vascular involvement
     Code also, if applicable, cerebral infarction (I63.-)
    •**D57.438   Sickle-cell thalassemia beta zero with crisis with other specified complication**
     HbS-beta zero with other specified complication
     Sickle-cell beta zero with other specified complication

[4th]   [5th]   [6th]   [7th]   Additional Character Required   ✔   3-character code   •=New Code   ▲=Revised Code   *Excludes1*—Not coded here, do not use together   *Excludes2*—Not included here

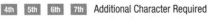

Left margin: CHAPTER 3. DISEASES OF THE BLOOD AND BLOOD-FORMING ORGANS AND CERTAIN DISORDERS INVOLVING THE IMMUNE MECHANISM   (D56.3–D57.438)

Use additional code to identify complications, such as:
cholelithiasis (K80.-)
priapism (N48.32)

- **D57.439** **Sickle-cell thalassemia beta zero with crisis, unspecified**
HbS-beta zero with other specified complication
Sickle-cell beta zero with crisis unspecified
Sickle-cell thalassemia beta zero with (painful) crisis NOS
Sickle-cell thalassemia beta zero with vasoocclusive pain

- **D57.44** **Sickle-cell thalassemia beta plus without crisis**
HbS-beta plus without crisis
Sickle-cell beta plus without crisis

- **D57.45** **Sickle-cell thalassemia beta plus**
`6th` HbS-beta plus with crisis
Sickle-cell beta plus with crisis

  - **D57.451** **Sickle-cell thalassemia beta plus with acute chest syndrome**
HbS-beta plus with acute chest syndrome
Sickle-cell beta plus with acute chest syndrome

  - **D57.452** **Sickle-cell thalassemia beta plus with splenic sequestration**
HbS-beta plus with splenic sequestration
Sickle-cell beta plus with splenic sequestration

  - **D57.453** **Sickle-cell thalassemia beta plus with cerebral vascular involvement**
HbS-beta plus with cerebral vascular involvement
Sickle-cell beta plus with cerebral vascular involvement
Code also, if applicable, cerebral infarction (I63.-)

  - **D57.458** **Sickle-cell thalassemia beta plus with crisis with other specified complication**
HbS-beta plus with crisis with other specified complication
Sickle-cell beta plus with crisis with other specified complication
Use additional code to identify complications, such as:
cholelithiasis (K80.-)
priapism (N48.32)

  - **D57.459** **Sickle-cell thalassemia beta plus with crisis, unspecified**
HbS-beta plus with crisis with unspecified complication
Sickle-cell beta plus with crisis with unspecified complication
Sickle-cell thalassemia beta plus with (painful) crisis NOS
Sickle-cell thalassemia beta plus with vasoocclusive pain

D57.8 **Other sickle-cell disorders**
`5th` Hb-SD disease
Hb-SE disease

D57.80 **Other sickle-cell disorders without crisis**
D57.81 **Other sickle-cell disorders with crisis**
`6th`
  D57.811 **Other sickle-cell disorders with acute chest syndrome**
  D57.812 **Other sickle-cell disorders with splenic sequestration**
  - **D57.813** **Other sickle-cell disorders with cerebral vascular involvement**
Code also, if applicable: cerebral infarction (I63.-)

- **D57.818** **Other sickle-cell disorders with crisis with other specified complication**
Use additional code to identify complications, such as:
cholelithiasis (K80.-)
priapism (N48.32)

  D57.819 **Other sickle-cell disorders with crisis, unspecified**
Other sickle-cell disorders with (vasooclusive pain) crisis NOS

D58 **OTHER HEREDITARY HEMOLYTIC ANEMIAS**
`4th` **Excludes1:** hemolytic anemia of the newborn (P55.-)
D58.0 **Hereditary spherocytosis**
Acholuric (familial) jaundice
Congenital (spherocytic) hemolytic icterus
Minkowski-Chauffard syndrome
D58.1 **Hereditary elliptocytosis**
Elliptocytosis (congenital)
Ovalocytosis (congenital) (hereditary)
D58.2 **Other hemoglobinopathies**
Abnormal hemoglobin NOS
Congenital Heinz body anemia
Hb-C disease
Hb-D disease
Hb-E disease
Hemoglobinopathy NOS
Unstable hemoglobin hemolytic disease
Excludes1: familial polycythemia (D75.0)
Hb-M disease (D74.0)
hemoglobin E-beta thalassemia (D56.5)
hereditary persistence of fetal hemoglobin [HPFH] (D56.4)
high-altitude polycythemia (D75.1)
methemoglobinemia (D74.-)
other hemoglobinopathies with thalassemia (D56.8)
D58.8 **Other specified hereditary hemolytic anemias**
Stomatocytosis
D58.9 **Hereditary hemolytic anemia, unspecified**

D59 **ACQUIRED HEMOLYTIC ANEMIA**
`4th` **D59.0** **Drug-induced autoimmune hemolytic anemia**
Use additional code for adverse effect, if applicable, to identify drug (T36-T50 with fifth or sixth character 5)
▲**D59.1** **Other autoimmune hemolytic anemias**
`5th` **Excludes2:** Evans syndrome (D69.41)
hemolytic disease of newborn (P55.-)
paroxysmal cold hemoglobinuria (D59.6)
- **D59.10** **Autoimmune hemolytic anemia, unspecified**
- **D59.11** **Warm autoimmune hemolytic anemia**
Warm type (primary) (secondary) (symptomatic) autoimmune hemolytic anemia
Warm type autoimmune hemolytic disease
- **D59.12** **Cold autoimmune hemolytic anemia**
Chronic cold hemagglutinin disease
Cold agglutinin disease
Cold agglutinin hemoglobinuria
Cold type (primary) (secondary) (symptomatic) autoimmune hemolytic anemia
Cold type autoimmune hemolytic disease
- **D59.13** **Mixed type autoimmune hemolytic anemia**
Mixed type autoimmune hemolytic disease
Mixed type, cold and warm, (primary) (secondary) (symptomatic) autoimmune hemolyticanemia
- **D59.19** **Other autoimmune hemolytic anemia**
D59.2 **Drug-induced nonautoimmune hemolytic anemia**
Drug-induced enzyme deficiency anemia
Use additional code for adverse effect, if applicable, to identify drug (T36-T50 with fifth or sixth character 5)
D59.3 **Hemolytic-uremic syndrome**
Use additional code to identify associated:
E. coli infection (B96.2-)
Pneumococcal pneumonia (J13)
Shigella dysenteriae (A03.9)

CHAPTER 3. DISEASES OF THE BLOOD AND BLOOD-FORMING ORGANS AND CERTAIN DISORDERS INVOLVING THE IMMUNE MECHANISM (D57.439–D59.3)

`4th` `5th` `6th` `7th` Additional Character Required ✔ 3-character code

•=New Code
▲=Revised Code

Excludes1—Not coded here, do not use together
Excludes2—Not included here

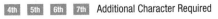 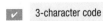

CHAPTER 3. DISEASES OF THE BLOOD AND BLOOD-FORMING ORGANS AND CERTAIN DISORDERS INVOLVING THE IMMUNE MECHANISM (D59.4–D64.9)

D59.4 Other nonautoimmune hemolytic anemias
Mechanical hemolytic anemia
Microangiopathic hemolytic anemia
Toxic hemolytic anemia

D59.5 Paroxysmal nocturnal hemoglobinuria [Marchiafava-Micheli]
Excludes1: hemoglobinuria NOS (R82.3)

D59.6 Hemoglobinuria due to hemolysis from other external causes
Hemoglobinuria from exertion
March hemoglobinuria
Paroxysmal cold hemoglobinuria
Use additional code (Chapter 20) to identify external cause
Excludes1: hemoglobinuria NOS (R82.3)

D59.8 Other acquired hemolytic anemias

D59.9 Acquired hemolytic anemia, unspecified
Idiopathic hemolytic anemia, chronic

(D60–D64) APLASTIC AND OTHER ANEMIAS AND OTHER BONE MARROW FAILURE SYNDROMES

D60 ACQUIRED PURE RED CELL APLASIA [ERYTHROBLASTOPENIA]
4th
Includes: red cell aplasia (acquired) (adult) (with thymoma)
Excludes1: congenital red cell aplasia (D61.01)

D60.0 Chronic acquired pure red cell aplasia

D60.1 Transient acquired pure red cell aplasia

D60.8 Other acquired pure red cell aplasias

D60.9 Acquired pure red cell aplasia, unspecified

D61 OTHER APLASTIC ANEMIAS AND OTHER BONE MARROW FAILURE SYNDROMES
4th
Excludes2: neutropenia (D70.-)

D61.0 Constitutional aplastic anemia

5th **D61.01 Constitutional (pure) red blood cell aplasia**
Blackfan-Diamond syndrome
Congenital (pure) red cell aplasia
Familial hypoplastic anemia
Primary (pure) red cell aplasia
Red cell (pure) aplasia of infants
Excludes1: acquired red cell aplasia (D60.9)

D61.09 Other constitutional aplastic anemia
Fanconi's anemia
Pancytopenia with malformations

D61.1 Drug-induced aplastic anemia
Use additional code for adverse effect, if applicable, to identify drug (T36–T50 with fifth or sixth character 5)

D61.2 Aplastic anemia due to other external agents
Code first, if applicable, toxic effects of substances chiefly nonmedicinal as to source (T51–T65)

D61.3 Idiopathic aplastic anemia

D61.8 Other specified aplastic anemias and other bone marrow failure syndromes
5th

5th **D61.81 Pancytopenia**
6th *Excludes1:* pancytopenia (due to) (with) aplastic anemia (D61.9)
pancytopenia (due to) (with) bone marrow infiltration (D61.82)
pancytopenia (due to) (with) congenital (pure) red cell aplasia (D61.01)
pancytopenia (due to) (with) hairy cell leukemia (C91.4-)
pancytopenia (due to) (with) HIV disease (B20.-)
pancytopenia (due to) (with) leukoerythroblastic anemia (D61.82)
pancytopenia (due to) (with) myeloproliferative disease (D47.1)
Excludes2: pancytopenia (due to) (with) myelodysplastic syndromes (D46.-)

D61.810 Antineoplastic chemotherapy induced pancytopenia
Excludes2: aplastic anemia due to antineoplastic chemotherapy (D61.1)

D61.811 Other drug-induced pancytopenia
Excludes2: aplastic anemia due to drugs (D61.1)

D61.818 Other pancytopenia

D61.82 Myelophthisis
Leukoerythroblastic anemia
Myelophthisic anemia
Panmyelophthisis
Code also the underlying disorder, such as: malignant neoplasm of breast (C50.-)
tuberculosis (A15.-)
Excludes1: idiopathic myelofibrosis (D47.1)
myelofibrosis NOS (D75.81)
myelofibrosis with myeloid metaplasia (D47.4)
primary myelofibrosis (D47.1)
secondary myelofibrosis (D75.81)

D61.89 Other specified aplastic anemias and other bone marrow failure syndromes

D61.9 Aplastic anemia, unspecified
Hypoplastic anemia NOS
Medullary hypoplasia

D62 ACUTE POSTHEMORRHAGIC ANEMIA
✔
Excludes1: anemia due to chronic blood loss (D50.0)
blood loss anemia NOS (D50.0)
congenital anemia from fetal blood loss (P61.3)

D63 ANEMIA IN CHRONIC DISEASES CLASSIFIED ELSEWHERE
4th

D63.0 Anemia in neoplastic disease
Code first neoplasm (C00–D49)
Excludes1: aplastic anemia due to antineoplastic chemotherapy (D61.1)
Excludes2: anemia due to antineoplastic chemotherapy (D64.81)

D63.1 Anemia in chronic kidney disease
Erythropoietin-resistant anemia (EPO-resistant anemia)
Code first underlying chronic kidney disease (CKD) (N18.-)

D63.8 Anemia in other chronic diseases classified elsewhere
Code first underlying disease

D64 OTHER ANEMIAS
4th
Excludes1: refractory anemia (D46.-)
refractory anemia with excess blasts in transformation [RAEB T] (C92.0-)

D64.0 Hereditary sideroblastic anemia
Sex-linked hypochromic sideroblastic anemia

D64.1 Secondary sideroblastic anemia due to disease
Code first underlying disease

D64.2 Secondary sideroblastic anemia due to drugs and toxins
Code first poisoning due to drug or toxin, if applicable (T36 –T65 with fifth or sixth character 1-4 or 6)
Use additional code for adverse effect, if applicable, to identify drug (T36-T50 with fifth or sixth character 5)

D64.3 Other sideroblastic anemias
Sideroblastic anemia NOS
Pyridoxine-responsive sideroblastic anemia NEC

D64.4 Congenital dyserythropoietic anemia
Dyshematopoietic anemia (congenital)
Excludes1: Blackfan-Diamond syndrome (D61.01)
Di Guglielmo's disease (C94.0)

D64.8 Other specified anemias
5th **D64.81 Anemia due to antineoplastic chemotherapy**
Antineoplastic chemotherapy induced anemia
Excludes1: aplastic anemia due to antineoplastic chemotherapy (D61.1)
Excludes2: anemia in neoplastic disease (D63.0)

D64.89 Other specified anemias
Infantile pseudoleukemia

D64.9 Anemia, unspecified

4th 5th 6th 7th Additional Character Required   ✔ 3-character code   •=New Code ▲=Revised Code

Excludes1—Not coded here, do not use together
Excludes2—Not included here

(D65–D69) COAGULATION DEFECTS, PURPURA AND OTHER HEMORRHAGIC CONDITIONS

D65 ✔ **DISSEMINATED INTRAVASCULAR COAGULATION [DEFIBRINATION SYNDROME]**
Afibrinogenemia, acquired
Consumption coagulopathy
Diffuse or disseminated intravascular coagulation [DIC]
Fibrinolytic hemorrhage, acquired
Fibrinolytic purpura
Purpura fulminans
Excludes1: disseminated intravascular coagulation (complicating):
  abortion or ectopic or molar pregnancy (O00–O07, O08.1)
  in newborn (P60)
  pregnancy, childbirth and the puerperium (O45.0, O46.0, O67.0, O72.3)

D66 ✔ **HEREDITARY FACTOR VIII DEFICIENCY**
Classical hemophilia
Deficiency factor VIII (with functional defect)
Hemophilia NOS
Hemophilia A
Excludes1: factor VIII deficiency with vascular defect (D68.0)

D67 ✔ **HEREDITARY FACTOR IX DEFICIENCY**
Christmas disease
Factor IX deficiency (with functional defect)
Hemophilia B
Plasma thromboplastin component [PTC] deficiency

D68 [4th] **OTHER COAGULATION DEFECTS**
Excludes1: abnormal coagulation profile (R79.1)
  coagulation defects complicating abortion or ectopic or molar pregnancy (O00–O07, O08.1)
  coagulation defects complicating pregnancy, childbirth and the puerperium (O45.0, O46.0, O67.0, O72.3)

D68.0 Von Willebrand's disease
Angiohemophilia
Factor VIII deficiency with vascular defect
Vascular hemophilia
Excludes1: capillary fragility (hereditary) (D69.8)
  factor VIII deficiency NOS (D66)
  factor VIII deficiency with functional defect (D66)

D68.1 Hereditary factor XI deficiency
Hemophilia C
Plasma thromboplastin antecedent [PTA] deficiency
Rosenthal's disease

D68.2 Hereditary deficiency of other clotting factors
AC globulin deficiency
Congenital afibrinogenemia
Deficiency of factor I [fibrinogen]
Deficiency of factor II [prothrombin]
Deficiency of factor V [labile]
Deficiency of factor VII [stable]
Deficiency of factor X [Stuart-Prower]
Deficiency of factor XII [Hageman]
Deficiency of factor XIII [fibrin stabilizing]
Dysfibrinogenemia (congenital)
Hypoproconvertinemia
Owren's disease
Proaccelerin deficiency

D68.3 Hemorrhagic disorder due to circulating anticoagulants
[5th] **D68.31** [6th] **Hemorrhagic disorder due to intrinsic circulating anticoagulants, antibodies, or inhibitors**
  D68.311 Acquired hemophilia
  Autoimmune hemophilia
  Autoimmune inhibitors to clotting factors
  Secondary hemophilia
  D68.312 Antiphospholipid antibody with hemorrhagic disorder
  LAC with hemorrhagic disorder
  SLE inhibitor with hemorrhagic disorder

Excludes1: antiphospholipid antibody, finding without diagnosis (R76.0)
  antiphospholipid antibody syndrome (D68.61)
  antiphospholipid antibody with hypercoagulable state (D68.61)
  LAC finding without diagnosis (R76.0)
  LAC with hypercoagulable state (D68.62)
  SLE inhibitor finding without diagnosis (R76.0)
  SLE inhibitor with hypercoagulable state (D68.62)

D68.318 Other hemorrhagic disorder due to intrinsic circulating anticoagulants, antibodies, or inhibitors
Antithromboplastinemia
Antithromboplastinogenemia
Hemorrhagic disorder due to intrinsic increase in antithrombin
Hemorrhagic disorder due to intrinsic increase in anti-VIIIa
Hemorrhagic disorder due to intrinsic increase in anti-IXa
Hemorrhagic disorder due to intrinsic increase in anti-Xia

D68.32 Hemorrhagic disorder due to extrinsic circulating anticoagulants
Drug-induced hemorrhagic disorder
Hemorrhagic disorder due to increase in anti-IIa
Hemorrhagic disorder due to increase in anti-Xa
Hyperheparinemia
Use additional code for adverse effect, if applicable, to identify drug (T45.515, T45.525)

D68.4 Acquired coagulation factor deficiency
Deficiency of coagulation factor due to liver disease
Deficiency of coagulation factor due to vitamin K deficiency
Excludes1: vitamin K deficiency of newborn (P53)

D68.5 Primary thrombophilia
[5th] Primary hypercoagulable states
Excludes1: antiphospholipid syndrome (D68.61)
  LAC (D68.62)
  secondary activated protein C resistance (D68.69)
  secondary antiphospholipid antibody syndrome (D68.69)
  secondary LAC with hypercoagulable state (D68.69)
  SLE inhibitor with hypercoagulable state (D68.69)
  SLE inhibitor finding without diagnosis (R76.0)
  SLE inhibitor with hemorrhagic disorder (D68.312)
  thrombotic thrombocytopenic purpura (M31.1)

D68.51 Activated protein C resistance
Factor V Leiden mutation
D68.52 Prothrombin gene mutation
D68.59 Other primary thrombophilia
Antithrombin III deficiency
Hypercoagulable state NOS
Primary hypercoagulable state NEC
Primary thrombophilia NEC
Protein C deficiency
Protein S deficiency
Thrombophilia NOS

D68.6 Other thrombophilia
[5th] Other hypercoagulable states
Excludes1: diffuse or disseminated intravascular coagulation [DIC] (D65)
  heparin induced thrombocytopenia (HIT) (D75.82)
  hyperhomocysteinemia (E72.11)

D68.61 Antiphospholipid syndrome
Anticardiolipin syndrome
Antiphospholipid antibody syndrome
Excludes1: anti-phospholipid antibody, finding without diagnosis (R76.0)
  anti-phospholipid antibody with hemorrhagic disorder (D68.312)
  LAC syndrome (D68.62)

[4th] [5th] [6th] [7th] Additional Character Required   ✔ 3-character code

•=New Code
▲=Revised Code

Excludes1—Not coded here, do not use together
Excludes2—Not included here

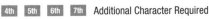

D68.62 LAC syndrome
LAC
Presence of SLE inhibitor
Excludes1: anticardiolipin syndrome (D68.61)
antiphospholipid syndrome (D68.61)
LAC finding without diagnosis (R76.0)
LAC with hemorrhagic disorder (D68.312)

D68.69 Other thrombophilia
Hypercoagulable states NEC
Secondary hypercoagulable state NOS

D68.8 Other specified coagulation defects
Excludes1: hemorrhagic disease of newborn (P53)

D68.9 Coagulation defect, unspecified

D69 PURPURA AND OTHER HEMORRHAGIC CONDITIONS
4th
Excludes1: benign hypergammaglobulinemic purpura (D89.0)
cryoglobulinemic purpura (D89.1)
essential (hemorrhagic) thrombocythemia (D47.3)
hemorrhagic thrombocythemia (D47.3)
purpura fulminans (D65)
thrombotic thrombocytopenic purpura (M31.1)
Waldenström hypergammaglobulinemic purpura (D89.0)

D69.0 Allergic purpura
Allergic vasculitis
Nonthrombocytopenic hemorrhagic purpura
Nonthrombocytopenic idiopathic purpura
Purpura anaphylactoid
Purpura Henoch(-Schönlein)
Purpura rheumatica
Vascular purpura
Excludes1: thrombocytopenic hemorrhagic purpura (D69.3)

D69.1 Qualitative platelet defects
Bernard-Soulier [giant platelet] syndrome
Glanzmann's disease
Grey platelet syndrome
Thromboasthenia (hemorrhagic) (hereditary)
Thrombocytopathy
Excludes1: von Willebrand's disease (D68.0)

D69.2 Other nonthrombocytopenic purpura
Purpura NOS
Purpura simplex
Senile purpura

D69.3 Immune thrombocytopenic purpura
Hemorrhagic (thrombocytopenic) purpura
Idiopathic thrombocytopenic purpura
Tidal platelet dysgenesis

D69.4 Other primary thrombocytopenia
5th
Excludes1: transient neonatal thrombocytopenia (P61.0)
Wiskott-Aldrich syndrome (D82.0)

D69.41 Evans syndrome

D69.42 Congenital and hereditary thrombocytopenia purpura
Congenital thrombocytopenia
Hereditary thrombocytopenia
Code first congenital or hereditary disorder, such as:
TAR syndrome (Q87.2)

D69.49 Other primary thrombocytopenia
Megakaryocytic hypoplasia
Primary thrombocytopenia NOS

D69.5 Secondary thrombocytopenia
5th
Excludes1: heparin induced thrombocytopenia (HIT) (D75.82)
transient thrombocytopenia of newborn (P61.0)

D69.51 Posttransfusion purpura
Posttransfusion purpura from whole blood (fresh) or
blood products
PTP

D69.59 Other secondary thrombocytopenia

D69.6 Thrombocytopenia, unspecified

D69.8 Other specified hemorrhagic conditions
Capillary fragility (hereditary)
Vascular pseudohemophilia

D69.9 Hemorrhagic condition, unspecified

(D70–D77) OTHER DISORDERS OF BLOOD AND BLOOD-FORMING ORGANS

D70 NEUTROPENIA
4th
Includes: agranulocytosis
decreased absolute neutrophil count (ANC)
Use additional code for any associated: fever (R50.81)
mucositis (J34.81, K12.3-, K92.81, N76.81)
Excludes1: neutropenic splenomegaly (D73.81)
transient neonatal neutropenia (P61.5)

D70.0 Congenital agranulocytosis
Congenital neutropenia
Infantile genetic agranulocytosis
Kostmann's disease

D70.1 Agranulocytosis secondary to cancer chemotherapy
Use additional code for adverse effect, if applicable, to identify
drug (T45.1X5)
Code also underlying neoplasm

D70.2 Other drug-induced agranulocytosis
Use additional code for adverse effect, if applicable, to identify
drug (T36–T50 with fifth or sixth character 5)

D70.3 Neutropenia due to infection

D70.4 Cyclic neutropenia
Cyclic hematopoiesis
Periodic neutropenia

D70.8 Other neutropenia

D70.9 Neutropenia, unspecified

D71 FUNCTIONAL DISORDERS OF POLYMORPHONUCLEAR NEUTROPHILS
✓
Cell membrane receptor complex [CR3] defect
Chronic (childhood) granulomatous disease
Congenital dysphagocytosis
Progressive septic granulomatosis

D72 OTHER DISORDERS OF WHITE BLOOD CELLS
4th
Excludes1: basophilia (D72.824)
immunity disorders (D80–D89)
neutropenia (D70)
preleukemia (syndrome) (D46.9)

D72.0 Genetic anomalies of leukocytes
Alder syndrome
Hereditary leukocytic hyper/hypo segmentation
Hereditary leukomelanopathy
May-Hegglin syndrome
Pelger-Huët syndrome

▲D72.1 Eosinophilia
5th
Excludes2: Löffler's syndrome (J82)
pulmonary eosinophilia (J82)

•**D72.10 Eosinophilia, unspecified**
6th
•**D72.110 Idiopathic hypereosinophilic syndrome [IHES]**

•**D72.111 Lymphocytic Variant Hypereosinophilic Syndrome [LHES]**
Lymphocyte variant hypereosinophilia
Code also, if applicable, any associated
lymphocytic neoplastic disorder

•**D72.118 Other hypereosinophilic syndrome**
Episodic angioedema with eosinophilia
Gleich's syndrome

•**D72.119 Hypereosinophilic syndrome [HES], unspecified**

•**D72.12 Drug rash with eosinophilia and systemic symptoms syndrome**
DRESS syndrome
Use additional code for adverse effect, if applicable, to
identify drug (T36–T50 with fifth or sixth character 5)

•**D72.18 Eosinophilia in diseases classified elsewhere**
Code first underlying disease, such as:
chronic myelomonocytic leukemia (C93.1-)

•**D72.19 Other eosinophilia**
Familial eosinophilia
Hereditary eosinophilia

4th	5th	6th	7th	Additional Character Required		✓	3-character code	•=New Code	*Excludes1*—Not coded here, do not use together
								▲=Revised Code	*Excludes2*—Not included here

D72.8 **Other specified disorders of white blood cells**
> `5th` *Excludes1:* leukemia (C91–C95)

    D72.81 **Decreased white blood cell count**
> `6th` *Excludes1:* neutropenia (D70.-)

        D72.810 **Lymphocytopenia**
Decreased lymphocytes

        D72.818 **Other decreased white blood cell count**
Basophilic leukopenia
Eosinophilic leukopenia
Monocytopenia
Other decreased leukocytes
Plasmacytopenia

        D72.819 **Decreased white blood cell count, unspecified**
Decreased leukocytes, unspecified
Leukocytopenia, unspecified
Leukopenia
Excludes1: malignant leukopenia (D70.9)

    D72.82 **Elevated white blood cell count**
> `6th` *Excludes1:* eosinophilia (D72.1)

        D72.820 **Lymphocytosis (symptomatic)**
Elevated lymphocytes

        D72.821 **Monocytosis (symptomatic)**
Excludes1: infectious mononucleosis (B27.-)

        D72.822 **Plasmacytosis**

        D72.823 **Leukemoid reaction**
Basophilic leukemoid reaction
Leukemoid reaction NOS
Lymphocytic leukemoid reaction
Monocytic leukemoid reaction
Myelocytic leukemoid reaction
Neutrophilic leukemoid reaction

        D72.824 **Basophilia**

        D72.825 **Bandemia**
Bandemia without diagnosis of specific infection
Excludes1: confirmed infection—code to infection
leukemia (C91.-, C92.-, C93.-, C94.-, C95.-)

        D72.828 **Other elevated white blood cell count**

        D72.829 **Elevated white blood cell count, unspecified**
Elevated leukocytes, unspecified
Leukocytosis, unspecified

    D72.89 **Other specified disorders of white blood cells**
Abnormality of white blood cells NEC

D72.9 **Disorder of white blood cells, unspecified**
Abnormal leukocyte differential NOS

D73 **DISEASES OF SPLEEN**
> `4th`

D73.0 **Hyposplenism**
Atrophy of spleen
Excludes1: asplenia (congenital) (Q89.01)
postsurgical absence of spleen (Z90.81)

D73.1 **Hypersplenism**
Excludes1: neutropenic splenomegaly (D73.81)
primary splenic neutropenia (D73.81)
splenitis, splenomegaly in late syphilis (A52.79)
splenitis, splenomegaly in tuberculosis (A18.85)
splenomegaly NOS (R16.1)
splenomegaly congenital (Q89.0)

D73.2 **Chronic congestive splenomegaly**

D73.3 **Abscess of spleen**

D73.4 **Cyst of spleen**

D73.5 **Infarction of spleen**
Splenic rupture, nontraumatic
Torsion of spleen
Excludes1: rupture of spleen due to Plasmodium vivax malaria (B51.0)
traumatic rupture of spleen (S36.03-)

D73.8 **Other diseases of spleen**
> `5th`

    D73.81 **Neutropenic splenomegaly**
Werner-Schultz disease

    D73.89 **Other diseases of spleen**
Fibrosis of spleen NOS
Perisplenitis
Splenitis NOS

D74 **METHEMOGLOBINEMIA**
> `4th`

D74.0 **Congenital methemoglobinemia**
Congenital NADH-methemoglobin reductase deficiency
Hemoglobin-M [Hb-M] disease
Methemoglobinemia, hereditary

D74.8 **Other methemoglobinemias**
Acquired methemoglobinemia (with sulfhemoglobinemia)
Toxic methemoglobinemia

D74.9 **Methemoglobinemia, unspecified**

D75 **OTHER AND UNSPECIFIED DISEASES OF BLOOD AND**
> `4th` **BLOOD-FORMING ORGANS**

Excludes2: acute lymphadenitis (L04.-)
chronic lymphadenitis (I88.1)
enlarged lymph nodes (R59.-)
hypergammaglobulinemia NOS (D89.2)
lymphadenitis NOS (I88.9)
mesenteric lymphadenitis (acute) (chronic) (I88.0)

D75.0 **Familial erythrocytosis**
Benign polycythemia
Familial polycythemia
Excludes1: hereditary ovalocytosis (D58.1)

D75.1 **Secondary polycythemia**
Acquired polycythemia
Emotional polycythemia
Erythrocytosis NOS
Hypoxemic polycythemia
Nephrogenous polycythemia
Polycythemia due to erythropoietin
Polycythemia due to fall in plasma volume
Polycythemia due to high altitude
Polycythemia due to stress
Polycythemia NOS
Relative polycythemia
Excludes1: polycythemia neonatorum (P61.1)
polycythemia vera (D45)

D75.8 **Other specified diseases of blood and blood-forming organs**
> `5th` **D75.81** **Myelofibrosis**
Myelofibrosis NOS
Secondary myelofibrosis NOS
Code first the underlying disorder
Use additional code, if applicable, for associated therapy-related myelodysplastic syndrome (D46.-)
Use additional code for adverse effect, if applicable, to identify drug (T45.1X5)
Excludes1: acute myelofibrosis (C94.4-)
idiopathic myelofibrosis (D47.1)
leukoerythroblastic anemia (D61.82)
myelofibrosis with myeloid metaplasia (D47.4)
myelophthisic anemia (D61.82)
myelophthisis (D61.82)
primary myelofibrosis (D47.1)

    D75.82 **Heparin-induced thrombocytopenia (HIT)**

    D75.89 **Other specified diseases of blood and blood-forming organs**

D75.9 **Disease of blood and blood-forming organs, unspecified**

D75.A **Glucose-6-phosphate dehydrogenase (G6PD) deficiency without anemia**
Excludes1: G6PD deficiency with anemia (D55.0)

D76 **OTHER SPECIFIED DISEASES WITH PARTICIPATION OF**
> `4th` **LYMPHORETICULAR AND RETICULOHISTIOCYTIC TISSUE**

Excludes1: (Abt-) Letterer-Siwe disease (C96.0)
eosinophilic granuloma (C96.6)
Hand-Schüller-Christian disease (C96.5)
histiocytic medullary reticulosis (C96.9)
histiocytic sarcoma (C96.A)
histiocytosis X, multifocal (C96.5)
histiocytosis X, unifocal (C96.6)
Langerhans-cell histiocytosis, multifocal (C96.5)

`4th` `5th` `6th` `7th` Additional Character Required   ✓ 3-character code   •=New Code   *Excludes1*—Not coded here, do not use together
▲=Revised Code   *Excludes2*—Not included here

Langerhans-cell histiocytosis NOS (C96.6)
Langerhans-cell histiocytosis, unifocal (C96.6)
leukemic reticuloendotheliosis (C91.4-)
lipomelanotic reticulosis (I89.8)
malignant histiocytosis (C96.A)
malignant reticulosis (C86.0)
nonlipid reticuloendotheliosis (C96.0)

D76.1 Hemophagocytic lymphohistiocytosis
Familial hemophagocytic reticulosis
Histiocytoses of mononuclear phagocytes

D76.2 Hemophagocytic syndrome, infection-associated
Use additional code to identify infectious agent or disease.

D76.3 Other histiocytosis syndromes
Reticulohistiocytoma (giant-cell)
Sinus histiocytosis with massive lymphadenopathy
Xanthogranuloma

D77 OTHER DISORDERS OF BLOOD AND BLOOD-FORMING ✔
ORGANS IN DISEASES CLASSIFIED ELSEWHERE
Code first underlying disease, such as:
amyloidosis (E85.-)
congenital early syphilis (A50.0)
echinococcosis (B67.0–B67.9)
malaria (B50.0–B54)
schistosomiasis [bilharziasis] (B65.0–B65.9)
vitamin C deficiency (E54)
Excludes1: rupture of spleen due to Plasmodium vivax malaria (B51.0)
splenitis, splenomegaly in late syphilis (A52.79)
splenitis, splenomegaly in tuberculosis (A18.85)

(D78) INTRAOPERATIVE AND POSTPROCEDURAL COMPLICATIONS OF THE SPLEEN

(D80–D89) CERTAIN DISORDERS INVOLVING THE IMMUNE MECHANISM

Includes: defects in the complement system
immunodeficiency disorders, except HIV disease
sarcoidosis
Excludes1: autoimmune disease (systemic) NOS (M35.9)
functional disorders of polymorphonuclear neutrophils (D71)
HIV disease (B20)

D80 IMMUNODEFICIENCY WITH PREDOMINANTLY ANTIBODY 4th **DEFECTS**

D80.0 Hereditary hypogammaglobulinemia
Autosomal recessive agammaglobulinemia (Swiss type)
X-linked agammaglobulinemia [Bruton] (with growth hormone deficiency)

D80.1 Nonfamilial hypogammaglobulinemia
Agammaglobulinemia with immunoglobulin-bearing B-lymphocytes
Common variable agammaglobulinemia [CVAgamma]
Hypogammaglobulinemia NOS

D80.2 Selective deficiency of immunoglobulin A [IgA]
D80.3 Selective deficiency of immunoglobulin G [IgG] subclasses
D80.4 Selective deficiency of immunoglobulin M [IgM]
D80.5 Immunodeficiency with increased immunoglobulin M [IgM]
D80.6 Antibody deficiency with near-normal immunoglobulins or with hypogammaglobulinemia
D80.7 Transient hypogammaglobulinemia of infancy
D80.8 Other immunodeficiencies with predominantly antibody defects
Kappa light chain deficiency
D80.9 Immunodeficiency with predominantly antibody defects, unspecified

D81 COMBINED IMMUNODEFICIENCIES
4th **Excludes1:** autosomal recessive agammaglobulinemia (Swiss type) (D80.0)
D81.0 SCID with reticular dysgenesis
D81.1 SCID with low T- and B-cell numbers
D81.2 SCID with low or normal B-cell numbers
D81.3 Adenosine deaminase [ADA] deficiency
5th

D81.30 Adenosine deaminase deficiency, unspecified
ADA deficiency NOS

D81.31 SCID due to adenosine deaminase deficiency
ADA deficiency with SCID
Adenosine deaminase [ADA] deficiency with SCID

D81.32 Adenosine deaminase 2 deficiency
ADA2 deficiency
Adenosine deaminase deficiency type 2
Code also, if applicable, any associated manifestations, such as:
polyarteritis nodosa (M30.0)
stroke (I63.-)

D81.39 Other adenosine deaminase deficiency
Adenosine deaminase [ADA] deficiency type 1, NOS
Adenosine deaminase [ADA] deficiency type 1, without SCID
Partial adenosine deaminase deficiency (type 1)

D81.4 Nezelof's syndrome
D81.5 Purine nucleoside phosphorylase [PNP] deficiency
D81.6 Major histocompatibility complex class I deficiency
Bare lymphocyte syndrome
D81.7 Major histocompatibility complex class II deficiency
D81.8 Other combined immunodeficiencies
5th **D81.81 Biotin-dependent carboxylase deficiency**
6th Multiple carboxylase deficiency
Excludes1: biotin-dependent carboxylase deficiency due to dietary deficiency of biotin (E53.8)

D81.810 Biotinidase deficiency
D81.818 Other biotin-dependent carboxylase deficiency
Holocarboxylase synthetase deficiency
Other multiple carboxylase deficiency
D81.819 Biotin-dependent carboxylase deficiency, unspecified
Multiple carboxylase deficiency, unspecified

D81.89 Other combined immunodeficiencies
D81.9 Combined immunodeficiency, unspecified
SCID NOS

D82 IMMUNODEFICIENCY ASSOCIATED WITH OTHER
4th **MAJOR DEFECTS**
Excludes1: ataxia telangiectasia [Louis-Bar] (G11.3)
D82.0 Wiskott-Aldrich syndrome
Immunodeficiency with thrombocytopenia and eczema
D82.1 Di George's syndrome
Pharyngeal pouch syndrome
Thymic alymphoplasia
Thymic aplasia or hypoplasia with immunodeficiency
D82.2 Immunodeficiency with short-limbed stature
D82.3 Immunodeficiency following hereditary defective response to Epstein-Barr virus
X-linked lymphoproliferative disease
D82.4 Hyperimmunoglobulin E [IgE] syndrome
D82.9 Immunodeficiency associated with major defect, unspecified

D83 COMMON VARIABLE IMMUNODEFICIENCY
4th **D83.0 Common variable immunodeficiency with predominant abnormalities of B-cell numbers and function**
D83.1 Common variable immunodeficiency with predominant immunoregulatory T-cell disorders
Code first underlying condition, such as:
chromosomal abnormalities (Q90–Q99)
diabetes mellitus (E08–E13)
malignant neoplasms (C00–C96)
Excludes1: certain disorders involving the immune mechanism (D80-D83, D84.0, D84.1,D84.9)
human immunodeficiency virus [HIV] disease (B20)
D83.2 Common variable immunodeficiency with autoantibodies to B- or T-cells
D83.8 Other common variable immunodeficiencies
D83.9 Common variable immunodeficiency, unspecified

D84 OTHER IMMUNODEFICIENCIES
4th **D84.0 Lymphocyte function antigen-1 [LFA-1] defect**

4th 5th 6th 7th Additional Character Required   ✔ 3-character code   •=New Code   **Excludes1**—Not coded here, do not use together
▲=Revised Code   **Excludes2**—Not included here

D84.1 Defects in the complement system
C1 esterase inhibitor [C1-INH] deficiency

▲**D84.8 Other specified immunodeficiencies**

5th • **D84.81   Immunodeficiency due to conditions classified elsewhere**
Code first underlying condition, such as:
chromosomal abnormalities (Q90–Q99)
diabetes mellitus (E08–E13)
malignant neoplasms (C00–C96)
Excludes1: certain disorders involving the immune mechanism (D80–D83, D84.0, D84.1,D84.9)
human immunodeficiency virus [HIV] disease (B20)

• **D84.82   Immunodeficiency due to other causes**

6th • **D84.821   Immunodeficiency due to drugs**
Immunodeficiency due to (current or past) medication
Use additional code for adverse effect, if applicable, to identify adverse effect ofdrug (T36–T50 with fifth or six character 5)
Use additional code, if applicable, for associated long term (current) drug therapy drug or medication such as:
long term (current) drug therapy systemic steroids (Z79.52)
other long term (current) drug therapy (Z79.899)

• **D84.822   Immunodeficiency due to external causes**
Code also, if applicable, radiological procedure and radiotherapy (Y84.2)
Use additional code for external cause such as:
exposure to ionizing radiation (W88)

• **D84.89   Other immunodeficiencies**

D84.9 Immunodeficiency, unspecified
Immunocompromised NOS
Immunodeficient NOS
Immunosuppressed NOS

D86   SARCOIDOSIS
4th **D86.0 Sarcoidosis of lung**
D86.1 Sarcoidosis of lymph nodes
D86.2 Sarcoidosis of lung with sarcoidosis of lymph nodes
D86.3 Sarcoidosis of skin
D86.8 Sarcoidosis of other sites
5th **D86.81   Sarcoid meningitis**
D86.82   Multiple cranial nerve palsies in sarcoidosis
D86.83   Sarcoid iridocyclitis
D86.84   Sarcoid pyelonephritis
Tubulo-interstitial nephropathy in sarcoidosis
D86.85   Sarcoid myocarditis
D86.86   Sarcoid arthropathy
Polyarthritis in sarcoidosis
D86.87   Sarcoid myositis
D86.89   Sarcoidosis of other sites
Hepatic granuloma
Uveoparotid fever [Heerfordt]

D86.9 Sarcoidosis, unspecified

D89   OTHER DISORDERS INVOLVING THE IMMUNE
4th **MECHANISM, NEC**
Excludes1: hyperglobulinemia NOS (R77.1)
monoclonal gammopathy (of undetermined significance) (D47.2)
Excludes2: transplant failure and rejection (T86.-)

D89.0 Polyclonal hypergammaglobulinemia
Benign hypergammaglobulinemic purpura
Polyclonal gammopathy NOS

D89.1 Cryoglobulinemia
Cryoglobulinemic purpura
Cryoglobulinemic vasculitis
Essential cryoglobulinemia
Idiopathic cryoglobulinemia
Mixed cryoglobulinemia
Primary cryoglobulinemia
Secondary cryoglobulinemia

D89.2 Hypergammaglobulinemia, unspecified
D89.3 Immune reconstitution syndrome
Immune reconstitution inflammatory syndrome [IRIS]
Use additional code for adverse effect, if applicable, to identify drug (T36-T50 with fifth or sixth character 5)

D89.4 Mast cell activation syndrome and related disorders
5th ***Excludes1:*** aggressive systemic mastocytosis (C96.21)
congenital cutaneous mastocytosis (Q82.2)
indolent systemic mastocytosis (D47.02)
malignant mast cell neoplasm (C96.2-)
mast cell leukemia (C94.3-)
malignant mastocytoma (C96.29)
systemic mastocytosis associated with a clonal hematologic non-mast cell lineage disease (SM-AHNMD) (D47.02)
mast cell sarcoma (C96.22)
mastocytoma NOS (D47.09)
other mast cell neoplasms of uncertain behavior (D47.09)

D89.40   Mast cell activation disorder, unspecified or NOS
D89.41   Monoclonal mast cell activation syndrome
D89.42   Idiopathic mast cell activation syndrome
D89.43   Secondary mast cell activation syndrome
Secondary mast cell activation syndrome
Code also underlying etiology, if known
D89.49   Other mast cell activation disorder

D89.8 Other specified disorders involving the immune mechanism,
5th **NEC**
D89.81   Graft-versus-host disease
6th **Code first** underlying cause, such as:
complications of transplanted organs and tissue (T86.-)
complications of blood transfusion (T80.89)
Use additional code to identify associated manifestations, such as:
desquamative dermatitis (L30.8)
diarrhea (R19.7)
elevated bilirubin (R17)
hair loss (L65.9)
D89.810   Acute graft-versus-host disease
D89.811   Chronic graft-versus-host disease
D89.812   Acute on chronic graft-versus-host disease
D89.813   Graft-versus-host disease, unspecified
D89.82   Autoimmune lymphoproliferative syndrome [ALPS]
• **D89.83   Cytokine release syndrome**
6th **Code first** underlying cause, such as:
complications following infusion, transfusion and therapeutic injection (T80.89-)
complications of transplanted organs and tissue (T86.-)
Use additional code to identify associated manifestations
• **D89.831   Cytokine release syndrome, grade 1**
• **D89.832   Cytokine release syndrome, grade 2**
• **D89.833   Cytokine release syndrome, grade 3**
• **D89.834   Cytokine release syndrome, grade 4**
• **D89.835   Cytokine release syndrome, grade 5**
• **D89.839   Cytokine release syndrome, grade unspecified**
D89.89   Other specified disorders involving the immune mechanism, NEC
Excludes1: HIV disease (B20)

D89.9 Disorder involving the immune mechanism, unspecified
Immune disease NOS

> PANDAS code to D89.89 plus manifestations

4th 5th 6th 7th Additional Character Required   ✓ 3-character code

•=New Code
▲=Revised Code

Excludes1—Not coded here, do not use together
Excludes2—Not included here

CHAPTER 3. DISEASES OF THE BLOOD AND BLOOD-FORMING ORGANS AND CERTAIN DISORDERS INVOLVING THE IMMUNE MECHANISM   (D84.1–D89.9)

Chapter 4. Endocrine, nutritional and metabolic diseases (E00–E89)

GUIDELINES

Diabetes Mellitus (DM)

Refer to categories E08–E13 for guidelines.
Note: All neoplasms, whether functionally active or not, are classified in Chapter 2. Appropriate codes in this chapter (ie, E05.8, E07.0, E16–E31, E34.-) may be used as additional codes to indicate either functional activity by neoplasms and ectopic endocrine tissue or hyperfunction and hypofunction of endocrine glands associated with neoplasms and other conditions classified elsewhere.
Excludes1: transitory endocrine and metabolic disorders specific to newborn (P70–P74)

(E00–E07) DISORDERS OF THYROID GLAND

E00   **CONGENITAL IODINE-DEFICIENCY SYNDROME**
`4th`   **Use additional code** (F70–F79) to identify associated intellectual disabilities.
    Excludes1: subclinical iodine-deficiency hypothyroidism (E02)
  E00.0 **Congenital iodine-deficiency syndrome, neurological type**
      Endemic cretinism, neurological type
  E00.1 **Congenital iodine-deficiency syndrome, myxedematous type**
      Endemic hypothyroid cretinism
      Endemic cretinism, myxedematous type
  E00.2 **Congenital iodine-deficiency syndrome, mixed type**
      Endemic cretinism, mixed type
  E00.9 **Congenital iodine-deficiency syndrome, unspecified**
      Congenital iodine-deficiency hypothyroidism NOS
      Endemic cretinism NOS

E01   **IODINE-DEFICIENCY RELATED THYROID DISORDERS**
`4th`   **AND ALLIED CONDITIONS**
    Excludes1: congenital iodine-deficiency syndrome (E00.-)
      subclinical iodine-deficiency hypothyroidism (E02)
  E01.0 **Iodine-deficiency related diffuse (endemic) goiter**
  E01.1 **Iodine-deficiency related multinodular (endemic) goiter**
      Iodine-deficiency related nodular goiter
  E01.2 **Iodine-deficiency related (endemic) goiter, unspecified**
      Endemic goiter NOS
  E01.8 **Other iodine-deficiency related thyroid disorders and allied conditions**
      Acquired iodine-deficiency hypothyroidism NOS

E02   **SUBCLINICAL IODINE-DEFICIENCY HYPOTHYROIDISM**
`✔`

E03   **OTHER HYPOTHYROIDISM**
`4th`   ***Excludes1:*** iodine-deficiency related hypothyroidism (E00–E02)
      postprocedural hypothyroidism (E89.0)
  E03.0 **Congenital hypothyroidism with diffuse goiter**
      Congenital parenchymatous goiter (nontoxic)
      Congenital goiter (nontoxic) NOS
      Excludes1: transitory congenital goiter with normal function (P72.0)
  E03.1 **Congenital hypothyroidism without goiter**
      Aplasia of thyroid (with myxedema)
      Congenital atrophy of thyroid
      Congenital hypothyroidism NOS
  E03.2 **Hypothyroidism due to medicines/drugs and other exogenous substances**
      Code first poisoning due to drug or toxin, if applicable (T36–T65 with fifth or sixth character 1–4 or 6)
      Use additional code for adverse effect, if applicable, to identify drug (T36–T50 with fifth or sixth character 5)
  E03.3 **Postinfectious hypothyroidism**
  E03.4 **Atrophy of thyroid (acquired)**
      Excludes1: congenital atrophy of thyroid (E03.1)
  E03.8 **Other specified hypothyroidism**
  E03.9 **Hypothyroidism, unspecified**
      Myxedema NOS

E04   **OTHER NONTOXIC GOITER**
`4th`   ***Excludes1:*** congenital goiter (NOS) (diffuse) (parenchymatous) (E03.0)
      iodine-deficiency related goiter (E00–E02)
  E04.0 **Nontoxic diffuse goiter**
      Diffuse (colloid) nontoxic goiter
      Simple nontoxic goiter
  E04.1 **Nontoxic single thyroid nodule**
      Colloid nodule (cystic) (thyroid)
      Nontoxic uninodular goiter
      Thyroid (cystic) nodule NOS
  E04.2 **Nontoxic multinodular goiter**
      Cystic goiter NOS
      Multinodular (cystic) goiter NOS
  E04.8 **Other specified nontoxic goiter**
  E04.9 **Nontoxic goiter, unspecified**
      Goiter NOS
      Nodular goiter (nontoxic) NOS

E05   **THYROTOXICOSIS [HYPERTHYROIDISM]**
`4th`   ***Excludes1:*** chronic thyroiditis with transient thyrotoxicosis (E06.2)
      neonatal thyrotoxicosis (P72.1)
  E05.0 **Thyrotoxicosis with diffuse goiter**
  `5th`   Exophthalmic or toxic goiter NOS
      Graves' disease
      Toxic diffuse goiter
     E05.00 **Thyrotoxicosis with diffuse goiter without thyrotoxic crisis or storm**
     E05.01 **Thyrotoxicosis with diffuse goiter with thyrotoxic crisis or storm**
  E05.9 **Thyrotoxicosis, unspecified**
  `5th`   Hyperthyroidism NOS
     E05.90 **Thyrotoxicosis, unspecified without thyrotoxic crisis or storm**
     E05.91 **Thyrotoxicosis, unspecified with thyrotoxic crisis or storm**

E06   **THYROIDITIS**
`4th`   ***Excludes1:*** postpartum thyroiditis (O90.5)
  E06.0 **Acute thyroiditis**
      Abscess of thyroid
      Pyogenic thyroiditis
      Suppurative thyroiditis
      Use additional code (B95–B97) to identify infectious agent.
  E06.1 **Subacute thyroiditis**
      de Quervain thyroiditis
      Giant-cell thyroiditis
      Granulomatous thyroiditis
      Nonsuppurative thyroiditis
      Viral thyroiditis
      Excludes1: autoimmune thyroiditis (E06.3)
  E06.2 **Chronic thyroiditis with transient thyrotoxicosis**
      Excludes1: autoimmune thyroiditis (E06.3)
  E06.3 **Autoimmune thyroiditis**
      Hashimoto's thyroiditis
      Hashitoxicosis (transient)
      Lymphadenoid goiter
      Lymphocytic thyroiditis
      Struma lymphomatosa
  E06.4 **Drug-induced thyroiditis**
      Use additional code for adverse effect, if applicable, to identify drug (T36-T50 with fifth or sixth character 5)
  E06.5 **Other chronic thyroiditis**
      Chronic fibrous thyroiditis
      Chronic thyroiditis NOS
      Ligneous thyroiditis
      Riedel thyroiditis
  E06.9 **Thyroiditis, unspecified**

E07   **OTHER DISORDERS OF THYROID**
`4th`   **E07.8** **Other specified disorders of thyroid**
  `5th`

`4th` `5th` `6th` `7th` Additional Character Required   `✔` 3-character code

•=New Code
▲=Revised Code

Excludes1—Not coded here, do not use together
Excludes2—Not included here

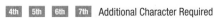

E07.89   Other specified disorders of thyroid
Abnormality of thyroid-binding globulin
Hemorrhage of thyroid
Infarction of thyroid
E07.9   Disorder of thyroid, unspecified

(E08–E13) DIABETES MELLITUS

GUIDELINES

The DM codes are combination codes that include the type of DM, the body system affected, and the complications affecting that body system. As many codes within a particular category as are necessary to describe all of the complications of the disease may be used. They should be sequenced based on the reason for a particular encounter. Assign as many codes from categories E08–E13 as needed to identify all of the associated conditions that the patient has.

Type of diabetes

The age of a patient is not the sole determining factor, though most type 1 diabetics develop the condition before reaching puberty. For this reason type 1 DM is also referred to as juvenile diabetes.

Type of DM not documented

If the type of DM is not documented in the medical record the default is E11.-, Type 2 DM.

DM and the use of insulin and oral hypoglycemics

If the documentation in a medical record does not indicate the type of diabetes but does indicate that the patient uses insulin, code E11-, Type 2 DM, should be assigned. An additional code should be assigned from category Z79 to identify the long-term (current) use of insulin or oral hypoglycemic drugs. If the patient is treated with both oral medications and insulin, only the code for long-term (current) use of insulin should be assigned. **If the patient is treated with both insulin and an injectable non-insulin antidiabetic drug, assign codes Z79.4, Long-term (current) use of insulin, and Z79.899, Other long term (current) drug therapy. If the patient is treated with both oral hypoglycemic drugs and an injectable non-insulin antidiabetic drug, assign codes Z79.84, Long-term (current) use of oral hypoglycemic drugs, and Z79.899, Other long-term (current) drug therapy.** Code Z79.4 should not be assigned if insulin is given temporarily to bring a type 2 patient's blood sugar under control during an encounter.

Complications due to insulin pump malfunction

UNDERDOSE OF INSULIN DUE TO INSULIN PUMP FAILURE
An underdose of insulin due to an insulin pump failure should be assigned to a code from subcategory T85.6, Mechanical complication of other specified internal and external prosthetic devices, implants and grafts, that specifies the type of pump malfunction, as the principal or first-listed code, followed by code T38.3x6-, Underdosing of insulin and oral hypoglycemic [antidiabetic] drugs. Additional codes for the type of DM and any associated complications due to the underdosing should also be assigned.

OVERDOSE OF INSULIN DUE TO INSULIN PUMP FAILURE
The principal or first-listed code for an encounter due to an insulin pump malfunction resulting in an overdose of insulin, should also be T85.6-, Mechanical complication of other specified internal and external prosthetic devices, implants and grafts, followed by code T38.3x1-, Poisoning by insulin and oral hypoglycemic [antidiabetic] drugs, accidental (unintentional).

Secondary DM

Codes under categories E08, DM due to underlying condition, E09, Drug or chemical induced DM, and E13, Other specified DM, identify complications/manifestations associated with secondary DM. Secondary diabetes is always caused by another condition or event (e.g., cystic fibrosis, malignant neoplasm of pancreas, pancreatectomy, adverse effect of drug, or poisoning).

SECONDARY DM AND THE USE OF INSULIN OR ORAL HYPOGLYCEMICS
For patients with secondary diabetes mellitus who routinely use insulin or oral hypoglycemic drugs, an additional code from category Z79 should be assigned to identify the long-term (current) use of insulin or oral hypoglycemic drugs. If

the patient is treated with both oral medications and insulin, only the code for long-term (current) use of insulin should be assigned. **If the patient is treated with both insulin and an injectable non-insulin antidiabetic drug, assign codes Z79.4, Long-term (current) use of insulin, and Z79.899, Other long term (current) drug therapy. If the patient is treated with both oral hypoglycemic drugs and an injectable non-insulin antidiabetic drug, assign codes Z79.84, Long-term (current) use of oral hypoglycemic drugs, and Z79.899, Other long-term (current) drug therapy.** Code Z79.4 should not be assigned if insulin is given temporarily to bring a type 2 patient's blood sugar under control during an encounter.

ASSIGNING AND SEQUENCING SECONDARY DIABETES CODES AND ITS CAUSES
The sequencing of the secondary diabetes codes in relationship to codes for the cause of the diabetes is based on the Tabular List instructions for categories E08, E09 and E13.

Secondary DM due to pancreatectomy
For postpancreatectomy DM (lack of insulin due to the surgical removal of all or part of the pancreas), assign code E89.1, Postprocedural hypoinsulinemia. Assign a code from category E13 and a code from subcategory Z90.41-, Acquired absence of pancreas, as additional codes.

Secondary diabetes due to drugs
Secondary diabetes may be caused by an adverse effect of correctly administered medications, poisoning or sequela of poisoning.
Refer to categories T36–T50 for coding of adverse effects and poisoning.
Note for hyperglycemia not caused by DM or for transient hyperglycemia, refer to code R73.9, hyperglycemia, NOS

E08   DM DUE TO UNDERLYING CONDITION
[4th]   **Code first** the underlying condition, such as:
congenital rubella (P35.0)
Cushing's syndrome (E24.-)
cystic fibrosis (E84.-)
malignant neoplasm (C00–C96)
malnutrition (E40–E46)
pancreatitis and other diseases of the pancreas (K85-K86.-)
Use additional code to identify control using:
insulin (Z79.4)
oral antidiabetic drugs (Z79.84)
oral hypoglycemic drugs (Z79.84)
Excludes1: drug or chemical induced DM (E09.-)
gestational diabetes (O24.4-)
neonatal DM (transient) (P70.2)
postpancreatectomy DM (E13.-)
postprocedural DM (E13.-)
secondary DM NEC (E13.-)
type 1 DM (E10.-)
type 2 DM (E11.-)

E08.0   DM due to underlying condition with hyperosmolarity;
[5th]   **E08.00   without NKHHC**
E08.01   with coma
E08.1   DM due to underlying condition with ketoacidosis;
[5th]   **E08.10   without coma**
E08.11   with coma
E08.2   DM due to underlying condition with; kidney complications
[5th]   **E08.21   diabetic nephropathy or intercapillary**
glomerulosclerosis or intracapillary glomerulonephrosis or Kimmelstiel-Wilson disease
E08.22   diabetic CKD
Use additional code to identify stage of CKD (N18.1–N18.6)
E08.29   other diabetic kidney complication
Renal tubular degeneration in DM due to underlying condition
E08.3   DM due to underlying condition with ophthalmic complications
[5th]   **E08.31   DM due to underlying condition with unspecified**
[6th]   **diabetic retinopathy;**
E08.311   with macular edema
[7th]
E08.319   without macular edema
[7th]

E08.32 `6th` **DM due to underlying condition with mild nonproliferative diabetic retinopathy (NOS);**

7th characters for subcategories E08.31, E08.32, E08.33, E08.34, E08.35
1—left eye
2—right eye
3—bilateral

    E08.321 `7th` **with macular edema**

    E08.329 `7th` **without macular edema**

E08.33 `6th` **DM due to underlying condition with moderate nonproliferative diabetic retinopathy;**

    E08.331 `7th` **with macular edema**

    E08.339 `7th` **without macular edema**

E08.34 `6th` **DM due to underlying condition with severe nonproliferative diabetic retinopathy;**

    E08.341 `7th` **with macular edema**

    E08.349 `7th` **without macular edema**

E08.35 `6th` **DM due to underlying condition with proliferative diabetic retinopathy;**

    E08.351 `7th` **with macular edema**

    E08.359 `7th` **without macular edema**

E08.36 **DM due to underlying condition with diabetic cataract**

E08.39 **DM due to underlying condition with other diabetic ophthalmic complication**
    Use additional code to identify manifestation, such as:
      diabetic glaucoma (H40–H42)

E08.4 `5th` **DM due to underlying condition with; neurological complications**

    E08.40 **diabetic neuropathy, unspecified**

    E08.41 **diabetic mononeuropathy**

    E08.42 **diabetic polyneuropathy**
      diabetic neuralgia

    E08.43 **diabetic autonomic (poly)neuropathy**
      diabetic gastroparesis

    E08.44 **diabetic amyotrophy**

    E08.49 **other diabetic neurological complication**

E08.5 `5th` **DM due to underlying condition with; circulatory complications**

    E08.51 **diabetic peripheral angiopathy without gangrene**

    E08.52 **diabetic peripheral angiopathy with gangrene**
      diabetic gangrene

    E08.59 **other circulatory complications**

E08.6 `5th` **DM due to underlying condition with other specified complications**

    E08.61 `6th` **DM due to underlying condition with; diabetic arthropathy**

      E08.610 **diabetic neuropathic arthropathy**
        Charcôt's joints

      E08.618 **other diabetic arthropathy**

    E08.62 `6th` **DM due to underlying condition with; skin complications**

      E08.620 **diabetic dermatitis**
        diabetic necrobiosis lipoidica

      E08.621 **foot ulcer**
        Use additional code to identify site of ulcer (L97.4-, L97.5-)

      E08.622 **other skin ulcer**
        Use additional code to identify site of ulcer (L97.1–L97.9, L98.41–L98.49)

      E08.628 **other skin complications**

    E08.63 `6th` **DM due to underlying condition with; oral complications**

      E08.630 **periodontal disease**

      E08.638 **other oral complications**

    E08.64 `6th` **DM due to underlying condition with hypoglycemia;**

      E08.641 **with coma**

      E08.649 **without coma**

    E08.65 **DM due to underlying condition with hyperglycemia**

E08.69 **DM due to underlying condition with other specified complication**
    Use additional code to identify complication

E08.8 **DM due to underlying condition with unspecified complications**

E08.9 **DM due to underlying condition without complications**

E09 `4th` **DRUG OR CHEMICAL INDUCED DM**
Refer to category E08 for guidelines
Code first poisoning due to drug or toxin, if applicable (T36–T65 with fifth or sixth character 1–4 or 6)
Use additional code for adverse effect, if applicable, to identify drug (T36–T50 with fifth or sixth character 5)
Use additional code to identify control using:
   insulin (Z79.4)
   oral antidiabetic drugs (Z79.84)
   oral hypoglycemic drugs (Z79.84)
Excludes1: DM due to underlying condition (E08.-)
   gestational diabetes (O24.4-)
   neonatal DM (P70.2)
   postpancreatectomy DM (E13.-)
   postprocedural DM (E13.-)
   secondary DM NEC (E13.-)
   type 1 DM (E10.-)
   type 2 DM (E11.-)

E09.0 **Drug or chemical induced DM with hyperosmolarity**

    `5th` **E09.00** **Drug or chemical induced DM with hyperosmolarity without NKHHC**

    E09.01 **Drug or chemical induced DM with hyperosmolarity with coma**

E09.1 **Drug or chemical induced DM with ketoacidosis;**

    `5th` **E09.10** **without coma**

    E09.11 **with coma**

E09.2 **Drug or chemical induced DM with; kidney complications**

    `5th` **E09.21** **diabetic nephropathy**
      Drug or chemical induced DM with intercapillary glomerulosclerosis or intracapillary glomerulonephrosis or Kimmelstiel-Wilson disease

    E09.22 **diabetic CKD**
      Use additional code to identify stage of CKD (N18.1–N18.6)

    E09.29 **other diabetic kidney complication**
      Drug or chemical induced DM with renal tubular degeneration

E09.3 **Drug or chemical induced DM with ophthalmic complications**

    `5th` **E09.31** `6th` **Drug or chemical induced DM with unspecified diabetic retinopathy;**

      E09.311 **with macular edema**

      E09.319 **without macular edema**

    E09.32 `6th` **Drug or chemical induced DM with mild nonproliferative diabetic retinopathy;** Drug or chemical induced DM with nonproliferative diabetic retinopathy NOS

7th characters for subcategory E09.32, E09.33, E09.34, E09.35
1—left eye
2—right eye
3—bilateral

      E09.321 `7th` **with macular edema**

      E09.329 `7th` **without macular edema**

    E09.33 `6th` **Drug or chemical induced DM with moderate nonproliferative diabetic retinopathy;**

      E09.331 `7th` **with macular edema**

      E09.339 `7th` **without macular edema**

    E09.34 `6th` **Drug or chemical induced DM with severe nonproliferative diabetic retinopathy;**

      E09.341 `7th` **with macular edema**

      E09.349 `7th` **without macular edema**

`4th` `5th` `6th` `7th` Additional Character Required   ✔ 3-character code

•=New Code   *Excludes1*—Not coded here, do not use together
▲=Revised Code   *Excludes2*—Not included here

E09.35 [6th] **Drug or chemical induced DM with proliferative diabetic retinopathy;**
    E09.351 [7th] **with macular edema**
    E09.353 [7th] **with traction retinal detachment not involving the macula**
    E09.354 [7th] **with combined traction retinal detachment and rhegmatogenous retinal detachment**
    E09.355 [7th] **stable**
    E09.359 [7th] **without macular edema**

E09.36 **Drug or chemical induced DM with diabetic cataract**
E09.39 **Drug or chemical induced DM with other diabetic ophthalmic complication**
    Use additional code to identify manifestation, such as: diabetic glaucoma (H40–H42)

E09.4 [5th] **Drug or chemical induced DM with neurological complications;**
  E09.40 **with diabetic neuropathy, unspecified**
  E09.41 **with diabetic mononeuropathy**
  E09.42 **with diabetic polyneuropathy**
    with diabetic neuralgia
  E09.43 **with diabetic autonomic (poly)neuropathy**
    with diabetic gastroparesis
  E09.44 **diabetic amyotrophy**
  E09.49 **with other diabetic neurological complication**

E09.5 [5th] **Drug or chemical induced DM with; circulatory complications**
  E09.51 **diabetic peripheral angiopathy without gangrene**
  E09.52 **diabetic peripheral angiopathy with gangrene**
    diabetic gangrene
  E09.59 **other circulatory complications**

E09.6 [5th] **Drug or chemical induced DM with other specified complications**
  E09.61 [6th] **Drug or chemical induced DM with; diabetic arthropathy**
    E09.610 **diabetic neuropathic arthropathy**
      Charcôt's joints
    E09.618 **other diabetic arthropathy**
  E09.62 [6th] **Drug or chemical induced DM with; skin complications**
    E09.620 **diabetic dermatitis**
      diabetic necrobiosis lipoidica
    E09.621 **foot ulcer**
      Use additional code to identify site of ulcer (L97.4-, L97.5-)
    E09.622 **other skin ulcer**
      Use additional code to identify site of ulcer (L97.1–L97.9, L98.41–L98.49)
    E09.628 **other skin complications**
  E09.63 [6th] **Drug or chemical induced DM with; oral complications**
    E09.630 **periodontal disease**
    E09.638 **other oral complications**
  E09.64 [6th] **Drug or chemical induced DM with hypoglycemia;**
    E09.641 **with coma**
    E09.649 **without coma**
  E09.65 **Drug or chemical induced DM with hyperglycemia**
  E09.69 **Drug or chemical induced DM with other specified complication**
    Use additional code to identify complication

E09.8 **Drug or chemical induced DM with unspecified complications**
E09.9 **Drug or chemical induced DM without complications**

E10 [4th] **TYPE 1 DM**
Refer to category E08 for guidelines
Includes: brittle diabetes (mellitus)
  diabetes (mellitus) due to autoimmune process
  diabetes (mellitus) due to immune mediated pancreatic islet beta-cell destruction
  idiopathic diabetes (mellitus)
  juvenile onset diabetes (mellitus)
  ketosis-prone diabetes (mellitus)
Excludes1: DM due to underlying condition (E08.-)
  drug or chemical induced DM (E09.-)
  gestational diabetes (O24.4-)

hyperglycemia NOS (R73.9)
neonatal DM (P70.2)
postpancreatectomy DM (E13.-)
postprocedural DM (E13.-)
secondary DM NEC (E13.-)
type 2 DM (E11.-)

E10.1 **Type 1 DM with ketoacidosis;**
  [5th] **E10.10** **Type 1 DM with ketoacidosis without coma**
  E10.11 **Type 1 DM with ketoacidosis with coma**

E10.2 **Type 1 DM with kidney complications**
  [5th] **E10.21** **Type 1 DM with diabetic nephropathy**
    Type 1 DM with intercapillary glomerulosclerosis or intracapillary glomerulonephrosis or Kimmelstiel-Wilson disease
  E10.22 **Type 1 DM with diabetic CKD**
    Use additional code to identify stage of CKD (N18.1–N18.6)
  E10.29 **Type 1 DM with other diabetic kidney complication**
    Type 1 DM with renal tubular degeneration

E10.3 **Type 1 DM with ophthalmic complications**
  [5th] **E10.31** [6th] **Type 1 DM with unspecified diabetic retinopathy;**
    E10.311 **with macular edema**
    E10.319 **without macular edema**
  E10.32 [6th] **Type 1 DM with mild nonproliferative diabetic retinopathy;**
    diabetic retinopathy NOS
    E10.321 [7th] **with macular edema**
    E10.329 [7th] **without macular edema**

> 7th characters for subcategory E10.32, E10.33, E10.34, E10.35
> 1—left eye
> 2—right eye
> 3—bilateral

  E10.33 [6th] **Type 1 DM with moderate nonproliferative diabetic retinopathy;**
    E10.331 [7th] **with macular edema**
    E10.339 [7th] **without macular edema**
  E10.34 [6th] **Type 1 DM with severe nonproliferative diabetic retinopathy;**
    E10.341 [7th] **with macular edema**
    E10.349 [7th] **without macular edema**
  E10.35 [6th] **Type 1 DM with proliferative diabetic retinopathy;**
    E10.351 [7th] **with macular edema**
    E10.359 [7th] **without macular edema**
  E10.36 **Type 1 DM with diabetic cataract**
  E10.39 **Type 1 DM with other diabetic ophthalmic complication**
    Use additional code to identify manifestation, such as: diabetic glaucoma (H40–H42)

E10.4 **Type 1 DM with neurological complications**
  [5th] **E10.40** **Type 1 DM with diabetic neuropathy, unspecified**
  E10.41 **Type 1 DM with diabetic mononeuropathy**
  E10.42 **Type 1 DM with diabetic polyneuropathy**
    Type 1 DM with diabetic neuralgia
  E10.43 **Type 1 DM with diabetic autonomic (poly)neuropathy**
  E10.44 **Type 1 DM with diabetic amyotrophy**
  E10.49 **Type 1 DM with other diabetic neurological complication**

E10.5 **Type 1 DM with circulatory complications**
  [5th] **E10.51** **Type 1 DM with diabetic peripheral angiopathy without gangrene**
  E10.52 **Type 1 DM with diabetic peripheral angiopathy with gangrene**
    Type 1 DM with diabetic gangrene
  E10.59 **Type 1 DM with other circulatory complications**

E10.6 **Type 1 DM with other specified complications**
  [5th] **E10.61** [6th] **Type 1 DM with diabetic arthropathy**

[4th] [5th] [6th] [7th] Additional Character Required   ✔ 3-character code

•=New Code   ***Excludes1***—Not coded here, do not use together
▲=Revised Code   ***Excludes2***—Not included here

E10.610 Type 1 DM with diabetic neuropathic arthropathy
Type 1 DM with Charcôt's joints
E10.618 Type 1 DM with other diabetic arthropathy
E10.62 Type 1 DM with skin complications
`6th` **E10.620** Type 1 DM with diabetic dermatitis
Type 1 DM with diabetic necrobiosis lipoidica
 E10.621 Type 1 DM with foot ulcer
Use additional code to identify site of ulcer (L97.4-, L97.5-)
 E10.622 Type 1 DM with other skin ulcer
Use additional code to identify site of ulcer (L97.1–L97.9, L98.41–L98.49)
 E10.628 Type 1 DM with other skin complications
E10.63 Type 1 DM with oral complications
`6th` **E10.630** Type 1 DM with periodontal disease
 E10.638 Type 1 DM with other oral complications
E10.64 Type 1 DM with hypoglycemia
`6th` **E10.641** Type 1 DM with hypoglycemia with coma
 E10.649 Type 1 DM with hypoglycemia without coma
E10.65 Type 1 DM with hyperglycemia
E10.69 Type 1 DM with other specified complication
Use additional code to identify complication
E10.8 Type 1 DM with unspecified complications
E10.9 Type 1 DM without complications

E11 **TYPE 2 DM**
`4th`
Refer to category E08 for guidelines
If the type of DM is not documented in the medical record the default is E11.-, Type 2 DM.
Includes: diabetes (mellitus) due to insulin secretory defect
 diabetes NOS
 insulin resistant diabetes (mellitus)
Use additional code to identify control using:
 insulin (Z79.4)
 oral antidiabetic drugs (Z79.84)
 oral hypoglycemic drugs (Z79.84)
Excludes1: DM due to underlying condition (E08.-)
 drug or chemical induced DM (E09.-)
 gestational diabetes (O24.4-)
 neonatal DM (P70.2)
 postpancreatectomy DM (E13.-)
 postprocedural DM (E13.-)
 secondary DM NEC (E13.-)
 type 1 DM (E10.-)
E11.0 Type 2 DM with hyperosmolarity;
`5th` **E11.00** without NKHHC
 E11.01 with coma
E11.1 Type 2 diabetes mellitus with ketoacidosis
`5th` **E11.10** Type 2 diabetes mellitus with ketoacidosis without coma
 E11.11 Type 2 diabetes mellitus with ketoacidosis with coma
E11.2 Type 2 DM with kidney complications
`5th` **E11.21** Type 2 DM with diabetic nephropathy or intercapillary glomerulosclerosis or intracapillary glomerulonephrosis or Kimmelstiel-Wilson disease
 E11.22 Type 2 DM with diabetic CKD
Use additional code to identify stage of CKD (N18.1–N18.6)
 E11.29 Type 2 DM with other diabetic kidney complication
Type 2 DM with renal tubular degeneration
E11.3 Type 2 DM with ophthalmic complications
`5th` **E11.31** Type 2 DM with unspecified diabetic retinopathy;
`6th`   **E11.311** with macular edema
  E11.319 without macular edema
 E11.32 Type 2 DM with mild nonproliferative diabetic retinopathy;
`6th`
Type 2 DM with nonproliferative diabetic retinopathy NOS

7th character for subcategories E11.32, E11.33, E11.34, E11.35
1—right eye
2—left eye
3—bilateral

  E11.321 with macular edema
`7th`
  E11.329 without macular edema
`7th`
 E11.33 Type 2 DM with moderate nonproliferative diabetic retinopathy;
`6th`   **E11.331** with macular edema
`7th`
  E11.339 without macular edema
`7th`
 E11.34 Type 2 DM with severe nonproliferative diabetic retinopathy;
`6th`   **E11.341** with macular edema
`7th`
  E11.349 without macular edema
`7th`
 E11.35 Type 2 DM with proliferative diabetic retinopathy;
`6th`   **E11.351** with macular edema
`7th`
  E11.359 without macular edema
`7th`
 E11.36 Type 2 DM with diabetic cataract
 E11.39 Type 2 DM with other diabetic ophthalmic complication
Use additional code to identify manifestation, such as: diabetic glaucoma (H40–H42)
E11.4 Type 2 DM with neurological complications
`5th` **E11.40** Type 2 DM with diabetic neuropathy, unspecified
 E11.41 Type 2 DM with diabetic mononeuropathy
 E11.42 Type 2 DM with diabetic polyneuropathy
Type 2 DM with diabetic neuralgia
 E11.43 Type 2 DM with diabetic autonomic (poly)neuropathy
Type 2 DM with diabetic gastroparesis
 E11.44 Type 2 DM with diabetic amyotrophy
 E11.49 Type 2 DM with other diabetic neurological complication
E11.5 Type 2 DM with circulatory complications
`5th` **E11.51** Type 2 DM with diabetic peripheral angiopathy without gangrene
 E11.52 Type 2 DM with diabetic peripheral angiopathy with gangrene
Type 2 DM with diabetic gangrene
 E11.59 Type 2 DM with other circulatory complications
E11.6 Type 2 DM with other specified complications
`5th` **E11.61** Type 2 DM with diabetic arthropathy
`6th`   **E11.610** Type 2 DM with diabetic neuropathic arthropathy
Type 2 DM with Charcôt's joints
  E11.618 Type 2 DM with other diabetic arthropathy
 E11.62 Type 2 DM with skin complications
`6th`   **E11.620** Type 2 DM with diabetic dermatitis
Type 2 DM with diabetic necrobiosis lipoidica
  E11.621 Type 2 DM with foot ulcer
Use additional code to identify site of ulcer (L97.4-, L97.5-)
  E11.622 Type 2 DM with other skin ulcer
Use additional code to identify site of ulcer (L97.1–L97.9, L98.41–L98.49)
  E11.628 Type 2 DM with other skin complications
 E11.63 Type 2 DM with oral complications
`6th`   **E11.630** Type 2 DM with periodontal disease
  E11.638 Type 2 DM with other oral complications
 E11.64 Type 2 DM with hypoglycemia
`6th`   **E11.641** Type 2 DM with hypoglycemia with coma
  E11.649 Type 2 DM with hypoglycemia without coma
 E11.65 Type 2 DM with hyperglycemia
 E11.69 Type 2 DM with other specified complication
Use additional code to identify complication
E11.8 Type 2 DM with unspecified complications
E11.9 Type 2 DM without complications

`4th` `5th` `6th` `7th` Additional Character Required	✓ 3-character code	•=New Code ▲=Revised Code	***Excludes1***—Not coded here, do not use together ***Excludes2***—Not included here

(E15–E16) OTHER DISORDERS OF GLUCOSE REGULATION AND PANCREATIC INTERNAL SECRETION

E15 ✔ **NONDIABETIC HYPOGLYCEMIC COMA**
Includes: drug-induced insulin coma in nondiabetic
hyperinsulinism with hypoglycemic coma
hypoglycemic coma NOS

E16 **4th** **OTHER DISORDERS OF PANCREATIC INTERNAL SECRETION**

E16.0 **Drug-induced hypoglycemia without coma**
Use additional code for adverse effect, if applicable, to identify drug (T36–T50 with fifth or sixth character 5)
Excludes 1: diabetes with hypoglycemia without coma (E09.649)

E16.1 **Other hypoglycemia**
Functional hyperinsulinism
Functional nonhyperinsulinemic hypoglycemia
Hyperinsulinism NOS
Hyperplasia of pancreatic islet beta cells NOS
Excludes1: diabetes with hypoglycemia (E08.649, E10.649, E11.649)
hypoglycemia in infant of diabetic mother (P70.1)
neonatal hypoglycemia (P70.4)

E16.2 **Hypoglycemia, unspecified**
Excludes 1: diabetes with hypoglycemia (E08.649, E10.649, E11.649)

E16.8 **Other specified disorders of pancreatic internal secretion**
Increased secretion from endocrine pancreas of growth hormone-releasing hormone or pancreatic polypeptide or somatostatin or vasoactive-intestinal polypeptide

E16.9 **Disorder of pancreatic internal secretion, unspecified**
Islet-cell hyperplasia NOS
Pancreatic endocrine cell hyperplasia NOS

(E20–E35) DISORDERS OF OTHER ENDOCRINE GLANDS

Excludes1: galactorrhea (N64.3)
gynecomastia (N62)

E20 **4th** **HYPOPARATHYROIDISM**
Excludes1: Di George's syndrome (D82.1)
postprocedural hypoparathyroidism (E89.2)
tetany NOS (R29.0)
transitory neonatal hypoparathyroidism (P71.4)

E20.0 **Idiopathic hypoparathyroidism**
E20.1 **Pseudohypoparathyroidism**
E20.8 **Other hypoparathyroidism**
E20.9 **Hypoparathyroidism, unspecified**
Parathyroid tetany

E22 **4th** **HYPERFUNCTION OF PITUITARY GLAND**
Excludes1: Cushing's syndrome (E24.-)
Nelson's syndrome (E24.1)
overproduction of ACTH not associated with Cushing's disease (E27.0)
overproduction of pituitary ACTH (E24.0)
overproduction of thyroid-stimulating hormone (E05.8-)

E22.0 **Acromegaly and pituitary gigantism**
Overproduction of growth hormone
Excludes1: constitutional gigantism (E34.4)
constitutional tall stature (E34.4)
increased secretion from endocrine pancreas of growth hormone-releasing hormone (E16.8)

E22.2 **Syndrome of inappropriate secretion of antidiuretic hormone**
E22.8 **Other hyperfunction of pituitary gland**
Central precocious puberty
E22.9 **Hyperfunction of pituitary gland, unspecified**

E23 **4th** **HYPOFUNCTION AND OTHER DISORDERS OF THE PITUITARY GLAND**
Includes: the listed conditions whether the disorder is in the pituitary or the hypothalamus
Excludes1: postprocedural hypopituitarism (E89.3)
E23.0 **Hypopituitarism**

E23.1 **Drug-induced hypopituitarism**
Use additional code for adverse effect, if applicable, to identify drug (T36-T50 with fifth or sixth character 5)
E23.2 **Diabetes insipidus**
Excludes1: nephrogenic diabetes insipidus (N25.1)
E23.3 **Hypothalamic dysfunction, not elsewhere classified**
Excludes1: Prader-Willi syndrome (Q87.11)
Russell-Silver syndrome (Q87.1)
E23.6 **Other disorders of pituitary gland**
Abscess of pituitary
Adiposogenital dystrophy
E24.8 **Other Cushing's syndrome**
E23.7 **Disorder of pituitary gland, unspecified**

E24 **4th** **CUSHING'S SYNDROME**
Excludes1: congenital adrenal hyperplasia (E25.0)
E24.0 **Pituitary-dependent Cushing's disease**
Overproduction of pituitary ACTH
Pituitary-dependent hypercorticalism
E24.2 **Drug-induced Cushing's syndrome**
Use additional code for adverse effect, if applicable, to identify drug (T36-T50 with fifth or sixth character 5)
E24.8 **Other Cushing's syndrome**
E24.9 **Cushing's syndrome, unspecified**

E25 **4th** **ADRENOGENITAL DISORDERS**
Includes: adrenogenital syndromes, virilizing or feminizing, whether acquired or due to adrenal hyperplasia consequent on inborn enzyme defects in hormone synthesis
Female adrenal pseudohermaphroditism
Female heterosexual precocious pseudopuberty
Male isosexual precocious pseudopuberty
Male macrogenitosomia praecox
Male sexual precocity with adrenal hyperplasia
Male virilization (female)
Excludes1: indeterminate sex and pseudohermaphroditism (Q56)
chromosomal abnormalities (Q90–Q99)
E25.0 **Congenital adrenogenital disorders associated with enzyme deficiency**
Congenital adrenal hyperplasia
21-Hydroxylase deficiency
Salt-losing congenital adrenal hyperplasia
E25.8 **Other adrenogenital disorders**
Idiopathic adrenogenital disorder
Use additional code for adverse effect, if applicable, to identify drug (T36-T50 with fifth or sixth character 5)
E25.9 **Adrenogenital disorder, unspecified**
Adrenogenital syndrome NOS

E27 **4th** **OTHER DISORDERS OF ADRENAL GLAND**
Refer to code C74, Malignant neoplasm of adrenal gland, to report neuroblastomas
E27.0 **Other adrenocortical overactivity**
Overproduction of ACTH, not associated with Cushing's disease
Premature adrenarche
Excludes1: Cushing's syndrome (E24.-)
E27.1 **Primary adrenocortical insufficiency**
Addison's disease
Autoimmune adrenalitis
Excludes1: Addison only phenotype adrenoleukodystrophy (E71.528)
amyloidosis (E85.-)
tuberculous Addison's disease (A18.7)
Waterhouse-Friderichsen syndrome (A39.1)
E27.2 **Addisonian crisis**
Adrenal crisis
Adrenocortical crisis
E27.3 **Drug-induced adrenocortical insufficiency**
Use additional code for adverse effect, if applicable, to identify drug (T36-T50 with fifth or sixth character 5)
E27.4 **Other and unspecified adrenocortical insufficiency**
5th **E27.40** **Unspecified adrenocortical insufficiency**
Adrenocortical insufficiency NOS

4th **5th** **6th** **7th** Additional Character Required   ✔ 3-character code   •=New Code   ▲=Revised Code   *Excludes1*—Not coded here, do not use together   *Excludes2*—Not included here

E27.49 **Other adrenocortical insufficiency**
Adrenal hemorrhage
Adrenal infarction

E27.8 **Other specified disorders of adrenal gland**
Abnormality of cortisol-binding globulin

E27.9 **Disorder of adrenal gland, unspecified**
Excludes1: adrenoleukodystrophy [Addison-Schilder] (E71.528)
Waterhouse-Friderichsen syndrome (A39.1)

E28 OVARIAN DYSFUNCTION
`4th` ***Excludes1:*** isolated gonadotropin deficiency (E23.0)
postprocedural ovarian failure (E89.4-)

E28.0 **Estrogen excess**
Use additional code for adverse effect, if applicable, to identify
drug (T36–T50 with fifth or sixth character 5)

E28.1 **Androgen excess**
Hypersecretion of ovarian androgens
Use additional code for adverse effect, if applicable, to identify
drug (T36–T50 with fifth or sixth character 5)

E28.2 **Polycystic ovarian syndrome**
Sclerocystic ovary syndrome
Stein-Leventhal syndrome

E28.3 **Primary ovarian failure**
`5th` ***Excludes1:*** pure gonadal dysgenesis (Q99.1)
Turner's syndrome (Q96.-)

E28.39 **Other primary ovarian failure**
Decreased estrogen
Resistant ovary syndrome

E30 DISORDERS OF PUBERTY, NEC
`4th` E30.0 **Delayed puberty**
Constitutional delay of puberty
Delayed sexual development

E30.1 **Precocious puberty**
Precocious menstruation
Excludes1: Albright (-McCune) (-Sternberg) syndrome (Q78.1)
central precocious puberty (E22.8)
congenital adrenal hyperplasia (E25.0)
female heterosexual precocious pseudopuberty (E25.-)
male isosexual precocious pseudopuberty (E25.-)

E30.8 **Other disorders of puberty**
Premature thelarche

E30.9 **Disorder of puberty, unspecified**

E31 POLYGLANDULAR DYSFUNCTION
`4th` ***Excludes1:*** ataxia telangiectasia [Louis-Bar] (G11.3)
dystrophia myotonica [Steinert] (G71.11)
pseudohypoparathyroidism (E20.1)

E31.2 **Multiple endocrine neoplasia [MEN] syndromes**
`5th` Multiple endocrine adenomatosis
Code also any associated malignancies and other conditions
associated with the syndromes

E31.20 **Multiple endocrine neoplasia [MEN] syndrome,
unspecified**
Multiple endocrine adenomatosis NOS
Multiple endocrine neoplasia [MEN] syndrome NOS

E31.21 **Multiple endocrine neoplasia [MEN] type I**
Wermer's syndrome

E31.22 **Multiple endocrine neoplasia [MEN] type IIA**
Sipple's syndrome

E31.23 **Multiple endocrine neoplasia [MEN] type IIB**

E34 OTHER ENDOCRINE DISORDERS
`4th` ***Excludes1:*** pseudohypoparathyroidism (E20.1)

E34.0 **Carcinoid syndrome**
Note: May be used as an additional code to identify functional
activity associated with a carcinoid tumor.

E34.3 **Short stature due to endocrine disorder**
Constitutional short stature
Laron-type short stature
Excludes1: achondroplastic short stature (Q77.4)
hypochondroplastic short stature (Q77.4)
nutritional short stature (E45)
pituitary short stature (E23.0)
progeria (E34.8)
renal short stature (N25.0)

Russell-Silver syndrome (Q87.19)
short-limbed stature with immunodeficiency (D82.2)
short stature in specific dysmorphic syndromes — **code to**
syndrome — **see** Alphabetical Index
short stature NOS (R62.52)

E34.4 **Constitutional tall stature**

E34.5 **Androgen insensitivity syndrome**
`5th` E34.50 **Androgen insensitivity syndrome, unspecified**
Androgen insensitivity NOS

E34.51 **Complete androgen insensitivity syndrome**
Complete androgen insensitivity
de Quervain syndrome
Goldberg-Maxwell syndrome

E34.52 **Partial androgen insensitivity syndrome**
Partial androgen insensitivity
Reifenstein syndrome

E34.8 **Other specified endocrine disorders**
Pineal gland dysfunction
Progeria
Excludes2: pseudohypoparathyroidism (E20.1)

E34.9 **Endocrine disorder, unspecified**
Endocrine disturbance NOS
Hormone disturbance NOS

(E36) INTRAOPERATIVE COMPLICATIONS OF ENDOCRINE SYSTEM

(E40–E46) MALNUTRITION

E40 KWASHIORKOR
`✔` Severe malnutrition with nutritional edema with dyspigmentation of skin
and hair
Excludes1: marasmic kwashiorkor (E42)

**E44 PROTEIN-CALORIE MALNUTRITION OF MODERATE
AND MILD DEGREE**
`4th` E44.0 **Moderate protein-calorie malnutrition**

E44.1 **Mild protein-calorie malnutrition**
Nutritional short stature
Nutritional stunting
Physical retardation due to malnutrition

**E45 RETARDED DEVELOPMENT FOLLOWING PROTEIN-
CALORIE MALNUTRITION**
`✔`

E46 UNSPECIFIED PROTEIN-CALORIE MALNUTRITION
`✔` Malnutrition NOS
Protein-calorie imbalance NOS
Excludes1: nutritional deficiency NOS (E63.9)

(E50–E64) OTHER NUTRITIONAL DEFICIENCIES

E55 VITAMIN D DEFICIENCY
`4th` ***Excludes1:*** adult osteomalacia (M83.-)
osteoporosis (M80.-)
sequelae of rickets (E64.3)

E55.0 **Rickets, active**
Infantile osteomalacia
Juvenile osteomalacia
Excludes1: celiac rickets (K90.0)
Crohn's rickets (K50.-)
hereditary vitamin D-dependent rickets (E83.32)
inactive rickets (E64.3)
renal rickets (N25.0)
sequelae of rickets (E64.3)
vitamin D-resistant rickets (E83.31)

E55.9 **Vitamin D deficiency, unspecified**
Avitaminosis D

E56 OTHER VITAMIN DEFICIENCIES
`4th` ***Excludes1:*** sequelae of other vitamin deficiencies (E64.8)

E56.0 **Deficiency of vitamin E**

`4th` `5th` `6th` `7th` Additional Character Required `✔` 3-character code

•=New Code ***Excludes1***—Not coded here, do not use together
▲=Revised Code ***Excludes2***—Not included here

E56.1 Deficiency of vitamin K
> *Excludes1:* deficiency of coagulation factor due to vitamin K
> deficiency (D68.4)
> vitamin K deficiency of newborn (P53)

E56.8 Deficiency of other vitamins

E56.9 Vitamin deficiency, unspecified

E58 DIETARY CALCIUM DEFICIENCY
✓
> *Excludes1:* disorders of calcium metabolism (E83.5-)
> sequelae of calcium deficiency (E64.8)

E63 OTHER NUTRITIONAL DEFICIENCIES
`4th`
> *Excludes1:* dehydration (E86.0)
> failure to thrive, adult (R62.7)
> failure to thrive, child (R62.51)
> feeding problems in newborn (P92.-)
> sequelae of malnutrition and other nutritional deficiencies (E64.-)

E63.0 Essential fatty acid [EFA] deficiency

E63.1 Imbalance of constituents of food intake

E63.8 Other specified nutritional deficiencies

E63.9 Nutritional deficiency, unspecified

(E65–E68) OVERWEIGHT, OBESITY AND OTHER HYPERALIMENTATION

E66 OVERWEIGHT AND OBESITY
`4th`
> **Use additional code** to identify body mass index (BMI), if known (Z68.-)
> *Excludes1:* adiposogenital dystrophy (E23.6)
> lipomatosis NOS (E88.2)
> lipomatosis dolorosa [Dercum] (E88.2)
> Prader-Willi syndrome (Q87.11)

E66.0 Obesity due to excess calories
`5th` **E66.01 Morbid (severe) obesity due to excess calories**
> *Excludes1:* morbid (severe) obesity with alveolar
> hypoventilation (E66.2)

      E66.09 Other obesity due to excess calories

E66.1 Drug-induced obesity
> **Use additional code** for adverse effect, if applicable, to identify
> drug (T36-T50 with fifth or sixth character 5)

E66.2 Morbid (severe) obesity with alveolar hypoventilation
> obesity hypoventilation syndrome (OHS)
> *Use with* Z68.30–Z68.45 (adults) or Z68.53 (pediatrics, 2–20 yrs)
> Pickwickian syndrome

E66.3 Overweight
> *Use with* Z68.25–Z68.29 (adults) or Z68.53 (pediatrics, 2–20 yrs)

E66.8 Other obesity
> *Use with* Z68.30–Z68.45 (adults) or Z68.53 (pediatrics, 2–20 yrs)

E66.9 Obesity, unspecified
> *Use with* Z68.30–Z68.45 (adults) or Z68.53 (pediatrics, 2–20 yrs)
> Obesity NOS

(E70–E88) METABOLIC DISORDERS

Excludes1: androgen insensitivity syndrome (E34.5-)
> congenital adrenal hyperplasia (E25.0)
> Ehlers-Danlos syndromes (Q79.6-)
> hemolytic anemias attributable to enzyme disorders (D55.-)
> Marfan's syndrome (Q87.4)
> 5-alpha-reductase deficiency (E29.1)

E70 DISORDERS OF AROMATIC AMINO-ACID METABOLISM
`4th`
E70.0 Classical phenylketonuria

E70.1 Other hyperphenylalaninemias

•**E70.8 Disorders of aromatic amino-acid metabolism**
`5th` •**E70.81 Aromatic L-amino acid decarboxylase deficiency**
> AADC deficiency

    •**E70.89 Other disorders of aromatic amino-acid metabolism**

E71 DISORDERS OF BRANCHED-CHAIN AMINO-ACID METABOLISM AND FATTY-ACID METABOLISM
`4th`
E71.0 Maple-syrup-urine disease

E71.1 Other disorders of branched-chain amino-acid metabolism
`5th` **E71.11 Branched-chain organic acidurias**
`6th` **E71.110 Isovaleric acidemia**
      E71.111 3-methylglutaconic aciduria
      E71.118 Other branched-chain organic acidurias

E71.12 Disorders of propionate metabolism
`6th` **E71.120 Methylmalonic acidemia**
      E71.121 Propionic acidemia
      E71.128 Other disorders of propionate metabolism

E71.19 Other disorders of branched-chain amino-acid metabolism
> Hyperleucine-isoleucinemia
> Hypervalinemia

E71.2 Disorder of branched-chain amino-acid metabolism, unspecified

E71.3 Disorders of fatty-acid metabolism
`5th`
> *Excludes1:* peroxisomal disorders (E71.5)
> Refsum's disease (G60.1)
> Schilder's disease (G37.0)
> *Excludes2:* carnitine deficiency due to inborn error of metabolism
> (E71.42)

E71.30 Disorder of fatty-acid metabolism, unspecified

E71.31 Disorders of fatty-acid oxidation
`6th` **E71.310 Long chain/very long chain acyl CoA dehydrogenase deficiency**
> LCAD
> VLCAD

      E71.311 Medium chain acyl CoA dehydrogenase deficiency
> MCAD

      E71.312 Short chain acyl CoA dehydrogenase deficiency
> SCAD

      E71.313 Glutaric aciduria type II
> Glutaric aciduria type II A
> Glutaric aciduria type II B
> Glutaric aciduria type II C
> *Excludes1:* glutaric aciduria (type 1) NOS
> (E72.3)

      E71.314 Muscle carnitine palmitoyltransferase deficiency

      E71.318 Other disorders of fatty-acid oxidation

E71.32 Disorders of ketone metabolism

E71.39 Other disorders of fatty-acid metabolism

E71.4 Disorders of carnitine metabolism
`5th`
> *Excludes1:* Muscle carnitine palmitoyltransferase deficiency
> (E71.314)

E71.40 Disorder of carnitine metabolism, unspecified

E71.41 Primary carnitine deficiency

E71.42 Carnitine deficiency due to inborn errors of metabolism
> **Code also** associated inborn error or metabolism

E71.43 Iatrogenic carnitine deficiency
> Carnitine deficiency due to hemodialysis
> Carnitine deficiency due to Valproic acid therapy

E71.44 Other secondary carnitine deficiency
`6th` **E71.440 Ruvalcaba-Myhre-Smith syndrome**
      E71.448 Other secondary carnitine deficiency

E71.5 Peroxisomal disorders
`5th`
> *Excludes1:* Schilder's disease (G37.0)

E71.50 Peroxisomal disorder, unspecified

E71.51 Disorders of peroxisome biogenesis
`6th`
> Group 1 peroxisomal disorders
> *Excludes1:* Refsum's disease (G60.1)

  E71.510 Zellweger syndrome

  E71.511 Neonatal adrenoleukodystrophy
> *Excludes1:* X-linked adrenoleukodystrophy
> (E71.42-)

  E71.518 Other disorders of peroxisome biogenesis

E71.52 X-linked adrenoleukodystrophy
`6th` **E71.520 Childhood cerebral X-linked adrenoleukodystrophy**

  E71.521 Adolescent X-linked adrenoleukodystrophy

  E71.522 Adrenomyeloneuropathy

  E71.528 Other X-linked adrenoleukodystrophy
> Addison only phenotype
> adrenoleukodystrophy
> Addison-Schilder adrenoleukodystrophy

`4th` `5th` `6th` `7th` Additional Character Required   ✓ 3-character code

•=New Code   *Excludes1*—Not coded here, do not use together
▲=Revised Code   *Excludes2*—Not included here

E71.529   **X-linked adrenoleukodystrophy, unspecified type**
E71.53   **Other group 2 peroxisomal disorders**
E71.54   **Other peroxisomal disorders**
6th   E71.540   **Rhizomelic chondrodysplasia punctata**
Excludes1: chondrodysplasia punctata NOS (Q77.3)
E71.541   **Zellweger-like syndrome**
E71.542   **Other group 3 peroxisomal disorders**
E71.548   **Other peroxisomal disorders**

E72   **OTHER DISORDERS OF AMINO-ACID METABOLISM**
4th   *Excludes1:* disorders of aromatic amino-acid metabolism (E70.-)
branched-chain amino-acid metabolism (E71.0–E71.2)
fatty-acid metabolism (E71.3)
purine and pyrimidine metabolism (E79.-)
gout (M1A.-, M10.-)
E72.0   **Disorders of amino-acid transport**
5th   *Excludes1:* disorders of tryptophan metabolism (E70.5)
E72.00   **Disorders of amino-acid transport, unspecified**
E72.01   **Cystinuria**
E72.02   **Hartnup's disease**
E72.03   **Lowe's syndrome**
Use additional code for associated glaucoma (H42)
E72.04   **Cystinosis**
E72.09   **Other disorders of amino-acid transport**
Fanconi (-de Toni) (-Debré) syndrome, unspecified
E72.5   **Disorders of glycine metabolism**
5th   E72.50   **Disorder of glycine metabolism, unspecified**
E72.51   **Non-ketotic hyperglycinemia**
E72.52   **Trimethylaminuria**
E72.53   **Primary hyperoxaluria**
Oxalosis
Oxaluria
E72.59   **Other disorders of glycine metabolism**
D-glycericacidemia
Hyperhydroxyprolinemia
Hyperprolinemia (types I, II)
Sarcosinemia
E72.8   **Other specified disorders of amino-acid metabolism**
5th   E72.81   **Disorders of gamma aminobutyric acid metabolism**
4-hydroxybutyric aciduria
Disorders of GABA metabolism
GABA metabolic defect
GABA transaminase deficiency
GABA-T deficiency
Gamma-hydroxybutyric aciduria
SSADHD
Succinic semialdehyde dehydrogenase deficiency
E72.89   **Other specified disorders of amino-acid metabolism**
Disorders of beta-amino-acid metabolism
Disorders of gamma-glutamyl cycle
E72.9   **Disorder of amino-acid metabolism, unspecified**
5th

E73   **LACTOSE INTOLERANCE**
4th   E73.0   **Congenital lactase deficiency**
E73.1   **Secondary lactase deficiency**
E73.8   **Other lactose intolerance**
E73.9   **Lactose intolerance, unspecified**

E74   **OTHER DISORDERS OF CARBOHYDRATE METABOLISM**
4th   *Excludes1:* DM (E08–E13)
hypoglycemia NOS (E16.2)
increased secretion of glucagon (E16.3)
mucopolysaccharidosis (E76.0–E76.3) E74.1
E74.1   **Disorders of fructose metabolism**
5th   *Excludes1:* muscle phosphofructokinase deficiency (E74.09)
E74.10   **Disorder of fructose metabolism, unspecified**
E74.11   **Essential fructosuria**
Fructokinase deficiency
E74.12   **Hereditary fructose intolerance**
Fructosemia
E74.19   **Other disorders of fructose metabolism**
Fructose-1, 6-diphosphatase deficiency

E74.2   **Disorders of galactose metabolism**
5th   E74.20   **Disorders of galactose metabolism, unspecified**
E74.21   **Galactosemia**
E74.29   **Other disorders of galactose metabolism**
Galactokinase deficiency
E74.3   **Other disorders of intestinal carbohydrate absorption**
5th   *Excludes2:* lactose intolerance (E73.-)
E74.31   **Sucrase-isomaltase deficiency**
E74.39   **Other disorders of intestinal carbohydrate absorption**
Disorder of intestinal carbohydrate absorption NOS
Glucose-galactose malabsorption
Sucrase deficiency
E74.4   **Disorders of pyruvate metabolism and gluconeogenesis**
Deficiency of phosphoenolpyruvate carboxykinase
Deficiency of pyruvate carboxylase
Deficiency of pyruvate dehydrogenase
Excludes1: disorders of pyruvate metabolism and gluconeogenesis with anemia (D55.-)
Leigh's syndrome (G31.82)
▲E74.8   **Disorders of carbohydrate metabolism**
5th   •E74.81   **Disorders of glucose transport**
6th   •E74.810   **Glucose transporter protein type 1 deficiency**
De Vivo syndrome
Glucose transport defect, blood-brain barrier
Glut1 deficiency
GLUT1 deficiency syndrome 1, infantile onset
GLUT1 deficiency syndrome 2, childhood onset
•E74.818   **Other disorders of glucose transport**
(Familial) renal glycosuria
•E74.819   **Disorders of glucose transport, unspecified**
•E74.89   **Other specified disorders of carbohydrate metabolism**
Essential pentosuria

E75   **DISORDERS OF SPHINGOLIPID METABOLISM AND**
4th   **OTHER LIPID STORAGE DISORDERS**
Excludes1: mucolipidosis, types I-III (E77.0-E77.1)
Refsum's disease (G60.1)
E75.0   **GM2 gangliosidosis**
5th   E75.00   **GM2 gangliosidosis, unspecified**
E75.01   **Sandhoff disease**
E75.02   **Tay-Sachs disease**
E75.2   **Other sphingolipidosis**
5th   *Excludes1:* adrenoleukodystrophy [Addison-Schilder] (E71.528)
E75.21   **Fabry (-Anderson) disease**
E75.22   **Gaucher disease**
E75.23   **Krabbe disease**
E75.24   **Niemann-Pick disease**
6th   E75.240   **Niemann-Pick disease type A**
E75.241   **Niemann-Pick disease type B**
E75.242   **Niemann-Pick disease type C**
E75.243   **Niemann-Pick disease type D**
E75.248   **Other Niemann-Pick disease**
E75.249   **Niemann-Pick disease, unspecified**
E75.25   **Metachromatic leukodystrophy**
E75.26   **Sulfatase deficiency**
Multiple sulfatase deficiency (MSD)
E75.29   **Other sphingolipidosis**
Farber's syndrome
Sulfatide lipidosis

E76   **DISORDERS OF GLYCOSAMINOGLYCAN METABOLISM**
4th   E76.0   **Mucopolysaccharidosis, type I**
5th   E76.01   **Hurler's syndrome**
E76.02   **Hurler-Scheie syndrome**
E76.03   **Scheie's syndrome**
E76.1   **Mucopolysaccharidosis, type II**
Hunter's syndrome
E76.2   **Other mucopolysaccharidoses**
5th   E76.21   **Morquio mucopolysaccharidosis**
6th

CHAPTER 4. ENDOCRINE, NUTRITIONAL AND METABOLIC DISEASES   (E71.529-E76.21)

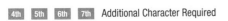 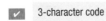

4th 5th 6th 7th   Additional Character Required   ✓   3-character code

•=New Code   *Excludes1*—Not coded here, do not use together
▲=Revised Code   *Excludes2*—Not included here

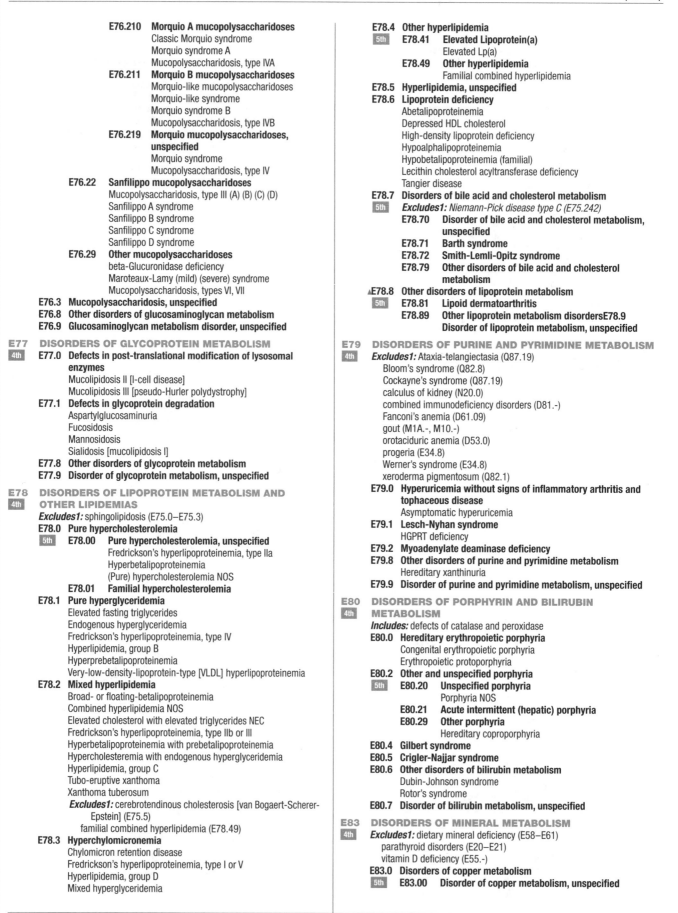

E76.210 **Morquio A mucopolysaccharidoses**
Classic Morquio syndrome
Morquio syndrome A
Mucopolysaccharidosis, type IVA

E76.211 **Morquio B mucopolysaccharidoses**
Morquio-like mucopolysaccharidoses
Morquio-like syndrome
Morquio syndrome B
Mucopolysaccharidosis, type IVB

E76.219 **Morquio mucopolysaccharidoses, unspecified**
Morquio syndrome
Mucopolysaccharidosis, type IV

E76.22 **Sanfilippo mucopolysaccharidoses**
Mucopolysaccharidosis, type III (A) (B) (C) (D)
Sanfilippo A syndrome
Sanfilippo B syndrome
Sanfilippo C syndrome
Sanfilippo D syndrome

E76.29 **Other mucopolysaccharidoses**
beta-Glucuronidase deficiency
Maroteaux-Lamy (mild) (severe) syndrome
Mucopolysaccharidosis, types VI, VII

E76.3 **Mucopolysaccharidosis, unspecified**
E76.8 **Other disorders of glucosaminoglycan metabolism**
E76.9 **Glucosaminoglycan metabolism disorder, unspecified**

E77 **DISORDERS OF GLYCOPROTEIN METABOLISM**
`4th`
E77.0 **Defects in post-translational modification of lysosomal enzymes**
Mucolipidosis II [I-cell disease]
Mucolipidosis III [pseudo-Hurler polydystrophy]

E77.1 **Defects in glycoprotein degradation**
Aspartylglucosaminuria
Fucosidosis
Mannosidosis
Sialidosis [mucolipidosis I]

E77.8 **Other disorders of glycoprotein metabolism**
E77.9 **Disorder of glycoprotein metabolism, unspecified**

E78 **DISORDERS OF LIPOPROTEIN METABOLISM AND OTHER LIPIDEMIAS**
`4th`
Excludes1: sphingolipidosis (E75.0–E75.3)

E78.0 **Pure hypercholesterolemia**
`5th` **E78.00** **Pure hypercholesterolemia, unspecified**
Fredrickson's hyperlipoproteinemia, type IIa
Hyperbetalipoproteinemia
(Pure) hypercholesterolemia NOS

E78.01 **Familial hypercholesterolemia**

E78.1 **Pure hyperglyceridemia**
Elevated fasting triglycerides
Endogenous hyperglyceridemia
Fredrickson's hyperlipoproteinemia, type IV
Hyperlipidemia, group B
Hyperprebetalipoproteinemia
Very-low-density-lipoprotein-type [VLDL] hyperlipoproteinemia

E78.2 **Mixed hyperlipidemia**
Broad- or floating-betalipoproteinemia
Combined hyperlipidemia NOS
Elevated cholesterol with elevated triglycerides NEC
Fredrickson's hyperlipoproteinemia, type IIb or III
Hyperbetalipoproteinemia with prebetalipoproteinemia
Hypercholesteremia with endogenous hyperglyceridemia
Hyperlipidemia, group C
Tubo-eruptive xanthoma
Xanthoma tuberosum
Excludes1: cerebrotendinous cholesterosis [van Bogaert-Scherer-Epstein] (E75.5)
familial combined hyperlipidemia (E78.49)

E78.3 **Hyperchylomicronemia**
Chylomicron retention disease
Fredrickson's hyperlipoproteinemia, type I or V
Hyperlipidemia, group D
Mixed hyperglyceridemia

E78.4 **Other hyperlipidemia**
`5th` **E78.41** **Elevated Lipoprotein(a)**
Elevated Lp(a)
E78.49 **Other hyperlipidemia**
Familial combined hyperlipidemia

E78.5 **Hyperlipidemia, unspecified**
E78.6 **Lipoprotein deficiency**
Abetalipoproteinemia
Depressed HDL cholesterol
High-density lipoprotein deficiency
Hypoalphalipoproteinemia
Hypobetalipoproteinemia (familial)
Lecithin cholesterol acyltransferase deficiency
Tangier disease

E78.7 **Disorders of bile acid and cholesterol metabolism**
`5th` **Excludes1:** Niemann-Pick disease type C (E75.242)
E78.70 **Disorder of bile acid and cholesterol metabolism, unspecified**
E78.71 **Barth syndrome**
E78.72 **Smith-Lemli-Opitz syndrome**
E78.79 **Other disorders of bile acid and cholesterol metabolism**

▲**E78.8** **Other disorders of lipoprotein metabolism**
`5th` **E78.81** **Lipoid dermatoarthritis**
E78.89 **Other lipoprotein metabolism disordersE78.9**
Disorder of lipoprotein metabolism, unspecified

E79 **DISORDERS OF PURINE AND PYRIMIDINE METABOLISM**
`4th`
Excludes1: Ataxia-telangiectasia (Q87.19)
Bloom's syndrome (Q82.8)
Cockayne's syndrome (Q87.19)
calculus of kidney (N20.0)
combined immunodeficiency disorders (D81.-)
Fanconi's anemia (D61.09)
gout (M1A.-, M10.-)
orotaciduric anemia (D53.0)
progeria (E34.8)
Werner's syndrome (E34.8)
xeroderma pigmentosum (Q82.1)

E79.0 **Hyperuricemia without signs of inflammatory arthritis and tophaceous disease**
Asymptomatic hyperuricemia

E79.1 **Lesch-Nyhan syndrome**
HGPRT deficiency

E79.2 **Myoadenylate deaminase deficiency**
E79.8 **Other disorders of purine and pyrimidine metabolism**
Hereditary xanthinuria

E79.9 **Disorder of purine and pyrimidine metabolism, unspecified**

E80 **DISORDERS OF PORPHYRIN AND BILIRUBIN METABOLISM**
`4th`
Includes: defects of catalase and peroxidase

E80.0 **Hereditary erythropoietic porphyria**
Congenital erythropoietic porphyria
Erythropoietic protoporphyria

E80.2 **Other and unspecified porphyria**
`5th` **E80.20** **Unspecified porphyria**
Porphyria NOS
E80.21 **Acute intermittent (hepatic) porphyria**
E80.29 **Other porphyria**
Hereditary coproporphyria

E80.4 **Gilbert syndrome**
E80.5 **Crigler-Najjar syndrome**
E80.6 **Other disorders of bilirubin metabolism**
Dubin-Johnson syndrome
Rotor's syndrome

E80.7 **Disorder of bilirubin metabolism, unspecified**

E83 **DISORDERS OF MINERAL METABOLISM**
`4th`
Excludes1: dietary mineral deficiency (E58–E61)
parathyroid disorders (E20–E21)
vitamin D deficiency (E55.-)

E83.0 **Disorders of copper metabolism**
`5th` **E83.00** **Disorder of copper metabolism, unspecified**

`4th` `5th` `6th` `7th` Additional Character Required   ✔ 3-character code   ●=New Code   **Excludes1**—Not coded here, do not use together
▲=Revised Code   **Excludes2**—Not included here

E83.01 Wilson's disease
Code also associated Kayser Fleischer ring (H18.04-)

E83.09 Other disorders of copper metabolism
Menkes' (kinky hair) (steely hair) disease

E83.1 Disorders of iron metabolism
5th **Excludes1:** iron deficiency anemia (D50.-)
sideroblastic anemia (D64.0–D64.3)

E83.10 Disorder of iron metabolism, unspecified

E83.11 Hemochromatosis
6th **Excludes1:** Gestational alloimmune liver disease/GALD (P78.84)
Neonatal hemochromatosis (P78.84)

E83.110 Hereditary hemochromatosis
Bronzed diabetes
Pigmentary cirrhosis (of liver)
Primary (hereditary) hemochromatosis

E83.111 Hemochromatosis due to repeated red blood cell transfusions
Iron overload due to repeated red blood cell transfusions
Transfusion (red blood cell) associated hemochromatosis

E83.118 Other hemochromatosis

E83.119 Hemochromatosis, unspecified

E83.19 Other disorders of iron metabolism
Use additional code, if applicable, for idiopathic pulmonary hemosiderosis (J84.03)

E83.2 Disorders of zinc metabolism
Acrodermatitis enteropathica

E83.3 Disorders of phosphorus metabolism and phosphatases
5th **Excludes1:** adult osteomalacia (M83.-)
osteoporosis (M80.-)

E83.30 Disorder of phosphorus metabolism, unspecified

E83.31 Familial hypophosphatemia
Vitamin D-resistant osteomalacia
Vitamin D-resistant rickets
Excludes1: vitamin D-deficiency rickets (E55.0)

E83.32 Hereditary vitamin D-dependent rickets (type 1) (type 2)
25-hydroxyvitamin D 1-alpha-hydroxylase deficiency
Pseudovitamin D deficiency
Vitamin D receptor defect

E83.39 Other disorders of phosphorus metabolism
Acid phosphatase deficiency
Hyperphosphatemia
Hypophosphatasia

E83.4 Disorders of magnesium metabolism
5th Refer to Category P71 for transitory neonatal disorders of magnesium metabolism

E83.40 Disorders of magnesium metabolism, unspecified

E83.41 Hypermagnesemia

E83.42 Hypomagnesemia

E83.49 Other disorders of magnesium metabolism

E83.5 Disorders of calcium metabolism
5th **Excludes1:** chondrocalcinosis (M11.1–M11.2)
Refer to Category P71 for transitory neonatal disorders of calcium metabolism
hungry bone syndrome (E83.81) hyperparathyroidism (E21.0–E21.3)

E83.50 Unspecified disorder of calcium metabolism

E83.51 Hypocalcemia
For associated tetany report R29.0

E83.52 Hypercalcemia
Familial hypocalciuric hypercalcemia

E83.59 Other disorders of calcium metabolism

E83.8 Other disorders of mineral metabolism
5th **E83.81 Hungry bone syndrome**

E83.89 Other disorders of mineral metabolism

E83.9 Disorder of mineral metabolism, unspecified

E84 CYSTIC FIBROSIS
4th **Includes:** mucoviscidosis
Code also exocrine pancreatic insufficiency (K86.81)

E84.0 Cystic fibrosis with pulmonary manifestations
Use additional code to identify any infectious organism present, such as: Pseudomonas (B96.5)

E84.1 Cystic fibrosis with intestinal manifestations
5th **E84.11 Meconium ileus in cystic fibrosis**
Excludes1: meconium ileus not due to cystic fibrosis (P76.0)

E84.19 Cystic fibrosis with other intestinal manifestations
Distal intestinal obstruction syndrome

E84.8 Cystic fibrosis with other manifestations

E84.9 Cystic fibrosis, unspecified

E86 VOLUME DEPLETION
4th **Use additional code(s)** for any associated disorders of electrolyte and acid-base balance (E87.-)
Excludes1: dehydration of newborn (P74.1)
postprocedural hypovolemic shock (T81.19)
traumatic hypovolemic shock (T79.4)
Excludes 2: hypovolemic shock NOS (R57.1)

E86.0 Dehydration

E86.1 Hypovolemia
Depletion of volume of plasma

E86.9 Volume depletion, unspecified

E87 OTHER DISORDERS OF FLUID, ELECTROLYTE AND ACID-BASE BALANCE
4th **Excludes1:** diabetes insipidus (E23.2)
electrolyte imbalance associated with hyperemesis gravidarum (O21.1)
electrolyte imbalance following ectopic or molar pregnancy (O08.5)
familial periodic paralysis (G72.3)

E87.0 Hyperosmolality and hypernatremia
Refer to code P74.2 for transitory neonatal sodium imbalance
Sodium [Na] excess
Sodium [Na] overload

E87.1 Hypo-osmolality and hyponatremia
Sodium [Na] deficiency
Excludes1: syndrome of inappropriate secretion of antidiuretic hormone (E22.2)

E87.2 Acidosis
Acidosis NOS
Lactic acidosis
Metabolic acidosis
Respiratory acidosis
Excludes1: diabetic acidosis — see categories E08–E10, E13 with ketoacidosis

E87.3 Alkalosis
Alkalosis NOS
Metabolic alkalosis
Respiratory alkalosis

E87.4 Mixed disorder of acid-base balance

E87.5 Hyperkalemia
Refer to code P74.3 for transitory neonatal potassium imbalance
Potassium [K] excess
Potassium [K] overload

E87.6 Hypokalemia
Potassium [K] deficiency

E87.7 Fluid overload
5th **Excludes1:** edema NOS (R60.9)
fluid retention (R60.9)

E87.70 Fluid overload, unspecified

E87.71 Transfusion associated circulatory overload
Fluid overload due to transfusion (blood) (blood components)
TACO

E87.79 Other fluid overload

E87.8 Other disorders of electrolyte and fluid balance, NEC
Electrolyte imbalance NOS
Hyperchloremia
Hypochloremia

E88 OTHER AND UNSPECIFIED METABOLIC DISORDERS
4th **Use additional codes** for associated conditions

| 4th | 5th | 6th | 7th | Additional Character Required | | ✔ | 3-character code |

•=New Code
▲=Revised Code

Excludes1—Not coded here, do not use together
Excludes2—Not included here

CHAPTER 4. ENDOCRINE, NUTRITIONAL AND METABOLIC DISEASES   (E88.0– E89.89)

E88.0 **Disorders of plasma-protein metabolism, NEC**
  `5th`   *Excludes1:* monoclonal gammopathy (of undetermined significance) (D47.2)
         polyclonal hypergammaglobulinemia (D89.0)
         Waldenström macroglobulinemia (C88.0)
     Excludes2: disorder of lipoprotein metabolism (E78.-)
     E88.01   **Alpha-1-antitrypsin deficiency**
           AAT deficiency
     E88.02   **Plasminogen deficiency**
           Dysplasminogenemia
           Hypoplasminogenemia
           Type 1 plasminogen deficiency
           Type 2 plasminogen deficiency
           Code also, if applicable, ligneous conjunctivitis (H10.51)
           Use additional code for associated findings, such as:
              hydrocephalus (G91.4)
              ligneous conjunctivitis (H10.51)
              otitis media (H67.-)
              respiratory disorder related to plasminogen deficiency (J99)
     E88.09   **Other disorders of plasma-protein metabolism, NEC**
           Bisalbuminemia
E88.1 **Lipodystrophy, NEC**
     Lipodystrophy NOS
E88.2 **Lipomatosis, NEC**
     Lipomatosis NOS
     Lipomatosis (Check) dolorosa [Dercum]
E88.3 **Tumor lysis syndrome**
     Tumor lysis syndrome (spontaneous)
     Tumor lysis syndrome following antineoplastic drug chemotherapy
     Use additional code for adverse effect, if applicable, to identify drug (T45.1X5)
E88.4 **Mitochondrial metabolism disorders**
  `5th`   *Excludes1:* disorders of pyruvate metabolism (E74.4)
         Kearns-Sayre syndrome (H49.81)
         Leber's disease (H47.22)
         Leigh's encephalopathy (G31.82)
         Mitochondrial myopathy, NEC (G71.3)
         Reye's syndrome (G93.7)
     E88.40   **Mitochondrial metabolism disorder, unspecified**
     E88.41   **MELAS syndrome**
           Mitochondrial myopathy, encephalopathy, lactic acidosis and stroke-like episodes
     E88.42   **MERRF syndrome**
           Myoclonic epilepsy associated with ragged-red fibers
           Code also progressive myoclonic epilepsy (G40.3-)
     E88.49   **Other mitochondrial metabolism disorders**

E88.8 **Other specified metabolic disorders**
  `5th`   **E88.81**   **Metabolic syndrome**
           Dysmetabolic syndrome X
           Use additional codes for associated manifestations, such as: obesity (E66.-)
     E88.89   **Other specified metabolic disorders**
           Launois-Bensaude adenolipomatosis
           Excludes1: adult pulmonary Langerhans cell histiocytosis (J84.82)
E88.9 **Metabolic disorder, unspecified**

(E89) POSTPROCEDURAL ENDOCRINE AND METABOLIC COMPLICATIONS AND DISORDERS, NOT ELSEWHERE CLASSIFIED

E89 **POSTPROCEDURAL ENDOCRINE AND METABOLIC**
  `4th`   **COMPLICATIONS AND DISORDERS, NOT ELSEWHERE CLASSIFIED**
     Excludes2: intraoperative complications of endocrine system organ or structure (E36.0-, E36.1-, E36.8)
E89.0 **Postprocedural hypothyroidism**
     Postirradiation hypothyroidism
     Postsurgical hypothyroidism
E89.1 **Postprocedural hypoinsulinemia**
     Postpancreatectomy hyperglycemia
     Postsurgical hypoinsulinemia
     Use additional code, if applicable, to identify:
         acquired absence of pancreas (Z90.41-)
         diabetes mellitus (postpancreatectomy) (postprocedural) (E13.-)
         insulin use (Z79.4)
     Excludes1: transient postprocedural hyperglycemia (R73.9)
         transient postprocedural hypoglycemia (E16.2)
E89.2 **Postprocedural hypoparathyroidism**
     Parathyroprival tetany
E89.3 **Postprocedural hypopituitarism**
     Postirradiation hypopituitarism
E89.8 **Other postprocedural endocrine and metabolic complications**
  `5th`   **and disorders**
     E89.89   **Other postprocedural endocrine and metabolic**
  `6th`   **complications and disorders**
           Use additional code, if applicable, to further specify disorder

    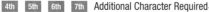   `4th` `5th` `6th` `7th`   Additional Character Required   ✓   3-character code   •=New Code   ▲=Revised Code   *Excludes1*—Not coded here, do not use together   *Excludes2*—Not included here

170   **PEDIATRIC ICD-10-CM 2021: A MANUAL FOR PROVIDER-BASED CODING**

Chapter 5. Mental, behavioral, and neurodevelopmental disorders (F01–F99)

Pain disorders related to psychological factors

Refer to category F45.

Mental and behavioral disorders due to psychoactive substance use

Refer to categories F10–F19
Includes: disorders of psychological development
Excludes2: symptoms, signs and abnormal clinical laboratory findings, not elsewhere classified (R00–R99)

(F01–F09) MENTAL DISORDERS DUE TO KNOWN PHYSIOLOGICAL CONDITIONS

Note: This block comprises a range of mental disorders grouped together on the basis of their having in common a demonstrable etiology in cerebral disease, brain injury, or other insult leading to cerebral dysfunction. The dysfunction may be primary, as in diseases, injuries, and insults that affect the brain directly and selectively; or secondary, as in systemic diseases and disorders that attack the brain only as one of the multiple organs or systems of the body that are involved.

F02 **DEMENTIA IN OTHER DISEASES CLASSIFIED ELSEWHERE**
4th **Code first** the underlying physiological condition, such as:
cerebral lipidosis (E75.4)
Creutzfeldt-Jakob disease (A81.0-)
dementia with Lewy bodies (G31.83)
dementia with Parkinsonism (G31.83)
epilepsy and recurrent seizures (G40.-)
frontotemporal dementia (G31.09)
hepatolenticular degeneration (E83.0)
HIV disease (B20)
Huntington's disease (G10)
hypercalcemia (E83.52)
hypothyroidism, acquired (E00-E03.-)
intoxications (T36-T65)
Jakob-Creutzfeldt disease (A81.0-)
multiple sclerosis (G35)
neurosyphilis (A52.17)
niacin deficiency [pellagra] (E52)
Parkinson's disease (G20)
Pick's disease (G31.01)
polyarteritis nodosa (M30.0)
SLE (M32.-)
traumatic brain injury (S06.-)
trypanosomiasis (B56.-, B57.-)
vitamin B deficiency (E53.8)
Includes: major neurocognitive disorders in other diseases classified elsewhere
Excludes2: dementia in alcohol and psychoactive substance disorders (F10–F19, with .17, .27, .97)
vascular dementia (F01.5-)
F02.8 **Dementia in other diseases classified elsewhere**
5th **F02.80** **Dementia in other diseases classified elsewhere without behavioral disturbance**
Dementia in other diseases classified elsewhere NOS
Major neurocognitive disorder in other diseases classified elsewhere
F02.81 **Dementia in other diseases classified elsewhere with behavioral disturbance**
Use additional code, if applicable, to identify wandering in dementia in conditions classified elsewhere (Z91.83)
Dementia in other diseases classified elsewhere with:
aggressive behavior
combative behavior
violent behavior
Major neurocognitive disorder in other diseases classified elsewhere with:
aggressive behavior
combative behavior
violent behavior

F07 **PERSONALITY AND BEHAVIORAL DISORDERS DUE TO**
4th **KNOWN PHYSIOLOGICAL CONDITION**
Code first the underlying physiological condition
F07.8 **Other personality and behavioral disorders due to known**
5th **physiological condition**
F07.81 **Postconcussional syndrome**
Postcontusional syndrome (encephalopathy)
Post-traumatic brain syndrome, nonpsychotic
Use additional code to identify associated post-traumatic headache, if applicable (G44.3-)
Excludes1: current concussion (brain) (S06.0-)
postencephalitic syndrome (F07.89)
F07.89 **Other personality and behavioral disorders due to known physiological condition**
Postencephalitic syndrome
Right hemispheric organic affective disorder
F07.9 **Unspecified personality and behavioral disorder due to known physiological condition**
Organic p syndrome

F09 **UNSPECIFIED MENTAL DISORDER DUE TO KNOWN**
✔ **PHYSIOLOGICAL CONDITION**
Mental disorder NOS due to known physiological condition
Organic brain syndrome NOS
Organic mental disorder NOS
Organic psychosis NOS
Symptomatic psychosis NOS
Code first the underlying physiological condition
Excludes1: psychosis NOS (F29)

(F10–F19) MENTAL AND BEHAVIORAL DISORDERS DUE TO PSYCHOACTIVE SUBSTANCE USE

Mental and behavioral disorders due to psychoactive substance use

IN REMISSION

Selection of codes for "in remission" for categories F10–F19, Mental and behavioral disorders due to psychoactive substance use (categories F10–F19 with -.21) requires the provider's clinical judgment. The appropriate codes for "in remission" are assigned only on the basis of provider documentation (as defined inthe Official Guidelines for Coding and Reporting) unless otherwise instructed by the classification. Mild substance use disorders in early or sustained remission are classified to the appropriate codes for substance abuse in remission, and moderate or severe substance use disorders in early or sustained remission are classified to the appropriate codes for substance dependence in remission.

PSYCHOACTIVE SUBSTANCE USE, ABUSE, AND DEPENDENCE

When the provider documentation refers to use, abuse and dependence of the same substance (e.g. alcohol, opioid, cannabis, etc.), only one code should be assigned to identify the pattern of use based on the following hierarchy:
• If both use and abuse are documented, assign only the code for abuse
• If both abuse and dependence are documented, assign only the code for dependence
• If use, abuse and dependence are all documented, assign only the code for dependence
• If both use and dependence are documented, assign only the code for dependence.

PSYCHOACTIVE SUBSTANCE USE, UNSPECIFIED

As with all other unspecified diagnoses, the codes for unspecified psychoactive substance use (F10.9-, F11.9-, F12.9-, F13.9-, F14.9-, F15.9-, F16.9-, F18.9-, F19.9-) should only be assigned based on provider documentation and when they meet the definition of a reportable diagnosis (see Section III, Reporting Additional Diagnoses). The codes are to be used only when the psychoactive substance use is associated with a physical, mental or behavioral disorder and when such a relationship is documented by the provider.

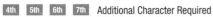 **4th** **5th** **6th** **7th** Additional Character Required 3-character code

• =New Code
▲ =Revised Code

Excludes1—Not coded here, do not use together
Excludes2—Not included here

F10   **ALCOHOL RELATED DISORDERS**
`4th`   **Use additional code** for blood alcohol level, if applicable (Y90.-)

F10.1   **Alcohol abuse**
`5th`   *Excludes1:* alcohol dependence (F10.2-)
     alcohol use, unspecified (F10.9-)

   F10.10   **Alcohol abuse, uncomplicated**
      Alcohol use disorder, mild

   F10.11   **Alcohol abuse, in remission**
      Alcohol use disorder, mild, in early remission
      Alcohol use disorder, mild, in sustained remission

   F10.12   **Alcohol abuse with intoxication**
    `6th`   **F10.120**   **Alcohol abuse with intoxication, uncomplicated**
        F10.121   **Alcohol abuse with intoxication delirium**
        F10.129   **Alcohol abuse with intoxication, unspecified**

   •**F10.13** **Alcohol abuse with withdrawal**
    `6th`   •**F10.130**   **Alcohol abuse with withdrawal, uncomplicated**
        •**F10.131**   **Alcohol abuse with withdrawal delirium**
        •**F10.132**   **Alcohol abuse with withdrawal with perceptual disturbance**
        •**F10.139**   **Alcohol abuse with withdrawal, unspecified**

F10.2   **Alcohol dependence**
`5th`   *Excludes1:* alcohol abuse (F10.1-)
     alcohol use, unspecified (F10.9-)
   Excludes2: toxic effect of alcohol (T51.0-)

   F10.20   **Alcohol dependence, uncomplicated**
      Alcohol use disorder, moderate
      Alcohol use disorder, severe

   F10.21   **Alcohol dependence, in remission**
      Alcohol use disorder, moderate or severe, in early remission
      Alcohol use disorder, moderate or severe, in sustained remission

   F10.22   **Alcohol dependence with intoxication**
    `6th`   Acute drunkenness (in alcoholism)
      Excludes2: alcohol dependence with withdrawal (F10.23-)
        F10.220   **Alcohol dependence with intoxication, uncomplicated**
        F10.221   **Alcohol dependence with intoxication delirium**
        F10.229   **Alcohol dependence with intoxication, unspecified**

   F10.23   **Alcohol dependence with withdrawal**
    `6th`   *Excludes2:* Alcohol dependence with intoxication (F10.22-)
        F10.230   **Alcohol dependence with withdrawal, uncomplicated**
        F10.231   **Alcohol dependence with withdrawal delirium**
        F10.232   **Alcohol dependence with withdrawal with perceptual disturbance**
        F10.239   **Alcohol dependence with withdrawal, unspecified**

   F10.24   **Alcohol dependence with alcohol-induced mood disorder**
      Alcohol use disorder, moderate or severe, with alcohol-induced bipolar or related disorder
      Alcohol use disorder, moderate or severe, with alcohol-induced depressive disorder

   F10.28   **Alcohol dependence with other alcohol-induced disorders**
    `6th`   **F10.280**   **Alcohol dependence with alcohol-induced anxiety disorder**
        F10.282   **Alcohol dependence with alcohol-induced sleep disorder**
        F10.288   **Alcohol dependence with other alcohol-induced disorder**
          Alcohol use disorder, moderate or severe, with alcohol-induced mild neurocognitive disorder

F10.9   **Alcohol use, unspecified**
`5th`   *Excludes1:* alcohol abuse (F10.1-)
     alcohol dependence (F10.2-)

   F10.92   **Alcohol use, unspecified with intoxication;**
    `6th`   **F10.920**   **uncomplicated**
        F10.921   **delirium**
        F10.929   **unspecified**

   •**F10.93**   **Alcohol use, unspecified with withdrawal**
    `6th`   •**F10.930**   **Alcohol use, unspecified with withdrawal, uncomplicated**
        •**F10.931**   **Alcohol use, unspecified with withdrawal delirium**
        •**F10.932**   **Alcohol use, unspecified with withdrawal with perceptual disturbance**
        •**F10.939**   **Alcohol use, unspecified with withdrawal, unspecified**

F11   **OPIOID RELATED DISORDERS**
`4th`

F11.1   **Opioid abuse**
`5th`   *Excludes1:* opioid dependence (F11.2-)
     opioid use, unspecified (F11.9-)

   F11.10   **Opioid abuse, uncomplicated**
      Opioid use disorder, mild

   F11.11   **Opioid abuse, in remission**
      Opioid use disorder, mild, in early or sustained remission

   •**F11.13**   **Opioid abuse with withdrawal**

F12   **CANNABIS RELATED DISORDERS**
`4th`   *Includes:* marijuana

F12.1   **Cannabis abuse**
`5th`   *Excludes1:* cannabis dependence (F12.2-)
     cannabis use, unspecified (F12.9-)

   F12.10   **Cannabis abuse, uncomplicated**
      cannabis use disorder, mild

   F12.11   **Cannabis abuse, in remission**
      Cannabis use disorder, mild, in early or sustained remission

   •**F12.13**   **Cannabis abuse with withdrawal**

F12.2   **Cannabis dependence**
`5th`   *Excludes1:* cannabis abuse (F12.1-)
     cannabis use, unspecified (F12.9-)
   Excludes2: cannabis poisoning (T40.7-)

   F12.20   **Cannabis dependence, uncomplicated**

   F12.21   **Cannabis dependence, in remission**
      Cannabis use disorder, moderate or severe, in early remission
      Cannabis use disorder, moderate or severe, in sustained remission

   F12.22   **Cannabis dependence with intoxication;**
    `6th`   **F12.220**   **uncomplicated**
          Cannabis use disorder, moderate
          Cannabis use disorder, severe
        F12.221   **delirium**
        F12.222   **with perceptual disturbance**
        F12.229   **unspecified**

   F12.23   **Cannabis dependence with withdrawal**

F12.9   **Cannabis use, unspecified**
`5th`   *Excludes1:* cannabis abuse (F12.1-)
     cannabis dependence (F12.2-)

   F12.90   **Cannabis use, unspecified, uncomplicated**
      Amphetamine type substance use disorder, moderate or severe, in early or sustained remission
      Other or unspecified stimulant use disorder, moderate or severe, in early or sustained remission

   F12.93   **Cannabis use, unspecified with withdrawal**

F13   **SEDATIVE, HYPNOTIC, OR ANIOLYTIC RELATED DISORDERS**
`4th`

F13.1   **Sedative, hypnotic or anxiolytic-related abuse**
`5th`   *Excludes1:* sedative, hypnotic or anxiolytic-related dependence (F13.2-)
     sedative, hypnotic, or anxiolytic use, unspecified (F13.9-)

   F13.10   **Sedative, hypnotic or anxiolytic abuse, uncomplicated**
      Sedative, hypnotic, or anxiolytic use disorder, mild

•=New Code   *Excludes1*—Not coded here, do not use together
▲=Revised Code   *Excludes2*—Not included here

Chapter side tab: (F10–F13.10) / CHAPTER 5. MENTAL, BEHAVIORAL, AND NEURODEVELOPMENTAL DISORDERS

F13.11   Sedative, hypnotic or anxiolytic abuse, in remission
Sedative, hypnotic or anxiolytic use disorder, mild, in early or sustained remission

• **F13.13   Sedative, hypnotic or anxiolytic abuse with withdrawal**
6th

 • **F13.130   Sedative, hypnotic or anxiolytic abuse with withdrawal, uncomplicated**
 • **F13.131   Sedative, hypnotic or anxiolytic abuse with withdrawal delirium**
 • **F13.132   Sedative, hypnotic or anxiolytic abuse with withdrawal with perceptual disturbance**
 • **F13.139   Sedative, hypnotic or anxiolytic abuse with withdrawal, unspecified**

F14   COCAINE RELATED DISORDERS
4th
Excludes2: other stimulant-related disorders (F15.-)

F14.1   Cocaine abuse
5th
Excludes1: cocaine dependence (F14.2-)
cocaine use, unspecified (F14.9-)

F14.10   Cocaine abuse, uncomplicated
Cocaine use disorder, mild

F14.11   Cocaine abuse, in remission
Cocaine use disorder, mild, in early or sustained remission

F14.12   Cocaine abuse with intoxication;
6th
F14.120   uncomplicated
F14.121   delirium
F14.122   with perceptual disturbance
F14.129   unspecified

• **F14.13   Cocaine abuse, unspecified with withdrawal**

F14.2   Cocaine dependence
5th
Excludes1: cocaine abuse (F14.1-)
cocaine use, unspecified (F14.9-)
Excludes2: cocaine poisoning (T40.5-)

F14.20   Cocaine dependence, uncomplicated
Cocaine use disorder, moderate
Cocaine use disorder, severe

F14.21   Cocaine dependence, in remission
Cocaine use disorder, moderate, in early or sustained remission
Cocaine use disorder, severe, in early or sustained remission

F14.22   Cocaine dependence with intoxication;
6th
Excludes1: cocaine dependence with withdrawal (F14.23)
F14.220   uncomplicated
F14.221   delirium
F14.222   with perceptual disturbance
F14.229   unspecified

F14.23   Cocaine dependence with withdrawal
Excludes1: cocaine dependence with intoxication (F14.22-)

F14.9   Cocaine use, unspecified
5th
Excludes1: cocaine abuse (F14.1-)
cocaine dependence (F14.2-)

F14.90   Cocaine use, unspecified, uncomplicated
F14.92   Cocaine use, unspecified with intoxication;
6th
F14.920   uncomplicated
F14.921   delirium
F14.922   with perceptual disturbance
F14.929   unspecified

• **F14.93   Cocaine use, unspecified with withdrawal**

F15   OTHER STIMULANT RELATED DISORDERS
4th
Includes: amphetamine-related disorders
caffeine
Excludes2: cocaine-related disorders (F14.-)

F15.1   Other stimulant abuse
5th
Excludes1: other stimulant dependence (F15.2-)
other stimulant use, unspecified (F15.9-)

F15.10   Other stimulant abuse, uncomplicated
Amphetamine type substance use disorder, mild
Other or unspecified stimulant use disorder, mild
Cocaine use disorder, moderate, in early or sustained remission
Cocaine use disorder, severe, in early or sustained remission

F15.11   Other stimulant abuse, in remission
Amphetamine type substance use disorder, mild, in early or sustained remission
Other or unspecified stimulant use disorder, mild, in early or sustained remission

F15.12   Other stimulant abuse with intoxication;
6th
F15.120   uncomplicated
F15.121   delirium
F15.122   perceptual disturbance
Amphetamine or other stimulant use disorder, mild, with amphetamine or other stimulant intoxication, with perceptual disturbances

F15.129   unspecified
Amphetamine or other stimulant use disorder, mild, with amphetamine or other stimulant intoxication, without perceptual disturbances

• **F15.13   Other stimulant abuse with withdrawal**

F15.2   Other stimulant dependence
5th
Excludes1: other stimulant abuse (F15.1-)
other stimulant use, unspecified (F15.9-)

F15.20   Other stimulant dependence, uncomplicated
Amphetamine type substance use disorder, moderate or severe
Other or unspecified stimulant use disorder, moderate or severe

F15.21   Other stimulant dependence, in remission
Amphetamine type substance use disorder, moderate or severe, in early or sustained remission
Other or unspecified stimulant use disorder, moderate or severe, in early or sustained remission

F15.22   Other stimulant dependence with intoxication;
6th
Excludes1: other stimulant dependence with withdrawal (F15.23)
F15.220   uncomplicated
F15.221   delirium
F15.222   with perceptual disturbance
Amphetamine or other stimulant use disorder, moderate, with amphetamine or other stimulant intoxication, with perceptual disturbances

F15.229   unspecified
Amphetamine or other stimulant use disorder, severe, with amphetamine or other stimulant intoxication, with perceptual disturbances

F15.23   Other stimulant dependence with withdrawal
Amphetamine or other stimulant withdrawal
Excludes1: other stimulant dependence with intoxication (F15.22-)

F15.9   Other stimulant use, unspecified
5th
Excludes1: other stimulant abuse (F15.1-)
other stimulant dependence (F15.2-)

F15.90   Other stimulant use, unspecified, uncomplicated
F15.93   Other stimulant use, unspecified with withdrawal
Caffeine withdrawal

F16   HALLUCINOGEN RELATED DISORDERS
4th
Includes: ecstasy
PCP
phencyclidine

F16.1   Hallucinogen abuse
5th
Excludes1: hallucinogen dependence (F16.2-)
hallucinogen use, unspecified (F16.9-)

F16.10   Hallucinogen abuse, uncomplicated
Other hallucinogen use disorder, mild
Phencyclidine use disorder, mild

4th 5th 6th 7th   Additional Character Required   ✔ 3-character code

•=New Code   *Excludes1*—Not coded here, do not use together
▲=Revised Code   *Excludes2*—Not included here

CHAPTER 5. MENTAL, BEHAVIORAL, AND NEURODEVELOPMENTAL DISORDERS   (F13.11–F16.10)

F16.11   Hallucinogen abuse, in remission
Other hallucinogen use disorder, mild, in early or sustained remission
Phencyclidine use disorder, mild, in early or sustained remission

F16.2   Hallucinogen dependence
`5th`   *Excludes1:* hallucinogen abuse (F16.1-)
    hallucinogen use, unspecified (F16.9-)

F16.20   Hallucinogen dependence, uncomplicated
Other hallucinogen use disorder, moderate
Other hallucinogen use disorder, severe
Phencyclidine use disorder, moderate
Phencyclidine use disorder, severe

F17   NICOTINE DEPENDENCE
`4th`   *Excludes1:* history of tobacco dependence (Z87.891)
    tobacco use NOS (Z72.0)
Excludes2: tobacco use (smoking) during pregnancy, childbirth and the puerperium (O99.33-)
    toxic effect of nicotine (T65.2-)

F17.2   Nicotine dependence
`5th`   **F17.20   Nicotine dependence, unspecified**
    `6th`   **F17.200   Nicotine dependence, unspecified; uncomplicated**
      Tobacco use disorder, mild
      Tobacco use disorder, moderate
      Tobacco use disorder, severe
    F17.201   in remission
      Tobacco use disorder, mild, in early or sustained remission
      Tobacco use disorder, moderate, in early or sustained remission
      Tobacco use disorder, severe, in early or sustained remission
    F17.203   with withdrawal
      Tobacco withdrawal
    F17.208   with other nicotine-induced disorders
    F17.209   with unspecified nicotine-induced disorders

F17.21   Nicotine dependence, cigarettes
    `6th`   **F17.210   Nicotine dependence, cigarettes; uncomplicated**
    F17.211   in remission
      Tobacco use disorder, cigarettes, mild, in early or sustained remission
      Tobacco use disorder, cigarettes, moderate, in early or sustained remission
      Tobacco use disorder, cigarettes, severe, in early or sustained remission
    F17.213   with withdrawal
    F17.218   with other nicotine-induced disorders
    F17.219   with unspecified nicotine-induced disorders

F17.22   Nicotine dependence, chewing tobacco
    `6th`   **F17.220   Nicotine dependence, chewing tobacco; uncomplicated**
    F17.221   in remission
      Tobacco use disorder, chewing tobacco, mild, in early or sustained remission
      Tobacco use disorder, chewing tobacco, moderate, in early or sustained remission
      Tobacco use disorder, chewing tobacco, severe, in early or sustained remission
    F17.223   with withdrawal
    F17.228   with other nicotine-induced disorders
    F17.229   with unspecified nicotine-induced disorders

F17.29   Nicotine dependence, other tobacco product
    `6th`   **F17.290   Nicotine dependence, other tobacco product; uncomplicated**

F17.291   in remission
Tobacco use disorder, other product, mild, in early or sustained remission
Tobacco use disorder, other product, moderate, in early or sustained remission
Tobacco use disorder, other product, severe, in early or sustained remission

F17.293   with withdrawal
F17.298   with other nicotine-induced disorders
F17.299   with unspecified nicotine-induced disorders

F18   INHALANT RELATED DISORDERS
`4th`   *Includes:* volatile solvents

F18.1   Inhalant abuse
`5th`   *Excludes1:* inhalant dependence (F18.2-)
    inhalant use, unspecified (F18.9-)

F18.10   Inhalant abuse, uncomplicated
    Inhalant use disorder, mild

F18.11   Inhalant abuse, in remission
    Inhalant use disorder, mild, in early or sustained remission

F18.12   Inhalant abuse with intoxication
    `6th`   **F18.120   Inhalant abuse with intoxication; uncomplicated**
    F18.121   delirium
    F18.129   unspecified

F18.2   Inhalant dependence
`5th`   *Excludes1:* inhalant abuse (F18.1-)
    inhalant use, unspecified (F18.9-)

F18.20   Inhalant dependence, uncomplicated
    Inhalant use disorder, moderate
    Inhalant use disorder, severe

F18.21   Inhalant dependence, in remission
F18.22   Inhalant dependence with intoxication
    `6th`   **F18.220   Inhalant dependence with intoxication; uncomplicated**
    F18.221   delirium
    F18.229   unspecified

F18.9   Inhalant use, unspecified
`5th`   *Excludes1:* inhalant abuse (F18.1-)
    inhalant dependence (F18.2-)

F18.90   Inhalant use, unspecified, uncomplicated
F18.92   Inhalant use, unspecified with intoxication
    `6th`   **F18.920   Inhalant use, unspecified with intoxication, uncomplicated**
    F18.921   Inhalant use, unspecified with intoxication with delirium
    F18.929   Inhalant use, unspecified with intoxication, unspecified

F19   OTHER PSYCHOACTIVE SUBSTANCE RELATED DISORDERS
`4th`   *Includes:* polysubstance drug use (indiscriminate drug use)

F19.1   Other psychoactive substance abuse
`5th`   *Excludes1:* other psychoactive substance dependence (F19.2-)
    other psychoactive substance use, unspecified (F19.9-)

F19.10   Other psychoactive substance abuse, uncomplicated
    Other (or unknown) substance use disorder, mild

F19.12   Other psychoactive substance abuse with intoxication
    `6th`   **F19.120   Other psychoactive substance abuse with intoxication; uncomplicated**
    F19.121   delirium
    F19.122   with perceptual disturbances
    F19.129   unspecified

•**F19.13   Other psychoactive substance abuse**
    `6th`   •**F19.130   Other psychoactive substance abuse with withdrawal, uncomplicated**
    •**F19.131   Other psychoactive substance abuse with withdrawal delirium**
    •**F19.132   Other psychoactive substance abuse with withdrawal with perceptual disturbance**
    •**F19.139   Other psychoactive substance abuse with withdrawal, unspecified**

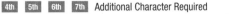 `4th` `5th` `6th` `7th`   Additional Character Required   ✔   3-character code

•=New Code   *Excludes1*—Not coded here, do not use together
▲=Revised Code   *Excludes2*—Not included here

CHAPTER 5. MENTAL, BEHAVIORAL, AND NEURODEVELOPMENTAL DISORDERS   (F16.11–F19.139)

F19.2   **Other psychoactive substance dependence**
> **5th**   *Excludes1:* other psychoactive substance abuse (F19.1-)
> other psychoactive substance use, unspecified (F19.9-)

    F19.20   **Other psychoactive substance dependence, uncomplicated**
> Other (or unknown) substance use disorder, moderate
> Other (or unknown) substance use disorder, severe

    F19.21   **Other psychoactive substance dependence, in remission**
> Other (or unknown) substance use disorder, moderate, in early remission or in sustained remission
> Other (or unknown) substance use disorder, severe, in early remission or in sustained remission

    F19.22   **Other psychoactive substance dependence with intoxication**
> **6th**
> *Excludes1:* psychoactive other substance dependence with withdrawal (F19.23-)

       F19.220   **Other psychoactive substance dependence with intoxication; uncomplicated**
       F19.221   **delirium**
       F19.222   **with perceptual disturbance**
       F19.229   **unspecified**

    F19.23   **Other psychoactive substance dependence with withdrawal**
> **6th**
> *Excludes1:* other psychoactive substance dependence with intoxication (F19.22-)

       F19.230   **Other psychoactive substance dependence with withdrawal; uncomplicated**
       F19.231   **delirium**
       F19.232   **with perceptual disturbance**
       F19.239   **unspecified**

F19.9   **Other psychoactive substance use, unspecified**
> **5th**   *Excludes1:* other psychoactive substance abuse (F19.1-)
> other psychoactive substance dependence (F19.2-)

    F19.90   **Other psychoactive substance use, unspecified, uncomplicated**

    F19.92   **Other psychoactive substance use, unspecified with intoxication**
> **6th**
> *Excludes1:* other psychoactive substance use, unspecified with withdrawal (F19.93)

       F19.920   **Other psychoactive substance use, unspecified with intoxication; uncomplicated**
       F19.921   **with delirium**
> Other (or unknown) substance-induced delirium
       F19.922   **with perceptual disturbance**
       F19.929   **unspecified**

(F20–F29) SCHIZOPHRENIA, SCHIZOTYPAL, DELUSIONAL, AND OTHER NON-MOOD PSYCHOTIC DISORDERS

(F30–F39) MOOD [AFFECTIVE] DISORDERS

F31   **BIPOLAR DISORDER**
> **4th**   *Includes:* bipolar I disorder
> bipolar type I disorder manic-depressive illness manic-depressive psychosis manic-depressive reaction
> *Excludes1:* bipolar disorder, single manic episode (F30.-)
> major depressive disorder, single episode (F32.-)
> major depressive disorder, recurrent (F33.-)

F31.0   **Bipolar disorder, current episode hypomanic**

F31.1   **Bipolar disorder, current episode manic without psychotic features**
> **5th**

    F31.10   **Bipolar disorder, current episode manic without psychotic features, unspecified**
    F31.11   **Bipolar disorder, current episode manic without psychotic features, mild**
    F31.12   **Bipolar disorder, current episode manic without psychotic features, moderate**
    F31.13   **Bipolar disorder, current episode manic without psychotic features, severe**

F31.3   **Bipolar disorder, current episode depressed, mild or moderate severity**
> **5th**

    F31.30   **Bipolar disorder, current episode depressed, mild or moderate severity, unspecified**
    F31.31   **Bipolar disorder, current episode depressed, mild**
    F31.32   **Bipolar disorder, current episode depressed, moderate**

F31.4   **Bipolar disorder, current episode depressed, severe, without psychotic features**

F31.6   **Bipolar disorder, current episode mixed**
> **5th**   **F31.60**   **Bipolar disorder, current episode mixed, unspecified**
    F31.61   **Bipolar disorder, current episode mixed, mild**
    F31.62   **Bipolar disorder, current episode mixed, moderate**
    F31.63   **Bipolar disorder, current episode mixed, severe, without psychotic features**

F31.8   **Other bipolar disorders**
> **5th**   **F31.81**   **Bipolar II disorder**
> Bipolar disorder, type 2
    F31.89   **Other bipolar disorder**
> Recurrent manic episodes NOS

F31.9   **Bipolar disorder, unspecified**
> Manic depression

F32   **MAJOR DEPRESSIVE DISORDER, SINGLE EPISODE**
> **4th**   *Includes:* single episode of agitated depression
> single episode of depressive reaction
> single episode of major depression
> single episode of psychogenic depression
> single episode of reactive depression
> single episode of vital depression
> *Excludes1:* bipolar disorder (F31.-)
> manic episode (F30.-)
> recurrent depressive disorder (F33.-)
> *Excludes2:* adjustment disorder (F43.2)

F32.0   **Major depressive disorder, single episode, mild**

F32.1   **Major depressive disorder, single episode, moderate**

F32.2   **Major depressive disorder, single episode, severe without psychotic features**

F32.3   **Major depressive disorder, single episode, severe with psychotic features**
> Single episode of major depression with mood-congruent psychotic symptoms
> Single episode of major depression with mood-incongruent psychotic symptoms
> Single episode of major depression with psychotic symptoms
> Single episode of psychogenic depressive psychosis
> Single episode of psychotic depression
> Single episode of reactive depressive psychosis

F32.4   **Major depressive disorder, single episode, in partial remission**

F32.5   **Major depressive disorder, single episode, in full remission**

F32.8   **Other depressive episodes**
> **5th**   **F32.81**   **Premenstrual dysphoric disorder**
> *Excludes1:* premenstrual tension syndrome (N94.3)
    F32.89   **Other specified depressive episodes**
> Atypical depression
> Post-schizophrenic depression
> Single episode of 'masked' depression NOS

F32.9   **Major depressive disorder, single episode, unspecified**
> Depression NOS
> Depressive disorder NOS
> Major depression NOS

F33   **MAJOR DEPRESSIVE DISORDER, RECURRENT**
> **4th**   *Includes:* recurrent episodes of depressive reaction
> recurrent episodes of endogenous depression
> recurrent episodes of major depression
> recurrent episodes of psychogenic depression
> recurrent episodes of reactive depression
> recurrent episodes of seasonal depressive disorder
> recurrent episodes of vital depression
> *Excludes1:* bipolar disorder (F31.-)
> manic episode (F30.-)

F33.0   **Major depressive disorder, recurrent, mild**

F33.1   **Major depressive disorder, recurrent, moderate**

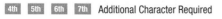   Additional Character Required   ✔   3-character code

•=New Code   *Excludes1*—Not coded here, do not use together
▲=Revised Code   *Excludes2*—Not included here

F33.2 **Major depressive disorder, recurrent severe without psychotic features**

F33.3 **Major depressive disorder, recurrent, severe with psychotic symptoms**
Major depressive disorder, recurrent, with psychotic features
Endogenous depression with psychotic symptoms
Recurrent severe episodes of major depression with mood-congruent psychotic symptoms
Major depression with mood-incongruent psychotic symptoms
Major depression with psychotic symptoms
Psychogenic depressive psychosis
Psychotic depression
Reactive depressive psychosis

F33.4 **Major depressive disorder, recurrent, in remission**
5th **F33.40** **Major depressive disorder, recurrent, in remission, unspecified**
F33.41 **in partial remission**
F33.42 **in full remission**

F33.8 **Other recurrent depressive disorders**
Recurrent brief depressive episodes

F33.9 **Major depressive disorder, recurrent, unspecified**
Monopolar depression NOS

F34 **PERSISTENT MOOD [AFFECTIVE] DISORDERS**
4th **F34.0** **Cyclothymic disorder**
Affective personality disorder
Cycloid personality
Cyclothymia
Cyclothymic personality

F34.1 **Dysthymic disorder**
Depressive neurosis
Depressive personality disorder
Dysthymia
Neurotic depression
Persistent anxiety depression
Persistent depressive disorder
Excludes2: anxiety depression (mild or not persistent) (F41.8)

F34.8 **Other persistent mood [affective] disorders**
5th **F34.81** **Disruptive mood dysregulation disorder**
F34.89 **Other specified persistent mood disorders**

F34.9 **Persistent mood [affective] disorder, unspecified**

F39 **UNSPECIFIED MOOD [AFFECTIVE] DISORDER**
✔ Affective psychosis NOS

(F40–F48) ANXIETY, DISSOCIATIVE, STRESS-RELATED, SOMATOFORM AND OTHER NONPSYCHOTIC MENTAL DISORDERS

F40 **PHOBIC ANXIETY DISORDERS**
4th **F40.0** **Agoraphobia**
5th **F40.00** **Agoraphobia, unspecified**
F40.01 **Agoraphobia with panic disorder**
Panic disorder with agoraphobia
Excludes1: panic disorder without agoraphobia (F41.0)
F40.02 **Agoraphobia without panic disorder**

F40.1 **Social phobias**
5th Anthropophobia
Social anxiety disorder
Social anxiety disorder of childhood
Social neurosis
F40.10 **Social phobia, unspecified**
F40.11 **Social phobia, generalized**

F40.8 **Other phobic anxiety disorders**
Phobic anxiety disorder of childhood

F40.9 **Phobic anxiety disorder, unspecified**
Phobia NOS
Phobic state NOS

F41 **OTHER ANXIETY DISORDERS**
4th *Excludes2:* anxiety in: acute stress reaction (F43.0)
transient adjustment reaction (F43.2)
neurasthenia (F48.8)

psychophysiologic disorders (F45.-)
separation anxiety (F93.0)

F41.0 **Panic disorder [episodic paroxysmal anxiety]**
Panic attack
Panic state
Excludes1: panic disorder with agoraphobia (F40.01)

F41.1 **Generalized anxiety disorder**
Anxiety neurosis
Anxiety reaction
Anxiety state
Overanxious disorder
Excludes2: neurasthenia (F48.8)

F41.3 **Other mixed anxiety disorders**

F41.8 **Other specified anxiety disorders**
Anxiety depression (mild or not persistent)
Anxiety hysteria
Mixed anxiety and depressive disorder

F41.9 **Anxiety disorder, unspecified**
Anxiety NOS

F42 **OBSESSIVE-COMPULSIVE DISORDER**
4th *Excludes2:* obsessive-compulsive personality (disorder) (F60.5)
obsessive-compulsive symptoms occurring in depression (F32–F33)
obsessive-compulsive symptoms occurring in schizophrenia (F20.-)

F42.2 **Mixed obsessional thoughts and acts**

F42.3 **Hoarding disorder**

F42.4 **Excoriation (skin-picking) disorder**
Excludes1: factitial dermatitis (L98.1)
other specified behavioral and emotional disorders with onset usually occurring in early childhood and adolescence (F98.8)

F42.8 **Other obsessive compulsive disorder**
Anancastic neurosis
Obsessive-compulsive neurosis

F42.9 **Obsessive-compulsive disorder, unspecified**

F43 **REACTION TO SEVERE STRESS, AND ADJUSTMENT DISORDERS**
4th **F43.0** **Acute stress reaction**
Acute crisis reaction
Acute reaction to stress
Combat and operational stress reaction
Combat fatigue
Crisis state
Psychic shock

F43.1 **Post-traumatic stress disorder (PTSD)**
5th Traumatic neurosis
F43.10 **Post-traumatic stress disorder, unspecified**
F43.11 **Post-traumatic stress disorder, acute**
F43.12 **Post-traumatic stress disorder, chronic**

F43.2 **Adjustment disorders**
5th Culture shock
Grief reaction
Hospitalism in children
Excludes2: separation anxiety disorder of childhood (F93.0)
F43.20 **Adjustment disorder, unspecified**
F43.21 **Adjustment disorder with depressed mood**
F43.22 **Adjustment disorder with anxiety**
F43.23 **Adjustment disorder with mixed anxiety and depressed mood**
F43.24 **Adjustment disorder with disturbance of conduct**
F43.25 **Adjustment disorder with mixed disturbance of emotions and conduct**
F43.29 **Adjustment disorder with other symptoms**

F43.8 **Other reactions to severe stress**
Other specified trauma and stressor-related disorder

F43.9 **Reaction to severe stress, unspecified**
Trauma and stressor-related disorder, NOS

F44 **DISSOCIATIVE AND CONVERSION DISORDERS**
4th *Includes:* conversion hysteria
conversion reaction
hysteria
hysterical psychosis
Excludes2: malingering [conscious simulation] (Z76.5)

4th 5th 6th 7th Additional Character Required   ✔ 3-character code

•=New Code   *Excludes1*—Not coded here, do not use together
▲=Revised Code   *Excludes2*—Not included here

F44.4 **Conversion disorder with motor symptom or deficit**
Conversion disorder with abnormal movement
Conversion disorder with speech symptoms
Conversion disorder with swallowing symptoms
Conversion disorder with weakness/paralysis
Psychogenic aphonia
Psychogenic dysphonia

F44.5 **Conversion disorder with seizures or convulsions**
Conversion disorder with attacks or seizures
Dissociative convulsions

F44.6 **Conversion disorder with sensory symptom or deficit**
Conversion disorder with anesthesia or sensory loss or with special sensory symptoms
Dissociative anesthesia and sensory loss
Psychogenic deafness

F44.7 **Conversion disorder with mixed symptom presentation**

F44.8 **Other dissociative and conversion disorders**
> **5th**   **F44.81**   **Dissociative identity disorder**
Multiple personality disorder
>   **F44.89**   **Other dissociative and conversion disorders**
Ganser's syndrome
Psychogenic confusion
Psychogenic twilight state
Trance and possession disorders

F44.9 **Dissociative and conversion disorder, unspecified**
Dissociative disorder NOS

F45 **SOMATOFORM DISORDERS**
> **4th**

   GUIDELINES

Pain disorders related to psychological factors
  Assign code F45.41, for pain that is exclusively related to psychological disorders. As indicated by the *Excludes1* note under category G89, a code from category G89 should not be assigned with code F45.41
  Code F45.42, Pain disorders with related psychological factors, should be used with a code from category G89, Pain, not elsewhere classified, if there is documentation of a psychological component for a patient with acute or chronic pain.
  See Chapter 6

Excludes2: dissociative and conversion disorders (F44.-)
  factitious disorders (F68.1-, F68.A)
  hair-plucking (F63.3)
  lalling (F80.0)
  lisping (F80.0)
  malingering [conscious simulation] (Z76.5)
  nail-biting (F98.8)
  psychological or behavioral factors associated with disorders or diseases classified elsewhere (F54)
  sexual dysfunction, not due to a substance or known physiological condition (F52.-)
  thumb-sucking (F98.8)
  tic disorders (in childhood and adolescence) (F95.-)
  Tourette's syndrome (F95.2)
  trichotillomania (F63.3)

F45.0 **Somatization disorder**
Briquet's disorder
Multiple psychosomatic disorders

F45.1 **Undifferentiated somatoform disorder**
Somatic symptom disorder
Undifferentiated psychosomatic disorder

F45.2 **Hypochondriacal disorders**
> **5th**   *Excludes2:* delusional dysmorphophobia (F22)
fixed delusions about bodily functions or shape (F22)
>   **F45.20**   **Hypochondriacal disorder, unspecified**
>   **F45.21**   **Hypochondriasis**
Hypochondriacal neurosis
Illness anxiety disorder
>   **F45.22**   **Body dysmorphic disorder**
Dysmorphophobia (nondelusional)
Nosophobia
>   **F45.29**   **Other hypochondriacal disorders**

F45.4 **Pain disorders related to psychological factors**
> **5th**   *Excludes1:* pain NOS (R52)

F45.41 **Pain disorder exclusively related to psychological factors**
Somatoform pain disorder (persistent)

F45.42 **Pain disorder with related psychological factors**
Code also associated acute or chronic pain (G89.-)

F45.8 **Other somatoform disorders**
Psychogenic dysmenorrhea
Psychogenic dysphagia, including 'globus hystericus'
Psychogenic pruritus
Psychogenic torticollis
Somatoform autonomic dysfunction
Teeth grinding
Excludes1: sleep related teeth grinding (G47.63)

F45.9 **Somatoform disorder, unspecified**
Psychosomatic disorder NOS

F48 **OTHER NONPSYCHOTIC MENTAL DISORDERS**
> **4th**   **F48.8**   **Other specified nonpsychotic mental disorders**
Dhat syndrome
Neurasthenia
Occupational neurosis, including writer's cramp
Psychasthenia
Psychasthenic neurosis
Psychogenic syncope

F48.9 **Nonpsychotic mental disorder, unspecified**
Neurosis NOS

(F50–F59) BEHAVIORAL SYNDROMES ASSOCIATED WITH PHYSIOLOGICAL DISTURBANCES AND PHYSICAL FACTORS

F50 **EATING DISORDERS**
> **4th**   *Excludes1:* anorexia NOS (R63.0)
feeding difficulties (R63.3)
polyphagia (R63.2)

Excludes2: feeding disorder in infancy or childhood (F98.2-)

F50.0 **Anorexia nervosa**
> **5th**   *Excludes1:* loss of appetite (R63.0)
psychogenic loss of appetite (F50.89)
>   **F50.00**   **Anorexia nervosa, unspecified**
>   **F50.01**   **Anorexia nervosa, restricting type**
>   **F50.02**   **Anorexia nervosa, binge eating/purging type**
Excludes1: bulimia nervosa (F50.2)

F50.2 **Bulimia nervosa**
Bulimia NOS
Hyperorexia nervosa
Excludes1: anorexia nervosa, binge eating/purging type (F50.02)

F50.8 **Other eating disorders**
> **5th**   **F50.81**   **Binge eating disorder**
>   **F50.82**   **Avoidant/restrictive food intake disorder**
>   **F50.89**   **Other specified eating disorder**
Pica in adults
Psychogenic loss of appetite
Excludes2: pica of infancy and childhood (F98.3)

F50.9 **Eating disorder, unspecified**
Atypical anorexia nervosa
Atypical bulimia nervosa | For picky eaters see R63.3 |
Feeding or eating disorder, unspecified
Other specified feeding disorder

F51 **SLEEP DISORDERS NOT DUE TO A SUBSTANCE OR KNOWN PHYSIOLOGICAL CONDITION**
> **4th**
Excludes2: organic sleep disorders (G47.-)

F51.0 **Insomnia not due to a substance or known physiological condition**
> **5th**
Excludes2: alcohol related insomnia
drug-related insomnia
insomnia NOS (G47.0-)
insomnia due to known physiological condition (G47.0-)
organic insomnia (G47.0-)
sleep deprivation (Z72.820)
>   **F51.01**   **Primary insomnia**
Idiopathic insomnia
>   **F51.02**   **Adjustment insomnia**

> **4th**   **5th**   **6th**   **7th**   Additional Character Required   ✔   3-character code

•=New Code   *Excludes1*—Not coded here, do not use together
▲=Revised Code   *Excludes2*—Not included here

F51.03 Paradoxical insomnia
F51.04 Psychophysiological insomnia
F51.05 Insomnia due to other mental disorder
Code also associated mental disorder
F51.09 Other insomnia not due to a substance or known physiological condition
F51.3 Sleepwalking [somnambulism]
Non-rapid eye movement sleep arousal disorders, sleepwalking type
F51.4 Sleep terrors [night terrors]
Non-rapid eye movement sleep arousal disorders, sleep terror type
F51.5 Nightmare disorder
Dream anxiety disorder
F51.8 Other sleep disorders not due to a substance or known physiological condition
F51.9 Sleep disorder not due to a substance or known physiological condition, unspecified
Emotional sleep disorder NOS

F54 ☑ **PSYCHOLOGICAL AND BEHAVIORAL FACTORS ASSOCIATED WITH DISORDERS OR DISEASES CLASSIFIED ELSEWHERE**
Psychological factors affecting physical conditions
Code first the associated physical disorder, such as:
asthma (J45.-)
dermatitis (L23-L25)
gastric ulcer (K25.-)
mucous colitis (K58.-)
ulcerative colitis (K51.-)
urticaria (L50.-)
Excludes2: tension-type headache (G44.2)

F55 4th **ABUSE OF NON-PSYCHOACTIVE SUBSTANCES**
Excludes2: abuse of psychoactive substances (F10-F19)
F55.0 Abuse of antacids
F55.1 Abuse of herbal or folk remedies
F55.2 Abuse of laxatives
F55.3 Abuse of steroids or hormones
F55.4 Abuse of vitamins
F55.8 Abuse of other non-psychoactive substances

F59 ☑ **UNSPECIFIED BEHAVIORAL SYNDROMES ASSOCIATED WITH PHYSIOLOGICAL DISTURBANCES AND PHYSICAL FACTORS**
Psychogenic physiological dysfunction NOS

(F60–F69) DISORDERS OF ADULT PERSONALITY AND BEHAVIOR

F60 **SPECIFIC PERSONALITY DISORDERS**
4th **F60.0** Paranoid personality disorder
Expansive paranoid personality (disorder)
Fanatic personality (disorder)
Paranoid personality (disorder)
Sensitive paranoid personality (disorder)
Excludes2: paranoia (F22)
paranoid schizophrenia (F20.0)
F60.1 Schizoid personality disorder
Excludes2: Asperger's syndrome (F84.5)
delusional disorder (F22)
schizoid disorder of childhood (F84.5)
schizophrenia (F20.-)
schizotypal disorder (F21)
F60.2 Antisocial personality disorder
Dissocial personality disorder
Excludes1: conduct disorders (F91.-)
Excludes2: borderline personality disorder (F60.3)
F60.3 Borderline personality disorder
Aggressive personality (disorder)
Explosive personality (disorder)
Excludes2: antisocial personality disorder (F60.2)
F60.4 Histrionic personality disorder
F60.5 Obsessive-compulsive personality disorder
Excludes2: obsessive-compulsive disorder (F42.-)

F60.6 Avoidant personality disorder
Anxious personality disorder
F60.9 Personality disorder, unspecified
Character disorder NOS
Character neurosis NOS
Pathological personality NOS

F63 4th **IMPULSE DISORDERS**
Excludes2: habitual excessive use of alcohol or psychoactive substances (F10–F19)
impulse disorders involving sexual behavior (F65.-)
F63.0 Pathological gambling
Compulsive gambling
Excludes1: gambling and betting NOS (Z72.6)
Excludes2: excessive gambling by manic patients (F30, F31)
gambling in antisocial personality disorder (F60.2)
F63.1 Pyromania
Pathological fire-setting
Excludes2: fire-setting (by) (in):
adult with antisocial personality disorder (F60.2)
alcohol or psychoactive substance intoxication (F10–F19)
conduct disorders (F91.-)
mental disorders due to known physiological condition (F01–F09)
schizophrenia (F20.-)
F63.2 Kleptomania
Pathological stealing
Excludes1: shoplifting as the reason for observation for suspected mental disorder (Z03.8)
Excludes2: depressive disorder with stealing (F31–F33)
stealing due to underlying mental condition-code to mental condition
stealing in mental disorders due to known physiological condition (F01–F09)
F63.3 Trichotillomania
Hair plucking
Excludes2: other stereotyped movement disorder (F98.4)
F63.8 Other impulse disorders
5th **F63.81** Intermittent explosive disorder
F63.89 Other impulse disorders
F63.9 Impulse disorder, unspecified
Impulse control disorder NOS

F64 4th **GENDER IDENTITY DISORDERS**
F64.0 Transsexualism
Gender identity disorder in adolescence and adulthood
Gender dysphoria in adolescents and adults
F64.1 Dual role transvestism
Use additional code to identify sex reassignment status (Z87.890)
Excludes1: gender identity disorder in childhood (F64.2)
Excludes2: fetishistic transvestism (F65.1)
F64.2 Gender identity disorder of childhood
Gender dysphoria in children
Excludes1: gender identity disorder in adolescence and adulthood (F64.0)
Excludes2: sexual maturation disorder (F66)
F64.8 Other gender identity disorders
F64.9 Gender identity disorder, unspecified
Gender dysphoria, unspecified
Gender-role disorder NOS

F66 ☑ **OTHER SEXUAL DISORDERS**
Sexual maturation disorder
Sexual relationship disorder

(F70–F79) INTELLECTUAL DISABILITIES

Code first any associated physical or developmental disorders
Excludes1: borderline intellectual functioning, IQ above 70 to 84 (R41.83)

F70 ☑ **MILD INTELLECTUAL DISABILITIES**
IQ level 50–55 to approximately 70
Mild mental subnormality

F71 ☑ **MODERATE INTELLECTUAL DISABILITIES**
IQ level 35–40 to 50–55
Moderate mental subnormality

4th 5th 6th 7th Additional Character Required   ☑ 3-character code

•=New Code   *Excludes1*—Not coded here, do not use together
▲=Revised Code   *Excludes2*—Not included here

CHAPTER 5. MENTAL, BEHAVIORAL, AND NEURODEVELOPMENTAL DISORDERS (F51.03–F71)

F72   SEVERE INTELLECTUAL DISABILITIES
✔   IQ 20–25 to 35–40
Severe mental subnormality

F73   PROFOUND INTELLECTUAL DISABILITIES
✔   IQ level below 20–25
Profound mental subnormality

F78   OTHER INTELLECTUAL DISABILITIES
✔

F79   UNSPECIFIED INTELLECTUAL DISABILITIES
✔   Mental deficiency NOS
Mental subnormality NOS

(F80–F89) PERVASIVE AND SPECIFIC DEVELOPMENTAL DISORDERS

F80   SPECIFIC DEVELOPMENTAL DISORDERS OF SPEECH
`4th`   **AND LANGUAGE**

F80.0   **Phonological disorder**
Dyslalia
Functional speech articulation disorder
Lalling
Lisping
Phonological developmental disorder
Speech articulation developmental disorder
Speech-sound disorder
Excludes1: speech articulation impairment due to aphasia NOS (R47.01)
speech articulation impairment due to apraxia (R48.2)
Excludes2: speech articulation impairment due to hearing loss (F80.4)
speech articulation impairment due to intellectual disabilities (F70–F79)
speech articulation impairment with expressive language developmental disorder (F80.1)
speech articulation impairment with mixed receptive expressive language developmental disorder (F80.2)

F80.1   **Expressive language disorder**
Developmental dysphasia or aphasia, expressive type
Excludes1: mixed receptive-expressive language disorder (F80.2)
dysphasia and aphasia NOS (R47.-)
Excludes2: acquired aphasia with epilepsy [Landau-Kleffner] (G40.80-)
selective mutism (F94.0)
intellectual disabilities (F70–F79)
pervasive developmental disorders (F84.-)

F80.2   **Mixed receptive-expressive language disorder**
Developmental dysphasia or aphasia, receptive type
Developmental Wernicke's aphasia
Excludes1: central auditory processing disorder (H93.25)
dysphasia or aphasia NOS (R47.-)
expressive language disorder (F80.1)
expressive type dysphasia or aphasia (F80.1)
word deafness (H93.25)
Excludes2: acquired aphasia with epilepsy [Landau-Kleffner] (G40.80-)
pervasive developmental disorders (F84.-)
selective mutism (F94.0)
intellectual disabilities (F70–F79)

F80.4   **Speech and language development delay due to hearing loss**
Code also type of hearing loss (H90.-, H91.-)

F80.8   **Other developmental disorders of speech and language**
`5th`   **F80.81   Childhood onset fluency disorder**
Cluttering NOS
Stuttering NOS
Excludes1: adult onset fluency disorder (F98.5)
fluency disorder in conditions classified elsewhere (R47.82)
fluency disorder (stuttering) following cerebrovascular disease (I69. with final characters -23)

F80.82   Social pragmatic communication disorder
Excludes1: Asperger's syndrome (F84.5)
autistic disorder (F84.0)

F80.89   Other developmental disorders of speech and language

F80.9   **Developmental disorder of speech and language, unspecified**
Communication disorder NOS
Language disorder NOS

F81   SPECIFIC DEVELOPMENTAL DISORDERS OF
`4th`   **SCHOLASTIC SKILLS**

F81.0   **Specific reading disorder**
'Backward reading'
Developmental dyslexia
Specific learning disorder, with impairment in reading
Excludes1: alexia NOS (R48.0)
dyslexia NOS (R48.0)

F81.2   **Mathematics disorder**
Developmental acalculia
Developmental arithmetical disorder
Developmental Gerstmann's syndrome
Specific learning disorder, with impairment in mathematics
Excludes1: acalculia NOS (R48.8)
Excludes2: arithmetical difficulties associated with a reading disorder (F81.0)
arithmetical difficulties associated with a spelling disorder (F81.81)
arithmetical difficulties due to inadequate teaching (Z55.8)

F81.8   **Other developmental disorders of scholastic skills**
`5th`   **F81.81   Disorder of written expression**
Specific spelling disorder
Specific learning disorder, with impairment in written expression

F81.89   Other developmental disorders of scholastic skills

F81.9   **Developmental disorder of scholastic skills, unspecified**
Knowledge acquisition disability NOS
Learning disability NOS
Learning disorder NOS

F82   SPECIFIC DEVELOPMENTAL DISORDER OF
✔   **MOTOR FUNCTION**
Clumsy child syndrome
Developmental coordination disorder
Developmental dyspraxia
Excludes1: abnormalities of gait and mobility (R26.-)
lack of coordination (R27.-)
Excludes2: lack of coordination secondary to intellectual disabilities (F70–F79)

F84   PERVASIVE DEVELOPMENTAL DISORDERS
`4th`   **Use additional code** to identify any associated medical condition and intellectual disabilities.

F84.0   **Autistic disorder**
Autism spectrum disorder
Infantile autism
Infantile psychosis
Kanner's syndrome
Excludes1: Asperger's syndrome (F84.5)

F84.2   **Rett's syndrome**
Excludes1: Asperger's syndrome (F84.5)
Autistic disorder (F84.0)
Other childhood disintegrative disorder (F84.3)

F84.3   **Other childhood disintegrative disorder**
Dementia infantilis
Disintegrative psychosis
Heller's syndrome
Symbiotic psychosis
Use additional code to identify any associated neurological condition.
Excludes1: Asperger's syndrome (F84.5)
Autistic disorder (F84.0)
Rett's syndrome (F84.2)

F84.5   **Asperger's syndrome**
Asperger's disorder
Autistic psychopathy
Schizoid disorder of childhood

`4th` `5th` `6th` `7th`   Additional Character Required   ✔   3-character code

•=New Code
▲=Revised Code

Excludes1—Not coded here, do not use together
Excludes2—Not included here

CHAPTER 5. MENTAL, BEHAVIORAL, AND NEURODEVELOPMENTAL DISORDERS   (F72–F84.5)

F84.8   Other pervasive developmental disorders
Overactive disorder associated with intellectual disabilities and stereotyped movements

F84.9   Pervasive developmental disorder, unspecified
Atypical autism

F88   OTHER DISORDERS OF PSYCHOLOGICAL DEVELOPMENT ✔
Developmental agnosia
Global developmental delay
Other specified neurodevelopmental disorder

F89   UNSPECIFIED DISORDER OF PSYCHOLOGICAL DEVELOPMENT ✔
Developmental disorder NOS
Neurodevelopmental disorder NOS

(F90–F98) BEHAVIORAL AND EMOTIONAL DISORDERS WITH ONSET USUALLY OCCURRING IN CHILDHOOD AND ADOLESCENCE

Note: Codes within categories F90–F98 may be used regardless of the age of a patient. These disorders generally have onset within the childhood or adolescent years, but may continue throughout life or not be diagnosed until adulthood

F90   ATTENTION-DEFICIT HYPERACTIVITY DISORDERS `4th`
Includes: attention deficit disorder with hyperactivity
    attention deficit syndrome with hyperactivity
Excludes2: anxiety disorders (F40.-, F41.-)
    mood [affective] disorders (F30–F39)
    pervasive developmental disorders (F84.-)
    schizophrenia (F20.-)

F90.0   Attention-deficit hyperactivity disorder, predominantly inattentive type
ADD without hyperactivity

F90.1   Attention-deficit hyperactivity disorder, predominantly hyperactive type

F90.2   Attention-deficit hyperactivity disorder, combined type

F90.8   Attention-deficit hyperactivity disorder, other type

F90.9   Attention-deficit hyperactivity disorder, unspecified type
Attention-deficit hyperactivity disorder of childhood or adolescence NOS
Attention-deficit hyperactivity disorder NOS

F91   CONDUCT DISORDERS `4th`
Excludes1: antisocial behavior (Z72.81-)
    antisocial personality disorder (F60.2)
Excludes2: conduct problems associated with attention-deficit hyperactivity disorder (F90.-)
    mood [affective] disorders (F30–F39)
    pervasive developmental disorders (F84.-)
    schizophrenia (F20.-)

F91.0   Conduct disorder confined to family context

F91.1   Conduct disorder, childhood-onset type
Unsocialized conduct disorder
Conduct disorder, solitary aggressive type
Unsocialized aggressive disorder

F91.2   Conduct disorder, adolescent-onset type
Socialized conduct disorder
Conduct disorder, group type

F91.3   Oppositional defiant disorder

F91.8   Other conduct disorders
Other specified conduct disorder
Other specified disruptive disorder

F91.9   Conduct disorder, unspecified
Behavioral disorder NOS
Conduct disorder NOS
Disruptive behavior disorder NOS

F93   EMOTIONAL DISORDERS WITH ONSET SPECIFIC TO CHILDHOOD `4th`

F93.0   Separation anxiety disorder of childhood
Excludes2: mood [affective] disorders (F30–F39)
    nonpsychotic mental disorders (F40–F48)
    phobic anxiety disorder of childhood (F40.8)
    social phobia (F40.1)

F93.8   Other childhood emotional disorders
Identity disorder
Excludes2: gender identity disorder of childhood (F64.2)

F93.9   Childhood emotional disorder, unspecified

F94   DISORDERS OF SOCIAL FUNCTIONING WITH ONSET SPECIFIC TO CHILDHOOD AND ADOLESCENCE `4th`

F94.0   Selective mutism
Elective mutism
Excludes2: pervasive developmental disorders (F84.-)
    schizophrenia (F20.-)
    specific developmental disorders of speech and language (F80.-)
    transient mutism as part of separation anxiety in young children (F93.0)

F94.1   Reactive attachment disorder of childhood
Use additional code to identify any associated failure to thrive or growth retardation
Excludes1: disinhibited attachment disorder of childhood (F94.2)
    normal variation in pattern of selective attachment
Excludes2: Asperger's syndrome (F84.5)
    maltreatment syndromes (T74.-)
    sexual or physical abuse in childhood, resulting in psychosocial problems (Z62.81-)

F94.2   Disinhibited attachment disorder of childhood
Affectionless psychopathy
Institutional syndrome
Excludes1: reactive attachment disorder of childhood (F94.1)
Excludes2: Asperger's syndrome (F84.5)
    attention-deficit hyperactivity disorders (F90.-)
    hospitalism in children (F43.2-)

F94.8   Other childhood disorders of social functioning

F94.9   Childhood disorder of social functioning, unspecified

F95   TIC DISORDER `4th`

F95.0   Transient tic disorder
Provisional tic disorder

F95.1   Chronic motor or vocal tic disorder

F95.2   Tourette's disorder
Combined vocal and multiple motor tic disorder [de la Tourette]
Tourette's syndrome

F95.8   Other tic disorders

F95.9   Tic disorder, unspecified
Tic NOS

F98   OTHER BEHAVIORAL AND EMOTIONAL DISORDERS WITH ONSET USUALLY OCCURRING IN CHILDHOOD AND ADOLESCENCE `4th`
Excludes2: breath-holding spells (R06.89)
    gender identity disorder of childhood (F64.2)
    Kleine-Levin syndrome (G47.13)
    obsessive-compulsive disorder (F42.-)
    sleep disorders not due to a substance or known physiological condition (F51.-)

F98.0   Enuresis not due to a substance or known physiological condition
Enuresis (primary) (secondary) of nonorganic origin
Functional enuresis
Psychogenic enuresis
Urinary incontinence of nonorganic origin
Excludes1: enuresis NOS (R32)

F98.1   Encopresis not due to a substance or known physiological condition
Functional encopresis
Incontinence of feces of nonorganic origin
Psychogenic encopresis
Use additional code to identify the cause of any coexisting constipation.
Excludes1: encopresis NOS (R15.-)

F98.2   Other feeding disorders of infancy and childhood `5th`
Excludes1: feeding difficulties (R63.3)
Excludes2: anorexia nervosa and other eating disorders (F50.-)
    feeding problems of newborn (P92.-)
    pica of infancy or childhood (F98.3)

F98.21   Rumination disorder of infancy

`4th` `5th` `6th` `7th` Additional Character Required   ✔ 3-character code

•=New Code   *Excludes1*—Not coded here, do not use together
▲=Revised Code   *Excludes2*—Not included here

F98.29   **Other feeding disorders of infancy and early childhood**

F98.3   **Pica of infancy and childhood**

F98.4   **Stereotyped movement disorders**

Stereotype/habit disorder

Excludes1: abnormal involuntary movements (R25.-)

Excludes2: compulsions in obsessive-compulsive disorder (F42.-)
- hair plucking (F63.3)
- movement disorders of organic origin (G20–G25)
- nail-biting (F98.8)
- nose-picking (F98.8)
- stereotypies that are part of a broader psychiatric condition (F01–F95)
- thumb-sucking (F98.8)
- tic disorders (F95.-)
- trichotillomania (F63.3)

F98.8   **Other specified behavioral and emotional disorders with onset usually occurring in childhood and adolescence**

Excessive masturbation Nail-biting

Nose-picking

Thumb-sucking

F98.9   **Unspecified behavioral and emotional disorders with onset usually occurring in childhood and adolescence**

(F99) UNSPECIFIED MENTAL DISORDER

F99   **MENTAL DISORDER, NOT OTHERWISE SPECIFIED**

☑ Mental illness NOS

Excludes1: unspecified mental disorder due to known physiological condition (F09)

| 4th | 5th | 6th | 7th | Additional Character Required | ☑ 3-character code | •=New Code   *Excludes1*—Not coded here, do not use together |
| ▲=Revised Code   *Excludes2*—Not included here |

PEDIATRIC ICD-10-CM 2021: A MANUAL FOR PROVIDER-BASED CODING   181

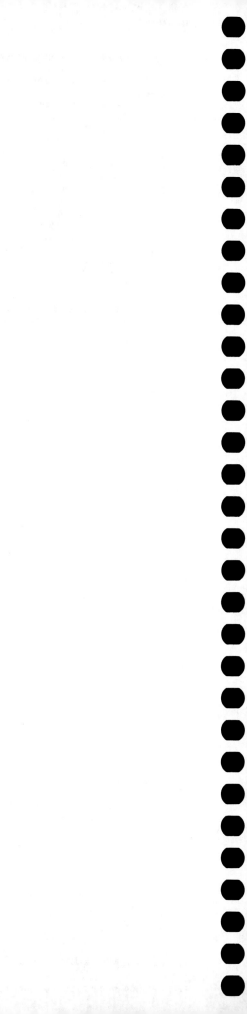

Chapter 6. Diseases of the nervous system (G00–G99)

GUIDELINES

Dominant/nondominant side

Refer to category G81 and subcategories G83.1 and G83.2.

Pain

Refer to category G89.

Excludes2: certain conditions originating in the perinatal period (P04–P96)
    certain infectious and parasitic diseases (A00–B99)
    complications of pregnancy, childbirth and the puerperium (O00–O9A)
    congenital malformations, deformations, and chromosomal abnormalities
      (Q00–Q99)
    endocrine, nutritional and metabolic diseases (E00–E88)
    injury, poisoning and certain other consequences of external causes (S00–T88)
    neoplasms (C00–D49)
    symptoms, signs and abnormal clinical and laboratory findings, not elsewhere
      classified (R00–R94)

(G00–G09) INFLAMMATORY DISEASES OF THE CENTRAL NERVOUS SYSTEM

G00   **BACTERIAL MENINGITIS, NOT ELSEWHERE CLASSIFIED**
`4th`   ***Includes:*** bacterial arachnoiditis
    bacterial leptomeningitis
    bacterial meningitis
    bacterial pachymeningitis
  Excludes1: bacterial meningoencephalitis (G04.2)
    bacterial meningomyelitis (G04.2)

G00.0   **Hemophilus meningitis**
    Meningitis due to H. influenzae

G00.1   **Pneumococcal meningitis**
    Meningitis due to streptococcus pneumoniae

G00.2   **Streptococcal meningitis**
    Use additional code to further identify organism (B95.0–B95.5)

G00.3   **Staphylococcal meningitis**
    Use additional code to further identify organism (B95.61–B95.8)

G00.8   **Other bacterial meningitis**
    Meningitis due to E. coli
    Meningitis due to Friedländer's bacillus
    Meningitis due to Klebsiella
    Use additional code to further identify organism (B96.-)

G00.9   **Bacterial meningitis, unspecified**
    Meningitis due to gram-negative bacteria, unspecified
    Purulent meningitis NOS
    Pyogenic meningitis NOS
    Suppurative meningitis NOS

G01   **MENINGITIS IN BACTERIAL DISEASES CLASSIFIED ELSEWHERE**
`✓`   **Code first** underlying disease
  Excludes1: meningitis (in): gonococcal (A54.81)
    leptospirosis (A27.81)
    listeriosis (A32.11)
    Lyme disease (A69.21)
    meningococcal (A39.0)
    neurosyphilis (A52.13)
    tuberculosis (A17.0)
    meningoencephalitis and meningomyelitis in bacterial diseases
      classified elsewhere (G05)

G02   **MENINGITIS IN OTHER INFECTIOUS AND PARASITIC DISEASES CLASSIFIED ELSEWHERE**
`✓`   **Code first** underlying disease, such as: African trypanosomiasis (B56.-)
    poliovirus infection (A80.-)
  Excludes1: candidal meningitis (B37.5)
    coccidioidomycosis meningitis (B38.4)
    cryptococcal meningitis (B45.1)
    herpesviral [herpes simplex] meningitis (B00.3)
    infectious mononucleosis complicated by meningitis (B27.- with 4th
      character 2)

    measles complicated by meningitis (B05.1)
    meningoencephalitis and meningomyelitis in other infectious and
    parasitic diseases classified elsewhere (G05)
    mumps meningitis (B26.1)
    rubella meningitis (B06.02)
    varicella [chickenpox] meningitis (B01.0)
    zoster meningitis (B02.1)

G03   **MENINGITIS DUE TO OTHER AND UNSPECIFIED CAUSES**
`4th`   ***Includes:*** arachnoiditis NOS
    leptomeningitis NOS
    meningitis NOS
    pachymeningitis NOS
  Excludes1: meningoencephalitis (G04.-)
    meningomyelitis (G04.-)

G03.0   **Nonpyogenic meningitis**
    Aseptic meningitis
    Nonbacterial meningitis

G03.1   **Chronic meningitis**

G03.2   **Benign recurrent meningitis [Mollaret]**

G03.8   **Meningitis due to other specified causes**

G03.9   **Meningitis, unspecified**
    Arachnoiditis (spinal) NOS

G04   **ENCEPHALITIS, MYELITIS AND ENCEPHALOMYELITIS**
`4th`   ***Includes:*** acute ascending myelitis
    meningoencephalitis
    meningomyelitis
  Excludes1: encephalopathy NOS (G93.40)
  Excludes2: acute transverse myelitis (G37.3-)
    alcoholic encephalopathy (G31.2)
    benign myalgic encephalomyelitis (G93.3)
    multiple sclerosis (G35)
    subacute necrotizing myelitis (G37.4)
    toxic encephalitis (G92)
    toxic encephalopathy (G92)

G04.0   **Acute disseminated encephalitis and encephalomyelitis**
`5th`   **(ADEM)**
    Excludes1: acute necrotizing hemorrhagic encephalopathy (G04.3-)
      other noninfectious acute disseminated encephalomyelitis
      (noninfectious ADEM) (G04.81)

    G04.00   **Acute disseminated encephalitis and
        encephalomyelitis, unspecified**

    G04.01   **Postinfectious acute disseminated encephalitis and
        encephalomyelitis (postinfectious ADEM)**
        Excludes1: post chickenpox encephalitis (B01.1)
          post measles encephalitis (B05.0)
          post measles myelitis (B05.1)

    G04.02   **Postimmunization acute disseminated encephalitis,
        myelitis and encephalomyelitis**
        Encephalitis, post immunization
        Encephalomyelitis, post immunization
        Use additional code to identify the vaccine (T50.A-,
          T50.B-, T50.Z-)

G04.2   **Bacterial meningoencephalitis and meningomyelitis, not
    elsewhere classified**

G04.3   **Acute necrotizing hemorrhagic encephalopathy**
`5th`   ***Excludes1:*** acute disseminated encephalitis and encephalomyelitis
      (G04.0-)

    G04.30   **Acute necrotizing hemorrhagic encephalopathy,
        unspecified**

    G04.31   **Postinfectious acute necrotizing hemorrhagic
        encephalopathy**

    G04.32   **Postimmunization acute necrotizing hemorrhagic
        encephalopathy**
        Use additional code to identify the vaccine (T50.A-,
          T50.B-, T50.Z-)

    G04.39   **Other acute necrotizing hemorrhagic encephalopathy**
        Code also underlying etiology, if applicable

G04.8   **Other encephalitis, myelitis and encephalomyelitis**
`5th`   **Code also** any associated seizure (G40.-, R56.9)

`4th` `5th` `6th` `7th`   Additional Character Required   `✓`   3-character code

•=New Code   ***Excludes1***—Not coded here, do not use together
▲=Revised Code   ***Excludes2***—Not included here

CHAPTER 6. DISEASES OF THE NERVOUS SYSTEM   (G04.81–G13.8)

G04.81 Other encephalitis and encephalomyelitis
Noninfectious acute disseminated encephalomyelitis (noninfectious ADEM)
G04.89 Other myelitis
G04.9 Encephalitis, myelitis and encephalomyelitis, unspecified
  5th   **G04.90 Encephalitis and encephalomyelitis, unspecified**
Ventriculitis (cerebral) NOS
G04.91 Myelitis, unspecified

G05   **ENCEPHALITIS, MYELITIS AND ENCEPHALOMYELITIS IN**
4th   **DISEASES CLASSIFIED ELSEWHERE**
Code first underlying disease, such as:
  HIV disease (B20)
  poliovirus (A80.-)
  suppurative otitis media (H66.01–H66.4)
  trichinellosis (B75)
Excludes1:
  adenoviral encephalitis, myelitis and encephalomyelitis (A85.1)
  congenital toxoplasmosis encephalitis, myelitis and encephalomyelitis (P37.1)
  cytomegaloviral encephalitis, myelitis and encephalomyelitis (B25.8)
  encephalitis, myelitis and encephalomyelitis (in) measles (B05.0)
  encephalitis, myelitis and encephalomyelitis (in) SLE (M32.19)
  enteroviral encephalitis, myelitis and encephalomyelitis (A85.0)
  eosinophilic meningoencephalitis (B83.2)
  herpesviral [herpes simplex] encephalitis, myelitis and encephalomyelitis (B00.4)
  listerial encephalitis, myelitis and encephalomyelitis (A32.12)
  meningococcal encephalitis, myelitis and encephalomyelitis (A39.81)
  mumps encephalitis, myelitis and encephalomyelitis (B26.2)
  postchickenpox encephalitis, myelitis and encephalomyelitis (B01.1-)
  rubella encephalitis, myelitis and encephalomyelitis (B06.01)
  toxoplasmosis encephalitis, myelitis and encephalomyelitis (B58.2)
  zoster encephalitis, myelitis and encephalomyelitis (B02.0)
G05.3 Encephalitis and encephalomyelitis in diseases classified elsewhere
Meningoencephalitis in diseases classified elsewhere
G05.4 Myelitis in diseases classified elsewhere
Meningomyelitis in diseases classified elsewhere

G06   **INTRACRANIAL AND INTRASPINAL ABSCESS AND**
4th   **GRANULOMA**
Use additional code (B95–B97) to identify infectious agent.
G06.0 Intracranial abscess and granuloma
Brain [any part] abscess (embolic)
Cerebellar abscess (embolic)
Cerebral abscess (embolic)
Intracranial epidural abscess or granuloma
Intracranial extradural abscess or granuloma
Intracranial subdural abscess or granuloma
Otogenic abscess (embolic)
Excludes1: tuberculous intracranial abscess and granuloma (A17.81)
G06.1 Intraspinal abscess and granuloma
Abscess (embolic) of spinal cord [any part]
Intraspinal epidural abscess or granuloma
Intraspinal extradural abscess or granuloma
Intraspinal subdural abscess or granuloma
Excludes1: tuberculous intraspinal abscess and granuloma (A17.81)
G06.2 Extradural and subdural abscess, unspecified

G08   **INTRACRANIAL AND INTRASPINAL PHLEBITIS AND**
✔   **THROMBOPHLEBITIS**
Septic embolism of intracranial or intraspinal venous sinuses and veins
Septic endophlebitis of intracranial or intraspinal venous sinuses and veins
Septic phlebitis of intracranial or intraspinal venous sinuses and veins
Septic thrombophlebitis of intracranial or intraspinal venous sinuses and veins
Septic thrombosis of intracranial or intraspinal venous sinuses and veins
Excludes1: intracranial phlebitis and thrombophlebitis complicating:
  abortion, ectopic or molar pregnancy (O00–O07, O08.7)
  pregnancy, childbirth and the puerperium (O22.5, O87.3)
  nonpyogenic intracranial phlebitis and thrombophlebitis (I67.6)

Excludes2: intracranial phlebitis and thrombophlebitis complicating nonpyogenic intraspinal phlebitis and thrombophlebitis (G95.1)

G09   **SEQUELAE OF INFLAMMATORY DISEASES OF CENTRAL**
✔   **NERVOUS SYSTEM**
Note: Category G09 is to be used to indicate conditions whose primary classification is to G00-G08 as the cause of sequelae, themselves classifiable elsewhere. The 'sequelae' include conditions specified as residuals.
Code first condition resulting from (sequela) of inflammatory diseases of central nervous system

(G10–G14) SYSTEMIC ATROPHIES PRIMARILY AFFECTING THE CENTRAL NERVOUS SYSTEM

G11   **HEREDITARY ATAXIA**
4th   **Excludes2:** cerebral palsy (G80.-)
  hereditary and idiopathic neuropathy (G60.-)
  metabolic disorders (E70–E88)
G11.0 Congenital nonprogressive ataxia
▲**G11.1 Early-onset cerebellar ataxia**
  5th   •**G11.10 Early-onset cerebellar ataxia, unspecified**
    •**G11.11 Friedreich ataxia**
      Autosomal recessive Friedreich ataxia
      Friedreich ataxia with retained reflexes
    •**G11.19 Other early-onset cerebellar ataxia**
      Early-onset cerebellar ataxia with essential tremor
      Early-onset cerebellar ataxia with myoclonus [Hunt's ataxia]
      Early-onset cerebellar ataxia with retained tendon reflexes
      X-linked recessive spinocerebellar ataxia
G11.2 Late-onset cerebellar ataxia
G11.3 Cerebellar ataxia with defective DNA repair
Ataxia telangiectasia [Louis-Bar]
Excludes2: Cockayne's syndrome (Q87.19)
  other disorders of purine and pyrimidine metabolism (E79.-)
  xeroderma pigmentosum (Q82.1)
G11.9 Hereditary ataxia, unspecified
Hereditary cerebellar ataxia NOS
Hereditary cerebellar degeneration
Hereditary cerebellar disease
Hereditary cerebellar syndrome

G12   **SPINAL MUSCULAR ATROPHY AND RELATED**
4th   **SYNDROMES**
G12.0 Infantile spinal muscular atrophy, type I [Werdnig-Hoffman]
G12.2 Motor neuron disease
  5th   **G12.20 Motor neuron disease, unspecified**
    G12.21 Amyotrophic lateral sclerosis
    G12.22 Progressive bulbar palsy
    G12.25 Progressive spinal muscle atrophy
    G12.29 Other motor neuron disease
G12.9 Spinal muscular atrophy, unspecified

G13   **SYSTEMIC ATROPHIES PRIMARILY AFFECTING**
4th   **CENTRAL NERVOUS SYSTEM IN DISEASES CLASSIFIED ELSEWHERE**
G13.0 Paraneoplastic neuromyopathy and neuropathy
Carcinomatous neuromyopathy
Sensorial paraneoplastic neuropathy [Denny Brown]
Code first underlying neoplasm (C00-D49)
G13.1 Other systemic atrophy primarily affecting central nervous system in neoplastic disease
Paraneoplastic limbic encephalopathy
Code first underlying neoplasm (C00-D49)
G13.2 Systemic atrophy primarily affecting the central nervous system in myxedema
Code first underlying disease, such as:
  hypothyroidism (E03.-)
  myxedematous congenital iodine deficiency (E00.1)
G13.8 Systemic atrophy primarily affecting central nervous system in other diseases classified elsewhere
Code first underlying disease

4th   **5th**   **6th**   **7th**   Additional Character Required   **✔**   3-character code   •=New Code   ▲=Revised Code   **Excludes1**—Not coded here, do not use together   **Excludes2**—Not included here

(G20–G26) EXTRAPYRAMIDAL AND MOVEMENT DISORDERS

G24   **DYSTONIA**
4th
Includes: dyskinesia
Excludes2: athetoid cerebral palsy (G80.3)

G24.0   Drug induced dystonia
5th   **Use additional code** for adverse effect, if applicable, to identify drug (T36-T50 with fifth or sixth character 5)

     G24.01   Drug induced subacute dyskinesia
          Drug induced blepharospasm
          Drug induced orofacial dyskinesia
          Neuroleptic induced tardive dyskinesia
          Tardive dyskinesia

     G24.02   Drug induced acute dystonia
          Acute dystonic reaction to drugs
          Neuroleptic induced acute dystonia

     G24.09   Other drug induced dystonia

G24.1   Genetic torsion dystonia
     Dystonia deformans progressiva
     Dystonia musculorum deformans
     Familial torsion dystonia
     Idiopathic familial dystonia
     Idiopathic (torsion) dystonia NOS
     (Schwalbe-) Ziehen-Oppenheim disease

G24.2   Idiopathic nonfamilial dystonia

G24.8   Other dystonia
     Acquired torsion dystonia NOS

G24.9   Dystonia, unspecified
     Dyskinesia NOS

G25   **OTHER EXTRAPYRAMIDAL AND MOVEMENT DISORDERS**
4th
Excludes2: sleep related movement disorders (G47.6-)

G25.0   Essential tremor
     Familial tremor
     Excludes1: tremor NOS (R25.1)

G25.1   Drug-induced tremor
     Use additional code for adverse effect, if applicable, to identify drug (T36-T50 with fifth or sixth character 5)

G25.2   Other specified forms of tremor
     Intention tremor

G25.3   Myoclonus
     Drug-induced myoclonus
     Palatal myoclonus
     Use additional code for adverse effect, if applicable, to identify drug (T36–T50 with fifth or sixth character 5)
     Excludes1: facial myokymia (G51.4)
         myoclonic epilepsy (G40.-)

G25.4   Drug-induced chorea
     Use additional code for adverse effect, if applicable, to identify drug (T36-T50 with fifth or sixth character 5)

G25.5   Other chorea
     Chorea NOS
     Excludes1: chorea NOS with heart involvement (I02.-)
         Huntington's chorea (G10)

G25.6   Drug induced tics and other tics of organic origin
5th   **G25.61   Drug induced tics**
         Use additional code for adverse effect, if applicable, to identify drug (T36-T50 with fifth or sixth character 5)

     G25.69   Other tics of organic origin
         Excludes1: habit spasm (F95.9)
           tic NOS (F95.9)
           Tourette's syndrome (F95.2)

G25.7   Other and unspecified drug induced movement disorders
5th   **Use additional code** for adverse effect, if applicable, to identify drug (T36-T50 with fifth or sixth character 5)

     G25.70   Drug induced movement disorder, unspecified
     G25.71   Drug induced akathisia
         Drug induced acathisia
         Neuroleptic induced acute akathisia
         Tardive akathisia

     G25.79   Other drug induced movement disorders

G25.8   Other specified extrapyramidal and movement disorders
5th   **G25.81   Restless legs syndrome**
     G25.83   Benign shuddering attacks

     G25.89   Other specified extrapyramidal and movement disorders

G25.9   Extrapyramidal and movement disorder, unspecified

(G30–G32) OTHER DEGENERATIVE DISEASES OF THE NERVOUS SYSTEM

G31   **OTHER DEGENERATIVE DISEASES OF NERVOUS**
4th   **SYSTEM, NOT ELSEWHERE CLASSIFIED**
For codes G31.0-G31.83, G31.85-G31.9, **use additional code** to identify:
     dementia with behavioral disturbance (F02.81)
     dementia without behavioral disturbance (F02.80)
Excludes2: Reye's syndrome (G93.7)

G31.8   Other specified degenerative diseases of nervous system
5th   **G31.89   Other specified degenerative diseases of nervous system**

G31.9   Degenerative disease of nervous system, unspecified

G32   **OTHER DEGENERATIVE DISORDERS OF NERVOUS**
4th   **SYSTEM IN DISEASES CLASSIFIED ELSEWHERE**
G32.0   Subacute combined degeneration of spinal cord in diseases classified elsewhere
     Dana-Putnam syndrome
     Sclerosis of spinal cord (combined) (dorsolateral) (posterolateral)
     Code first underlying disease, such as:
         anemia (D51.9)
         dietary (D51.3)
         pernicious (D51.0)
         vitamin B12 deficiency (E53.8)
     Excludes1: syphilitic combined degeneration of spinal cord (A52.11)

G32.8   Other specified degenerative disorders of nervous system in
5th   **diseases classified elsewhere**
     Code first underlying disease, such as:
         amyloidosis cerebral degeneration (E85.-)
         cerebral degeneration (due to) hypothyroidism (E00.0-E03.9)
         cerebral degeneration (due to) neoplasm (C00-D49)
         cerebral degeneration (due to) vitamin B deficiency, except thiamine (E52-E53.-)
     Excludes1: superior hemorrhagic polioencephalitis [Wernicke's encephalopathy] (E51.2)

     G32.81   Cerebellar ataxia in diseases classified elsewhere
         Code first underlying disease, such as:
           celiac disease (with gluten ataxia) (K90.0)
           cerebellar ataxia (in) neoplastic disease (paraneoplastic cerebellar degeneration) (C00-D49)
           non-celiac gluten ataxia (M35.9)
         Excludes1: systemic atrophy primarily affecting the central nervous system in alcoholic cerebellarataxia (G31.2)
           systemic atrophy primarily affecting the central nervous system in myxedema (G13.2)

     G32.89   Other specified degenerative disorders of nervous system in diseases classified elsewhere
         Degenerative encephalopathy in diseases classified elsewhere

(G35–G37) DEMYELINATING DISEASES OF THE CENTRAL NERVOUS SYSTEM

G35   **MULTIPLE SCLEROSIS**
✔   Disseminated multiple sclerosis
     Generalized multiple sclerosis
     Multiple sclerosis NOS
     Multiple sclerosis of brain stem
     Multiple sclerosis of cord

G36   **OTHER ACUTE DISSEMINATED DEMYELINATION**
4th
Excludes1: postinfectious encephalitis and encephalomyelitis NOS (G04.01)

G36.0   Neuromyelitis optica [Devic]
     Demyelination in optic neuritis
     Excludes1: optic neuritis NOS (H46)

G36.1   Acute and subacute hemorrhagic leukoencephalitis [Hurst]

4th   **5th**   **6th**   **7th**   Additional Character Required   ✔   3-character code

•=New Code   *Excludes1*—Not coded here, do not use together
▲=Revised Code   *Excludes2*—Not included here

G36.8 Other specified acute disseminated demyelination
G36.9 Acute disseminated demyelination, unspecified

G37   **OTHER DEMYELINATING DISEASES OF CENTRAL**
4th   **NERVOUS SYSTEM**
    G37.1 Central demyelination of corpus callosum
    G37.8 Other specified demyelinating diseases of central nervous
            system
    G37.9 Demyelinating disease of central nervous system, unspecified

(G40–G47) EPISODIC AND PAROXYSMAL DISORDERS

G40   **EPILEPSY AND RECURRENT SEIZURES**
4th   **Note:** the following terms are to be considered equivalent to intractable:
      pharmacoresistant (pharmacologically resistant), treatment resistant,
      refractory (medically) and poorly controlled
    Excludes1: conversion disorder with seizures (F44.5)
      convulsions NOS (R56.9)
      post traumatic seizures (R56.1)
      seizure (convulsive) NOS (R56.9)
      seizure of newborn (P90)
    Excludes2: hippocampal sclerosis (G93.81)
      mesial temporal sclerosis (G93.81)
      temporal sclerosis (G93.81)
      Todd's paralysis (G83.8)

> G40.0-, G40.1-, G40.2-, G40.3-,
> G40.40-, G40.41-, G40.B-, G40.A-,
> G40.91- Codes require a 6th
> character:
> 1 — with status epilepticus
> 9 — without status epilepticus
> or NOS

G40.0 **Localization-related (focal)**
5th   **(partial) idiopathic epilepsy**
    and epileptic syndromes with
    seizures of localized onset
    Benign childhood epilepsy with
      centrotemporal EEG spikes
    Childhood epilepsy with occipital EEG paroxysms
    Excludes1: adult onset localization-related epilepsy (G40.1-,
      G40.2-)
    G40.00 **Localization-related (focal) (partial) idiopathic**
    6th   **epilepsy and epileptic syndromes with seizures**
           of localized onset, not intractable (without
           intractability)
    G40.01 **Localization-related (focal) (partial) idiopathic**
    6th   **epilepsy and epileptic syndromes with seizures of**
           localized onset, intractable

G40.1 **Localization-related (focal) (partial) symptomatic epilepsy and**
5th   **epileptic syndromes with simple partial seizures**
    Attacks without alteration of consciousness
    Epilepsia partialis continua [Kozhevnikof]
    Simple partial seizures developing into secondarily generalized
      seizures
    G40.10 **Localization-related (focal) (partial) symptomatic**
    6th   **epilepsy and epileptic sydromes with simple partial**
           seizures, not intractable (without intractability)
    G40.11 **Localization-related (focal) (partial) symptomatic**
    6th   **epilepsy and epileptic syndromes with simple partial**
           seizures, intractable

G40.2 **Localization-related (focal) (partial) symptomatic epilepsy and**
5th   **epileptic syndromes with complex partial seizures**
    Attacks with alteration of consciousness, often with automatisms
    Complex partial seizures developing into secondarily generalized
      seizures
    G40.20 **Localization-related (focal) (partial) symptomatic**
    6th   **epilepsy and epileptic syndromes with complex**
           partial seizures, not intractable (without
           intractability)
    G40.21 **Localization-related (focal) (partial) symptomatic**
    6th   **epilepsy and epileptic syndromes with complex**
           partial seizures, intractable

G40.3 **Generalized idiopathic epilepsy and epileptic syndromes**
5th   **Code also** MERRF syndrome, if applicable (E88.42)
    G40.30 **Generalized idiopathic epilepsy and epileptic**
    6th   **syndromes, not intractable (without intractability)**
    G40.31 **Generalized idiopathic epilepsy and epileptic**
    6th   **syndromes, intractable**

G40.A **Absence epileptic syndrome**
5th   Childhood absence epilepsy [pyknolepsy]
    Juvenile absence epilepsy
    Absence epileptic syndrome, NOS

G40.A0 **Absence epileptic syndrome, not intractable**
6th
G40.A1 **Absence epileptic syndrome, intractable**
6th

G40.B **Juvenile myoclonic epilepsy [impulsive petit mal]**
5th   G40.B0 **Juvenile myoclonic epilepsy, not intractable**
    6th
    G40.B1 **Juvenile myoclonic epilepsy, intractable**
    6th

G40.4 **Other generalized epilepsy and epileptic syndromes**
5th   Epilepsy with grand mal seizures on awakening
    Epilepsy with myoclonic absences
    Epilepsy with myoclonic-astatic seizures
    Grand mal seizure NOS
    Nonspecific atonic epileptic seizures
    Nonspecific clonic epileptic seizures
    Nonspecific myoclonic epileptic seizures
    Nonspecific tonic epileptic seizures
    Nonspecific tonic-clonic epileptic seizures
    Symptomatic early myoclonic encephalopathy
    G40.40 **Other generalized epilepsy and epileptic syndromes,**
    6th   **not intractable**
           Other generalized epilepsy and epileptic syndromes
             without intractability
           Other generalized epilepsy and epileptic syndromes NOS
    G40.41 **Other generalized epilepsy and epileptic syndromes,**
    6th   **intractable**
    •G40.42 **Cyclin-Dependent Kinase-Like 5 Deficiency Disorder**
           CDKL5
           Use additional code, if known, to identify associated
             manifestations, such as:
             cortical blindness (H47.61-)
             global developmental delay (F88)

G40.5 **Epileptic seizures related to external causes**
5th   Epileptic seizures related to alcohol
    Epileptic seizures related to drugs
    Epileptic seizures related to hormonal changes
    Epileptic seizures related to sleep deprivation
    Epileptic seizures related to stress
    Code also, if applicable, associated epilepsy and recurrent seizures
      (G40.-)
    Use additional code for adverse effect, if applicable, to identify
      drug (T36–T50 with fifth or sixth character 5)
    G40.50 **Epileptic seizures related to external causes, not**
    6th   **intractable**
           G40.501 **Epileptic seizures related to external**
                 causes, not intractable, with status
                 epilepticus
           G40.509 **Epileptic seizures related to external**
                 causes, not intractable, without status
                 epilepticus
                 Epileptic seizures related to external
                   causes,
                      NOS

G40.8 **Other epilepsy and recurrent seizures**
5th   Epilepsies and epileptic syndromes undetermined as to whether
      they are focal or generalized
    Landau-Kleffner syndrome
    G40.80 **Other epilepsy**
    6th   G40.801 **Other epilepsy, not intractable, with status**
                 epilepticus
                 Other epilepsy without intractability with
                   status epilepticus
           G40.802 **Other epilepsy, not intractable, without**
                 status epilepticus
                 Other epilepsy NOS
                 Other epilepsy without intractability without
                   status epilepticus
           G40.803 **Other epilepsy, intractable, with status**
                 epilepticus
           G40.804 **Other epilepsy, intractable, without status**
                 epilepticus
    G40.81 **Lennox-Gastaut syndrome**
    6th

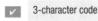

| 4th | 5th | 6th | 7th | Additional Character Required | ✓ 3-character code | •=New Code ▲=Revised Code | *Excludes1*—Not coded here, do not use together *Excludes2*—Not included here |

G40.811 Lennox-Gastaut syndrome, not intractable, with status epilepticus

G40.812 Lennox-Gastaut syndrome, not intractable, without status epilepticus

G40.813 Lennox-Gastaut syndrome, intractable, with status epilepticus

G40.814 Lennox-Gastaut syndrome, intractable, without status epilepticus

G40.82 Epileptic spasms `6th`
Infantile spasms
Salaam attacks
West's syndrome

G40.821 Epileptic spasms, not intractable, with status epilepticus

G40.822 Epileptic spasms, not intractable, without status epilepticus

G40.823 Epileptic spasms, intractable, with status epilepticus

G40.824 Epileptic spasms, intractable, without status epilepticus

• **G40.83 Dravet syndrome** `6th`
Polymorphic epilepsy in infancy (PMEI)
Severe myoclonic epilepsy in infancy (SMEI)

• **G40.833 Dravet syndrome, intractable, with status epilepticus**

• **G40.834 Dravet syndrome, intractable, without status epilepticus**
Dravet syndrome NOS

G40.89 Other seizures
Excludes1: post traumatic seizures (R56.1)
recurrent seizures NOS (G40.909)
seizure NOS (R56.9)

G40.9 Epilepsy, unspecified `5th`

G40.90 Epilepsy, unspecified, not intractable `6th`
Epilepsy, unspecified, without intractability

G40.901 Epilepsy, unspecified, not intractable, with status epilepticus

G40.909 Epilepsy, unspecified, not intractable, without status epilepticus
Epilepsy NOS
Epileptic convulsions NOS
Epileptic fits NOS
Epileptic seizures NOS
Recurrent seizures NOS
Seizure disorder NOS

G40.91 Epilepsy, unspecified, intractable `6th`
Intractable seizure disorder NOS

G43 MIGRAINE `4th`
Note: the following terms are to be considered equivalent to intractable: pharmacoresistant (pharmacologically resistant), treatment resistant, refractory (medically) and poorly controlled
Use additional code for adverse effect, if applicable, to identify drug (T36–T50 with fifth or sixth character 5)
Excludes1: headache NOS (R51.9)
lower half migraine (G44.00)
Excludes2: headache syndromes (G44.-)

G43.0 Migraine without aura `5th`
Common migraine
Excludes1: chronic migraine without aura (G43.7-)

G43.00 Migraine without aura, not intractable `6th`
Migraine without aura without mention of refractory migraine

G43.001 Migraine without aura, not intractable, with status migrainosus

G43.009 Migraine without aura, not intractable, without status migrainosus
Migraine without aura NOS

G43.01 Migraine without aura, intractable `6th`
Migraine without aura with refractory migraine

G43.011 Migraine without aura, intractable, with status migrainosus

G43.019 Migraine without aura, intractable, without status migrainosus

G43.1 Migraine with aura `5th`
Basilar migraine
Classical migraine
Migraine equivalents
Migraine preceded or accompanied by transient focal neurological phenomena
Migraine triggered seizures
Migraine with acute-onset aura
Migraine with aura without headache (migraine equivalents)
Migraine with prolonged aura
Migraine with typical aura
Retinal migraine
Code also any associated seizure (G40.-, R56.9)
Excludes1: persistent migraine aura (G43.5-, G43.6-)

G43.10 Migraine with aura, not intractable `6th`
Migraine with aura without mention of refractory migraine

G43.101 Migraine with aura, not intractable, with status migrainosus

G43.109 Migraine with aura, not intractable, without status migrainosus
Migraine with aura NOS

G43.11 Migraine with aura, intractable `6th`
Migraine with aura with refractory migraine

G43.111 Migraine with aura, intractable, with status migrainosus

G43.119 Migraine with aura, intractable, without status migrainosus

G43.A Cyclical vomiting `5th`
Excludes 1: cyclical vomiting syndrome unrelated to migraine (R11.15)

G43.A0 Cyclical vomiting, in migraine not intractable
Cyclical vomiting, without refractory migraine

G43.A1 Cyclical vomiting, in migraine intractable
Cyclical vomiting, with refractory migraine

G43.C Periodic headache syndromes in child or adult `5th`

G43.C0 Periodic headache syndromes in child or adult, not intractable
Periodic headache syndromes in child or adult, without refractory migraine

G43.C1 Periodic headache syndromes in child or adult, intractable
Periodic headache syndromes in child or adult, with refractory migraine

G43.8 Other migraine `5th`

G43.80 Other migraine, not intractable `6th`
Other migraine, without refractory migraine

G43.801 Other migraine, not intractable, with status migrainosus

G43.809 Other migraine, not intractable, without status migrainosus

G43.81 Other migraine, intractable `6th`
Other migraine, with refractory migraine

G43.811 Other migraine, intractable, with status migrainosus

G43.819 Other migraine, intractable, without status migrainosus

G43.82 Menstrual migraine, not intractable `6th`
Menstrual migraine, without refractory migraine
Menstrually related migraine, not intractable
Pre-menstrual migraine/headache, not intractable
Pure menstrual migraine, not intractable
Code also associated premenstrual tension syndrome (N94.3)

G43.821 Menstrual migraine, not intractable, with status migrainosus

G43.829 Menstrual migraine, not intractable, without status migrainosus
Menstrual migraine NOS

`4th` `5th` `6th` `7th` Additional Character Required   ✔ `3-character code`

• =New Code
▲ =Revised Code

Excludes1—Not coded here, do not use together
Excludes2—Not included here

G43.83   **Menstrual migraine, intractable**
[6th]
Menstrual headache, intractable
Menstrual migraine, with refractory migraine
Menstrually related migraine, intractable
Pre-menstrual migraine/headache, intractable
Pure menstrual migraine, intractable
Code also associated premenstrual tension syndrome (N94.3)

G43.831   **Menstrual migraine, intractable, with status migrainosus**

G43.839   **Menstrual migraine, intractable, without status migrainosus**

G43.9   **Migraine, unspecified**
[5th]
G43.90   **Migraine, unspecified, not intractable**
[6th]
Migraine, unspecified, without refractory migraine

G43.901   **Migraine, unspecified, not intractable, with status migrainosus**
Status migrainosus NOS

G43.909   **Migraine, unspecified, not intractable, without status migrainosus**
Migraine NOS

G43.91   **Migraine, unspecified, intractable**
[6th]
Migraine, unspecified, with refractory migraine

G43.911   **Migraine, unspecified, intractable, with status migrainosus**

G43.919   **Migraine, unspecified, intractable, without status migrainosus**

G44   **OTHER HEADACHE SYNDROMES**
[4th]
Excludes1: headache NOS (R51.9)
Excludes2: atypical facial pain (G50.1)
     headache due to lumbar puncture (G97.1)
     migraines (G43.-)
     trigeminal neuralgia (G50.0)

G44.0   **Cluster headaches and other trigeminal autonomic cephalgias (TAC)**
[5th]
G44.00   **Cluster headache syndrome, unspecified**
[6th]
Ciliary neuralgia
Cluster headache NOS
Histamine cephalgia
Lower half migraine
Migrainous neuralgia

G44.001   **Cluster headache syndrome, unspecified, intractable**

G44.009   **Cluster headache syndrome, unspecified, not intractable**
Cluster headache syndrome NOS

G44.2   **Tension-type headache**
[5th]
G44.20   **Tension-type headache, unspecified**
[6th]
G44.201   **Tension-type headache, unspecified, intractable**

G44.209   **Tension-type headache, unspecified, not intractable**
Tension headache NOS

G44.21   **Episodic tension-type headache**
[6th]
G44.211   **Episodic tension-type headache, intractable**

G44.219   **Episodic tension-type headache, not intractable**
Episodic tension-type headache NOS

G44.22   **Chronic tension-type headache**
[6th]
G44.221   **Chronic tension-type headache, intractable**

G44.229   **Chronic tension-type headache, not intractable**
Chronic tension-type headache NOS

G44.3   **Post-traumatic headache**
[5th]
G44.30   **Post-traumatic headache, unspecified**
[6th]
G44.301   **Post-traumatic headache, unspecified, intractable**

G44.309   **Post-traumatic headache, unspecified, not intractable**
Post-traumatic headache NOS

G44.31   **Acute post-traumatic headache**
[6th]
G44.311   **Acute post-traumatic headache, intractable**

G44.319   **Acute post-traumatic headache, not intractable**
Acute post-traumatic headache NOS

G44.32   **Chronic post-traumatic headache**
[6th]
G44.321   **Chronic post-traumatic headache, intractable**

G44.329   **Chronic post-traumatic headache, not intractable**
Chronic post-traumatic headache NOS

G45   **TRANSIENT CEREBRAL ISCHEMIC ATTACKS AND RELATED SYNDROMES**
[4th]
Excludes1: neonatal cerebral ischemia (P91.0)
     transient retinal artery occlusion (H34.0-)

G45.8   **Other transient cerebral ischemic attacks and related syndromes**

G45.9   **Transient cerebral ischemic attack, unspecified**
Spasm of cerebral artery
TIA
Transient cerebral ischemia NOS

G47   **SLEEP DISORDERS**
[4th]
Excludes2: nightmares (F51.5)
     nonorganic sleep disorders (F51.-)
     sleep terrors (F51.4)
     sleepwalking (F51.3)

G47.0   **Insomnia**
[5th]
Excludes2: alcohol or drug-related insomnia
     idiopathic insomnia (F51.01)
     insomnia due to a mental disorder (F51.05)
     insomnia not due to a substance or known physiological condition (F51.0-)
     nonorganic insomnia (F51.0-)
     primary insomnia (F51.01)
     sleep apnea (G47.3-)

G47.00   **Insomnia, unspecified**
Insomnia NOS

G47.01   **Insomnia due to medical condition**
Code also associated medical condition

G47.09   **Other insomnia**

G47.2   **Circadian rhythm sleep disorders**
[5th]
Disorders of the sleep wake schedule
Inversion of nyctohemeral rhythm
Inversion of sleep rhythm

G47.20   **Circadian rhythm sleep disorder, unspecified type**
Sleep wake schedule disorder NOS

G47.21   **Circadian rhythm sleep disorder, delayed sleep phase type**
Delayed sleep phase syndrome

G47.22   **Circadian rhythm sleep disorder, advanced sleep phase type**

G47.23   **Circadian rhythm sleep disorder, irregular sleep wake type**
Irregular sleep-wake pattern

G47.24   **Circadian rhythm sleep disorder, free running type**
Circadian rhythm sleep disorder, non-24-hour sleep-wake type

G47.25   **Circadian rhythm sleep disorder, jet lag type**

G47.27   **Circadian rhythm sleep disorder in conditions classified elsewhere**
Code first underlying condition

G47.29   **Other circadian rhythm sleep disorder**

G47.3   **Sleep apnea**
[5th]
Code also any associated underlying condition
Excludes1: apnea NOS (R06.81)
     Cheyne-Stokes breathing (R06.3)
     pickwickian syndrome (E66.2)
     sleep apnea of newborn (P28.3)

G47.30   **Sleep apnea, unspecified**
Sleep apnea NOS

G47.31   **Primary central sleep apnea**
Idiopathic central sleep apnea

[4th] [5th] [6th] [7th] Additional Character Required   ✓ 3-character code   •=New Code   ▲=Revised Code   *Excludes1*—Not coded here, do not use together   *Excludes2*—Not included here

G47.32   **High altitude periodic breathing**

G47.33   **Obstructive sleep apnea (adult) (pediatric)**
Obstructive sleep apnea hypopnea
Excludes1: obstructive sleep apnea of newborn (P28.3)

G47.37   **Central sleep apnea in conditions classified elsewhere**
Code first underlying condition

G47.39   **Other sleep apnea**

G47.5   **Parasomnia**
[5th] *Excludes1:* alcohol induced parasomnia
drug induced parasomnia
parasomnia not due to a substance or known physiological condition

G47.50   **Parasomnia, unspecified**
Parasomnia NOS

G47.51   **Confusional arousals**

G47.52   **REM sleep behavior disorder**

G47.53   **Recurrent isolated sleep paralysis**

G47.54   **Parasomnia in conditions classified elsewhere**
Code first underlying condition

G47.59   **Other parasomnia**

G47.6   **Sleep related movement disorders**
[5th] *Excludes2:* restless legs syndrome (G25.81)

G47.61   **Periodic limb movement disorder**

G47.62   **Sleep related leg cramps**

G47.63   **Sleep related bruxism**
Excludes1: psychogenic bruxism (F45.8)

G47.69   **Other sleep related movement disorders**

G47.8   **Other sleep disorders**
Other specified sleep-wake disorder

G47.9   **Sleep disorder, unspecified**
Sleep disorder NOS

(G50–G59) NERVE, NERVE ROOT AND PLEXUS DISORDERS

Excludes1: current traumatic nerve, nerve root and plexus disorders — see Injury, nerve by body region
neuralgia NOS (M79.2)
neuritis NOS (M79.2)
peripheral neuritis in pregnancy (O26.82-)
radiculitis NOS (M54.1-)

G51   **FACIAL NERVE DISORDERS**
[4th] *Includes:* disorders of 7th cranial nerve

G51.0   **Bell's palsy**
Facial palsy

G51.8   **Other disorders of facial nerve**

G51.9   **Disorder of facial nerve, unspecified**

G52   **DISORDERS OF OTHER CRANIAL NERVES**
[4th] *Excludes2:* disorders of acoustic [8th] nerve (H93.3)
disorders of optic [2nd] nerve (H46, H47.0)
paralytic strabismus due to nerve palsy (H49.0–H49.2)

G52.2   **Disorders of vagus nerve**
Disorders of pneumogastric [10th] nerve

G52.7   **Disorders of multiple cranial nerves**
Polyneuritis cranialis

G52.9   **Cranial nerve disorder, unspecified**

G53   **CRANIAL NERVE DISORDERS IN DISEASES CLASSIFIED ELSEWHERE**
[✔]
Code first underlying disease, such as:
neoplasm (C00-D49)
Excludes1: multiple cranial nerve palsy in sarcoidosis (D86.82)
multiple cranial nerve palsy in syphilis (A52.15)
postherpetic geniculate ganglionitis (B02.21)
postherpetic trigeminal neuralgia (B02.22)

G54   **NERVE ROOT AND PLEXUS DISORDERS**
[4th] *Excludes1:* current traumatic nerve root and plexus disorders—see nerve injury by body region
intervertebral disc disorders (M50-M51)
neuralgia or neuritis NOS (M79.2)
neuritis or radiculitis brachial NOS (M54.13)
neuritis or radiculitis lumbar NOS (M54.16)
neuritis or radiculitis lumbosacral NOS (M54.17)

neuritis or radiculitis thoracic NOS (M54.14)
radiculitis NOS (M54.10)
radiculopathy NOS (M54.10)
spondylosis (M47.-)

G54.0   **Brachial plexus disorders**
Thoracic outlet syndrome

G54.1   **Lumbosacral plexus disorders**

G54.9   **Nerve root and plexus disorder, unspecified**

G55   **NERVE ROOT AND PLEXUS COMPRESSIONS IN DISEASES CLASSIFIED ELSEWHERE**
[✔]
Code first underlying disease, such as:
neoplasm (C00-D49)
Excludes1: nerve root compression (due to) (in) ankylosing spondylitis (M45.-)
nerve root compression (due to) (in) dorsopathies (M53.-, M54.-)
nerve root compression (due to) (in) intervertebral disc disorders (M50.1-, M51.1-)
nerve root compression (due to) (in) spondylopathies (M46.-, M48.-)
nerve root compression (due to) (in) spondylosis (M47.0–M47.2.-)

G58   **OTHER MONONEUROPATHIES**
[4th] **G58.9**   **Mononeuropathy, unspecified**

(G60–G65) POLYNEUROPATHIES AND OTHER DISORDERS OF THE PERIPHERAL NERVOUS SYSTEM

Excludes1: neuralgia NOS (M79.2)
neuritis NOS (M79.2)
peripheral neuritis in pregnancy (O26.82-)
radiculitis NOS (M54.10)

G60   **HEREDITARY AND IDIOPATHIC NEUROPATHY**
[4th] **G60.0**   **Hereditary motor and sensory neuropathy**
Charcot-Marie-Tooth disease
Déjérine-Sottas disease
Hereditary motor and sensory neuropathy, types I-IV
Hypertrophic neuropathy of infancy
Peroneal muscular atrophy (axonal type) (hypertrophic type)
Roussy-Levy syndrome

G60.3   **Idiopathic progressive neuropathy**

G60.8   **Other hereditary and idiopathic neuropathies**
Dominantly inherited sensory neuropathy
Morvan's disease
Nelaton's syndrome
Recessively inherited sensory neuropathy

G60.9   **Hereditary and idiopathic neuropathy, unspecified**

G61   **INFLAMMATORY POLYNEUROPATHY**
[4th] **G61.0**   **Guillain-Barre syndrome**
Acute (post-) infective polyneuritis
Miller Fisher Syndrome

G61.9   **Inflammatory polyneuropathy, unspecified**

G62   **OTHER AND UNSPECIFIED POLYNEUROPATHIES**
[4th] **G62.9**   **Polyneuropathy, unspecified**
Neuropathy NOS

G63   **POLYNEUROPATHY IN DISEASES CLASSIFIED ELSEWHERE**
[✔]
Code first underlying disease, such as:
amyloidosis (E85.-)
endocrine disease, except diabetes (E00-E07, E15-E16, E20-E34)
metabolic diseases (E70-E88)
neoplasm (C00-D49)
nutritional deficiency (E40-E64)
Excludes1: polyneuropathy (in):
diabetes mellitus (E08-E13 with .42)
diphtheria (A36.83)
infectious mononucleosis (B27.0-B27.9 with 1)
Lyme disease (A69.22)
mumps (B26.84)
postherpetic (B02.23)
rheumatoid arthritis (M05.5-)
scleroderma (M34.83)
systemic lupus erythematosus (M32.19)

(G70–G73) DISEASES OF MYONEURAL JUNCTION AND MUSCLE

G70 **MYASTHENIA GRAVIS AND OTHER MYONEURAL DISORDERS** `4th`
> *Excludes1:* botulism (A05.1, A48.51–A48.52)
> transient neonatal myasthenia gravis (P94.0)

G70.0 Myasthenia gravis
> `5th` **G70.00** **Myasthenia gravis without (acute) exacerbation**
> Myasthenia gravis NOS
> **G70.01** **Myasthenia gravis with (acute) exacerbation**
> Myasthenia gravis in crisis

G70.1 Toxic myoneural disorders
> **Code first** (T51–T65) to identify toxic agent

G70.2 Congenital and developmental myasthenia

G70.8 Other specified myoneural disorders
> `5th` **G70.80** **Lambert-Eaton syndrome, unspecified**
> Lambert-Eaton syndrome NOS
> **G70.81** **Lambert-Eaton syndrome in disease classified elsewhere**
> **Code first** underlying disease
> *Excludes1:* Lambert-Eaton syndrome in neoplastic disease (G73.1)
> **G70.89** **Other specified myoneural disorders**

G70.9 Myoneural disorder, unspecified

G71 **PRIMARY DISORDERS OF MUSCLES** `4th`
> *Excludes2:* arthrogryposis multiplex congenita (Q74.3)
> metabolic disorders (E70–E88)
> myositis (M60.-)

G71.0 Muscular dystrophy
> `5th` **G71.00** **Muscular dystrophy, unspecified**
> **G71.01** **Duchenne or Becker muscular dystrophy**
> Autosomal recessive, childhood type, muscular dystrophy resembling Duchenne or Becker muscular dystrophy
> Benign [Becker] muscular dystrophy
> Severe [Duchenne] muscular dystrophy
> **G71.02** **Facioscapulohumeral muscular dystrophy**
> Scapulohumeral muscular dystrophy
> **G71.09** **Other specified muscular dystrophies**
> Benign scapuloperoneal muscular dystrophy with early contractures [Emery-Dreifuss]
> Congenital muscular dystrophy NOS
> Congenital muscular dystrophy with specific morphological abnormalities of the muscle fiber
> Distal muscular dystrophy
> Limb-girdle muscular dystrophy
> Ocular muscular dystrophy
> Oculopharyngeal muscular dystrophy
> Scapuloperoneal muscular dystrophy

G71.1 Myotonic disorders
> `5th` **G71.11** **Myotonic muscular dystrophy**
> Dystrophia myotonica [Steinert]
> Myotonia atrophica
> **G71.12** **Myotonia congenita**
> Acetazolamide responsive myotonia congenita
> Dominant myotonia congenita [Thomsen disease]
> Myotonia levior
> Recessive myotonia congenita [Becker disease]
> **G71.13** **Myotonic chondrodystrophy**
> Chondrodystrophic myotonia
> Congenital myotonic chondrodystrophy
> Schwartz-Jampel disease

▲G71.2 Congenital myopathies
> `5th` *Excludes2:* arthrogryposis multiplex congenita (Q74.3)
> •**G71.20** **Congenital myopathy, unspecified**
> •**G71.21** **Nemaline myopathy**
> •**G71.22** **Centronuclear myopathy**
> `6th` •**G71.220** **X-linked myotubular myopathy**
> Myotubular (centronuclear) myopathy
> •**G71.228** **Other centronuclear myopathy**
> Autosomal centronuclear myopathy
> Autosomal dominant centronuclear myopathy
> Autosomal recessive centronuclear myopathy
> Centronuclear myopathy, NOS

> •**G71.29** **Other congenital myopathy**
> Central core disease
> Minicore disease
> Multicore disease
> Multiminicore disease

G71.9 Primary disorder of muscle, unspecified
> Hereditary myopathy NOS

G72 **OTHER AND UNSPECIFIED MYOPATHIES** `4th`
> *Excludes1:* arthrogryposis multiplex congenita (Q74.3)
> dermatopolymyositis (M33.-)
> ischemic infarction of muscle (M62.2-)
> myositis (M60.-)
> polymyositis (M33.2.-)

G72.8 Other specified myopathies
> `5th` **G72.81** **Critical illness myopathy**
> Acute necrotizing myopathy
> Acute quadriplegic myopathy
> Intensive care (ICU) myopathy
> Myopathy of critical illness
> **G72.89** **Other specified myopathies**

G72.9 Myopathy, unspecified

G73 **DISORDERS OF MYONEURAL JUNCTION AND MUSCLE IN DISEASES CLASSIFIED ELSEWHERE** `4th`

G73.1 Lambert-Eaton syndrome in neoplastic disease
> **Code first** underlying neoplasm (C00–D49)
> *Excludes1:* Lambert-Eaton syndrome not associated with neoplasm (G70.80–G70.81)

G73.3 Myasthenic syndromes in other diseases classified elsewhere
> **Code first** underlying disease, such as:
> neoplasm (C00-D49)
> thyrotoxicosis (E05.-)

G73.7 Myopathy in diseases classified elsewhere
> **Code first** underlying disease, such as:
> hyperparathyroidism (E21.0, E21.3)
> hypoparathyroidism (E20.-)
> glycogen storage disease (E74.0)
> lipid storage disorders (E75.-)
> *Excludes1:* myopathy in:
> rheumatoid arthritis (M05.32)
> sarcoidosis (D86.87)
> scleroderma (M34.82)
> sicca syndrome [Sjögren] (M35.03)
> systemic lupus erythematosus (M32.19)

(G80–G83) CEREBRAL PALSY AND OTHER PARALYTIC SYNDROMES

G80 **CEREBRAL PALSY** `4th`
> *Excludes1:* hereditary spastic paraplegia (G11.4)

G80.0 Spastic quadriplegic cerebral palsy
> Congenital spastic paralysis (cerebral)

G80.1 Spastic diplegic cerebral palsy
> Spastic cerebral palsy NOS

G80.2 Spastic hemiplegic cerebral palsy

G80.3 Athetoid cerebral palsy
> Double athetosis (syndrome)
> Dyskinetic cerebral palsy
> Dystonic cerebral palsy
> Vogt disease

G80.4 Ataxic cerebral palsy

G80.8 Other cerebral palsy
> Mixed cerebral palsy syndromes

G80.9 Cerebral palsy, unspecified
> Cerebral palsy NOS

G81 **HEMIPLEGIA AND HEMIPARESIS** `4th`

GUIDELINES

Codes from category G81, identify whether the dominant or nondominant side is affected. Should the affected side be documented, but not specified as dominant or nondominant, and the classification system does not indicate a default, code selection is as follows:
For ambidextrous patients, the default should be dominant.
If the left side is affected, the default is non-dominant.

`4th` `5th` `6th` `7th` Additional Character Required   ✔ 3-character code

•=New Code   *Excludes1*—Not coded here, do not use together
▲=Revised Code   *Excludes2*—Not included here

If the right side is affected, the default is dominant.

Note: This category is to be used only when hemiplegia (complete) (incomplete) is reported without further specification, or is stated to be old or longstanding but of unspecified cause. The category is also for use in multiple coding to identify these types of hemiplegia resulting from any cause.

Excludes1: congenital cerebral palsy (G80.-)

hemiplegia and hemiparesis due to sequela of cerebrovascular disease (I69.05-, I69.15-, I69.25-, I69.35-, I69.85-, I69.95-)

G81.0 Flaccid hemiplegia
| 5th |
- G81.01 Flaccid hemiplegia affecting right dominant side
- G81.02 Flaccid hemiplegia affecting left dominant side
- G81.03 Flaccid hemiplegia affecting right nondominant side
- G81.04 Flaccid hemiplegia affecting left nondominant side

G81.1 Spastic hemiplegia
| 5th |
- G81.11 Spastic hemiplegia affecting right dominant side
- G81.12 Spastic hemiplegia affecting left dominant side
- G81.13 Spastic hemiplegia affecting right nondominant side
- G81.14 Spastic hemiplegia affecting left nondominant side

G81.9 Hemiplegia, unspecified
| 5th |
- G81.91 Hemiplegia, unspecified affecting right dominant side
- G81.92 Hemiplegia, unspecified affecting left dominant side
- G81.93 Hemiplegia, unspecified affecting right nondominant side
- G81.94 Hemiplegia, unspecified affecting left nondominant side

G82 PARAPLEGIA (PARAPARESIS) AND QUADRIPLEGIA (QUADRIPARESIS)
| 4th |

Note: This category is to be used only when the listed conditions are reported without further specification, or are stated to be old or longstanding but of unspecified cause. The category is also for use in multiple coding to identify these conditions resulting from any cause

Excludes1: congenital cerebral palsy (G80.-)

functional quadriplegia (R53.2)

hysterical paralysis (F44.4)

G82.2 Paraplegia
| 5th |
Paralysis of both lower limbs NOS

Paraparesis (lower) NOS

Paraplegia (lower) NOS
- G82.20 Paraplegia, unspecified
- G82.21 Paraplegia, complete
- G82.22 Paraplegia, incomplete

G82.5 Quadriplegia
| 5th |
- G82.50 Quadriplegia, unspecified
- G82.51 Quadriplegia, C1-C4 complete
- G82.52 Quadriplegia, C1-C4 incomplete
- G82.53 Quadriplegia, C5-C7 complete
- G82.54 Quadriplegia, C5-C7 incomplete

G83 OTHER PARALYTIC SYNDROMES
| 4th |

GUIDELINES

Codes from subcategories, G83.1, G83.2, and G83.3, identify whether the dominant or nondominant side is affected. Should the affected side be documented, but not specified as dominant or nondominant, and the classification system does not indicate a default, code selection is as follows:

For ambidextrous patients, the default should be dominant.

If the left side is affected, the default is non-dominant.

If the right side is affected, the default is dominant.

Note: This category is to be used only when the listed conditions are reported without further specification, or are stated to be old or longstanding but of unspecified cause. The category is also for use in multiple coding to identify these conditions resulting from any cause.

Includes: paralysis (complete) (incomplete), except as in G80–G82

G83.0 Diplegia of upper limbs
Diplegia (upper)

Paralysis of both upper limbs

G83.1 Monoplegia of lower limb
| 5th |
Paralysis of lower limb

Excludes1: monoplegia of lower limbs due to sequela of cerebrovascular disease (I69.04-, I69.14-, I69.24-, I69.34-, I69.84-, I69.94-)

- G83.10 Monoplegia of lower limb affecting; unspecified side
- G83.11   right dominant side
- G83.12   left dominant side
- G83.13   right nondominant side
- G83.14   left nondominant side

G83.2 Monoplegia of upper limb
| 5th |
Paralysis of upper limb

Excludes1: monoplegia of upper limbs due to sequela of cerebrovascular disease (I69.03-, I69.13-, I69.23-, I69.33-, I69.83-, I69.93-)

- G83.21 Monoplegia of upper limb affecting; right dominant side
- G83.22   left dominant side
- G83.23   right nondominant side
- G83.24   left nondominant side

G83.3 Monoplegia, unspecified
| 5th |
- G83.31 Monoplegia, unspecified affecting; right dominant side
- G83.32   left dominant side
- G83.33   right nondominant side
- G83.34   left nondominant side

G83.4 Cauda equina syndrome
Neurogenic bladder due to cauda equina syndrome

Excludes1: cord bladder NOS (G95.89)

neurogenic bladder NOS (N31.9)

G83.9 Paralytic syndrome, unspecified

(G89–G99) OTHER DISORDERS OF THE NERVOUS SYSTEM

G89 PAIN, NOT ELSEWHERE CLASSIFIED
| 4th |

GUIDELINES

General coding information

Codes in category G89, Pain, not elsewhere classified, may be used in conjunction with codes from other categories and chapters to provide more detail about acute or chronic pain and neoplasm-related pain, unless otherwise indicated below.

If the pain is not specified as acute or chronic, post-thoracotomy, post-procedural, or neoplasm-related, do not assign codes from category G89.

A code from category G89 should not be assigned if the underlying (definitive) diagnosis is known, unless the reason for the encounter is pain control/management and not management of the underlying condition.

When an admission or encounter is for a procedure aimed at treating the underlying condition (e.g., spinal fusion, kyphoplasty), a code for the underlying condition (e.g., vertebral fracture, spinal stenosis) should be assigned as the principal diagnosis. No code from category G89 should be assigned.

CATEGORY G89 CODES AS PRINCIPAL OR FIRST-LISTED DIAGNOSIS

Category G89 codes are acceptable as principal diagnosis or the first-listed code:

- When pain control or pain management is the reason for the admission/encounter. The underlying cause of the pain should be reported as an additional diagnosis, if known.
- When a patient is admitted for the insertion of a neurostimulator for pain control. When an admission or encounter is for a procedure aimed at treating the underlying condition and a neurostimulator is inserted for pain control during the same admission/encounter, a code for the underlying condition should be assigned as the principal diagnosis and the appropriate pain code should be assigned as a secondary diagnosis.

USE OF CATEGORY G89 CODES IN CONJUNCTION WITH SITE-SPECIFIC PAIN CODES

Assigning Category G89 and Site-Specific Pain Codes

Codes from category G89 may be used in conjunction with codes that identify the site of pain (including codes from Chapter 18) if the category G89 code provides additional information. For example, if the code describes the site of the pain, but does not fully describe whether the pain is acute or chronic, then both codes should be assigned.

| 4th | 5th | 6th | 7th | Additional Character Required   ✔ 3-character code

•=New Code   *Excludes1*—Not coded here, do not use together
▲=Revised Code   *Excludes2*—Not included here

Sequencing of Category G89 Codes with Site-Specific Pain Codes

The sequencing of category G89 codes with site-specific pain codes (including Chapter 18 codes), is dependent on the circumstances of the encounter/admission as follows:

- If the encounter is for pain control or pain management, assign the code from category G89 followed by the code identifying the specific site of pain (e.g., encounter for pain management for acute neck pain from trauma is assigned code G89.11, Acute pain due to trauma, followed by code M54.2, Cervicalgia, to identify the site of pain).
- If the encounter is for any other reason except pain control or pain management, and a related definitive diagnosis has not been established (confirmed) by the provider, assign the code for the specific site of pain first, followed by the appropriate code from category G89.

Pain due to devices, implants, and grafts
Refer to Chapter 19 for pain due to medical devices.

Postoperative Pain
The provider's documentation should be used to guide the coding of postoperative pain, as well as Section IV. Diagnostic Coding and Reporting in the Outpatient Setting (page XIX).

The default for post-thoracotomy and other postoperative pain not specified as acute or chronic is the code for the acute form.

Routine or expected postoperative pain immediately after surgery should not be coded.

- Postoperative pain not associated with a specific postoperative complication is assigned to the appropriate postoperative pain code in category G89.
- Postoperative pain associated with a specific postoperative complication (such as painful wire sutures) is assigned to the appropriate code(s) found in Chapter 19. If appropriate, use additional code(s) from category G89 to identify acute or chronic pain (G89.18 or G89.28).

Chronic Pain
Chronic pain is classified to subcategory G89.2. There is no time frame defining when pain becomes chronic pain. The provider's documentation should be used to guide use of these codes.

Neoplasm Related Pain
Code G89.3 is assigned to pain documented as being related, associated or due to cancer, primary or secondary malignancy, or tumor. This code is assigned regardless of whether the pain is acute or chronic. This code may be assigned as the principal or first-listed code when the stated reason for the admission/encounter is documented as pain control/pain management. The underlying neoplasm should be reported as an additional diagnosis.

When the reason for the admission/encounter is management of the neoplasm and the pain associated with the neoplasm is also documented, code G89.3 may be assigned as an additional diagnosis. It is not necessary to assign an additional code for the site of the pain.

Refer to Chapter 2 for instructions on the sequencing of neoplasms for all other stated reasons for the admission/encounter (except for pain control/pain management).

Chronic Pain Syndrome
Central pain syndrome (G89.0) and chronic pain syndrome (G89.4) are different than the term "chronic pain," and therefore codes should only be used when the provider has specifically documented this condition.

See Chapter 5 for pain disorders related to psychological factors
Code also related psychological factors associated with pain (F45.42)
Excludes1: generalized pain NOS (R52)
     pain disorders exclusively related to psychological factors (F45.41)
     pain NOS (R52)
Excludes2: atypical face pain (G50.1)
     headache syndromes (G44.-)
     localized pain, unspecified type — code to pain by site, such as:
     abdomen pain (R10.-)
     back pain (M54.9)
     breast pain (N64.4)
     chest pain (R07.1–R07.9)
     ear pain (H92.0-)
     eye pain (H57.1)
     headache (R51.9)

     joint pain (M25.5-)
     limb pain (M79.6-)
     lumbar region pain (M54.5)
     painful urination (R30.9)
     pelvic and perineal pain (R10.2)
     shoulder pain (M25.51-)
     spine pain (M54.-)
     throat pain (R07.0)
     tongue pain (K14.6)
     tooth pain (K08.8)
     renal colic (N23)
     migraines (G43.-)
     myalgia (M79.1-)
     pain from prosthetic devices, implants, and grafts (T82.84, T83.84, T84.84, T85.84-)
     phantom limb syndrome with pain (G54.6)
     vulvar vestibulitis (N94.810)
     vulvodynia (N94.81-)

G89.1 Acute pain, not elsewhere classified
     `5th` **G89.11 Acute pain due to trauma**
       G89.12 Acute post-thoracotomy pain
         Post-thoracotomy pain NOS
       G89.18 Other acute postprocedural pain
         Postoperative pain NOS
         Postprocedural pain NOS

G89.2 Chronic pain, NEC
     `5th` ***Excludes1:*** causalgia, lower limb (G57.7-)
       causalgia, upper limb (G56.4-)
       central pain syndrome (G89.0)
       chronic pain syndrome (G89.4)
       complex regional pain syndrome II, lower limb (G57.7-)
       complex regional pain syndrome II, upper limb (G56.4-)
       neoplasm related chronic pain (G89.3)
       reflex sympathetic dystrophy (G90.5-)
     G89.21 Chronic pain due to trauma
     G89.22 Chronic post-thoracotomy pain
     G89.28 Other chronic postprocedural pain
       Other chronic postoperative pain

G89.3 Neoplasm related pain (acute) (chronic)
     Cancer associated pain
     Pain due to malignancy (primary) (secondary)
     Tumor associated pain

G90 DISORDERS OF AUTONOMIC NERVOUS SYSTEM
     `4th` ***Excludes1:*** dysfunction of the autonomic nervous system due to alcohol (G31.2)
G90.5 Complex regional pain syndrome I (CRPS I)
     `5th` Reflex sympathetic dystrophy
     Excludes1: causalgia of lower limb (G57.7-)
       causalgia of upper limb (G56.4-)
       complex regional pain syndrome II of lower limb (G57.7-)
       complex regional pain syndrome II of upper limb (G56.4-)
     G90.51 Complex regional pain syndrome I of upper limb
       `6th` **G90.511 Complex regional pain syndrome I of; right upper limb**
         G90.512 left upper limb
         G90.513 bilateral
         G90.519 unspecified upper limb
     G90.52 Complex regional pain syndrome I of lower limb
       `6th` **G90.521 Complex regional pain syndrome I of; right lower limb**
         G90.522 left lower limb
         G90.523 bilateral
         G90.529 unspecified lower limb
     G90.59 Complex regional pain syndrome I of other specified site
G90.8 Other disorders of autonomic nervous system
G90.9 Disorder of the autonomic nervous system, unspecified

G91 HYDROCEPHALUS
     `4th` **Includes:** acquired hydrocephalus
     Excludes1: Arnold-Chiari syndrome with hydrocephalus (Q07.-)
       congenital hydrocephalus (Q03.-)
       spina bifida with hydrocephalus (Q05.-)

`4th` `5th` `6th` `7th` Additional Character Required   ✔ 3-character code

•=New Code   ***Excludes1***—Not coded here, do not use together
▲=Revised Code   ***Excludes2***—Not included here

G91.0   **Communicating hydrocephalus**
Secondary normal pressure hydrocephalus
G91.1   **Obstructive hydrocephalus**
G91.2   **(Idiopathic) normal pressure hydrocephalus**
Normal pressure hydrocephalus NOS
G91.3   **Post-traumatic hydrocephalus, unspecified**
G91.4   **Hydrocephalus in diseases classified elsewhere**
Code first underlying condition, such as:
plasminogen deficiency E88.02
Excludes1: hydrocephalus due to congenital toxoplasmosis (P37.1)
G91.8   **Other hydrocephalus**
G91.9   **Hydrocephalus, unspecified**

G92   **TOXIC ENCEPHALOPATHY**
☑ Toxic encephalitis
Toxic metabolic encephalopathy
Code first if applicable, drug induced (T36-T50) or use (T51–T65) to identify toxic agent

G93   **OTHER DISORDERS OF BRAIN**
4th   **G93.0**   **Cerebral cysts**
Arachnoid cyst
Porencephalic cyst, acquired
Excludes1: acquired periventricular cysts of newborn (P91.1)
congenital cerebral cysts (Q04.6)
G93.1   **Anoxic brain damage, not elsewhere classified**
Excludes1: cerebral anoxia due to anesthesia during labor and delivery (O74.3)
cerebral anoxia due to anesthesia during the puerperium (O89.2)
neonatal anoxia (P84)
G93.2   **Benign intracranial hypertension**
Pseudotumor
Excludes1: hypertensive encephalopathy (I67.4)
obstructive hydrocephalus (G91.1)
G93.4   **Other and unspecified encephalopathy**
5th   *Excludes1*: alcoholic encephalopathy (G31.2)
encephalopathy in diseases classified elsewhere (G94)
hypertensive encephalopathy (I67.4)
Excludes2: toxic (metabolic) encephalopathy (G92)
    G93.40   **Encephalopathy, unspecified**
    G93.41   **Metabolic encephalopathy**
Septic encephalopathy
    G93.49   **Other encephalopathy**
Encephalopathy NEC
G93.5   **Compression of brain**
Arnold-Chiari type 1 compression of brain
Compression of brain (stem)
Herniation of brain (stem)
Excludes1: diffuse traumatic compression of brain (S06.2-)
focal traumatic compression of brain (S06.3-)
G93.6   **Cerebral edema**
Excludes1: cerebral edema due to birth injury (P11.0)
traumatic cerebral edema (S06.1-)
G93.7   **Reye's syndrome**
Code first poisoning due to salicylates, if applicable (T39.0-, with 6th character 1–4)
Use additional code for adverse effect due to salicylates, if applicable (T39.0-, with 6th character 5)
G93.8   **Other specified disorders of brain**
5th   **G93.81**   **Temporal sclerosis**
Hippocampal sclerosis
Mesial temporal sclerosis
    G93.82   **Brain death**
    G93.89   **Other specified disorders of brain**
Post-radiation encephalopathy
G93.9   **Disorder of brain, unspecified**

G94   **OTHER DISORDERS OF BRAIN IN DISEASES CLASSIFIED ELSEWHERE**
☑ **Code first** underlying disease

G95   **OTHER AND UNSPECIFIED DISEASES OF SPINAL CORD**
4th   *Excludes2*: myelitis (G04.-)
G95.1   **Vascular myelopathies**
5th   *Excludes2*: intraspinal phlebitis and thrombophlebitis, except non-pyogenic (G08)
    G95.11   **Acute infarction of spinal cord (embolic) (nonembolic)**
Anoxia of spinal cord
Arterial thrombosis of spinal cord
    G95.19   **Other vascular myelopathies**
Edema of spinal cord
Hematomyelia
Nonpyogenic intraspinal phlebitis and thrombophlebitis
Subacute necrotic myelopathy
G95.8   **Other specified diseases of spinal cord**
5th   *Excludes1*: neurogenic bladder NOS (N31.9)
neurogenic bladder due to cauda equina syndrome (G83.4)
neuromuscular dysfunction of bladder without spinal cord lesion (N31.-)
    G95.89   **Other specified diseases of spinal cord**
Cord bladder NOS
Drug-induced myelopathy
Radiation-induced myelopathy
Excludes1: myelopathy NOS (G95.9)
G95.9   **Disease of spinal cord, unspecified**
Myelopathy NOS

G96   **OTHER DISORDERS OF THE CENTRAL NERVOUS**
4th   **SYSTEM**
▲**G96.0**   **Cerebrospinal fluid leak**
5th   *Excludes1*: cerebrospinal fluid leak from spinal puncture (G97.0)
Code also, if applicable:
intracranial hypotension (G96.81-)
 •**G96.00**   **Cerebrospinal fluid leak, unspecified**
Code also, if applicable:
head injury (S00.- to S09.-)
 •**G96.01**   **Cranial cerebrospinal fluid leak, spontaneous**
Otorrhea due to spontaneous cerebrospinal fluid CSF leak
Rhinorrhea due to spontaneous cerebrospinal fluid CSF leak
Spontaneous cerebrospinal fluid leak from skull base
 •**G96.02**   **Spinal cerebrospinal fluid leak, spontaneous**
Spontaneous cerebrospinal fluid leak from spine
 •**G96.08**   **Other cranial cerebrospinal fluid leak**
Postoperative cranial cerebrospinal fluid leak
Traumatic cranial cerebrospinal fluid leak
Code also, if applicable:
head injury (S00.- to S09.-)
 •**G96.09**   **Other spinal cerebrospinal fluid leak**
Other spinal CSF leak
Postoperative spinal cerebrospinal fluid leak
Traumatic spinal cerebrospinal fluid leak
Code also, if applicable:
head injury (S00.- to S09.-)
G96.1   **Disorders of meninges, not elsewhere classified**
5th   **G96.11**   **Dural tear**
Excludes1: accidental puncture or laceration of dura during a procedure (G97.41)
Code also intracranial hypotension, if applicable (G96.81-)
    G96.12   **Meningeal adhesions (cerebral) (spinal)**
▲**G96.19**   **Other disorders of meninges, NEC**
6th •**G96.191**   **Perineural cyst**
Cervical nerve root cyst
Lumbar nerve root cyst
Sacral nerve root cyst
Tarlov cyst
Thoracic nerve root cyst
 •**G96.198**   **Other disorders of meninges, not elsewhere classified**

 4th 5th 6th 7th   Additional Character Required   ☑   3-character code

•=New Code   ***Excludes1***—Not coded here, do not use together
▲=Revised Code   ***Excludes2***—Not included here

▲G96.8 Other specified disorders of central nervous system

    [5th] •**G96.81 Intracranial hypotension**

        [6th] **Code also** any associated diagnoses, such as:

          Brachial amyotrophy (G54.5)

          Cerebrospinal fluid leak from spine (G96.02)

          Cranial nerve disorders in diseases classified elsewhere (G53)

          Nerve root and compressions in diseases classified elsewhere (G55)

          Nonpyogenic thrombosis of intracranial venous system (I67.6)

          Nontraumatic intracerebral hemorrhage (I61.-)

          Nontraumatic subdural hemorrhage (I62.0-)

          Other and unspecified cord compression (G95.2-)

          Other secondary parkinsonism (G21.8)

          Reversible cerebrovascular vasoconstriction syndrome (I67.841)

          Spinal cord herniation (G95.89)

          Stroke (I63.-)

          Syringomyelia (G95.0)

          •**G96.810 Intracranial hypotension, unspecified**

          •**G96.811 Intracranial hypotension, spontaneous**

          •**G96.819 Other intracranial hypotension**

    •**G96.89 Other specified disorders of central nervous system**

G96.9 Disorder of central nervous system, unspecified

G98 OTHER DISORDERS OF NERVOUS SYSTEM NOT

[4th] **ELSEWHERE CLASSIFIED**

Includes: nervous system disorder NOS

G98.0 Neurogenic arthritis, not elsewhere classified

    Nonsyphilitic neurogenic arthropathy NEC

    Nonsyphilitic neurogenic spondylopathy NEC

    Excludes1: spondylopathy (in):

        syringomyelia and syringobulbia (G95.0)

        tabes dorsalis (A52.11)

G98.8 Other disorders of nervous system

    Nervous system disorder NOS

G99 OTHER DISORDERS OF NERVOUS SYSTEM IN DISEASES

[4th] **CLASSIFIED ELSEWHERE**

G99.0 Autonomic neuropathy in diseases classified elsewhere

    Code first underlying disease, such as:

        amyloidosis (E85.-)

        gout (M1A.-, M10.-)

        hyperthyroidism (E05.-)

    Excludes1: diabetic autonomic neuropathy (E08-E13 with .43)

G99.2 Myelopathy in diseases classified elsewhere

    Code first underlying disease, such as:

        neoplasm (C00–D49)

    Excludes1: myelopathy in:

        intervertebral disease (M50.0-, M51.0-)

        spondylosis (M47.0-, M47.1-)

CHAPTER 6. DISEASES OF THE NERVOUS SYSTEM   (G96.8–G99.2)

[4th] [5th] [6th] [7th]   Additional Character Required   ✔   3-character code   •=New Code   **Excludes1**—Not coded here, do not use together

                                                ▲=Revised Code   **Excludes2**—Not included here

Chapter 7. Diseases of the eye and adnexa (H00–H59)

GUIDELINES

Refer to ICD-10-CM Official Guidelines for Coding and Reporting for reporting adult glaucoma

Note: Use an external cause code following the code for the eye condition, if applicable, to identify the cause of the eye condition

Excludes2: certain conditions originating in the perinatal period (P04–P96)
   certain infectious and parasitic diseases (A00–B99)
   complications of pregnancy, childbirth and the puerperium (O00–O9A)
   congenital malformations, deformations, and chromosomal abnormalities
     (Q00–Q99)
   DM related eye conditions (E09.3-, E10.3-, E11.3-, E13.3-)
   endocrine, nutritional and metabolic diseases (E00–E88)
   injury (trauma) of eye and orbit (S05.-)
   injury, poisoning and certain other consequences of external causes (S00–T88)
   neoplasms (C00–D49)
   symptoms, signs and abnormal clinical and laboratory findings, not elsewhere
     classified (R00–R94)
   syphilis related eye disorders (A50.01, A50.3-, A51.43, A52.71)

(H00–H05) DISORDERS OF EYELID, LACRIMAL SYSTEM AND ORBIT

H00 **HORDEOLUM AND CHALAZION**
`4th` **H00.0** **Hordeolum (externum) (internum) of eyelid**
   `5th` **H00.01** **Hordeolum externum**
     `6th` Hordeolum NOS
       Stye
       H00.011 **Hordeolum externum right upper eyelid**
       H00.012 **Hordeolum externum right lower eyelid**
       H00.013 **Hordeolum externum right eye, unspecified eyelid**
       H00.014 **Hordeolum externum left upper eyelid**
       H00.015 **Hordeolum externum left lower eyelid**
       H00.016 **Hordeolum externum left eye, unspecified eyelid**
   `5th` **H00.02** **Hordeolum internum**
     `6th` Infection of meibomian gland
       H00.021 **Hordeolum internum right upper eyelid**
       H00.022 **Hordeolum internum right lower eyelid**
       H00.023 **Hordeolum internum right eye, unspecified eyelid**
       H00.024 **Hordeolum internum left upper eyelid**
       H00.025 **Hordeolum internum left lower eyelid**
       H00.026 **Hordeolum internum left eye, unspecified eyelid**
   H00.03 **Abscess of eyelid**
     `6th` Furuncle of eyelid
       H00.031 **Abscess of right upper eyelid**
       H00.032 **Abscess of right lower eyelid**
       H00.033 **Abscess of eyelid right eye, unspecified eyelid**
       H00.034 **Abscess of left upper eyelid**
       H00.035 **Abscess of left lower eyelid**
       H00.036 **Abscess of eyelid left eye, unspecified eyelid**
  H00.1 **Chalazion**
   `5th` Meibomian (gland) cyst
     Excludes2: infected meibomian gland (H00.02-)
     H00.11 **Chalazion right upper eyelid**
     H00.12 **Chalazion right lower eyelid**
     H00.13 **Chalazion right eye, unspecified eyelid**
     H00.14 **Chalazion left upper eyelid**
     H00.15 **Chalazion left lower eyelid**
     H00.16 **Chalazion left eye, unspecified eyelid**

H01 **OTHER INFLAMMATION OF EYELID**
`4th` **H01.0** **Blepharitis**
   Excludes1: blepharoconjunctivitis (H10.5-)
   H01.00 **Unspecified blepharitis**
     `6th` **H01.001** **Unspecified blepharitis right upper eyelid**
       H01.002 **Unspecified blepharitis right lower eyelid**

       H01.003 **Unspecified blepharitis right eye, unspecified eyelid**
       H01.004 **Unspecified blepharitis left upper eyelid**
       H01.005 **Unspecified blepharitis left lower eyelid**
       H01.006 **Unspecified blepharitis left eye, unspecified eyelid**
       H01.00A **Unspecified blepharitis right eye, upper and lower eyelids**
       H01.00B **Unspecified blepharitis left eye, upper and lower eyelids**
  H01.1 **Noninfectious dermatoses of eyelid**
   `5th` **H01.11** **Allergic dermatitis of eyelid**
     `6th` Contact dermatitis of eyelid
       H01.111 **Allergic dermatitis of right upper eyelid**
       H01.112 **Allergic dermatitis of right lower eyelid**
       H01.113 **Allergic dermatitis of right eye, unspecified eyelid**
       H01.114 **Allergic dermatitis of left upper eyelid**
       H01.115 **Allergic dermatitis of left lower eyelid**
       H01.116 **Allergic dermatitis of left eye, unspecified eyelid**
  H01.8 **Other specified inflammations of eyelid**
  H01.9 **Unspecified inflammation of eyelid**
   Inflammation of eyelid NOS

H02 **OTHER DISORDERS OF EYELID**
`4th` **Excludes1:** congenital malformations of eyelid (Q10.0–Q10.3)
  H02.4 **Ptosis of eyelid**
   `5th` **H02.40** **Unspecified ptosis of eyelid**
     `6th` **H02.401** **Unspecified ptosis of right eyelid**
       H02.402 **Unspecified ptosis of left eyelid**
       H02.403 **Unspecified ptosis of bilateral eyelids**
       H02.409 **Unspecified ptosis of unspecified eyelid**
  H02.8 **Other specified disorders of eyelid**
   `5th` **H02.82** **Cysts of eyelid**
     `6th` Sebaceous cyst of eyelid
       H02.821 **Cysts of right upper eyelid**
       H02.822 **Cysts of right lower eyelid**
       H02.823 **Cysts of right eye, unspecified eyelid**
       H02.824 **Cysts of left upper eyelid**
       H02.825 **Cysts of left lower eyelid**
       H02.826 **Cysts of left eye, unspecified eyelid**
   H02.84 **Edema of eyelid**
     `6th` Hyperemia of eyelid
       H02.841 **Edema of right upper eyelid**
       H02.842 **Edema of right lower eyelid**
       H02.843 **Edema of right eye, unspecified eyelid**
       H02.844 **Edema of left upper eyelid**
       H02.845 **Edema of left lower eyelid**
       H02.846 **Edema of left eye, unspecified eyelid**
   H02.88 **Meibomian gland dysfunction**
     `6th` **H02.881** **Meibomian gland dysfunction right upper eyelid**
       H02.882 **Meibomian gland dysfunction right lower eyelid**
       H02.883 **Meibomian gland dysfunction of right eye, unspecified eyelid**
       H02.884 **Meibomian gland dysfunction left upper eyelid**
       H02.885 **Meibomian gland dysfunction left lower eyelid**
       H02.886 **Meibomian gland dysfunction of left eye, unspecified eyelid**
       H02.889 **Meibomian gland dysfunction of unspecified eye, unspecified eyelid**
       H02.88A **Meibomian gland dysfunction right eye, upper and lower eyelids**
       H02.88B **Meibomian gland dysfunction left eye, upper and lower eyelids**
   H02.89 **Other specified disorders of eyelid**
     Hemorrhage of eyelid

`4th` `5th` `6th` `7th` Additional Character Required ✔ 3-character code   Unspecified laterality codes were excluded here. •=New Code ▲=Revised Code **Excludes1**—Not coded here, do not use together **Excludes2**—Not included here

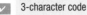

CHAPTER 7. DISEASES OF THE EYE AND ADNEXA   (H02.9–H18.503)

H02.9   **Unspecified disorder of eyelid**
     Disorder of eyelid NOS

H04   **DISORDERS OF LACRIMAL SYSTEM**
   `4th`   *Excludes1:* congenital malformations of lacrimal system (Q10.4-Q10.6)
   H04.1   **Other disorders of lacrimal gland**
    `5th`   **H04.12**   **Dry eye syndrome**
     `6th`   Tear film insufficiency, NOS
      H04.121   Dry eye syndrome of right lacrimal gland
      H04.122   Dry eye syndrome of left lacrimal gland
      H04.123   Dry eye syndrome of bilateral lacrimal glands
   H04.5   **Stenosis and insufficiency of lacrimal passages**
    `5th`   **H04.53**   **Neonatal obstruction of nasolacrimal duct**
     `6th`   *Excludes1:* congenital stenosis and stricture of lacrimal duct (Q10.5)
      H04.531   Neonatal obstruction of right nasolacrimal duct
      H04.532   Neonatal obstruction of left nasolacrimal duct
      H04.533   Neonatal obstruction of bilateral nasolacrimal duct
    H04.55   **Acquired stenosis of nasolacrimal duct**
     `6th`   **H04.551**   Acquired stenosis of right nasolacrimal duct
      H04.552   Acquired stenosis of left nasolacrimal duct
      H04.553   Acquired stenosis of bilateral nasolacrimal duct
    H04.57   **Stenosis of lacrimal sac**
     `6th`   **H04.571**   Stenosis of right lacrimal sac
      H04.572   Stenosis of left lacrimal sac
      H04.573   Stenosis of bilateral lacrimal sac
   H04.9   **Disorder of lacrimal system, unspecified**

H05   **DISORDERS OF ORBIT**
   `4th`   *Excludes1:* congenital malformation of orbit (Q10.7)
   H05.0   **Acute inflammation of orbit**
    `5th`   **H05.00**   **Unspecified acute inflammation of orbit**
    H05.01   **Cellulitis of orbit**
     `6th`   Abscess of orbit
      H05.011   Cellulitis of right orbit
      H05.012   Cellulitis of left orbit
      H05.013   Cellulitis of bilateral orbits
    H05.11   **Granuloma of orbit**
     `6th`   Pseudotumor (inflammatory) of orbit
      H05.111   Granuloma of right orbit
      H05.112   Granuloma of left orbit
      H05.113   Granuloma of bilateral orbits

(H10–H11) DISORDERS OF CONJUNCTIVA

H10   **CONJUNCTIVITIS**
   `4th`   *Excludes1:* keratoconjunctivitis (H16.2-)
   H10.0   **Mucopurulent conjunctivitis**
    `5th`   **H10.01**   **Acute follicular conjunctivitis**
     `6th`   **H10.011**   Acute follicular conjunctivitis, right eye
      H10.012   Acute follicular conjunctivitis, left eye
      H10.013   Acute follicular conjunctivitis, bilateral
    H10.02   **Other mucopurulent conjunctivitis**
     `6th`   **H10.021**   Other mucopurulent conjunctivitis, right eye
      H10.022   Other mucopurulent conjunctivitis, left eye
      H10.023   Other mucopurulent conjunctivitis, bilateral
   H10.1   **Acute atopic conjunctivitis**
    `5th`   Acute papillary conjunctivitis
    H10.11   Acute atopic conjunctivitis, right eye
    H10.12   Acute atopic conjunctivitis, left eye
    H10.13   Acute atopic conjunctivitis, bilateral
   H10.2   **Other acute conjunctivitis**
    `5th`   **H10.21**   **Acute toxic conjunctivitis**
     `6th`   Acute chemical conjunctivitis
     Code first (T51–T65) to identify chemical and intent
     Excludes1: burn and corrosion of eye and adnexa (T26.-)

H10.211   Acute toxic conjunctivitis, right eye
H10.212   Acute toxic conjunctivitis, left eye
H10.213   Acute toxic conjunctivitis, bilateral
  H10.22   **Pseudomembranous conjunctivitis**
   `6th`   **H10.221**   Pseudomembranous conjunctivitis, right eye
    H10.222   Pseudomembranous conjunctivitis, left eye
    H10.223   Pseudomembranous conjunctivitis, bilateral
  H10.23   **Serous conjunctivitis, except viral**
   `6th`   *Excludes1:* viral conjunctivitis (B30.-)
    H10.231   Serous conjunctivitis, except viral, right eye
    H10.232   Serous conjunctivitis, except viral, left eye
    H10.233   Serous conjunctivitis, except viral, bilateral
    H10.239   Serous conjunctivitis, except viral, unspecified eye
H10.3   **Unspecified acute conjunctivitis**
  `5th`   *Excludes1:* ophthalmia neonatorum NOS (P39.1)
   H10.31   Unspecified acute conjunctivitis, right eye
   H10.32   Unspecified acute conjunctivitis, left eye
   H10.33   Unspecified acute conjunctivitis, bilateral
H10.5   **Blepharoconjunctivitis**
  `5th`   **H10.50**   **Unspecified blepharoconjunctivitis**
   `6th`   **H10.501**   Unspecified blepharoconjunctivitis, right eye
    H10.502   Unspecified blepharoconjunctivitis, left eye
    H10.503   Unspecified blepharoconjunctivitis, bilateral
H10.8   **Other conjunctivitis**
  `5th`   **H10.82**   **Rosacea conjunctivitis**
   `6th`   **Code first** underlying rosacea dermatitis (L71.-)
    H10.821   Rosacea conjunctivitis, right eye
    H10.822   Rosacea conjunctivitis, left eye
    H10.823   Rosacea conjunctivitis, bilateral
H10.9   **Unspecified conjunctivitis**

H11   **OTHER DISORDERS OF CONJUNCTIVA**
  `4th`   *Excludes1:* keratoconjunctivitis (H16.2-)
  H11.3   **Conjunctival hemorrhage**
   `5th`   Subconjunctival hemorrhage
   H11.31   Conjunctival hemorrhage, right eye
   H11.32   Conjunctival hemorrhage, left eye
   H11.33   Conjunctival hemorrhage, bilateral
  H11.4   **Other conjunctival vascular disorders and cysts**
   `5th`   **H11.42**   **Conjunctival edema**
    `6th`   **H11.421**   Conjunctival edema, right eye
     H11.422   Conjunctival edema, left eye
     H11.423   Conjunctival edema, bilateral
  H11.9   **Unspecified disorder of conjunctiva**

(H15–H22) DISORDERS OF SCLERA, CORNEA, IRIS AND CILIARY BODY

H16.2   **Keratoconjunctivitis**
  `5th`   **H16.20**   **Unspecified keratoconjunctivitis**
   `6th`   Superficial keratitis with conjunctivitis NOS
    H16.201   Unspecified keratoconjunctivitis, right eye
    H16.202   Unspecified keratoconjunctivitis, left eye
    H16.203   Unspecified keratoconjunctivitis, bilateral
H16.9   **Unspecified keratitis**

H18   **OTHER DISORDERS OF CORNEA**
  `4th`   **H18.5 Hereditary corneal dystrophies**
   `5th`   ▲**H18.50**   **Unspecified hereditary corneal dystrophies**
    `6th`   •**H18.501**   Unspecified hereditary corneal dystrophies, right eye
     •**H18.502**   Unspecified hereditary corneal dystrophies, left eye
     •**H18.503**   Unspecified hereditary corneal dystrophies, bilateral

---

`4th` `5th` `6th` `7th` Additional Character Required   ✔ 3-character code

Unspecified laterality codes were excluded here.   •=New Code   ▲=Revised Code   *Excludes1*—Not coded here, do not use together   *Excludes2*—Not included here

▴H18.51 **Endothelial corneal dystrophy** `6th`
Fuchs' dystrophy
•H18.511   **Endothelial corneal dystrophy, right eye**
•H18.512   **Endothelial corneal dystrophy, left eye**
•H18.513   **Endothelial corneal dystrophy, bilateral**

▴H18.52 **Epithelial (juvenile) corneal dystrophy** `6th`
•H18.521   **Epithelial (juvenile) corneal dystrophy, right eye**
•H18.522   **Epithelial (juvenile) corneal dystrophy, left eye**
•H18.523   **Epithelial (juvenile) corneal dystrophy, bilateral**

▴H18.59 **Other hereditary corneal dystrophies** `6th`
•H18.591   **Other hereditary corneal dystrophies, right eye**
•H18.592   **Other hereditary corneal dystrophies, left eye**
•H18.593   **Other hereditary corneal dystrophies, bilateral**

H18.79   **Other corneal deformities** `6th`
H18.791   **Other corneal deformities, right eye**
H18.792   **Other corneal deformities, left eye**
H18.793   **Other corneal deformities, bilateral**

H18.8   **Other specified disorders of cornea** `5th`
H18.82   **Corneal disorder due to contact lens** `6th`
Excludes2: corneal edema due to contact lens (H18.21-)
H18.821   **Corneal disorder due to contact lens, right eye**
H18.822   **Corneal disorder due to contact lens, left eye**
H18.823   **Corneal disorder due to contact lens, bilateral**

H18.9   **Unspecified disorder of cornea**

(H25–H28) DISORDERS OF LENS

H26   OTHER CATARACT `4th`
Excludes1: congenital cataract (Q12.0)

H26.0   **Infantile and juvenile cataract** `5th`
H26.00   **Unspecified infantile and juvenile cataract** `6th`
H26.001   **Unspecified infantile and juvenile cataract, right eye**
H26.002   **Unspecified infantile and juvenile cataract, left eye**
H26.003   **Unspecified infantile and juvenile cataract, bilateral**

H26.01   **Infantile and juvenile cortical, lamellar, or zonular cataract** `6th`
H26.011   **Infantile and juvenile cortical, lamellar, or zonular cataract, right eye**
H26.012   **Infantile and juvenile cortical, lamellar, or zonular cataract, left eye**
H26.013   **Infantile and juvenile cortical, lamellar, or zonular cataract, bilateral**

H26.03   **Infantile and juvenile nuclear cataract** `6th`
H26.031   **Infantile and juvenile nuclear cataract, right eye**
H26.032   **Infantile and juvenile nuclear cataract, left eye**
H26.033   **Infantile and juvenile nuclear cataract, bilateral**

H26.04   **Anterior subcapsular polar infantile and juvenile cataract** `6th`
H26.041   **Anterior subcapsular polar infantile and juvenile cataract, right eye**
H26.042   **Anterior subcapsular polar infantile and juvenile cataract, left eye**
H26.043   **Anterior subcapsular polar infantile and juvenile cataract, bilateral**

H26.05   **Posterior subcapsular polar infantile and juvenile cataract** `6th`
H26.051   **Posterior subcapsular polar infantile and juvenile cataract, right eye**

H26.052   **Posterior subcapsular polar infantile and juvenile cataract, left eye**
H26.053   **Posterior subcapsular polar infantile and juvenile cataract, bilateral**

H26.06   **Combined forms of infantile and juvenile cataract** `6th`
H26.061   **Combined forms of infantile and juvenile cataract, right eye**
H26.062   **Combined forms of infantile and juvenile cataract, left eye**
H26.063   **Combined forms of infantile and juvenile cataract, bilateral**

H26.09   **Other infantile and juvenile cataract**

H26.9   **Unspecified cataract**

H27   OTHER DISORDERS OF LENS `4th`
Excludes1: congenital lens malformations (Q12.-)
mechanical complications of intraocular lens implant (T85.2)
pseudophakia (Z96.1)

H27.0   **Aphakia** `5th`
Acquired absence of lens
Acquired aphakia
Aphakia due to trauma
Excludes1: cataract extraction status (Z98.4-)
congenital absence of lens (Q12.3)
congenital aphakia (Q12.3)
H27.01   **Aphakia, right eye**
H27.02   **Aphakia, left eye**
H27.03   **Aphakia, bilateral**

H27.1   **Dislocation of lens** `5th`
H27.10   **Unspecified dislocation of lens**
H27.11   **Subluxation of lens** `6th`
H27.111   **Subluxation of lens, right eye**
H27.112   **Subluxation of lens, left eye**
H27.113   **Subluxation of lens, bilateral**
H27.12   **Anterior dislocation of lens** `6th`
H27.121   **Anterior dislocation of lens, right eye**
H27.122   **Anterior dislocation of lens, left eye**
H27.123   **Anterior dislocation of lens, bilateral**
H27.13   **Posterior dislocation of lens** `6th`
H27.131   **Posterior dislocation of lens, right eye**
H27.132   **Posterior dislocation of lens, left eye**
H27.133   **Posterior dislocation of lens, bilateral**

H27.8   **Other specified disorders of lens**
H27.9   **Unspecified disorder of lens**

H28   CATARACT IN DISEASES CLASSIFIED ELSEWHERE ✔
Code first underlying disease, such as:
hypoparathyroidism (E20.-)
myotonia (G71.1-)
myxedema (E03.-)
protein-calorie malnutrition (E40-E46)
Excludes1: cataract in diabetes mellitus

(H30–H36) DISORDERS OF CHOROID AND RETINA

H32   CHORIORETINAL DISORDERS IN DISEASES CLASSIFIED ELSEWHERE ✔
Code first underlying disease, such as:
congenital toxoplasmosis (P37.1)
histoplasmosis (B39.-)
leprosy (A30.-)
Excludes1: chorioretinitis (in):
toxoplasmosis (acquired) (B58.01)
tuberculosis (A18.53)

H35   OTHER RETINAL DISORDERS `4th`
Excludes2: diabetic retinal disorders (E08.311–E08.359, E09.311–E09.359, E10.311–E10.359, E11.311–E11.359, E13.311–E13.359)

H35.1   **Retinopathy of prematurity [ROP]** `5th`
H35.10   **Retinopathy of prematurity, unspecified** `6th`
Retinopathy of prematurity NOS
H35.101   **ROP, unspecified, right eye**
H35.102   **ROP, unspecified, left eye**
H35.103   **ROP, unspecified, bilateral**

CHAPTER 7. DISEASES OF THE EYE AND ADNEXA   (H18.51–H35.103)

`4th` `5th` `6th` `7th` Additional Character Required   ✔ 3-character code

Unspecified laterality codes were excluded here.   •=New Code   ▴=Revised Code

Excludes1—Not coded here, do not use together
Excludes2—Not included here

CHAPTER 7. DISEASES OF THE EYE AND ADNEXA   (H35.11–H49.812)

H35.11   **Retinopathy of prematurity, stage 0**
6th
    H35.111   ROP, stage 0, right eye
    H35.112   ROP, stage 0, left eye
    H35.113   ROP, stage 0, bilateral

H35.12   **Retinopathy of prematurity, stage 1**
6th
    H35.121   ROP, stage 1, right eye
    H35.122   ROP, stage 1, left eye
    H35.123   ROP, stage 1, bilateral

H35.13   **Retinopathy of prematurity, stage 2**
6th
    H35.131   ROP, stage 2, right eye
    H35.132   ROP, stage 2, left eye
    H35.133   ROP, stage 2, bilateral

H35.14   **Retinopathy of prematurity, stage 3**
6th
    H35.141   ROP, stage 3, right eye
    H35.142   ROP, stage 3, left eye
    H35.143   ROP, stage 3, bilateral

H35.15   **Retinopathy of prematurity, stage 4**
6th
    H35.151   ROP, stage 4, right eye
    H35.152   ROP, stage 4, left eye
    H35.153   ROP, stage 4, bilateral

H35.16   **Retinopathy of prematurity, stage 5**
6th
    H35.161   ROP, stage 5, right eye
    H35.162   ROP, stage 5, left eye
    H35.163   ROP, stage 5, bilateral

H35.17   **Retrolental fibroplasia**
6th
    H35.171   Retrolental fibroplasia, right eye
    H35.172   Retrolental fibroplasia, left eye
    H35.173   Retrolental fibroplasia, bilateral
    H35.179   Retrolental fibroplasia, unspecified eye

H35.5   **Hereditary retinal dystrophy**
5th
    Excludes1: dystrophies primarily involving Bruch's membrane (H31.1-)

    H35.50   **Unspecified hereditary retinal dystrophy**
    H35.51   **Vitreoretinal dystrophy**
    H35.52   **Pigmentary retinal dystrophy**
       Albipunctate retinal dystrophy
       Retinitis pigmentosa
       Tapetoretinal dystrophy
    H35.53   **Other dystrophies primarily involving the sensory retina**
       Stargardt's disease
    H35.54   **Dystrophies primarily involving the retinal pigment epithelium**
       Vitelliform retinal dystrophy

(H40–H42) GLAUCOMA

H40   **GLAUCOMA**
4th
Excludes1: absolute glaucoma (H44.51-)
    congenital glaucoma (Q15.0)
    traumatic glaucoma due to birth injury (P15.3)

H40.3   **Glaucoma secondary to eye trauma**
5th
    Code also underlying condition
    H40.31X   **Glaucoma secondary to eye trauma, right eye**
    7th
       H40.31X0   Glaucoma secondary to eye trauma, right eye; stage unspecified
       H40.31X1   mild stage
       H40.31X2   moderate stage
       H40.31X3   severe stage
       H40.31X4   indeterminate stage
    H40.32X   **Glaucoma secondary to eye trauma, left eye**
    7th
       H40.32X0   Glaucoma secondary to eye trauma, left eye; stage unspecified
       H40.32X1   mild stage
       H40.32X2   moderate stage
       H40.32X3   severe stage
       H40.32X4   indeterminate stage
    H40.33X   **Glaucoma secondary to eye trauma, bilateral**
    7th
       H40.33X0   Glaucoma secondary to eye trauma, bilateral; stage unspecified
       H40.33X1   mild stage
       H40.33X2   moderate stage

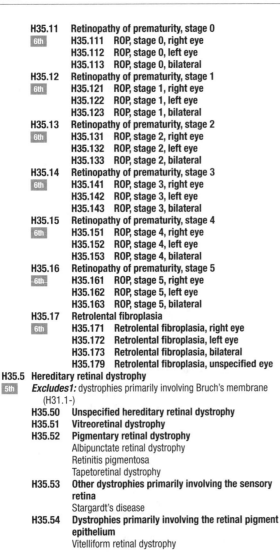

       H40.33X3   severe stage
       H40.33X4   indeterminate stage

H42   **GLAUCOMA IN DISEASES CLASSIFIED ELSEWHERE**
✔
    Code first underlying condition, such as: amyloidosis (E85.-)
       aniridia (Q13.1)
       Lowe's syndrome (E72.03)
       glaucoma in DM (E08.39, E09.39, E10.39, E11.39, E13.39) Reiger's anomaly (Q13.81)
       specified metabolic disorder (E70–E88)
    Excludes1: glaucoma (in):
       onchocerciasis (B73.02)
       syphilis (A52.71)
       tuberculous (A18.59)

(H43–H44) DISORDERS OF VITREOUS BODY AND GLOBE

(H46–H47) DISORDERS OF OPTIC NERVE AND VISUAL PATHWAYS

H47   **OTHER DISORDERS OF OPTIC [2ND] NERVE AND VISUAL PATHWAYS**
4th
H47.0   **Disorders of optic nerve, not elsewhere classified**
5th
    H47.03   **Optic nerve hypoplasia**
    6th
       H47.031   Optic nerve hypoplasia, right eye
       H47.032   Optic nerve hypoplasia, left eye
       H47.033   Optic nerve hypoplasia, bilateral
       H47.039   Optic nerve hypoplasia, unspecified eye
H47.1   **Papilledema**
5th
    H47.10   **Unspecified papilledema**
    H47.11   **Papilledema associated with increased intracranial pressure**
    H47.12   **Papilledema associated with decreased ocular pressure**
    H47.13   **Papilledema associated with retinal disorder**

(H49–H52) DISORDERS OF OCULAR MUSCLES, BINOCULAR MOVEMENT, ACCOMMODATION AND REFRACTION

H49   **PARALYTIC STRABISMUS**
4th
Excludes2: internal ophthalmoplegia (H52.51-)
    internuclear ophthalmoplegia (H51.2-)
    progressive supranuclear ophthalmoplegia (G23.1)
H49.0   **Third [oculomotor] nerve palsy**
5th
    H49.00   **Third [oculomotor] nerve palsy, unspecified eye**
    H49.01   **Third [oculomotor] nerve palsy, right eye**
    H49.02   **Third [oculomotor] nerve palsy, left eye**
    H49.03   **Third [oculomotor] nerve palsy, bilateral**
H49.1   **Fourth [trochlear] nerve palsy**
5th
    H49.11   **Fourth [trochlear] nerve palsy, right eye**
    H49.12   **Fourth [trochlear] nerve palsy, left eye**
    H49.13   **Fourth [trochlear] nerve palsy, bilateral**
H49.2   **Sixth [abducent] nerve palsy**
5th
    H49.21   **Sixth [abducent] nerve palsy, right eye**
    H49.22   **Sixth [abducent] nerve palsy, left eye**
    H49.23   **Sixth [abducent] nerve palsy, bilateral**
H49.3   **Total (external) ophthalmoplegia**
5th
    H49.31   **Total (external) ophthalmoplegia, right eye**
    H49.32   **Total (external) ophthalmoplegia, left eye**
    H49.33   **Total (external) ophthalmoplegia, bilateral**
H49.4   **Progressive external ophthalmoplegia**
5th
    Excludes1: Kearns-Sayre syndrome (H49.81-)
    H49.41   **Progressive external ophthalmoplegia, right eye**
    H49.42   **Progressive external ophthalmoplegia, left eye**
    H49.43   **Progressive external ophthalmoplegia, bilateral**
H49.8   **Other paralytic strabismus**
5th
    H49.81   **Kearns-Sayre syndrome**
    6th
       Progressive external ophthalmoplegia with pigmentary retinopathy
       Use additional code for other manifestation, such as: heart block (I45.9)
       H49.811   **Kearns-Sayre syndrome, right eye**
       H49.812   **Kearns-Sayre syndrome, left eye**

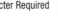 4th   5th   6th   7th   Additional Character Required   ✔   3-character code

Unspecified laterality codes were excluded here.   •=New Code   ▲=Revised Code   *Excludes1*—Not coded here, do not use together   *Excludes2*—Not included here

            H49.813   **Kearns-Sayre syndrome, bilateral**
     H49.88   **Other paralytic strabismus**
       6th   External ophthalmoplegia NOS
            H49.881   **Other paralytic strabismus, right eye**
            H49.882   **Other paralytic strabismus, left eye**
            H49.883   **Other paralytic strabismus, bilateral**
   H49.9   **Unspecified paralytic strabismus**

H50   **OTHER STRABISMUS**
4th   **H50.0**   **Esotropia**
     5th   Convergent concomitant strabismus
     Excludes1: intermittent esotropia (H50.31-, H50.32)
     H50.00   **Unspecified esotropia**
     H50.01   **Monocular esotropia**
       6th   **H50.011**   **Monocular esotropia, right eye**
            H50.012   **Monocular esotropia, left eye**
     H50.02   **Monocular esotropia with A pattern**
       6th   **H50.021**   **Monocular esotropia with A pattern, right eye**
            H50.022   **Monocular esotropia with A pattern, left eye**
     H50.03   **Monocular esotropia with V pattern**
       6th   **H50.031**   **Monocular esotropia with V pattern, right eye**
            H50.032   **Monocular esotropia with V pattern, left eye**
     H50.04   **Monocular esotropia with other noncomitancies**
       6th   **H50.041**   **Monocular esotropia with other noncomitancies, right eye**
            H50.042   **Monocular esotropia with other noncomitancies, left eye**
     H50.05   **Alternating esotropia**
     H50.06   **Alternating esotropia with A pattern**
     H50.07   **Alternating esotropia with V pattern**
     H50.08   **Alternating esotropia with other noncomitancies**
   H50.1   **Exotropia**
     5th   Divergent concomitant strabismus
     Excludes1: intermittent exotropia (H50.33-, H50.34)
     H50.10   **Unspecified exotropia**
     H50.11   **Monocular exotropia**
       6th   **H50.111**   **Monocular exotropia, right eye**
            H50.112   **Monocular exotropia, left eye**
     H50.12   **Monocular exotropia with A pattern**
       6th   **H50.121**   **Monocular exotropia with A pattern, right eye**
            H50.122   **Monocular exotropia with A pattern, left eye**
     H50.13   **Monocular exotropia with V pattern**
       6th   **H50.131**   **Monocular exotropia with V pattern, right eye**
            H50.132   **Monocular exotropia with V pattern, left eye**
     H50.14   **Monocular exotropia with other noncomitancies**
       6th   **H50.141**   **Monocular exotropia with other noncomitancies, right eye**
            H50.142   **Monocular exotropia with other noncomitancies, left eye**
     H50.15   **Alternating exotropia**
     H50.16   **Alternating exotropia with A pattern**
     H50.17   **Alternating exotropia with V pattern**
     H50.18   **Alternating exotropia with other noncomitancies**
   H50.2   **Vertical strabismus**
     5th   Hypertropia
     H50.21   **Vertical strabismus, right eye**
     H50.22   **Vertical strabismus, left eye**
   H50.3   **Intermittent heterotropia**
     5th   **H50.30**   **Unspecified intermittent heterotropia**
     H50.31   **Intermittent monocular esotropia**
       6th   **H50.311**   **Intermittent monocular esotropia, right eye**
            H50.312   **Intermittent monocular esotropia, left eye**
     H50.32   **Intermittent alternating esotropia**
     H50.33   **Intermittent monocular exotropia**
       6th

            H50.331   **Intermittent monocular exotropia, right eye**
            H50.332   **Intermittent monocular exotropia, left eye**
     H50.34   **Intermittent alternating exotropia**
   H50.4   **Other and unspecified heterotropia**
     5th   **H50.40**   **Unspecified heterotropia**
     H50.41   **Cyclotropia**
       6th   **H50.411**   **Cyclotropia, right eye**
            H50.412   **Cyclotropia, left eye**
     H50.42   **Monofixation syndrome**
     H50.43   **Accommodative component in esotropia**
   H50.5   **Heterophoria**
     5th   **H50.50**   **Unspecified heterophoria**
     H50.51   **Esophoria**
     H50.52   **Exophoria**
     H50.53   **Vertical heterophoria**
     H50.54   **Cyclophoria**
     H50.55   **Alternating heterophoria**
   H50.6   **Mechanical strabismus**
     5th   **H50.60**   **Mechanical strabismus, unspecified**
     H50.61   **Brown's sheath syndrome**
       6th   **H50.611**   **Brown's sheath syndrome, right eye**
            H50.612   **Brown's sheath syndrome, left eye**
     H50.69   **Other mechanical strabismus**
         Strabismus due to adhesions
         Traumatic limitation of duction of eye muscle
   H50.8   **Other specified strabismus**
     5th   **H50.81**   **Duane's syndrome**
       6th   **H50.811**   **Duane's syndrome, right eye**
            H50.812   **Duane's syndrome, left eye**
     H50.89   **Other specified strabismus**
   H50.9   **Unspecified strabismus**

H51   **OTHER DISORDERS OF BINOCULAR MOVEMENT**
4th   **H51.0**   **Palsy (spasm) of conjugate gaze**
   H51.8   **Other specified disorders of binocular movement**
   H51.9   **Unspecified disorder of binocular movement**

H52   **DISORDERS OF REFRACTION AND ACCOMMODATION**
4th   **H52.0**   **Hypermetropia**
     5th   **H52.01**   **Hypermetropia, right eye**
     H52.02   **Hypermetropia, left eye**
     H52.03   **Hypermetropia, bilateral**
   H52.1   **Myopia**
     5th   **Excludes1:** degenerative myopia (H44.2-)
     H52.11   **Myopia, right eye**
     H52.12   **Myopia, left eye**
     H52.13   **Myopia, bilateral**
   H52.2   **Astigmatism**
     5th   **H52.20**   **Unspecified astigmatism**
       6th   **H52.201**   **Unspecified astigmatism, right eye**
            H52.202   **Unspecified astigmatism, left eye**
            H52.203   **Unspecified astigmatism, bilateral**
     H52.21   **Irregular astigmatism**
       6th   **H52.211**   **Irregular astigmatism, right eye**
            H52.212   **Irregular astigmatism, left eye**
            H52.213   **Irregular astigmatism, bilateral**
     H52.22   **Regular astigmatism**
       6th   **H52.221**   **Regular astigmatism, right eye**
            H52.222   **Regular astigmatism, left eye**
            H52.223   **Regular astigmatism, bilateral**
   H52.3   **Anisometropia and aniseikonia**
     5th   **H52.31**   **Anisometropia**
     H52.32   **Aniseikonia**
   H52.4   **Presbyopia**
   H52.5   **Disorders of accommodation**
     5th   **H52.51**   **Internal ophthalmoplegia (complete) (total)**
       6th   **H52.511**   **right eye**
            H52.512   **left eye**
            H52.513   **bilateral**
     H52.52   **Paresis of accommodation**
       6th   **H52.521**   **Paresis of accommodation, right eye**
            H52.522   **Paresis of accommodation, left eye**
            H52.523   **Paresis of accommodation, bilateral**

| 4th | 5th | 6th | 7th | Additional Character Required | ✔ 3-character code |

Unspecified laterality codes were excluded here.   •=New Code   ▲=Revised Code

Excludes1—Not coded here, do not use together
Excludes2—Not included here

CHAPTER 7. DISEASES OF THE EYE AND ADNEXA   (H52.53–H54.42A4)

H52.53   **Spasm of accommodation**
- **6th** H52.531   **Spasm of accommodation, right eye**
- H52.532   **Spasm of accommodation, left eye**
- H52.533   **Spasm of accommodation, bilateral**

H52.6   **Other disorders of refraction**

H52.7   **Unspecified disorder of refraction**

(H53–H54) VISUAL DISTURBANCES AND BLINDNESS

H53   VISUAL DISTURBANCES

4th   H53.0   **Amblyopia ex anopsia**
- **5th**   *Excludes1:* amblyopia due to vitamin A deficiency (E50.5)

H53.00   **Unspecified amblyopia**
- **6th** H53.001   **Unspecified amblyopia, right eye**
- H53.002   **Unspecified amblyopia, left eye**
- H53.003   **Unspecified amblyopia, bilateral**

H53.01   **Deprivation amblyopia**
- **6th** H53.011   **Deprivation amblyopia, right eye**
- H53.012   **Deprivation amblyopia, left eye**
- H53.013   **Deprivation amblyopia, bilateral**

H53.02   **Refractive amblyopia**
- **6th** H53.021   **Refractive amblyopia, right eye**
- H53.022   **Refractive amblyopia, left eye**
- H53.023   **Refractive amblyopia, bilateral**

H53.04   **Amblyopia suspect**
- **6th** H53.041   **Amblyopia suspect, right eye**
- H53.042   **Amblyopia suspect, left eye**
- H53.043   **Amblyopia suspect, bilateral eye**

H53.2   **Diplopia**
Double vision

H53.3   **Other and unspecified disorders of binocular vision**
- **5th** H53.30   **Unspecified disorder of binocular vision**
- H53.31   **Abnormal retinal correspondence**

H53.8   **Other visual disturbances**

H53.9   **Unspecified visual disturbance**

H54   BLINDNESS AND LOW VISION

4th

GUIDELINES

If "blindness" or "low vision" of both eyes is documented but the visual impairment category is not documented, assign code H54.3, Unqualified visual loss, both eyes. If "blindness" or "low vision" in one eye is documented but the visual impairment category is not documented, assign a code from H54.6-, Unqualified visual loss, one eye. If "blindness" or "visual loss" is documented without any information about whether one or both eyes are affected, assign code H54.7, Unspecified visual loss. **Note:** For definition of visual impairment categories see table below
Code first any associated underlying cause of the blindness
Excludes1: amaurosis fugax (G45.3)

H54.0   **Blindness, both eyes**
- **5th**   Visual impairment categories 3, 4, 5 in both eyes.

H54.0X   **Blindness, both eyes, different category levels**
- **6th** H54.0X3   **Blindness right eye, category 3**
  - **7th** H54.0X33   **Blindness right eye category 3, blindness left eye category 3**
  - H54.0X34   **Blindness right eye category 3, blindness left eye category 4**
  - H54.0X35   **Blindness right eye category 3, blindness left eye category 5**
- H54.0X4   **Blindness right eye, category 4**
  - **7th** H54.0X43   **Blindness right eye category 4, blindness left eye category 3**
  - H54.0X44   **Blindness right eye category 4, blindness left eye category 4**
  - H54.0X45   **Blindness right eye category 4, blindness left eye category 5**
- H54.0X5   **Blindness right eye, category 5**
  - **7th** H54.0X53   **Blindness right eye category 5, blindness left eye category 3**
  - H54.0X54   **Blindness right eye category 5, blindness left eye category 4**
  - H54.0X55   **Blindness right eye category 5, blindness left eye category 5**

H54.1   **Blindness, one eye, low vision other eye**
- **5th**   Visual impairment categories 3, 4, 5 in one eye, with categories 1 or 2 in the other eye.

H54.11   **Blindness, right eye, low vision left eye**
- **6th** H54.113   **Blindness right eye category 3, low vision left eye**
  - **7th** H54.1131   **Blindness right eye category 3, low vision left eye category 1**
  - H54.1132   **Blindness right eye category 3, low vision left eye category 2**
- H54.114   **Blindness right eye category 4, low vision left eye**
  - **7th** H54.1141   **Blindness right eye category 4, low vision left eye category 1**
  - H54.1142   **Blindness right eye category 4, low vision left eye category 2**
- H54.115   **Blindness right eye category 5, low vision left eye**
  - **7th** H54.1151   **Blindness right eye category 5, low vision left eye category 1**
  - H54.1152   **Blindness right eye category 5, low vision left eye category 2**

H54.12   **Blindness, left eye, low vision right eye**
- **6th** H54.121   **Low vision right eye category 1, blindness left eye**
  - **7th** H54.1213   **Low vision right eye category 1, blindness left eye category 3**
  - H54.1214   **Low vision right eye category 1, blindness left eye category 4**
  - H54.1215   **Low vision right eye category 1, blindness left eye category 5**
- H54.122   **Low vision right eye category 2, blindness left eye**
  - **7th** H54.1223   **Low vision right eye category 2, blindness left eye category 3**
  - H54.1224   **Low vision right eye category 2, blindness left eye category 4**
  - H54.1225   **Low vision right eye category 2, blindness left eye category 5**

H54.2   **Low vision, both eyes**
- **5th**   Visual impairment categories 1 or 2 in both eyes.

H54.2X   **Low vision, both eyes, different category levels**
- **6th** H54.2X1   **Low vision, right eye, category 1**
  - **7th** H54.2X11   **Low vision right eye category 1, low vision left eye category 1**
  - H54.2X12   **Low vision right eye category 1, low vision left eye category 2**
- H54.2X2   **Low vision, right eye, category 2**
  - **7th** H54.2X21   **Low vision right eye category 2, low vision left eye category 1**
  - H54.2X22   **Low vision right eye category 2, low vision left eye category 2**

H54.3   **Unqualified visual loss, both eyes**
Visual impairment category 9 in both eyes.

H54.4   **Blindness, one eye**
- **5th**   Visual impairment categories 3, 4, 5 in one eye [normal vision in other eye].

H54.41   **Blindness, right eye, normal vision left eye**
- **6th** H54.413   **Blindness, right eye, category 3**
  - **7th** H54.413A   **Blindness right eye category 3, normal vision left eye**
- H54.414   **Blindness, right eye, category 4**
  - **7th** H54.414A   **Blindness right eye category 4, normal vision left eye**
- H54.415   **Blindness, right eye, category 5**
  - **7th** H54.415A   **Blindness right eye category 5, normal vision left eye**

H54.42   **Blindness, left eye, normal vision right eye**
- **6th** H54.42A   **Blindness, left eye, category 3-5**
  - **7th** H54.42A3   **Blindness left eye category 3, normal vision right eye**
  - H54.42A4   **Blindness left eye category 4, normal vision right eye**

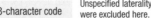

4th **5th** **6th** **7th** Additional Character Required   ✔ 3-character code   Unspecified laterality codes were excluded here.   •=New Code   ▲=Revised Code   *Excludes1*—Not coded here, do not use together   *Excludes2*—Not included here

H54.42A5   Blindness left eye category 5, normal vision right eye

H54.5 Low vision, one eye
5th Visual impairment categories 1 or 2 in one eye [normal vision in other eye].

H54.51   Low vision, right eye, normal vision left eye
     6th   **H54.511**   Low vision, right eye, category 1-2
        7th   **H54.511A**   Low vision right eye category 1, normal vision left eye
             H54.512A   Low vision right eye category 2, normal vision left eye

H54.52   Low vision, left eye, normal vision right eye
     6th   **H54.52A**   Low vision, left eye, category 1-2
        7th   **H54.52A1**   Low vision left eye category 1, normal vision right eye
             H54.52A2   Low vision left eye category 2, normal vision right eye

H54.6 Unqualified visual loss, one eye
5th Visual impairment category 9 in one eye [normal vision in other eye].

H54.61   Unqualified visual loss, right eye, normal vision left eye
H54.62   Unqualified visual loss, left eye, normal vision right eye

H54.7 Unspecified visual loss
Visual impairment category 9 NOS

H54.8 Legal blindness, as defined in USA
Blindness NOS according to USA definition

Excludes1: legal blindness with specification of impairment level (H54.0–H54.7)

Note: The term 'low vision' in category H54 comprises categories 1 and 2 of the table, the term 'blindness' categories 3, 4, and 5, and the term 'unqualified visual loss' category 9.

If the extent of the visual field is taken into account, patients with a field no greater than 10 but greater than 5 around central fixation should be placed in category 3 and patients with a field no greater than 5 around central fixation should be placed in category 4, even if the central acuity is not impaired.

Category of visual impairment	Visual acuity with best possible correction	
	Maximum less than:	**Minimum equal to or better than:**
	6/18	6/60
3/10 (0.3)	1/10 (0.1)	
20/70	20/200	
	6/60	3/60
1/10 (0.1)	1/20 (0.05)	
20/200	20/400	
	3/60	1/60 (finger counting at one meter)
1/20 (0.05)	1/50 (0.02)	
20/400	5/300 (20/1200)	
	1/60 (finer counting at one meter)	Light perception
1/50 (0.02)		
5/300		
	No light perception	
	Undetermined or unspecified	

(H55–H57) OTHER DISORDERS OF EYE AND ADNEXA

H55   **NYSTAGMUS AND OTHER IRREGULAR EYE MOVEMENTS**
4th   **H55.0 Nystagmus**
   5th   **H55.00**   Unspecified nystagmus
        H55.01   Congenital nystagmus
        H55.02   Latent nystagmus
        H55.03   Visual deprivation nystagmus
        H55.04   Dissociated nystagmus
        H55.09   Other forms of nystagmus

H57   **OTHER DISORDERS OF EYE AND ADNEXA**
4th   **H57.0 Anomalies of pupillary function**
   5th   **H57.00**   Unspecified anomaly of pupillary function
            Excludes1: syphilitic Argyll Robertson pupil (A52.19)
        H57.02   Anisocoria
        H57.09   Other anomalies of pupillary function

   H57.1 Ocular pain
   5th   **H57.11**   Ocular pain, right eye
        H57.12   Ocular pain, left eye
        H57.13   Ocular pain, bilateral

   H57.8 Other specified disorders of eye and adnexa
   5th   **H57.81**   Brow ptosis acquired
     6th   **H57.811**   Brow ptosis, right
            H57.812   Brow ptosis, left
            H57.813   Brow ptosis, bilateral
            H57.819   Brow ptosis, unspecified
        H57.89   Other specified disorders of eye and adnexa

   H57.9 Unspecified disorder of eye and adnexa

(H59) INTRAOPERATIVE AND POSTPROCEDURAL COMPLICATIONS AND DISORDERS OF EYE AND ADNEXA, NOT ELSEWHERE CLASSIFIED

4th **5th** **6th** **7th** Additional Character Required   ✓   3-character code   Unspecified laterality codes were excluded here.   •=New Code   ▲=Revised Code   *Excludes1*—Not coded here, do not use together   *Excludes2*—Not included here

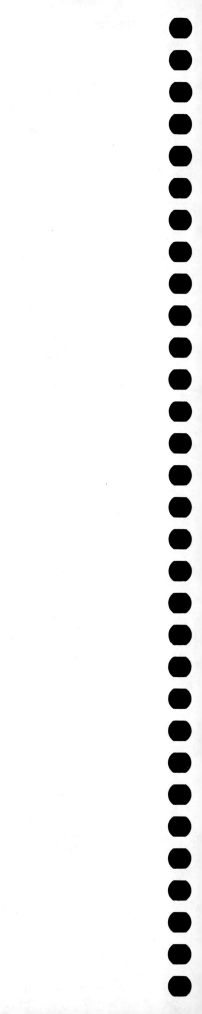

Chapter 8. Diseases of the ear and mastoid process (H60–H95)

GUIDELINES

Note: Use an external cause code following the code for the ear condition, if applicable, to identify the cause of the ear condition

Excludes2: certain conditions originating in the perinatal period (P04–P96)
     certain infectious and parasitic diseases (A00–B99)
     complications of pregnancy, childbirth and the puerperium (O00–O9A)
     congenital malformations, deformations and chromosomal abnormalities (Q00–Q99)
     endocrine, nutritional and metabolic diseases (E00–E88)
     injury, poisoning and certain other consequences of external causes (S00–T88)
     neoplasms (C00–D49)
     symptoms, signs and abnormal clinical and laboratory findings, not elsewhere classified (R00–R94)

(H60–H62) DISEASES OF EXTERNAL EAR

H60   OTITIS EXTERNA

[4th] H60.0   Abscess of external ear
[5th] Boil of external ear
Carbuncle of auricle or external auditory canal
Furuncle of external ear
H60.01   Abscess of right external ear
H60.02   Abscess of left external ear
H60.03   Abscess of external ear, bilateral

H60.1   Cellulitis of external ear
[5th] Cellulitis of auricle
Cellulitis of external auditory canal
H60.11   Cellulitis of right external ear
H60.12   Cellulitis of left external ear
H60.13   Cellulitis of external ear, bilateral

H60.3   Other infective otitis externa
[5th] H60.31   Diffuse otitis externa
[6th]   H60.311   Diffuse otitis externa, right ear
     H60.312   Diffuse otitis externa, left ear
     H60.313   Diffuse otitis externa, bilateral
H60.32   Hemorrhagic otitis externa
[6th]   H60.321   Hemorrhagic otitis externa, right ear
     H60.322   Hemorrhagic otitis externa, left ear
     H60.323   Hemorrhagic otitis externa, bilateral
H60.33   Swimmer's ear
[6th]   H60.331   Swimmer's ear, right ear
     H60.332   Swimmer's ear, left ear
     H60.333   Swimmer's ear, bilateral
H60.39   Other infective otitis externa
[6th]   H60.391   Other infective otitis externa, right ear
     H60.392   Other infective otitis externa, left ear
     H60.393   Other infective otitis externa, bilateral

H60.5   Acute noninfective otitis externa
[5th] H60.50   Unspecified acute noninfective otitis externa
[6th] Acute otitis externa NOS
     H60.501   Unspecified acute noninfective otitis externa, right ear
     H60.502   Unspecified acute noninfective otitis externa, left ear
     H60.503   Unspecified acute noninfective otitis externa, bilateral

H60.8   Other otitis externa
[5th] H60.8X   Other otitis externa
[6th]   H60.8X1   Other otitis externa, right ear
     H60.8X2   Other otitis externa, left ear
     H60.8X3   Other otitis externa, bilateral
     H60.8X9   Other otitis externa, unspecified ear

H60.9   Unspecified otitis externa
[5th]   H60.91   Unspecified otitis externa, right ear
     H60.92   Unspecified otitis externa, left ear
     H60.93   Unspecified otitis externa, bilateral

H61   OTHER DISORDERS OF EXTERNAL EAR

[4th] H61.0   Chondritis and perichondritis of external ear
[5th] Chondrodermatitis nodularis chronica helicis
Perichondritis of auricle
Perichondritis of pinna
H61.00   Unspecified perichondritis of external ear
[6th]   H61.001   Unspecified perichondritis of right external ear
     H61.002   Unspecified perichondritis of left external ear
     H61.003   Unspecified perichondritis of external ear, bilateral
H61.01   Acute perichondritis of external ear
[6th]   H61.011   Acute perichondritis of right external ear
     H61.012   Acute perichondritis of left external ear
     H61.013   Acute perichondritis of external ear, bilateral
H61.02   Chronic perichondritis of external ear
[6th]   H61.021   Chronic perichondritis of right external ear
     H61.022   Chronic perichondritis of left external ear
     H61.023   Chronic perichondritis of external ear, bilateral

H61.1   Noninfective disorders of pinna
[5th] ***Excludes2:*** cauliflower ear (M95.1-)
     gouty tophi of ear (M1A.-)
H61.10   Unspecified noninfective disorders of pinna
[6th] Disorder of pinna NOS
     H61.101   Unspecified noninfective disorders of pinna, right ear
     H61.102   Unspecified noninfective disorders of pinna, left ear
     H61.103   Unspecified noninfective disorders of pinna, bilateral
H61.11   Acquired deformity of pinna
[6th] Acquired deformity of auricle
Excludes2: cauliflower ear (M95.1-)
     H61.111   Acquired deformity of pinna, right ear
     H61.112   Acquired deformity of pinna, left ear
     H61.113   Acquired deformity of pinna, bilateral
H61.12   Hematoma of pinna
[6th] Hematoma of auricle
     H61.121   Hematoma of pinna, right ear
     H61.122   Hematoma of pinna, left ear
     H61.123   Hematoma of pinna, bilateral
H61.19   Other noninfective disorders of pinna
[6th]   H61.191   Noninfective disorders of pinna, right ear
     H61.192   Noninfective disorders of pinna, left ear
     H61.193   Noninfective disorders of pinna, bilateral

H61.2   Impacted cerumen
[5th] Wax in ear
H61.21   Impacted cerumen, right ear
H61.22   Impacted cerumen, left ear
H61.23   Impacted cerumen, bilateral

H62   DISORDERS OF EXTERNAL EAR IN DISEASES
[4th]   CLASSIFIED ELSEWHERE

H62.4   Otitis externa in other diseases classified elsewhere
[5th] **Code first** underlying disease, such as: erysipelas (A46)
     impetigo (L01.0)
Excludes1: otitis externa (in):
     candidiasis (B37.84)
     herpes viral [herpes simplex] (B00.1)
     herpes zoster (B02.8)
H62.41   Otitis externa in other diseases classified elsewhere, right ear
H62.42   Otitis externa in other diseases classified elsewhere, left ear
H62.43   Otitis externa in other diseases classified elsewhere, bilateral

  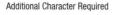 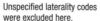

[4th] [5th] [6th] [7th]   Additional Character Required   ✔   3-character code   Unspecified laterality codes were excluded here.   • =New Code   ▲ =Revised Code   ***Excludes1***—Not coded here, do not use together   ***Excludes2***—Not included here

PEDIATRIC ICD-10-CM 2021: A MANUAL FOR PROVIDER-BASED CODING   203

CHAPTER 8. DISEASES OF THE EAR AND MASTOID PROCESS   (H65–H66.3X3)

(H65–H75) DISEASES OF MIDDLE EAR AND MASTOID

H65 NONSUPPURATIVE OTITIS MEDIA
4th
   Includes: nonsuppurative otitis media with myringitis
   Use additional code for any associated perforated tympanic membrane (H72.-)
   Use additional code, if applicable, to identify:
     exposure to environmental tobacco smoke (Z77.22)
     exposure to tobacco smoke in the perinatal period (P96.81)
     history of tobacco dependence (Z87.891)
     infectious agent (B95–B97)
     occupational exposure to environmental tobacco smoke (Z57.31)
     tobacco dependence (F17.-)
     tobacco use (Z72.0)

H65.0 Acute serous otitis media
5th
   Acute and subacute secretory otitis
   H65.01   Acute serous otitis media, right ear
   H65.02   Acute serous otitis media, left ear
   H65.03   Acute serous otitis media, bilateral
   H65.04   Acute serous otitis media, recurrent, right ear
   H65.05   Acute serous otitis media, recurrent, left ear
   H65.06   Acute serous otitis media, recurrent, bilateral

H65.1 Other acute nonsuppurative otitis media
5th
   Excludes1: otitic barotrauma (T70.0)
     otitis media (acute) NOS (H66.9)
   H65.11   Acute and subacute allergic otitis media (mucoid)
   6th   **(sanguinous) (serous)**
     H65.111   Acute and subacute allergic otitis media (mucoid) (sanguinous) (serous), right ear
     H65.112   Acute and subacute allergic otitis media (mucoid) (sanguinous) (serous), left ear
     H65.113   Acute and subacute allergic otitis media (mucoid) (sanguinous) (serous), bilateral
     H65.114   Acute and subacute allergic otitis media (mucoid) (sanguinous) (serous), recurrent, right ear
     H65.115   Acute and subacute allergic otitis media (mucoid) (sanguinous) (serous), recurrent, left ear
     H65.116   Acute and subacute allergic otitis media (mucoid) (sanguinous) (serous), recurrent, bilateral

H65.2 Chronic serous otitis media
5th
   Chronic tubotympanal catarrh
   H65.21   Chronic serous otitis media, right ear
   H65.22   Chronic serous otitis media, left ear
   H65.23   Chronic serous otitis media, bilateral

H65.3 Chronic mucoid otitis media
5th
   Chronic mucinous otitis media
   Chronic secretory otitis media
   Chronic transudative otitis media
   Glue ear
   Excludes1: adhesive middle ear disease (H74.1)
   H65.31   Chronic mucoid otitis media, right ear
   H65.32   Chronic mucoid otitis media, left ear
   H65.33   Chronic mucoid otitis media, bilateral

H65.4 Other chronic nonsuppurative otitis media
5th
   H65.41   Chronic allergic otitis media
   6th
     H65.411   Chronic allergic otitis media, right ear
     H65.412   Chronic allergic otitis media, left ear
     H65.413   Chronic allergic otitis media, bilateral
   H65.49   Other chronic nonsuppurative otitis media
   6th
     Chronic exudative otitis media
     Chronic nonsuppurative otitis media NOS
     Chronic otitis media with effusion (nonpurulent)
     Chronic seromucinous otitis media
     H65.491   Other chronic nonsuppurative otitis media, right ear
     H65.492   Other chronic nonsuppurative otitis media, left ear
     H65.493   Other chronic nonsuppurative otitis media, bilateral

H65.9 Unspecified nonsuppurative otitis media
5th
   Allergic otitis media NOS
   Catarrhal otitis media NOS
   Exudative otitis media NOS
   Mucoid otitis media NOS
   Otitis media with effusion (nonpurulent) NOS
   Secretory otitis media NOS
   Seromucinous otitis media NOS
   Serous otitis media NOS
   Transudative otitis media NOS
   H65.91   Unspecified nonsuppurative otitis media, right ear
   H65.92   Unspecified nonsuppurative otitis media, left ear
   H65.93   Unspecified nonsuppurative otitis media, bilateral

H66 SUPPURATIVE AND UNSPECIFIED OTITIS MEDIA
4th
   Includes: suppurative and unspecified otitis media with myringitis
   Use additional code to identify: exposure to environmental tobacco smoke (Z77.22)
     exposure to tobacco smoke in the perinatal period (P96.81)
     history of tobacco dependence (Z87.891)
     occupational exposure to environmental tobacco smoke (Z57.31)
     tobacco dependence (F17.-)
     tobacco use (Z72.0)

H66.0 Acute suppurative otitis media
5th
   H66.00   Acute suppurative otitis media without spontaneous
   6th   **rupture of; ear drum**
     H66.001   right ear drum
     H66.002   left ear drum
     H66.003   bilateral ear drums
     H66.004   recurrent, right ear drum
     H66.005   recurrent, left ear drum
     H66.006   recurrent, bilateral ear drums
   H66.01   Acute suppurative otitis media with spontaneous
   6th   **rupture of; ear drum**
     H66.011   right ear drum
     H66.012   left ear drum
     H66.013   bilateral ear drums
     H66.014   recurrent, right ear drum
     H66.015   recurrent, left ear drum
     H66.016   recurrent, bilateral ear drums

H66.1 Chronic tubotympanic suppurative otitis media
5th
   Benign chronic suppurative otitis media
   Chronic tubotympanic disease
   Use additional code for any associated perforated tympanic membrane (H72.-)
   H66.11   Chronic tubotympanic suppurative otitis media, right ear
   H66.12   Chronic tubotympanic suppurative otitis media, left ear
   H66.13   Chronic tubotympanic suppurative otitis media, bilateral

H66.2 Chronic atticoantral suppurative otitis media
5th
   Chronic atticoantral disease
   Use additional code for any associated perforated tympanic membrane(H72.-)
   H66.21   Chronic atticoantral suppurative otitis media, right ear
   H66.22   Chronic atticoantral suppurative otitis media, left ear
   H66.23   Chronic atticoantral suppurative otitis media, bilateral

H66.3 Other chronic suppurative otitis media
5th
   Chronic suppurative otitis media NOS
   Use additional code for any associated perforated tympanic membrane (H72.-)
   Excludes1: tuberculous otitis media (A18.6)
   H66.3X   Other chronic suppurative otitis media
   6th
     H66.3X1   Other chronic suppurative otitis media, right ear
     H66.3X2   Other chronic suppurative otitis media, left ear
     H66.3X3   Other chronic suppurative otitis media, bilateral

---

   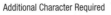   **4th** **5th** **6th** **7th**   Additional Character Required   ✔   3-character code   Unspecified laterality codes were excluded here.   •=New Code   ▲=Revised Code   ***Excludes1***—Not coded here, do not use together   ***Excludes2***—Not included here

H66.4   **Suppurative otitis media, unspecified**
[5th]   Purulent otitis media NOS
Use additional code for any associated perforated tympanic membrane (H72.-)

   H66.41   **Suppurative otitis media, unspecified, right ear**
   H66.42   **Suppurative otitis media, unspecified, left ear**
   H66.43   **Suppurative otitis media, unspecified, bilateral**

H66.9   **Otitis media, unspecified**
[5th]   Otitis media NOS
Acute otitis media NOS
Chronic otitis media NOS
Use additional code for any associated perforated tympanic membrane (H72.-)

   H66.91   **Otitis media, unspecified, right ear**
   H66.92   **Otitis media, unspecified, left ear**
   H66.93   **Otitis media, unspecified, bilateral**

H67 [4th]   **OTITIS MEDIA IN DISEASES CLASSIFIED ELSEWHERE**
Code first underlying disease, such as:
plasminogen deficiency (E88.02)
viral disease NEC (B00–B34)
Use additional code for any associated perforated tympanic membrane (H72.-)
Excludes1: otitis media in: influenza (J09.X9, J10.83, J11.83)
measles (B05.3)
scarlet fever (A38.0)
tuberculosis (A18.6)

H67.1   **Otitis media in diseases classified elsewhere, right ear**
H67.2   **Otitis media in diseases classified elsewhere, left ear**
H67.3   **Otitis media in diseases classified elsewhere, bilateral**

H69 [4th]   **OTHER AND UNSPECIFIED DISORDERS OF EUSTACHIAN TUBE**

H69.8   **Other specified disorders of Eustachian tube**
[5th]   Use for Eustachian tube dysfunction

   H69.81   **Other specified disorders of Eustachian tube, right ear**
   H69.82   **Other specified disorders of Eustachian tube, left ear**
   H69.83   **Other specified disorders of Eustachian tube, bilateral**

H69.9   **Unspecified Eustachian tube disorder**
[5th]
   H69.91   **Unspecified Eustachian tube disorder, right ear**
   H69.92   **Unspecified Eustachian tube disorder, left ear**
   H69.93   **Unspecified Eustachian tube disorder, bilateral**

H72 [4th]   **PERFORATION OF TYMPANIC MEMBRANE**
Includes: persistent post-traumatic perforation of ear drum
postinflammatory perforation of ear drum
Code first any associated otitis media
Excludes1: acute suppurative otitis media with rupture of the tympanic membrane
traumatic rupture of ear drum

H72.0   **Central perforation of tympanic membrane**
[5th]
   H72.01   **Central perforation of tympanic membrane, right ear**
   H72.02   **Central perforation of tympanic membrane, left ear**
   H72.03   **Central perforation of tympanic membrane, bilateral**

H72.1   **Attic perforation of tympanic membrane**
[5th]   Perforation of pars flaccida

   H72.11   **Attic perforation of tympanic membrane, right ear**
   H72.12   **Attic perforation of tympanic membrane, left ear**
   H72.13   **Attic perforation of tympanic membrane, bilateral**

H72.2   **Other marginal perforations of tympanic membrane**
[5th]   **H72.2X**   **Other marginal perforations of tympanic membrane**
[6th]
    H72.2X1   **Other marginal perforations of tympanic membrane, right ear**
    H72.2X2   **Other marginal perforations of tympanic membrane, left ear**
    H72.2X3   **Other marginal perforations of tympanic membrane, bilateral**

H72.8   **Other perforations of tympanic membrane**
[5th]   **H72.81**   **Multiple perforations of tympanic membrane**
[6th]
    H72.811   **Multiple perforations of tympanic membrane, right ear**
    H72.812   **Multiple perforations of tympanic membrane, left ear**

    H72.813   **Multiple perforations of tympanic membrane, bilateral**
   H72.82   **Total perforations of tympanic membrane**
[6th]
    H72.821   **Total perforations of tympanic membrane, right ear**
    H72.822   **Total perforations of tympanic membrane, left ear**
    H72.823   **Total perforations of tympanic membrane, bilateral**

H72.9   **Unspecified perforation of tympanic membrane**
[5th]   **H72.91**   **Unspecified perforation of tympanic membrane, right ear**
   H72.92   **Unspecified perforation of tympanic membrane, left ear**
   H72.93   **Unspecified perforation of tympanic membrane, bilateral**

H73 [4th]   **OTHER DISORDERS OF TYMPANIC MEMBRANE**

H73.0   **Acute myringitis**
[5th]   *Excludes1:* acute myringitis with otitis media (H65, H66)

   H73.00   **Unspecified acute myringitis**
[6th]   Acute tympanitis NOS
    H73.001   **Acute myringitis, right ear**
    H73.002   **Acute myringitis, left ear**
    H73.003   **Acute myringitis, bilateral**

   H73.01   **Bullous myringitis**
[6th]
    H73.011   **Bullous myringitis, right ear**
    H73.012   **Bullous myringitis, left ear**
    H73.013   **Bullous myringitis, bilateral**

H73.1   **Chronic myringitis**
[5th]   Chronic tympanitis
Excludes1: chronic myringitis with otitis media (H65, H66)

   H73.11   **Chronic myringitis, right ear**
   H73.12   **Chronic myringitis, left ear**
   H73.13   **Chronic myringitis, bilateral**

H73.2   **Unspecified myringitis**
[5th]
   H73.21   **Unspecified myringitis, right ear**
   H73.22   **Unspecified myringitis, left ear**
   H73.23   **Unspecified myringitis, bilateral**

H73.8   **Other specified disorders of tympanic membrane**

(H80–H83) DISEASES OF INNER EAR

H81 [4th]   **DISORDERS OF VESTIBULAR FUNCTION**
Excludes1: epidemic vertigo (A88.1)
vertigo NOS (R42)

H81.0   **Ménière's disease**
[5th]   Labyrinthine hydrops
Ménière's syndrome or vertigo
   H81.01   **Ménière's disease, right ear**
   H81.02   **Ménière's disease, left ear**
   H81.03   **Ménière's disease, bilateral**

H81.1   **Benign paroxysmal vertigo**
[5th]
   H81.11   **Benign paroxysmal vertigo, right ear**
   H81.12   **Benign paroxysmal vertigo, left ear**
   H81.13   **Benign paroxysmal vertigo, bilateral**

H81.3   **Other peripheral vertigo**
[5th]   **H81.31**   **Aural vertigo**
[6th]
    H81.311   **Aural vertigo, right ear**
    H81.312   **Aural vertigo, left ear**
    H81.313   **Aural vertigo, bilateral**

   H81.39   **Other peripheral vertigo**
[6th]   Lermoyez' syndrome
Otogenic vertigo
Peripheral vertigo NOS
    H81.391   **Other peripheral vertigo, right ear**
    H81.392   **Other peripheral vertigo, left ear**
    H81.393   **Other peripheral vertigo, bilateral**

H81.4   **Vertigo of central origin**
Central positional nystagmus

H81.8   **Other disorders of vestibular function**
[5th]   **H81.8X**   **Other disorders of vestibular function**
[6th]   **H81.8X1**   **Other disorders of vestibular function, right ear**

[4th] [5th] [6th] [7th] Additional Character Required   ✓ 3-character code   Unspecified laterality codes were excluded here.   •=New Code   ▲=Revised Code   *Excludes1*—Not coded here, do not use together   *Excludes2*—Not included here

CHAPTER 8. DISEASES OF THE EAR AND MASTOID PROCESS   (H81.8X2–H93.2)

H81.8X2 Other disorders of vestibular function, left ear

H81.8X3 Other disorders of vestibular function, bilateral

H81.9 Unspecified disorder of vestibular function
- 5th   Vertiginous syndrome NOS
- **H81.91** Unspecified disorder of vestibular function, right ear
- **H81.92** Unspecified disorder of vestibular function, left ear
- **H81.93** Unspecified disorder of vestibular function, bilateral

H83   OTHER DISEASES OF INNER EAR
4th

H83.0 Labyrinthitis
- 5th
- **H83.01** Labyrinthitis, right ear
- **H83.02** Labyrinthitis, left ear
- **H83.03** Labyrinthitis, bilateral
- **H83.09** Labyrinthitis, unspecified ear

H83.3 Noise effects on inner ear
- 5th   Acoustic trauma of inner ear
- Noise-induced hearing loss of inner ear
- **H83.3X** Noise effects on inner ear
  - 6th
  - **H83.3X1** Noise effects on right inner ear
  - **H83.3X2** Noise effects on left inner ear
  - **H83.3X3** Noise effects on inner ear, bilateral

(H90–H94) OTHER DISORDERS OF EAR

H90   CONDUCTIVE AND SENSORINEURAL HEARING LOSS
4th

Excludes1: deaf nonspeaking NEC (H91.3)
- deafness NOS (H91.9-)
- hearing loss NOS (H91.9-)
- noise-induced hearing loss (H83.3-)
- ototoxic hearing loss (H91.0-)
- sudden (idiopathic) hearing loss (H91.2-)

H90.0 Conductive hearing loss, bilateral

H90.1 Conductive hearing loss, unilateral with unrestricted hearing
- 5th   on the contralateral side
- **H90.11** Conductive hearing loss, unilateral, right ear, with unrestricted hearing on the contralateral side
- **H90.12** Conductive hearing loss, unilateral, left ear, with unrestricted hearing on the contralateral side

H90.2 Conductive hearing loss, unspecified
- Conductive deafness NOS

H90.3 Sensorineural hearing loss, bilateral

H90.4 Sensorineural hearing loss, unilateral with unrestricted
- 5th   hearing on the contralateral side
- **H90.41** Sensorineural hearing loss, unilateral, right ear, with unrestricted hearing on the contralateral side
- **H90.42** Sensorineural hearing loss, unilateral, left ear, with unrestricted hearing on the contralateral side

H90.5 Unspecified sensorineural hearing loss
- Central hearing loss NOS
- Congenital deafness NOS
- Neural hearing loss NOS
- Perceptive hearing loss NOS
- Sensorineural deafness NOS
- Sensory hearing loss NOS
- ***Excludes1:*** abnormal auditory perception (H93.2-)
  - psychogenic deafness (F44.6)

H90.6 Mixed conductive and sensorineural hearing loss, bilateral

H90.7 Mixed conductive and sensorineural hearing loss, unilateral
- 5th   with unrestricted hearing on the contralateral side
- **H90.71** Mixed conductive and sensorineural hearing loss, unilateral, right ear, with unrestricted hearing on the contralateral side
- **H90.72** Mixed conductive and sensorineural hearing loss, unilateral, left ear, with unrestricted hearing on the contralateral side

H90.8 Mixed conductive and sensorineural hearing loss, unspecified

H90.A Hearing loss, unilateral, with restricted hearing on the
- 5th   contralateral side
- **H90.A1** Conductive hearing loss, unilateral, with restricted
  - 6th   hearing on the contralateral side

H90.A11 Conductive hearing loss, unilateral, right ear with restricted hearing on the contralateral side

H90.A12 Conductive hearing loss, unilateral, left ear with restricted hearing on the contralateral side

H90.A2 Sensorineural hearing loss, unilateral, with restricted
- 6th   hearing on the contralateral side
- **H90.A21** Sensorineural hearing loss, unilateral, right ear, with restricted hearing on the contralateral side
- **H90.A22** Sensorineural hearing loss, unilateral, left ear, with restricted hearing on the contralateral side

H90.A3 Mixed conductive and sensorineural hearing
- 6th   loss, unilateral, with restricted hearing on the contralateral side
- **H90.A31** Mixed conductive and sensorineural hearing loss, unilateral, right ear with restricted hearing on the contralateral side
- **H90.A32** Mixed conductive and sensorineural hearing, unilateral, left ear with restricted hearing on the contralateral side

H91   OTHER AND UNSPECIFIED HEARING LOSS
4th

Excludes1: abnormal auditory perception (H93.2-)
- hearing loss as classified in H90.-
- impacted cerumen (H61.2-)
- noise-induced hearing loss (H83.3-)
- psychogenic deafness (F44.6)
- transient ischemic deafness (H93.01-)

H91.2 Sudden idiopathic hearing loss
- 5th   Sudden hearing loss NOS
- **H91.21** Sudden idiopathic hearing loss, right ear
- **H91.22** Sudden idiopathic hearing loss, left ear
- **H91.23** Sudden idiopathic hearing loss, bilateral

H91.3 Deaf nonspeaking, not elsewhere classified

H91.8 Other specified hearing loss
- 5th   **H91.8X** Other specified hearing loss
  - 6th   **H91.8X1** Other specified hearing loss, right ear
  - **H91.8X2** Other specified hearing loss, left ear
  - **H91.8X3** Other specified hearing loss, bilateral

H91.9 Unspecified hearing loss
- 5th   Deafness NOS
- High frequency deafness
- Low frequency deafness
- **H91.91** Unspecified hearing loss, right ear
- **H91.92** Unspecified hearing loss, left ear
- **H91.93** Unspecified hearing loss, bilateral

H92   OTALGIA AND EFFUSION OF EAR
4th

H92.0 Otalgia
- 5th
- **H92.01** Otalgia, right ear
- **H92.02** Otalgia, left ear
- **H92.03** Otalgia, bilateral

H92.1 Otorrhea
- 5th   ***Excludes1:*** leakage of cerebrospinal fluid through ear (G96.0)
- **H92.11** Otorrhea, right ear
- **H92.12** Otorrhea, left ear
- **H92.13** Otorrhea, bilateral

H93   OTHER DISORDERS OF EAR, NOT ELSEWHERE
4th   CLASSIFIED

H93.1 Tinnitus
- 5th
- **H93.11** Tinnitus, right ear
- **H93.12** Tinnitus, left ear
- **H93.13** Tinnitus, bilateral

H93.A Pulsatile tinnitus
- 5th
- **H93.A1** Pulsatile tinnitus, right ear
- **H93.A2** Pulsatile tinnitus, left ear
- **H93.A3** Pulsatile tinnitus, bilateral

H93.2 Other abnormal auditory perceptions
- 5th   auditory hallucinations (R44.0)

  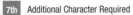 Additional Character Required   ✔ 3-character code   Unspecified laterality codes were excluded here.   •=New Code   ▲=Revised Code   ***Excludes1***—Not coded here, do not use together   ***Excludes2***—Not included here

H93.25 **Central auditory processing disorder**
Congenital auditory imperception
Word deafness

H93.29 **Other abnormal auditory perceptions**

6th   H93.291   **Other abnormal auditory perceptions, right ear**

H93.292   **Other abnormal auditory perceptions, left ear**

H93.293   **Other abnormal auditory perceptions, bilateral**

H93.8 **Other specified disorders of ear**

5th   H93.8X   **Other specified disorders of ear**

6th   H93.8X1   **Other specified disorders of right ear**

H93.8X2   **Other specified disorders of left ear**

H93.8X3   **Other specified disorders of ear, bilateral**

(H95) INTRAOPERATIVE AND POSTPROCEDURAL COMPLICATIONS AND DISORDERS OF EAR AND MASTOID PROCESS, NOT ELSEWHERE CLASSIFIED

| 4th | 5th | 6th | 7th | Additional Character Required | ✔ | 3-character code | Unspecified laterality codes were excluded here. | •=New Code ▲=Revised Code | **Excludes1**—Not coded here, do not use together **Excludes2**—Not included here |

Chapter 9. Diseases of the circulatory system (I00–I99)

GUIDELINES

a. Hypertension

The classification presumes a causal relationship between hypertension and heart involvement and between hypertension and kidney involvement, as the two conditions are linked by the term "with" in the Alphabetic Index. These conditions should be coded as related even in the absence of provider documentation explicitly linking them, unless the documentation clearly states the conditions are unrelated.

For hypertension and conditions not specifically linked by relational terms such as "with," "associated with" or "due to" in the classification, provider documentation must link the conditions in order to code them as related.

1) Hypertension with Heart Disease

Hypertension with heart conditions classified to I50.- or I51.4–I51.7, I51.89, I51.9, are assigned to a code from category I11, Hypertensive heart disease. Use additional code(s) from category I50, Heart failure, to identify the type(s) of heart failure in those patients with heart failure.

The same heart conditions (I50.-, I51.4–I51.7, I51.89, I51.9) with hypertension are coded separately if the provider has documented they are unrelated to the hypertension. Sequence according to the circumstances of the admission/encounter.

Refer to ICD-10-CM Official Guidelines for Coding and Reporting for instructions for reporting atherosclerotic coronary artery disease, cerebrovascular accident, and/or myocardial infarction

Excludes2:

certain conditions originating in the perinatal period (P04–P96)

certain infectious and parasitic diseases (A00–B99)

complications of pregnancy, childbirth and the puerperium (O00–O9A)

congenital malformations, deformations, and chromosomal abnormalities (Q00–Q99)

endocrine, nutritional and metabolic diseases (E00–E88)

injury, poisoning and certain other consequences of external causes (S00–T88)

neoplasms (C00–D49)

symptoms, signs and abnormal clinical and laboratory findings, not elsewhere classified (R00–R94)

systemic connective tissue disorders (M30–M36)

transient cerebral ischemic attacks and related syndromes (G45.-)

(I00–I02) ACUTE RHEUMATIC FEVER

I00 **RHEUMATIC FEVER WITHOUT HEART INVOLVEMENT**

[✓] ***Includes:*** arthritis, rheumatic, acute or subacute
Excludes1: rheumatic fever with heart involvement (I01.0–I01.9)

I01 **RHEUMATIC FEVER WITH HEART INVOLVEMENT**

[4th] ***Excludes1:*** chronic diseases of rheumatic origin (I05–I09) unless rheumatic fever is also present or there is evidence of reactivation or activity of the rheumatic process.

I01.0 **Acute rheumatic pericarditis**
Any condition in I00 with pericarditis
Rheumatic pericarditis (acute)
Excludes1: acute pericarditis not specified as rheumatic (I30.-)

I01.1 **Acute rheumatic endocarditis**
Any condition in I00 with endocarditis or valvulitis
Acute rheumatic valvulitis

I01.2 **Acute rheumatic myocarditis**
Any condition in I00 with myocarditis

I01.8 **Other acute rheumatic heart disease**
Any condition in I00 with other or multiple types of heart involvement
Acute rheumatic pancarditis

I01.9 **Acute rheumatic heart disease, unspecified**
Any condition in I00 with unspecified type of heart involvement
Rheumatic carditis, acute
Rheumatic heart disease, active or acute

I02 **RHEUMATIC CHOREA**

[4th] ***Includes:*** Sydenham's chorea
Excludes1: chorea NOS (G25.5)
Huntington's chorea (G10)

I02.0 **Rheumatic chorea with heart involvement**
Chorea NOS with heart involvement
Rheumatic chorea with heart involvement of any type classifiable under I01.-

I02.9 **Rheumatic chorea without heart involvement**
Rheumatic chorea NOS
Rheumatic heart disease, active or acute

(I05–I09) CHRONIC RHEUMATIC HEART DISEASES

I05 **RHEUMATIC MITRAL VALVE DISEASES**

[4th] ***Includes:*** conditions classifiable to both I05.0 and I05.2–I05.9, whether specified as rheumatic or not
Excludes1: mitral valve disease specified as nonrheumatic (I34.-)
mitral valve disease with aortic and/or tricuspid valve involvement (I08.-)

I05.0 **Rheumatic mitral stenosis**
Mitral (valve) obstruction (rheumatic)

I05.1 **Rheumatic mitral insufficiency**
Rheumatic mitral incompetence
Rheumatic mitral regurgitation
Excludes1: mitral insufficiency not specified as rheumatic (I34.0)

I05.2 **Rheumatic mitral stenosis with insufficiency**
Rheumatic mitral stenosis with incompetence or regurgitation

I05.8 **Other rheumatic mitral valve diseases**
Rheumatic mitral (valve) failure

I05.9 **Rheumatic mitral valve disease, unspecified**
Rheumatic mitral (valve) disorder (chronic) NOS

I06 **RHEUMATIC AORTIC VALVE DISEASES**

[4th] ***Excludes1:*** aortic valve disease not specified as rheumatic (I35.-)
aortic valve disease with mitral and/or tricuspid valve involvement (I08.-)

I06.0 **Rheumatic aortic stenosis**
Rheumatic aortic (valve) obstruction

I06.1 **Rheumatic aortic insufficiency**
Rheumatic aortic incompetence
Rheumatic aortic regurgitation

I06.2 **Rheumatic aortic stenosis with insufficiency**
Rheumatic aortic stenosis with incompetence or regurgitation

I06.8 **Other rheumatic aortic valve diseases**

I06.9 **Rheumatic aortic valve disease, unspecified**
Rheumatic aortic (valve) disease NOS

I07 **RHEUMATIC TRICUSPID VALVE DISEASES**

[4th] ***Includes:*** rheumatic tricuspid valve diseases specified as rheumatic or unspecified
Excludes1: tricuspid valve disease specified as nonrheumatic (I36.-)
tricuspid valve disease with aortic and/or mitral valve involvement (I08.-)

I07.0 **Rheumatic tricuspid stenosis**
Tricuspid (valve) stenosis (rheumatic)

I07.1 **Rheumatic tricuspid insufficiency**
Tricuspid (valve) insufficiency (rheumatic)

I07.2 **Rheumatic tricuspid stenosis and insufficiency**

I07.8 **Other rheumatic tricuspid valve diseases**

I07.9 **Rheumatic tricuspid valve disease, unspecified**
Rheumatic tricuspid valve disorder NOS

I08 **MULTIPLE VALVE DISEASES**

[4th] ***Includes:*** multiple valve diseases specified as rheumatic or unspecified
Excludes1: endocarditis, valve unspecified (I38)
multiple valve disease specified a nonrheumatic (I34.-, I35.-, I36.-, I37.-, I38.-, Q22.-, Q23.-, Q24.8-)
rheumatic valve disease NOS (I09.1)

I08.0 **Rheumatic disorders of both mitral and aortic valves**
Involvement of both mitral and aortic valves specified as rheumatic or unspecified

I08.1 **Rheumatic disorders of both mitral and tricuspid valves**

I08.2 **Rheumatic disorders of both aortic and tricuspid valves**

I08.3 **Combined rheumatic disorders of mitral, aortic and tricuspid valves**

I08.8 **Other rheumatic multiple valve diseases**

I08.9 **Rheumatic multiple valve disease, unspecified**

[4th] [5th] [6th] [7th] Additional Character Required   3-character code

•=New Code   ***Excludes1***—Not coded here, do not use together
▲=Revised Code   ***Excludes2***—Not included here

I09 OTHER RHEUMATIC HEART DISEASES

`4th`

I09.0 **Rheumatic myocarditis**
Excludes1: myocarditis not specified as rheumatic (I51.4)

I09.1 **Rheumatic diseases of endocardium, valve unspecified**
Rheumatic endocarditis (chronic)
Rheumatic valvulitis (chronic)
Excludes1: endocarditis, valve unspecified (I38)

I09.2 **Chronic rheumatic pericarditis**
Adherent pericardium, rheumatic
Chronic rheumatic mediastinopericarditis
Chronic rheumatic myopericarditis
Excludes1: chronic pericarditis not specified as rheumatic (I31.-)

I09.8 **Other specified rheumatic heart diseases**
`5th` **I09.81** **Rheumatic heart failure**
Use additional code to identify type of heart failure (I50.-)

I09.89 **Other specified rheumatic heart diseases**
Rheumatic disease of pulmonary valve

I09.9 **Rheumatic heart disease, unspecified**
Rheumatic carditis
Excludes1: rheumatoid carditis (M05.31)

(I10–I16) HYPERTENSIVE DISEASES

Use additional code to identify: exposure to environmental tobacco smoke (Z77.22)
history of tobacco dependence (Z87.891)
occupational exposure to environmental tobacco smoke (Z57.31)
tobacco dependence (F17.-)
tobacco use (Z72.0)
Excludes1: neonatal hypertension (P29.2)
primary pulmonary hypertension (I27.0)
Excludes2: hypertensive disease complicating pregnancy, childbirth and the puerperium (O10–O11, O13–O16)

I10 ESSENTIAL (PRIMARY) HYPERTENSION

`✓`

Includes: high blood pressure
hypertension (arterial) (benign) (essential) (malignant) (primary) (systemic)
Excludes1: hypertensive disease complicating pregnancy, childbirth and the puerperium (O10–O11, O13–O16)
Excludes2: essential (primary) hypertension involving vessels of brain (I60–I69)
essential (primary) hypertension involving vessels of eye (H35.0-)

I11 HYPERTENSIVE HEART DISEASE

`4th`

Includes: any condition in I50.-, or I51.4-, I51.7, I51.89, I51.9 due to hypertension

I11.0 **Hypertensive heart disease with heart failure**
Hypertensive heart failure
Use additional code to identify type of heart failure (I50.-)

I11.9 **Hypertensive heart disease without heart failure**
Hypertensive heart disease NOS

I12 HYPERTENSIVE CHRONIC KIDNEY DISEASE

`4th`

GUIDELINES

Assign codes from category I12, Hypertensive chronic kidney disease, when both hypertension and a condition classifiable to category N18, Chronic kidney disease (CKD), are present. CKD should not be coded as hypertensive if the provider indicates the CKD is not related to the hypertension.

The appropriate code from category N18 should be used as a secondary code with a code from category I12 to identify the stage of chronic kidney disease.

If a patient has hypertensive chronic kidney disease and acute renal failure, an additional code for the acute renal failure is required.

Includes: any condition in N18 and N26 - due to hypertension
arteriosclerosis of kidney
arteriosclerotic nephritis (chronic) (interstitial)
hypertensive nephropathy
nephrosclerosis
Excludes1: hypertension due to kidney disease (I15.0, I15.1)
renovascular hypertension (I15.0)
secondary hypertension (I15.-)
Excludes2: acute kidney failure (N17.-)

I12.0 **Hypertensive chronic kidney disease with stage 5 chronic kidney disease or end stage renal disease**
Use additional code to identify the stage of chronic kidney disease (N18.5, N18.6)

I12.9 **Hypertensive chronic kidney disease with stage 1 through stage 4 chronic kidney disease, or unspecified chronic kidney disease**
Hypertensive chronic kidney disease NOS
Hypertensive renal disease NOS
Use additional code to identify the stage of chronic kidney disease (N18.1-N18.4, N18.9)

I16 HYPERTENSIVE CRISIS

`4th`

GUIDELINES

Assign a code from category I16, Hypertensive crisis, for documented hypertensive urgency, hypertensive emergency or unspecified hypertensive crisis. Code also any identified hypertensive disease (I10-I15). The sequencing is based on the reason for the encounter.
Code also any identified hypertensive disease (I10–I15)

I16.0 **Hypertensive urgency**
I16.1 **Hypertensive emergency**
I16.9 **Hypertensive crisis, unspecified**

(I20–I25) ISCHEMIC HEART DISEASES

Use additional code to identify presence of hypertension (I10–I16)
Please see full ICD-10-CM manual for cardiovascular disease with symptoms or infarction.

I20 ANGINA PECTORIS

`4th`

Use additional code to identify:
exposure to environmental tobacco smoke (Z77.22)
history of tobacco dependence (Z87.891)
occupational exposure to environmental tobacco smoke (Z57.31)
tobacco dependence (F17.-)
tobacco use (Z72.0)
Excludes1: angina pectoris with atherosclerotic heart disease of native coronary arteries (I25.1-)
atherosclerosis of coronary artery bypass graft(s) and coronary artery of transplanted heart with anginapectoris (I25.7-)
postinfarction angina (I23.7)

I20.9 **Angina pectoris, unspecified**
Angina NOS
Anginal syndrome
Cardiac angina
Ischemic chest pain

I23 CERTAIN CURRENT COMPLICATIONS FOLLOWING ST ELEVATION (STEMI) AND NON-ST ELEVATION (NSTEMI) MYOCARDIALINFARCTION (WITHIN THE 28 DAY PERIOD)

`4th`

I23.0 **Hemopericardium as current complication following acute myocardial infarction**
Excludes1: hemopericardium not specified as current complication following acute myocardial infarction (I31.2)

I23.3 **Rupture of cardiac wall without hemopericardium as current complication following acute myocardial infarction**

I24 OTHER ACUTE ISCHEMIC HEART DISEASES

`4th`

Excludes1: angina pectoris (I20.-)
transient myocardial ischemia in newborn (P29.4)

I24.1 **Dressler's syndrome**
Postmyocardial infarction syndrome
Excludes1: postinfarction angina (I23.7)

I24.9 **Acute ischemic heart disease, unspecified**
Excludes1: ischemic heart disease (chronic) NOS (I25.9)

I25 CHRONIC ISCHEMIC HEART DISEASE

`4th`

Use additional history of tobacco dependence (Z87.891)

I25.1 **Atherosclerotic cardiovascular disease**
`5th` Coronary (artery) atheroma
Coronary (artery) atherosclerosis
Coronary (artery) disease
Coronary (artery) sclerosis

I25.10 **Atherosclerotic heart disease of native coronary artery without angina pectoris**
Atherosclerotic heart disease NOS

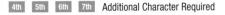 `4th` `5th` `6th` `7th` Additional Character Required   `✓` 3-character code

•=New Code   *Excludes1*—Not coded here, do not use together
▲=Revised Code   *Excludes2*—Not included here

(I26–I28) PULMONARY HEART DISEASE AND DISEASES OF PULMONARY CIRCULATION

I27   **OTHER PULMONARY HEART DISEASES**

4th

GUIDELINES

Pulmonary hypertension is classified to category I27, Other pulmonary heart diseases. For secondary pulmonary hypertension (I27.1, I27.2-), code also any associated conditions or adverse effects of drugs or toxins. The sequencing is based on the reason for the encounter.

I27.0   **Primary pulmonary hypertension**
Heritable pulmonary arterial hypertension
Idiopathic pulmonary arterial hypertension
Primary group 1 pulmonary hypertension
Primary pulmonary arterial hypertension
Excludes1: persistent pulmonary hypertension of newborn (P29.30)
   pulmonary hypertension NOS (I27.20)
   secondary pulmonary arterial hypertension (I27.21)
   secondary pulmonary hypertension (I27.29)

I27.1   **Kyphoscoliotic heart disease**

I27.2   **Other secondary pulmonary hypertension**

5th   **Code also** associated underlying condition
Excludes1: Eisenmenger's syndrome (I27.83)

     I27.20   **Pulmonary hypertension, unspecified**
         Pulmonary hypertension NOS

     I27.21   **Secondary pulmonary arterial hypertension**
         (Associated) (drug-induced) (toxin-induced) pulmonary arterial hypertension NOS
         (Associated) (drug-induced) (toxin-induced) (secondary) group 1 pulmonary hypertension
         Code also associated conditions if applicable, or adverse effects of drugs or toxins, such as:
           adverse effect of appetite depressants (T50.5X5)
           congenital heart disease (Q20-Q28)
           human immunodeficiency virus [HIV] disease (B20)
           polymyositis (M33.2-)
           portal hypertension (K76.6)
           rheumatoid arthritis (M05.-)
           schistosomiasis (B65.-)
         Sjögren syndrome (M35.0-)
         systemic sclerosis (M34.-)

     I27.22   **Pulmonary hypertension due to left heart disease**
         Group 2 pulmonary hypertension
         Code also associated left heart disease, if known, such as:
           multiple valve disease (I08.-)
           rheumatic mitral valve diseases (I05.-)
           rheumatic aortic valve diseases (I06.-)

     I27.23   **Pulmonary hypertension due to lung diseases and hypoxia**
         Group 3 pulmonary hypertension
         Code also associated lung disease, if known, such as:
           bronchiectasis (J47.-)
           cystic fibrosis with pulmonary manifestations (E84.0)
           interstitial lung disease (J84.-)
           pleural effusion (J90)
           sleep apnea (G47.3-)

     I27.24   **Chronic thromboembolic pulmonary hypertension**
         Group 4 pulmonary hypertension
         Code also associated pulmonary embolism, if applicable (I26.-, I27.82)

     I27.29   **Other secondary pulmonary hypertension**
         Group 5 pulmonary hypertension
         Pulmonary hypertension with unclear multifactorial mechanisms
         Pulmonary hypertension due to hematologic disorders
         Pulmonary hypertension due to metabolic disorders
         Pulmonary hypertension due to other systemic disorders
         Code also other associated disorders, if known, such as:
           chronic myeloid leukemia (C92.10–C92.22)
           essential thrombocythemia (D47.3)
           Gaucher disease (E75.22)

         hypertensive chronic kidney disease with end stage renal disease (I12.0, I13.11, I13.2)
         hyperthyroidism (E05.-)
         hypothyroidism (E00-E03)
         polycythemia vera (D45)
         sarcoidosis (D86.-)

I27.8   **Other specified pulmonary heart diseases**

5th   **I27.81**   **Cor pulmonale (chronic)**
         Cor pulmonale NOS
         Excludes1: acute cor pulmonale (I26.0-)

     I27.82   **Chronic pulmonary embolism**
         Use additional code, if applicable, for associated long-term (current) use of anticoagulants (Z79.01)
         Excludes1: personal history of pulmonary embolism (Z86.711)

     I27.83   **Eisenmenger's syndrome**
         Eisenmenger's complex
         (Irreversible) Eisenmenger's disease
         Pulmonary hypertension with right to left shunt related to congenital heart disease
         Code also underlying heart defect, if known, such as:
           atrial septal defect (Q21.1)
           Eisenmenger's defect (Q21.8)
           patent ductus arteriosus (Q25.0)
           ventricular septal defect (Q21.0)

     I27.89   **Other specified pulmonary heart diseases**
         Excludes1: Eisenmenger's defect (Q21.8)

I27.9   **Pulmonary heart disease, unspecified**
Chronic cardiopulmonary disease

I28   **OTHER DISEASES OF PULMONARY VESSELS**

4th   **I28.0**   **Arteriovenous fistula of pulmonary vessels**
         Excludes1: congenital arteriovenous fistula (Q25.72)

     I28.1   **Aneurysm of pulmonary artery**
         Excludes1: congenital aneurysm (Q25.79)
           congenital arteriovenous aneurysm (Q25.72)

     I28.8   **Other diseases of pulmonary vessels**
         Pulmonary arteritis
         Pulmonary endarteritis
         Rupture of pulmonary vessels
         Stenosis of pulmonary vessels
         Stricture of pulmonary vessels

     I28.9   **Disease of pulmonary vessels, unspecified**

(I30–I52) OTHER FORMS OF HEART DISEASE

I30   **ACUTE PERICARDITIS**

4th   *Includes:* acute mediastinopericarditis
     acute myopericarditis
     acute pericardial effusion
     acute pleuropericarditis
     acute pneumopericarditis
   Excludes1: Dressler's syndrome (I24.1)
     rheumatic pericarditis (acute) (I01.0)
     viral pericarditis due to Coxsakie virus (B33.23)

     I30.0   **Acute nonspecific idiopathic pericarditis**

     I30.1   **Infective pericarditis**
         Pneumococcal pericarditis
         Pneumopyopericardium
         Purulent pericarditis
         Pyopericarditis
         Pyopericardium
         Pyopneumopericardium
         Staphylococcal pericarditis
         Streptococcal pericarditis
         Suppurative pericarditis
         Viral pericarditis
         Use additional code (B95–B97) to identify infectious agent

     I30.8   **Other forms of acute pericarditis**

     I30.9   **Acute pericarditis, unspecified**

I31   **OTHER DISEASES OF PERICARDIUM**

4th   *Excludes1:* diseases of pericardium specified as rheumatic (I09.2)
     postcardiotomy syndrome (I97.0)
     traumatic injury to pericardium (S26.-)

4th **5th** **6th** **7th**   Additional Character Required   ✔   3-character code

•=New Code   *Excludes1*—Not coded here, do not use together
▲=Revised Code   *Excludes2*—Not included here

CHAPTER 9. DISEASES OF THE CIRCULATORY SYSTEM   (I31.0–I44.1)

I31.0   **Chronic adhesive pericarditis**
Accretio cordis
Adherent pericardium
Adhesive mediastinopericarditis

I31.1   **Chronic constrictive pericarditis**
Concretio cordis
Pericardial calcification

I31.2   **Hemopericardium, not elsewhere classified**
Excludes1: hemopericardium as current complication following acute myocardial infarction (I23.0)

I31.3   **Pericardial effusion (noninflammatory)**
Chylopericardium
Excludes1: acute pericardial effusion (I30.9)

I31.4   **Cardiac tamponade**
Code first underlying cause

I31.8   **Other specified diseases of pericardium**
Epicardial plaques
Focal pericardial adhesions

I31.9   **Disease of pericardium, unspecified**
Pericarditis (chronic) NOS

I33   **ACUTE AND SUBACUTE ENDOCARDITIS**
`4th`   *Excludes1:* acute rheumatic endocarditis (I01.1)
endocarditis NOS (I38)

I33.0   **Acute and subacute infective endocarditis**
Bacterial endocarditis (acute) (subacute)
Infective endocarditis (acute) (subacute) NOS
Endocarditis lenta (acute) (subacute)
Malignant endocarditis (acute) (subacute)
Purulent endocarditis (acute) (subacute)
Septic endocarditis (acute) (subacute)
Ulcerative endocarditis (acute) (subacute)
Vegetative endocarditis (acute) (subacute)
Use additional code (B95–B97) to identify infectious agent

I33.9   **Acute and subacute endocarditis, unspecified**
Acute endocarditis NOS
Acute myoendocarditis NOS
Acute periendocarditis NOS
Subacute endocarditis NOS
Subacute myoendocarditis NOS
Subacute periendocarditis NOS

I34   **NONRHEUMATIC MITRAL VALVE DISORDERS**
`4th`   *Excludes1:* mitral valve disease (I05.9)
mitral valve failure (I05.8)
mitral valve stenosis (I05.0)
mitral valve disorder of unspecified cause with diseases of aortic and/or tricuspid valve(s) (I08.-)
mitral valve disorder of unspecified cause with mitral stenosis or obstruction (I05.0)
mitral valve disorder specified as congenital (Q23.2, Q23.9)
mitral valve disorder specified as rheumatic (I05.-)

I34.0   **Nonrheumatic mitral (valve) insufficiency**
Nonrheumatic mitral (valve) incompetence NOS
Nonrheumatic mitral (valve) regurgitation NOS

I35   **NONRHEUMATIC AORTIC VALVE DISORDERS**
`4th`   *Excludes1:* aortic valve disorder of unspecified cause but with diseases of mitral and/or tricuspid valve(s) (I08.-)
aortic valve disorder specified as congenital (Q23.0, Q23.1)
aortic valve disorder specified as rheumatic (I06.-)
hypertrophic subaortic stenosis (I42.1)

I35.0   **Nonrheumatic aortic (valve) stenosis**

I35.1   **Nonrheumatic aortic (valve) insufficiency**
Nonrheumatic aortic (valve) incompetence NOS
Nonrheumatic aortic (valve) regurgitation NOS

I35.2   **Nonrheumatic aortic (valve) stenosis with insufficiency**

I35.8   **Other nonrheumatic aortic valve disorders**

I35.9   **Nonrheumatic aortic valve disorder, unspecified**

I36   **NONRHEUMATIC TRICUSPID VALVE DISORDERS**
`4th`   *Excludes1:* tricuspid valve disorders of unspecified cause (I07.-)
tricuspid valve disorders specified as congenital (Q22.4, Q22.8, Q22.9)
tricuspid valve disorders specified as rheumatic (I07.-)
tricuspid valve disorders with aortic and/or mitral valve involvement (I08.-)

I36.0   **Nonrheumatic tricuspid (valve) stenosis**

I36.1   **Nonrheumatic tricuspid (valve) insufficiency**
Nonrheumatic tricuspid (valve) incompetence
Nonrheumatic tricuspid (valve) regurgitation

I36.2   **Nonrheumatic tricuspid (valve) stenosis with insufficiency**

I36.8   **Other nonrheumatic tricuspid valve disorders**

I36.9   **Nonrheumatic tricuspid valve disorder, unspecified**

I37   **NONRHEUMATIC PULMONARY VALVE DISORDERS**
`4th`   *Excludes1:* pulmonary valve disorder specified as congenital (Q22.1, Q22.2, Q22.3)
pulmonary valve disorder specified as rheumatic (I09.89)

I37.0   **Nonrheumatic pulmonary valve stenosis**

I37.1   **Nonrheumatic pulmonary valve insufficiency**
Nonrheumatic pulmonary valve incompetence
Nonrheumatic pulmonary valve regurgitation

I37.2   **Nonrheumatic pulmonary valve stenosis with insufficiency**

I37.8   **Other nonrheumatic pulmonary valve disorders**

I37.9   **Nonrheumatic pulmonary valve disorder, unspecified**

I38   **ENDOCARDITIS, VALVE UNSPECIFIED**
`✔`   *Includes:* endocarditis (chronic) NOS
valvular incompetence NOS
valvular insufficiency NOS
valvular regurgitation NOS
valvular stenosis NOS
valvulitis (chronic) NOS
Excludes1: congenital insufficiency of cardiac valve NOS (Q24.8)
congenital stenosis of cardiac valve NOS (Q24.8)
endocardial fibroelastosis (I42.4)
endocarditis specified as rheumatic (I09.1)

I40   **ACUTE MYOCARDITIS**
`4th`   *Includes:* subacute myocarditis
Excludes1: acute rheumatic myocarditis (I01.2)

I40.0   **Infective myocarditis**
Septic myocarditis
Use additional code (B95–B97) to identify infectious agent

I40.8   **Other acute myocarditis**

I40.9   **Acute myocarditis, unspecified**

I42   **CARDIOMYOPATHY**
`4th`   *Includes:* myocardiopathy
Code first pre-existing cardiomyopathy complicating pregnancy and puerperium (O99.4)
Excludes2: ischemic cardiomyopathy (I25.5)
peripartum cardiomyopathy (O90.3)
ventricular hypertrophy (I51.7)

I42.1   **Obstructive hypertrophic cardiomyopathy**
Hypertrophic subaortic stenosis (idiopathic)

I42.2   **Other hypertrophic cardiomyopathy**
Nonobstructive hypertrophic cardiomyopathy

I42.5   **Other restrictive cardiomyopathy**
Constrictive cardiomyopathy NOS

I42.9   **Cardiomyopathy, unspecified**
Cardiomyopathy (primary) (secondary) NOS

I43   **CARDIOMYOPATHY IN DISEASES CLASSIFIED ELSEWHERE**
`✔`   **Code first** underlying disease, such as:
amyloidosis (E85.-)
glycogen storage disease (E74.0)
gout (M10.0-)
thyrotoxicosis (E05.0-E05.9-)
Excludes1: cardiomyopathy (in):
infectious diseases
sarcoidosis (D86.85)

I44   **ATRIOVENTRICULAR AND LEFT BUNDLE-BRANCH BLOCK**
`4th`
I44.0   **Atrioventricular block, first degree**

I44.1   **Atrioventricular block, second degree**
Atrioventricular block, type I and II
Möbitz block, type I and II
Second degree block, type I and II
Wenckebach's block

`4th` `5th` `6th` `7th` Additional Character Required   `✔` 3-character code

●=New Code   *Excludes1*—Not coded here, do not use together
▲=Revised Code   *Excludes2*—Not included here

I44.2 Atrioventricular block, complete
Complete heart block NOS
Third degree block

I45 OTHER CONDUCTION DISORDERS

`4th` **I45.6 Pre-excitation syndrome**
Accelerated atrioventricular conduction
Accessory atrioventricular conduction
Anomalous atrioventricular excitation
Lown-Ganong-Levine syndrome
Pre-excitation atrioventricular conduction
Wolff-Parkinson-White syndrome

I45.8 Other specified conduction disorders
`5th` **I45.81 Long QT syndrome**
I45.89 Other specified conduction disorders
Atrioventricular [AV] dissociation
Interference dissociation
Isorhythmic dissociation
Nonparoxysmal AV nodal tachycardia

I45.9 Conduction disorder, unspecified
Heart block NOS
Stokes-Adams syndrome

I46 CARDIAC ARREST

`4th` ***Excludes2:*** cardiogenic shock (R57.0)

I46.2 Cardiac arrest due to underlying cardiac condition
Code first underlying cardiac condition

I46.8 Cardiac arrest due to other underlying condition
Code first underlying condition

I46.9 Cardiac arrest, cause unspecified

I47 PAROXYSMAL TACHYCARDIA

`4th` **Code first** tachycardia complicating: abortion or ectopic or molar
pregnancy (O00–O07, O08.8)
obstetric surgery and procedures (O75.4)

Excludes1: tachycardia NOS (R00.0)
sinoauricular tachycardia NOS (R00.0)
sinus [sinusal] tachycardia NOS (R00.0)

I47.1 Supraventricular tachycardia
Atrial (paroxysmal) tachycardia
Atrioventricular [AV] (paroxysmal) tachycardia
Atrioventricular re-entrant (nodal) tachycardia [AVNRT] [AVRT]
Junctional (paroxysmal) tachycardia
Nodal (paroxysmal) tachycardia

I48 ATRIAL FIBRILLATION AND FLUTTER

`4th` **I48.0 Paroxysmal atrial fibrillation**
I48.1 Persistent atrial fibrillation
`5th` ***Excludes1:*** Permanent atrial fibrillation (I48.21)
I48.11 Longstanding persistent atrial fibrillation
I48.19 Other persistent atrial fibrillation
Chronic persistent atrial fibrillation
Persistent atrial fibrillation, NOS

I48.2 Chronic atrial fibrillation
`5th` **I48.20 Chronic atrial fibrillation, unspecified**
Excludes1: Chronic persistent atrial fibrillation (I48.19)
I48.21 Permanent atrial fibrillation

I48.3 Typical atrial flutter
Type I atrial flutter

I48.4 Atypical atrial flutter
Type II atrial flutter

I48.9 Unspecified atrial fibrillation and atrial flutter
`5th` **I48.91 Unspecified atrial fibrillation**
I48.92 Unspecified atrial flutter

I49 OTHER CARDIAC ARRHYTHMIAS

`4th` **Code first** cardiac arrhythmia complicating: abortion or ectopic or molar
pregnancy (O00–O07, O08.8)
obstetric surgery and procedures (O75.4)

Excludes1: neonatal dysrhythmia (P29.1-)
sinoatrial bradycardia (R00.1)
sinus bradycardia (R00.1)
vagal bradycardia (R00.1)

Excludes2: bradycardia NOS (R00.1)

I49.0 Ventricular fibrillation and flutter
`5th` **I49.01 Ventricular fibrillation**
I49.02 Ventricular flutter

I49.1 Atrial premature depolarization
Atrial premature beats

I49.5 Sick sinus syndrome
Tachycardia-bradycardia syndrome

I49.9 Cardiac arrhythmia, unspecified
Arrhythmia (cardiac) NOS

I50 HEART FAILURE

`4th` **Code first:** heart failure complicating abortion or ectopic or molar
pregnancy (O00–O07, O08.8)
heart failure due to hypertension (I11.0)
heart failure due to hypertension with CKD (I13.-)
heart failure following surgery (I97.13-)
obstetric surgery and procedures (O75.4)
rheumatic heart failure (I09.81)

Excludes1: neonatal cardiac failure (P29.0)
Excludes2: cardiac arrest (I46.-)

I50.1 Left ventricular failure, unspecified
Cardiac asthma
Edema of lung with heart disease NOS
Edema of lung with heart failure
Left heart failure
Pulmonary edema with heart disease NOS
Pulmonary edema with heart failure
Excludes1: edema of lung without heart disease or heart failure
(J81.-)
pulmonary edema without heart disease or failure (J81.-)

I50.2 Systolic (congestive) heart failure
`5th` Heart failure with reduced ejection fraction [HFrEF]
Systolic left ventricular heart failure
Code also end stage heart failure, if applicable (I50.84)
Excludes1: combined systolic (congestive) and diastolic
(congestive) heart failure (I50.4-)
I50.20 Unspecified systolic (congestive) heart failure
I50.21 Acute systolic (congestive) heart failure
I50.22 Chronic systolic (congestive) heart failure
I50.23 Acute on chronic systolic (congestive) heart failure

I50.3 Diastolic (congestive) heart failure
`5th` Diastolic left ventricular heart failure
Heart failure with normal ejection fraction
Heart failure with preserved ejection fraction [HFpEF]
Code also end stage heart failure, if applicable (I50.84)
Excludes1: combined systolic (congestive) and diastolic
(congestive) heart failure (I50.4-)
I50.30 Unspecified diastolic (congestive) heart failure
I50.31 Acute diastolic (congestive) heart failure
I50.32 Chronic diastolic (congestive) heart failure
I50.33 Acute on chronic diastolic (congestive) heart failure

I50.4 Combined systolic (congestive) and diastolic (congestive)
`5th` **heart failure**
I50.40 Unspecified combined systolic (congestive) and
diastolic (congestive) heart failure
I50.41 Acute combined systolic (congestive) and diastolic
(congestive) heart failure
I50.42 Chronic combined systolic (congestive) and diastolic
(congestive) heart failure
I50.43 Acute on chronic combined systolic (congestive) and
diastolic (congestive) heart failure

I50.8 Other heart failure
`5th` **I50.82 Biventricular heart failure**
Code also the type of left ventricular failure as systolic,
diastolic, or combined, if known (I50.2-I50.43)
I50.83 High output heart failure
I50.84 End stage heart failure
Stage D heart failure
Code also the type of heart failure as systolic, diastolic,
or combined, if known (I50.2-I50.43)
I50.89 Other heart failure

CHAPTER 9. DISEASES OF THE CIRCULATORY SYSTEM   (I44.2-I50.89)

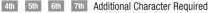

`4th` `5th` `6th` `7th` Additional Character Required   ✔ 3-character code

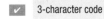

•=New Code   ***Excludes1***—Not coded here, do not use together
▲=Revised Code   ***Excludes2***—Not included here

I50.9   Heart failure, unspecified
Biventricular (heart) failure NOS
Cardiac, heart or myocardial failure NOS
Congestive heart disease
Congestive heart failure NOS
Right ventricular failure (secondary to left heart failure)
Excludes2: fluid overload unrelated to congestive heart failure
(E87.70)

I51   COMPLICATIONS AND ILL-DEFINED DESCRIPTIONS OF
`4th`   **HEART DISEASE**
Excludes1: any condition in I51.4–I51.9 due to hypertension (I11.-)
any condition in I51.4–I51.9 due to hypertension and CKD (I13.-)
heart disease specified as rheumatic (I00–I09)

I51.4   Myocarditis, unspecified
Chronic (interstitial) myocarditis
Myocardial fibrosis
Myocarditis NOS
Excludes1: acute or subacute myocarditis (I40.-)

I51.5   Myocardial degeneration
Fatty degeneration of heart or myocardium
Myocardial disease
Senile degeneration of heart or myocardium

I51.7   Cardiomegaly
Cardiac dilatation
Cardiac hypertrophy
Ventricular dilatation

I51.8   Other ill-defined heart diseases
`5th`   **I51.81   Takotsubo syndrome**
Reversible left ventricular dysfunction following sudden
emotional stress
Stress induced cardiomyopathy
Takotsubo cardiomyopathy
Transient left ventricular apical ballooning syndrome
I51.89   Other ill-defined heart diseases
Carditis (acute)(chronic)
Pancarditis (acute)(chronic)

I51.9   Heart disease, unspecified

I52   OTHER HEART DISORDERS IN DISEASES CLASSIFIED
`✔`   **ELSEWHERE**
Code first underlying disease, such as:
congenital syphilis (A50.5)
mucopolysaccharidosis (E76.3)
schistosomiasis (B65.0-B65.9)
Excludes1: heart disease (in):
gonococcal infection (A54.83)
meningococcal infection (A39.50)
rheumatoid arthritis (M05.31)
syphilis (A52.06)

(I60–I69) CEREBROVASCULAR DISEASES

Use additional code to identify presence of:
alcohol abuse and dependence (F10.-)
exposure to environmental tobacco smoke (Z77.22)
history of tobacco dependence (Z87.891)
hypertension (I10–I16)
occupational exposure to environmental tobacco smoke (Z57.31)
tobacco dependence (F17.-)
tobacco use (Z72.0)
Excludes1: traumatic intracranial hemorrhage (S06.-)

I60   NONTRAUMATIC SUBARACHNOID HEMORRHAGE
`4th`   *Excludes1:* syphilitic ruptured cerebral aneurysm (A52.05)
Excludes2: sequelae of subarachnoid hemorrhage (I69.0-)
I60.0   Nontraumatic subarachnoid hemorrhage from; carotid siphon
`5th`   **and bifurcation**
I60.00   unspecified carotid siphon and bifurcation
I60.01   right carotid siphon and bifurcation
I60.02   left carotid siphon and bifurcation
I60.1   Nontraumatic subarachnoid hemorrhage from; middle
cerebral artery
I60.2   Nontraumatic subarachnoid hemorrhage from; anterior
communicating artery

I60.3   Nontraumatic subarachnoid hemorrhage from; posterior
`5th`   **communicating artery**
I60.30   unspecified posterior communicating artery
I60.31   right posterior communicating artery
I60.32   left posterior communicating artery
I60.4   Nontraumatic subarachnoid hemorrhage from basilar artery
I60.5   Nontraumatic subarachnoid hemorrhage from; vertebral artery
`5th`   **I60.50   unspecified vertebral artery**
I60.51   from right vertebral artery
I60.52   from left vertebral artery
I60.6   Nontraumatic subarachnoid hemorrhage from other
intracranial arteries
I60.7   Nontraumatic subarachnoid hemorrhage from unspecified
intracranial artery
Ruptured (congenital) berry aneurysm
Ruptured (congenital) cerebral aneurysm
Subarachnoid hemorrhage (nontraumatic) from cerebral artery NOS
Subarachnoid hemorrhage (nontraumatic) from communicating
artery NOS
Excludes1: berry aneurysm, nonruptured (I67.1)
I60.8   Other nontraumatic subarachnoid hemorrhage
Meningeal hemorrhage
Rupture of cerebral arteriovenous malformation
I60.9   Nontraumatic subarachnoid hemorrhage, unspecified

I61   NONTRAUMATIC INTRACEREBRAL HEMORRHAGE
`4th`   *Excludes2:* sequelae of intracerebral hemorrhage (I69.1-)
I61.0   Nontraumatic intracerebral hemorrhage in hemisphere,
subcortical
Deep intracerebral hemorrhage (nontraumatic)
I61.1   Nontraumatic intracerebral hemorrhage; in hemisphere,
cortical
Cerebral lobe hemorrhage (nontraumatic)
Superficial intracerebral hemorrhage (nontraumatic)
I61.2   in hemisphere, unspecified
I61.3   in brain stem
I61.4   in cerebellum
I61.5   intraventricular
I61.6   multiple localized
I61.8   Other nontraumatic intracerebral hemorrhage
I61.9   Nontraumatic intracerebral hemorrhage, unspecified

I62   OTHER AND UNSPECIFIED NONTRAUMATIC
`4th`   **INTRACRANIAL HEMORRHAGE**
Excludes2: sequelae of intracranial hemorrhage (I69.2)
I62.0   Nontraumatic subdural hemorrhage
`5th`   **I62.00   Nontraumatic subdural hemorrhage, unspecified**
I62.01   Nontraumatic acute subdural hemorrhage
I62.02   Nontraumatic subacute subdural hemorrhage
I62.03   Nontraumatic chronic subdural hemorrhage
I62.1   Nontraumatic extradural hemorrhage
Nontraumatic epidural hemorrhage
I62.9   Nontraumatic intracranial hemorrhage, unspecified

I67   OTHER CEREBROVASCULAR DISEASES
`4th`   *Excludes2:* sequelae of the listed conditions (I69.8)
I67.1   Cerebral aneurysm, nonruptured
Cerebral aneurysm NOS
Cerebral arteriovenous fistula, acquired
Internal carotid artery aneurysm, intracranial portion
Internal carotid artery aneurysm, NOS
Excludes1: congenital cerebral aneurysm, nonruptured (Q28.-)
ruptured cerebral aneurysm (I60.7)
I67.4   Hypertensive encephalopathy
Excludes2: insufficiency, NOS, of precerebral arteries (G45.2)
I67.7   Cerebral arteritis, not elsewhere classified
Granulomatous angiitis of the nervous system
Excludes1: allergic granulomatous angiitis (M30.1)
I67.8   Other specified cerebrovascular diseases
`5th`   **I67.81   Acute cerebrovascular insufficiency**
Acute cerebrovascular insufficiency unspecified as to
location or reversibility
I67.82   Cerebral ischemia
Chronic cerebral ischemia

`4th` `5th` `6th` `7th` Additional Character Required   `✔` 3-character code

•=New Code   *Excludes1*—Not coded here, do not use together
▲=Revised Code   *Excludes2*—Not included here

I67.83 Posterior reversible encephalopathy syndrome
PRES

I67.84 Cerebral vasospasm and vasoconstriction

6th **I67.841 Reversible cerebrovascular vasoconstriction syndrome**
Call-Fleming syndrome
Code first underlying condition, if applicable, such as eclampsia (O15.00-O15.9)

I67.848 Other cerebrovascular vasospasm and vasoconstriction

I67.85 Hereditary cerebrovascular diseases

6th **I67.850 Cerebral autosomal dominant arteriopathy with subcortical infarcts and leukoencephalopathy CADASIL**
Code also any associated diagnoses, such as:
epilepsy (G40.-)
stroke (I63.-)
vascular dementia (F01.-)

I67.858 Other hereditary cerebrovascular disease

I67.89 Other cerebrovascular disease

I67.9 Cerebrovascular disease, unspecified

(I70–I79) DISEASES OF ARTERIES, ARTERIOLES AND CAPILLARIES

I70 ATHEROSCLEROSIS
4th
Includes: arteriolosclerosis
arterial degeneration
arteriosclerosis
arteriosclerotic vascular disease
arteriovascular degeneration
atheroma
endarteritis deformans or obliterans
senile arteritis
senile endarteritis
vascular degeneration
Use additional code to identify:
exposure to environmental tobacco smoke (Z77.22)
history of tobacco dependence (Z87.891)
occupational exposure to environmental tobacco smoke (Z57.31)
tobacco dependence (F17.-)
tobacco use (Z72.0)
Excludes2: arteriosclerotic cardiovascular disease (I25.1-)
arteriosclerotic heart disease (I25.1-)
atheroembolism (I75.-)
cerebral atherosclerosis (I67.2)
coronary atherosclerosis (I25.1-)
mesenteric atherosclerosis (K55.1)
precerebral atherosclerosis (I67.2)
primary pulmonary atherosclerosis (I27.0)

I70.0 Atherosclerosis of aorta

I70.8 Atherosclerosis of other arteries

I70.9 Other and unspecified atherosclerosis

5th **I70.90 Unspecified atherosclerosis**
I70.91 Generalized atherosclerosis
I70.92 Chronic total occlusion of artery of the extremities
Complete occlusion of artery of the extremities
Total occlusion of artery of the extremities
Code first atherosclerosis of arteries of the extremities (I70.2-, I70.3-, I70.4-, I70.5-, I70.6-, I70.7-)

I71 AORTIC ANEURYSM AND DISSECTION
4th
Excludes1: aortic ectasia (I77.81-)
syphilitic aortic aneurysm (A52.01)
traumatic aortic aneurysm (S25.09, S35.09)

I71.8 Aortic aneurysm of unspecified site, ruptured
Rupture of aorta NOS

I71.9 Aortic aneurysm of unspecified site, without rupture
Aneurysm of aorta
Dilatation of aorta
Hyaline necrosis of aorta

I73 OTHER PERIPHERAL VASCULAR DISEASES
4th
Excludes2: chilblains (T69.1)
frostbite (T33–T34)
immersion hand or foot (T69.0-)
spasm of cerebral artery (G45.9)

I73.8 Other specified peripheral vascular diseases
5th **Excludes1:** diabetic (peripheral) angiopathy (E08–E13 with .51–.52)
I73.89 Other specified peripheral vascular diseases
Acrocyanosis
Erythrocyanosis
Simple acroparesthesia [Schultze's type]
Vasomotor acroparesthesia [Nothnagel's type]

I73.9 Peripheral vascular disease, unspecified
Intermittent claudication
Peripheral angiopathy NOS
Spasm of artery
Excludes1: atherosclerosis of the extremities (I70.2–I70.7-)

I74 ARTERIAL EMBOLISM AND THROMBOSIS
4th
Includes: embolic infarction
embolic occlusion
thrombotic infarction
thrombotic occlusion
Code first embolism and thrombosis complicating abortion or ectopic or molar pregnancy (O00–O07, O08.2)
embolism and thrombosis complicating pregnancy, childbirth and the puerperium (O88.-)
Excludes2: atheroembolism (I75.-)
basilar embolism and thrombosis (I63.0–I63.2, I65.1)
carotid embolism and thrombosis (I63.0–I63.2, I65.2)
cerebral embolism and thrombosis (I63.3–I63.5, I66.-)
coronary embolism and thrombosis (I21–I25)
mesenteric embolism and thrombosis (K55.0-)
ophthalmic embolism and thrombosis (H34.-)
precerebral embolism and thrombosis NOS (I63.0–I63.2, I65.9)
pulmonary embolism and thrombosis (I26.-)
renal embolism and thrombosis (N28.0)
retinal embolism and thrombosis (H34.-)
septic embolism and thrombosis (I76)
vertebral embolism and thrombosis (I63.0–I63.2, I65.0)

I74.8 Embolism and thrombosis of other arteries

I74.9 Embolism and thrombosis of unspecified artery

I76 SEPTIC ARTERIAL EMBOLISM
✔ **Code first** underlying infection, such as:
infective endocarditis (I33.0)
lung abscess (J85.-)
Use additional code to identify the site of the embolism (I74.-)
Excludes2: septic pulmonary embolism (I26.01, I26.90)

I77 OTHER DISORDERS OF ARTERIES AND ARTERIOLES
4th
Excludes2: collagen (vascular) diseases (M30–M36)
hypersensitivity angiitis (M31.0)
pulmonary artery (I28.-)

I77.1 Stricture of artery
Narrowing of artery

I77.6 Arteritis, unspecified
Aortitis NOS
Endarteritis NOS
Excludes1: arteritis or endarteritis:
aortic arch (M31.4)
cerebral NEC (I67.7)
coronary (I25.89)
deformans (I70.-)
giant cell (M31.5, M31.6)
obliterans (I70.-)
senile (I70.-)

I78 DISEASES OF CAPILLARIES
4th **I78.0 Hereditary hemorrhagic telangiectasia**
Rendu-Osler-Weber disease

•=New Code
▲=Revised Code

Excludes1—Not coded here, do not use together
Excludes2—Not included here

CHAPTER 9. DISEASES OF THE CIRCULATORY SYSTEM   (I67.83–I78.0)

I78.1   **Nevus, non-neoplastic**
Araneus nevus
Senile nevus
Spider nevus
Stellar nevus
Excludes1: nevus NOS (D22.-)
     vascular NOS (Q82.5)
Excludes2: blue nevus (D22.-)
     flammeus nevus (Q82.5)
     hairy nevus (D22.-)
     melanocytic nevus (D22.-)
     pigmented nevus (D22.-)
     portwine nevus (Q82.5)
     sanguineous nevus (Q82.5)
     strawberry nevus (Q82.5)
     verrucous nevus (Q82.5)
I78.8   **Other diseases of capillaries**
I78.9   **Disease of capillaries, unspecified**

(I80–I89) DISEASES OF VEINS, LYMPHATIC VESSELS AND LYMPH NODES, NOT ELSEWHERE CLASSIFIED

I80   **PHLEBITIS AND THROMBOPHLEBITIS**
[4th]
Includes: endophlebitis
     inflammation, vein
     periphlebitis
     suppurative phlebitis
Code first phlebitis and thrombophlebitis complicating abortion, ectopic
     or molar pregnancy (O00–O07, O08.7) phlebitis and thrombophlebitis
     complicating pregnancy, childbirth and the puerperium (O22.-, O87.-)
Excludes1: venous embolism and thrombosis of lower extremities (I82.4-,
     I82.5-, I82.81-)
I80.0   **Phlebitis and thrombophlebitis of superficial vessels of; lower**
[5th]   **extremities**
Phlebitis and thrombophlebitis of femoropopliteal vein
     I80.00   **unspecified lower extremity**
     I80.01   **right lower extremity**
     I80.02   **left lower extremity**
     I80.03   **lower extremities, bilateral**
I80.1   **Phlebitis and thrombophlebitis of; femoral vein**
[5th]   Phlebitis and thrombophlebitis of common femoral vein
Phlebitis and thrombophlebitis of deep femoral vein
     I80.10   **unspecified femoral vein**
     I80.11   **right femoral vein**
     I80.12   **left femoral vein**
     I80.13   **femoral vein, bilateral**
I80.2   **Phlebitis and thrombophlebitis of other and unspecified deep**
[5th]   **vessels of lower extremities**
     I80.20   **Phlebitis and thrombophlebitis of unspecified deep**
     [6th]   **vessels of; lower extremities**
       I80.201   **right lower extremity**
       I80.202   **left lower extremity**
       I80.203   **lower extremities, bilateral**
       I80.209   **unspecified lower extremity**
     I80.21   **Phlebitis and thrombophlebitis of; iliac vein**
     [6th]   Phlebitis and thrombophlebitis of common iliac vein
       Phlebitis and thrombophlebitis of external iliac vein
       Phlebitis and thrombophlebitis of internal iliac vein
       I80.211   **right iliac vein**
       I80.212   **left iliac vein**
       I80.213   **iliac vein, bilateral**
       I80.219   **unspecified iliac vein**
     I80.22   **Phlebitis and thrombophlebitis of; popliteal vein**
     [6th]   **I80.221**   **right popliteal vein**
       I80.222   **left popliteal vein**
       I80.223   **popliteal vein, bilateral**
       I80.229   **unspecified popliteal vein**
     I80.23   **Phlebitis and thrombophlebitis of; tibial vein**
     [6th]   Phlebitis and thrombophlebitis of anterior tibial vein
       Phlebitis and thrombophlebitis of posterior tibial vein
       I80.231   **right tibial vein**
       I80.232   **left tibial vein**

I80.233   **tibial vein, bilateral**
I80.239   **unspecified tibial vein**
I80.24   **Phlebitis and thrombophlebitis of peroneal vein**
[6th]   **I80.241**   **Phlebitis and thrombophlebitis of right**
       peroneal vein
     I80.242   **Phlebitis and thrombophlebitis of left**
       peroneal vein
     I80.243   **Phlebitis and thrombophlebitis of peroneal**
       vein, bilateral
     I80.249   **Phlebitis and thrombophlebitis of**
       unspecified peroneal vein
I80.25   **Phlebitis and thrombophlebitis of calf muscular vein**
[6th]   Phlebitis and thrombophlebitis of calf muscular vein,
       NOS
Phlebitis and thrombophlebitis of gastrocnemial vein
Phlebitis and thrombophlebitis of soleal vein
     I80.251   **Phlebitis and thrombophlebitis of right**
       calf muscular vein
     I80.252   **Phlebitis and thrombophlebitis of left calf**
       muscular vein
     I80.253   **Phlebitis and thrombophlebitis of calf**
       muscular vein, bilateral
     I80.259   **Phlebitis and thrombophlebitis of**
       unspecified calf muscular vein
I80.29   **Phlebitis and thrombophlebitis of other deep vessels**
[6th]   **of; lower extremities**
     I80.291   **right lower extremity**
     I80.292   **left lower extremity**
     I80.293   **lower extremity, bilateral**
     I80.299   **unspecified lower extremity**
I80.3   **Phlebitis and thrombophlebitis of lower extremities,**
unspecified
I80.8   **Phlebitis and thrombophlebitis of other sites**
I80.9   **Phlebitis and thrombophlebitis of unspecified site**

I81   **PORTAL VEIN THROMBOSIS**
[✔]
Portal (vein) obstruction
Excludes2: hepatic vein thrombosis (I82.0)
     phlebitis of portal vein (K75.1)

I82   **OTHER VENOUS EMBOLISM AND THROMBOSIS**
[4th]
Code first venous embolism and thrombosis complicating:
     abortion, ectopic or molar pregnancy (O00–O07, O08.7)
     pregnancy, childbirth and the puerperium (O22.-, O87.-)
Excludes2: venous embolism and thrombosis (of):
     cerebral (I63.6, I67.6)
     coronary (I21–I25)
     intracranial and intraspinal, septic or NOS (G08)
     intracranial, nonpyogenic (I67.6)
     intraspinal, nonpyogenic (G95.1)
     mesenteric (K55.0-)
     portal (I81)
     pulmonary (I26.-)
I82.0   **Budd-Chiari syndrome**
Hepatic vein thrombosis
I82.3   **Embolism and thrombosis of renal vein**
I82.9   **Embolism and thrombosis of unspecified vein**
[5th]   **I82.90**   **Acute embolism and thrombosis of unspecified vein**
     Embolism of vein NOS
     Thrombosis (vein) NOS

I83   **VARICOSE VEINS OF LOWER EXTREMITIES**
[4th]
Excludes1: varicose veins complicating pregnancy (O22.0-)
     varicose veins complicating the puerperium (O87.4)
I83.9   **Asymptomatic varicose veins of lower extremities**
[5th]   Phlebectasia of lower extremities
Varicose veins of lower extremities
Varix of lower extremities
     I83.91   **Asymptomatic varicose veins of right lower**
       extremity
     I83.92   **Asymptomatic varicose veins of left lower extremity**
     I83.93   **Asymptomatic varicose veins of bilateral lower**
       extremities

[4th] [5th] [6th] [7th]   Additional Character Required   [✔]   3-character code   •=New Code   *Excludes1*—Not coded here, do not use together
     ▲=Revised Code   *Excludes2*—Not included here

 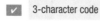

I85 ESOPHAGEAL VARICES
`4th`
Use additional code to identify:
  alcohol abuse and dependence (F10.-)
  I85.0 Esophageal varices
  `5th` Idiopathic esophageal varices
    Primary esophageal varices
    I85.00 Esophageal varices without bleeding
      Esophageal varices NOS
    I85.01 Esophageal varices with bleeding

I86 VARICOSE VEINS OF OTHER SITES
`4th`
Excludes1: varicose veins of unspecified site (I83.9-)
Excludes2: retinal varices (H35.0-)
  I86.1 Scrotal varices
    Varicocele

I88 NONSPECIFIC LYMPHADENITIS
`4th`
Excludes1: acute lymphadenitis, except mesenteric (L04.-)
  enlarged lymph nodes NOS (R59.-)
  HIV disease resulting in generalized lymphadenopathy (B20)
  I88.0 Nonspecific mesenteric lymphadenitis
    Mesenteric lymphadenitis (acute)(chronic)
  I88.1 Chronic lymphadenitis, except mesenteric
    Adenitis
    Lymphadenitis
  I88.8 Other nonspecific lymphadenitis
  I88.9 Nonspecific lymphadenitis, unspecified
    Lymphadenitis NOS

I89 OTHER NONINFECTIVE DISORDERS OF LYMPHATIC
`4th` **VESSELS AND LYMPH NODES**
Excludes1: chylocele, tunica vaginalis (nonfilarial) NOS (N50.89)
enlarged lymph nodes NOS (R59.-)
filarial chylocele (B74.-)
hereditary lymphedema (Q82.0)
  I89.1 Lymphangitis
    Chronic lymphangitis
    Lymphangitis NOS
    Subacute lymphangitis
    Excludes1: acute lymphangitis (L03.-)
  I89.8 Other specified noninfective disorders of lymphatic vessels and lymph nodes
    Chylocele (nonfilarial)
    Chylous ascites
    Chylous cyst
    Lipomelanotic reticulosis
    Lymph node or vessel fistula
    Lymph node or vessel infarction
    Lymph node or vessel rupture
  I89.9 Noninfective disorder of lymphatic vessels and lymph nodes, unspecified
    Disease of lymphatic vessels NOS

(I95–I99) OTHER AND UNSPECIFIED DISORDERS OF THE CIRCULATORY SYSTEM

I95 HYPOTENSION
`4th`
Excludes1: cardiovascular collapse (R57.9)
  maternal hypotension syndrome (O26.5-)
  nonspecific low blood pressure reading NOS (R03.1)
  I95.1 Orthostatic hypotension
    Hypotension, postural
    Excludes1: neurogenic orthostatic hypotension [Shy-Drager] (G90.3)
      orthostatic hypotension due to drugs (I95.2)
  I95.9 Hypotension, unspecified

I97 INTRAOPERATIVE AND POSTPROCEDURAL
`4th` **COMPLICATIONS AND DISORDERS OF CIRCULATORY SYSTEM, NOT ELSEWHERE CLASSIFIED**
Excludes2: postprocedural shock (T81.1-)
  I97.0 Postcardiotomy syndrome
  I97.1 Other postprocedural cardiac functional disturbances
  `5th` *Excludes2:* acute pulmonary insufficiency following thoracic surgery (J95.1)
    intraoperative cardiac functional disturbances (I97.7-)
    I97.11 Postprocedural cardiac insufficiency
    `6th` **I97.110 Postprocedural cardiac insufficiency following cardiac surgery**
      I97.111 Postprocedural cardiac insufficiency following other surgery
    I97.12 Postprocedural cardiac arrest
    `6th` **I97.120 Postprocedural cardiac arrest following cardiac surgery**
      I97.121 Postprocedural cardiac arrest following other surgery
    I97.13 Postprocedural heart failure
    `6th` Use additional code to identify the heart failure (I50.-)
      I97.130 Postprocedural heart failure following cardiac surgery
      I97.131 Postprocedural heart failure following other surgery
    I97.19 Other postprocedural cardiac functional
    `6th` **disturbances**
      Use additional code, if applicable, to further specify disorder
      I97.190 Other postprocedural cardiac functional disturbances following cardiac surgery
      I97.191 Other postprocedural cardiac functional disturbances following other surgery
  I97.8 Other intraoperative and postprocedural complications and disorders of the circulatory system, not elsewhere classified
    Use additional code, if applicable, to further specify disorder
    I97.88 Other intraoperative complications of the circulatory system, NEC
    I97.89 Other postprocedural complications and disorders of the circulatory system, NEC

I99 OTHER AND UNSPECIFIED DISORDERS OF
`4th` **CIRCULATORY SYSTEM**
  I99.8 Other disorder of circulatory system
  I99.9 Unspecified disorder of circulatory system

| `4th` | `5th` | `6th` | `7th` | Additional Character Required | ✔ 3-character code | •=New Code ▲=Revised Code | *Excludes1*—Not coded here, do not use together *Excludes2*—Not included here |

PEDIATRIC ICD-10-CM 2021: A MANUAL FOR PROVIDER-BASED CODING

217

CHAPTER 9. DISEASES OF THE CIRCULATORY SYSTEM (I85–I99.9)

Chapter 10. Diseases of the respiratory system (J00–J99)

GUIDELINES

Acute Respiratory Failure

ACUTE RESPIRATORY FAILURE AS PRINCIPAL DIAGNOSIS
Refer to category J96 for guidelines.

ACUTE RESPIRATORY FAILURE AS SECONDARY DIAGNOSIS
Respiratory failure may be listed as a secondary diagnosis if it occurs after admission, or if it is present on admission, but does not meet the definition of principal diagnosis.

SEQUENCING OF ACUTE RESPIRATORY FAILURE AND ANOTHER ACUTE CONDITION
When a patient is admitted with respiratory failure and another acute condition, (e.g., myocardial infarction, cerebrovascular accident, aspiration pneumonia), the principal diagnosis will not be the same in every situation. This applies whether the other acute condition is a respiratory or nonrespiratory condition. Selection of the principal diagnosis will be dependent on the circumstances of admission. If both the respiratory failure and the other acute condition are equally responsible for occasioning the admission to the hospital, and there are no chapter-specific sequencing rules, the guideline regarding two or more diagnoses that equally meet the definition for principal diagnosis may be applied in these situations.

Influenza due to certain identified influenza viruses

See categories J09–J18 for guidelines.

Ventilator associated Pneumonia

DOCUMENTATION OF VENTILATOR ASSOCIATED PNEUMONIA
Refer to category J95 for guidelines.

VENTILATOR ASSOCIATED PNEUMONIA DEVELOPS AFTER ADMISSION
Refer to category J95 for guidelines.

VAPING-RELATED DISORDERS
Refer to code U07.0 for guidelines.

Note: When a respiratory condition is described as occurring in more than one site and is not specifically indexed, it should be classified to the lower anatomic site (e.g. tracheobronchitis to bronchitis in J40).

Use additional code, where applicable, to identify:
exposure to environmental tobacco smoke (Z77.22)
exposure to tobacco smoke in the perinatal period (P96.81)
history of tobacco dependence (Z87.891)
occupational exposure to environmental tobacco smoke (Z57.31)
tobacco dependence (F17.-)
tobacco use (Z72.0)
Excludes2: certain conditions originating in the perinatal period (P04–P96)
certain infectious and parasitic diseases (A00–B99)
complications of pregnancy, childbirth and the puerperium (O00–O9A)
congenital malformations, deformations and chromosomal abnormalities (Q00–Q99)
endocrine, nutritional and metabolic diseases (E00–E88)
injury, poisoning and certain other consequences of external causes (S00–T88)
neoplasms (C00–D49)
smoke inhalation (T59.81-)
symptoms, signs and abnormal clinical and laboratory findings, NEC (R00–R94)

(J00–J06) ACUTE UPPER RESPIRATORY INFECTIONS

Excludes1: COPD with acute lower respiratory
infection (J44.0)

J00   ACUTE NASOPHARYNGITIS [COMMON COLD]
☑   Acute rhinitis
Coryza (acute)
Infective nasopharyngitis NOS
Infective rhinitis
Nasal catarrh, acute
Nasopharyngitis NOS

Excludes1: acute pharyngitis (J02.-)
acute sore throat NOS (J02.9)
influenza virus with other respiratory manifestations (J09.X2, J10.1, J11.1)
pharyngitis NOS (J02.9)
rhinitis NOS (J31.0)
sore throat NOS (J02.9)
Excludes2: allergic rhinitis (J30.1–J30.9)
chronic pharyngitis (J31.2)
chronic rhinitis (J31.0)
chronic sore throat (J31.2)
nasopharyngitis, chronic (J31.1)
vasomotor rhinitis (J30.0)

J01   ACUTE SINUSITIS
4th   *Includes:* acute abscess of sinus
acute empyema of sinus
acute infection of sinus
acute inflammation of sinus
acute suppuration of sinus
Use additional code (B95–B97) to identify infectious agent.
Excludes1: sinusitis NOS (J32.9)
Excludes2: chronic sinusitis (J32.0–J32.8)

J01.0   Acute maxillary sinusitis
5th   Acute antritis
     J01.00   Acute maxillary sinusitis, unspecified
     J01.01   Acute recurrent maxillary sinusitis
J01.1   Acute frontal sinusitis
5th   **J01.10   Acute frontal sinusitis, unspecified**
     J01.11   Acute recurrent frontal sinusitis
J01.2   Acute ethmoidal sinusitis
5th   **J01.20   Acute ethmoidal sinusitis, unspecified**
     J01.21   Acute recurrent ethmoidal sinusitis
J01.3   Acute sphenoidal sinusitis
5th   **J01.30   Acute sphenoidal sinusitis, unspecified**
     J01.31   Acute recurrent sphenoidal sinusitis
J01.4   Acute pansinusitis
5th   **J01.40   Acute pansinusitis, unspecified**
     J01.41   Acute recurrent pansinusitis
J01.8   Other acute sinusitis
5th   **J01.80   Other acute sinusitis**
          Acute sinusitis involving more than one sinus but not pansinusitis
     J01.81   Other acute recurrent sinusitis
          Acute recurrent sinusitis involving more than one sinus but not pansinusitis
J01.9   Acute sinusitis, unspecified
5th   **J01.90   Acute sinusitis, unspecified**
     J01.91   Acute recurrent sinusitis, unspecified

J02   ACUTE PHARYNGITIS
4th   *Includes:* acute sore throat
Excludes1: acute laryngopharyngitis (J06.0)
peritonsillar abscess (J36)
pharyngeal abscess (J39.1)
retropharyngeal abscess (J39.0)
Excludes2: chronic pharyngitis (J31.2)
J02.0   Streptococcal pharyngitis
     Septic pharyngitis
     Streptococcal sore throat
     Excludes2: scarlet fever (A38.-)
J02.8   Acute pharyngitis due to other specified organisms
     Use additional code (B95–B97) to identify infectious agent
     Excludes1: acute pharyngitis due to coxsackie virus (B08.5)
          acute pharyngitis due to gonococcus (A54.5)
          acute pharyngitis due to herpes [simplex] virus (B00.2)
          acute pharyngitis due to infectious mononucleosis (B27.-)
          enteroviral vesicular pharyngitis (B08.5)

4th   5th   6th   7th   Additional Character Required   ☑   3-character code

• =New Code   ***Excludes1***—Not coded here, do not use together
▲ =Revised Code   ***Excludes2***—Not included here

J02.9 Acute pharyngitis, unspecified
Gangrenous pharyngitis (acute)
Infective pharyngitis (acute) NOS
Pharyngitis (acute) NOS
Sore throat (acute) NOS
Suppurative pharyngitis (acute)
Ulcerative pharyngitis (acute)
Excludes1: influenza virus with other respiratory manifestations (J09.X2, J10.1, J11.1)

J03 ACUTE TONSILLITIS
4th
Excludes1: acute sore throat (J02.-)
hypertrophy of tonsils (J35.1)
peritonsillar abscess (J36)
sore throat NOS (J02.9)
streptococcal sore throat (J02.0)
Excludes2: chronic tonsillitis (J35.0)

J03.0 Streptococcal tonsillitis
5th
J03.00 Acute streptococcal tonsillitis, unspecified
J03.01 Acute recurrent streptococcal tonsillitis

J03.8 Acute tonsillitis due to other specified organisms
5th
Use additional code (B95–B97) to identify infectious agent.
Excludes1: diphtheritic tonsillitis (A36.0)
herpesviral pharyngotonsillitis (B00.2)
streptococcal tonsillitis (J03.0)
tuberculous tonsillitis (A15.8)
Vincent's tonsillitis (A69.1)
J03.80 Acute tonsillitis due to other specified organisms
J03.81 Acute recurrent tonsillitis due to other specified organisms

J03.9 Acute tonsillitis, unspecified
5th
Follicular tonsillitis (acute)
Gangrenous tonsillitis (acute)
Infective tonsillitis (acute)
Tonsillitis (acute) NOS
Ulcerative tonsillitis (acute)
Excludes1: influenza virus with other respiratory manifestations (J09.X2, J10.1, J11.1)
J03.90 Acute tonsillitis, unspecified
J03.91 Acute recurrent tonsillitis, unspecified

J04 ACUTE LARYNGITIS AND TRACHEITIS
4th
Use additional code (B95–B97) to identify infectious agent.
Code also influenza, if present, such as:
influenza due to identified novel influenza A virus with other respiratory manifestations (J09.X2)
influenza due to other identified influenza virus with other respiratory manifestations (J10.1)
influenza due to unidentified influenza virus with other respiratory manifestations (J11.1)
Excludes1: acute obstructive laryngitis [croup] and epiglottitis (J05.-)
Excludes2: laryngismus (stridulus) (J38.5)

J04.0 Acute laryngitis
Edematous laryngitis (acute)
Laryngitis (acute) NOS
Subglottic laryngitis (acute)
Suppurative laryngitis (acute)
Ulcerative laryngitis (acute)
Excludes1: acute obstructive laryngitis (J05.0)
Excludes2: chronic laryngitis (J37.0)

J04.1 Acute tracheitis
5th
Acute viral tracheitis
Catarrhal tracheitis (acute)
Tracheitis (acute) NOS
Excludes2: chronic tracheitis (J42)
J04.10 Acute tracheitis without obstruction
J04.11 Acute tracheitis with obstruction

J04.2 Acute laryngotracheitis
Laryngotracheitis NOS
Tracheitis (acute) with laryngitis (acute)
Excludes1: acute obstructive laryngotracheitis (J05.0)
Excludes2: chronic laryngotracheitis (J37.1)

J04.3 Supraglottitis, unspecified
5th
J04.30 Supraglottitis, unspecified, without obstruction

J04.31 Supraglottitis, unspecified, with obstruction

J05 ACUTE OBSTRUCTIVE LARYNGITIS [CROUP] AND EPIGLOTTITIS
4th
Use additional code (B95–B97) to identify infectious agent.
Code also, if present, such as:
influenza due to identified novel influenza A virus with other respiratory manifestations (J09.X2)
influenza due to other identified influenza virus with other respiratory manifestations (J10.1)
influenza due to unidentified influenza virus with other respiratory manifestations (J11.1)

J05.0 Acute obstructive laryngitis [croup]
Obstructive laryngitis (acute) NOS
Obstructive laryngotracheitis NOS

J05.1 Acute epiglottitis
5th
Excludes2: epiglottitis, chronic (J37.0)
J05.10 Acute epiglottitis without obstruction
Epiglottitis NOS
J05.11 Acute epiglottitis with obstruction

J06 ACUTE UPPER RESPIRATORY INFECTIONS OF MULTIPLE AND UNSPECIFIED SITES
4th
Excludes1: acute respiratory infection NOS (J22)
influenza virus with other respiratory manifestations (J09.X2, J10.1, J11.1)
streptococcal pharyngitis (J02.0)
J06.0 Acute laryngopharyngitis
J06.9 Acute upper respiratory infection, unspecified
Use additional code (B95-B97) to identify infectious agent, if known, such as:
respiratory syncytial virus (RSV) (B97.4)
Upper respiratory disease, acute
Upper respiratory infection NOS

(J09–J18) INFLUENZA AND PNEUMONIA

GUIDELINES

Code only confirmed cases of influenza due to certain identified influenza viruses (category J09), and due to other identified influenza virus (category J10). This is an exception to the hospital inpatient guideline Section II, H. (Uncertain Diagnosis).

In this context, "confirmation" does not require documentation of positive laboratory testing specific for avian or other novel influenza A or other identified influenza virus. However, coding should be based on the provider's diagnostic statement that the patient has avian influenza, or other novel influenza A, for category J09, or has another particular identified strain of influenza, such as H1N1 or H3N2, but not identified as novel or variant, for category J10.

If the provider records "suspected" or "possible" or "probable" avian influenza, or novel influenza, or other identified influenza, then the appropriate influenza code from category J11, Influenza due to unidentified influenza virus, should be assigned. A code from category J09, Influenza due to certain identified influenza viruses, should not be assigned nor should a code from category J10, Influenza due to other identified influenza virus.

Excludes2: allergic or eosinophilic pneumonia (J82)
aspiration pneumonia NOS (J69.0)
meconium pneumonia (P24.01)
neonatal aspiration pneumonia (P24.-)
pneumonia due to solids and liquids (J69.-)
congenital pneumonia (P23.9)
lipid pneumonia (J69.1)
rheumatic pneumonia (I00)
ventilator associated pneumonia (J95.851)

J09 INFLUENZA DUE TO CERTAIN IDENTIFIED INFLUENZA VIRUSES
4th
Excludes1: influenza A/H1N1 (J10.-)
influenza due to other identified influenza virus (J10.-)
influenza due to unidentified influenza virus (J11.-)
seasonal influenza due to other identified influenza virus (J10.-)
seasonal influenza due to unidentified influenza virus (J11.-)

4th 5th 6th 7th Additional Character Required   ✔ 3-character code

•=New Code   *Excludes1*—Not coded here, do not use together
▲=Revised Code   *Excludes2*—Not included here

J09.X **Influenza due to identified novel influenza A virus**
5th
Avian influenza
Bird influenza
Influenza A/H5N1
Influenza of other animal origin, not bird or swine
Swine influenza virus (viruses that normally cause infections in pigs)

J09.X1 **Influenza due to identified novel influenza A virus with pneumonia**
Code also, if applicable, associated: lung abscess (J85.1)
other specified type of pneumonia

J09.X2 **Influenza due to identified novel influenza A virus with other respiratory manifestations**
Influenza due to identified novel influenza A virus NOS
Influenza due to identified novel influenza A virus with laryngitis
Influenza due to identified novel influenza A virus with pharyngitis
Influenza due to identified novel influenza A virus with upper respiratory symptoms
Use additional code, if applicable, for associated: pleural effusion (J91.8) sinusitis (J01.-)

J09.X3 **Influenza due to identified novel influenza A virus with gastrointestinal manifestations**
Influenza due to identified novel influenza A virus gastroenteritis
Excludes1: 'intestinal flu' [viral gastroenteritis] (A08.-)

J09.X9 **Influenza due to identified novel influenza A virus with other manifestations**
Influenza due to identified novel influenza A virus with encephalopathy
Influenza due to identified novel influenza A virus with myocarditis
Influenza due to identified novel influenza A virus with otitis media
Use additional code to identify manifestation

J10 **INFLUENZA DUE TO OTHER IDENTIFIED INFLUENZA VIRUS**
4th
Includes: influenza A (non-novel)
influenza B
influenza C
Excludes1: influenza due to avian influenza virus (J09.X-)
influenza due to swine flu (J09.X-)
influenza due to unidentified influenza virus (J11.-)

J10.0 **Influenza due to other identified influenza virus with pneumonia**
5th
Code also associated lung abscess, if applicable (J85.1)

J10.00 **Influenza due to other identified influenza virus with unspecified type of pneumonia**

J10.01 **Influenza due to other identified influenza virus with the same other identified influenza virus pneumonia**

J10.08 **Influenza due to other identified influenza virus with other specified pneumonia**
Code also other specified type of pneumonia

J10.1 **Influenza due to other identified influenza virus with other respiratory manifestations**
Influenza due to other identified influenza virus NOS
Influenza due to other identified influenza virus with laryngitis
Influenza due to other identified influenza virus with pharyngitis
Influenza due to other identified influenza virus with upper respiratory symptoms
Use additional code for associated pleural effusion, if applicable (J91.8)
Use additional code for associated sinusitis, if applicable (J01.-)

J10.2 **Influenza due to other identified influenza virus with gastrointestinal manifestations**
Influenza due to other identified influenza virus gastroenteritis
Excludes1: 'intestinal flu' [viral gastroenteritis] (A08.-)

J10.8 **Influenza due to other identified influenza virus with other manifestations**
5th

J10.81 **Influenza due to other identified influenza virus with encephalopathy**

J10.82 **Influenza due to other identified influenza virus with myocarditis**

J10.83 **Influenza due to other identified influenza virus with otitis media**
Use additional code for any associated perforated tympanic membrane (H72.-)

J10.89 **Influenza due to other identified influenza virus with other manifestations**
Use additional codes to identify the manifestations

J11 **INFLUENZA DUE TO UNIDENTIFIED INFLUENZA VIRUS**
4th

J11.0 **Influenza due to unidentified influenza virus with pneumonia**
5th
Code also associated lung abscess, if applicable (J85.1)

J11.00 **Influenza due to unidentified influenza virus with unspecified type of pneumonia**
Influenza with pneumonia NOS

J11.08 **Influenza due to unidentified influenza virus with specified pneumonia**
Code also other specified type of pneumonia

J11.1 **Influenza due to unidentified influenza virus with other respiratory manifestations**
Influenza NOS
Influenzal laryngitis NOS
Influenzal pharyngitis NOS
Influenza with upper respiratory symptoms NOS
Use additional code for associated pleural effusion, if applicable (J91.8)
Use additional code for associated sinusitis, if applicable (J01.-)

J11.2 **Influenza due to unidentified influenza virus with gastrointestinal manifestations**
Influenza gastroenteritis NOS
Excludes1: 'intestinal flu' [viral gastroenteritis] (A08.-)

J11.8 **Influenza due to unidentified influenza virus with other manifestations**
5th

J11.81 **Influenza due to unidentified influenza virus with encephalopathy**
Influenzal encephalopathy NOS

J11.82 **Influenza due to unidentified influenza virus with myocarditis**
Influenzal myocarditis NOS

J11.83 **Influenza due to unidentified influenza virus with otitis media**
Influenzal otitis media NOS
Use additional code for any associated perforated tympanic membrane (H72.-)

J11.89 **Influenza due to unidentified influenza virus with other manifestations**
Use additional codes to identify the manifestations

J12 **VIRAL PNEUMONIA, NEC**
4th
Includes: bronchopneumonia due to viruses other than influenza viruses
Code first associated influenza, if applicable (J09.X1, J10.0-, J11.0-)
Code also associated abscess, if applicable (J85.1)
Excludes1: aspiration pneumonia due to solids and liquids (J69.-)
aspiration pneumonia NOS (J69.0)
congenital pneumonia (P23.0)
congenital rubella pneumonitis (P35.0)
interstitial pneumonia NOS (J84.9)
lipid pneumonia (J69.1)
neonatal aspiration pneumonia (P24.-)

J12.0 **Adenoviral pneumonia**

J12.1 **RSV pneumonia**

J12.2 **Parainfluenza virus pneumonia**

J12.3 **Human metapneumovirus pneumonia**

J12.8 **Other viral pneumonia**
5th
J12.81 **Pneumonia due to SARS-associated coronavirus**
SARS NOS

J12.89 **Other viral pneumonia**

J12.9 **Viral pneumonia, unspecified**

4th   5th   6th   7th   Additional Character Required   ✔   3-character code

•=New Code
▲=Revised Code

Excludes1—Not coded here, do not use together
Excludes2—Not included here

J13 PNEUMONIA DUE TO STREPTOCOCCUS PNEUMONIAE

✔ Bronchopneumonia due to S. pneumoniae
Code first associated influenza, if applicable (J09.X1, J10.0-, J11.0-)
Code also associated abscess, if applicable (J85.1)
Excludes1: congenital pneumonia due to S. pneumoniae (P23.6)
    lobar pneumonia, unspecified organism (J18.1)
    pneumonia due to other streptococci (J15.3-J15.4)

J14 PNEUMONIA DUE TO H. INFLUENZAE

✔ Bronchopneumonia due to H. influenzae
Code first associated influenza, if applicable (J09.X1, J10.0-, J11.0-)
Code also associated abscess, if applicable (J85.1)
Excludes1: congenital pneumonia due to H. influenzae (P23.6)

J15 BACTERIAL PNEUMONIA, NEC

4th *Includes:* bronchopneumonia due to bacteria other than S. pneumoniae
and H. influenzae
Code first associated influenza, if applicable (J09.X1, J10.0-, J11.0-)
Code also associated abscess, if applicable (J85.1)
Excludes1: chlamydial pneumonia (J16.0)
    congenital pneumonia (P23.-)
    Legionnaires' disease (A48.1)
    spirochetal pneumonia (A69.8)
J15.0 Pneumonia due to K. pneumoniae
J15.1 Pneumonia due to Pseudomonas
J15.2 Pneumonia due to staphylococcus
   5th **J15.20 Pneumonia due to staphylococcus, unspecified**
        J15.21 Pneumonia due to staphylococcus aureus
       6th **J15.211 Pneumonia due to MSSA**
            MSSA pneumonia
            Pneumonia due to Staphylococcus aureus
            NOS
        J15.212 Pneumonia due to MRSA
     J15.29 Pneumonia due to other staphylococcus
J15.3 Pneumonia due to streptococcus, group B
J15.4 Pneumonia due to other streptococci
    Excludes1: pneumonia due to streptococcus, group B (J15.3)
        pneumonia due to Streptococcus pneumoniae (J13)
J15.5 Pneumonia due to E. coli
J15.6 Pneumonia due to other (aerobic) Gram-negative bacteria
    Pneumonia due to Serratia marcescens
J15.7 Pneumonia due to M. pneumoniae
J15.8 Pneumonia due to other specified bacteria
J15.9 Unspecified bacterial pneumonia
    Pneumonia due to gram-positive bacteria

J16 PNEUMONIA DUE TO OTHER INFECTIOUS ORGANISMS, NEC

4th
Code first associated influenza, if applicable (J09.X1, J10.0-, J11.0-)
Code also associated abscess, if applicable (J85.1)
Excludes1: congenital pneumonia (P23.-)
    ornithosis (A70)
    pneumocystosis (B59)
    pneumonia NOS (J18.9)
J16.0 Chlamydial pneumonia
J16.8 Pneumonia due to other specified infectious organisms

J17 PNEUMONIA IN DISEASES CLASSIFIED ELSEWHERE

✔ **Code first** underlying disease, such as:
    Q fever (A78)
    rheumatic fever (I00)
    schistosomiasis (B65.0–B65.9)
Excludes1: candidial pneumonia (B37.1)
    chlamydial pneumonia (J16.0)
    gonorrheal pneumonia (A54.84)
    histoplasmosis pneumonia (B39.0–B39.2)
    measles pneumonia (B05.2)
    nocardiosis pneumonia (A43.0)
    pneumocystosis (B59)
    pneumonia due to Pneumocystis carinii (B59)
    pneumonia due to Pneumocystis jiroveci (B59)
    pneumonia in actinomycosis (A42.0)
    pneumonia in anthrax (A22.1)
    pneumonia in ascariasis (B77.81)

pneumonia in aspergillosis (B44.0–B44.1)
pneumonia in coccidioidomycosis (B38.0–B38.2)
pneumonia in cytomegalovirus disease (B25.0)
pneumonia in toxoplasmosis (B58.3)
rubella pneumonia (B06.81)
salmonella pneumonia (A02.22)
spirochetal infection NEC with pneumonia (A69.8)
tularemia pneumonia (A21.2)
typhoid fever with pneumonia (A01.03)
varicella pneumonia (B01.2)
whooping cough with pneumonia (A37 with fifth-character 1)

J18 PNEUMONIA, UNSPECIFIED ORGANISM

4th **Code first** associated influenza, if applicable (J09.X1, J10.0-, J11.0-)
Excludes1: abscess of lung with pneumonia (J85.1)
    aspiration pneumonia due to solids and liquids (J69.-)
    aspiration pneumonia NOS (J69.0)
    congenital pneumonia (P23.0)
    drug-induced interstitial lung disorder (J70.2–J70.4)
    interstitial pneumonia NOS (J84.9)
    lipid pneumonia (J69.1)
    neonatal aspiration pneumonia (P24.-)
    pneumonitis due to external agents (J67–J70)
    pneumonitis due to fumes and vapors (J68.0)
    usual interstitial pneumonia (J84.178)
J18.0 Bronchopneumonia, unspecified organism
    Excludes1: hypostatic bronchopneumonia (J18.2)
        lipid pneumonia (J69.1)
    Excludes2: acute bronchiolitis (J21.-)
        chronic bronchiolitis (J44.9)
J18.1 Lobar pneumonia, unspecified organism
J18.8 Other pneumonia, unspecified organism
J18.9 Pneumonia, unspecified organism

(J20–J22) OTHER ACUTE LOWER RESPIRATORY INFECTIONS

Excludes2: COPD with acute lower respiratory infection (J44.0)

J20 ACUTE BRONCHITIS

4th *Includes:* acute and subacute bronchitis (with) bronchospasm
    acute and subacute bronchitis (with) tracheitis
    acute and subacute bronchitis (with) tracheobronchitis, acute
    acute and subacute fibrinous bronchitis
    acute and subacute membranous bronchitis
    acute and subacute purulent bronchitis
    acute and subacute septic bronchitis
Excludes1: bronchitis NOS (J40)
    tracheobronchitis NOS
Excludes2: acute bronchitis with bronchiectasis (J47.0)
    acute bronchitis with chronic obstructive asthma (J44.0)
    acute bronchitis with COPD (J44.0)
    allergic bronchitis NOS (J45.909-)
    bronchitis due to chemicals, fumes and vapors (J68.0)
    chronic bronchitis NOS (J42)
    chronic mucopurulent bronchitis (J41.1)
    chronic obstructive bronchitis (J44.-)
    chronic obstructive tracheobronchitis (J44.-)
    chronic simple bronchitis (J41.0)
    chronic tracheobronchitis (J42)
J20.0 Acute bronchitis due to M. pneumoniae
J20.1 Acute bronchitis due to H. influenzae
J20.2 Acute bronchitis due to streptococcus
J20.3 Acute bronchitis due to coxsackievirus
J20.4 Acute bronchitis due to parainfluenza virus
J20.5 Acute bronchitis due to RSV
J20.6 Acute bronchitis due to rhinovirus
J20.7 Acute bronchitis due to echovirus
J20.8 Acute bronchitis due to other specified organisms
J20.9 Acute bronchitis, unspecified

J21 ACUTE BRONCHIOLITIS

4th *Includes:* acute bronchiolitis with bronchospasm
Excludes2: respiratory bronchiolitis interstitial lung disease (J84.115)
J21.0 Acute bronchiolitis due to RSV
J21.1 Acute bronchiolitis due to human metapneumovirus
J21.8 Acute bronchiolitis due to other specified organisms

4th 5th 6th 7th Additional Character Required   ✔ 3-character code

•=New Code   *Excludes1*—Not coded here, do not use together
▲=Revised Code   *Excludes2*—Not included here

J21.9 Acute bronchiolitis, unspecified
Bronchiolitis (acute)
Excludes1: chronic bronchiolitis (J44.-)

J22 UNSPECIFIED ACUTE LOWER RESPIRATORY INFECTION
Acute (lower) respiratory (tract) infection NOS
Excludes1: upper respiratory infection (acute) (J06.9)

(J30–J39) OTHER DISEASES OF UPPER RESPIRATORY TRACT

J30 VASOMOTOR AND ALLERGIC RHINITIS
Includes: spasmodic rhinorrhea
Excludes1: allergic rhinitis with asthma (bronchial) (J45.909)
   rhinitis NOS (J31.0)
  J30.1 Allergic rhinitis due to pollen
    Allergy NOS due to pollen
    Hay fever
    Pollinosis
  J30.2 Other seasonal allergic rhinitis
  J30.5 Allergic rhinitis due to food
  J30.8 Other allergic rhinitis
    J30.81 Allergic rhinitis due to animal (cat) (dog) hair and dander
    J30.89 Other allergic rhinitis
      Perennial allergic rhinitis
  J30.9 Allergic rhinitis, unspecified

J31 CHRONIC RHINITIS, NASOPHARYNGITIS AND PHARYNGITIS
Use additional code to identify: (Refer to Chapter 10 guidelines for codes)
  J31.0 Chronic rhinitis
    Atrophic rhinitis (chronic)
    Granulomatous rhinitis (chronic)
    Hypertrophic rhinitis (chronic)
    Obstructive rhinitis (chronic)
    Ozena
    Purulent rhinitis (chronic)
    Rhinitis (chronic) NOS
    Ulcerative rhinitis (chronic)
    Excludes1: allergic rhinitis (J30.1–J30.9)
      vasomotor rhinitis (J30.0)
  J31.1 Chronic nasopharyngitis
    Excludes2: acute nasopharyngitis (J00)
  J31.2 Chronic pharyngitis
    Chronic sore throat
    Atrophic pharyngitis (chronic)
    Granular pharyngitis (chronic)
    Hypertrophic pharyngitis (chronic)
    Excludes2 acute pharyngitis (J02.9)

J32 CHRONIC SINUSITIS
Includes: sinus abscess
  sinus empyema
  sinus infection
  sinus suppuration
Use additional code to identify: (Refer to Chapter 10 guidelines for codes)
Excludes2: acute sinusitis (J01.-)
  J32.0 Chronic maxillary sinusitis
    Antritis (chronic)
    Maxillary sinusitis NOS
  J32.1 Chronic frontal sinusitis
    Frontal sinusitis NOS
  J32.2 Chronic ethmoidal sinusitis
    Ethmoidal sinusitis NOS
    Excludes1: Woakes' ethmoiditis (J33.1)
  J32.3 Chronic sphenoidal sinusitis
    Sphenoidal sinusitis NOS
  J32.4 Chronic pansinusitis
    Pansinusitis NOS
  J32.8 Other chronic sinusitis
    Sinusitis (chronic) involving more than one sinus but not pansinusitis
  J32.9 Chronic sinusitis, unspecified
    Sinusitis (chronic) NOS

J33 NASAL POLYP
Use additional code to identify: (Refer to Chapter 10 guidelines for codes)
Excludes1: adenomatous polyps (D14.0)
  J33.0 Polyp of nasal cavity
    Choanal polyp
    Nasopharyngeal polyp
  J33.8 Other polyp of sinus
    Accessory polyp of sinus
    Ethmoidal polyp of sinus
    Maxillary polyp of sinus
    Sphenoidal polyp of sinus
  J33.9 Nasal polyp, unspecified

J34 OTHER AND UNSPECIFIED DISORDERS OF NOSE AND NASAL SINUSES
Excludes2: varicose ulcer of nasal septum (I86.8)
  J34.0 Abscess, furuncle and carbuncle of nose
    Cellulitis of nose
    Necrosis of nose
    Ulceration of nose
  J34.1 Cyst and mucocele of nose and nasal sinus
  J34.2 Deviated nasal septum
    Deflection or deviation of septum (nasal) (acquired)
    Excludes1: congenital deviated nasal septum (Q67.4)
  J34.3 Hypertrophy of nasal turbinates
  J34.8 Other specified disorders of nose and nasal sinuses
    J34.81 Nasal mucositis (ulcerative)
      Code also type of associated therapy, such as:
        antineoplastic and immunosuppressive drugs (T45.1X-)
        radiological procedure and radiotherapy (Y84.2)
      Excludes2: gastrointestinal mucositis (ulcerative) (K92.81)
        mucositis (ulcerative) of vagina and vulva (N76.81)
        oral mucositis (ulcerative) (K12.3-)
    J34.89 Other specified disorders of nose and nasal sinuses
      Perforation of nasal septum NOS
      Rhinolith
  J34.9 Unspecified disorder of nose and nasal sinuses

J35 CHRONIC DISEASES OF TONSILS AND ADENOIDS
Use additional code to identify: (Refer to Chapter 10 guidelines for codes)
  J35.0 Chronic tonsillitis and adenoiditis
    Excludes2: acute tonsillitis (J03.-)
    J35.01 Chronic tonsillitis
    J35.02 Chronic adenoiditis
    J35.03 Chronic tonsillitis and adenoiditis
  J35.1 Hypertrophy of tonsils
    Enlargement of tonsils
    Excludes1: hypertrophy of tonsils with tonsillitis (J35.0-)
  J35.2 Hypertrophy of adenoids
    Enlargement of adenoids
    Excludes1: hypertrophy of adenoids with adenoiditis (J35.0-)
  J35.3 Hypertrophy of tonsils with hypertrophy of adenoids
    Excludes1: hypertrophy of tonsils and adenoids with tonsillitis and adenoiditis (J35.03)
  J35.8 Other chronic diseases of tonsils and adenoids
    Adenoid vegetations
    Amygdalolith
    Calculus, tonsil
    Cicatrix of tonsil (and adenoid)
    Tonsillar tag
    Ulcer of tonsil
  J35.9 Chronic disease of tonsils and adenoids, unspecified
    Disease (chronic) of tonsils and adenoids NOS

J36 PERITONSILLAR ABSCESS
Includes: abscess of tonsil
  peritonsillar cellulitis
  quinsy
Use additional code (B95-B97) to identify infectious agent.
Excludes1: acute tonsillitis (J03.-)
  chronic tonsillitis (J35.0)
  retropharyngeal abscess (J39.0)
  tonsillitis NOS (J03.9-)

4th 5th 6th 7th Additional Character Required   ✔ 3-character code

•=New Code   *Excludes1*—Not coded here, do not use together
▲=Revised Code   *Excludes2*—Not included here

CHAPTER 10. DISEASES OF THE RESPIRATORY SYSTEM (J37–J69)

J37 `4th` **CHRONIC LARYNGITIS AND LARYNGOTRACHEITIS**
Use additional code to identify: (Refer to Chapter 10 guidelines for codes)

J37.0 Chronic laryngitis
Catarrhal laryngitis
Hypertrophic laryngitis
Sicca laryngitis
Excludes2: acute laryngitis (J04.0)
    obstructive (acute) laryngitis (J05.0)

J37.1 Chronic laryngotracheitis
Laryngitis, chronic, with tracheitis (chronic)
Tracheitis, chronic, with laryngitis
Excludes1: chronic tracheitis (J42)
Excludes2: acute laryngotracheitis (J04.2)
    acute tracheitis (J04.1)

J38 `4th` **DISEASES OF VOCAL CORDS AND LARYNX, NEC**
Use additional code to identify: (Refer to Chapter 10 guidelines for codes)
Excludes1: congenital laryngeal stridor (P28.89)
    obstructive laryngitis (acute) (J05.0)
    postprocedural subglottic stenosis (J95.5)
    stridor (R06.1)
    ulcerative laryngitis (J04.0)

J38.0 Paralysis of vocal cords and larynx
`5th` Laryngoplegia
Paralysis of glottis
  J38.00 Paralysis of vocal cords and larynx, unspecified
  J38.01 Paralysis of vocal cords and larynx, unilateral
  J38.02 Paralysis of vocal cords and larynx, bilateral

J38.4 Edema of larynx
Edema (of) glottis
Subglottic edema
Supraglottic edema
Excludes1: acute obstructive laryngitis [croup] (J05.0)
    edematous laryngitis (J04.0)

J38.5 Laryngeal spasm
Laryngismus (stridulus)

J39 `4th` **OTHER DISEASES OF UPPER RESPIRATORY TRACT**
Excludes1: acute respiratory infection NOS (J22)
    acute upper respiratory infection (J06.9)
    upper respiratory inflammation due to chemicals, gases, fumes or vapors (J68.2)

J39.0 Retropharyngeal and parapharyngeal abscess
Peripharyngeal abscess
Excludes1: peritonsillar abscess (J36)

J39.2 Other diseases of pharynx
Cyst of pharynx
Edema of pharynx
Excludes2: chronic pharyngitis (J31.2)
    ulcerative pharyngitis (J02.9)

J39.8 Other specified diseases of upper respiratory tract
J39.9 Disease of upper respiratory tract, unspecified

(J40–J47) CHRONIC LOWER RESPIRATORY DISEASES

Excludes1: bronchitis due to chemicals, gases, fumes and vapors (J68.0)
Excludes2: cystic fibrosis (E84.-)

J40 ✔ **BRONCHITIS, NOT SPECIFIED AS ACUTE OR CHRONIC**
Bronchitis NOS
Bronchitis with tracheitis NOS
Catarrhal bronchitis
Tracheobronchitis NOS
Use additional code to identify: (Refer to Chapter 10 guidelines for codes)
Excludes1: acute bronchitis (J20.-)
    allergic bronchitis NOS (J45.909-)
    asthmatic bronchitis NOS (J45.9-)
    bronchitis due to chemicals, gases, fumes and vapors (J68.0)

J42 ✔ **UNSPECIFIED CHRONIC BRONCHITIS**
Chronic bronchitis NOS
Chronic tracheitis
Chronic tracheobronchitis
Use additional code to identify any associated tobacco use or exposure

Excludes1: chronic asthmatic bronchitis (J44.-)
    chronic bronchitis with airways obstruction (J44.-)
    chronic emphysematous bronchitis (J44.-)
    chronic obstructive pulmonary disease NOS (J44.9)
    simple and mucopurulent chronic bronchitis (J41.-)

J45 `4th` **ASTHMA**
Includes: allergic (predominantly) asthma
allergic bronchitis NOS
allergic rhinitis with asthma
atopic asthma
extrinsic allergic asthma
hay fever with asthma
idiosyncratic asthma
intrinsic nonallergic asthma
nonallergic asthma
Use additional code to identify: (Refer to Chapter 10 guidelines for codes)
eosinophilic asthma (J82.83)
Excludes1: detergent asthma (J69.8)
    eosinophilic asthma (J82)
    miner's asthma (J60)
    wheezing NOS (R06.2)
    wood asthma (J67.8)
Excludes2: asthma with COPD (J44.9)
    chronic asthmatic (obstructive) bronchitis (J44.9)
    chronic obstructive asthma (J44.9)

J45.2 Mild intermittent asthma
`5th`   **J45.20 Mild intermittent asthma, uncomplicated**
    Mild intermittent asthma NOS
  J45.21 Mild intermittent asthma with (acute) exacerbation
  J45.22 Mild intermittent asthma with status asthmaticus

J45.3 Mild persistent asthma
`5th`   **J45.30 Mild persistent asthma, uncomplicated**
    Mild persistent asthma NOS
  J45.31 Mild persistent asthma with (acute) exacerbation
  J45.32 Mild persistent asthma with status asthmaticus

J45.4 Moderate persistent asthma
`5th`   **J45.40 Moderate persistent asthma, uncomplicated**
    Moderate persistent asthma NOS
  J45.41 Moderate persistent asthma with (acute) exacerbation
  J45.42 Moderate persistent asthma with status asthmaticus

J45.5 Severe persistent asthma
`5th`   **J45.50 Severe persistent asthma, uncomplicated**
    Severe persistent asthma NOS
  J45.51 Severe persistent asthma with (acute) exacerbation
  J45.52 Severe persistent asthma with status asthmaticus

J45.9 Other and unspecified asthma
`5th`   **J45.90 Unspecified asthma**
`6th`   Asthmatic bronchitis NOS
    Childhood asthma NOS
    Late onset asthma
    J45.901 Unspecified asthma with (acute) exacerbation
    J45.902 Unspecified asthma with status asthmaticus
    J45.909 Unspecified asthma, uncomplicated
      Asthma NOS
      Excludes2: lung diseases due to external agents (J60–J70)
  J45.99 Other asthma
`6th`   **J45.990 Exercise induced bronchospasm**
    J45.991 Cough variant asthma
    J45.998 Other asthma

(J60–J70) LUNG DISEASES DUE TO EXTERNAL AGENTS

Excludes2: asthma (J45.-)
    malignant neoplasm of bronchus and lung (C34.-)

J69 `4th` **PNEUMONITIS DUE TO SOLIDS AND LIQUIDS**
Excludes1: neonatal aspiration syndromes (P24.-)
    postprocedural pneumonitis (J95.4)

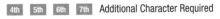 `4th` `5th` `6th` `7th` Additional Character Required   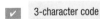 ✔ 3-character code

•=New Code   *Excludes1*—Not coded here, do not use together
▲=Revised Code   *Excludes2*—Not included here

J69.0 Pneumonitis due to inhalation of food and vomit
Aspiration pneumonia NOS
Aspiration pneumonia (due to) food (regurgitated)
Aspiration pneumonia (due to) gastric secretions
Aspiration pneumonia (due to) milk
Aspiration pneumonia (due to) vomit
Code also any associated FB in respiratory tract (T17.-)
Excludes1: chemical pneumonitis due to anesthesia (J95.4)

J69.1 Pneumonitis due to inhalation of oils and essences
Exogenous lipoid pneumonia
Lipid pneumonia NOS
Code first (T51–T65) to identify substance
Excludes1: endogenous lipoid pneumonia (J84.89)

J69.8 Pneumonitis due to inhalation of other solids and liquids
Pneumonitis due to aspiration of blood
Pneumonitis due to aspiration of detergent
Code first (T51–T65) to identify substance

J70 `4th` **RESPIRATORY CONDITIONS DUE TO OTHER EXTERNAL AGENTS**

J70.5 Respiratory conditions due to smoke inhalation
Code first smoke inhalation (T59.81-)
Excludes2: smoke inhalation due to chemicals, gases, fumes and vapors (J68.9)

J70.9 Respiratory conditions due to unspecified external agent
Code first (T51–T65) to identify the external agent

(J80–J84) OTHER RESPIRATORY DISEASES PRINCIPALLY AFFECTING THE INTERSTITIUM

J80 ✔ **ACUTE RESPIRATORY DISTRESS SYNDROME**
Acute respiratory distress syndrome in adult or child
Adult hyaline membrane disease
Excludes1: respiratory distress syndrome in newborn (perinatal) (P22.0)

J81 `4th` **PULMONARY EDEMA**
Use additional code to identify: (Refer to Chapter 10 guidelines for codes)
Excludes1: chemical (acute) pulmonary edema (J68.1)
hypostatic pneumonia (J18.2)
passive pneumonia (J18.2)
pulmonary edema due to external agents (J60-J70)
pulmonary edema with heart disease NOS (I50.1)
pulmonary edema with heart failure (I50.1)

J81.0 Acute pulmonary edema
Acute edema of lung

J82 `4th` **PULMONARY EOSINOPHILIA, NOT ELSEWHERE CLASSIFIED**
•**J82.8 Pulmonary eosinophilia, NEC**
`5th` •**J82.81 Chronic eosinophilic pneumonia**
Eosinophilic pneumonia, NOS
•**J82.82 Acute eosinophilic pneumonia**
•**J82.83 Eosinophilic asthma**
Code first asthma, by type, such as:
mild intermittent asthma (J45.2-)
mild persistent asthma (J45.3-)
moderate persistent asthma (J45.4-)
severe persistent asthma (J45.5-)
•**J82.89 Other pulmonary eosinophilia, not elsewhere classified**
Allergic pneumonia
Löffler's pneumonia
Tropical (pulmonary) eosinophilia NOS

J84 `4th` **OTHER INTERSTITIAL PULMONARY DISEASES**
Excludes1: drug-induced interstitial lung disorders (J70.2-J70.4)
interstitial emphysema (J98.2)
Excludes2: lung diseases due to external agents (J60-J70)
J84.0 Alveolar and parieto-alveolar conditions
`5th` **J84.01 Alveolar proteinosis**
J84.02 Pulmonary alveolar microlithiasis
J84.03 Idiopathic pulmonary hemosiderosis
Essential brown induration of lung
Code first underlying disease, such as:
disorders of iron metabolism (E83.1-)

Excludes1: acute idiopathic pulmonary hemorrhage in infants [AIPHI] (R04.81)
J84.09 Other alveolar and parieto-alveolar conditions
J84.8 Other specified interstitial pulmonary diseases
`5th` *Excludes1:* exogenous or unspecified lipoid pneumonia (J69.1)
J84.83 Surfactant mutations of the lung
J84.84 Other interstitial lung diseases of childhood
`6th` **J84.841 Neuroendocrine cell hyperplasia of infancy**
J84.842 Pulmonary interstitial glycogenosis
J84.843 Alveolar capillary dysplasia with vein misalignment
J84.848 Other interstitial lung diseases of childhood
J84.89 Other specified interstitial pulmonary disease
J84.9 Interstitial pulmonary disease, unspecified
Interstitial pneumonia NOS

(J85–J86) SUPPURATIVE AND NECROTIC CONDITIONS OF THE LOWER RESPIRATORY TRACT

J86 `4th` **PYOTHORAX**
Use additional code (B95–B97) to identify infectious agent.
Excludes1: abscess of lung (J85.-)
pyothorax due to tuberculosis (A15.6)
J86.0 Pyothorax with fistula
Bronchocutaneous fistula
Bronchopleural fistula
Hepatopleural fistula
Mediastinal fistula
Pleural fistula
Thoracic fistula
Any condition classifiable to J86.9 with fistula
J86.9 Pyothorax without fistula
Abscess of pleura
Abscess of thorax
Empyema (chest) (lung) (pleura)
Fibrinopurulent pleurisy
Purulent pleurisy
Pyopneumothorax
Septic pleurisy
Seropurulent pleurisy
Suppurative pleurisy

(J90–J94) OTHER DISEASES OF THE PLEURA

J90 ✔ **PLEURAL EFFUSION, NEC**
Encysted pleurisy
Pleural effusion NOS
Pleurisy with effusion (exudative) (serous)
Excludes1: chylous (pleural) effusion (J94.0)
malignant pleural effusion (J91.0))
pleurisy NOS (R09.1)
tuberculous pleural effusion (A15.6)

J91 `4th` **PLEURAL EFFUSION IN CONDITIONS CLASSIFIED ELSEWHERE**
Excludes2: pleural effusion in heart failure (I50.-)
pleural effusion in SLE (M32.13)
J91.0 Malignant pleural effusion
Code first underlying neoplasm
J91.8 Pleural effusion in other conditions classified elsewhere
Code first underlying disease, such as:
filariasis (B74.0-B74.9)
influenza (J09.X2, J10.1, J11.1)

J93 `4th` **PNEUMOTHORAX AND AIR LEAK**
Excludes1: congenital or perinatal pneumothorax (P25.1)
postprocedural air leak (J95.812)
postprocedural pneumothorax (J95.811)
traumatic pneumothorax (S27.0)
tuberculous (current disease) pneumothorax (A15.-)
pyopneumothorax (J86.-)
J93.0 Spontaneous tension pneumothorax

CHAPTER 10. DISEASES OF THE RESPIRATORY SYSTEM   (J69.0–J93.0)

`4th` `5th` `6th` `7th` Additional Character Required   ✔ 3-character code

•=New Code   *Excludes1*—Not coded here, do not use together
▲=Revised Code   *Excludes2*—Not included here

CHAPTER 10. DISEASES OF THE RESPIRATORY SYSTEM   (J93.1–J96)

J93.1   Other spontaneous pneumothorax
[5th]   J93.11   Primary spontaneous pneumothorax
        J93.12   Secondary spontaneous pneumothorax
            Code first underlying condition, such as:
                catamenial pneumothorax due to endometriosis (N80.8)
                cystic fibrosis (E84.-)
                eosinophilic pneumonia (J82)
                lymphangioleiomyomatosis (J84.81)
                malignant neoplasm of bronchus and lung (C34.-)
                Marfan's syndrome (Q87.4)
                pneumonia due to Pneumocystis carinii (B59)
                secondary malignant neoplasm of lung (C78.0-)
                spontaneous rupture of the esophagus (K22.3)
J93.8   Other pneumothorax and air leak
[5th]   J93.81   Chronic pneumothorax
        J93.82   Other air leak
            Persistent air leak
        J93.83   Other pneumothorax
            Acute pneumothorax
            Spontaneous pneumothorax NOS
J93.9   Pneumothorax, unspecified
        Pneumothorax NOS

(J95) INTRAOPERATIVE AND POSTPROCEDURAL COMPLICATIONS AND DISORDERS OF RESPIRATORY SYSTEM, NEC

GUIDELINES

As with all procedural or postprocedural complications, code assignment is based on the provider's documentation of the relationship between the condition and the procedure.

Code J95.851, Ventilator associated pneumonia (VAP), should be assigned only when the provider has documented VAP. An additional code to identify the organism (e.g., Pseudomonas aeruginosa, code B96.5) should also be assigned. Do not assign an additional code from categories J12-J18 to identify the type of pneumonia.

Code J95.851 should not be assigned for cases where the patient has pneumonia and is on a mechanical ventilator and the provider has not specifically stated that the pneumonia is ventilator-associated pneumonia. If the documentation is unclear as to whether the patient has a pneumonia that is a complication attributable to the mechanical ventilator, query the provider.

A patient may be admitted with one type of pneumonia (e.g., code J13, Pneumonia due to Streptococcus pneumonia) and subsequently develop VAP. In this instance, the principal diagnosis would be the appropriate code from categories J12-J18 for the pneumonia diagnosed at the time of admission. Code J95.851, Ventilator associated pneumonia, would be assigned as an additional diagnosis when the provider has also documented the presence of ventilator associated pneumonia.

J95   INTRAOPERATIVE AND POSTPROCEDURAL
[4th]   COMPLICATIONS AND DISORDERS OF RESPIRATORY SYSTEM, NEC
        Excludes2: aspiration pneumonia (J69.-)
            emphysema (subcutaneous) resulting from a procedure (T81.82)
            hypostatic pneumonia (J18.2)
            pulmonary manifestations due to radiation (J70.0-J70.1)
J95.8   Other intraoperative and postprocedural complications and
[5th]   disorders of respiratory system, NEC
        J95.81   Postprocedural pneumothorax and air leak
        [6th]   J95.811   Postprocedural pneumothorax
                J95.812   Postprocedural air leak
        J95.82   Postprocedural respiratory failure
        [6th]   *Excludes1:* Respiratory failure in other conditions (J96.-)
                J95.821   Acute postprocedural respiratory failure
                    Postprocedural respiratory failure NOS
                J95.822   Acute and chronic post–procedural respiratory failure
        J95.83   Postprocedural hemorrhage of a respiratory system
        [6th]   organ or structure; following a procedure
                J95.830   following a respiratory system procedure
                J95.831   following other procedure
        J95.84   Transfusion-related acute lung injury (TRALI)

J95.85   Complication of respirator [ventilator]
[6th]   J95.850   Mechanical complication of respirator
                Excludes1: encounter for respirator [ventilator] dependence during power failure (Z99.12)
        J95.851   Ventilator associated pneumonia
                Ventilator associated pneumonitis
                Use additional code to identify organism, if known (B95.-, B96.-, B97.-)
                Excludes1: ventilator lung in newborn (P27.8)
        J95.859   Other complication of respirator [ventilator]
J95.86   Postprocedural hematoma and seroma of a respiratory
[6th]   system organ or structure following a procedure
        J95.860   Postprocedural hematoma of a respiratory system organ or structure following a respiratory system procedure
        J95.861   Postprocedural hematoma of a respiratory system organ or structure following other procedure
        J95.862   Postprocedural seroma of a respiratory system organ or structure following a respiratory system procedure
        J95.863   Postprocedural seroma of a respiratory system organ or structure following other procedure
J95.88   Other intraoperative complications of respiratory system, NEC
J95.89   Other postprocedural complications and disorders of respiratory system, NEC
        Use additional code to identify disorder, such as:
            aspiration pneumonia (J69.-)
            bacterial or viral pneumonia (J12-J18)
        Excludes2: acute pulmonary insufficiency following thoracic surgery (J95.1)
            postprocedural subglottic stenosis (J95.5)

(J96–J99) OTHER DISEASES OF THE RESPIRATORY SYSTEM

J96   RESPIRATORY FAILURE, NEC
[4th]   GUIDELINES

Acute Respiratory Failure

AS PRINCIPAL DIAGNOSIS
A code from subcategory J96.0, Acute respiratory failure, or subcategory J96.2, Acute and chronic respiratory failure, may be assigned as a principal diagnosis when it is the condition established after study to be chiefly responsible for occasioning the admission to the hospital, and the selection is supported by the Alphabetic Index and Tabular List. However, chapter-specific coding guidelines (such as obstetrics, poisoning, HIV, newborn) that provide sequencing direction take precedence.

AS SECONDARY DIAGNOSIS
Respiratory failure may be listed as a secondary diagnosis if it occurs after admission, or if it is present on admission, but does not meet the definition of principal diagnosis.

SEQUENCING OF ACUTE RESPIRATORY FAILURE AND ANOTHER ACUTE CONDITION
When a patient is admitted with respiratory failure and another acute condition, (eg, myocardial infarction, cerebrovascular accident, aspiration pneumonia), the principal diagnosis will not be the same in every situation. This applies whether the other acute condition is a respiratory or nonrespiratory condition. Selection of the principal diagnosis will be dependent on the circumstances of admission. If both the respiratory failure and the other acute condition are equally responsible for occasioning the admission to the hospital, and there are no chapter-specific sequencing rules, the guideline regarding two or more diagnoses that equally meet the definition for principal diagnosis may be applied in these situations.

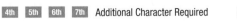

| **[4th] [5th] [6th] [7th]** Additional Character Required | ✔ 3-character code | •=New Code ▲=Revised Code | ***Excludes1***—Not coded here, do not use together ***Excludes2***—Not included here |

Excludes1: acute respiratory distress syndrome (J80)
　　cardiorespiratory failure (R09.2)
　　newborn respiratory distress syndrome (P22.0)
　　postprocedural respiratory failure (J95.82-)
　　respiratory arrest (R09.2)
　　respiratory arrest of newborn (P28.81)
　　respiratory failure of newborn (P28.5)

J96.0　Acute respiratory failure
- **5th** **J96.00　Acute respiratory failure, unspecified whether with hypoxia or hypercapnia**
- **J96.01　Acute respiratory failure with hypoxia**
- **J96.02　Acute respiratory failure with hypercapnia**

J96.1　Chronic respiratory failure
- **5th** **J96.10　Chronic respiratory failure, unspecified whether with hypoxia or hypercapnia**
- **J96.11　Chronic respiratory failure with hypoxia**
- **J96.12　Chronic respiratory failure with hypercapnia**

J96.2　Acute and chronic respiratory failure
- **5th** Acute on chronic respiratory failure
- **J96.20　Acute and chronic respiratory failure, unspecified whether with hypoxia or hypercapnia**
- **J96.21　Acute and chronic respiratory failure with hypoxia**
- **J96.22　Acute and chronic respiratory failure with hypercapnia**

J96.9　Respiratory failure, unspecified
- **5th** **J96.90　Respiratory failure, unspecified, unspecified whether with hypoxia or hypercapnia**
- **J96.91　Respiratory failure, unspecified with hypoxia**
- **J96.92　Respiratory failure, unspecified with hypercapnia**

J98　OTHER RESPIRATORY DISORDERS
4th **Use additional code** to identify (Refer to Chapter 10 guidelines for codes)
Excludes1: newborn apnea (P28.4)
　　newborn sleep apnea (P28.3)
Excludes2: apnea NOS (R06.81)
　　sleep apnea (G47.3-)

J98.0　Diseases of bronchus, NEC
- **5th** **J98.01　Acute bronchospasm**
  - *Excludes1:* acute bronchiolitis with bronchospasm (J21.-)
    acute bronchitis with bronchospasm (J20.-)
    asthma (J45.-)
    exercise induced bronchospasm (J45.990)
- **J98.09　Other diseases of bronchus, not elsewhere classified**
  - Broncholithiasis
  - Calcification of bronchus
  - Stenosis of bronchus
  - Tracheobronchial collapse
  - Tracheobronchial dyskinesia
  - Ulcer of bronchus

J98.1　Pulmonary collapse
- **5th** *Excludes1:* therapeutic collapse of lung status (Z98.3)
- **J98.11　Atelectasis**
  - *Excludes1:* newborn atelectasis
    tuberculous atelectasis (current disease) (A15)

J98.2　Interstitial emphysema
Mediastinal emphysema
Excludes1: emphysema NOS (J43.9)
　　emphysema in newborn (P25.0)
　　surgical emphysema (subcutaneous) (T81.82)
　　traumatic subcutaneous emphysema (T79.7)

J98.4　Other disorders of lung
Calcification of lung
Cystic lung disease (acquired)
Lung disease NOS
Pulmolithiasis

J98.6　Disorders of diaphragm
Diaphragmatitis
Paralysis of diaphragm
Relaxation of diaphragm
Excludes1: congenital malformation of diaphragm NEC (Q79.1)
　　congenital diaphragmatic hernia (Q79.0)
Excludes2: diaphragmatic hernia (K44.-)

J98.8　Other specified respiratory disorders

J98.9　Respiratory disorder, unspecified
Respiratory disease (chronic) NOS

J99　RESPIRATORY DISORDERS IN DISEASES CLASSIFIED ELSEWHERE
✓
Code first underlying disease, such as:
　amyloidosis (E85.-)
　ankylosing spondylitis (M45)
　congenital syphilis (A50.5)
　cryoglobulinemia (D89.1)
　early congenital syphilis (A50.0)
　plasminogen deficiency (E88.02)
　schistosomiasis (B65.0-B65.9)
Excludes1: respiratory disorders in:
　amebiasis (A06.5)
　blastomycosis (B40.0-B40.2)
　candidiasis (B37.1)
　coccidioidomycosis (B38.0-B38.2)
　cystic fibrosis with pulmonary manifestations (E84.0)
　dermatomyositis (M33.01, M33.11)
　histoplasmosis (B39.0-B39.2)
　late syphilis (A52.72, A52.73)
　polymyositis (M33.21)
　sicca syndrome (M35.02)
　SLE (M32.13)
　systemic sclerosis (M34.81)
　Wegener's granulomatosis (M31.30-M31.31)

4th **5th** **6th** **7th** Additional Character Required　　**✓** 3-character code

•=New Code
▲=Revised Code

Excludes1—Not coded here, do not use together
Excludes2—Not included here

PEDIATRIC ICD-10-CM 2021: A MANUAL FOR PROVIDER-BASED CODING　　227

Chapter 11. Diseases of the digestive system (K00–K95)

GUIDELINES

None currently.

Excludes2: certain conditions originating in the perinatal period (P04–P96)
certain infectious and parasitic diseases (A00–B99)
complications of pregnancy, childbirth and the puerperium (O00–O9A)
congenital malformations, deformations and chromosomal abnormalities (Q00–Q99)
endocrine, nutritional and metabolic diseases (E00–E88)
injury, poisoning and certain other consequences of external causes (S00–T88)
neoplasms (C00–D49)
symptoms, signs and abnormal clinical and laboratory findings, NEC (R00–R94)

(K00–K14) DISEASES OF ORAL CAVITY AND SALIVARY GLANDS

K00 **DISORDERS OF TOOTH DEVELOPMENT AND ERUPTION**
`4th` **Excludes2:** embedded and impacted teeth (K01.-)

K00.0 **Anodontia**
Hypodontia
Oligodontia
Excludes1: acquired absence of teeth (K08.1-)

K00.1 **Supernumerary teeth**
Distomolar
Fourth molar
Mesiodens
Paramolar
Supplementary teeth
Excludes2: supernumerary roots (K00.2)

K00.3 **Mottled teeth**
Dental fluorosis
Mottling of enamel
Nonfluoride enamel opacities
Excludes2: deposits [accretions] on teeth (K03.6)

K00.6 **Disturbances in tooth eruption**
Dentia praecox
Natal tooth
Neonatal tooth
Premature eruption of tooth
Premature shedding of primary [deciduous] tooth
Prenatal teeth
Retained [persistent] primary tooth
Excludes2: embedded and impacted teeth (K01.-)

K00.7 **Teething syndrome**

K00.8 **Other disorders of tooth development**
Color changes during tooth formation
Intrinsic staining of teeth NOS
Excludes2: posteruptive color changes (K03.7)

K00.9 **Disorder of tooth development, unspecified**
Disorder of odontogenesis NOS

K02 **DENTAL CARIES**
`4th` **Includes:** caries of dentine
early childhood caries
pre-eruptive caries
recurrent caries (dentino enamel junction) (enamel) (to the pulp)
dental cavities
tooth decay

K02.9 **Dental caries, unspecified**

K03 **OTHER DISEASES OF HARD TISSUES OF TEETH**
`4th` **Excludes2:** bruxism (F45.8)
dental caries (K02.-)
teeth-grinding NOS (F45.8)

K03.1 **Abrasion of teeth**
Dentifrice abrasion of teeth
Habitual abrasion of teeth
Occupational abrasion of teeth
Ritual abrasion of teeth
Traditional abrasion of teeth
Wedge defect NOS

K03.8 **Other specified diseases of hard tissues of teeth**
`5th` **K03.81** **Cracked tooth**
Excludes1: broken or fractured tooth due to trauma (S02.5)
K03.89 **Other specified diseases of hard tissues of teeth**
K03.9 **Disease of hard tissues of teeth, unspecified**

K04 **DISEASES OF PULP AND PERIAPICAL TISSUES**
`4th` **K04.7** **Periapical abscess without sinus**
Dental abscess without sinus
Dentoalveolar abscess without sinus
Periapical abscess without sinus

K04.8 **Radicular cyst**
Apical (periodontal) cyst
Periapical cyst
Residual radicular cyst
Excludes2: lateral periodontal cyst (K09.0)

K05 **GINGIVITIS AND PERIODONTAL DISEASES**
`4th` **Use additional code** to identify:
alcohol abuse and dependence (F10.-)
exposure to environmental tobacco smoke (Z77.22)
exposure to tobacco smoke in the perinatal period (P96.81)
history of tobacco dependence (Z87.891)
occupational exposure to environmental tobacco smoke (Z57.31)
tobacco dependence (F17.-)
tobacco use (Z72.0)

K05.0 **Acute gingivitis**
`5th` **Excludes1:** acute necrotizing ulcerative gingivitis (A69.1)
herpesviral [herpes simplex] gingivostomatitis (B00.2)
K05.00 **Acute gingivitis, plaque induced**
Acute gingivitis NOS
Plaque-induced gingival disease

K06 **OTHER DISORDERS OF GINGIVA AND EDENTULOUS ALVEOLAR RIDGE**
`4th` **Excludes2:** acute gingivitis (K05.0)
atrophy of edentulous alveolar ridge (K08.2)
chronic gingivitis (K05.1)
gingivitis NOS (K05.1)

K06.1 **Gingival enlargement**
Gingival fibromatosis

K08 **OTHER DISORDERS OF TEETH AND SUPPORTING STRUCTURES**
`4th` **Excludes2:** dentofacial anomalies [including malocclusion] (M26.-)
disorders of jaw (M27.-)

K08.1 **Complete loss of teeth**
`5th` Acquired loss of teeth, complete
Excludes1: congenital absence of teeth (K00.0)
exfoliation of teeth due to systemic causes (K08.0)
partial loss of teeth (K08.4-)

K08.10	**Complete loss of teeth, unspecified cause**	
`6th`	**K08.101**	**Complete loss of teeth, unspecified cause; class I**
	K08.102	**class II**
	K08.103	**class III**
	K08.104	**class IV**
	K08.109	**unspecified class**
		Edentulism NOS
K08.11	**Complete loss of teeth due to trauma**	
`6th`	**K08.111**	**Complete loss of teeth due to trauma; class I**
	K08.112	**class II**
	K08.113	**class III**
	K08.114	**class IV**
	K08.119	**unspecified class**
K08.12	**Complete loss of teeth due to periodontal diseases**	
`6th`	**K08.121**	**Complete loss of teeth due to periodontal diseases, class I**
	K08.122	**class II**
	K08.123	**class III**
	K08.124	**class IV**
	K08.129	**unspecified class**

CHAPTER 11. DISEASES OF THE DIGESTIVE SYSTEM   (K08.13–K12)

K08.13   **Complete loss of teeth due to caries**
- 6th   **K08.131**   **Complete loss of teeth due to caries; class I**
- **K08.132**   **class II**
- **K08.133**   **class III**
- **K08.134**   **class IV**
- **K08.139**   **unspecified class**

K08.19   **Complete loss of teeth due to other specified cause**
- 6th   **K08.191**   **Complete loss of teeth due to other specified cause, class I**
- **K08.192**   **class II**
- **K08.193**   **class III**
- **K08.194**   **class IV**
- **K08.199**   **unspecified class**

K08.4   **Partial loss of teeth**
5th   Acquired loss of teeth, partial
Excludes1: complete loss of teeth (K08.1-)
     congenital absence of teeth (K00.0)
Excludes2: exfoliation of teeth due to systemic causes (K08.0)

K08.40   **Partial loss of teeth, unspecified cause**
- 6th   **K08.401**   **Partial loss of teeth, unspecified cause; class I**
- **K08.402**   **class II**
- **K08.403**   **class III**
- **K08.404**   **class IV**
- **K08.409**   **unspecified class**
     Tooth extraction status NOS

K08.41   **Partial loss of teeth due to trauma**
- 6th   **K08.411**   **Partial loss of teeth due to trauma; class I**
- **K08.412**   **class II**
- **K08.413**   **class III**
- **K08.414**   **class IV**
- **K08.419**   **unspecified class**

K08.42   **Partial loss of teeth due to periodontal diseases**
- 6th   **K08.421**   **Partial loss of teeth due to periodontal diseases, class I**
- **K08.422**   **class II**
- **K08.423**   **class III**
- **K08.424**   **class IV**
- **K08.429**   **unspecified class**

K08.43   **Partial loss of teeth due to caries**
- 6th   **K08.431**   **Partial loss of teeth due to caries; class I**
- **K08.432**   **class II**
- **K08.433**   **class III**
- **K08.434**   **class IV**
- **K08.439**   **unspecified class**

K08.49   **Partial loss of teeth due to other specified cause**
- 6th   **K08.491**   **class I**
- **K08.492**   **class II**
- **K08.493**   **class III**
- **K08.494**   **class IV**
- **K08.499**   **unspecified class**

K08.8   **Other specified disorders of teeth and supporting structures**
- 5th   **K08.81**   **Primary occlusal trauma**
- **K08.82**   **Secondary occlusal trauma**
- **K08.89**   **Other specified disorders of teeth and supporting structures**
     Enlargement of alveolar ridge NOS
     Insufficient anatomic crown height
     Insufficient clinical crown length
     Irregular alveolar process
     Toothache NOS

K08.9   **Disorder of teeth and supporting structures, unspecified**

K09   **CYSTS OF ORAL REGION, NEC**
4th   *Includes:* lesions showing histological features both of aneurysmal cyst and of another fibro-osseous lesion
Excludes2: cysts of jaw (M27.0-, M27.4-)
     radicular cyst (K04.8)

K09.0   **Developmental odontogenic cysts**
     Dentigerous cyst
     Eruption cyst
     Follicular cyst
     Gingival cyst
     Lateral periodontal cyst
     Primordial cyst
     Excludes2: keratocysts (D16.4, D16.5)
         odontogenic keratocystic tumors (D16.4, D16.5)

K09.1   **Developmental (nonodontogenic) cysts of oral region**
     Cyst (of) incisive canal or palatine of papilla
     Globulomaxillary cyst
     Median palatal cyst
     Nasoalveolar cyst
     Nasolabial cyst
     Nasopalatine duct cyst

K09.8   **Other cysts of oral region, NEC**
     Dermoid cyst
     Epidermoid cyst
     Lymphoepithelial cyst
     Epstein's pearl

K09.9   **Cyst of oral region, unspecified**

K11   **DISEASES OF SALIVARY GLANDS**
4th   **Use additional code** to identify:
     alcohol abuse and dependence (F10.-)
     exposure to environmental tobacco smoke (Z77.22)
     exposure to tobacco smoke in the perinatal period (P96.81)
     history of tobacco dependence (Z87.891)
     occupational exposure to environmental tobacco smoke (Z57.31)
     tobacco dependence (F17.-)
     tobacco use (Z72.0)

K11.2   **Sialoadenitis**
5th   Parotitis
Excludes1: epidemic parotitis (B26.-)
     mumps (B26.-)
     uveoparotid fever [Heerfordt] (D86.89)
- **K11.20**   **Sialoadenitis, unspecified**
- **K11.21**   **Acute sialoadenitis**
     Excludes1: acute recurrent sialoadenitis (K11.22)
- **K11.22**   **Acute recurrent sialoadenitis**
- **K11.23**   **Chronic sialoadenitis**

K11.3   **Abscess of salivary gland**

K11.4   **Fistula of salivary gland**
Excludes1: congenital fistula of salivary gland (Q38.4)

K11.7   **Disturbances of salivary secretion**
     Hypoptyalism
     Ptyalism
     Xerostomia
     Excludes2: dry mouth NOS (R68.2)

K11.8   **Other diseases of salivary glands**
     Benign lymphoepithelial lesion of salivary gland
     Mikulicz' disease
     Necrotizing sialometaplasia
     Sialectasia
     Stenosis of salivary duct
     Stricture of salivary duct
     Excludes1: sicca syndrome [Sjögren] (M35.0-)

K11.9   **Disease of salivary gland, unspecified**
     Sialoadenopathy NOS

K12   **STOMATITIS AND RELATED LESIONS**
4th   **Use additional code** to identify: alcohol abuse and dependence (F10.-)
     exposure to environmental tobacco smoke (Z77.22)
     exposure to tobacco smoke in the perinatal period (P96.81)
     history of tobacco dependence (Z87.891)
     occupational exposure to environmental tobacco smoke (Z57.31)
     tobacco dependence (F17.-)
     tobacco use (Z72.0)
Excludes1: cancrum oris (A69.0)
     cheilitis (K13.0)
     gangrenous stomatitis (A69.0)
     herpesviral [herpes simplex] gingivostomatitis (B00.2)
     noma (A69.0)

4th   5th   6th   7th   Additional Character Required   ✓   3-character code   •=New Code   ▲=Revised Code   *Excludes1*—Not coded here, do not use together   *Excludes2*—Not included here

K12.0 Recurrent oral aphthae
Aphthous stomatitis (major) (minor)
Bednar's aphthae
Periadenitis mucosa necrotica recurrens
Recurrent aphthous ulcer
Stomatitis herpetiformis

K12.1 Other forms of stomatitis
Stomatitis NOS
Denture stomatitis
Ulcerative stomatitis
Vesicular stomatitis
Excludes1: acute necrotizing ulcerative stomatitis (A69.1)

K12.2 Cellulitis and abscess of mouth
Cellulitis of mouth (floor)
Submandibular abscess
Excludes2: abscess of salivary gland (K11.3)
abscess of tongue (K14.0)
periapical abscess (K04.6–K04.7)
periodontal abscess (K05.21)
peritonsillar abscess (J36)

K12.3 Oral mucositis (ulcerative)
`5th` Mucositis (oral) (oropharyngeal)
Excludes2: gastrointestinal mucositis (ulcerative) (K92.81)
mucositis (ulcerative) of vagina and vulva (N76.81)
nasal mucositis (ulcerative) (J34.81)
K12.30   Oral mucositis (ulcerative), unspecified

K13 OTHER DISEASES OF LIP AND ORAL MUCOSA
`4th` *Includes:* epithelial disturbances of tongue
Use additional code to identify:
alcohol abuse and dependence (F10.-)
exposure to environmental tobacco smoke (Z77.22)
exposure to tobacco smoke in the perinatal period (P96.81)
history of tobacco dependence (Z87.891)
occupational exposure to environmental tobacco smoke (Z57.31)
tobacco dependence (F17.-)
tobacco use (Z72.0)
Excludes2: certain disorders of gingiva and edentulous alveolar ridge (K05–K06)
cysts of oral region (K09.-)
diseases of tongue (K14.-)
stomatitis and related lesions (K12.-)

K13.0 Diseases of lips
Abscess of lips
Angular cheilitis
Cellulitis of lips
Cheilitis NOS
Cheilodynia
Cheilosis
Exfoliative cheilitis
Fistula of lips
Glandular cheilitis
Hypertrophy of lips
Perlèche NEC
Excludes1: ariboflavinosis (E53.0)
cheilitis due to radiation-related disorders (L55–L59)
congenital fistula of lips (Q38.0)
congenital hypertrophy of lips (Q18.6)
Perlèche due to candidiasis (B37.83)
Perlèche due to riboflavin deficiency (E53.0)

K13.1 Cheek and lip biting
K13.7 Other and unspecified lesions of oral mucosa
`5th` **K13.70   Unspecified lesions of oral mucosa**
K13.79   Other lesions of oral mucosa
Focal oral mucinosis

K14 DISEASES OF TONGUE
`4th` **Use additional code** to identify: alcohol abuse and dependence (F10.-)
exposure to environmental tobacco smoke (Z77.22)
history of tobacco dependence (Z87.891)
occupational exposure to environmental tobacco smoke (Z57.31)
tobacco dependence (F17.-)
tobacco use (Z72.0)

Excludes2: erythroplakia (K13.29)
focal epithelial hyperplasia (K13.29)
leukedema of tongue (K13.29)
leukoplakia of tongue (K13.21)
hairy leukoplakia (K13.3)
macroglossia (congenital) (Q38.2)
submucous fibrosis of tongue (K13.5)

K14.0 Glossitis
Abscess of tongue
Ulceration (traumatic) of tongue
Excludes1: atrophic glossitis (K14.4)

K14.1 Geographic tongue
Benign migratory glossitis
Glossitis areata exfoliativa

K14.3 Hypertrophy of tongue papillae
Black hairy tongue
Coated tongue
Hypertrophy of foliate papillae
Lingua villosa nigra

K14.8 Other diseases of tongue
Atrophy of tongue
Crenated tongue
Enlargement of tongue
Glossocele
Glossoptosis
Hypertrophy of tongue

(K20–K31) DISEASES OF ESOPHAGUS, STOMACH AND DUODENUM

Excludes2: hiatus hernia (K44.-)

K20 ESOPHAGITIS
`4th` **Use additional code** to identify: alcohol abuse and dependence (F10.-)
Excludes1: erosion of esophagus (K22.1-)
esophagitis with gastro-esophageal reflux disease (K21.0-)
reflux esophagitis (K21.0-)
ulcerative esophagitis (K22.1-)
Excludes2: eosinophilic gastritis or gastroenteritis (K52.81)
K20.0 Eosinophilic esophagitis
▲**K20.8 Other esophagitis**
`5th` •**K20.80   Other esophagitis without bleeding**
Abscess of esophagus
Other esophagitis NOS
•**K20.81   Other esophagitis with bleeding**
▲**K20.9 Esophagitis, unspecified**
`5th` •**K20.90   Esophagitis, unspecified without bleeding**
Esophagitis, NOS
•**K20.91   Esophagitis, unspecified with bleeding**

K21 GASTRO-ESOPHAGEAL REFLUX DISEASE
`4th` *Excludes1:* newborn esophageal reflux (P78.83)
▲**K21.0 Gastro-esophageal reflux disease (GERD) with esophagitis**
`5th` •**K21.00   GERD with esophagitis, without bleeding**
Reflux esophagitis
•**K21.01   GERD with esophagitis, with bleeding**
K21.9 GERD without esophagitis
Esophageal reflux NOS

K22 OTHER DISEASES OF ESOPHAGUS
`4th` *Excludes2:* esophageal varices (I85.-)
K22.0 Achalasia of cardia
Achalasia NOS
Cardiospasm
Excludes1: congenital cardiospasm (Q39.5)
K22.1 Ulcer of esophagus
`5th` Barrett's ulcer
Erosion of esophagus
Fungal ulcer of esophagus
Peptic ulcer of esophagus
Ulcer of esophagus due to ingestion of chemicals
Ulcer of esophagus due to ingestion of drugs and medicaments
Ulcerative esophagitis
Code first poisoning due to drug or toxin, if applicable (T36-T65 with fifth or sixth character 1-4 or 6)

`4th` `5th` `6th` `7th` Additional Character Required   ✔ `3-character code`

•=New Code   *Excludes1*—Not coded here, do not use together
▲=Revised Code   *Excludes2*—Not included here

CHAPTER 11. DISEASES OF THE DIGESTIVE SYSTEM   (K12.0–K22.1)

Use additional code for adverse effect, if applicable, to identify drug (T36–T50 with fifth or sixth character 5)
Excludes1: Barrett's esophagus (K22.7-)

K22.10   Ulcer of esophagus without bleeding
Ulcer of esophagus NOS

K22.11   Ulcer of esophagus with bleeding
Excludes2: bleeding esophageal varices (I85.01, I85.11)

K22.4   Dyskinesia of esophagus
Corkscrew esophagus
Diffuse esophageal spasm
Spasm of esophagus
Excludes1: cardiospasm (K22.0)

K22.8   Other specified diseases of esophagus
Hemorrhage of esophagus NOS
Excludes2: esophageal varices (I85.-)
Paterson-Kelly syndrome (D50.1)

K22.9   Disease of esophagus, unspecified

K25   GASTRIC ULCER
`4th`
Includes: erosion (acute) of stomach
pylorus ulcer (peptic)
stomach ulcer (peptic)
Use additional code to identify: alcohol abuse and dependence (F10.-)
Excludes1: acute gastritis (K29.0-)
peptic ulcer NOS (K27.-)

K25.0   Acute gastric ulcer; with hemorrhage
K25.1   with perforation
K25.2   with both hemorrhage and perforation
K25.3   without hemorrhage or perforation
K25.4   Chronic or unspecified gastric ulcer; with hemorrhage
K25.5   with perforation
K25.6   with both hemorrhage and perforation
K25.7   without hemorrhage or perforation
K25.9   Gastric ulcer, unspecified as acute or chronic, without hemorrhage or perforation

K26   DUODENAL ULCER
`4th`
Includes: erosion (acute) of duodenum
duodenum ulcer (peptic)
postpyloric ulcer (peptic)
Use additional code to identify: alcohol abuse and dependence (F10.-)
Excludes1: peptic ulcer NOS (K27.-)

K26.0   Acute duodenal ulcer; with hemorrhage
K26.1   with perforation
K26.2   with both hemorrhage and perforation
K26.3   without hemorrhage or perforation
K26.4   Chronic or unspecified duodenal ulcer; with hemorrhage
K26.5   with perforation
K26.6   with both hemorrhage and perforation
K26.7   without hemorrhage or perforation
K26.9   Duodenal ulcer, unspecified as acute or chronic, without hemorrhage or perforation

K27   PEPTIC ULCER, SITE UNSPECIFIED
`4th`
Includes: gastroduodenal ulcer NOS
peptic ulcer NOS
Use additional code to identify: alcohol abuse and dependence (F10.-)
Excludes1: peptic ulcer of newborn (P78.82)

K27.0   Acute peptic ulcer, site unspecified; with hemorrhage
K27.1   with perforation
K27.2   with both hemorrhage and perforation
K27.3   without hemorrhage or perforation
K27.4   Chronic or unspecified peptic ulcer, site unspecified; with hemorrhage
K27.5   with perforation
K27.6   with both hemorrhage and perforation
K27.7   without hemorrhage or perforation
K27.9   Peptic ulcer, site unspecified, unspecified as acute or chronic, without hemorrhage or perforation

K29   GASTRITIS AND DUODENITIS
`4th`
Excludes1: eosinophilic gastritis or gastroenteritis (K52.81)
Zollinger-Ellison syndrome (E16.4)

K29.0   Acute gastritis
`5th`   **Use additional code** to identify: alcohol abuse and dependence (F10.-)
Excludes1: erosion (acute) of stomach (K25.-)

K29.00   Acute gastritis without bleeding
K29.01   Acute gastritis with bleeding
K29.7   Gastritis, unspecified
`5th`   **K29.70   Gastritis, unspecified, without bleeding**
K29.71   Gastritis, unspecified, with bleeding
K29.8   Duodenitis
`5th`   **K29.80   Duodenitis without bleeding**
K29.81   Duodenitis with bleeding
K29.9   Gastroduodenitis, unspecified
`5th`   **K29.90   Gastroduodenitis, unspecified, without bleeding**
K29.91   Gastroduodenitis, unspecified, with bleeding

K30   FUNCTIONAL DYSPEPSIA
`✔`
Indigestion
Excludes1: dyspepsia NOS (R10.13)
heartburn (R12)
nervous dyspepsia (F45.8)
neurotic dyspepsia (F45.8)
psychogenic dyspepsia (F45.8)

K31   OTHER DISEASES OF STOMACH AND DUODENUM
`4th`
Includes: functional disorders of stomach
Excludes2: diabetic gastroparesis (E08.43, E09.43, E10.43, E11.43, E13.43)
diverticulum of duodenum (K57.00–K57.13)

K31.0   Acute dilatation of stomach
Acute distention of stomach
K31.1   Adult hypertrophic pyloric stenosis
Pyloric stenosis NOS
Excludes1: congenital or infantile pyloric stenosis (Q40.0)
K31.3   Pylorospasm, NEC
Excludes1: congenital or infantile pylorospasm (Q40.0)
neurotic pylorospasm (F45.8)
psychogenic pylorospasm (F45.8)
K31.5   Obstruction of duodenum
Constriction of duodenum
Duodenal ileus (chronic)
Stenosis of duodenum
Stricture of duodenum
Volvulus of duodenum
Excludes 1: congenital stenosis of duodenum (Q41.0)
K31.8   Other specified diseases of stomach and duodenum
`5th`   **K31.83   Achlorhydria**
K31.84   Gastroparesis
Gastroparalysis
Code first underlying disease, if known, such as:
anorexia nervosa (F50.0-)
diabetes mellitus (E08.43, E09.43, E10.43, E11.43, E13.43)
scleroderma (M34.-)
K31.89   Other diseases of stomach and duodenum
K31.9   Disease of stomach and duodenum, unspecified

(K35–K38) DISEASES OF APPENDIX

K35   ACUTE APPENDICITIS
`4th`   **K35.2   Acute appendicitis with generalized peritonitis**
`5th`   **K35.20   Acute appendicitis with generalized peritonitis, without abscess**
(Acute) appendicitis with generalized peritonitis NOS
K35.21   Acute appendicitis with generalized peritonitis, with abscess
K35.3   Acute appendicitis with localized peritonitis
`5th`   **K35.30   Acute appendicitis with localized peritonitis, without perforation or gangrene**
Acute appendicitis with localized peritonitis NOS
K35.31   Acute appendicitis with localized peritonitis and gangrene, without perforation
K35.32   Acute appendicitis with perforation and localized peritonitis, without abscess
(Acute) appendicitis with perforation NOS
Perforated appendix NOS
Ruptured appendix (with localized peritonitis) NOS

`4th` `5th` `6th` `7th`   Additional Character Required   `✔`   3-character code

•=New Code   *Excludes1*—Not coded here, do not use together
▲=Revised Code   *Excludes2*—Not included here

K35.33 **Acute appendicitis with perforation and localized peritonitis, with abscess**
(Acute) appendicitis with (peritoneal) abscess NOS
Ruptured appendix with localized peritonitis and abscess

K35.8 **Other and unspecified acute appendicitis**
5th **K35.80** **Unspecified acute appendicitis**
Acute appendicitis NOS
Acute appendicitis without (localized) (generalized) peritonitis

K35.89 **Other acute appendicitis**
6th **K35.890** **Other acute appendicitis without perforation or gangrene**
K35.891 **Other acute appendicitis without perforation, with gangrene**

K37 **UNSPECIFIED APPENDICITIS**
☑ **Excludes1:** -unspecified appendicitis with peritonitis (K35.2-, K35.3-)

(K40–K46) HERNIA

Note: Hernia with both gangrene and obstruction is classified to hernia with gangrene.
Includes: acquired hernia
congenital [except diaphragmatic or hiatus] hernia
recurrent hernia

K40 **INGUINAL HERNIA**
4th **Includes:** bubonocele
direct inguinal hernia
double inguinal hernia
indirect inguinal hernia
inguinal hernia NOS
oblique inguinal hernia
scrotal hernia

K40.0 **Bilateral inguinal hernia, with obstruction, without gangrene**
5th Inguinal hernia (bilateral) causing obstruction without gangrene
Incarcerated or Irreducible or Strangulated inguinal hernia (bilateral) without gangrene
K40.00 **Bilateral inguinal hernia, with obstruction, without gangrene, not specified as recurrent**
Bilateral inguinal hernia, with obstruction, without gangrene NOS
K40.01 **Bilateral inguinal hernia, with obstruction, without gangrene, recurrent**

K40.1 **Bilateral inguinal hernia, with gangrene**
5th **K40.10** **Bilateral inguinal hernia, with gangrene, not specified as recurrent**
Bilateral inguinal hernia, with gangrene NOS
K40.11 **Bilateral inguinal hernia, with gangrene, recurrent**

K40.2 **Bilateral inguinal hernia, without obstruction or gangrene**
5th **K40.20** **Bilateral inguinal hernia, without obstruction or gangrene, not specified as recurrent**
Bilateral inguinal hernia NOS
K40.21 **Bilateral inguinal hernia, without obstruction or gangrene, recurrent**

K40.3 **Unilateral inguinal hernia, with obstruction, without gangrene**
5th Inguinal hernia (unilateral) causing obstruction without gangrene
Incarcerated or Irreducible or Strangulated inguinal hernia (unilateral) without gangrene
K40.30 **Unilateral inguinal hernia, with obstruction, without gangrene, not specified as recurrent**
Inguinal hernia, with obstruction NOS
Unilateral inguinal hernia, with obstruction, without gangrene NOS
K40.31 **Unilateral inguinal hernia, with obstruction, without gangrene, recurrent**

K40.4 **Unilateral inguinal hernia, with gangrene**
5th **K40.40** **Unilateral inguinal hernia, with gangrene, not specified as recurrent**
Inguinal hernia with gangrene NOS
Unilateral inguinal hernia with gangrene NOS
K40.41 **Unilateral inguinal hernia, with gangrene, recurrent**

K40.9 **Unilateral inguinal hernia, without obstruction or gangrene**
5th

K40.90 **Unilateral inguinal hernia, without obstruction or gangrene, not specified as recurrent**
Inguinal hernia NOS
Unilateral inguinal hernia NOS
K40.91 **Unilateral inguinal hernia, without obstruction or gangrene, recurrent**

K42 **UMBILICAL HERNIA**
4th **Includes:** paraumbilical hernia
Excludes1: omphalocele (Q79.2)
K42.0 **Umbilical hernia with obstruction, without gangrene**
Umbilical hernia causing obstruction, without gangrene
Incarcerated or Irreducible or Strangulated umbilical hernia, without gangrene
K42.1 **Umbilical hernia with gangrene**
Gangrenous umbilical hernia
K42.9 **Umbilical hernia without obstruction or gangrene**
Umbilical hernia NOS

K43 **VENTRAL HERNIA**
4th **K43.0** **Incisional hernia with obstruction, without gangrene**
Incisional hernia causing obstruction, without gangrene
Incarcerated or Irreducible or Strangulated incisional hernia, without gangrene
K43.1 **Incisional hernia with gangrene**
Gangrenous incisional hernia
K43.2 **Incisional hernia without obstruction or gangrene**
Incisional hernia NOS
K43.9 **Ventral hernia without obstruction or gangrene**
Epigastric hernia
Ventral hernia NOS

K44 **DIAPHRAGMATIC HERNIA**
4th **Includes:** hiatus hernia (esophageal) (sliding)
paraesophageal hernia
Excludes1: congenital diaphragmatic hernia (Q79.0)
congenital hiatus hernia (Q40.1)
K44.0 **Diaphragmatic hernia with obstruction, without gangrene**
Diaphragmatic hernia causing obstruction
Incarcerated or Irreducible or Strangulated diaphragmatic hernia
K44.1 **Diaphragmatic hernia with gangrene**
Gangrenous diaphragmatic hernia
K44.9 **Diaphragmatic hernia without obstruction or gangrene**
Diaphragmatic hernia NOS

K46 **UNSPECIFIED ABDOMINAL HERNIA**
4th **Includes:** enterocele
epiplocele
hernia NOS
interstitial hernia
intestinal hernia
intra-abdominal hernia
Excludes1: vaginal enterocele (N81.5)
K46.0 **Unspecified abdominal hernia with obstruction, without gangrene**
Unspecified abdominal hernia causing obstruction
Unspecified incarcerated abdominal hernia
Unspecified irreducible abdominal hernia
Unspecified strangulated abdominal hernia
K46.1 **Unspecified abdominal hernia with gangrene**
Any condition listed under K46 specified as gangrenous
K46.9 **Unspecified abdominal hernia without obstruction or gangrene**
Abdominal hernia NOS

(K50–K52) NONINFECTIVE ENTERITIS AND COLITIS

Includes: noninfective inflammatory bowel disease
Excludes1: irritable bowel syndrome (K58.-)
megacolon (K59.3-)

K50 **CROHN'S DISEASE [REGIONAL ENTERITIS]**
4th **Includes:** granulomatous enteritis
Use additional code to identify manifestations, such as: pyoderma gangrenosum (L88)
Excludes1: ulcerative colitis (K51.-)

4th **5th** **6th** **7th**   Additional Character Required   ☑   3-character code

•=New Code   **Excludes1**—Not coded here, do not use together
▲=Revised Code   **Excludes2**—Not included here

CHAPTER 11. DISEASES OF THE DIGESTIVE SYSTEM   (K50.0–K51.919)

K50.0   **Crohn's disease of small intestine**
`5th`   Crohn's disease [regional enteritis] of duodenum or ileum or jejunum
    Regional ileitis
    Terminal ileitis
    Excludes1: Crohn's disease of both small and large intestine
      (K50.8-)
    K50.00   **Crohn's disease of small intestine without complications**
    K50.01   **Crohn's disease of small intestine with**
    `6th`   **complications**
       K50.011   **Crohn's disease of small intestine; with rectal bleeding**
       K50.012   **with intestinal obstruction**
       K50.013   **with fistula**
       K50.014   **with abscess**
       K50.018   **with other complication**
       K50.019   **with unspecified complications**

K50.1   **Crohn's disease of large intestine**
`5th`   Crohn's disease [regional enteritis] of colon or large bowel or
     rectum
    Granulomatous colitis
    Regional colitis
    Excludes1: Crohn's disease of both small and large intestine
      (K50.8)
    K50.10   **Crohn's disease of large intestine without complications**
    K50.11   **Crohn's disease of large intestine with complications**
    `6th`   **K50.111**   **Crohn's disease of large intestine; with rectal bleeding**
       K50.112   **with intestinal obstruction**
       K50.113   **with fistula**
       K50.114   **with abscess**
       K50.118   **with other complication**
       K50.119   **with unspecified complications**

K50.8   **Crohn's disease of both small and large intestine**
`5th`   **K50.80**   **Crohn's disease of both small and large intestine without complications**
    K50.81   **Crohn's disease of both small and large intestine**
    `6th`   **with complications**
       K50.811   **Crohn's disease of both small and large intestine; with rectal bleeding**
       K50.812   **with intestinal obstruction**
       K50.813   **with fistula**
       K50.814   **with abscess**
       K50.818   **with other complication**
       K50.819   **with unspecified complications**

K50.9   **Crohn's disease, unspecified**
`5th`   **K50.90**   **Crohn's disease, unspecified, without complications**
       Crohn's disease NOS
       Regional enteritis NOS
    K50.91   **Crohn's disease, unspecified, with complications**
    `6th`   **K50.911**   **Crohn's disease, unspecified; with rectal bleeding**
       K50.912   **with intestinal obstruction**
       K50.913   **with fistula**
       K50.914   **with abscess**
       K50.918   **with other complication**
       K50.919   **with unspecified complications**

K51   **ULCERATIVE COLITIS**
`4th`   **Use additional code** to identify manifestations, such as: pyoderma
     gangrenosum (L88)
    Excludes1: Crohn's disease [regional enteritis] (K50.-)
    K51.0   **Ulcerative (chronic) pancolitis**
    `5th`   Backwash ileitis
      K51.00   **Ulcerative (chronic) pancolitis without complications**
        Ulcerative (chronic) pancolitis NOS
      K51.01   **Ulcerative (chronic) pancolitis with complications**
      `6th`   **K51.011**   **Ulcerative (chronic) pancolitis; with rectal bleeding**
        K51.012   **with intestinal obstruction**
        K51.013   **with fistula**
        K51.014   **with abscess**

        K51.018   **with other complication**
        K51.019   **with unspecified complications**
K51.2   **Ulcerative (chronic) proctitis**
`5th`   **K51.20**   **Ulcerative (chronic) proctitis without complications**
        Ulcerative (chronic) proctitis NOS
    K51.21   **Ulcerative (chronic) proctitis with complications**
    `6th`   **K51.211**   **Ulcerative (chronic) proctitis; with rectal bleeding**
        K51.212   **with intestinal obstruction**
        K51.213   **with fistula**
        K51.214   **with abscess**
        K51.218   **with other complication**
        K51.219   **with unspecified complications**

K51.3   **Ulcerative (chronic) rectosigmoiditis**
`5th`   **K51.30**   **Ulcerative (chronic) rectosigmoiditis without complications**
        Ulcerative (chronic) rectosigmoiditis NOS
    K51.31   **Ulcerative (chronic) rectosigmoiditis with**
    `6th`   **complications**
        K51.311   **Ulcerative (chronic) rectosigmoiditis; with rectal bleeding**
        K51.312   **with intestinal obstruction**
        K51.313   **with fistula**
        K51.314   **with abscess**
        K51.318   **with other complication**
        K51.319   **with unspecified complications**

K51.4   **Inflammatory polyps of colon**
`5th`   **Excludes1:** adenomatous polyp of colon (D12.6)
      polyposis of colon (D12.6)
      polyps of colon NOS (K63.5)
    K51.40   **Inflammatory polyps of colon without complications**
        Inflammatory polyps of colon NOS
    K51.41   **Inflammatory polyps of colon with complications**
    `6th`   **K51.411**   **Inflammatory polyps of colon; with rectal bleeding**
        K51.412   **with intestinal obstruction**
        K51.413   **with fistula**
        K51.414   **with abscess**
        K51.418   **with other complication**
        K51.419   **with unspecified complications**

K51.5   **Left sided colitis**
`5th`   Left hemicolitis
    K51.50   **Left sided colitis without complications**
        Left sided colitis NOS
    K51.51   **Left sided colitis with complications**
    `6th`   **K51.511**   **Left sided colitis; with rectal bleeding**
        K51.512   **with intestinal obstruction**
        K51.513   **with fistula**
        K51.514   **with abscess**
        K51.518   **with other complication**
        K51.519   **with unspecified complications**

K51.8   **Other ulcerative colitis**
`5th`   **K51.80**   **Other ulcerative colitis without complications**
    K51.81   **Other ulcerative colitis with complications**
    `6th`   **K51.811**   **Other ulcerative colitis; with rectal bleeding**
        K51.812   **with intestinal obstruction**
        K51.813   **with fistula**
        K51.814   **with abscess**
        K51.818   **with other complication**
        K51.819   **with unspecified complications**

K51.9   **Ulcerative colitis, unspecified**
`5th`   **K51.90**   **Ulcerative colitis, unspecified, without complications**
    K51.91   **Ulcerative colitis, unspecified, with complications**
    `6th`   **K51.911**   **Ulcerative colitis, unspecified; with rectal bleeding**
        K51.912   **with intestinal obstruction**
        K51.913   **with fistula**
        K51.914   **with abscess**
        K51.918   **with other complication**
        K51.919   **with unspecified complications**

`4th` `5th` `6th` `7th`   Additional Character Required   ✔   3-character code   •=New Code   ▲=Revised Code   **Excludes1**—Not coded here, do not use together   **Excludes2**—Not included here

K52 OTHER AND UNSPECIFIED NONINFECTIVE
`4th` GASTROENTERITIS AND COLITIS

K52.2 **Allergic and dietetic gastroenteritis and colitis**
`5th` Food hypersensitivity gastroenteritis or colitis
Use additional code to identify type of food allergy (Z91.01-, Z91.02-)
Excludes2: allergic eosinophilic colitis (K52.82)
allergic eosinophilic esophagitis (K20.0)
allergic eosinophilic gastritis (K52.81)
allergic eosinophilic gastroenteritis (K52.81)
food protein–induced proctocolitis (K52.82)

K52.21 **Food protein–induced enterocolitis syndrome (FPIES)**
Use additional code for hypovolemic shock, if present (R57.1)

K52.22 **Food protein–induced enteropathy**

K52.29 **Other allergic and dietetic gastroenteritis and colitis**
Food hypersensitivity gastroenteritis or colitis
Immediate gastrointestinal hypersensitivity

K52.3 **Indeterminate colitis**
Colonic inflammatory bowel disease unclassified (IBDU)
Excludes1: unspecified colitis (K52.9)

K52.8 **Other specified noninfective gastroenteritis and colitis**
`5th` **K52.81** **Eosinophilic gastritis or gastroenteritis**
Eosinophilic enteritis
Excludes2: eosinophilic esophagitis (K20.0)

K52.82 **Eosinophilic colitis**
Allergic proctocolitis
Food-induced eosinophilic proctocolitis
Food protein-induced proctocolitis
Milk protein-induced proctocolitis

K52.83 **Microscopic colitis**
`6th` **K52.831** **Collagenous colitis**
K52.832 **Lymphocytic colitis**
K52.838 **Other microscopic colitis**
K52.839 **Microscopic colitis, unspecified**

K52.89 **Other specified noninfective gastroenteritis and colitis**

K52.9 **Noninfective gastroenteritis and colitis, unspecified**
Colitis or Enteritis or Gastroenteritis NOS
Ileitis or Jejunitis or Sigmoiditis NOS
Excludes1: diarrhea NOS (R19.7)
functional diarrhea (K59.1)
infectious gastroenteritis and colitis NOS (A09)
neonatal diarrhea (noninfective) (P78.3)
psychogenic diarrhea (F45.8)

(K55–K64) OTHER DISEASES OF INTESTINES

K55 VASCULAR DISORDERS OF INTESTINES
`4th` **K55.0** **Acute vascular disorders of intestine**
`5th` Infarction of appendices epiploicae
Mesenteric (artery) (vein) embolism
Mesenteric (artery) (vein) infarction
Mesenteric (artery) (vein) thrombosis

K55.01 **Ischemia of small intestines**
`6th` **K55.011** **Focal (segmental) acute (reversible) ischemia of small intestine**
K55.012 **Diffuse acute (reversible) ischemia of small intestine**
K55.019 **Acute (reversible) ischemia of small intestine, extent unspecified**

K55.02 **Infarction of small intestines**
`6th` Gangrene or necrosis of small intestine
K55.021 **Focal (segmental) acute infarction of small intestine**
K55.022 **Diffuse acute infarction of small intestine**
K55.029 **Acute infarction of small intestine, extent unspecified**

K55.03 **Ischemia of small intestine**
`6th` Acute fulminant ischemic colitis
Subacute ischemic colitis
K55.031 **Focal (segmental) acute (reversible) ischemia of large intestine**

K55.032 **Diffuse acute (reversible) ischemia of large intestine**
K55.039 **Acute (reversible) ischemia of large intestine, extent unspecified**

K55.04 **Infarction of intestine, part unspecified**
`6th` Gangrene or necrosis of large intestine
K55.041 **Focal (segmental) acute infarction of large intestine**
K55.042 **Diffuse acute infarction of large intestine**
K55.049 **Acute infarction of large intestine, extent unspecified**

K55.05 **Ischemia of intestine, part unspecified**
`6th` **K55.051** **Focal (segmental) acute (reversible) ischemia of intestine, part unspecified**
K55.052 **Diffuse acute (reversible) ischemia of intestine, part unspecified**
K55.059 **Acute (reversible) ischemia of intestine, part and extent unspecified**

K55.06 **Infarction of intestine, part unspecified**
`6th` **K55.061** **Focal (segmental) acute infarction of intestine, part unspecified**
K55.062 **Diffuse acute infarction of intestine, part unspecified**
K55.069 **Acute infarction of intestine, part and extent unspecified**

K55.1 **Chronic vascular disorders of intestine**
Chronic ischemic colitis
Chronic ischemic enteritis
Chronic ischemic enterocolitis
Ischemic stricture of intestine
Mesenteric atherosclerosis
Mesenteric vascular insufficiency

K55.3 **Necrotizing enterocolitis**
`5th` *Excludes1:* necrotizing enterocolitis of newborn (P77.-)
Excludes2: necrotizing enterocolitis due to Clostridium difficile (A04.7-)

K55.30 **Necrotizing enterocolitis, unspecified**
Necrotizing enterocolitis, NOS

K55.31 **Stage 1 necrotizing enterocolitis**
Necrotizing enterocolitis without pneumonia or perforation

K55.32 **Stage 2 necrotizing enterocolitis**
Necrotizing enterocolitis with pneumonia, without perforation

K55.33 **Stage 3 necrotizing enterocolitis**
Necrotizing enterocolitis with perforation
Necrotizing enterocolitis with pneumatosis and perforation

K55.9 **Vascular disorder of intestine, unspecified**
Ischemic colitis
Ischemic enteritis
Ischemic enterocolitis

K56 PARALYTIC ILEUS AND INTESTINAL OBSTRUCTION
`4th` WITHOUT HERNIA
Excludes1: congenital stricture or stenosis of intestine (Q41–Q42)
cystic fibrosis with meconium ileus (E84.11)
ischemic stricture of intestine (K55.1)
meconium ileus NOS (P76.0)
neonatal intestinal obstructions classifiable to P76.-
obstruction of duodenum (K31.5)
postprocedural intestinal obstruction (K91.3-)
Excludes2: stenosis of anus or rectum (K62.4)

K56.0 **Paralytic ileus**
Paralysis of bowel or colon or intestine
Excludes1: gallstone ileus (K56.3)
ileus NOS (K56.7)
obstructive ileus NOS (K56.69-)

K56.1 **Intussusception**
Intussusception or invagination of bowel or colon or intestine or rectum
Excludes2: intussusception of appendix (K38.8)

`4th` `5th` `6th` `7th` Additional Character Required   ✓   3-character code

● =New Code
▲ =Revised Code

Excludes1—Not coded here, do not use together
Excludes2—Not included here

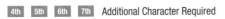

K56.2 Volvulus
Strangulation of colon or intestine
Torsion or Twist of colon or intestine
Excludes2: volvulus of duodenum (K31.5)
K56.4 Other impaction of intestine
- 5th **K56.41 Fecal impaction**
  - *Excludes1:* constipation (K59.0-)
    - incomplete defecation (R15.0)
  - **K56.49 Other impaction of intestine**
K56.6 Other and unspecified intestinal obstruction
- 5th **K56.60 Unspecified intestinal obstruction**
  - 6th Intestinal obstruction NOS
    - **K56.600 Partial intestinal obstruction, unspecified as to cause**
      - Incomplete intestinal obstruction, NOS
    - **K56.601 Complete intestinal obstruction, unspecified as to cause**
    - **K56.609 Unspecified intestinal obstruction, unspecified as to partial versus complete obstruction**
      - Intestinal obstruction NOS
  - **K56.69 Other intestinal obstruction**
    - 6th Enterostenosis NOS
      - Obstructive ileus NOS
      - Occlusion or Stenosis or Stricture of colon or intestine NOS
      - *Excludes1:* intestinal obstruction due to specified condition-code to condition
    - **K56.690 Other partial intestinal obstruction**
      - Other incomplete intestinal obstruction
    - **K56.691 Other complete intestinal obstruction**
    - **K56.699 Other intestinal obstruction unspecified as to partial versus complete obstruction**
      - Other intestinal obstruction, NEC
K56.7 Ileus, unspecified
Excludes1: obstructive ileus (K56.69-)
Excludes2: intestinal obstruction with hernia (K40-K46)

K58 IRRITABLE BOWEL SYNDROME
- 4th *Includes:* irritable colon
  - spastic colon
K58.0 Irritable bowel syndrome with diarrhea
K58.1 Irritable bowel syndrome with constipation
K58.2 Mixed irritable bowel syndrome
K58.8 Other Irritable bowel syndrome
K58.9 Irritable bowel syndrome without diarrhea
Irritable bowel syndrome NOS

K59 OTHER FUNCTIONAL INTESTINAL DISORDERS
- 4th *Excludes1:* change in bowel habit NOS (R19.4)
  - intestinal malabsorption (K90.-)
  - psychogenic intestinal disorders (F45.8)
Excludes2: functional disorders of stomach (K31.-)
K59.0 Constipation
- 5th *Excludes1:* fecal impaction (K56.41)
  - incomplete defecation (R15.0)
  - **K59.00 Constipation, unspecified**
  - **K59.01 Slow transit constipation**
  - **K59.02 Outlet dysfunction constipation**
  - **K59.03 Drug-induced constipation**
    - **Use additional code** for adverse effect, if applicable, to identify drug (T36 –T50) with fifth or sixth character 5
  - **K59.04 Chronic Idiopathic constipation**
    - Functional constipation
  - **K59.09 Other constipation**
    - Chronic constipation
K59.1 Functional diarrhea
Excludes1: diarrhea NOS (R19.7)
irritable bowel syndrome with diarrhea (K58.0)
K59.2 Neurogenic bowel, not elsewhere classified

K59.3 Megacolon, NEC
- 5th Dilatation of colon
  - *Excludes1:* congenital megacolon (aganglionic) (Q43.1)
    - megacolon (due to) (in) Chagas' disease (B57.32)
    - megacolon (due to) (in) Clostridium difficile (A04.7-)
    - megacolon (due to) (in) Hirschsprung's disease (Q43.1)
  - **K59.31 Toxic megacolon**
    - **Code first** (T51–T65) to identify toxic agent, if applicable
  - **K59.39 Other megacolon**
    - Megacolon NOS
K59.4 Anal spasm
Proctalgia fugax
▲**K59.8 Other specified functional intestinal disorders**
- •**K59.81 Ogilvie syndrome**
  - Acute colonic pseudo-obstruction (ACPO)
- •**K59.89 Other specified functional intestinal disorders**
  - Atony of colon
  - Pseudo-obstruction (acute) (chronic) of intestine
K59.9 Functional intestinal disorder, unspecified

K60 FISSURE AND FISTULA OF ANAL AND RECTAL REGIONS
- 4th *Excludes1:* fissure and fistula of anal and rectal regions with abscess or cellulitis (K61.-)
Excludes2: anal sphincter tear (healed) (nontraumatic) (old) (K62.81)
K60.0 Acute anal fissure
K60.1 Chronic anal fissure
K60.2 Anal fissure, unspecified
K60.3 Anal fistula
K60.4 Rectal fistula
Fistula of rectum to skin
Excludes1: rectovaginal fistula (N82.3)
vesicorectal fistula (N32.1)

K61 ABSCESS OF ANAL AND RECTAL REGIONS
- 4th *Includes:* abscess of anal and rectal regions
  - cellulitis of anal and rectal regions
K61.0 Anal abscess
Perianal abscess
Excludes2: intrasphincteric abscess (K61.4)
K61.1 Rectal abscess
Perirectal abscess
Excludes1: ischiorectal abscess (K61.39)
K61.2 Anorectal abscess
K61.3 Ischiorectal abscess
- 5th **K61.31 Horseshoe abscess**
  - **K61.39 Other ischiorectal abscess**
    - Abscess of ischiorectal fossa
    - Ischiorectal abscess, NOS
K61.4 Intrasphincteric abscess
Intersphincteric abscess
K61.5 Supralevator abscess

K62 OTHER DISEASES OF ANUS AND RECTUM
- 4th *Includes:* anal canal
Excludes2: colostomy and enterostomy malfunction (K94.0-, K94.1-)
fecal incontinence (R15.-)
hemorrhoids (K64.-)
K62.0 Anal polyp
K62.1 Rectal polyp
Excludes1: adenomatous polyp (D12.8)
K62.2 Anal prolapse
Prolapse of anal canal
K62.3 Rectal prolapse
Prolapse of rectal mucosa
K62.4 Stenosis of anus and rectum
Stricture of anus (sphincter)
K62.5 Hemorrhage of anus and rectum
Excludes1: gastrointestinal bleeding NOS (K92.2)
melena (K92.1)
neonatal rectal hemorrhage (P54.2)
K62.6 Ulcer of anus and rectum
Solitary ulcer of anus and rectum
Stercoral ulcer of anus and rectum
K62.8 Other specified diseases of anus and rectum
- 5th *Excludes2:* ulcerative proctitis (K51.2)

4th 5th 6th 7th Additional Character Required   ✔ 3-character code

•=New Code   *Excludes1*—Not coded here, do not use together
▲=Revised Code   *Excludes2*—Not included here

K62.81   **Anal sphincter tear (healed) (nontraumatic) (old)**
Tear of anus, nontraumatic
Use additional code for any associated fecal
   incontinence (R15.-)
Excludes2: anal fissure (K60.-)
   anal sphincter tear (healed) (old) complicating delivery
     (O34.7-)
   traumatic tear of anal sphincter (S31.831)

K62.82   **Dysplasia of anus**
Anal intraepithelial neoplasia I and II (AIN I and II)
   (histologically confirmed)
Dysplasia of anus NOS
Mild and moderate dysplasia of anus (histologically
   confirmed)
Excludes1: abnormal results from anal cytologic
   examination without histologic confirmation (R85.61-)
   anal intraepithelial neoplasia III (D01.3)
   carcinoma in situ of anus (D01.3)
   HGSIL of anus (R85.613)
   severe dysplasia of anus (D01.3)

K62.89   **Other specified diseases of anus and rectum**
Proctitis NOS
Use additional code for any associated fecal
   incontinence (R15.-)

K62.9   Disease of anus and rectum, unspecified

K63   **OTHER DISEASES OF INTESTINE**
`4th`
  K63.0   **Abscess of intestine**
Excludes1: abscess of intestine with Crohn's disease (K50.014,
   K50.114, K50.814, K50.914)
   abscess of intestine with diverticular disease (K57.0, K57.2,
    K57.4, K57.8)
   abscess of intestine with ulcerative colitis (K51.014, K51.214,
    K51.314, K51.414, K51.514,K51.814, K51.914)
Excludes2: abscess of anal and rectal regions (K61.-)
   abscess of appendix (K35.3-)

  K63.3   **Ulcer of intestine**
Primary ulcer of small intestine
Excludes1: duodenal ulcer (K26.-)
   gastrointestinal ulcer (K28.-)
   gastrojejunal ulcer (K28.-)
   jejunal ulcer (K28.-)
   peptic ulcer, site unspecified (K27.-)
   ulcer of intestine with perforation (K63.1)
   ulcer of anus or rectum (K62.6)
   ulcerative colitis (K51.-)

  K63.5   **Polyp of colon**
Excludes1: adenomatous polyp of colon (D12.-)
   inflammatory polyp of colon (K51.4-)
   polyposis of colon (D12.6)

  K63.8   **Other specified diseases of intestine**
   `5th`   **K63.81**   **Dieulafoy lesion of intestine**
     Excludes2: Dieulafoy lesion of stomach and duodenum
       (K31.82)
    K63.89   **Other specified diseases of intestine**

  K63.9   Disease of intestine, unspecified

K64   **HEMORRHOIDS AND PERIANAL VENOUS THROMBOSIS**
`4th`
Includes: piles
Excludes1: hemorrhoids complicating childbirth and the puerperium
   (O87.2)
   hemorrhoids complicating pregnancy (O22.4)

  K64.0   **First degree hemorrhoids**
Grade/stage I hemorrhoids
Hemorrhoids (bleeding) without prolapse outside of anal canal

  K64.1   **Second degree hemorrhoids**
Grade/stage II hemorrhoids
Hemorrhoids (bleeding) that prolapse with straining, but retract
   spontaneously

  K64.2   **Third degree hemorrhoids**
Grade/stage III hemorrhoids
Hemorrhoids (bleeding) that prolapse with straining and require
   manual replacement back inside anal canal

K64.3   **Fourth degree hemorrhoids**
Grade/stage IV hemorrhoids
Hemorrhoids (bleeding) with prolapsed tissue that cannot be
   manually replaced

K64.4   **Residual hemorrhoidal skin tags**
External hemorrhoids, NOS
Skin tags of anus

K64.5   **Perianal venous thrombosis**
External hemorrhoids with thrombosis
Perianal hematoma
Thrombosed hemorrhoids NOS

K64.8   **Other hemorrhoids**
Internal hemorrhoids, without mention of degree
Prolapsed hemorrhoids, degree not specified

K64.9   **Unspecified hemorrhoids**
Hemorrhoids (bleeding) NOS
Hemorrhoids (bleeding) without mention of degree

(K65–K68) DISEASES OF PERITONEUM AND RETROPERITONEUM

K65   **PERITONITIS**
`4th`
Use additional code (B95–B97), to identify infectious agent, if known
Code also if applicable diverticular disease of intestine (K57.-)
Excludes1: acute appendicitis with generalized peritonitis (K35.2-)
   aseptic peritonitis (T81.6)
   benign paroxysmal peritonitis (E85.0)
   chemical peritonitis (T81.6)
   gonococcal peritonitis (A54.85)
   neonatal peritonitis (P78.0–P78.1)
   pelvic peritonitis, female (N73.3–N73.5)
   periodic familial peritonitis (E85.0)
   peritonitis due to talc or other foreign substance (T81.6)
   peritonitis in chlamydia (A74.81) or in diphtheria (A36.89) or syphilis
    (late) (A52.74)
   peritonitis in tuberculosis (A18.31)
   peritonitis with or following appendicitis (K35.-)
   retroperitoneal infections (K68.-)

  K65.0   **Generalized (acute) peritonitis**
Pelvic peritonitis (acute), male
Subphrenic peritonitis (acute)
Suppurative peritonitis (acute)

  K65.1   **Peritoneal abscess**
Abdominopelvic abscess
Abscess (of) omentum
Abscess (of) peritoneum
Mesenteric abscess
Retrocecal abscess
Subdiaphragmatic abscess
Subhepatic abscess
Subphrenic abscess

  K65.2   **Spontaneous bacterial peritonitis**
Excludes1: bacterial peritonitis NOS (K65.9)

  K65.8   **Other peritonitis**
Chronic proliferative peritonitis
Peritonitis due to urine

  K65.9   **Peritonitis, unspecified**
Bacterial peritonitis NOS

(K70–K77) DISEASES OF LIVER

Excludes1: jaundice NOS (R17)
Excludes2: hemochromatosis (E83.11-)
  Reye's syndrome (G93.7)
  viral hepatitis (B15–B19)
  Wilson's disease (E83.0)

K73   **CHRONIC HEPATITIS, NEC**
`4th`
Excludes1: alcoholic hepatitis (chronic) (K70.1-)
   drug-induced hepatitis (chronic) (K71.-)
   granulomatous hepatitis (chronic) NEC (K75.3)
   reactive, nonspecific hepatitis (chronic) (K75.2)
   viral hepatitis (chronic) (B15–B19)

  K73.0   **Chronic persistent hepatitis, NEC**

`4th`   `5th`   `6th`   `7th`   Additional Character Required   ✓   3-character code   •=New Code   *Excludes1*—Not coded here, do not use together
                                                          ▲=Revised Code   *Excludes2*—Not included here

K73.1 Chronic lobular hepatitis, NEC
K73.2 Chronic active hepatitis, NEC
K73.8 Other chronic hepatitis, NEC
K73.9 Chronic hepatitis, unspecified

K74 FIBROSIS AND CIRRHOSIS OF LIVER
4th
    Code also, if applicable, viral hepatitis (acute) (chronic) (B15-B19)
    Excludes1: alcoholic cirrhosis (of liver) (K70.3)
       alcoholic fibrosis of liver (K70.2)
       cardiac sclerosis of liver (K76.1)
       cirrhosis (of liver) with toxic liver disease (K71.7)
       congenital cirrhosis (of liver) (P78.81)
       pigmentary cirrhosis (of liver) (E83.110)
    K74.5 Biliary cirrhosis, unspecified
    K74.6 Other and unspecified cirrhosis of liver
      5th **K74.60 Unspecified cirrhosis of liver**
                   Cirrhosis (of liver) NOS
           K74.69 Other cirrhosis of liver
                   Cryptogenic cirrhosis (of liver)
                   Macronodular cirrhosis (of liver)
                   Micronodular cirrhosis (of liver)
                   Mixed type cirrhosis (of liver)
                   Portal cirrhosis (of liver)
                   Postnecrotic cirrhosis (of liver)

K75 OTHER INFLAMMATORY LIVER DISEASES
4th
    Excludes2: toxic liver disease (K71.-)
    K75.2 Nonspecific reactive hepatitis
       Excludes1: acute or subacute hepatitis (K72.0-)
          chronic hepatitis NEC (K73.-)
          viral hepatitis (B15-B19)
    K75.3 Granulomatous hepatitis, not elsewhere classified
       Excludes1: acute or subacute hepatitis (K72.0-)
          chronic hepatitis NEC (K73.-)
          viral hepatitis (B15-B19)
    K75.9 Inflammatory liver disease, unspecified
       Hepatitis NOS
       Excludes1: acute or subacute hepatitis (K72.0-)
          chronic hepatitis NEC (K73.-)
          viral hepatitis (B15-B19)

K76 OTHER DISEASES OF LIVER
4th
    Excludes2: alcoholic liver disease (K70.-)
       amyloid degeneration of liver (E85.-)
       cystic disease of liver (congenital) (Q44.6)
       hepatic vein thrombosis (I82.0)
       hepatomegaly NOS (R16.0)
       pigmentary cirrhosis (of liver) (E83.110)
       portal vein thrombosis (I81)
       toxic liver disease (K71.-)
    K76.0 Fatty (change of) liver, not elsewhere classified
       Nonalcoholic fatty liver disease (NAFLD)
       Excludes1: nonalcoholic steatohepatitis (NASH) (K75.81)
    K76.8 Other specified diseases of liver
      5th **K76.81 Hepatopulmonary syndrome**
             Code first underlying liver disease, such as:
                alcoholic cirrhosis of liver (K70.3-)
                cirrhosis of liver without mention of alcohol (K74.6-)
           K76.89 Other specified diseases of liver
                   Cyst (simple) of liver
                   Focal nodular hyperplasia of liver
                   Hepatoptosis
    K76.9 Liver disease, unspecified

K77 LIVER DISORDERS IN DISEASES CLASSIFIED ELSEWHERE
☑
    Code first underlying disease, such as: amyloidosis (E85.-)
       congenital syphilis (A50.0, A50.5)
       congenital toxoplasmosis (P37.1)
       schistosomiasis (B65.0–B65.9)
    Excludes1: alcoholic hepatitis (K70.1-)
       alcoholic liver disease (K70.-)
       cytomegaloviral hepatitis (B25.1)
       herpesviral [herpes simplex] hepatitis (B00.81)
       infectious mononucleosis with liver disease (B27.0–B27.9 with .9)
       mumps hepatitis (B26.81)

       sarcoidosis with liver disease (D86.89)
       secondary syphilis with liver disease (A51.45)
       syphilis (late) with liver disease (A52.74)
       toxoplasmosis (acquired) hepatitis (B58.1)
       tuberculosis with liver disease (A18.83)

(K80–K87) DISORDERS OF GALLBLADDER, BILIARY TRACT AND PANCREAS

K80 CHOLELITHIASIS
4th
    Excludes1: retained cholelithiasis following cholecystectomy (K91.86)
    Use additional code if applicable for associated gangrene of gallbladder (K82.A1), or perforationof gallbladder (K82.A2) for sub-categories K80.0-, K80.1-, K80.4-, K80.6-
    K80.0 Calculus of gallbladder with acute cholecystitis
      5th Any condition listed in K80.2 with acute cholecystitis
          K80.00 Calculus of gallbladder with acute cholecystitis without obstruction
          K80.01 Calculus of gallbladder with acute cholecystitis with obstruction
    K80.1 Calculus of gallbladder; with other cholecystitis
      5th **K80.10 with chronic cholecystitis without obstruction**
                 Cholelithiasis with cholecystitis NOS
          K80.11 with chronic cholecystitis with obstruction
          K80.12 with acute and chronic cholecystitis without obstruction
          K80.13 with acute and chronic cholecystitis with obstruction
          K80.18 with other cholecystitis without obstruction
          K80.19 with other cholecystitis with obstruction
    K80.2 Calculus of gallbladder without cholecystitis
      5th Cholecystolithiasis with cholecystitis
          Cholelithiasis (without cholecystitis)
          Colic (recurrent) of gallbladder (without cholecystitis)
          Gallstone (impacted) of cystic duct (without cholecystitis)
          Gallstone (impacted) of gallbladder (without cholecystitis)
          K80.20 Calculus of gallbladder without cholecystitis without obstruction
          K80.21 Calculus of gallbladder without cholecystitis with obstruction
    K80.5 Calculus of bile duct without cholangitis or cholecystitis
      5th Choledocholithiasis (without cholangitis or cholecystitis)
          Gallstone (impacted) of bile duct NOS (without cholangitis or cholecystitis)
          Gallstone (impacted) of common duct (without cholangitis or cholecystitis)
          Gallstone (impacted) of hepatic duct (without cholangitis or cholecystitis)
          Hepatic cholelithiasis (without cholangitis or cholecystitis)
          Hepatic colic (recurrent) (without cholangitis or cholecystitis)
          K80.50 Calculus of bile duct without cholangitis or cholecystitis without obstruction
          K80.51 Calculus of bile duct without cholangitis or cholecystitis with obstruction
    K80.8 Other cholelithiasis
      5th **K80.80 Other cholelithiasis without obstruction**
          K80.81 Other cholelithiasis with obstruction

K81 CHOLECYSTITIS
4th
    Use additional code if applicable for associated gangrene of gallbladder (K82.A1), or perforation of gallbladder (K82.A2)
    Excludes1: cholecystitis with cholelithiasis (K80.-)
    K81.0 Acute cholecystitis
       Abscess of gallbladder
       Angiocholecystitis
       Emphysematous (acute) cholecystitis
       Empyema of gallbladder
       Gangrene of gallbladder
       Gangrenous cholecystitis
       Suppurative cholecystitis
    K81.1 Chronic cholecystitis
    K81.2 Acute cholecystitis with chronic cholecystitis
    K81.9 Cholecystitis, unspecified

4th *5th* *6th* *7th* Additional Character Required   ☑ 3-character code

•=New Code   **Excludes1**—Not coded here, do not use together
▲=Revised Code   **Excludes2**—Not included here

K82   **OTHER DISEASES OF GALLBLADDER**
4th

Excludes1: nonvisualization of gallbladder (R93.2)
    postcholecystectomy syndrome (K91.5)

K82.0   **Obstruction of gallbladder**
Occlusion of cystic duct or gallbladder without cholelithiasis
Stenosis of cystic duct or gallbladder without cholelithiasis
Stricture of cystic duct or gallbladder without cholelithiasis
Excludes1: obstruction of gallbladder with cholelithiasis (K80.-)

K82.8   **Other specified diseases of gallbladder**
Adhesions of cystic duct or gallbladder
Atrophy of cystic duct or gallbladder
Cyst of cystic duct or gallbladder
Dyskinesia of cystic duct or gallbladder
Hypertrophy of cystic duct or gallbladder
Nonfunctioning of cystic duct or gallbladder
Ulcer of cystic duct or gallbladder

K82.9   **Disease of gallbladder, unspecified**

K82.A   **Disorders of gallbladder in diseases classified elsewhere**
5th   **Code first** the type of cholecystitis (K81.-), or cholelithiasis with cholecystitis (K80.00-K80.19, K80.40-K80.47,K80.60-K80.67)

    K82.A1   **Gangrene of gallbladder in cholecystitis**
    K82.A2   **Perforation of gallbladder in cholecystitis**

K83   **OTHER DISEASES OF BILIARY TRACT**
4th

Excludes1: postcholecystectomy syndrome (K91.5)
Excludes2: conditions involving the gallbladder (K81-K82)
    conditions involving the cystic duct (K81-K82)

K83.1   **Obstruction of bile duct**
Occlusion of bile duct without cholelithiasis
Stenosis of bile duct without cholelithiasis
Stricture of bile duct without cholelithiasis
Excludes1: congenital obstruction of bile duct (Q44.3)
    obstruction of bile duct with cholelithiasis (K80.-)

K83.8   **Other specified diseases of biliary tract**
Adhesions of biliary tract
Atrophy of biliary tract
Hypertrophy of biliary tract
Ulcer of biliary tract

K83.9   **Disease of biliary tract, unspecified**

K85   **ACUTE PANCREATITIS**
4th

Includes: acute (recurrent) pancreatitis
    subacute pancreatitis

K85.0   **Idiopathic acute pancreatitis**
5th   **K85.00**   **Idiopathic acute pancreatitis without necrosis or infection**
    K85.01   **Idiopathic acute pancreatitis with uninfected necrosis**
    K85.02   **Idiopathic acute pancreatitis with infected necrosis**

K85.8   **Other acute pancreatitis**
5th   **K85.80**   **Other acute pancreatitis without necrosis or infection**
    K85.81   **Other acute pancreatitis with uninfected necrosis**
    K85.82   **Other acute pancreatitis with infected necrosis**

K85.9   **Acute pancreatitis, unspecified**
5th   Pancreatitis NOS
    K85.90   **Acute pancreatitis without necrosis or infection, unspecified**
    K85.91   **Acute pancreatitis with uninfected necrosis, unspecified**
    K85.92   **Acute pancreatitis with infected necrosis, unspecified**

K86   **OTHER DISEASES OF PANCREAS**
4th

Excludes2: fibrocystic disease of pancreas (E84.-)
    islet cell tumor (of pancreas) (D13.7)
    pancreatic steatorrhea (K90.3)

K86.2   **Cyst of pancreas**

K86.8   **Other specified diseases of pancreas**
5th   **K86.81**   **Exocrine pancreatic insufficiency**
    K86.89   **Other specified diseases of pancreas**
       Aseptic pancreatic necrosis, unrelated to acute pancreatitis
       Atrophy of pancreas
       Calculus of pancreas

Cirrhosis of pancreas
Fibrosis of pancreas
Pancreatic fat necrosis, unrelated to acute pancreatitis
Pancreatic infantilism
Pancreatic necrosis NOS, unrelated to acute pancreatitis

K86.9   **Disease of pancreas, unspecified**

(K90–K95) OTHER DISEASES OF THE DIGESTIVE SYSTEM

K90   **INTESTINAL MALABSORPTION**
4th

Excludes1: intestinal malabsorption following gastrointestinal surgery (K91.2)

K90.0   **Celiac disease**
Celiac disease with steatorrhea
Celiac gluten-sensitive enteropathy
Nontropical sprue
Code also exocrine pancreatic insufficiency (K86.81)
Use additional code *for associated disorders including:*
    dermatitis herpetiformis (L13.0)
    gluten ataxia (G32.81)

K90.1   **Tropical sprue**
Sprue NOS
Tropical steatorrhea

K90.2   **Blind loop syndrome, not elsewhere classified**
Blind loop syndrome NOS
Excludes1: congenital blind loop syndrome (Q43.8)
    postsurgical blind loop syndrome (K91.2)

K90.3   **Pancreatic steatorrhea**

K90.4   **Other malabsorption due to intolerance**
5th   *Excludes2:* celiac gluten-sensitive enteropathy (K90.0)
    lactose intolerance (E73.-)

    K90.41   **Non-celiac gluten sensitivity**
       Gluten sensitivity NOS
       Non-celiac gluten sensitive enteropathy

    K90.49   **Malabsorption due to intolerance, NEC**
       Malabsorption due to intolerance to carbohydrate or fat or protein or starch

K90.8   **Other intestinal malabsorption**
5th   **K90.81**   **Whipple's disease**
    K90.89   **Other intestinal malabsorption**

K90.9   **Intestinal malabsorption, unspecified**

K91   **INTRAOPERATIVE AND POSTPROCEDURAL**
4th   **COMPLICATIONS AND DISORDERS OF DIGESTIVE SYSTEM, NEC**

Excludes2: complications of artificial opening of digestive system (K94.-)
    complications of bariatric procedures (K95.-)
    gastrojejunal ulcer (K28.-)
    postprocedural (radiation) retroperitoneal abscess (K68.11)
    radiation colitis (K52.0)
    radiation gastroenteritis (K52.0)
    radiation proctitis (K62.7)

K91.2   **Postsurgical malabsorption, NEC**
Postsurgical blind loop syndrome
Excludes1: malabsorption osteomalacia in adults (M83.2)
    malabsorption osteoporosis, postsurgical (M80.8-, M81.8)

K91.3   **Postprocedural intestinal obstruction**
5th   **K91.30**   **Postprocedural intestinal obstruction, unspecified as to partial versus complete**
       Postprocedural intestinal obstruction NOS
    K91.31   **Postprocedural partial intestinal obstruction**
       Postprocedural incomplete intestinal obstruction
    K91.32   **Postprocedural complete intestinal obstruction**

K91.8   **Other intraoperative and postprocedural complications and**
5th   **disorders of digestive system**
    K91.89   **Other postprocedural complications and disorders of digestive system**
       Use additional code, if applicable, to further specify disorder
       Excludes2: postprocedural retroperitoneal abscess (K68.11)

K92   **OTHER DISEASES OF DIGESTIVE SYSTEM**
4th

Excludes1: neonatal gastrointestinal hemorrhage (P54.0–P54.3)

K92.0   **Hematemesis**

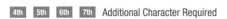

K92.1 Melena
> *Excludes1:* occult blood in feces (R19.5)

K92.2 Gastrointestinal hemorrhage, unspecified
Gastric hemorrhage NOS
Intestinal hemorrhage NOS
> *Excludes1:* acute hemorrhagic gastritis (K29.01)
> hemorrhage of anus and rectum (K62.5)
> angiodysplasia of stomach with hemorrhage (K31.811)
> diverticular disease with hemorrhage (K57.-)
> gastritis and duodenitis with hemorrhage (K29.-)
> peptic ulcer with hemorrhage (K25–K28)

K92.8 Other specified diseases of the digestive system

`5th` **K92.81 Gastrointestinal mucositis (ulcerative)**
> **Code also** type of associated therapy, such as:
> antineoplastic and immunosuppressive drugs (T45.1X-)
> radiological procedure and radiotherapy (Y84.2)
> *Excludes2:* mucositis (ulcerative) of vagina and vulva
> (N76.81)
> nasal mucositis (ulcerative) (J34.81)
> oral mucositis (ulcerative) (K12.3-)

     K92.89 Other specified diseases of the digestive system

K92.9 Disease of digestive system, unspecified

`K94` `4th` **COMPLICATIONS OF ARTIFICIAL OPENINGS OF THE DIGESTIVE SYSTEM**

K94.0 Colostomy complications

`5th` **K94.00 Colostomy complication, unspecified**

     K94.01 Colostomy hemorrhage

     K94.02 Colostomy infection
> **Use additional code** to specify type of infection, such as:
> cellulitis of abdominal wall (L03.311)
> sepsis (A40.-, A41.-)

     K94.03 Colostomy malfunction
> Mechanical complication of colostomy

     K94.09 Other complications of colostomy

K94.2 Gastrostomy complications

`5th` **K94.20 Gastrostomy complication, unspecified**

     K94.21 Gastrostomy hemorrhage

     K94.22 Gastrostomy infection
> **Use additional code** *to specify type of infection, such as:* sepsis (A40.-, A41.-)
> cellulitis of abdominal wall (L03.311)

     K94.23 Gastrostomy malfunction
> Mechanical complication of gastrostomy

     K94.29 Other complications of gastrostomy

`4th` `5th` `6th` `7th` Additional Character Required   ✔ 3-character code

•=New Code   *Excludes1*—Not coded here, do not use together
▲=Revised Code   *Excludes2*—Not included here

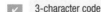

Chapter 12. Diseases of the skin and subcutaneous tissue (L00–L99)

GUIDELINES

Pressure ulcer stages

Refer to category L89.

Excludes2: certain conditions originating in the perinatal period (P04–P96)
    certain infectious and parasitic diseases (A00–B99)
    complications of pregnancy, childbirth and the puerperium (O00–O9A)
    congenital malformations, deformations, and chromosomal abnormalities
      (Q00–Q99)
    endocrine, nutritional and metabolic diseases (E00–E88)
    lipomelanotic reticulosis (I89.8)
    neoplasms (C00–D49)
    symptoms, signs and abnormal clinical and laboratory findings, NEC (R00–R94)
    systemic connective tissue disorders (M30–M36)
    viral warts (B07.-)

(L00–L08) INFECTIONS OF THE SKIN AND SUBCUTANEOUS TISSUE

Use additional code (B95–B97) to identify infectious agent.

Excludes2: hordeolum (H00.0)
    infective dermatitis (L30.3)
    local infections of skin classified in Chapter 1
    lupus panniculitis (L93.2)
    panniculitis NOS (M79.3)
    panniculitis of neck and back (M54.0-)
    Perlèche NOS (K13.0)
    Perlèche due to candidiasis (B37.0)
    Perlèche due to riboflavin deficiency (E53.0)
    pyogenic granuloma (L98.0)
    relapsing panniculitis [Weber-Christian] (M35.6)
    viral warts (B07.-)
    zoster (B02.-)

L00   **STAPHYLOCOCCAL SCALDED SKIN SYNDROME**
    Ritter's disease
    Use additional code to identify percentage of skin exfoliation (L49.-)
    Excludes1: bullous impetigo (L01.03)
      pemphigus neonatorum (L01.03)
      toxic epidermal necrolysis [Lyell] (L51.2)

L01   **IMPETIGO**
     [4th]   ***Excludes1:*** impetigo herpetiformis (L40.1)
    L01.0   **Impetigo**
       [5th]   Impetigo contagiosa
         Impetigo vulgaris
        L01.00   **Impetigo, unspecified**
             Impetigo NOS
        L01.01   **Non-bullous impetigo**
        L01.02   **Bockhart's impetigo**
             Impetigo follicularis
             Perifolliculitis NOS
             Superficial pustular perifolliculitis
        L01.03   **Bullous impetigo**
             Impetigo neonatorum
             Pemphigus neonatorum
        L01.09   **Other impetigo**
             Ulcerative impetigo
    L01.1   **Impetiginization of other dermatoses**

L02   **CUTANEOUS ABSCESS, FURUNCLE AND CARBUNCLE**
     [4th]   **Use additional code** to identify organism (B95–B96)
    Excludes2: abscess of anus and rectal regions (K61.-)
      abscess of female genital organs (external) (N76.4)
      abscess of male genital organs (external) (N48.2, N49.-)
    L02.0   **Cutaneous abscess, furuncle and carbuncle of face**
       [5th]   ***Excludes2:*** abscess of ear, external (H60.0)
         abscess of eyelid (H00.0)
         abscess of head [any part, except face] (L02.8)
         abscess of lacrimal gland (H04.0)
         abscess of lacrimal passages (H04.3)
         abscess of mouth (K12.2)
         abscess of nose (J34.0)
         abscess of orbit (H05.0)
         submandibular abscess (K12.2)
      L02.01   **Cutaneous abscess of face**
      L02.02   **Furuncle of face**
         Boil of face
         Folliculitis of face
      L02.03   **Carbuncle of face**
    L02.1   **Cutaneous abscess, furuncle and carbuncle of neck**
       [5th]   **L02.11**   **Cutaneous abscess of neck**
      L02.12   **Furuncle of neck**
         Boil of neck
         Folliculitis of neck
      L02.13   **Carbuncle of neck**
    L02.2   **Cutaneous abscess, furuncle and carbuncle of trunk**
       [5th]   ***Excludes1:*** non-newborn omphalitis (L08.82)
         omphalitis of newborn (P38.-)
      Excludes2: abscess of breast (N61.1)
         abscess of buttocks (L02.3)
         abscess of female external genital organs (N76.4)
         abscess of male external genital organs (N48.2, N49.-)
         abscess of hip (L02.4)
      L02.21   **Cutaneous abscess of trunk**
         [6th]   **L02.211**   **Cutaneous abscess of; abdominal wall**
        L02.212   **back [any part, except buttock]**
        L02.213   **chest wall**
        L02.214   **groin**
        L02.215   **perineum**
        L02.216   **umbilicus**
        L02.219   **trunk, unspecified**
      L02.22   **Furuncle of trunk**
         [6th]   Boil of trunk
         Folliculitis of trunk
        L02.221   **Furuncle of; abdominal wall**
        L02.222   **back [any part, except buttock]**
        L02.223   **chest wall**
        L02.224   **groin**
        L02.225   **perineum**
        L02.226   **umbilicus**
        L02.229   **trunk, unspecified**
      L02.23   **Carbuncle of trunk**
         [6th]   **L02.231**   **Carbuncle of; abdominal wall**
        L02.232   **back [any part, except buttock]**
        L02.233   **chest wall**
        L02.234   **groin**
        L02.235   **perineum**
        L02.236   **umbilicus**
        L02.239   **trunk, unspecified**
    L02.3   **Cutaneous abscess, furuncle and carbuncle of buttock**
       [5th]   ***Excludes1:*** pilonidal cyst with abscess (L05.01)
      L02.31   **Cutaneous abscess of buttock**
         Cutaneous abscess of gluteal region
      L02.32   **Furuncle of buttock**
         Boil of buttock
         Folliculitis of buttock
         Furuncle of gluteal region
      L02.33   **Carbuncle of buttock**
         Carbuncle of gluteal region
    L02.4   **Cutaneous abscess, furuncle and carbuncle of limb**
       [5th]   ***Excludes2:*** Cutaneous abscess, furuncle and carbuncle of groin
         (L02.214, L02.224, L02.234)
         Cutaneous abscess, furuncle and carbuncle of hand (L02.5-)
         Cutaneous abscess, furuncle and carbuncle of foot (L02.6-)
      L02.41   **Cutaneous abscess of; limb**
         [6th]   **L02.411**   **right axilla**
        L02.412   **left axilla**
        L02.413   **right upper limb**
        L02.414   **left upper limb**
        L02.415   **right lower limb**
        L02.416   **left lower limb**

[4th] [5th] [6th] [7th] Additional Character Required   ☑   3-character code

Unspecified laterality codes were excluded here.   •=New Code   ▲=Revised Code
Excludes1—Not coded here, do not use together
Excludes2—Not included here

L02.42   **Furuncle of; limb**
   6th   Boil of limb
     Folliculitis of limb
     L02.421   **right axilla**
     L02.422   **left axilla**
     L02.423   **right upper limb**
     L02.424   **left upper limb**
     L02.425   **right lower limb**
     L02.426   **left lower limb**

L02.43   **Carbuncle of; limb**
   6th   **L02.431**   **right axilla**
     L02.432   **left axilla**
     L02.433   **right upper limb**
     L02.434   **left upper limb**
     L02.435   **right lower limb**
     L02.436   **left lower limb**

L02.5   **Cutaneous abscess, furuncle and carbuncle of hand**
   5th   **L02.51**   **Cutaneous abscess of; hand**
     6th   **L02.511**   **right hand**
     L02.512   **left hand**

   L02.52   **Furuncle; hand**
     6th   Boil of hand
       Folliculitis of hand
       L02.521   **right hand**
       L02.522   **left hand**

   L02.53   **Carbuncle of; hand**
     6th   **L02.531**   **right hand**
     L02.532   **left hand**

L02.6   **Cutaneous abscess, furuncle and carbuncle of foot**
   5th   **L02.61**   **Cutaneous abscess of; foot**
     6th   **L02.611**   **right foot**
     L02.612   **left foot**

   L02.62   **Furuncle of; foot**
     6th   Boil of foot
       Folliculitis of foot
       L02.621   **right foot**
       L02.622   **left foot**

   L02.63   **Carbuncle of; foot**
     6th   **L02.631**   **right foot**
     L02.632   **left foot**

L02.8   **Cutaneous abscess, furuncle and carbuncle of other sites**
   5th   **L02.81**   **Cutaneous abscess of; other sites**
     6th   **L02.811**   **head [any part, except face]**
     L02.818   **other sites**

   L02.82   **Furuncle of; other sites**
     6th   Boil of other sites
       Folliculitis of other sites
       L02.821   **head [any part, except face]**
       L02.828   **other sites**

   L02.83   **Carbuncle of; other sites**
     6th   **L02.831**   **head [any part, except face]**
     L02.838   **other sites**

L02.9   **Cutaneous abscess, furuncle and carbuncle, unspecified**
   5th   **L02.91**   **Cutaneous abscess, unspecified**
   L02.92   **Furuncle, unspecified**
     Boil NOS
     Furunculosis NOS
   L02.93   **Carbuncle, unspecified**

L03   **CELLULITIS AND ACUTE LYMPHANGITIS**
   4th   *Excludes2:* cellulitis of anal and rectal region (K61.-)
     cellulitis of external auditory canal (H60.1)
     cellulitis of eyelid (H00.0)
     cellulitis of female external genital organs (N76.4)
     cellulitis of lacrimal apparatus (H04.3)
     cellulitis of male external genital organs (N48.2, N49.-)
     cellulitis of mouth (K12.2)
     cellulitis of nose (J34.0)
     eosinophilic cellulitis [Wells] (L98.3)
     febrile neutrophilic dermatosis [Sweet] (L98.2)
     lymphangitis (chronic) (subacute) (I89.1)

L03.0   **Cellulitis and acute lymphangitis of finger and toe**
   5th   Infection of nail
     Onychia
     Paronychia
     Perionychia
   L03.01   **Cellulitis of; finger**
     6th   Felon
       Whitlow
       Excludes1: herpetic whitlow (B00.89)
       L03.011   **right finger**
       L03.012   **left finger**

   L03.02   **Acute lymphangitis of; finger**
     6th   Hangnail with lymphangitis of finger
       L03.021   **right finger**
       L03.022   **left finger**

   L03.03   **Cellulitis of; toe**
     6th   **L03.031**   **right toe**
     L03.032   **left toe**

   L03.04   **Acute lymphangitis of; toe**
     6th   Hangnail with lymphangitis of toe
       L03.041   **right toe**
       L03.042   **left toe**

L03.1   **Cellulitis and acute lymphangitis of other parts of limb**
   5th   **L03.11**   **Cellulitis of other parts of limb**
     6th   *Excludes2:* cellulitis of fingers (L03.01-)
       cellulitis of toes (L03.03-)
       groin (L03.314)
     L03.111   **Cellulitis of; right axilla**
     L03.112   **left axilla**
     L03.113   **right upper limb**
     L03.114   **left upper limb**
     L03.115   **right lower limb**
     L03.116   **left lower limb**

   L03.12   **Acute lymphangitis of other parts of limb**
     6th   *Excludes2:* acute lymphangitis of fingers (L03.2-)
       acute lymphangitis of toes (L03.04-)
       acute lymphangitis of groin (L03.324)
     L03.121   **Acute lymphangitis of; right axilla**
     L03.122   **left axilla**
     L03.123   **right upper limb**
     L03.124   **left upper limb**
     L03.125   **right lower limb**
     L03.126   **left lower limb**

L03.2   **Cellulitis and acute lymphangitis of face and neck**
   5th   **L03.21**   **Cellulitis and acute lymphangitis of face**
     6th   **L03.211**   **Cellulitis of face**
       Excludes2: abscess of orbit (H05.01-)
         cellulitis of ear (H60.1-)
         cellulitis of eyelid (H00.0-)
         cellulitis of head or scalp (L03.81)
         cellulitis of lacrimal apparatus (H04.3)
         cellulitis of lip (K13.0)
         cellulitis of mouth (K12.2)
         cellulitis of nose (internal) (J34.0)
         cellulitis of orbit (H05.01-)
     L03.212   **Acute lymphangitis of face**
     L03.213   **Periorbital cellulitis**
       Preseptal cellulitis

   L03.22   **Cellulitis and acute lymphangitis of neck**
     6th   **L03.221**   **Cellulitis of neck**
     L03.222   **Acute lymphangitis of neck**

L03.3   **Cellulitis and acute lymphangitis of trunk**
   5th   **L03.31**   **Cellulitis of trunk**
     6th   *Excludes2:* cellulitis of anal and rectal regions (K61.-)
       cellulitis of breast NOS (N61.0)
       cellulitis of female external genital organs (N76.4)
       cellulitis of male external genital organs (N48.2, N49.-)
       omphalitis of newborn (P38.-)
       puerperal cellulitis of breast (O91.2)
     L03.311   **Cellulitis of; abdominal wall**
       Excludes2: cellulitis of umbilicus (L03.316)
         cellulitis of groin (L03.314)
     L03.312   **back [any part except buttock]**

Unspecified laterality codes   •=New Code   *Excludes1*—Not coded here, do not use together
were excluded here.   ▲=Revised Code   *Excludes2*—Not included here

	L03.313	chest wall	
	L03.314	groin	
	L03.315	perineum	
	L03.316	umbicus	
	L03.317	buttock	
	L03.319	trunk, unspecified	

L03.32 Acute lymphangitis of; trunk

6th
- **L03.321** abdominal wall
- **L03.322** back [any part except buttock]
- **L03.323** chest wall
- **L03.324** groin
- **L03.325** perineum
- **L03.326** umbilicus
- **L03.327** buttock
- **L03.329** trunk, unspecified

L03.8 Cellulitis and acute lymphangitis of other sites

5th **L03.81** Cellulitis of; other sites

6th **L03.811** head [any part, except face]
Cellulitis of scalp
Excludes2: cellulitis of face (L03.211)
L03.818 other sites

L03.89 Acute lymphangitis of; other sites

6th **L03.891** head [any part, except face]
L03.898 other sites

L03.9 Cellulitis and acute lymphangitis, unspecified

5th **L03.90** Cellulitis, unspecified
L03.91 Acute lymphangitis, unspecified
Excludes1: lymphangitis NOS (I89.1)

L04 **ACUTE LYMPHADENITIS**

4th *Includes:* abscess (acute) of lymph nodes, except mesenteric
acute lymphadenitis, except mesenteric
Excludes1: chronic or subacute lymphadenitis, except mesenteric (I88.1)
enlarged lymph nodes (R59.-)
HIV disease resulting in generalized lymphadenopathy (B20)
lymphadenitis NOS (I88.9)
nonspecific mesenteric lymphadenitis (I88.0)

L04.0 Acute lymphadenitis of; face, head and neck
L04.1 trunk
L04.2 upper limb
Acute lymphadenitis of axilla or shoulder
L04.3 lower limb
Acute lymphadenitis of hip
Excludes2: acute lymphadenitis of groin (L04.1)
L04.8 other sites
L04.9 unspecified

L05 **PILONIDAL CYST AND SINUS**

4th **L05.0** Pilonidal cyst and sinus with abscess

5th **L05.01** Pilonidal cyst with abscess
Parasacral dimple with abscess
Excludes 2: congenital sacral dimple (Q82.6)
parasacral dimple (Q82.6)
L05.02 Pilonidal sinus with abscess

L05.9 Pilonidal cyst and sinus without abscess

5th **L05.91** Pilonidal cyst without abscess
Parasacral or Pilonidal or Postanal dimple
Pilonidal cyst NOS
Excludes 2: congenital sacral dimple (Q82.6)
parasacral dimple (Q82.6)
L05.92 Pilonidal sinus without abscess
Coccygeal fistula
Coccygeal sinus without abscess
Pilonidal fistula

L08 **OTHER LOCAL INFECTIONS OF SKIN AND**
4th **SUBCUTANEOUS TISSUE**

L08.0 Pyoderma
Dermatitis gangrenosa
Purulent or Septic or Suppurative dermatitis
Excludes1: pyoderma gangrenosum (L88)
pyoderma vegetans (L08.81)
L08.9 Local infection of the skin and subcutaneous tissue,
unspecified

(L10–L14) BULLOUS DISORDERS

Excludes1: benign familial pemphigus [Hailey-Hailey] (Q82.8)
staphylococcal scalded skin syndrome (L00)
toxic epidermal necrolysis [Lyell] (L51.2)

(L20–L30) DERMATITIS AND ECZEMA

Note: In this block the terms dermatitis and eczema are used synonymously and interchangeably.
Excludes2: chronic (childhood) granulomatous disease (D71)
dermatitis gangrenosa (L08.0)
dermatitis herpetiformis (L13.0)
dry skin dermatitis (L85.3)
factitial dermatitis (L98.1)
perioral dermatitis (L71.0)
radiation-related disorders of the skin and subcutaneous tissue (L55–L59)
stasis dermatitis (I87.2)

L20 **ATOPIC DERMATITIS**

4th **L20.0** Besnier's prurigo
L20.8 Other atopic dermatitis

5th *Excludes2:* circumscribed neurodermatitis (L28.0)
L20.81 Atopic neurodermatitis
Diffuse neurodermatitis
L20.82 Flexural eczema
L20.83 Infantile (acute) (chronic) eczema
L20.84 Intrinsic (allergic) eczema
L20.89 Other atopic dermatitis
L20.9 Atopic dermatitis, unspecified

L21 **SEBORRHEIC DERMATITIS**

4th *Excludes2:* infective dermatitis (L30.3)
seborrheic keratosis (L82.-)
L21.0 Seborrhea capitis
Cradle cap
L21.1 Seborrheic infantile dermatitis
L21.8 Other seborrheic dermatitis
L21.9 Seborrheic dermatitis, unspecified
Seborrhea NOS

L22 **DIAPER DERMATITIS**

✓ Diaper erythema
Diaper rash
Psoriasiform diaper rash

L23 **ALLERGIC CONTACT DERMATITIS**

4th *Excludes1:* allergy NOS (T78.40)
contact dermatitis NOS (L25.9)
dermatitis NOS (L30.9)
Excludes2: dermatitis due to substances taken internally (L27.-)
dermatitis of eyelid (H01.1-)
diaper dermatitis (L22)
eczema of external ear (H60.5-)
irritant contact dermatitis (L24.-)
perioral dermatitis (L71.0)
radiation-related disorders of the skin and subcutaneous tissue
(L55–L59)
L23.0 Allergic contact dermatitis due to; metals
Allergic contact dermatitis due to chromium or nickel
L23.1 adhesives
L23.2 cosmetics
L23.3 drugs in contact with skin
Use additional code for adverse effect, if applicable, to identify
drug (T36–T50 with fifth or sixth character 5)
Excludes2: dermatitis due to ingested drugs and medicaments
(L27.0–L27.1)
L23.4 Allergic contact dermatitis due to; dyes
L23.5 other chemical products
Allergic contact dermatitis due to cement or to insecticide
L23.6 food in contact with the skin
Excludes2: dermatitis due to ingested food (L27.2)
L23.7 plants, except food
Excludes2: allergy NOS due to pollen (J30.1)

Right margin: CHAPTER 12. DISEASES OF THE SKIN AND SUBCUTANEOUS TISSUE (L03.313–L23.7)

4th **5th** **6th** **7th** Additional Character Required · **✓** 3-character code

Unspecified laterality codes were excluded here. · ●=New Code ▲=Revised Code · *Excludes1*—Not coded here, do not use together · *Excludes2*—Not included here

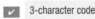

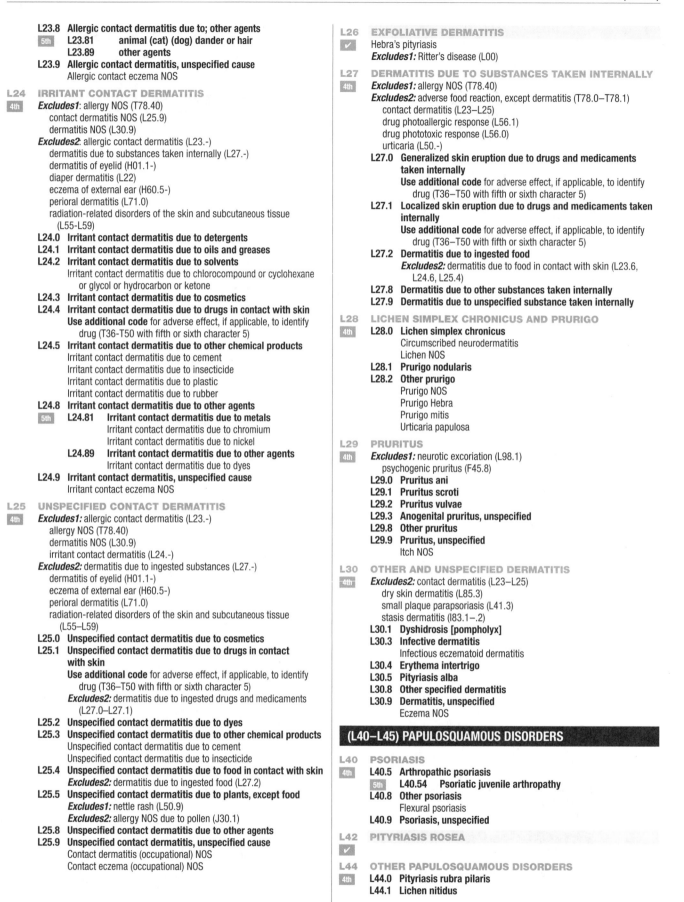

CHAPTER 12. DISEASES OF THE SKIN AND SUBCUTANEOUS TISSUE (L23.8–L44)

L23.8 Allergic contact dermatitis due to; other agents
- 5th **L23.81** animal (cat) (dog) dander or hair
- **L23.89** other agents

L23.9 Allergic contact dermatitis, unspecified cause
  Allergic contact eczema NOS

L24 IRRITANT CONTACT DERMATITIS
- 4th *Excludes1*: allergy NOS (T78.40)
  contact dermatitis NOS (L25.9)
  dermatitis NOS (L30.9)

Excludes2: allergic contact dermatitis (L23.-)
  dermatitis due to substances taken internally (L27.-)
  dermatitis of eyelid (H01.1-)
  diaper dermatitis (L22)
  eczema of external ear (H60.5-)
  perioral dermatitis (L71.0)
  radiation-related disorders of the skin and subcutaneous tissue
    (L55-L59)

L24.0 Irritant contact dermatitis due to detergents

L24.1 Irritant contact dermatitis due to oils and greases

L24.2 Irritant contact dermatitis due to solvents
  Irritant contact dermatitis due to chlorocompound or cyclohexane
    or glycol or hydrocarbon or ketone

L24.3 Irritant contact dermatitis due to cosmetics

L24.4 Irritant contact dermatitis due to drugs in contact with skin
  Use additional code for adverse effect, if applicable, to identify
    drug (T36-T50 with fifth or sixth character 5)

L24.5 Irritant contact dermatitis due to other chemical products
  Irritant contact dermatitis due to cement
  Irritant contact dermatitis due to insecticide
  Irritant contact dermatitis due to plastic
  Irritant contact dermatitis due to rubber

L24.8 Irritant contact dermatitis due to other agents
- 5th **L24.81** Irritant contact dermatitis due to metals
    Irritant contact dermatitis due to chromium
    Irritant contact dermatitis due to nickel
- **L24.89** Irritant contact dermatitis due to other agents
    Irritant contact dermatitis due to dyes

L24.9 Irritant contact dermatitis, unspecified cause
  Irritant contact eczema NOS

L25 UNSPECIFIED CONTACT DERMATITIS
- 4th *Excludes1*: allergic contact dermatitis (L23.-)
  allergy NOS (T78.40)
  dermatitis NOS (L30.9)
  irritant contact dermatitis (L24.-)

Excludes2: dermatitis due to ingested substances (L27.-)
  dermatitis of eyelid (H01.1-)
  eczema of external ear (H60.5-)
  perioral dermatitis (L71.0)
  radiation-related disorders of the skin and subcutaneous tissue
    (L55–L59)

L25.0 Unspecified contact dermatitis due to cosmetics

L25.1 Unspecified contact dermatitis due to drugs in contact
  with skin
  Use additional code for adverse effect, if applicable, to identify
    drug (T36–T50 with fifth or sixth character 5)
  Excludes2: dermatitis due to ingested drugs and medicaments
    (L27.0–L27.1)

L25.2 Unspecified contact dermatitis due to dyes

L25.3 Unspecified contact dermatitis due to other chemical products
  Unspecified contact dermatitis due to cement
  Unspecified contact dermatitis due to insecticide

L25.4 Unspecified contact dermatitis due to food in contact with skin
  Excludes2: dermatitis due to ingested food (L27.2)

L25.5 Unspecified contact dermatitis due to plants, except food
  Excludes1: nettle rash (L50.9)
  Excludes2: allergy NOS due to pollen (J30.1)

L25.8 Unspecified contact dermatitis due to other agents

L25.9 Unspecified contact dermatitis, unspecified cause
  Contact dermatitis (occupational) NOS
  Contact eczema (occupational) NOS

L26 EXFOLIATIVE DERMATITIS
- ✔ Hebra's pityriasis
Excludes1: Ritter's disease (L00)

L27 DERMATITIS DUE TO SUBSTANCES TAKEN INTERNALLY
- 4th *Excludes1*: allergy NOS (T78.40)
Excludes2: adverse food reaction, except dermatitis (T78.0–T78.1)
  contact dermatitis (L23–L25)
  drug photoallergic response (L56.1)
  drug phototoxic response (L56.0)
  urticaria (L50.-)

L27.0 Generalized skin eruption due to drugs and medicaments
  taken internally
  Use additional code for adverse effect, if applicable, to identify
    drug (T36–T50 with fifth or sixth character 5)

L27.1 Localized skin eruption due to drugs and medicaments taken
  internally
  Use additional code for adverse effect, if applicable, to identify
    drug (T36–T50 with fifth or sixth character 5)

L27.2 Dermatitis due to ingested food
  Excludes2: dermatitis due to food in contact with skin (L23.6,
    L24.6, L25.4)

L27.8 Dermatitis due to other substances taken internally

L27.9 Dermatitis due to unspecified substance taken internally

L28 LICHEN SIMPLEX CHRONICUS AND PRURIGO
- 4th **L28.0** Lichen simplex chronicus
  Circumscribed neurodermatitis
  Lichen NOS

L28.1 Prurigo nodularis

L28.2 Other prurigo
  Prurigo NOS
  Prurigo Hebra
  Prurigo mitis
  Urticaria papulosa

L29 PRURITUS
- 4th *Excludes1*: neurotic excoriation (L98.1)
  psychogenic pruritus (F45.8)

L29.0 Pruritus ani

L29.1 Pruritus scroti

L29.2 Pruritus vulvae

L29.3 Anogenital pruritus, unspecified

L29.8 Other pruritus

L29.9 Pruritus, unspecified
  Itch NOS

L30 OTHER AND UNSPECIFIED DERMATITIS
- 4th *Excludes2*: contact dermatitis (L23–L25)
  dry skin dermatitis (L85.3)
  small plaque parapsoriasis (L41.3)
  stasis dermatitis (I83.1–.2)

L30.1 Dyshidrosis [pompholyx]

L30.3 Infective dermatitis
  Infectious eczematoid dermatitis

L30.4 Erythema intertrigo

L30.5 Pityriasis alba

L30.8 Other specified dermatitis

L30.9 Dermatitis, unspecified
  Eczema NOS

(L40–L45) PAPULOSQUAMOUS DISORDERS

L40 PSORIASIS
- 4th **L40.5** Arthropathic psoriasis
  - 5th **L40.54** Psoriatic juvenile arthropathy
L40.8 Other psoriasis
  Flexural psoriasis

L40.9 Psoriasis, unspecified

L42 PITYRIASIS ROSEA
- ✔

L44 OTHER PAPULOSQUAMOUS DISORDERS
- 4th **L44.0** Pityriasis rubra pilaris
L44.1 Lichen nitidus

4th 5th 6th 7th Additional Character Required   ✔ 3-character code

Unspecified laterality codes were excluded here. •=New Code ▲=Revised Code *Excludes1*—Not coded here, do not use together *Excludes2*—Not included here

L44.2   **Lichen striatus**
L44.3   **Lichen ruber moniliformis**
L44.4   **Infantile papular acrodermatitis [Gianotti-Crosti]**
L44.8   **Other specified papulosquamous disorders**
L44.9   **Papulosquamous disorder, unspecified**

(L49–L54) URTICARIA AND ERYTHEMA

Excludes1: Lyme disease (A69.2-)
  rosacea (L71.-)

L50   **URTICARIA**
`4th`   ***Excludes1:*** allergic contact dermatitis (L23.-)
    angioneurotic edema or giant urticarial or Quincke's edema (T78.3)
    hereditary angio-edema (D84.1)
    serum urticaria (T80.6-)
    solar urticaria (L56.3)
    urticaria neonatorum (P83.8)
    urticaria papulosa (L28.2)
    urticaria pigmentosa (D47.01)
  L50.0   **Allergic urticaria**
  L50.1   **Idiopathic urticaria**
  L50.2   **Urticaria due to cold and heat**
    Excludes2: familial cold urticaria (M04.2)
  L50.3   **Dermatographic urticaria**
  L50.4   **Vibratory urticaria**
  L50.5   **Cholinergic urticaria**
  L50.6   **Contact urticaria**
  L50.8   **Other urticaria**
    Chronic urticaria
    Recurrent periodic urticaria
  L50.9   **Urticaria, unspecified**

L51   **ERYTHEMA MULTIFORME**
`4th`   **Use additional code** for adverse effect, if applicable, to identify drug
    (T36–T50 with fifth or sixth character 5)
  Use additional code to identify associated manifestations, such as:
    arthropathy associated with dermatological disorders (M14.8-)
    conjunctival edema (H11.42)
    conjunctivitis (H10.22-)
    corneal scars and opacities (H17.-)
    corneal ulcer (H16.0-)
    edema of eyelid (H02.84-)
    inflammation of eyelid (H01.8)
    keratoconjunctivitis sicca (H16.22-)
    mechanical lagophthalmos (H02.22-)
    stomatitis (K12.-)
    symblepharon (H11.23-)
  Use additional code to identify percentage of skin exfoliation (L49.-)
  Excludes1: staphylococcal scalded skin syndrome (L00)
    Ritter's disease (L00)
  L51.0   **Nonbullous erythema multiforme**
  L51.1   **Stevens-Johnson syndrome**
  L51.2   **Toxic epidermal necrolysis [Lyell]**
  L51.3   **Stevens-Johnson syndrome-toxic epidermal necrolysis overlap syndrome**
    SJS-TEN overlap syndrome
  L51.8   **Other erythema multiforme**
  L51.9   **Erythema multiforme, unspecified**
    Erythema iris
    Erythema multiforme major NOS
    Erythema multiforme minor NOS
    Herpes iris

L52   **ERYTHEMA NODOSUM**
`✓`   ***Excludes1:*** tuberculous erythema nodosum (A18.4)

L53   **OTHER ERYTHEMATOUS CONDITIONS**
`4th`   ***Excludes1:*** erythema ab igne (L59.0)
    erythema due to external agents in contact with skin (L23-L25)
    erythema intertrigo (L30.4)

L53.0   **Toxic erythema**
  Code first poisoning due to drug or toxin, if applicable (T36-T65 with fifth or sixth character 1-4 or 6)
  Use additional code for adverse effect, if applicable, to identify drug (T36-T50 with fifth or sixth character 5)
  Excludes1: neonatal erythema toxicum (P83.1)
L53.1   **Erythema annulare centrifugum**
L53.2   **Erythema marginatum**
L53.8   **Other specified erythematous conditions**
L53.9   **Erythematous condition, unspecified**
  Erythema NOS
  Erythroderma NOS

(L55–L59) RADIATION-RELATED DISORDERS OF THE SKIN AND SUBCUTANEOUS TISSUE

L55   **SUNBURN**
`4th`   L55.0   **Sunburn of first degree**
  L55.1   **Sunburn of second degree**
  L55.2   **Sunburn of third degree**
  L55.9   **Sunburn, unspecified**

L56   **OTHER ACUTE SKIN CHANGES DUE TO ULTRAVIOLET**
`4th`   **RADIATION**
  Use additional code to identify the source of the ultraviolet radiation (W89, X32)
  L56.0   **Drug phototoxic response**
    Use additional code for adverse effect, if applicable, to identify drug (T36-T50 with fifth or sixth character 5)
  L56.1   **Drug photoallergic response**
    Use additional code for adverse effect, if applicable, to identify drug (T36-T50 with fifth or sixth character 5)
  L56.3   **Solar urticaria**
  L56.8   **Other specified acute skin changes due to ultraviolet radiation**
  L56.9   **Acute skin change due to ultraviolet radiation, unspecified**

(L60–L75) DISORDERS OF SKIN APPENDAGES

Excludes1: congenital malformations of integument (Q84.-)

L60   **NAIL DISORDERS**
`4th`   ***Excludes2:*** clubbing of nails (R68.3)
    onychia and paronychia (L03.0-)
  L60.0   **Ingrowing nail**
  L60.1   **Onycholysis**
  L60.3   **Nail dystrophy**
  L60.8   **Other nail disorders**
  L60.9   **Nail disorder, unspecified**

L65   **OTHER NON-SCARRING HAIR LOSS**
`4th`   **Use additional code** for adverse effect, if applicable, to identify drug (T36–T50 with fifth or sixth character 5)
  Excludes1: trichotillomania (F63.3)
  L65.8   **Other specified non-scarring hair loss**
  L65.9   **Non-scarring hair loss, unspecified**
    Alopecia NOS

L68   **HYPERTRICHOSIS**
`4th`   ***Includes:*** excess hair
  Excludes1: congenital hypertrichosis (Q84.2)
    persistent lanugo (Q84.2)
  L68.0   **Hirsutism**

L70   **ACNE**
`4th`   ***Excludes2:*** acne keloid (L73.0)
  L70.0   **Acne vulgaris**
  L70.1   **Acne conglobata**
  L70.2   **Acne varioliformis**
    Acne necrotica miliaris
  L70.3   **Acne tropica**
  L70.4   **Infantile acne**
  L70.5   **Acné excoriée**
    Acné excoriée des jeunes filles
    Picker's acne
  L70.8   **Other acne**
  L70.9   **Acne, unspecified**

`4th` `5th` `6th` `7th` Additional Character Required   `✓` 3-character code

Unspecified laterality codes   •=New Code   ***Excludes1***—Not coded here, do not use together
were excluded here.   ▲=Revised Code   ***Excludes2***—Not included here

CHAPTER 12. DISEASES OF THE SKIN AND SUBCUTANEOUS TISSUE   (L72–L89)

L72 **FOLLICULAR CYSTS OF SKIN AND SUBCUTANEOUS**
`4th`   **TISSUE**
L72.0   **Epidermal cyst**
L72.1   **Pilar and trichodermal cyst**
    `5th`   L72.11   **Pilar cyst**
    L72.12   **Trichodermal cyst**
        Trichilemmal (proliferating) cyst
L72.3   **Sebaceous cyst**
    Excludes2: pilar cyst (L72.11)
        trichilemmal (proliferating) cyst (L72.12)
L72.8   **Other follicular cysts of the skin and subcutaneous tissue**
L72.9   **Follicular cyst of the skin and subcutaneous tissue, unspecified**

L73 **OTHER FOLLICULAR DISORDERS**
`4th`
L73.0   **Acne keloid**
L73.1   **Pseudofolliculitis barbae**
L73.2   **Hidradenitis suppurativa**
L73.8   **Other specified follicular disorders**
    Sycosis barbae
L73.9   **Follicular disorder, unspecified**

L74 **ECCRINE SWEAT DISORDERS**
`4th`   *Excludes2:* generalized hyperhidrosis (R61)
L74.0   **Miliaria rubra**
L74.1   **Miliaria crystallina**
L74.3   **Miliaria, unspecified**
L74.5   **Focal hyperhidrosis**
    `5th`   L74.51   **Primary focal hyperhidrosis**
        `6th`   L74.510   **Primary focal hyperhidrosis, axilla**
        L74.511   **Primary focal hyperhidrosis, face**
        L74.512   **Primary focal hyperhidrosis, palms**
        L74.513   **Primary focal hyperhidrosis, soles**
        L74.519   **Primary focal hyperhidrosis, unspecified**
    L74.52   **Secondary focal hyperhidrosis**
        Frey's syndrome

(L76) INTRAOPERATIVE AND POSTPROCEDURAL COMPLICATIONS OF SKIN AND SUBCUTANEOUS TISSUE

(L80–L99) OTHER DISORDERS OF THE SKIN AND SUBCUTANEOUS TISSUE

L80 **VITILIGO**
`✓`   *Excludes2:* vitiligo of eyelids (H02.73-)
        vitiligo of vulva (N90.89)

L81 **OTHER DISORDERS OF PIGMENTATION**
`4th`   *Excludes1:* birthmark NOS (Q82.5)
        Peutz-Jeghers syndrome (Q85.8)
    Excludes2: nevus — see Alphabetical Index
L81.2   **Freckles**
L81.3   **Café au lait spots**
L81.4   **Other melanin hyperpigmentation**
        Lentigo
L81.6   **Other disorders of diminished melanin formation**
L81.7   **Pigmented purpuric dermatosis**
        Angioma serpiginosum
L81.8   **Other specified disorders of pigmentation**
        Iron pigmentation
        Tattoo pigmentation
L81.9   **Disorder of pigmentation, unspecified**

L82 **SEBORRHEIC KERATOSIS**
`4th`   *Includes:* basal cell papilloma
        dermatosis papulosa nigra
        Leser-Trélat disease
    Excludes2: seborrheic dermatitis (L21.-)
L82.0   **Inflamed seborrheic keratosis**
L82.1   **Other seborrheic keratosis**
        Seborrheic keratosis NOS

L83 **ACANTHOSIS NIGRICANS**
`✓`   Confluent and reticulated papillomatosis

L84 **CORNS AND CALLOSITIES**
`✓`   Callus
    Clavus

L85 **OTHER EPIDERMAL THICKENING**
`4th`   *Excludes2:* hypertrophic disorders of the skin (L91.-)
L85.0   **Acquired ichthyosis**
    Excludes1: congenital ichthyosis (Q80.-)
L85.1   **Acquired keratosis [keratoderma] palmaris et plantaris**
    Excludes1: inherited keratosis palmaris et plantaris (Q82.8)
L85.2   **Keratosis punctata (palmaris et plantaris)**
L85.3   **Xerosis cutis**
        Dry skin dermatitis
L85.8   **Other specified epidermal thickening**
        Cutaneous horn
L85.9   **Epidermal thickening, unspecified**

L88 **PYODERMA GANGRENOSUM**
`✓`   Phagedenic pyoderma
    Excludes1: dermatitis gangrenosa (L08.0)

L89 **PRESSURE ULCER**
`4th`   **GUIDELINES**

Pressure ulcer stages

Codes in category L89, Pressure ulcer, are combination codes that identify the site and stage of the pressure ulcer as well as the stage of the ulcer. The *ICD-10-CM* classifies pressure ulcer stages based on severity, which is designated by stages 1–4, deep tissue pressure injury, unspecified stage and unstageable. Assign as many codes from category L89 as needed to identify all the pressure ulcers the patient has, if applicable. *See Section I.B.14 for pressure ulcer stage documentation by clinicians other than patient's provider.*

Unstageable pressure ulcers
Refer to the ICD-10-CM manual.

Documented pressure ulcer stage

Assignment of the pressure ulcer stage code should be guided by clinical documentation of the stage or documentation of the terms found in the Alphabetic Index. For clinical terms describing the stage that are not found in the Alphabetic Index, and there is no documentation of the stage, the provider should be queried.

Patients admitted with pressure ulcers documented as healed
No code is assigned if the documentation states that the pressure ulcer is completely healed.

Patients admitted with pressure ulcers documented as healing
Refer to the ICD-10-CM manual.

Patient admitted with pressure ulcer evolving into another stage during the admission
Refer to the ICD-10-CM manual.

Pressure-induced deep tissue damage

For pressure-induced deep tissue damage or deep tissue pressure injury, assign only the appropriate code for pressure-induced deep tissue damage (L89.--6).

Includes: bed sore
    decubitus ulcer
    plaster ulcer
    pressure area
    pressure sore
Code first any associated gangrene (I96)
Excludes2: decubitus (trophic) ulcer of
    cervix (uteri) (N86)
    diabetic ulcers (E08.621, E08.622, E09.621, E09.622, E10.621, E10.622, E11.621, E11.622, E13.621, E13.622)

Stage 1 — Pressure pre-ulcer skin changes limited to persistent focal edema
Stage 2 — Pressure ulcer with abrasion, blister, partial thickness skin loss involving epidermis and/or dermis
Stage 3 — Pressure ulcer with full thickness skin loss involving damage or necrosis of subcutaneous tissue
Stage 4 — Pressure ulcer with necrosis of soft tissues through to underlying muscle, tendon, or bone

---

`4th` `5th` `6th` `7th` Additional Character Required   `✓` 3-character code

non-pressure chronic ulcer of skin (L97.-)
skin infections (L00–L08)
varicose ulcer (I83.0, I83.2)

L89.0 Pressure ulcer of elbow

`5th` **L89.01 Pressure ulcer of right elbow**

`6th` Healing pressure ulcer of right elbow

L89.010 **Pressure ulcer of right elbow; unstageable**

L89.011 **stage 1**

L89.012 **stage 2**

L89.013 **stage 3**

L89.014 **stage 4**

L89.016 **Pressure-induced deep tissue damage of right elbow**

L89.019 **unspecified stage**

Healing pressure right of elbow NOS

L89.02 Pressure ulcer of left elbow

`6th` Healing pressure ulcer of left elbow

L89.020 **Pressure ulcer of left elbow; unstageable**

L89.021 **stage 1**

L89.022 **stage 2**

L89.023 **stage 3**

L89.024 **stage 4**

L89.026 **Pressure-induced deep tissue damage of left elbow**

L89.029 **Pressure ulcer of left elbow, unspecified stage**

Healing pressure ulcer of left of elbow NOS
Healing pressure ulcer of left elbow, unspecified stage

L89.1 Pressure ulcer of back

`5th` **L89.10 Pressure ulcer of unspecified part of back**

`6th` Healing pressure ulcer of unspecified part of back
Pressure pre-ulcer skin changes limited to persistent focal edema, unspecified part of back

L89.100 **Pressure ulcer of unspecified part of back; unstageable**

L89.101 **stage 1**

L89.102 **stage 2**

L89.103 **stage 3**

L89.104 **stage 4**

L89.106 **Pressure-induced deep tissue damage of unspecified part of back**

L89.109 **unspecified stage**

Healing pressure ulcer of unspecified part of back NOS

L89.11 Pressure ulcer of right upper back

`6th` Pressure ulcer of right shoulder blade
Healing pressure ulcer of right upper back

L89.110 **Pressure ulcer of right upper back; unstageable**

L89.111 **stage 1**

L89.112 **stage 2**

L89.113 **stage 3**

L89.114 **stage 4**

L89.116 **Pressure-induced deep tissue damage of right upper back**

L89.119 **unspecified stage**

Healing pressure ulcer of right upper back NOS

L89.12 Pressure ulcer of left upper back

`6th` Healing pressure ulcer of left upper back,
Pressure ulcer of left shoulder blade

L89.120 **Pressure ulcer of left upper back; unstageable**

L89.121 **stage 1**

L89.122 **stage 2**

L89.123 **stage 3**

L89.124 **stage 4**

L89.126 **Pressure-induced deep tissue damage of left upper back**

L89.129 **unspecified stage**

Healing pressure ulcer of left upper back NOS
Healing pressure ulcer of left upper back, unspecified stage

L89.13 Pressure ulcer of right lower back

`6th` Healing pressure ulcer of right lower back

L89.130 **Pressure ulcer of right lower back; unstageable**

L89.131 **stage 1**

L89.132 **stage 2**

L89.133 **stage 3**

L89.134 **stage 4**

L89.136 **Pressure-induced deep tissue damage of right lower back**

L89.139 **unspecified stage**

Healing pressure ulcer of right lower back NOS

L89.14 Pressure ulcer of left lower back

`6th` Healing pressure ulcer of left lower back

L89.140 **Pressure ulcer of left lower back; unstageable**

L89.141 **stage 1**

L89.142 **stage 2**

L89.143 **stage 3**

L89.144 **stage 4**

L89.146 **Pressure-induced deep tissue damage of left lower back**

L89.149 **unspecified stage**

Healing pressure ulcer of left lower back NOS

L89.15 Pressure ulcer of sacral region

`6th` Healing pressure ulcer of sacral region,
Pressure ulcer of coccyx
Pressure ulcer of tailbone

L89.150 **Pressure ulcer of sacral region; unstageable**

L89.151 **stage 1**

L89.152 **stage 2**

L89.153 **stage 3**

L89.154 **stage 4**

L89.156 **Pressure-induced deep tissue damage of sacral region**

L89.159 **unspecified stage**

Healing pressure ulcer of sacral region NOS

L89.2 Pressure ulcer of hip

`5th` **L89.21 Pressure ulcer of right hip**

`6th` Healing pressure ulcer of right hip

L89.210 **Pressure ulcer of right hip; unstageable**

L89.211 **stage 1**

L89.212 **stage 2**

L89.213 **stage 3**

L89.214 **stage 4**

L89.216 **Pressure-induced deep tissue damage of right hip**

L89.219 **unspecified stage**

Healing pressure ulcer of right hip NOS

L89.22 Pressure ulcer of left hip

`6th` Healing pressure ulcer of left hip back

L89.220 **Pressure ulcer of left hip; unstageable**

L89.221 **stage 1**

L89.222 **stage 2**

L89.223 **stage 3**

L89.224 **stage 4**

L89.226 **Pressure-induced deep tissue damage of left hip**

L89.229 **unspecified stage**

Healing pressure ulcer of left hip NOS

L89.3 Pressure ulcer of buttock

`5th` **L89.31 Pressure ulcer of right buttock**

`6th` Healing pressure ulcer of right buttock

L89.310 **Pressure ulcer of right buttock; unstageable**

`4th` `5th` `6th` `7th` Additional Character Required   ✔   3-character code

Unspecified laterality codes were excluded here.

•=New Code
▲=Revised Code

Excludes1—Not coded here, do not use together
Excludes2—Not included here

L89.311   stage 1
L89.312   stage 2
L89.313   stage 3
L89.314   stage 4
L89.316   **Pressure-induced deep tissue damage of right buttock**
L89.319   **unspecified stage**
         Healing pressure ulcer of right buttock NOS

L89.32   Pressure ulcer of left buttock
`6th`   Healing pressure ulcer of left buttock
L89.320   **Pressure ulcer of left buttock; unstageable**
L89.321   stage 1
L89.322   stage 2
L89.323   stage 3
L89.324   stage 4
L89.326   **Pressure-induced deep tissue damage of left buttock**
L89.329   **Pressure ulcer of left buttock, unspecified stage**
         Healing pressure ulcer of left buttock NOS

L89.4 Pressure ulcer of contiguous site of back, buttock and hip
`5th` Healing pressure ulcer of contiguous site of back, buttock and hip
L89.40   **Pressure ulcer of contiguous site of back, buttock and hip; unspecified stage**
        Healing pressure ulcer of contiguous site of back, buttock and hip NOS
L89.41   stage 1
L89.42   stage 2
L89.43   stage 3
L89.44   stage 4
L89.45   unstageable
L89.46   **Pressure-induced deep tissue damage of contiguous site of back, buttock and hip**

L89.5 Pressure ulcer of ankle
`5th` **L89.51 Pressure ulcer of right ankle**
   `6th` Healing pressure ulcer of right ankle
L89.510   **Pressure ulcer of right ankle; unstageable**
L89.511   stage 1
L89.512   stage 2
L89.513   stage 3
L89.514   stage 4
L89.516   **Pressure-induced deep tissue damage of right ankle**
L89.519   **unspecified stage**
        Healing pressure ulcer of right ankle NOS

L89.52 Pressure ulcer of left ankle
`6th` Healing pressure ulcer of left ankle
L89.520   **Pressure ulcer of left ankle; unstageable**
L89.521   stage 1
        Pressure pre-ulcer skin changes limited to persistent focal edema, left ankle
L89.522   stage 2
L89.523   stage 3
L89.524   stage 4
L89.526   **Pressure-induced deep tissue damage of left ankle**
L89.529   **unspecified stage**
        Healing pressure ulcer of left ankle NOS

L89.6 Pressure ulcer of heel
`5th` **L89.61 Pressure ulcer of right heel**
   `6th` Healing pressure ulcer of right heel
L89.610   **Pressure ulcer of right heel; unstageable**
L89.611   stage 1
L89.612   stage 2
L89.613   stage 3
L89.614   stage 4
L89.616   **Pressure-induced deep tissue damage of right heel**
L89.619   **unspecified stage**
        Healing pressure ulcer of right heel NOS

L89.62 Pressure ulcer of left heel
`6th` Healing pressure ulcer of left heel

L89.620   **Pressure ulcer of left heel; unstageable**
L89.621   stage 1
L89.622   stage 2
L89.623   stage 3
L89.624   stage 4
L89.626   **Pressure-induced deep tissue damage of left heel**
L89.629   **unspecified stage**
        Healing pressure ulcer of left heel NOS

L89.8 Pressure ulcer of other site
`5th` **L89.81 Pressure ulcer of head**
   `6th` Pressure ulcer of face
       Healing pressure ulcer of head
L89.810   **Pressure ulcer of head; unstageable**
L89.811   stage 1
L89.812   stage 2
L89.813   stage 3
L89.814   stage 4
L89.816   **Pressure-induced deep tissue damage of head**
L89.819   **unspecified stage**
        Healing pressure ulcer of head NOS

L89.89 Pressure ulcer of other site
`6th` Healing pressure ulcer of other site
L89.890   **Pressure ulcer of other site; unstageable**
L89.891   stage 1
L89.892   stage 2
L89.893   stage 3
L89.894   stage 4
L89.896   **Pressure-induced deep tissue damage of other site**
L89.899   **unspecified stage**
        Healing pressure ulcer of other site NOS

L89.9 Pressure ulcer of unspecified site
`5th` Healing pressure ulcer of unspecified site
L89.90   **Pressure ulcer of unspecified site; unspecified stage**
L89.91   stage 1
L89.92   stage 2
L89.93   stage 3
L89.94   stage 4
L89.95   unstageable
L89.96   **Pressure-induced deep tissue damage of unspecified site**

L90 ATROPHIC DISORDERS OF SKIN
`4th` **L90.5 Scar conditions and fibrosis of skin**
     Adherent scar (skin)
     Cicatrix
     Disfigurement of skin due to scar
     Fibrosis of skin NOS

L91 HYPERTROPHIC DISORDERS OF SKIN
`4th` **L91.0 Hypertrophic scar**
     Keloid
     Keloid scar
     Excludes2: acne keloid (L73.0)
         scar NOS (L90.5)
L91.8 Other hypertrophic disorders of the skin
L91.9 Hypertrophic disorder of the skin, unspecified

L92 GRANULOMATOUS DISORDERS OF SKIN AND SUBCUTANEOUS TISSUE
`4th` ***Excludes2:*** actinic granuloma (L57.5)
L92.0 Granuloma annulare
     Perforating granuloma annulare
L92.3 FB granuloma of the skin and subcutaneous tissue
     Use additional code to identify the type of retained FB (Z18.-)
L92.9 Granulomatous disorder of the skin and subcutaneous tissue, unspecified
     Excludes2: umbilical granuloma (P83.81)

L94 OTHER LOCALIZED CONNECTIVE TISSUE DISORDERS
`4th` ***Excludes1:*** systemic connective tissue disorders (M30–M36)
L94.2 Calcinosis cutis

`4th` `5th` `6th` `7th` Additional Character Required   ☑ 3-character code

Unspecified laterality codes were excluded here. ●=New Code ▲=Revised Code

Excludes1—Not coded here, do not use together
Excludes2—Not included here

L98 **OTHER DISORDERS OF SKIN AND SUBCUTANEOUS**
4th **TISSUE, NOT ELSEWHERE CLASSIFIED**

L98.0 **Pyogenic granuloma**
Excludes2: pyogenic granuloma of gingiva (K06.8)
pyogenic granuloma of maxillary alveolar ridge (K04.5)
pyogenic granuloma of oral mucosa (K13.4)

L98.1 **Factitial dermatitis**
Neurotic excoriation
Excludes1: excoriation (skin-picking) disorder (F42.4)

L98.5 **Mucinosis of the skin**
Focal mucinosis
Lichen myxedematosus
Reticular erythematous mucinosis
Excludes1: focal oral mucinosis (K13.79)
myxedema (E03.9)

L98.7 **Excessive and redundant skin and subcutaneous tissue**
Loose or sagging skin following bariatric surgery weight loss
Loose or sagging skin following dietary weight loss
Loose or sagging skin, NOS
Excludes2: acquired excess or redundant skin of eyelid (H02.3-)
congenital excess or redundant skin of eyelid (Q10.3)
skin changes due to chronic exposure to nonionizing
radiation (L57.-)

L98.8 **Other specified disorders of the skin and subcutaneous tissue**

L98.9 **Disorder of the skin and subcutaneous tissue, unspecified**

L99 **OTHER DISORDERS OF SKIN AND SUBCUTANEOUS**
✔ **TISSUE IN DISEASES CLASSIFIED ELSEWHERE**
Code first underlying disease, such as:
amyloidosis (E85.-)
Excludes1: skin disorders in diabetes (E08–E13 with .62)
skin disorders in gonorrhea (A54.89)
skin disorders in syphilis (A51.31, A52.79)

CHAPTER 12. DISEASES OF THE SKIN AND SUBCUTANEOUS TISSUE (L98–L99)

4th **5th** **6th** **7th** Additional Character Required **✔** 3-character code

Unspecified laterality codes •=New Code ***Excludes1***—Not coded here, do not use together
were excluded here. ▲=Revised Code ***Excludes2***—Not included here

Chapter 13. Diseases of the musculoskeletal system and connective tissue (M00–M99)

An "X" may be listed at the end of the code to indicate a placeholder digit(s). The X will be required in order to get to the 7th character, which indicates the type of encounter. Be sure to use all indicated placeholder digits prior to the appropriate 7th character digit.

GUIDELINES

Site and laterality

Most of the codes within Chapter 13 have site and laterality designations. The site represents the bone, joint or the muscle involved. For some conditions where more than one bone, joint or muscle is usually involved, such as osteoarthritis, there is a "multiple sites" code available. For categories where no multiple site code is provided and more than one bone, joint or muscle is involved, multiple codes should be used to indicate the different sites involved.

BONE VERSUS JOINT

For certain conditions, the bone may be affected at the upper or lower end. Though the portion of the bone affected may be at the joint, the site designation will be the bone, not the joint.

Acute traumatic versus chronic or recurrent musculoskeletal conditions

Many musculoskeletal conditions are a result of previous injury or trauma to a site, or are recurrent conditions. Bone, joint or muscle conditions that are the result of a healed injury are usually found in Chapter 13. Recurrent bone, joint or muscle conditions are also usually found in Chapter 13. Any current, acute injury should be coded to the appropriate injury code from Chapter 19. Chronic or recurrent conditions should generally be coded with a code from Chapter 13. If it is difficult to determine from the documentation in the record which code is best to describe a condition, query the provider.

Coding of Pathologic Fractures

Refer to category M84.

Note: Use an external cause code following the code for the musculoskeletal condition, if applicable, to identify the cause of the musculoskeletal condition

Excludes2: arthropathic psoriasis (L40.5-)
    certain conditions originating in the perinatal period (P04–P96)
    certain infectious and parasitic diseases (A00–B99)
    compartment syndrome (traumatic) (T79.A-)
    complications of pregnancy, childbirth and the puerperium (O00–O9A)
    congenital malformations, deformations, and chromosomal abnormalities (Q00–Q99)
    endocrine, nutritional and metabolic diseases (E00–E88)
    injury, poisoning and certain other consequences of external causes (S00–T88)
    neoplasms (C00–D49)
    symptoms, signs and abnormal clinical and laboratory findings, NEC (R00–R94)

(M00–M25) ARTHROPATHIES

Includes: disorders affecting predominantly peripheral (limb) joints

(M00–M02) INFECTIOUS ARTHROPATHIES

Note: This block comprises arthropathies due to microbiological agents. Distinction is made between the following types of etiological relationship:
a) direct infection of joint, where organisms invade synovial tissue and microbial antigen is present in the joint;
b) indirect infection, which may be of two types: a reactive arthropathy, where microbial infection of the body is established but neither organisms nor antigens can be identified in the joint, and a postinfective arthropathy, where microbial antigen is present but recovery of an organism is inconstant and evidence of local multiplication is lacking.

M00   **PYOGENIC ARTHRITIS**
`4th`   *Excludes2:* infection and inflammatory reaction due to internal joint prosthesis (T84.5-)

   M00.0 Staphylococcal arthritis and polyarthritis
     `5th`   Use additional code (B95.61–B95.8) to identify bacterial agent
     M00.00   Staphylococcal arthritis, unspecified joint
     M00.01   Staphylococcal arthritis, shoulder
     `6th`   **M00.011**   Staphylococcal arthritis, right shoulder

      M00.012   Staphylococcal arthritis, left shoulder
   M00.02   **Staphylococcal arthritis, elbow**
     `6th`
      M00.021   Staphylococcal arthritis, right elbow
      M00.022   Staphylococcal arthritis, left elbow
   M00.03   **Staphylococcal arthritis, wrist**
     `6th` phylococcal arthritis of carpal bones
      M00.031   Staphylococcal arthritis, right wrist
      M00.032   Staphylococcal arthritis, left wrist
   M00.04   **Staphylococcal arthritis, hand**
     `6th`   Staphylococcal arthritis of metacarpus and phalanges
      M00.041   Staphylococcal arthritis, right hand
      M00.042   Staphylococcal arthritis, left hand
   M00.05   **Staphylococcal arthritis, hip**
     `6th`
      M00.051   Staphylococcal arthritis, right hip
      M00.052   Staphylococcal arthritis, left hip
   M00.06   **Staphylococcal arthritis, knee**
     `6th`
      M00.061   Staphylococcal arthritis, right knee
      M00.062   Staphylococcal arthritis, left knee
   M00.07   **Staphylococcal arthritis, ankle and foot**
     `6th`   Staphylococcal arthritis, tarsus, metatarsus and phalanges
      M00.071   Staphylococcal arthritis, right ankle and foot
      M00.072   Staphylococcal arthritis, left ankle and foot
   M00.08   **Staphylococcal arthritis, vertebrae**
   M00.09   **Staphylococcal polyarthritis**
M00.1   **Pneumococcal arthritis and polyarthritis**
`5th`   **M00.10**   Pneumococcal arthritis, unspecified joint
   M00.11   **Pneumococcal arthritis, shoulder**
     `6th`
      M00.111   Pneumococcal arthritis, right shoulder
      M00.112   Pneumococcal arthritis, left shoulder
   M00.12   **Pneumococcal arthritis, elbow**
     `6th`
      M00.121   Pneumococcal arthritis, right elbow
      M00.122   Pneumococcal arthritis, left elbow
   M00.13   **Pneumococcal arthritis, wrist**
     `6th`   Pneumococcal arthritis of carpal bones
      M00.131   Pneumococcal arthritis, right wrist
      M00.132   Pneumococcal arthritis, left wrist`
   M00.14   **Pneumococcal arthritis, hand**
     `6th`   Pneumococcal arthritis of metacarpus and phalanges
      M00.141   Pneumococcal arthritis, right hand
      M00.142   Pneumococcal arthritis, left hand
   M00.15   **Pneumococcal arthritis, hip**
     `6th`
      M00.151   Pneumococcal arthritis, right hip
      M00.152   Pneumococcal arthritis, left hip
   M00.16   **Pneumococcal arthritis, knee**
     `6th`
      M00.161   Pneumococcal arthritis, right knee
      M00.162   Pneumococcal arthritis, left knee
   M00.17   **Pneumococcal arthritis, ankle and foot**
     `6th`   Pneumococcal arthritis, tarsus, metatarsus and phalanges
      M00.171   Pneumococcal arthritis, right ankle and foot
      M00.172   Pneumococcal arthritis, left ankle and foot
   M00.18   **Pneumococcal arthritis, vertebrae**
   M00.19   **Pneumococcal polyarthritis**
M00.2   **Other streptococcal arthritis and polyarthritis**
`5th`   Use additional code (B95.0–B95.2, B95.4–B95.5) to identify bacterial agent
   M00.20   **Other streptococcal arthritis, unspecified joint**
   M00.21   **Other streptococcal arthritis, shoulder**
     `6th`   **M00.211**   Other streptococcal arthritis, right shoulder
      M00.212   Other streptococcal arthritis, left shoulder
   M00.22   **Other streptococcal arthritis, elbow**
     `6th`   **M00.221**   Other streptococcal arthritis, right elbow
      M00.222   Other streptococcal arthritis, left elbow
   M00.23   **Other streptococcal arthritis, wrist**
     `6th`   Other streptococcal arthritis of carpal bones
      M00.231   Other streptococcal arthritis, right wrist
      M00.232   Other streptococcal arthritis, left wrist

| `4th` `5th` `6th` `7th` Additional Character Required   ✔   `3-character code` | Unspecified laterality codes were excluded here.   • =New Code   ▲ =Revised Code | *Excludes1*—Not coded here, do not use together *Excludes2*—Not included here |

CHAPTER 13. DISEASES OF THE MUSCULOSKELETAL SYSTEM AND CONNECTIVE TISSUE   (M00.24–M01.X9)

M00.24 **Other streptococcal arthritis, hand**
6th   Other streptococcal arthritis metacarpus and phalanges
     M00.241 **Other streptococcal arthritis, right hand**
     M00.242 **Other streptococcal arthritis, left hand**

M00.25 **Other streptococcal arthritis, hip**
6th   **M00.251** **Other streptococcal arthritis, right hip**
     M00.252 **Other streptococcal arthritis, left hip**

M00.26 **Other streptococcal arthritis, knee**
6th   **M00.261** **Other streptococcal arthritis, right knee**
     M00.262 **Other streptococcal arthritis, left knee**

M00.27 **Other streptococcal arthritis, ankle and foot**
6th   Other streptococcal arthritis, tarsus, metatarsus and phalanges
     M00.271 **Other streptococcal arthritis, right ankle and foot**
     M00.272 **Other streptococcal arthritis, left ankle and foot**

M00.28 **Other streptococcal arthritis, vertebrae**

M00.29 **Other streptococcal polyarthritis**

M00.8 **Arthritis and polyarthritis due to other bacteria**
5th   **Use additional code** (B96) to identify bacteria

M00.80 **Arthritis due to other bacteria, unspecified joint**

M00.81 **Arthritis due to other bacteria, shoulder**
6th   **M00.811** **Arthritis due to other bacteria, right shoulder**
     M00.812 **Arthritis due to other bacteria, left shoulder**

M00.82 **Arthritis due to other bacteria, elbow**
6th   **M00.821** **Arthritis due to other bacteria, right elbow**
     M00.822 **Arthritis due to other bacteria, left elbow**

M00.83 **Arthritis due to other bacteria, wrist**
6th   Arthritis due to other bacteria, carpal bones
     M00.831 **Arthritis due to other bacteria, right wrist**
     M00.832 **Arthritis due to other bacteria, left wrist**

M00.84 **Arthritis due to other bacteria, hand**
6th   Arthritis due to other bacteria, metacarpus and phalanges
     M00.841 **Arthritis due to other bacteria, right hand**
     M00.842 **Arthritis due to other bacteria, left hand**

M00.85 **Arthritis due to other bacteria, hip**
6th   **M00.851** **Arthritis due to other bacteria, right hip**
     M00.852 **Arthritis due to other bacteria, left hip**

M00.86 **Arthritis due to other bacteria, knee**
6th   **M00.861** **Arthritis due to other bacteria, right knee**
     M00.862 **Arthritis due to other bacteria, left knee**

M00.87 **Arthritis due to other bacteria, ankle and foot**
6th   Arthritis due to other bacteria, tarsus, metatarsus, and phalanges
     M00.871 **Arthritis due to other bacteria, right ankle and foot**
     M00.872 **Arthritis due to other bacteria, left ankle and foot**

M00.88 **Arthritis due to other bacteria, vertebrae**

M00.89 **Polyarthritis due to other bacteria**

M00.9 **Pyogenic arthritis, unspecified**
Infective arthritis NOS
Autoinflammatory syndromes (M04)

M01 **DIRECT INFECTIONS OF JOINT IN INFECTIOUS AND**
4th   **PARASITIC DISEASES CLASSIFIED ELSEWHERE**
Code first underlying disease, such as:
   leprosy [Hansen's disease] (A30.-)
   mycoses (B35-B49)
   O'nyong-nyong fever (A92.1)
   paratyphoid fever (A01.1-A01.4)
Excludes1: arthropathy in Lyme disease (A69.23)
   gonococcal arthritis (A54.42)
   meningococcal arthritis (A39.83)
   mumps arthritis (B26.85)
   postinfective arthropathy (M02.-)
   postmeningococcal arthritis (A39.84)
   reactive arthritis (M02.3)
   rubella arthritis (B06.82)

   sarcoidosis arthritis (D86.86)
   typhoid fever arthritis (A01.04)
   tuberculosis arthritis (A18.01-A18.02)

M01.X **Direct infection of joint in infectious and parasitic diseases**
5th   **classified elsewhere**

M01.X0 **Direct infection of unspecified joint in infectious and parasitic diseases classified elsewhere**

M01.X1 **Direct infection of shoulder joint in infectious and**
6th   **parasitic diseases classified elsewhere**
     M01.X11 **Direct infection of right shoulder in infectious and parasitic diseases classified elsewhere**
     M01.X12 **Direct infection of left shoulder in infectious and parasitic diseases classified elsewhere**

M01.X2 **Direct infection of elbow in infectious and parasitic**
6th   **diseases classified elsewhere**
     M01.X21 **Direct infection of right elbow in infectious and parasitic diseases classified elsewhere**
     M01.X22 **Direct infection of left elbow in infectious and parasitic diseases classified elsewhere**

M01.X3 **Direct infection of wrist in infectious and parasitic**
6th   **diseases classified elsewhere**
   Direct infection of carpal bones in infectious and parasitic diseases classified elsewhere
     M01.X31 **Direct infection of right wrist in infectious and parasitic diseases classified elsewhere**
     M01.X32 **Direct infection of left wrist in infectious and parasitic diseases classified elsewhere**

M01.X4 **Direct infection of hand in infectious and parasitic**
6th   **diseases classified elsewhere**
   Direct infection of metacarpus and phalanges in infectious and parasitic diseases classified elsewhere
     M01.X41 **Direct infection of right hand in infectious and parasitic diseases classified elsewhere**
     M01.X42 **Direct infection of left hand in infectious and parasitic diseases classified elsewhere**

M01.X5 **Direct infection of hip in infectious and parasitic**
6th   **diseases classified elsewhere**
     M01.X51 **Direct infection of right hip in infectious and parasitic diseases classified elsewhere**
     M01.X52 **Direct infection of left hip in infectious and parasitic diseases classified elsewhere**

M01.X6 **Direct infection of knee in infectious and parasitic**
6th   **diseases classified elsewhere**
     M01.X61 **Direct infection of right knee in infectious and parasitic diseases classified elsewhere**
     M01.X62 **Direct infection of left knee in infectious and parasitic diseases classified elsewhere**

M01.X7 **Direct infection of ankle and foot in infectious and**
6th   **parasitic diseases classified elsewhere**
   Direct infection of tarsus, metatarsus and phalanges in infectious and parasitic diseases classified elsewhere
     M01.X71 **Direct infection of right ankle and foot in infectious and parasitic diseases classified elsewhere**
     M01.X72 **Direct infection of left ankle and foot in infectious and parasitic diseases classified elsewhere**

M01.X8 **Direct infection of vertebrae in infectious and parasitic diseases classified elsewhere**

M01.X9 **Direct infection of multiple joints in infectious and parasitic diseases classified elsewhere**

4th   5th   6th   7th   Additional Character Required   ✔   3-character code

Unspecified laterality codes were excluded here.   •=New Code   ▲=Revised Code   ***Excludes1***—Not coded here, do not use together   ***Excludes2***—Not included here

(M04) AUTOINFLAMMATORY SYNDROMES

M04 **AUTOINFLAMMATORY SYNDROMES**
`4th`   *Excludes2:* Crohn's disease (K50.-)

M04.1 Periodic fever syndromes
Familial Mediterranean fever
Hyperimmunoglobin D syndrome
Mevalonate kinase deficiency
Tumor necrosis factor receptor associated periodic syndrome [TRAPS]

M04.2 Cryopyrin-associated periodic syndromes
Chronic infantile neurological, cutaneous and articular syndrome [CINCA]
Familial cold autoinflammatory syndrome
Familial cold urticaria
Muckle-Wells syndrome
Neonatal onset multisystemic inflammatory disorder [NOMID]

M04.8 Other autoinflammatory syndromes
Blau syndrome
Deficiency of interleukin 1 receptor antagonist [DIRA]
Majeed syndrome
Periodic fever, aphthous stomatitis, pharyngitis, and adenopathy syndrome [PFAPA]
Pyogenic arthritis, pyoderma gangrenosum, and acne syndrome [PAPA]

M04.9 Autoinflammatory syndrome, unspecified

(M05–M14) INFLAMMATORY POLYARTHROPATHIES

M06 **OTHER RHEUMATOID ARTHRITIS**
`4th`   **M06.9 Rheumatoid arthritis, unspecified**

M08 **JUVENILE ARTHRITIS**
`4th`   Code also any associated underlying condition, such as: regional enteritis [Crohn's disease] (K50.-)
ulcerative colitis (K51.-)
Excludes1: arthropathy in Whipple's disease (M14.8)
Felty's syndrome (M05.0)
juvenile dermatomyositis (M33.0-)
psoriatic juvenile arthropathy (L40.54)

M08.0 Unspecified juvenile rheumatoid arthritis
`5th`   Juvenile rheumatoid arthritis with or without rheumatoid factor

M08.00 Unspecified juvenile rheumatoid arthritis of unspecified site
M08.01 Unspecified juvenile rheumatoid arthritis, shoulder
`6th`   **M08.011** Unspecified juvenile rheumatoid arthritis, right shoulder
M08.012 Unspecified juvenile rheumatoid arthritis, left shoulder
M08.02 Unspecified juvenile rheumatoid arthritis of elbow
`6th`   **M08.021** right elbow
M08.022 left elbow
M08.03 Unspecified juvenile rheumatoid arthritis, wrist
`6th`   **M08.031** right wrist
M08.032 left wrist
M08.04 Unspecified juvenile rheumatoid arthritis, hand
`6th`   **M08.041** right hand
M08.042 left hand
M08.05 Unspecified juvenile rheumatoid arthritis, hip
`6th`   **M08.051** right hip
M08.052 left hip
M08.06 Unspecified juvenile rheumatoid arthritis, knee
`6th`   **M08.061** right knee
M08.062 left knee
M08.07 Unspecified juvenile rheumatoid arthritis, ankle and foot
`6th`   **M08.071** right ankle and foot
M08.072 left ankle and foot
M08.08 Unspecified juvenile rheumatoid arthritis, vertebrae
M08.09 Unspecified juvenile rheumatoid arthritis, multiple sites
• **M08.0A** Unspecified juvenile rheumatoid arthritis, other specified site

M08.1 Juvenile ankylosing spondylitis
Excludes1: ankylosing spondylitis in adults (M45.0-)
M08.2 Juvenile rheumatoid arthritis with systemic onset
`5th`   Still's disease NOS
Excludes1: adult-onset Still's disease (M06.1-)
M08.20 Juvenile rheumatoid arthritis with systemic onset, unspecified site
M08.21 Juvenile rheumatoid arthritis with systemic onset, shoulder
`6th`   **M08.211** right shoulder
M08.212 left shoulder
M08.22 Juvenile rheumatoid arthritis with systemic onset, elbow
`6th`   **M08.221** right elbow
M08.222 left elbow
M08.23 Juvenile rheumatoid arthritis with systemic onset, wrist
`6th`   **M08.231** right wrist
M08.232 left wrist
M08.24 Juvenile rheumatoid arthritis with systemic onset, hand
`6th`   **M08.241** right hand
M08.242 left hand
M08.25 Juvenile rheumatoid arthritis with systemic onset, hip
`6th`   **M08.251** right hip
M08.252 left hip
M08.26 Juvenile rheumatoid arthritis with systemic onset, knee
`6th`   **M08.261** right knee
M08.262 left knee
M08.27 Juvenile rheumatoid arthritis with systemic onset, ankle and foot
`6th`   **M08.271** right ankle and foot
M08.272 left ankle and foot
M08.28 Juvenile rheumatoid arthritis with systemic onset, vertebrae
M08.29 Juvenile rheumatoid arthritis with systemic onset, multiple sites
• **M08.2A** Juvenile rheumatoid arthritis with systemic onset, other specified site
M08.3 Juvenile rheumatoid polyarthritis (seronegative)
M08.4 Pauciarticular juvenile rheumatoid arthritis
`5th`   **M08.40** Pauciarticular juvenile rheumatoid arthritis, unspecified site
M08.41 Pauciarticular juvenile rheumatoid arthritis, shoulder
`6th`   **M08.411** right shoulder
M08.412 left shoulder
M08.42 Pauciarticular juvenile rheumatoid arthritis, elbow
`6th`   **M08.421** right elbow
M08.422 left elbow
M08.43 Pauciarticular juvenile rheumatoid arthritis, wrist
`6th`   **M08.431** right wrist
M08.432 left wrist
M08.44 Pauciarticular juvenile rheumatoid arthritis, hand
`6th`   **M08.441** right hand
M08.442 left hand
M08.45 Pauciarticular juvenile rheumatoid arthritis, hip
`6th`   **M08.451** right hip
M08.452 left hip
M08.46 Pauciarticular juvenile rheumatoid arthritis, knee
`6th`   **M08.461** right knee
M08.462 left knee
M08.47 Pauciarticular juvenile rheumatoid arthritis, ankle and foot
`6th`   **M08.471** right ankle and foot
M08.472 left ankle and foot
M08.48 Pauciarticular juvenile rheumatoid arthritis, vertebrae
• **M08.4A** Pauciarticular juvenile rheumatoid arthritis, other specified site
M08.8 Other juvenile arthritis
`5th`   **M08.81** Other juvenile arthritis, shoulder
`6th`

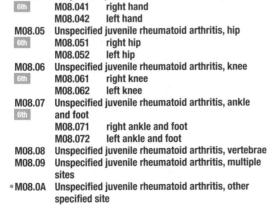

`4th` `5th` `6th` `7th` Additional Character Required   ✔ 3-character code

Unspecified laterality codes were excluded here.
•=New Code
▲=Revised Code

Excludes1—Not coded here, do not use together
Excludes2—Not included here

M08.811   right shoulder
M08.812   left shoulder
M08.82 Other juvenile arthritis, elbow
  `6th`   M08.821   right elbow
            M08.822   left elbow
M08.83 Other juvenile arthritis, wrist
  `6th`   M08.831   right wrist
            M08.832   left wrist
M08.84 Other juvenile arthritis, hand
  `6th`   M08.841   right hand
            M08.842   left hand
M08.85 Other juvenile arthritis, hip
  `6th`   M08.851   right hip
            M08.852   left hip
M08.86 Other juvenile arthritis, knee
  `6th`   M08.861   right knee
            M08.862   left knee
M08.87 Other juvenile arthritis, ankle and foot
  `6th`   M08.871   right ankle and foot
            M08.872   left ankle and foot
M08.88 Other juvenile arthritis, other specified site
            Other juvenile arthritis, vertebrae
M08.89 Other juvenile arthritis, multiple sites
M08.9 Juvenile arthritis, unspecified
  `5th`   *Excludes1:* juvenile rheumatoid arthritis, unspecified (M08.0-)
M08.90   Juvenile arthritis, unspecified, unspecified site
M08.91   Juvenile arthritis, unspecified, shoulder
  `6th`   M08.911   right shoulder
            M08.912   left shoulder
M08.92   Juvenile arthritis, unspecified, elbow
  `6th`   M08.921   right elbow
            M08.922   left elbow
M08.93   Juvenile arthritis, unspecified, wrist
  `6th`   M08.931   right wrist
            M08.932   left wrist
M08.94   Juvenile arthritis, unspecified, hand
  `6th`   M08.941   right hand
            M08.942   left hand
M08.95   Juvenile arthritis, unspecified, hip
  `6th`   M08.951   right hip
            M08.952   left hip
M08.96   Juvenile arthritis, unspecified, knee
  `6th`   M08.961   right knee
            M08.962   left knee
M08.97   Juvenile arthritis, unspecified, ankle and foot
  `6th`   M08.971   right ankle and foot
            M08.972   left ankle and foot
M08.98   Juvenile arthritis, unspecified, vertebrae
M08.99   Juvenile arthritis, unspecified, multiple sites
•**M08.9A   Juvenile arthritis, unspecified, other specified site**

M10 GOUT
  `4th`   Acute gout
          Gout attack
          Gout flare
          Podagra
          Use additional code to identify:
            Autonomic neuropathy in diseases classified elsewhere (G99.0)
            Calculus of urinary tract in diseases classified elsewhere (N22)
            Cardiomyopathy in diseases classified elsewhere (I43)
            Disorders of external ear in diseases classified elsewhere (H61.1-, H62.8-)
            Disorders of iris and ciliary body in diseases classified elsewhere (H22)
            Glomerular disorders in diseases classified elsewhere (N08)
          Excludes2: chronic gout (M1A.-)
M10.0 Idiopathic gout
  `5th`   Gouty bursitis
          Primary gout
M10.01   Idiopathic gout, shoulder
  `6th`   M10.011   right shoulder
            M10.012   left shoulder
M10.02   Idiopathic gout, elbow
  `6th`   M10.021   right elbow
            M10.022   left elbow

M10.03   Idiopathic gout, wrist
  `6th`   M10.031   right wrist
            M10.032   left wrist
M10.04   Idiopathic gout, hand
  `6th`   M10.041   right hand
            M10.042   left hand
M10.05   Idiopathic gout, hip
  `6th`   M10.051   right hip
            M10.052   left hip
M10.06   Idiopathic gout, knee
  `6th`   M10.061   right knee
            M10.062   left knee
M10.07   Idiopathic gout, ankle and foot
  `6th`   M10.071   right ankle and foot
            M10.072   left ankle and foot
M10.08   Idiopathic gout, vertebrae
M10.09   Idiopathic gout, multiple sites
M10.9 Gout, unspecified
          Gout NOS

M12 OTHER AND UNSPECIFIED ARTHROPATHY
  `4th`   *Excludes1:* arthrosis (M15-M19)
            cricoarytenoid arthropathy (J38.7)
M12.4 Intermittent hydrarthrosis
  `5th`   **M12.41   Intermittent hydrarthrosis, shoulder**
  `6th`   M12.411   right shoulder
            M12.412   left shoulder
M12.42   Intermittent hydrarthrosis, elbow
  `6th`   M12.421   right elbow
            M12.422   left elbow
M12.43   Intermittent hydrarthrosis, wrist
  `6th`   M12.431   right wrist
            M12.432   left wrist
M12.44   Intermittent hydrarthrosis, hand
  `6th`   M12.441   right hand
            M12.442   left hand
M12.45   Intermittent hydrarthrosis, hip
  `6th`   M12.451   right hip
            M12.452   left hip
M12.46   Intermittent hydrarthrosis, knee
  `6th`   M12.461   right knee
            M12.462   left knee
M12.47   Intermittent hydrarthrosis, ankle and foot
  `6th`   M12.471   right ankle and foot
            M12.472   left ankle and foot
M12.48   Intermittent hydrarthrosis, other site
M12.49   Intermittent hydrarthrosis, multiple sites
M12.5 Traumatic arthropathy
  `5th`   *Excludes1:* current injury — see Alphabetic Index
            post-traumatic osteoarthritis of first carpometacarpal joint (M18.2–M18.3)
            post-traumatic osteoarthritis of hip (M16.4–M16.5)
            post-traumatic osteoarthritis of knee (M17.2–M17.3)
            post-traumatic osteoarthritis NOS (M19.1-)
            post-traumatic osteoarthritis of other single joints (M19.1-)
M12.50   Traumatic arthropathy, unspecified site
M12.51   Traumatic arthropathy, shoulder
  `6th`   M12.511   right shoulder
            M12.512   left shoulder
M12.52   Traumatic arthropathy, elbow
  `6th`   M12.521   right elbow
            M12.522   left elbow
M12.53   Traumatic arthropathy, wrist
  `6th`   M12.531   right wrist
            M12.532   left wrist
M12.54   Traumatic arthropathy, hand
  `6th`   M12.541   right hand
            M12.542   left hand
M12.55   Traumatic arthropathy, hip
  `6th`   M12.551   right hip
            M12.552   left hip
M12.56   Traumatic arthropathy, knee
  `6th`   M12.561   right knee
            M12.562   left knee

`4th` `5th` `6th` `7th` Additional Character Required   ✔ 3-character code

Unspecified laterality codes were excluded here.   •=New Code   ▲=Revised Code   *Excludes1*—Not coded here, do not use together   *Excludes2*—Not included here

M12.57 Traumatic arthropathy, ankle and foot
`6th` M12.571 right ankle and foot
M12.572 left ankle and foot
M12.58 Traumatic arthropathy, other specified site
Traumatic arthropathy, vertebrae
M12.59 Traumatic arthropathy, multiple sites
M12.9 Arthropathy, unspecified

M14 ARTHROPATHIES IN OTHER DISEASES CLASSIFIED
`4th` **ELSEWHERE**
Excludes1: arthropathy in:
DM (E08-E13 with .61-)
hematological disorders (M36.2-M36.3)
hypersensitivity reactions (M36.4)
neoplastic disease (M36.1)
neurosyphillis (A52.16)
sarcoidosis (D86.86)
enteropathic arthropathies (M07.-)
juvenile psoriatic arthropathy (L40.54)
lipoid dermatoarthritis (E78.81)
M14.8 Arthropathies in other specified diseases classified elsewhere
`5th` **Code first:** underlying disease, such as:
amyloidosis (E85.-)
erythema multiforme (L51.-)
erythema nodosum (L52)
hemochromatosis (E83.11-)
hyperparathyroidism (E21.-)
hypothyroidism (E00–E03)
sickle-cell disorders (D57.-)
thyrotoxicosis [hyperthyroidism] (E05.-)
Whipple's disease (K90.81)
M14.80 Arthropathies in other specified diseases classified elsewhere, unspecified site
M14.81 Arthropathies in other specified diseases classified
`6th` **elsewhere; shoulder**
M14.811 right shoulder
M14.812 left shoulder
M14.82 Arthropathies in other specified diseases classified
`6th` **elsewhere; elbow**
M14.821 right elbow
M14.822 left elbow
M14.83 Arthropathies in other specified diseases classified
`6th` **elsewhere; wrist**
M14.831 right wrist
M14.832 left wrist
M14.84 Arthropathies in other specified diseases classified
`6th` **elsewhere; hand**
M14.841 right hand
M14.842 left hand
M14.85 Arthropathies in other specified diseases classified
`6th` **elsewhere; hip**
M14.851 right hip
M14.852 left hip
M14.86 Arthropathies in other specified diseases classified
`6th` **elsewhere; knee**
M14.861 right knee
M14.862 left knee
M14.87 Arthropathies in other specified diseases classified
`6th` **elsewhere; ankle and foot**
M14.871 right ankle and foot
M14.872 left ankle and foot
M14.88 Arthropathies in other specified diseases classified elsewhere, vertebrae
M14.89 Arthropathies in other specified diseases classified elsewhere, multiple sites

(M15–M19) OSTEOARTHRITIS

Excludes2: osteoarthritis of spine (M47.-)

(M20–M25) OTHER JOINT DISORDERS

Excludes2: joints of the spine (M40–M54)

M20 ACQUIRED DEFORMITIES OF FINGERS AND TOES
`4th` *Excludes1:* acquired absence of fingers and toes (Z89.-)
congenital absence of fingers and toes (Q71.3-, Q72.3-)
congenital deformities and malformations of fingers and toes (Q66.-, Q68–Q70, Q74.-)
M20.0 Deformity of finger(s)
`5th` *Excludes1:* clubbing of fingers (R68.3)
palmar fascial fibromatosis [Dupuytren] (M72.0)
trigger finger (M65.3)
M20.00 Unspecified deformity of finger(s)
`6th` M20.001 Unspecified deformity of right finger(s)
M20.002 Unspecified deformity of left finger(s)
M20.01 Mallet finger
`6th` M20.011 Mallet finger of right finger(s)
M20.012 Mallet finger of left finger(s)
M20.09 Other deformity of finger(s)
`6th` M20.091 Other deformity of right finger(s)
M20.092 Other deformity of left finger(s)
M20.1 Hallux valgus (acquired)
`5th` *Excludes2:* bunion (M21.6-)
M20.11 Hallux valgus (acquired), right foot
M20.12 Hallux valgus (acquired), left foot
M20.5 Other deformities of toe(s) (acquired)
`5th` **M20.5X Other deformities of toe(s) (acquired)**
`6th` M20.5X1 right foot
M20.5X2 left foot
M20.6 Acquired deformities of toe(s), unspecified
`5th` **M20.61 Acquired deformities of toe(s), unspecified, right foot**
M20.62 Acquired deformities of toe(s), unspecified, left foot

M21 OTHER ACQUIRED DEFORMITIES OF LIMBS
`4th` *Excludes1:* acquired absence of limb (Z89.-)
congenital absence of limbs (Q71–Q73)
congenital deformities and malformations of limbs (Q65–Q66, Q68–Q74)
Excludes2: acquired deformities of fingers or toes (M20.-)
coxa plana (M91.2)
M21.0 Valgus deformity, NEC
`5th` *Excludes1:* metatarsus valgus (Q66.6)
talipes calcaneovalgus (Q66.4-)
M21.06 Valgus deformity, NEC, knee
`6th` Genu valgum
Knock knee
M21.061 right knee
M21.062 left knee
M21.1 Varus deformity, NEC
`5th` *Excludes1:* metatarsus varus (Q66.22-)
tibia vara (M92.51-)
M21.16 Varus deformity, NEC, knee
`6th` Bow leg
Genu varum
M21.161 right knee
M21.162 left knee
M21.2 Flexion deformity
`5th` **M21.21 Flexion deformity, shoulder**
`6th` M21.211 right shoulder
M21.212 left shoulder
M21.22 Flexion deformity, elbow
`6th` M21.221 right elbow
M21.222 left elbow
M21.23 Flexion deformity, wrist
`6th` M21.231 right wrist
M21.232 left wrist
M21.24 Flexion deformity, finger joints
`6th` M21.241 right finger joints
M21.242 left finger joints
M21.25 Flexion deformity, hip
`6th` M21.251 right hip
M21.252 left hip
M21.26 Flexion deformity, knee
`6th` M21.261 right knee
M21.262 left knee
M21.27 Flexion deformity, ankle and toes
`6th` M21.271 right ankle and toes

`4th` `5th` `6th` `7th` Additional Character Required ✔ 3-character code

Unspecified laterality codes were excluded here. •=New Code ▲=Revised Code *Excludes1*—Not coded here, do not use together *Excludes2*—Not included here

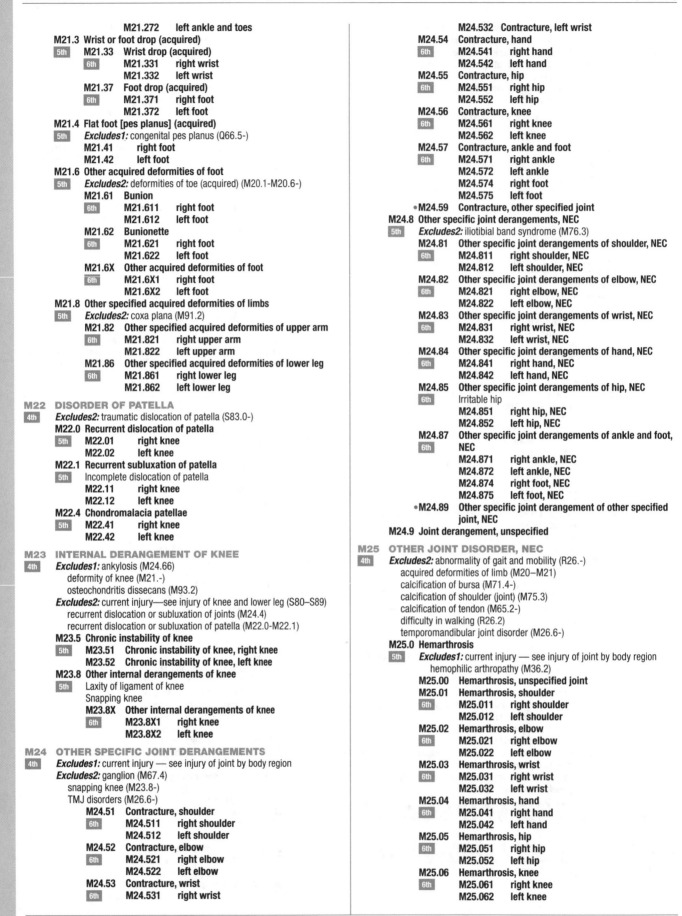

CHAPTER 13. DISEASES OF THE MUSCULOSKELETAL SYSTEM AND CONNECTIVE TISSUE (M21.272–M25.062)

M21.272   left ankle and toes

M21.3 Wrist or foot drop (acquired)
- `5th` M21.33   **Wrist drop (acquired)**
  - `6th` M21.331   **right wrist**
  - M21.332   **left wrist**
- M21.37   **Foot drop (acquired)**
  - `6th` M21.371   **right foot**
  - M21.372   **left foot**

M21.4 Flat foot [pes planus] (acquired)
- `5th` *Excludes1:* congenital pes planus (Q66.5-)
- M21.41   **right foot**
- M21.42   **left foot**

M21.6 Other acquired deformities of foot
- `5th` *Excludes2:* deformities of toe (acquired) (M20.1-M20.6-)
- M21.61   **Bunion**
  - `6th` M21.611   **right foot**
  - M21.612   **left foot**
- M21.62   **Bunionette**
  - `6th` M21.621   **right foot**
  - M21.622   **left foot**
- M21.6X   **Other acquired deformities of foot**
  - `6th` M21.6X1   **right foot**
  - M21.6X2   **left foot**

M21.8 Other specified acquired deformities of limbs
- `5th` *Excludes2:* coxa plana (M91.2)
- M21.82   **Other specified acquired deformities of upper arm**
  - `6th` M21.821   **right upper arm**
  - M21.822   **left upper arm**
- M21.86   **Other specified acquired deformities of lower leg**
  - `6th` M21.861   **right lower leg**
  - M21.862   **left lower leg**

M22 DISORDER OF PATELLA
- `4th` *Excludes2:* traumatic dislocation of patella (S83.0-)

M22.0 Recurrent dislocation of patella
- `5th` M22.01   **right knee**
- M22.02   **left knee**

M22.1 Recurrent subluxation of patella
- `5th` Incomplete dislocation of patella
- M22.11   **right knee**
- M22.12   **left knee**

M22.4 Chondromalacia patellae
- `5th` M22.41   **right knee**
- M22.42   **left knee**

M23 INTERNAL DERANGEMENT OF KNEE
- `4th` *Excludes1:* ankylosis (M24.66)
  - deformity of knee (M21.-)
  - osteochondritis dissecans (M93.2)
- *Excludes2:* current injury—see injury of knee and lower leg (S80–S89)
  - recurrent dislocation or subluxation of joints (M24.4)
  - recurrent dislocation or subluxation of patella (M22.0-M22.1)

M23.5 Chronic instability of knee
- `5th` M23.51   **Chronic instability of knee, right knee**
- M23.52   **Chronic instability of knee, left knee**

M23.8 Other internal derangements of knee
- `5th` Laxity of ligament of knee
- Snapping knee
- M23.8X   **Other internal derangements of knee**
  - `6th` M23.8X1   **right knee**
  - M23.8X2   **left knee**

M24 OTHER SPECIFIC JOINT DERANGEMENTS
- `4th` *Excludes1:* current injury — see injury of joint by body region
- *Excludes2:* ganglion (M67.4)
  - snapping knee (M23.8-)
  - TMJ disorders (M26.6-)
- M24.51   **Contracture, shoulder**
  - `6th` M24.511   **right shoulder**
  - M24.512   **left shoulder**
- M24.52   **Contracture, elbow**
  - `6th` M24.521   **right elbow**
  - M24.522   **left elbow**
- M24.53   **Contracture, wrist**
  - `6th` M24.531   **right wrist**

M24.532   **Contracture, left wrist**
- M24.54   **Contracture, hand**
  - `6th` M24.541   **right hand**
  - M24.542   **left hand**
- M24.55   **Contracture, hip**
  - `6th` M24.551   **right hip**
  - M24.552   **left hip**
- M24.56   **Contracture, knee**
  - `6th` M24.561   **right knee**
  - M24.562   **left knee**
- M24.57   **Contracture, ankle and foot**
  - `6th` M24.571   **right ankle**
  - M24.572   **left ankle**
  - M24.574   **right foot**
  - M24.575   **left foot**
- •M24.59   **Contracture, other specified joint**

M24.8 Other specific joint derangements, NEC
- `5th` *Excludes2:* iliotibial band syndrome (M76.3)
- M24.81   **Other specific joint derangements of shoulder, NEC**
  - `6th` M24.811   **right shoulder, NEC**
  - M24.812   **left shoulder, NEC**
- M24.82   **Other specific joint derangements of elbow, NEC**
  - `6th` M24.821   **right elbow, NEC**
  - M24.822   **left elbow, NEC**
- M24.83   **Other specific joint derangements of wrist, NEC**
  - `6th` M24.831   **right wrist, NEC**
  - M24.832   **left wrist, NEC**
- M24.84   **Other specific joint derangements of hand, NEC**
  - `6th` M24.841   **right hand, NEC**
  - M24.842   **left hand, NEC**
- M24.85   **Other specific joint derangements of hip, NEC**
  - `6th` Irritable hip
  - M24.851   **right hip, NEC**
  - M24.852   **left hip, NEC**
- M24.87   **Other specific joint derangements of ankle and foot, NEC**
  - `6th` M24.871   **right ankle, NEC**
  - M24.872   **left ankle, NEC**
  - M24.874   **right foot, NEC**
  - M24.875   **left foot, NEC**
- •M24.89   **Other specific joint derangement of other specified joint, NEC**

M24.9 Joint derangement, unspecified

M25 OTHER JOINT DISORDER, NEC
- `4th` *Excludes2:* abnormality of gait and mobility (R26.-)
  - acquired deformities of limb (M20–M21)
  - calcification of bursa (M71.4-)
  - calcification of shoulder (joint) (M75.3)
  - calcification of tendon (M65.2-)
  - difficulty in walking (R26.2)
  - temporomandibular joint disorder (M26.6-)

M25.0 Hemarthrosis
- `5th` *Excludes1:* current injury — see injury of joint by body region
  - hemophilic arthropathy (M36.2)
- M25.00   **Hemarthrosis, unspecified joint**
- M25.01   **Hemarthrosis, shoulder**
  - `6th` M25.011   **right shoulder**
  - M25.012   **left shoulder**
- M25.02   **Hemarthrosis, elbow**
  - `6th` M25.021   **right elbow**
  - M25.022   **left elbow**
- M25.03   **Hemarthrosis, wrist**
  - `6th` M25.031   **right wrist**
  - M25.032   **left wrist**
- M25.04   **Hemarthrosis, hand**
  - `6th` M25.041   **right hand**
  - M25.042   **left hand**
- M25.05   **Hemarthrosis, hip**
  - `6th` M25.051   **right hip**
  - M25.052   **left hip**
- M25.06   **Hemarthrosis, knee**
  - `6th` M25.061   **right knee**
  - M25.062   **left knee**

`4th` `5th` `6th` `7th` Additional Character Required   ✓ 3-character code

Unspecified laterality codes were excluded here.   •=New Code   ▲=Revised Code   *Excludes1*—Not coded here, do not use together *Excludes2*—Not included here

M25.07 Hemarthrosis, ankle and foot
> 6th   M25.071   right ankle
> M25.072   left ankle
> M25.074   right foot
> M25.075   left foot

M25.08 Hemarthrosis, other specified site
> Hemarthrosis, vertebrae

M25.2 Flail joint
> 5th   **M25.21 Flail joint, shoulder**
>> 6th   M25.211   right shoulder
>> M25.212   left shoulder
> **M25.22 Flail joint, elbow**
>> 6th   M25.221   right elbow
>> M25.222   left elbow
> **M25.23 Flail joint, wrist**
>> 6th   M25.231   right wrist
>> M25.232   left wrist
> **M25.24 Flail joint, hand**
>> 6th   M25.241   right hand
>> M25.242   left hand
> **M25.25 Flail joint, hip**
>> 6th   M25.251   right hip
>> M25.252   left hip
> **M25.26 Flail joint, knee**
>> 6th   M25.261   right knee
>> M25.262   left knee
> **M25.27 Flail joint, ankle and foot**
>> 6th   M25.271   right ankle and foot
>> M25.272   left ankle and foot
> **M25.28 Flail joint, other site**

M25.3 Other instability of joint
> 5th   *Excludes1:* instability of joint secondary to old ligament injury (M24.2-)
> instability of joint secondary to removal of joint prosthesis (M96.8-)
> *Excludes2:* spinal instabilities (M53.2-)
> **M25.30 Other instability, unspecified joint**
> **M25.31 Other instability, shoulder**
>> 6th   M25.311   right shoulder
>> M25.312   left shoulder
> **M25.32 Other instability, elbow**
>> 6th   M25.321   right elbow
>> M25.322   left elbow
> **M25.33 Other instability, wrist**
>> 6th   M25.331   right wrist
>> M25.332   left wrist
> **M25.34 Other instability, hand**
>> 6th   M25.341   right hand
>> M25.342   left hand
> **M25.35 Other instability, hip**
>> 6th   M25.351   right hip
>> M25.352   left hip
> **M25.36 Other instability, knee**
>> 6th   M25.361   right knee
>> M25.362   left knee
> **M25.37 Other instability, ankle and foot**
>> 6th   M25.371   right ankle
>> M25.372   left ankle
>> M25.374   right foot
>> M25.375   left foot
> **•M25.39 Other instability, other specified joint**

M25.4 Effusion of joint
> 5th   *Excludes1:* hydrarthrosis in yaws (A66.6)
> intermittent hydrarthrosis (M12.4-)
> other infective (teno)synovitis (M65.1-)
> **M25.40 Effusion, unspecified joint**
> **M25.41 Effusion, shoulder**
>> 6th   M25.411   right shoulder
>> M25.412   left shoulder
> **M25.42 Effusion, elbow**
>> 6th   M25.421   right elbow
>> M25.422   left elbow
> **M25.43 Effusion, wrist**
>> 6th   M25.431   right wrist

> M25.432   left wrist
> **M25.44 Effusion, hand**
>> 6th   M25.441   right hand
>> M25.442   left hand
> **M25.45 Effusion, hip**
>> 6th   M25.451   right hip
>> M25.452   left hip
> **M25.46 Effusion, knee**
>> 6th   M25.461   right knee
>> M25.462   left knee
> **M25.47 Effusion, ankle and foot**
>> 6th   M25.471   right ankle
>> M25.472   left ankle
>> M25.474   right foot
>> M25.475   left foot
> **M25.48 Effusion, other site**

M25.5 Pain in joint
> 5th   *Excludes2:* pain in hand (M79.64-)
> pain in fingers (M79.64-)
> pain in foot (M79.67-)
> pain in limb (M79.6-)
> pain in toes (M79.67-)
> **M25.50 Pain in unspecified joint**
> **M25.51 Pain in shoulder**
>> 6th   M25.511   right shoulder
>> M25.512   left shoulder
> **M25.52 Pain in elbow**
>> 6th   M25.521   right elbow
>> M25.522   left elbow
> **M25.53 Pain in wrist**
>> 6th   M25.531   right wrist
>> M25.532   left wrist
> **M25.54 Pain in hand joints**
>> 6th   M25.541   right hand
>> M25.542   left hand
> **M25.55 Pain in hip**
>> 6th   M25.551   right hip
>> M25.552   left hip
> **M25.56 Pain in knee**
>> 6th   M25.561   right knee
>> M25.562   left knee
> **M25.57 Pain in ankle and joints of foot**
>> 6th   M25.571   Pain in right ankle and joints of right foot
>> M25.572   Pain in left ankle and joints of left foot
> **•M25.59 Pain in other specified joint**

M25.6 Stiffness of joint, NEC
> 5th   *Excludes1:* ankylosis of joint (M24.6-)
> contracture of joint (M24.5-)
> **M25.60 Stiffness of unspecified joint, NEC**
> **M25.61 Stiffness of shoulder, NEC**
>> 6th   M25.611   Stiffness of right shoulder, NEC
>> M25.612   Stiffness of left shoulder, NEC
> **M25.62 Stiffness of elbow, NEC**
>> 6th   M25.621   Stiffness of right elbow, NEC
>> M25.622   Stiffness of left elbow, NEC
> **M25.63 Stiffness of wrist, NEC**
>> 6th   M25.631   Stiffness of right wrist, NEC
>> M25.632   Stiffness of left wrist, NEC
> **M25.64 Stiffness of hand, NEC**
>> 6th   M25.641   Stiffness of right hand, NEC
>> M25.642   Stiffness of left hand, NEC
> **M25.65 Stiffness of hip, NEC**
>> 6th   M25.651   Stiffness of right hip, NEC
>> M25.652   Stiffness of left hip, NEC
> **M25.66 Stiffness of knee, NEC**
>> 6th   M25.661   Stiffness of right knee, NEC
>> M25.662   Stiffness of left knee, NEC
> **M25.67 Stiffness of ankle and foot, NEC**
>> 6th   M25.671   Stiffness of right ankle, NEC
>> M25.672   Stiffness of left ankle, NEC
>> M25.674   Stiffness of right foot, NEC
>> M25.675   Stiffness of left foot, NEC
> **•M25.69 Stiffness of other specified joint, NEC**

| 4th | 5th | 6th | 7th | Additional Character Required | ✓ | 3-character code | Unspecified laterality codes were excluded here. | •=New Code ▲=Revised Code | *Excludes1*—Not coded here, do not use together *Excludes2*—Not included here |

M25.7 Osteophyte
- **5th** **M25.70 Osteophyte, unspecified joint**
- **M25.71 Osteophyte, shoulder**
  - **6th** **M25.711 right shoulder**
  - **M25.712 left shoulder**
- **M25.72 Osteophyte, elbow**
  - **6th** **M25.721 right elbow**
  - **M25.722 left elbow**
- **M25.73 Osteophyte, wrist**
  - **6th** **M25.731 right wrist**
  - **M25.732 left wrist**
- **M25.74 Osteophyte, hand**
  - **6th** **M25.741 right hand**
  - **M25.742 left hand**
- **M25.75 Osteophyte, hip**
  - **6th** **M25.751 right hip**
  - **M25.752 left hip**
- **M25.76 Osteophyte, knee**
  - **6th** **M25.761 right knee**
  - **M25.762 left knee**
- **M25.77 Osteophyte, ankle and foot**
  - **6th** **M25.771 right ankle**
  - **M25.772 left ankle**
  - **M25.774 right foot**
  - **M25.775 left foot**
- **M25.78 Osteophyte, vertebrae**

M25.9 Joint disorder, unspecified

(M26–M27) DENTOFACIAL ANOMALIES [INCLUDING MALOCCLUSION] AND OTHER DISORDERS OF JAW

Excludes1: hemifacial atrophy or hypertrophy (Q67.4)
   unilateral condylar hyperplasia or hypoplasia (M27.8)

M26 DENTOFACIAL ANOMALIES [INCLUDING
4th MALOCCLUSION]
- **M26.0 Major anomalies of jaw size**
  - **5th** *Excludes1:* acromegaly (E22.0)
    - Robin's syndrome (Q87.0)
  - **M26.00 Unspecified anomaly of jaw size**
  - **M26.04 Mandibular hypoplasia**
  - **M26.09 Other specified anomalies of jaw size**
- **M26.2 Anomalies of dental arch relationship**
  - **5th** **M26.20 Unspecified anomaly of dental arch relationship**
  - **M26.29 Other anomalies of dental arch relationship**
    - Midline deviation of dental arch
    - Overbite (excessive) deep
    - Overbite (excessive) horizontal
    - Overbite (excessive) vertical
    - Posterior lingual occlusion of mandibular teeth
- **M26.4 Malocclusion, unspecified**
- **M26.6 Temporomandibular joint disorders**
  - **5th** *Excludes2:* current temporomandibular joint dislocation (S03.0)
    - current temporomandibular joint sprain (S03.4)
  - **M26.60 Temporomandibular joint disorder, unspecified**
    - **6th** **M26.601 Right temporomandibular joint disorder**
    - **M26.602 Left temporomandibular joint disorder**
    - **M26.603 Bilateral temporomandibular joint disorder**
  - **M26.61 Adhesions and ankylosis of temporomandibular joint**
    - **6th** **M26.611 Adhesions and ankylosis of right temporomandibular joint**
    - **M26.612 Adhesions and ankylosis of left temporomandibular joint**
    - **M26.613 Adhesions and ankylosis of bilateral temporomandibular joint**
  - **M26.62 Arthralgia of temporomandibular joint**
    - **6th** **M26.621 Arthralgia of right temporomandibular joint**
    - **M26.622 Arthralgia of left temporomandibular joint**
    - **M26.623 Arthralgia of bilateral temporomandibular joint**
  - **M26.63 Articular disc disorder of temporomandibular joint**
    - **6th** **M26.631 Articular disc disorder of right temporomandibular joint**
    - **M26.632 Articular disc disorder of left temporomandibular joint**
    - **M26.633 Articular disc disorder of bilateral temporomandibular joint**
  - **M26.69 Other specified disorders of temporomandibular joint**

M27 OTHER DISEASES OF JAWS
- **4th** **M27.0 Developmental disorders of jaws**
  - Latent bone cyst of jaw
  - Stafne's cyst
  - Torus mandibularis
  - Torus palatinus
- **M27.2 Inflammatory conditions of jaws**
  - Osteitis of jaw(s)
  - Osteomyelitis (neonatal) jaw(s)
  - Osteoradionecrosis jaw(s)
  - Periostitis jaw(s)
  - Sequestrum of jaw bone
  - **Use additional code** (W88–W90, X39.0) to identify radiation, if radiation-induced
  - *Excludes2:* osteonecrosis of jaw due to drug (M87.180)
- **M27.4 Other and unspecified cysts of jaw**
  - **5th** *Excludes1:* cysts of oral region (K09.-)
    - latent bone cyst of jaw (M27.0)
    - Stafne's cyst (M27.0)
  - **M27.40 Unspecified cyst of jaw**
    - Cyst of jaw NOS
  - **M27.49 Other cysts of jaw**
    - Aneurysmal cyst of jaw
    - Hemorrhagic cyst of jaw
    - Traumatic cyst of jaw
- **M27.8 Other specified diseases of jaws**
  - Cherubism
  - Exostosis
  - Fibrous dysplasia
  - Unilateral condylar hyperplasia
  - Unilateral condylar hypoplasia
  - *Excludes1:* jaw pain (R68.84)

(M30–M36) SYSTEMIC CONNECTIVE TISSUE DISORDERS

Includes: autoimmune disease NOS
   collagen (vascular) disease NOS
   systemic autoimmune disease
   systemic collagen (vascular) disease
Excludes1: autoimmune disease, single organ or single cell type—code to relevant condition category

M30 POLYARTERITIS NODOSA AND RELATED CONDITIONS
- **4th** *Excludes1:* microscopic polyarteritis (M31.7)
- **M30.2 Juvenile polyarteritis**
- **M30.3 Mucocutaneous lymph node syndrome [Kawasaki]**
- **M30.8 Other conditions related to polyarteritis nodosa**
  - Polyangiitis overlap syndrome

M31 OTHER NECROTIZING VASCULOPATHIES
- **4th** **M31.0 Hypersensitivity angiitis**
  - Goodpasture's syndrome
- **M31.1 Thrombotic microangiopathy**
  - Thrombotic thrombocytopenic purpura
- **M31.3 Wegener's granulomatosis**
  - **5th** Granulomatosis with polyangiitis
    - Necrotizing respiratory granulomatosis
  - **M31.30 Wegener's granulomatosis without renal involvement**
    - Wegener's granulomatosis NOS
  - **M31.31 Wegener's granulomatosis with renal involvement**
- **M31.4 Aortic arch syndrome [Takayasu]**
- **M31.8 Other specified necrotizing vasculopathies**
  - Hypocomplementemic vasculitis
  - Septic vasculitis
- **M31.9 Necrotizing vasculopathy, unspecified**

M32 SLE
- **4th** *Excludes1:* lupus erythematosus (discoid) (NOS) (L93.0)
- **M32.0 Drug-induced systemic lupus erythematosus**
  - **Use additional code** for adverse effect, if applicable, to identify drug (T36–T50 with fifth or sixth character 5)

4th **5th** **6th** **7th** Additional Character Required   ✓   3-character code

Unspecified laterality codes were excluded here.   •=New Code   ▲=Revised Code   *Excludes1*—Not coded here, do not use together   *Excludes2*—Not included here

M32.1 SLE with organ or system involvement
> **5th** **M32.10** SLE, organ or system involvement unspecified
> **M32.11 Endocarditis in SLE**
> Libman-Sacks disease
> **M32.12 Pericarditis in SLE**
> Lupus pericarditis
> **M32.13 Lung involvement in SLE**
> Pleural effusion due to SLE
> **M32.14 Glomerular disease in SLE**
> Lupus renal disease NOS
> **M32.15 Tubulo-interstitial nephropathy in SLE**
> **M32.19 Other organ or system involvement in SLE**

M32.8 Other forms of SLE

M32.9 SLE, unspecified
> SLE NOS
> SLE NOS
> SLE without organ involvement

M33 DERMATOPOLYMYOSITIS (4th)
> **M33.0 Juvenile dermatomyositis**
>> **5th** **M33.00 Juvenile dermatomyositis, organ involvement unspecified**
>> **M33.01 Juvenile dermatomyositis with respiratory involvement**
>> **M33.02 Juvenile dermatomyositis with myopathy**
>> **M33.03 Juvenile dermatomyositis without myopathy**
>> **M33.09 Juvenile dermatomyositis with other organ involvement**

> **M33.1 Other dermatomyositis**
>> **5th** Adult dermatomyositis
>> **M33.10 Other dermatomyositis, organ involvement unspecified**
>> **M33.11 Other dermatomyositis with respiratory involvement**
>> **M33.12 Other dermatomyositis with myopathy**
>> **M33.13 Other dermatomyositis without myopathy**
>> Dermatomyositis NOS
>> **M33.19 Other dermatomyositis with other organ involvement**

> **M33.9 Dermatopolymyositis, unspecified**
>> **5th** **M33.90 Dermatopolymyositis, unspecified, organ involvement unspecified**
>> **M33.91 Dermatopolymyositis, unspecified with respiratory involvement**
>> **M33.92 Dermatopolymyositis, unspecified with myopathy**
>> **M33.93 Dermatopolymyositis, unspecified without myopathy**
>> **M33.99 Dermatopolymyositis, unspecified with other organ involvement**

M35 OTHER SYSTEMIC INVOLVEMENT OF CONNECTIVE TISSUE (4th)
> *Excludes1:* reactive perforating collagenosis (L87.1)
> **M35.7 Hypermobility syndrome**
> Familial ligamentous laxity
> *Excludes1:* Ehlers-Danlos syndromes (Q79.6-)
> ligamentous laxity, NOS (M24.2-)
> **M35.8 Other specified systemic involvement of connective tissue**
> **M35.9 Systemic involvement of connective tissue, unspecified**
> Autoimmune disease (systemic) NOS
> Collagen (vascular) disease NOS

M36 SYSTEMIC DISORDERS OF CONNECTIVE TISSUE IN DISEASES CLASSIFIED ELSEWHERE (4th)
> *Excludes2:* arthropathies in diseases classified elsewhere (M14.-)
> **M36.0 Dermato(poly)myositis in neoplastic disease**
> Code first underlying neoplasm (C00-D49)
> **M36.1 Arthropathy in neoplastic disease**
> Code first underlying neoplasm, such as:
> leukemia (C91-C95)
> malignant histiocytosis (C96.A)
> multiple myeloma (C90.0)
> **M36.2 Hemophilic arthropathy**
> Hemarthrosis in hemophilic arthropathy
> Code first: underlying disease, such as: factor VIII deficiency (D66)
> with vascular defect (D68.0)
> factor IX deficiency (D67)

hemophilia (classical) (D66)
hemophilia B (D67)
hemophilia C (D68.1)
M36.3 Arthropathy in other blood disorders
M36.4 Arthropathy in hypersensitivity reactions classified elsewhere
> Code first underlying disease, such as Henoch (-Schönlein) purpura (D69.0)
> serum sickness (T80.6-)

M36.8 Systemic disorders of connective tissue in other diseases classified elsewhere
> Code first underlying disease, such as:
> alkaptonuria (E70.2)
> hypogammaglobulinemia (D80.-)
> ochronosis (E70.2)

(M40–M43) DEFORMING DORSOPATHIES

M40 KYPHOSIS AND LORDOSIS (4th)
> *Excludes1:* congenital kyphosis and lordosis (Q76.4)
> kyphoscoliosis (M41.-)
> postprocedural kyphosis and lordosis (M96.-)

> **M40.2 Other and unspecified kyphosis**
>> **5th** **M40.20 Unspecified kyphosis**
>>> **6th** M40.202 cervical region
>>> M40.203 cervicothoracic region
>>> M40.204 thoracic region
>>> M40.205 thoracolumbar region
>>> M40.209 site unspecified
>> **M40.29 Other kyphosis**
>>> **6th** M40.292 cervical region
>>> M40.293 cervicothoracic region
>>> M40.294 thoracic region
>>> M40.295 thoracolumbar region
>>> M40.299 site unspecified

> **M40.4 Postural lordosis**
>> **5th** Acquired lordosis
>> M40.40 site unspecified
>> M40.45 thoracolumbar region
>> M40.46 lumbar region
>> M40.47 lumbosacral region

> **M40.5 Lordosis, unspecified**
>> **5th** M40.50 site unspecified
>> M40.55 thoracolumbar region
>> M40.56 lumbar region
>> M40.57 lumbosacral region

M41 SCOLIOSIS (4th)
> *Includes:* kyphoscoliosis
> *Excludes1:* congenital scoliosis NOS (Q67.5)
> congenital scoliosis due to bony malformation (Q76.3)
> postural congenital scoliosis (Q67.5)
> kyphoscoliotic heart disease (I27.1)
> postprocedural scoliosis (M96.-)

> **M41.0 Infantile idiopathic scoliosis**
>> **5th** M41.00 site unspecified
>> M41.02 cervical region
>> M41.03 cervicothoracic region
>> M41.04 thoracic region
>> M41.05 thoracolumbar region
>> M41.06 lumbar region
>> M41.07 lumbosacral region
>> M41.08 sacral and sacrococcygeal region

> **M41.1 Juvenile and adolescent idiopathic scoliosis**
>> **5th** **M41.11 Juvenile idiopathic scoliosis**
>>> **6th** M41.112 cervical region
>>> M41.113 cervicothoracic region
>>> M41.114 thoracic region
>>> M41.115 thoracolumbar region
>>> M41.116 lumbar region
>>> M41.117 lumbosacral region
>>> M41.119 site unspecified
>> **M41.12 Adolescent scoliosis**
>>> **6th** **M41.122 Adolescent idiopathic scoliosis, cervical region**

4th **5th** **6th** **7th** Additional Character Required   ✓ 3-character code

Unspecified laterality codes were excluded here.
●=New Code
▲=Revised Code
Excludes1—Not coded here, do not use together
Excludes2—Not included here

M41.123 **Adolescent idiopathic scoliosis, cervicothoracic region**
M41.124 **Adolescent idiopathic scoliosis, thoracic region**
M41.125 **Adolescent idiopathic scoliosis, thoracolumbar region**
M41.126 **Adolescent idiopathic scoliosis, lumbar region**
M41.127 **Adolescent idiopathic scoliosis, lumbosacral region**
M41.129 **Adolescent idiopathic scoliosis, site unspecified**

M41.2 **Other idiopathic scoliosis**
[5th] M41.20 **Other idiopathic scoliosis, site unspecified**
M41.22 **Other idiopathic scoliosis, cervical region**
M41.23 **Other idiopathic scoliosis, cervicothoracic region**
M41.24 **Other idiopathic scoliosis, thoracic region**
M41.25 **Other idiopathic scoliosis, thoracolumbar region**
M41.26 **Other idiopathic scoliosis, lumbar region**
M41.27 **Other idiopathic scoliosis, lumbosacral region**

M41.9 **Scoliosis, unspecified**

M43 **OTHER DEFORMING DORSOPATHIES**
[4th] *Excludes1:* congenital spondylolysis and spondylolisthesis (Q76.2)
hemivertebra (Q76.3–Q76.4)
Klippel-Feil syndrome (Q76.1)
lumbarization and sacralization (Q76.4)
platyspondylisis (Q76.4)
spina bifida occulta (Q76.0)
spinal curvature in osteoporosis (M80.-)
spinal curvature in Paget's disease of bone [osteitis deformans] (M88.-)

M43.0 **Spondylolysis**
[5th] *Excludes1:* congenital spondylolysis (Q76.2)
spondylolisthesis (M43.1)
M43.00 **Spondylolysis, site unspecified**
M43.01 **Spondylolysis, occipito-atlanto-axial region**
M43.02 **Spondylolysis, cervical region**
M43.03 **Spondylolysis, cervicothoracic region**
M43.04 **Spondylolysis, thoracic region**
M43.05 **Spondylolysis, thoracolumbar region**
M43.06 **Spondylolysis, lumbar region**
M43.07 **Spondylolysis, lumbosacral region**
M43.08 **Spondylolysis, sacral and sacrococcygeal region**
M43.09 **Spondylolysis, multiple sites in spine**

M43.1 **Spondylolisthesis**
[5th] *Excludes1:* acute traumatic of lumbosacral region (S33.1)
acute traumatic of sites other than lumbosacral- code to Fracture, vertebra, by region
congenital spondylolisthesis (Q76.2)
M43.10 **Spondylolisthesis, site unspecified**
M43.11 **Spondylolisthesis, occipito-atlanto-axial region**
M43.12 **Spondylolisthesis, cervical region**
M43.13 **Spondylolisthesis, cervicothoracic region**
M43.14 **Spondylolisthesis, thoracic region**
M43.15 **Spondylolisthesis, thoracolumbar region**
M43.16 **Spondylolisthesis, lumbar region**
M43.17 **Spondylolisthesis, lumbosacral region**
M43.18 **Spondylolisthesis, sacral and sacrococcygeal region**
M43.19 **Spondylolisthesis, multiple sites in spine**

M43.6 **Torticollis**
Excludes1: congenital (sternomastoid) torticollis (Q68.0)
current injury — see Injury, of spine, by body region
ocular torticollis (R29.891)
psychogenic torticollis (F45.8)
spasmodic torticollis (G24.3)
torticollis due to birth injury (P15.2)

(M45–M49) SPONDYLOPATHIES

M48 **OTHER SPONDYLOPATHIES**
[4th] M48.0 **Spinal stenosis**
[5th] Caudal stenosis
M48.00 **Spinal stenosis, site unspecified**
M48.01 **Spinal stenosis, occipito-atlanto-axial region**

M48.02 **Spinal stenosis, cervical region**
M48.03 **Spinal stenosis, cervicothoracic region**
M48.04 **Spinal stenosis, thoracic region**
M48.05 **Spinal stenosis, thoracolumbar region**
M48.06 **Spinal stenosis, lumbar region**
[6th] M48.061 **Spinal stenosis, lumbar region without neurogenic claudication**
Spinal stenosis, lumbar region NOS
M48.062 **Spinal stenosis, lumbar region with neurogenic claudication**
M48.07 **Spinal stenosis, lumbosacral region**
M48.08 **Spinal stenosis, sacral and sacrococcygeal region**

(M50–M54) OTHER DORSOPATHIES

Excludes1: current injury — see injury of spine by body region
discitis NOS (M46.4-)

M53 **OTHER AND UNSPECIFIED DORSOPATHIES, NOT**
[4th] **ELSEWHERE CLASSIFIED**
M53.3 **Sacrococcygeal disorders, not elsewhere classified**
Coccygodynia
M53.9 **Dorsopathy, unspecified**

M54 **DORSALGIA**
[4th] *Excludes1:* psychogenic dorsalgia (F45.41)
M54.2 **Cervicalgia**
Excludes1: cervicalgia due to intervertebral cervical disc disorder (M50.-)
M54.4 **Lumbago with sciatica**
[5th] *Excludes1:* lumbago with sciatica due to intervertebral disc disorder (M51.1-)
M54.40 **Lumbago with sciatica, unspecified side**
M54.41 **Lumbago with sciatica, right side**
M54.42 **Lumbago with sciatica, left side**
M54.5 **Low back pain**
Loin pain
Lumbago NOS
Excludes1: low back strain (S39.012)
lumbago due to intervertebral disc displacement (M51.2-)
lumbago with sciatica (M54.4-)
M54.9 **Dorsalgia, unspecified**
Backache NOS
Back pain NOS

(M60–M79) Soft tissue disorders

(M60–M63) DISORDERS OF MUSCLES

M60 **MYOSITIS**
[4th] *Excludes2:* inclusion body myositis [IBM] (G72.41)
M60.0 **Infective myositis**
[5th] Tropical pyomyositis
Use additional code (B95–B97) to identify infectious agent
M60.00 **Infective myositis, unspecified site**
[6th] M60.000 **Infective myositis, unspecified right arm**
Infective myositis, right upper limb NOS
M60.001 **Infective myositis, unspecified left arm**
Infective myositis, left upper limb NOS
M60.003 **Infective myositis, unspecified right leg**
Infective myositis, right lower limb NOS
M60.004 **Infective myositis, unspecified left leg**
Infective myositis, left lower limb NOS
M60.009 **Infective myositis, unspecified site**
M60.01 **Infective myositis, shoulder**
[6th] M60.011 **right shoulder**
M60.012 **left shoulder**
M60.02 **Infective myositis, upper arm**
[6th] M60.021 **right upper arm**
M60.022 **left upper arm**
M60.03 **Infective myositis, forearm**
[6th] M60.031 **right forearm**
M60.032 **left forearm**
M60.04 **Infective myositis, hand and fingers**
[6th] M60.041 **right hand**

[4th] [5th] [6th] [7th] Additional Character Required ✓ 3-character code

Unspecified laterality codes were excluded here.
*=New Code
▲=Revised Code
Excludes1—Not coded here, do not use together
Excludes2—Not included here

M60.042   left hand
M60.044   right finger(s)
M60.045   left finger(s)

M60.05   **Infective myositis, thigh**
  6th   M60.051   right thigh
       M60.052   left thigh

M60.06   **Infective myositis, lower leg**
  6th   M60.061   right lower leg
       M60.062   left lower leg

M60.07   **Infective myositis, ankle, foot and toes**
  6th   M60.070   right ankle
       M60.071   left ankle
       M60.073   right foot
       M60.074   left foot
       M60.076   right toe(s)
       M60.077   left toe(s)

M60.08   **Infective myositis, other site**
M60.09   **Infective myositis, multiple sites**

M60.1   **Interstitial myositis**
 5th   M60.10   **Interstitial myositis of unspecified site**
       M60.11   **Interstitial myositis, shoulder**
    6th   M60.111   right shoulder
         M60.112   left shoulder
       M60.12   **Interstitial myositis, upper arm**
    6th   M60.121   right upper arm
         M60.122   left upper arm
       M60.13   **Interstitial myositis, forearm**
    6th   M60.131   right forearm
         M60.132   left forearm
       M60.14   **Interstitial myositis, hand**
    6th   M60.141   right hand
         M60.142   left hand
       M60.15   **Interstitial myositis, thigh**
    6th   M60.151   right thigh
         M60.152   left thigh
       M60.16   **Interstitial myositis, lower leg**
    6th   M60.161   right lower leg
         M60.162   left lower leg

M60.2   **Foreign body granuloma of soft tissue, not elsewhere**
 5th   **classified**
       Use additional code to identify the type of retained foreign body
       (Z18.-)
       Excludes1: foreign body granuloma of skin and subcutaneous
       tissue (L92.3)
       M60.21   **Foreign body granuloma of soft tissue, NEC, shoulder**
    6th   M60.211   right shoulder
         M60.212   left shoulder
       M60.22   **Foreign body granuloma of soft tissue, NEC, upper**
    6th   **arm**
         M60.221   right upper arm
         M60.222   left upper arm
       M60.23   **Foreign body granuloma of soft tissue, NEC, forearm**
    6th   M60.231   right forearm
         M60.232   left forearm
       M60.24   **Foreign body granuloma of soft tissue, NEC, hand**
    6th   M60.241   right hand
         M60.242   left hand
       M60.25   **Foreign body granuloma of soft tissue, NEC, thigh**
    6th   M60.251   right thigh
         M60.252   left thigh
       M60.26   **Foreign body granuloma of soft tissue, NEC, lower**
    6th   **leg**
         M60.261   right lower leg
         M60.262   left lower leg
       M60.27   **Foreign body granuloma of soft tissue, NEC, ankle**
    6th   **and foot**
         M60.271   right ankle and foot
         M60.272   left ankle and foot
       M60.28   **Foreign body granuloma of soft tissue, NEC, other**
       site

M60.9   **Myositis, unspecified**

M62   **OTHER DISORDERS OF MUSCLE**
 4th   ***Excludes1:*** alcoholic myopathy (G72.1)
       cramp and spasm (R25.2)
       drug-induced myopathy (G72.0)
       myalgia (M79.1-)
       stiff-man syndrome (G25.82)
       Excludes2: nontraumatic hematoma of muscle (M79.81)

M62.4   **Contracture of muscle**
 5th   Contracture of tendon (sheath)
       Excludes1: contracture of joint (M24.5-)
       M62.40   **Contracture of muscle, unspecified site**
       M62.41   **Contracture of muscle, shoulder**
    6th   M62.411   right shoulder
         M62.412   left shoulder
       M62.42   **Contracture of muscle, upper arm**
    6th   M62.421   right upper arm
         M62.422   left upper arm
       M62.43   **Contracture of muscle, forearm**
    6th   M62.431   right forearm
         M62.432   left forearm
       M62.44   **Contracture of muscle, hand**
    6th   M62.441   right hand
         M62.442   left hand
       M62.45   **Contracture of muscle, thigh**
    6th   M62.451   right thigh
         M62.452   left thigh
       M62.46   **Contracture of muscle, lower leg**
    6th   M62.461   right lower leg
         M62.462   left lower leg
       M62.47   **Contracture of muscle, ankle and foot**
    6th   M62.471   right ankle and foot
         M62.472   left ankle and foot
       M62.48   **Contracture of muscle, other site**
       M62.49   **Contracture of muscle, multiple sites**

M62.8   **Other specified disorders of muscle**
 5th   ***Excludes2:*** nontraumatic hematoma of muscle (M79.81)
       M62.81   **Muscle weakness (generalized)**
         Excludes1: muscle weakness in sarcopenia (M62.84)
       M62.82   **Rhabdomyolysis**
         Excludes1: traumatic rhabdomyolysis (T79.6)
       M62.83   **Muscle spasm**
    6th   M62.830   **Muscle spasm of back**
         M62.831   **Muscle spasm of calf**
            Charley-horse
         M62.838   **Other muscle spasm**
       M62.89   **Other specified disorders of muscle**
         Muscle (sheath) hernia

M62.9   **Disorder of muscle, unspecified**

(M65–M67) DISORDERS OF SYNOVIUM AND TENDON

M65   **SYNOVITIS AND TENOSYNOVITIS**
 4th   ***Excludes1:*** chronic crepitant synovitis of hand and wrist (M70.0-)
       current injury — see injury of ligament or tendon by body region
       soft tissue disorders related to use, overuse and pressure (M70.-)

M65.4   **Radial styloid tenosynovitis [de Quervain]**

M65.8   **Other synovitis and tenosynovitis**
 5th   M65.80   **Other synovitis and tenosynovitis, unspecified site**
       M65.81   **Other synovitis and tenosynovitis; shoulder**
    6th   M65.811   right shoulder
         M65.812   left shoulder
       M65.82   **Other synovitis and tenosynovitis; upper arm**
    6th   M65.821   right upper arm
         M65.822   left upper arm
       M65.83   **Other synovitis and tenosynovitis; forearm**
    6th   M65.831   right forearm
         M65.832   left forearm
       M65.84   **Other synovitis and tenosynovitis; hand**
    6th   M65.841   right hand
         M65.842   left hand
       M65.85   **Other synovitis and tenosynovitis; thigh**
    6th   M65.851   right thigh
         M65.852   left thigh

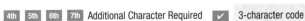

4th   **5th**   **6th**   **7th**   Additional Character Required   ✔   3-character code

Unspecified laterality codes
were excluded here.

•=New Code
▲=Revised Code

Excludes1—Not coded here, do not use together
Excludes2—Not included here

CHAPTER 13. DISEASES OF THE MUSCULOSKELETAL SYSTEM AND CONNECTIVE TISSUE (M65.86–M76)

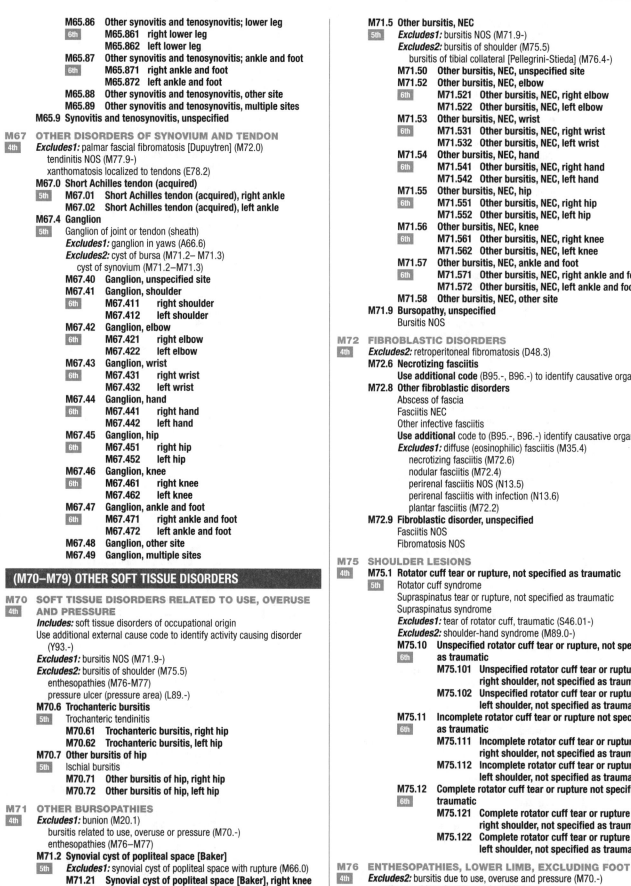

M65.86 **Other synovitis and tenosynovitis; lower leg**
6th
    M65.861 right lower leg
    M65.862 left lower leg
M65.87 **Other synovitis and tenosynovitis; ankle and foot**
6th
    M65.871 right ankle and foot
    M65.872 left ankle and foot
M65.88 **Other synovitis and tenosynovitis, other site**
M65.89 **Other synovitis and tenosynovitis, multiple sites**
M65.9 **Synovitis and tenosynovitis, unspecified**

M67 **OTHER DISORDERS OF SYNOVIUM AND TENDON**
4th
Excludes1: palmar fascial fibromatosis [Dupuytren] (M72.0)
    tendinitis NOS (M77.9-)
    xanthomatosis localized to tendons (E78.2)
M67.0 **Short Achilles tendon (acquired)**
5th
    M67.01 **Short Achilles tendon (acquired), right ankle**
    M67.02 **Short Achilles tendon (acquired), left ankle**
M67.4 **Ganglion**
5th
    Ganglion of joint or tendon (sheath)
    Excludes1: ganglion in yaws (A66.6)
    Excludes2: cyst of bursa (M71.2– M71.3)
        cyst of synovium (M71.2–M71.3)
    M67.40 **Ganglion, unspecified site**
    M67.41 **Ganglion, shoulder**
    6th
        M67.411 right shoulder
        M67.412 left shoulder
    M67.42 **Ganglion, elbow**
    6th
        M67.421 right elbow
        M67.422 left elbow
    M67.43 **Ganglion, wrist**
    6th
        M67.431 right wrist
        M67.432 left wrist
    M67.44 **Ganglion, hand**
    6th
        M67.441 right hand
        M67.442 left hand
    M67.45 **Ganglion, hip**
    6th
        M67.451 right hip
        M67.452 left hip
    M67.46 **Ganglion, knee**
    6th
        M67.461 right knee
        M67.462 left knee
    M67.47 **Ganglion, ankle and foot**
    6th
        M67.471 right ankle and foot
        M67.472 left ankle and foot
    M67.48 **Ganglion, other site**
    M67.49 **Ganglion, multiple sites**

(M70–M79) OTHER SOFT TISSUE DISORDERS

M70 **SOFT TISSUE DISORDERS RELATED TO USE, OVERUSE**
4th **AND PRESSURE**
Includes: soft tissue disorders of occupational origin
Use additional external cause code to identify activity causing disorder
    (Y93.-)
Excludes1: bursitis NOS (M71.9-)
Excludes2: bursitis of shoulder (M75.5)
    enthesopathies (M76-M77)
    pressure ulcer (pressure area) (L89.-)
M70.6 **Trochanteric bursitis**
5th
    Trochanteric tendinitis
    M70.61 **Trochanteric bursitis, right hip**
    M70.62 **Trochanteric bursitis, left hip**
M70.7 **Other bursitis of hip**
5th
    Ischial bursitis
    M70.71 **Other bursitis of hip, right hip**
    M70.72 **Other bursitis of hip, left hip**

M71 **OTHER BURSOPATHIES**
4th
Excludes1: bunion (M20.1)
    bursitis related to use, overuse or pressure (M70.-)
    enthesopathies (M76–M77)
M71.2 **Synovial cyst of popliteal space [Baker]**
5th
    Excludes1: synovial cyst of popliteal space with rupture (M66.0)
    M71.21 **Synovial cyst of popliteal space [Baker], right knee**
    M71.22 **Synovial cyst of popliteal space [Baker], left knee**

M71.5 **Other bursitis, NEC**
5th
Excludes1: bursitis NOS (M71.9-)
Excludes2: bursitis of shoulder (M75.5)
    bursitis of tibial collateral [Pellegrini-Stieda] (M76.4-)
    M71.50 **Other bursitis, NEC, unspecified site**
    M71.52 **Other bursitis, NEC, elbow**
    6th
        M71.521 **Other bursitis, NEC, right elbow**
        M71.522 **Other bursitis, NEC, left elbow**
    M71.53 **Other bursitis, NEC, wrist**
    6th
        M71.531 **Other bursitis, NEC, right wrist**
        M71.532 **Other bursitis, NEC, left wrist**
    M71.54 **Other bursitis, NEC, hand**
    6th
        M71.541 **Other bursitis, NEC, right hand**
        M71.542 **Other bursitis, NEC, left hand**
    M71.55 **Other bursitis, NEC, hip**
    6th
        M71.551 **Other bursitis, NEC, right hip**
        M71.552 **Other bursitis, NEC, left hip**
    M71.56 **Other bursitis, NEC, knee**
    6th
        M71.561 **Other bursitis, NEC, right knee**
        M71.562 **Other bursitis, NEC, left knee**
    M71.57 **Other bursitis, NEC, ankle and foot**
    6th
        M71.571 **Other bursitis, NEC, right ankle and foot**
        M71.572 **Other bursitis, NEC, left ankle and foot**
    M71.58 **Other bursitis, NEC, other site**
M71.9 **Bursopathy, unspecified**
    Bursitis NOS

M72 **FIBROBLASTIC DISORDERS**
4th
Excludes2: retroperitoneal fibromatosis (D48.3)
M72.6 **Necrotizing fasciitis**
    Use additional code (B95.-, B96.-) to identify causative organism
M72.8 **Other fibroblastic disorders**
    Abscess of fascia
    Fasciitis NEC
    Other infective fasciitis
    Use additional code to (B95.-, B96.-) identify causative organism
    Excludes1: diffuse (eosinophilic) fasciitis (M35.4)
        necrotizing fasciitis (M72.6)
        nodular fasciitis (M72.4)
        perirenal fasciitis NOS (N13.5)
        perirenal fasciitis with infection (N13.6)
        plantar fasciitis (M72.2)
M72.9 **Fibroblastic disorder, unspecified**
    Fasciitis NOS
    Fibromatosis NOS

M75 **SHOULDER LESIONS**
4th
M75.1 **Rotator cuff tear or rupture, not specified as traumatic**
5th
    Rotator cuff syndrome
    Supraspinatus tear or rupture, not specified as traumatic
    Supraspinatus syndrome
    Excludes1: tear of rotator cuff, traumatic (S46.01-)
    Excludes2: shoulder-hand syndrome (M89.0-)
    M75.10 **Unspecified rotator cuff tear or rupture, not specified**
    6th **as traumatic**
        M75.101 **Unspecified rotator cuff tear or rupture of right shoulder, not specified as traumatic**
        M75.102 **Unspecified rotator cuff tear or rupture of left shoulder, not specified as traumatic**
    M75.11 **Incomplete rotator cuff tear or rupture not specified**
    6th **as traumatic**
        M75.111 **Incomplete rotator cuff tear or rupture of right shoulder, not specified as traumatic**
        M75.112 **Incomplete rotator cuff tear or rupture of left shoulder, not specified as traumatic**
    M75.12 **Complete rotator cuff tear or rupture not specified as**
    6th **traumatic**
        M75.121 **Complete rotator cuff tear or rupture of right shoulder, not specified as traumatic**
        M75.122 **Complete rotator cuff tear or rupture of left shoulder, not specified as traumatic**

M76 **ENTHESOPATHIES, LOWER LIMB, EXCLUDING FOOT**
4th
Excludes2: bursitis due to use, overuse and pressure (M70.-)
    enthesopathies of ankle and foot (M77.5-)

4th 5th 6th 7th Additional Character Required   ✓ 3-character code

Unspecified laterality codes •=New Code   *Excludes1*—Not coded here, do not use together
were excluded here. ▲=Revised Code   *Excludes2*—Not included here

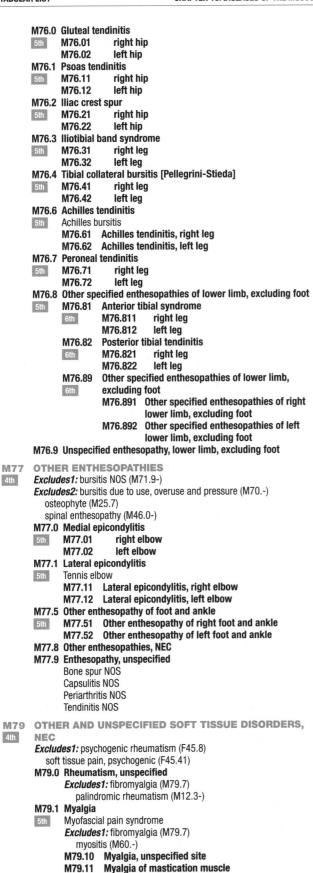

M76.0 Gluteal tendinitis
- **5th**   **M76.01**   right hip
- **M76.02**   left hip

M76.1 Psoas tendinitis
- **5th**   **M76.11**   right hip
- **M76.12**   left hip

M76.2 Iliac crest spur
- **5th**   **M76.21**   right hip
- **M76.22**   left hip

M76.3 Iliotibial band syndrome
- **5th**   **M76.31**   right leg
- **M76.32**   left leg

M76.4 Tibial collateral bursitis [Pellegrini-Stieda]
- **5th**   **M76.41**   right leg
- **M76.42**   left leg

M76.6 Achilles tendinitis
- **5th**   Achilles bursitis
- **M76.61**   Achilles tendinitis, right leg
- **M76.62**   Achilles tendinitis, left leg

M76.7 Peroneal tendinitis
- **5th**   **M76.71**   right leg
- **M76.72**   left leg

M76.8 Other specified enthesopathies of lower limb, excluding foot
- **5th**   **M76.81**   Anterior tibial syndrome
  - **6th**   **M76.811**   right leg
  - **M76.812**   left leg
- **M76.82**   Posterior tibial tendinitis
  - **6th**   **M76.821**   right leg
  - **M76.822**   left leg
- **M76.89**   Other specified enthesopathies of lower limb, excluding foot
  - **6th**
  - **M76.891**   Other specified enthesopathies of right lower limb, excluding foot
  - **M76.892**   Other specified enthesopathies of left lower limb, excluding foot

M76.9 Unspecified enthesopathy, lower limb, excluding foot

M77 OTHER ENTHESOPATHIES
- **4th**
- ***Excludes1:*** bursitis NOS (M71.9-)
- ***Excludes2:*** bursitis due to use, overuse and pressure (M70.-)
  - osteophyte (M25.7)
  - spinal enthesopathy (M46.0-)

M77.0 Medial epicondylitis
- **5th**   **M77.01**   right elbow
- **M77.02**   left elbow

M77.1 Lateral epicondylitis
- **5th**   Tennis elbow
- **M77.11**   Lateral epicondylitis, right elbow
- **M77.12**   Lateral epicondylitis, left elbow

M77.5 Other enthesopathy of foot and ankle
- **5th**   **M77.51**   Other enthesopathy of right foot and ankle
- **M77.52**   Other enthesopathy of left foot and ankle

M77.8 Other enthesopathies, NEC

M77.9 Enthesopathy, unspecified
- Bone spur NOS
- Capsulitis NOS
- Periarthritis NOS
- Tendinitis NOS

M79 OTHER AND UNSPECIFIED SOFT TISSUE DISORDERS, NEC
- **4th**
- ***Excludes1:*** psychogenic rheumatism (F45.8)
  - soft tissue pain, psychogenic (F45.41)

M79.0 Rheumatism, unspecified
- ***Excludes1:*** fibromyalgia (M79.7)
  - palindromic rheumatism (M12.3-)

M79.1 Myalgia
- **5th**   Myofascial pain syndrome
- ***Excludes1:*** fibromyalgia (M79.7)
  - myositis (M60.-)
- **M79.10**   Myalgia, unspecified site
- **M79.11**   Myalgia of mastication muscle
- **M79.12**   Myalgia of auxiliary muscles, head and neck
- **M79.18**   Myalgia, other site

M79.2 Neuralgia and neuritis, unspecified
- ***Excludes1:*** brachial radiculitis NOS (M54.1)
  - lumbosacral radiculitis NOS (M54.1)
  - mononeuropathies (G56-G58)
  - radiculitis NOS (M54.1)
  - sciatica (M54.3-M54.4)

M79.5 Residual foreign body in soft tissue
- ***Excludes1:*** foreign body granuloma of skin and subcutaneous tissue (L92.3)
  - foreign body granuloma of soft tissue (M60.2-)

M79.6 Pain in limb, hand, foot, fingers and toes
- **5th**   ***Excludes2:*** pain in joint (M25.5-)
- **M79.60**   Pain in limb, unspecified
  - **6th**
  - **M79.601**   Pain in right arm
    - Pain in right upper limb NOS
  - **M79.602**   Pain in left arm
    - Pain in left upper limb NOS
  - **M79.604**   Pain in right leg
    - Pain in right lower limb NOS
  - **M79.605**   Pain in left leg
    - Pain in left lower limb NOS
- **M79.62**   Pain in upper arm
  - **6th**   Pain in axillary region
  - **M79.621**   Pain in right upper arm
  - **M79.622**   Pain in left upper arm
- **M79.63**   Pain in forearm
  - **6th**   **M79.631**   Pain in right forearm
  - **M79.632**   Pain in left forearm
- **M79.64**   Pain in hand and fingers
  - **6th**   **M79.641**   Pain in right hand
  - **M79.642**   Pain in left hand
  - **M79.644**   Pain in right finger(s)
  - **M79.645**   Pain in left finger(s)
- **M79.65**   Pain in thigh
  - **6th**   **M79.651**   Pain in right thigh
  - **M79.652**   Pain in left thigh
- **M79.66**   Pain in lower leg
  - **6th**   **M79.661**   Pain in right lower leg
  - **M79.662**   Pain in left lower leg
- **M79.67**   Pain in foot and toes
  - **6th**   **M79.671**   Pain in right foot
  - **M79.672**   Pain in left foot
  - **M79.674**   Pain in right toe(s)
  - **M79.675**   Pain in left toe(s)

M79.8 Other specified soft tissue disorders
- **5th**   **M79.81**   Nontraumatic hematoma of soft tissue
  - Nontraumatic hematoma of muscle
  - Nontraumatic seroma of muscle and soft tissue
- **M79.89**   Other specified soft tissue disorders
  - Polyalgia

M79.9 Soft tissue disorder, unspecified

(M80–M94) OSTEOPATHIES AND CHONDROPATHIES
(M80–M85) DISORDERS OF BONE DENSITY AND STRUCTURE

M84 DISORDER OF CONTINUITY OF BONE
- **4th**   **GUIDELINES**

Coding of Pathologic Fractures

7th character A is for use as long as the patient is receiving active treatment for the fracture. Examples of active treatment are: surgical treatment, emergency department encounter, evaluation and continuing treatment by the same or a different physician. While the patient may be seen by a new or different provider over the course of treatment for a pathological fracture, assignment of the 7th character is based on whether the patient is undergoing active treatment and not whether the provider is seeing the patient for the first time. 7th character, D is to be used for encounters after the patient has completed active treatment for the fracture and is receiving routine care for the fracture during the healing or recovery phase. The other 7th characters, listed under each subcategory in the Tabular List, are to be used for subsequent encounters for treatment

---

4th	5th	6th	7th	Additional Character Required

✓ 3-character code

Unspecified laterality codes were excluded here.

•=New Code
▲=Revised Code

Excludes1—Not coded here, do not use together
Excludes2—Not included here

of problems associated with the healing, such as malunions, nonunions, and sequelae.

Care for complications of surgical treatment for fracture repairs during the healing or recovery phase should be coded with the appropriate complication codes.

Excludes2: traumatic fracture of bone-see fracture, by site

M84.3 **Stress fracture**
`5th`
Fatigue fracture
March fracture
Stress fracture NOS
Stress reaction
Use additional external cause code(s) to identify the cause of the stress fracture

Excludes1: pathological fracture NOS (M84.4.-)
    pathological fracture due to osteoporosis (M80.-)
    traumatic fracture (S12.-, S22.-, S32.-, S42.-, S52.-, S62.-, S72.-, S82.-, S92.-)

Excludes2: personal history of (healed) stress (fatigue) fracture (Z87.312)
    stress fracture of vertebra (M48.4-)

> M84 requires 7th character to identify the encounter type
> A—initial encounter for fracture care
> D—subsequent encounter with routine healing
> G—subsequent encounter for fracture with delayed healing
> K—subsequent encounter for fracture with nonunion
> P—subsequent encounter for fracture with malunion
> S—sequela

    M84.30X **Stress fracture, unspecified site** `7th`

M84.31 **Stress fracture, shoulder**
`6th`
    M84.311 **Stress fracture, right shoulder** `7th`
    M84.312 **Stress fracture, left shoulder** `7th`

M84.32 **Stress fracture, humerus**
`6th`
    M84.321 **Stress fracture, right humerus** `7th`
    M84.322 **Stress fracture, left humerus** `7th`

M84.33 **Stress fracture, ulna and radius**
`6th`
    M84.331 **Stress fracture, right ulna** `7th`
    M84.332 **Stress fracture, left ulna** `7th`
    M84.333 **Stress fracture, right radius** `7th`
    M84.334 **Stress fracture, left radius** `7th`

M84.34 **Stress fracture, hand and fingers**
`6th`
    M84.341 **Stress fracture, right hand** `7th`
    M84.342 **Stress fracture, left hand** `7th`
    M84.344 **Stress fracture, right finger(s)** `7th`
    M84.345 **Stress fracture, left finger(s)** `7th`

M84.35 **Stress fracture, pelvis and femur**
`6th`
Stress fracture, hip
    M84.350 **Stress fracture, pelvis** `7th`
    M84.351 **Stress fracture, right femur** `7th`
    M84.352 **Stress fracture, left femur** `7th`
    M84.359 **Stress fracture, hip, unspecified** `7th`

M84.36 **Stress fracture, tibia and fibula**
`6th`
    M84.361 **Stress fracture, right tibia** `7th`
    M84.362 **Stress fracture, left tibia** `7th`
    M84.363 **Stress fracture, right fibula** `7th`
    M84.364 **Stress fracture, left fibula** `7th`

M84.37 **Stress fracture, ankle, foot and toes**
`6th`
    M84.371 **Stress fracture, right ankle** `7th`
    M84.372 **Stress fracture, left ankle** `7th`
    M84.374 **Stress fracture, right foot** `7th`
    M84.375 **Stress fracture, left foot** `7th`
    M84.377 **Stress fracture, right toe(s)** `7th`
    M84.378 **Stress fracture, left toe(s)** `7th`

M84.38X **Stress fracture, other site** `7th`
    Excludes2: stress fracture of vertebra (M48.4-)
M84.88 **Other disorders of continuity of bone, other site**

M85 **OTHER DISORDERS OF BONE DENSITY AND STRUCTURE**
`4th`
Excludes1: osteogenesis imperfecta (Q78.0)
    osteopetrosis (Q78.2)
    osteopoikilosis (Q78.8)
    polyostotic fibrous dysplasia (Q78.1)
M85.2 **Hyperostosis of skull**
M85.6 **Other cyst of bone**
`5th`
Excludes1: cyst of jaw NEC (M27.4)
    osteitis fibrosa cystica generalisata [von Recklinghausen's disease of bone] (E21.0)
    M85.60 **Other cyst of bone, unspecified site**
    M85.61 **Other cyst of bone, shoulder**
`6th`
        M85.611 right shoulder
        M85.612 left shoulder
    M85.62 **Other cyst of bone, upper arm**
`6th`
        M85.621 right upper arm
        M85.622 left upper arm
    M85.63 **Other cyst of bone, forearm**
`6th`
        M85.631 right forearm
        M85.632 left forearm
    M85.64 **Other cyst of bone, hand**
`6th`
        M85.641 right hand
        M85.642 left hand
    M85.65 **Other cyst of bone, thigh**
`6th`
        M85.651 right thigh
        M85.652 left thigh
    M85.66 **Other cyst of bone, lower leg**
`6th`
        M85.661 right lower leg
        M85.662 left lower leg
    M85.67 **Other cyst of bone, ankle and foot**
`6th`
        M85.671 right ankle and foot
        M85.672 left ankle and foot
    M85.68 **Other cyst of bone, other site**
    M85.69 **Other cyst of bone, multiple sites**

(M86–M90) OTHER OSTEOPATHIES

Excludes1: postprocedural osteopathies (M96.-)

M86 **OSTEOMYELITIS**
`4th`
Use additional code (B95–B97) to identify infectious agent
Use additional code to identify major osseous defect, if applicable (M89.7-)
Excludes1: osteomyelitis due to:
    Echinococcus (B67.2)
    gonococcus (A54.43)
    Salmonella (A02.24)
Excludes2: osteomyelitis of:
    orbit (H05.0-)
    petrous bone (H70.2-)
    vertebra (M46.2-)
M86.1 **Other acute osteomyelitis**
`5th`
    M86.10 **Other acute osteomyelitis, unspecified site**
    M86.11 **Other acute osteomyelitis, shoulder**
`6th`
        M86.111 right shoulder
        M86.112 left shoulder
    M86.12 **Other acute osteomyelitis, humerus**
`6th`
        M86.121 right humerus

CHAPTER 13. DISEASES OF THE MUSCULOSKELETAL SYSTEM AND CONNECTIVE TISSUE (M84.3–M86.121)

`4th` `5th` `6th` `7th` Additional Character Required   ✓ 3-character code   Unspecified laterality codes were excluded here.   •=New Code   ▲=Revised Code   *Excludes1*—Not coded here, do not use together   *Excludes2*—Not included here

M86.122   left humerus
M86.13   Other acute osteomyelitis, radius and ulna
   6th   M86.131   right radius and ulna
     M86.132   left radius and ulna
M86.14   Other acute osteomyelitis, hand
   6th   M86.141   right hand
     M86.142   left hand
M86.15   Other acute osteomyelitis, femur
   6th   M86.151   right femur
     M86.152   left femur
M86.16   Other acute osteomyelitis, tibia and fibula
   6th   M86.161   right tibia and fibula
     M86.162   left tibia and fibula
M86.17   Other acute osteomyelitis, ankle and foot
   6th   M86.171   right ankle and foot
     M86.172   left ankle and foot
M86.18   Other acute osteomyelitis, other site
M86.19   Other acute osteomyelitis, multiple sites
M86.9 Osteomyelitis, unspecified
Infection of bone NOS
Periostitis without osteomyelitis

M88   **OSTEITIS DEFORMANS [PAGET'S DISEASE OF BONE]**
4th   *Excludes1:* osteitis deformans in neoplastic disease (M90.6)
M88.0 Osteitis deformans of skull
M88.1 Osteitis deformans of vertebrae
M88.8 Osteitis deformans of other bones
  5th   **M88.81**   Osteitis deformans of shoulder
   6th   M88.811   right shoulder
     M88.812   left shoulder
   M88.82   Osteitis deformans of upper arm
   6th   M88.821   right upper arm
     M88.822   left upper arm
   M88.83   Osteitis deformans of forearm
   6th   M88.831   right forearm
     M88.832   left forearm
   M88.84   Osteitis deformans of hand
   6th   M88.841   right hand
     M88.842   left hand
   M88.85   Osteitis deformans of thigh
   6th   M88.851   right thigh
     M88.852   left thigh
   M88.86   Osteitis deformans of lower leg
   6th   M88.861   right lower leg
     M88.862   left lower leg
   M88.87   Osteitis deformans of ankle and foot
   6th   M88.871   right ankle and foot
     M88.872   left ankle and foot
   M88.88   Osteitis deformans of other bones
     Excludes2: osteitis deformans of skull (M88.0)
      osteitis deformans of vertebrae (M88.1)
   M88.89   Osteitis deformans of multiple sites
M88.9   Osteitis deformans of unspecified bone

M89   **OTHER DISORDERS OF BONE**
4th   **M89.1 Physeal arrest**
  5th   Arrest of growth plate
    Epiphyseal arrest
    Growth plate arrest
   M89.12   Physeal arrest, humerus
   6th   M89.121   Complete physeal arrest, right proximal humerus
     M89.122   Complete physeal arrest, left proximal humerus
     M89.123   Partial physeal arrest, right proximal humerus
     M89.124   Partial physeal arrest, left proximal humerus
     M89.125   Complete physeal arrest, right distal humerus
     M89.126   Complete physeal arrest, left distal humerus
     M89.127   Partial physeal arrest, right distal humerus
     M89.128   Partial physeal arrest, left distal humerus
     M89.129   Physeal arrest, humerus, unspecified

M89.13   Physeal arrest, forearm
   6th   M89.131   Complete physeal arrest, right distal radius
     M89.132   Complete physeal arrest, left distal radius
     M89.133   Partial physeal arrest, right distal radius
     M89.134   Partial physeal arrest, left distal radius
     M89.138   Other physeal arrest of forearm
     M89.139   Physeal arrest, forearm, unspecified
M89.15   Physeal arrest, femur
   6th   M89.151   Complete physeal arrest, right proximal femur
     M89.152   Complete physeal arrest, left proximal femur
     M89.153   Partial physeal arrest, right proximal femur
     M89.154   Partial physeal arrest, left proximal femur
     M89.155   Complete physeal arrest, right distal femur
     M89.156   Complete physeal arrest, left distal femur
     M89.157   Partial physeal arrest, right distal femur
     M89.158   Partial physeal arrest, left distal femur
     M89.159   Physeal arrest, femur, unspecified
M89.16   Physeal arrest, lower leg
   6th   M89.160   Complete physeal arrest, right proximal tibia
     M89.161   Complete physeal arrest, left proximal tibia
     M89.162   Partial physeal arrest, right proximal tibia
     M89.163   Partial physeal arrest, left proximal tibia
     M89.164   Complete physeal arrest, right distal tibia
     M89.165   Complete physeal arrest, left distal tibia
     M89.166   Partial physeal arrest, right distal tibia
     M89.167   Partial physeal arrest, left distal tibia
     M89.168   Other physeal arrest of lower leg
     M89.169   Physeal arrest, lower leg, unspecified
M89.18   Physeal arrest, other site

M90   **OSTEOPATHIES IN DISEASES CLASSIFIED ELSEWHERE**
4th   *Excludes1:* osteochondritis, osteomyelitis, and osteopathy (in):
    cryptococcosis (B45.3)
    DM (E08–E13 with .69-)
    gonococcal (A54.43)
    neurogenic syphilis (A52.11)
    renal osteodystrophy (N25.0)
    salmonellosis (A02.24)
    secondary syphilis (A51.46)
    syphilis (late) (A52.77)
M90.5 Osteonecrosis in diseases classified elsewhere
  5th   *Code first* underlying disease, such as: caisson disease (T70.3)
     hemoglobinopathy (D50–D64)
   M90.50   Osteonecrosis in diseases classified elsewhere, unspecified site
   M90.51   Osteonecrosis in diseases classified elsewhere; shoulder
   6th   M90.511   right shoulder
     M90.512   left shoulder
   M90.52   Osteonecrosis in diseases classified elsewhere; upper arm
   6th   M90.521   right upper arm
     M90.522   left upper arm
   M90.53   Osteonecrosis in diseases classified elsewhere; forearm
   6th   M90.531   right forearm
     M90.532   left forearm
   M90.54   Osteonecrosis in diseases classified elsewhere; hand
   6th   M90.541   right hand
     M90.542   left hand
   M90.55   Osteonecrosis in diseases classified elsewhere; thigh
   6th   M90.551   right thigh
     M90.552   left thigh
   M90.56   Osteonecrosis in diseases classified elsewhere; lower leg
   6th   M90.561   right lower leg
     M90.562   left lower leg

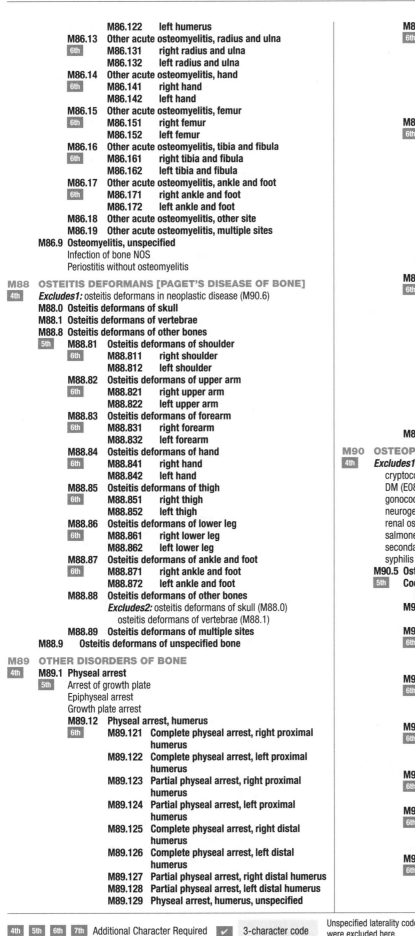

4th   **5th**   **6th**   **7th**   Additional Character Required   ✔   3-character code

Unspecified laterality codes were excluded here.   •=New Code   ▲=Revised Code

Excludes1—Not coded here, do not use together
Excludes2—Not included here

CHAPTER 13. DISEASES OF THE MUSCULOSKELETAL SYSTEM AND CONNECTIVE TISSUE (M90.57–M93.012)

M90.57 [6th] Osteonecrosis in diseases classified elsewhere; ankle and foot
     M90.571   right ankle and foot
     M90.572   left ankle and foot
M90.58 Osteonecrosis in diseases classified elsewhere, other site
M90.59 Osteonecrosis in diseases classified elsewhere, multiple sites
M90.6 **Osteitis deformans in neoplastic diseases**
[5th] Osteitis deformans in malignant neoplasm of bone
Code first the neoplasm (C40.-, C41.-)
Excludes1: osteitis deformans [Paget's disease of bone] (M88.-)
Refer to the full *ICD-10-CM* manual for full codes
M90.8 **Osteopathy in diseases classified elsewhere**
[5th] **Code first** underlying disease, such as:
     rickets (E55.0)
     vitamin-D-resistant rickets (E83.3)
     M90.80   Osteopathy in diseases classified elsewhere, unspecified site

(M91–M94) CHONDROPATHIES

Excludes1: postprocedural chondropathies (M96.-)

M91   **JUVENILE OSTEOCHONDROSIS OF HIP AND PELVIS**
[4th]   ***Excludes1:*** slipped upper femoral epiphysis (nontraumatic) (M93.0)
M91.0 **Juvenile osteochondrosis of pelvis**
     Osteochondrosis (juvenile) of acetabulum
     Osteochondrosis (juvenile) of iliac crest [Buchanan]
     Osteochondrosis (juvenile) of ischiopubic synchondrosis [van Neck]
     Osteochondrosis (juvenile) of symphysis pubis [Pierson]
M91.1 **Juvenile osteochondrosis of head of femur [Legg-Calvé-Perthes]**
[5th]   **M91.11**   Juvenile osteochondrosis of head of femur [Legg-Calvé-Perthes], right leg
     M91.12   Juvenile osteochondrosis of head of femur [Legg-Calvé-Perthes], left leg
M91.2 **Coxa plana**
[5th]   Hip deformity due to previous juvenile osteochondrosis
     M91.21   Coxa plana, right hip
     M91.22   Coxa plana, left hip
M91.3 **Pseudocoxalgia**
[5th]   **M91.31**   Pseudocoxalgia, right hip
     M91.32   Pseudocoxalgia, left hip
M91.4 **Coxa magna**
[5th]   **M91.41**   Coxa magna, right hip
     M91.42   Coxa magna, left hip
M91.8 **Other juvenile osteochondrosis of hip and pelvis**
[5th]   Juvenile osteochondrosis after reduction of congenital dislocation of hip
     M91.81   Other juvenile osteochondrosis of hip and pelvis, right leg
     M91.82   Other juvenile osteochondrosis of hip and pelvis, left leg
M91.9 **Juvenile osteochondrosis of hip and pelvis, unspecified**
[5th]   **M91.91**   Juvenile osteochondrosis of hip and pelvis, unspecified, right leg
     M91.92   Juvenile osteochondrosis of hip and pelvis, unspecified, left leg

M92   **OTHER JUVENILE OSTEOCHONDROSIS**
[4th]   **M92.0** **Juvenile osteochondrosis of humerus**
[5th]   Osteochondrosis (juvenile) of capitulum of humerus [Panner]
     Osteochondrosis (juvenile) of head of humerus [Haas]
     M92.01   Juvenile osteochondrosis of humerus, right arm
     M92.02   Juvenile osteochondrosis of humerus, left arm
M92.1 **Juvenile osteochondrosis of radius and ulna**
[5th]   Osteochondrosis (juvenile) of lower ulna [Burns]
     Osteochondrosis (juvenile) of radial head [Brailsford]
     M92.11   Juvenile osteochondrosis of radius and ulna, right arm
     M92.12   Juvenile osteochondrosis of radius and ulna, left arm
M92.2 **Juvenile osteochondrosis, hand**
[5th]   **M92.20**   Unspecified juvenile osteochondrosis; hand
[6th]   **M92.201**   right hand
        M92.202   left hand

M92.21 [6th] Osteochondrosis (juvenile) of carpal lunate [Kienböck];
     M92.211   right hand
     M92.212   left hand
M92.22 [6th] Osteochondrosis (juvenile) of metacarpal heads [Mauclaire];
     M92.221   right hand
     M92.222   left hand
M92.29 [6th] Other juvenile osteochondrosis; hand
     M92.291   right hand
     M92.292   left hand
M92.3 **Other juvenile osteochondrosis; upper limb**
[5th]   **M92.31**   right upper limb
     M92.32   left upper limb
M92.4 **Juvenile osteochondrosis of patella;**
[5th]   Osteochondrosis (juvenile) of primary patellar center [Köhler]
     Osteochondrosis (juvenile) of secondary patellar centre [Sinding Larsen]
     M92.41   right knee
     M92.42   left knee
M92.5 **Juvenile osteochondrosis of tibia and fibula;**
[5th] ▲**M92.50**   Unspecified juvenile osteochondrosis of tibia and fibula
[6th]   •**M92.501**   right leg
        •**M92.502**   left leg
        •**M92.503**   bilateral leg
     ▲**M92.51**   Juvenile osteochondrosis of proximal tibia
[6th]   Blount disease
        Tibia vara
        •**M92.511**   right leg
        •**M92.512**   left leg
        •**M92.513**   bilateral
     ▲**M92.52**   Juvenile osteochondrosis of tibia tubercle
[6th]   Osgood-Schlatter disease
        •**M92.521**   right leg
        •**M92.522**   left leg
        •**M92.523**   bilateral
     •**M92.59**   Other juvenile osteochondrosis of tibia and fibula
[6th]   •**M92.591**   right leg
        •**M92.592**   left leg
        •**M92.593**   bilateral
M92.6 **Juvenile osteochondrosis of tarsus;**
[5th]   Osteochondrosis (juvenile) of calcaneum [Sever]
     Osteochondrosis (juvenile) of os tibiale externum [Haglund]
     Osteochondrosis (juvenile) of talus [Diaz]
     Osteochondrosis (juvenile) of tarsal navicular [Köhler]
     M92.61   right ankle
     M92.62   left ankle
M92.7 **Juvenile osteochondrosis of metatarsus;**
[5th]   Osteochondrosis (juvenile) of fifth metatarsus [Iselin]
     Osteochondrosis (juvenile) of second metatarsus [Freiberg]
     M92.71   right foot
     M92.72   left foot
M92.8 **Other specified juvenile osteochondrosis**
     Calcaneal apophysitis
M92.9 **Juvenile osteochondrosis, unspecified**
     Juvenile apophysitis NOS
     Juvenile epiphysitis NOS
     Juvenile osteochondritis NOS
     Juvenile osteochondrosis NOS

M93   **OTHER OSTEOCHONDROPATHIES**
[4th]   ***Excludes2:*** osteochondrosis of spine (M42.-)
M93.0 **Slipped upper femoral epiphysis (nontraumatic)**
[5th]   **Use additional code** for associated chondrolysis (M94.3)
     M93.00   Unspecified slipped upper femoral epiphysis (nontraumatic);
[6th]   **M93.001**   right hip
        M93.002   left hip
     M93.01   Acute slipped upper femoral epiphysis (nontraumatic);
[6th]   **M93.011**   right hip
        M93.012   left hip

[4th] [5th] [6th] [7th] Additional Character Required   ✓   3-character code   Unspecified laterality codes were excluded here.   •=New Code   ▲=Revised Code   ***Excludes1***—Not coded here, do not use together   ***Excludes2***—Not included here

M93.02 Chronic slipped upper femoral epiphysis
`6th` (nontraumatic);
     M93.021 right hip
     M93.022 left hip

M93.03 Acute on chronic slipped upper femoral epiphysis
`6th` (nontraumatic);
     M93.031 right hip
     M93.032 left hip

M93.9 Osteochondropathy, unspecified
`5th`
Apophysitis NOS
Epiphysitis NOS
Osteochondritis NOS
Osteochondrosis NOS
Refer to full *ICD-10-CM* Manual for codes

M94 **OTHER DISORDERS OF CARTILAGE**
`4th`
M94.0 Chondrocostal junction syndrome [Tietze]
Costochondritis

M94.2 Chondromalacia
`5th` **M94.26** Chondromalacia, knee
    `6th` **M94.261** Chondromalacia, right knee
       M94.262 Chondromalacia, left knee

M94.8 Other specified disorders of cartilage
`5th` **M94.8X** Other specified disorders of cartilage
    `6th` **M94.8X0** multiple sites
       M94.8X1 shoulder
       M94.8X2 upper arm
       M94.8X3 forearm
       M94.8X4 hand
       M94.8X5 thigh
       M94.8X6 lower leg
       M94.8X7 ankle and foot
       M94.8X8 other site
       M94.8X9 unspecified sites

(M95) OTHER DISORDERS OF MUSCULOSKELETAL SYSTEM AND CONNECTIVE TISSUE

M95 **OTHER ACQUIRED DEFORMITIES OF**
`4th` **MUSCULOSKELETAL SYSTEM AND CONNECTIVE TISSUE**
Excludes2: acquired absence of limbs and organs (Z89–Z90)
    acquired deformities of limbs (M20–M21)
    congenital malformations and deformations of the musculoskeletal
      system (Q65–Q79)
    deforming dorsopathies (M40–M43)
    dentofacial anomalies [including malocclusion] (M26.-)
    postprocedural musculoskeletal disorders (M96.-)

M95.0 Acquired deformity of nose
    Excludes2: deviated nasal septum (J34.2)

M95.2 Other acquired deformity of head

M95.3 Acquired deformity of neck

M95.4 Acquired deformity of chest and rib

M95.5 Acquired deformity of pelvis

M95.8 Other specified acquired deformities of musculoskeletal system

M95.9 Acquired deformity of musculoskeletal system, unspecified

---

 `4th` `5th` `6th` `7th` Additional Character Required ☑ 3-character code

Unspecified laterality codes were excluded here. •=New Code ▲=Revised Code

Excludes1—Not coded here, do not use together
Excludes2—Not included here

Chapter 14. Diseases of the genitourinary system (N00–N99)

Chronic kidney disease

STAGES OF CKD
Refer to category N18 for guidelines.

CKD AND KIDNEY TRANSPLANT STATUS
Refer to category N18 for guidelines.

CKD WITH OTHER CONDITIONS
Patients with CKD may also suffer from other serious conditions, most commonly DM and hypertension (in adults). The sequencing of the CKD code in relationship to codes for other contributing conditions is based on the conventions in the Tabular List.
  Refer to Chapter 19. CKD and kidney transplant complications.
Excludes2: certain conditions originating in the perinatal period (P04–P96)
  certain infectious and parasitic diseases (A00–B99)
  complications of pregnancy, childbirth and the puerperium (O00–O9A)
  congenital malformations, deformations and chromosomal abnormalities
    (Q00–Q99)
  endocrine, nutritional and metabolic diseases (E00–E88)
  injury, poisoning and certain other consequences of external causes (S00–T88)
  neoplasms (C00–D49)
  symptoms, signs and abnormal clinical and laboratory findings, NEC (R00–R94)

(N00–N08) GLOMERULAR DISEASES

Code also any associated kidney failure (N17–N19).
Excludes1: hypertensive CKD (I12.-)

N00   **ACUTE NEPHRITIC SYNDROME**
4th   ***Includes:*** acute glomerular disease
     acute glomerulonephritis
     acute nephritis
   Excludes1: acute tubulo-interstitial nephritis (N10)
     nephritic syndrome NOS (N05.-)
   N00.0   **Acute nephritic syndrome with; minor glomerular abnormality**
     Acute nephritic syndrome with minimal change lesion
   N00.1   **focal and segmental glomerular lesions**
     Acute nephritic syndrome with focal and segmental hyalinosis or with focal and segmental sclerosis or with focal glomerulonephritis
   N00.2   **diffuse membranous glomerulonephritis**
   N00.3   **diffuse mesangial proliferative glomerulonephritis**
   N00.4   **diffuse endocapillary proliferative glomerulonephritis**
   N00.5   **diffuse mesangiocapillary glomerulonephritis**
     Acute nephritic syndrome with MPGN, types 1 and 3, or NOS
     Excludes1: Acute nephritic syndrome with C3 glomerulonephritis or glomerulopathy (N00.A)
   N00.6   **dense deposit disease**
     Acute nephritic syndrome with C3 glomerulopathy with dense deposit disease
     Acute nephritic syndrome with MPGN, type 2
   N00.7   **diffuse crescentic glomerulonephritis**
     Acute nephritic syndrome with extracapillary glomerulonephritis
   N00.8   **other morphologic changes**
     Acute nephritic syndrome with proliferative glomerulonephritis NOS
   N00.9   **unspecified morphologic changes**
   •**N00.A** **Acute nephritic syndrome with C3 glomerulonephritis**
     Acute nephritic syndrome with C3 glomerulopathy, NOS
     Excludes1: Acute nephritic syndrome (with C3 glomerulopathy) with dense deposit disease(N00.6)

N01   **RAPIDLY PROGRESSIVE NEPHRITIC SYNDROME**
4th   ***Includes:*** rapidly progressive glomerular disease
     rapidly progressive glomerulonephritis
     rapidly progressive nephritis
   Excludes1: nephritic syndrome NOS (N05.-)
   N01.0   **Rapidly progressive nephritic syndrome with; minor glomerular abnormality**
     Rapidly progressive nephritic syndrome with minimal change lesion

   N01.1   **focal and segmental glomerular lesions**
     Rapidly progressive nephritic syndrome with focal and segmental hyalinosis or with focal and segmental sclerosis or with focal glomerulonephritis
   N01.2   **diffuse membranous glomerulonephritis**
   N01.3   **diffuse mesangial proliferative glomerulonephritis**
   N01.4   **diffuse endocapillary proliferative glomerulonephritis**
   N01.5   **diffuse mesangiocapillary glomerulonephritis**
     Rapidly progressive nephritic syndrome with MPGN, types 1 and 3, or NOS
     Excludes1: Rapidly progressive nephritic syndrome with C3 glomerulonephritis or glomerulopathy (N01.A)
   N01.6   **dense deposit disease**
     Rapidly progressive nephritic syndrome with C3 glomerulopathy with dense deposit disease
     Rapidly progressive nephritic syndrome with MPGN, type 2
   N01.7   **diffuse crescentic glomerulonephritis**
     Rapidly progressive nephritic syndrome with extracapillary glomerulonephritis
   N01.8   **other morphologic changes**
     Rapidly progressive nephritic syndrome with proliferative glomerulonephritis NOS
   N01.9   **unspecified morphologic changes**
   •**N01.A** **Rapidly progressive nephritic syndrome with C3 glomerulonephritis**
     Rapidly progressive nephritic syndrome with C3 glomerulopathy, NOS
     Excludes1: Rapidly progressive nephritic syndrome (with C3 glomerulopathy) with dense depositdisease (N01.6)

N03   **CHRONIC NEPHRITIC SYNDROME**
4th   ***Includes:*** chronic glomerular disease
     chronic glomerulonephritis
     chronic nephritis
   Excludes1: chronic tubulo-interstitial nephritis (N11.-)
     diffuse sclerosing glomerulonephritis (N05.8-)
     nephritic syndrome NOS (N05.-)
   N03.0   **Chronic nephritic syndrome with; minor glomerular abnormality**
     Chronic nephritic syndrome with minimal change lesion
   N03.1   **focal and segmental glomerular lesions**
     Chronic nephritic syndrome with focal and segmental hyalinosis or with focal and segmental sclerosis or with focal glomerulonephritis
   N03.2   **diffuse membranous glomerulonephritis**
   N03.3   **diffuse mesangial proliferative glomerulonephritis**
   N03.4   **diffuse endocapillary proliferative glomerulonephritis**
   N03.5   **diffuse mesangiocapillary glomerulonephritis**
     Chronic nephritic syndrome with MPGN, types 1 and 3, or NOS
     Excludes1: Chronic nephritic syndrome with C3 glomerulonephritis or glomerulopathy (N03.A)
   N03.6   **dense deposit disease**
     Chronic nephritic syndrome with MPGN, type 2
   N03.7   **diffuse crescentic glomerulonephritis**
     Chronic nephritic syndrome with C3 glomerulopathy with dense deposit disease
     Chronic nephritic syndrome with extracapillary glomerulonephritis
   N03.8   **other morphologic changes**
     Chronic nephritic syndrome with proliferative glomerulonephritis NOS
   N03.9   **unspecified morphologic changes**
   •**N03.A** **Chronic nephritic syndrome with C3 glomerulonephritis**
     Chronic nephritic syndrome with C3 glomerulopathy
     Excludes1: Chronic nephritic syndrome (with C3 glomerulopathy) with dense deposit disease (N03.6)

N04   **NEPHROTIC SYNDROME**
4th   ***Includes:*** congenital nephrotic syndrome
     lipoid nephrosis

4th **5th** **6th** **7th**   Additional Character Required   ✔   3-character code   •=New Code   ***Excludes1***—Not coded here, do not use together
                                                     ▲=Revised Code   ***Excludes2***—Not included here

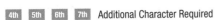 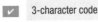

CHAPTER 14. DISEASES OF THE GENITOURINARY SYSTEM (N04.0–N13.1)

N04.0 Nephrotic syndrome with; minor glomerular abnormality
Nephrotic syndrome with minimal change lesion

N04.1 focal and segmental glomerular lesions
Nephrotic syndrome with focal and segmental hyalinosis or with focal and segmental sclerosis or with focal glomerulonephritis

N04.2 diffuse membranous glomerulonephritis

N04.3 diffuse mesangial proliferative glomerulonephritis

N04.4 diffuse endocapillary proliferative glomerulonephritis

N04.5 diffuse mesangiocapillary glomerulonephritis
Nephrotic syndrome with MPGN, types 1 and 3, or NOS
Excludes1: Nephrotic syndrome with C3 glomerulonephritis or glomerulopathy (N04.A)

N04.6 dense deposit disease
Nephrotic syndrome with C3 glomerulopathy with dense deposit disease
Nephrotic syndrome with MPGN, type 2

N04.7 diffuse crescentic glomerulonephritis
Nephrotic syndrome with extracapillary glomerulonephritis

N04.8 other morphologic changes
Nephrotic syndrome with proliferative glomerulonephritis NOS

N04.9 unspecified morphologic changes

•**N04.A Nephrotic syndrome with C3 glomerulonephritis**
Nephrotic syndrome with C3 glomerulopathy
Excludes1: Nephrotic syndrome (with C3 glomerulopathy) with dense deposit disease (N04.6)

N05 UNSPECIFIED NEPHRITIC SYNDROME
`4th`
Includes: glomerular disease NOS
glomerulonephritis NOS
nephritis NOS
nephropathy NOS and renal disease NOS with morphological lesion specified in .0–.8
Excludes1: nephropathy NOS with no stated morphological lesion (N28.9)
renal disease NOS with no stated morphological lesion (N28.9)
tubulo-interstitial nephritis NOS (N12)

N05.0 Unspecified nephritic syndrome with minor glomerular abnormality
Unspecified nephritic syndrome with minimal change lesion

N05.1 Unspecified nephritic syndrome with focal and segmental glomerular lesions
Unspecified nephritic syndrome with focal and segmental hyalinosis
Unspecified nephritic syndrome with focal and segmental sclerosis
Unspecified nephritic syndrome with focal glomerulonephritis

N05.2 Unspecified nephritic syndrome with diffuse membranous glomerulonephritis

N05.3 Unspecified nephritic syndrome with diffuse mesangial proliferative glomerulonephritis

N05.4 Unspecified nephritic syndrome with diffuse endocapillary proliferative glomerulonephritis

N05.5 Unspecified nephritic syndrome with diffuse mesangiocapillary glomerulonephritis
Unspecified nephritic syndrome with membranoproliferative glomerulonephritis, types 1 and 3, or NOS
Excludes1: Unspecified nephritic syndrome with C3 glomerulonephritis or glomerulopathy (N05.A)

N05.6 Unspecified nephritic syndrome with dense deposit disease
Unspecified nephritic syndrome with membranoproliferative glomerulonephritis, type 2
Unspecified nephritic syndrome with C3 glomerulopathy with dense deposit disease

N05.7 Unspecified nephritic syndrome with diffuse crescentic glomerulonephritis
Unspecified nephritic syndrome with extracapillary glomerulonephritis

N05.8 Unspecified nephritic syndrome with other morphologic changes
Unspecified nephritic syndrome with proliferative glomerulonephritis NOS

N05.9 Unspecified nephritic syndrome with unspecified morphologic changes

•**N05.A Unspecified nephritic syndrome with C3 glomerulonephritis**
Unspecified nephritic syndrome with C3 glomerulopathy
Excludes1: Unspecified nephritic syndrome (with C3 glomerulopathy) with dense deposit disease (N05.6)

N08 GLOMERULAR DISORDERS IN DISEASES
✓ **CLASSIFIED ELSEWHERE**
Glomerulonephritis
Nephritis
Nephropathy
Code first underlying disease, such as:
amyloidosis (E85.-)
congenital syphilis (A50.5)
cryoglobulinemia (D89.1)
disseminated intravascular coagulation (D65)
gout (M1A.-, M10.-)
microscopic polyangiitis (M31.7)
multiple myeloma (C90.0-)
sepsis (A40.0–A41.9)
sickle-cell disease (D57.0–D57.8)
Excludes1: glomerulonephritis, nephritis and nephropathy (in):
antiglomerular basement membrane disease (M31.0)
diabetes (E08–E13 with .21)
gonococcal (A54.21)
Goodpasture's syndrome (M31.0)
hemolytic-uremic syndrome (D59.3)
lupus (M32.14)
mumps (B26.83)
syphilis (A52.75)
SLE (M32.14)
Wegener's granulomatosis (M31.31)
pyelonephritis in diseases classified elsewhere (N16)
renal tubulo-interstitial disorders classified elsewhere (N16)

> Please note the numerous exclusions below.

(N10–N16) RENAL TUBULO-INTERSTITIAL DISEASES

Includes: pyelonephritis
Excludes1: pyeloureteritis cystica (N28.85)

N10 ACUTE PYELONEPHRITIS
✓
Acute infectious interstitial nephritis
Acute pyelitis
Hemoglobin nephrosis
Myoglobin nephrosis
Use additional code (B95–B97), to identify infectious agent.

N11 CHRONIC TUBULO-INTERSTITIAL NEPHRITIS
`4th`
Includes: chronic infectious interstitial nephritis
chronic pyelitis
chronic pyelonephritis
Use additional code (B95–B97), to identify infectious agent
N11.9 Chronic tubulo-interstitial nephritis, unspecified
Chronic interstitial nephritis NOS
Chronic pyelitis NOS
Chronic pyelonephritis NOS

N12 TUBULO-INTERSTITIAL NEPHRITIS, NOT SPECIFIED AS
✓ **ACUTE OR CHRONIC**
Interstitial nephritis NOS
Pyelitis NOS
Pyelonephritis NOS
Excludes1: calculus pyelonephritis (N20.9)

N13 OBSTRUCTIVE AND REFLUX UROPATHY
`4th`
Excludes2: calculus of kidney and ureter without hydronephrosis (N20.-)
congenital obstructive defects of renal pelvis and ureter (Q62.0–Q62.3)
hydronephrosis with ureteropelvic junction obstruction (Q62.11)
obstructive pyelonephritis (N11.1)
N13.0 Hydronephrosis with ureteropelvic junction obstruction
Hydronephrosis due to acquired occlusion ureteropelvic junction
Excludes2: hydronephrosis with ureteropelvic junction obstruction due to calculus (N13.2)
N13.1 Hydronephrosis with ureteral stricture, NEC
Excludes1: hydronephrosis with ureteral stricture with infection (N13.6)

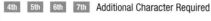 `4th` `5th` `6th` `7th` Additional Character Required   ✓ 3-character code

•=New Code   **Excludes1**—Not coded here, do not use together
▲=Revised Code   **Excludes2**—Not included here

N13.2 Hydronephrosis with renal and ureteral calculous obstruction
Excludes1: hydronephrosis with renal and ureteral calculous obstruction with infection (N13.6)

N13.3 Other and unspecified hydronephrosis
5th *Excludes1:* hydronephrosis with infection (N13.6)
    N13.30 Unspecified hydronephrosis
    N13.39 Other hydronephrosis

N13.5 Crossing vessel and stricture of ureter without hydronephrosis
Kinking and stricture of ureter without hydronephrosis
Excludes1: Crossing vessel and stricture of ureter without hydronephrosis with infection (N13.6)

N13.6 Pyonephrosis
Conditions in N13.0–N13.5 with infection
Obstructive uropathy with infection
Use additional code (B95–B97), to identify infectious agent.

N13.7 Vesicoureteral-reflux
5th *Excludes1:* reflux-associated pyelonephritis (N11.0)
    N13.70 Vesicoureteral-reflux, unspecified
    Vesicoureteral-reflux NOS
    N13.71 Vesicoureteral-reflux without reflux nephropathy

N13.8 Other obstructive and reflux uropathy
Urinary tract obstruction due to specified cause
Code first, if applicable, any causal condition, such as:
    enlarged prostate (N40.1)

N13.9 Obstructive and reflux uropathy, unspecified
Urinary tract obstruction NOS

N14 DRUG- AND HEAVY-METAL-INDUCED TUBULO-INTERSTITIAL AND TUBULAR CONDITIONS
4th
Code first poisoning due to drug or toxin, if applicable (T36–T65 with fifth or sixth character 1–4 or 6)
Use additional code for adverse effect, if applicable, to identify drug (T36–T50 with fifth or sixth character 5)

N14.0 Analgesic nephropathy

(N17–N19) ACUTE KIDNEY FAILURE AND CKD

Excludes2: congenital renal failure (P96.0)
drug- and heavy-metal–induced tubulo-interstitial and tubular conditions (N14.-)
extrarenal uremia (R39.2)
hemolytic-uremic syndrome (D59.3)
hepatorenal syndrome (K76.7)
postpartum hepatorenal syndrome (O90.4)
posttraumatic renal failure (T79.5)
prerenal uremia (R39.2)
renal failure complicating abortion or ectopic or molar pregnancy (O00–O07, O08.4)
renal failure following labor and delivery (O90.4)
renal failure postprocedural (N99.0)

N16 RENAL TUBULO-INTERSTITIAL DISORDERS IN DISEASES CLASSIFIED ELSEWHERE
✓
Pyelonephritis
Tubulo-interstitial nephritis
Code first underlying disease, such as:
    brucellosis (A23)
    cryoglobulinemia (D89.1)
    glycogen storage disease (E74.0)
    leukemia (C91-C95)
    lymphoma (C81.0-C85.9, C96.0-C96.9)
    multiple myeloma (C90.0-)
    sepsis (A40.0-A41.9)
    Wilson's disease (E83.0)
Excludes1: diphtheritic pyelonephritis and tubulo-interstitial nephritis (A36.84)
pyelonephritis and tubulo-interstitial nephritis in candidiasis (B37.49)
in cystinosis (E72.04)
in Salmonella infection (A02.25)
in sarcoidosis (D86.84)
in sicca syndrome [Sjogren's] (M35.04)
in systemic lupus erythematosus (M32.15)
in toxoplasmosis (B58.83)
renal tubular degeneration in diabetes (E08-E13 with .29)
syphilitic pyelonephritis and tubulo-interstitial nephritis (A52.75)

N17 ACUTE KIDNEY FAILURE
4th
Code also associated underlying condition
Excludes1: posttraumatic renal failure (T79.5)

N17.0 Acute kidney failure with tubular necrosis
Acute tubular necrosis
Renal tubular necrosis
Tubular necrosis NOS

N17.1 Acute kidney failure with acute cortical necrosis
Acute cortical necrosis
Cortical necrosis NOS
Renal cortical necrosis

N17.2 Acute kidney failure with medullary necrosis
Medullary [papillary] necrosis NOS
Acute medullary [papillary] necrosis
Renal medullary [papillary] necrosis

N17.8 Other acute kidney failure

N17.9 Acute kidney failure, unspecified
Acute kidney injury (nontraumatic)
Excludes2: traumatic kidney injury (S37.0-)

N18 CHRONIC KIDNEY DISEASE (CKD)
4th
GUIDELINES

Stages of CKD

The *ICD-10-CM* classifies CKD based on severity. The severity of CKD is designated by stages 1–5. Stage 2, code N18.2, equates to mild CKD; stage 3, code N18.3, equates to moderate CKD; and stage 4, code N18.4, equates to severe CKD. Code N18.6, ESRD, is assigned when the provider has documented ESRD.

If both a stage of CKD and ESRD are documented by the provider, only assign code N18.6 for ESRD (CKD requiring dialysis) only.

Patients who have undergone kidney transplant may still have some form of CKD because the kidney transplant may not fully restore kidney function. Therefore, the presence of CKD alone does not constitute a transplant complication. Assign the appropriate N18 code for the patient's stage of CKD and code Z94.0, Kidney transplant status. If a transplant complication such as failure or rejection or other transplant complication is documented, refer to code T86.1 for information on coding complications of a kidney transplant. If the documentation is unclear as to whether the patient has a complication of the transplant, query the provider.

Code first any associated diabetic CKD (E08.22, E09.22, E10.22, E11.22, E13.22)
    hypertensive chronic kidney disease (I12.-, I13.-)
Use additional code to identify kidney transplant status, if applicable, (Z94.0)

N18.1 CKD stage 1
N18.2 CKD stage 2 (mild)
▲**N18.3 CKD stage 3 (moderate)**
5th •**N18.30 CKD, stage 3 unspecified**
    •**N18.31 CKD, stage 3a**
    •**N18.32 CKD, stage 3b**
N18.4 CKD stage 4 (severe)
N18.5 CKD stage 5
Excludes1: CKD, stage 5 requiring chronic dialysis (N18.6)
N18.6 ESRD
CKD requiring chronic dialysis
Use additional code to identify dialysis status (Z99.2)
N18.9 CKD, unspecified
Chronic renal disease
Chronic renal failure NOS
Chronic renal insufficiency
Chronic uremia NOS

N19 UNSPECIFIED KIDNEY FAILURE
✓
Uremia NOS
Excludes1: acute kidney failure (N17.-)
chronic kidney disease (N18.-)
chronic uremia (N18.9)
extrarenal uremia (R39.2)
prerenal uremia (R39.2)
renal insufficiency (acute) (N28.9)
uremia of newborn (P96.0)

4th	5th	6th	7th	Additional Character Required	✓ 3-character code

•=New Code
▲=Revised Code

Excludes1—Not coded here, do not use together
Excludes2—Not included here

CHAPTER 14. DISEASES OF THE GENITOURINARY SYSTEM (N13.2–N19)

CHAPTER 14. DISEASES OF THE GENITOURINARY SYSTEM (N20–N32.2)

(N20–N23) UROLITHIASIS

N20 **CALCULUS OF KIDNEY AND URETER**
`4th`
Calculous pyelonephritis
Excludes1: nephrocalcinosis (E83.5)
   that with hydronephrosis (N13.2)

N20.0 **Calculus of kidney**
Nephrolithiasis NOS
Renal calculus
Renal stone
Staghorn calculus
Stone in kidney

N20.1 **Calculus of ureter**
Ureteric stone
Calculus of the ureteropelvic junction

N20.2 **Calculus of kidney with calculus of ureter**

N20.9 **Urinary calculus, unspecified**

N21 **CALCULUS OF LOWER URINARY TRACT**
`4th`
Includes: calculus of lower urinary tract with cystitis and urethritis

N21.0 **Calculus in bladder**
Calculus in diverticulum of bladder
Urinary bladder stone
Excludes2: staghorn calculus (N20.0)

N21.1 **Calculus in urethra**
Excludes2: calculus of prostate (N42.0)

N22 **CALCULUS OF URINARY TRACT IN DISEASES**
`✔` **CLASSIFIED ELSEWHERE**
Code first underlying disease, such as:
   gout (M1A.-, M10.-)
   schistosomiasis (B65.0-B65.9)

N23 **UNSPECIFIED RENAL COLIC**
`✔`

(N25–N29) OTHER DISORDERS OF KIDNEY AND URETER

Excludes2: disorders of kidney and ureter with urolithiasis (N20–N23)

N25 **DISORDERS RESULTING FROM IMPAIRED RENAL**
`4th` **TUBULAR FUNCTION**

N25.0 **Renal osteodystrophy**
Azotemic osteodystrophy
Phosphate-losing tubular disorders
Renal rickets
Renal short stature
Excludes2: metabolic disorders classifiable to E70–E88

N25.1 **Nephrogenic diabetes insipidus**
Excludes1: diabetes insipidus NOS (E23.2)

N27 **SMALL KIDNEY OF UNKNOWN CAUSE**
`4th`
Includes: oligonephronia

N27.0 **Small kidney, unilateral**

N27.1 **Small kidney, bilateral**

N28 **OTHER DISORDERS OF KIDNEY AND URETER, NEC**
`4th`
N28.0 **Ischemia and infarction of kidney**
Renal artery embolism or obstruction or occlusion or thrombosis
Renal infarct
Excludes1: atherosclerosis of renal artery (extrarenal part) (I70.1)
   congenital stenosis of renal artery (Q27.1)
   Goldblatt's kidney (I70.1)

N28.1 **Cyst of kidney, acquired**
Cyst (multiple)(solitary) of kidney (acquired)
Excludes1: cystic kidney disease (congenital) (Q61.-)

N28.8 **Other specified disorders of kidney and ureter**
`5th` *Excludes1:* hydroureter (N13.4)
   ureteric stricture with hydronephrosis (N13.1)
   ureteric stricture without hydronephrosis (N13.5)

N28.85 **Pyeloureteritis cystica**

N28.89 **Other specified disorders of kidney and ureter**

N28.9 **Disorder of kidney and ureter, unspecified**
Nephropathy NOS
Renal disease (acute) NOS
Renal insufficiency (acute)
Excludes1: chronic renal insufficiency (N18.9)
   unspecified nephritic syndrome (N05.-)

N29 **OTHER DISORDERS OF KIDNEY AND URETER IN**
`✔` **DISEASES CLASSIFIED ELSEWHERE**
Code first underlying disease, such as:
   amyloidosis (E85.-)
   nephrocalcinosis (E83.5)
   schistosomiasis (B65.0-B65.9)
Excludes1: disorders of kidney and ureter in:
   cystinosis (E72.0)
   gonorrhea (A54.21)
   syphilis (A52.75)
   tuberculosis (A18.11)

(N30–N39) OTHER DISEASES OF THE URINARY SYSTEM

Excludes1: urinary infection (complicating): abortion or ectopic or molar pregnancy (O00–O07, O08.8)
pregnancy, childbirth and the puerperium (O23.-, O75.3, O86.2-)

N30 **CYSTITIS**
`4th` **Use additional code** to identify infectious agent (B95–B97)
Excludes1: prostatocystitis (N41.3)

N30.0 **Acute cystitis**
`5th` *Excludes1:* irradiation cystitis (N30.4-)
   trigonitis (N30.3-)
N30.00 **Acute cystitis without hematuria**
N30.01 **Acute cystitis with hematuria**

N30.3 **Trigonitis**
`5th` Urethrotrigonitis
N30.30 **Trigonitis without hematuria**
N30.31 **Trigonitis with hematuria**

N30.4 **Irradiation cystitis**
`5th` **N30.40** **Irradiation cystitis without hematuria**
N30.41 **Irradiation cystitis with hematuria**

N30.8 **Other cystitis**
`5th` Abscess of bladder
N30.80 **Other cystitis without hematuria**
N30.81 **Other cystitis with hematuria**

N30.9 **Cystitis, unspecified**
`5th` **N30.90** **Cystitis, unspecified without hematuria**
N30.91 **Cystitis, unspecified with hematuria**

N31 **NEUROMUSCULAR DYSFUNCTION OF BLADDER, NEC**
`4th` **Use additional code** to identify any associated urinary incontinence (N39.3–N39.4-)
Excludes1: cord bladder NOS (G95.89)
   neurogenic bladder due to cauda equina syndrome (G83.4)
   neuromuscular dysfunction due to spinal cord lesion (G95.89)

N31.0 **Uninhibited neuropathic bladder, NEC**

N31.1 **Reflex neuropathic bladder, NEC**

N31.2 **Flaccid neuropathic bladder, NEC**
Atonic (motor) (sensory) neuropathic bladder
Autonomous neuropathic bladder
Nonreflex neuropathic bladder

N31.8 **Other neuromuscular dysfunction of bladder**

N31.9 **Neuromuscular dysfunction of bladder, unspecified**
Neurogenic bladder dysfunction NOS

N32 **OTHER DISORDERS OF BLADDER**
`4th` *Excludes2:* calculus of bladder (N21.0)
   cystocele (N81.1-)
   hernia or prolapse of bladder, female (N81.1-)

N32.0 **Bladder-neck obstruction**
Bladder-neck stenosis (acquired)
Excludes1: congenital bladder-neck obstruction (Q64.3-)

N32.1 **Vesicointestinal fistula**
Vesicorectal fistula

N32.2 **Vesical fistula, NEC**
Excludes1: fistula between bladder and female genital tract (N82.0–N82.1)

`4th` `5th` `6th` `7th` Additional Character Required   3-character code   •=New Code   *Excludes1*—Not coded here, do not use together
                                          ▲=Revised Code   *Excludes2*—Not included here

N32.3 Diverticulum of bladder
Excludes1: congenital diverticulum of bladder (Q64.6)
diverticulitis of bladder (N30.8-)

N32.8 Other specified disorders of bladder
5th **N32.81 Overactive bladder**
Detrusor muscle hyperactivity
Excludes1: frequent urination due to specified bladder
condition — code to condition

N32.89 Other specified disorders of bladder
Bladder hemorrhage
Bladder hypertrophy
Calcified bladder
Contracted bladder

N32.9 Bladder disorder, unspecified

N34 URETHRITIS AND URETHRAL SYNDROME
4th **Use additional code** (B95–B97), to identify infectious agent.
Excludes2: Reiter's disease (M02.3-)
urethritis in diseases with a predominantly sexual mode of transmission
(A50–A64)
urethrotrigonitis (N30.3-)

N34.0 Urethral abscess
Abscess (of) Cowper's gland
Abscess (of) Littré's gland
Abscess (of) urethral (gland)
Periurethral abscess
Excludes1: urethral caruncle (N36.2)

N34.1 Nonspecific urethritis
Nongonococcal urethritis
Nonvenereal urethritis

N34.2 Other urethritis
Meatitis, urethral
Postmenopausal urethritis
Ulcer of urethra (meatus)
Urethritis NOS

N34.3 Urethral syndrome, unspecified

N35 URETHRAL STRICTURE
4th *Excludes1:* congenital urethral stricture (Q64.3-)
postprocedural urethral stricture (N99.1-)

N35.0 Post-traumatic urethral stricture
5th Urethral stricture due to injury
Excludes1: postprocedural urethral stricture (N99.1-)

N35.01 Post-traumatic urethral stricture, male
6th **N35.010 Post-traumatic urethral stricture, male, meatal**
N35.011 Post-traumatic bulbous urethral stricture
N35.012 Post-traumatic membranous urethral stricture
N35.013 Post-traumatic anterior urethral stricture
N35.014 Post-traumatic urethral stricture, male, unspecified
N35.016 Post-traumatic urethral stricture, male, overlapping sites

N35.02 Post-traumatic urethral stricture, female
6th **N35.021 Urethral stricture due to childbirth**
N35.028 Other post-traumatic urethral stricture, female

N35.1 Postinfective urethral stricture, NEC
5th *Excludes1:* urethral stricture associated with schistosomiasis
(B65.-, N29)
gonococcal urethral stricture (A54.01)
syphilitic urethral stricture (A52.76)

N35.11 Postinfective urethral stricture, NEC, male
6th **N35.111 Postinfective urethral stricture, NEC, male, meatal**
N35.112 Postinfective bulbous urethral stricture, NEC, male
N35.113 Postinfective membranous urethral stricture, NEC, male
N35.114 Postinfective anterior urethral stricture, NEC, male
N35.116 Postinfective urethral stricture, NEC, male, overlapping sites
N35.119 Postinfective urethral stricture, NEC, male,

unspecified
N35.12 Postinfective urethral stricture, NEC, female
N35.8 Other urethral stricture
5th *Excludes1:* postprocedural urethral stricture (N99.1-)
N35.81 Other urethral stricture, male
6th **N35.811 Other urethral stricture, male, meatal**
N35.812 Other urethral bulbous stricture, male
N35.813 Other membranous urethral stricture, male
N35.814 Other anterior urethral stricture, male
N35.816 Other urethral stricture, male, overlapping sites
N35.819 Other urethral stricture, male, unspecified site
N35.82 Other urethral stricture, female
N35.9 Urethral stricture, unspecified
5th **N35.91 Urethral stricture, unspecified, male**
6th **N35.911 Unspecified urethral stricture, male, meatal**
N35.912 Unspecified bulbous urethral stricture, male
N35.913 Unspecified membranous urethral stricture, male
N35.914 Unspecified anterior urethral stricture, male
N35.916 Unspecified urethral stricture, male, overlapping sites
N35.919 Unspecified urethral stricture, male, unspecified site
N35.92 Unspecified urethral stricture, female

N39 OTHER DISORDERS OF URINARY SYSTEM
4th *Excludes2:* hematuria NOS (R31.-)
recurrent or persistent hematuria (N02.-)
recurrent or persistent hematuria with specified morphological lesion
(N02.-)
proteinuria NOS (R80.-)

N39.0 Urinary tract infection, site not specified
Use additional code (B95–B97), to identify infectious agent.
Excludes1: candidiasis of urinary tract (B37.4-)
neonatal urinary tract infection (P39.3)
pyuria (R82.81)
urinary tract infection of specified site, such as:
cystitis (N30.-)
urethritis (N34.-)

N39.4 Other specified urinary incontinence
5th **Code also any associated** overactive bladder (N32.81)
Excludes1: enuresis NOS (R32)
functional urinary incontinence (R39.81)
urinary incontinence associated with cognitive impairment
(R39.81)
urinary incontinence NOS (R32)
urinary incontinence of nonorganic origin (F98.0)

N39.44 Nocturnal enuresis
N39.8 Other specified disorders of urinary system
N39.9 Disorder of urinary system, unspecified

(N40–N53) DISEASES OF MALE GENITAL ORGANS

N41 INFLAMMATORY DISEASES OF PROSTATE
4th **Use additional code** (B95–B97), to identify infectious agent.
N41.0 Acute prostatitis
N41.9 Inflammatory disease of prostate, unspecified
Prostatitis NOS

N43 HYDROCELE AND SPERMATOCELE
4th *Includes:* hydrocele of spermatic cord, testis or tunica vaginalis
Excludes1: congenital hydrocele (P83.5)
N43.0 Encysted hydrocele
N43.1 Infected hydrocele
Use additional code (B95–B97), to identify infectious agent
N43.2 Other hydrocele
N43.3 Hydrocele, unspecified
N43.4 Spermatocele of epididymis
5th Spermatic cyst

4th 5th 6th 7th Additional Character Required   ✔ 3-character code

•=New Code   *Excludes1*—Not coded here, do not use together
▲=Revised Code   *Excludes2*—Not included here

CHAPTER 14. DISEASES OF THE GENITOURINARY SYSTEM   (N32.3–N43.4)

CHAPTER 14. DISEASES OF THE GENITOURINARY SYSTEM (N43.40–N64.4)

N43.40 Spermatocele of epididymis, unspecified
N43.41 Spermatocele of epididymis, single
N43.42 Spermatocele of epididymis, multiple

N44 NONINFLAMMATORY DISORDERS OF TESTIS
`4th`
  N44.0 Torsion of testis
  `5th` **N44.00** Torsion of testis, unspecified
    N44.01 Extravaginal torsion of spermatic cord
    N44.02 Intravaginal torsion of spermatic cord
      Torsion of spermatic cord NOS
    N44.03 Torsion of appendix testis
    N44.04 Torsion of appendix epididymis
  N44.1 Cyst of tunica albuginea testis
  N44.2 Benign cyst of testis
  N44.8 Other noninflammatory disorders of the testis

N45 ORCHITIS AND EPIDIDYMITIS
`4th`
  Use additional code (B95–B97), to identify infectious agent.
  N45.1 Epididymitis
  N45.2 Orchitis
  N45.3 Epididymo-orchitis
  N45.4 Abscess of epididymis or testis

N47 DISORDERS OF PREPUCE
`4th`
  N47.0 Adherent prepuce, newborn
  N47.1 Phimosis
  N47.2 Paraphimosis
  N47.4 Benign cyst of prepuce
  N47.5 Adhesions of prepuce and glans penis
  N47.6 Balanoposthitis
  N47.7 Other inflammatory diseases of prepuce
    Use additional code (B95–B97), to identify infectious agent.
  N47.8 Other disorders of prepuce
    Use additional code (B95–B97), to identify infectious agent.
    Excludes1: balanitis (N48.1)

N48 OTHER DISORDERS OF PENIS
`4th`
  N48.1 Balanitis
    Use additional code (B95–B97), to identify infectious agent
    Excludes1: amebic balanitis (A06.8)
      balanitis xerotica obliterans (N48.0)
      candidal balanitis (B37.42)
      gonococcal balanitis (A54.23)
      herpesviral [herpes simplex] balanitis (A60.01)
  N48.3 Priapism
  `5th` Painful erection
    Code first underlying cause
    N48.30 Priapism, unspecified
    N48.31 Priapism due to trauma
    N48.32 Priapism due to disease classified elsewhere
    N48.33 Priapism, drug-induced
    N48.39 Other priapism
  N48.8 Other specified disorders of penis
  `5th` **N48.82** Acquired torsion of penis
      Acquired torsion of penis NOS
      Excludes1: congenital torsion of penis (Q55.63)
    N48.89 Other specified disorders of penis
  N48.9 Disorder of penis, unspecified

N49 INFLAMMATORY DISORDERS OF MALE GENITAL ORGANS, NOT ELSEWHERE CLASSIFIED
`4th`
  Use additional code (B95–B97), to identify infectious agent
  Excludes1: inflammation of penis (N48.1, N48.2-)
    orchitis and epididymitis (N45.-)
  N49.0 Inflammatory disorders of seminal vesicle
    Vesiculitis NOS

N50 OTHER AND UNSPECIFIED DISORDERS OF MALE GENITAL ORGANS
`4th`
  Excludes2: torsion of testis (N44.0-)
  N50.0 Atrophy of testis
  N50.8 Other specified disorders of male genital organs
  `5th` **N50.81** Testicular pain
    `6th`

N50.811 Right testicular pain
N50.812 Left testicular pain
N50.82 Scrotal pain
N50.89 Other specified disorders of the male genital organs
  Atrophy or edema or hypertrophy or ulcer of scrotum, seminal vesicle, spermatic cord, tunica vaginalis and vas deferens
  Chylocele, tunica vaginalis (nonfilarial) NOS
  Urethroscrotal fistula
  Stricture of spermatic cord, tunica vaginalis, and vas deferens
N50.9 Disorder of male genital organs, unspecified

(N60–N65) DISORDERS OF BREAST

Excludes1: disorders of breast associated with childbirth (O91–O92)

N60 BENIGN MAMMARY DYSPLASIA
`4th`
  Includes: fibrocystic mastopathy
  N60.0 Solitary cyst of breast
  `5th` Cyst of breast
    N60.01 Solitary cyst of right breast
    N60.02 Solitary cyst of left breast
    N60.09 Solitary cyst of unspecified breast

N61 INFLAMMATORY DISORDERS OF BREAST
`4th`
  Excludes1: inflammatory carcinoma of breast (C50.9)
    inflammatory disorder of breast associated with childbirth (O91.-)
    neonatal infective mastitis (P39.0)
    thrombophlebitis of breast [Mondor's disease] (I80.8)
  N61.0 Mastitis without abscess
    Infective mastitis (acute) (subacute) (nonpuerperal)
    Mastitis (acute) (subacute) (nonpuerperal) NOS
    Cellulitis (acute) (nonpuerperal) (subacute) of breast or nipple NOS
  N61.1 Abscess of the breast and nipple
    Abscess (acute) (chronic) (nonpuerperal) of areola or breast
    Carbuncle of breast
    Mastitis with abscess

N62 HYPERTROPHY OF BREAST
`✔`
  Gynecomastia
  Hypertrophy of breast NOS
  Massive pubertal hypertrophy of breast
  Excludes1: breast engorgement of newborn (P83.4)
    disproportion of reconstructed breast (N65.1)

N63 UNSPECIFIED LUMP IN BREAST
`4th`
  Nodule(s) NOS in breast
  N63.0 Unspecified lump in unspecified breast
  N63.1 Unspecified lump in the right breast
  `5th` **N63.10** Unspecified lump in the right breast, unspecified quadrant
    N63.11 upper outer quadrant
    N63.12 upper inner quadrant
    N63.13 lower outer quadrant
    N63.14 lower inner quadrant
    N63.15 overlapping quadrants
  N63.2 Unspecified lump in the left breast
  `5th` **N63.20** Unspecified lump in the left breast, unspecified quadrant
    N63.21 upper outer quadrant
    N63.22 upper inner quadrant
    N63.23 lower outer quadrant
    N63.24 lower inner quadrant
    N63.25 overlapping quadrants
  N63.3 Unspecified lump in axillary tail
  `5th` **N63.31** Unspecified lump in axillary tail of the right breast
    N63.32 Unspecified lump in axillary tail of the left breast
  N63.4 Unspecified lump in breast, subareolar
  `5th` **N63.41** Unspecified lump in right breast, subareolar
    N63.42 Unspecified lump in left breast, subareolar

N64 OTHER DISORDERS OF BREAST
`4th`
  Excludes2: mechanical complication of breast prosthesis and implant (T85.4-)
  N64.3 Galactorrhea not associated with childbirth
  N64.4 Mastodynia

`4th` `5th` `6th` `7th` Additional Character Required   `✔` 3-character code

•=New Code   *Excludes1*—Not coded here, do not use together
▲=Revised Code   *Excludes2*—Not included here

N64.5 **Other signs and symptoms in breast**
  [5th]   *Excludes2:* abnormal findings on diagnostic imaging of breast (R92.-)
     N64.51   **Induration of breast**
     N64.52   **Nipple discharge**
       Excludes1: abnormal findings in nipple discharge (R89.-)
     N64.53   **Retraction of nipple**
     N64.59   **Other signs and symptoms in breast**
N64.8 **Other specified disorders of breast**
  [5th]   N64.89   **Other specified disorders of breast**
       Galactocele
       Subinvolution of breast (postlactational)

(N70–N77) INFLAMMATORY DISEASES OF FEMALE PELVIC ORGANS

Excludes1: inflammatory diseases of female pelvic organs complicating:
   abortion or ectopic or molar pregnancy (O00–O07, O08.0)
   pregnancy, childbirth and the puerperium (O23.-, O75.3, O85, O86.-)

N70   **SALPINGITIS AND OOPHORITIS**
[4th]   *Includes:* abscess (of) fallopian tube
     abscess (of) ovary
     pyosalpinx
     salpingo-oophoritis
     tubo-ovarian abscess
     tubo-ovarian inflammatory disease
Use additional code (B95–B97), to identify infectious agent
Excludes1: gonococcal infection (A54.24)
     tuberculous infection (A18.17)
N70.0 **Acute salpingitis and oophoritis**
  [5th]   N70.01   **Acute salpingitis**
     N70.02   **Acute oophoritis**
     N70.03   **Acute salpingitis and oophoritis**
N70.1 **Chronic salpingitis and oophoritis**
  [5th]   Hydrosalpinx
     N70.11   **Chronic salpingitis**
     N70.12   **Chronic oophoritis**
     N70.13   **Chronic salpingitis and oophoritis**
N70.9 **Salpingitis and oophoritis, unspecified**
  [5th]   N70.91   **Salpingitis, unspecified**
     N70.92   **Oophoritis, unspecified**
     N70.93   **Salpingitis and oophoritis, unspecified**

N71   **INFLAMMATORY DISEASE OF UTERUS, EXCEPT CERVIX**
[4th]   *Includes:* endo (myo) metritis
     metritis
     myometritis
     pyometra
     uterine abscess
Use additional code (B95–B97), to identify infectious agent
Excludes1: hyperplastic endometritis (N85.0-)
     infection of uterus following delivery (O85, O86.-)
N71.0 **Acute inflammatory disease of uterus**
N71.9 **Inflammatory disease of uterus, unspecified**

N72   **INFLAMMATORY DISEASE OF CERVIX UTERI**
[✓]   *Includes:* cervicitis or endocervicitis or exocervicitis (all with or without erosion or ectropion)
Use additional code (B95–B97), to identify infectious agent
Excludes1: erosion and ectropion of cervix without cervicitis (N86)

N73   **OTHER FEMALE PELVIC INFLAMMATORY DISEASES**
[4th]   **Use additional code** (B95–B97), to identify infectious agent.
N73.0 **Acute parametritis and pelvic cellulitis**
     Abscess of broad ligament
     Abscess of parametrium
     Pelvic cellulitis, female
N73.1 **Chronic parametritis and pelvic cellulitis**
     Any condition in N73.0 specified as chronic
     Excludes1: tuberculous parametritis and pelvic cellultis (A18.17)
N73.3 **Female acute pelvic peritonitis**
N73.4 **Female chronic pelvic peritonitis**
     Excludes1: tuberculous pelvic (female) peritonitis (A18.17)

N73.5 **Female pelvic peritonitis, unspecified**
N73.6 **Female pelvic peritoneal adhesions (postinfective)**
     Excludes2: postprocedural pelvic peritoneal adhesions (N99.4)
N73.8 **Other specified female pelvic inflammatory diseases**
N73.9 **Female pelvic inflammatory disease, unspecified**
     Female pelvic infection or inflammation NOS

N75   **DISEASES OF BARTHOLIN'S GLAND**
[4th]   N75.0   **Cyst of Bartholin's gland**
     N75.1   **Abscess of Bartholin's gland**

N76   **OTHER INFLAMMATION OF VAGINA AND VULVA**
[4th]   **Use additional code** (B95–B97), to identify infectious agent
Excludes2: vulvar vestibulitis (N94.810)
N76.0 **Acute vaginitis**
     Acute vulvovaginitis
N76.1 **Subacute and chronic vaginitis**
     Chronic vulvovaginitis
     Subacute vulvovaginitis
N76.2 **Acute vulvitis**
     Vulvitis NOS
N76.4 **Abscess of vulva**
     Furuncle of vulva
N76.8 **Other specified inflammation of vagina and vulva**
  [5th]   N76.89   **Other specified inflammation of vagina and vulva**

N77   **VULVOVAGINAL ULCERATION AND INFLAMMATION IN**
[4th]   **DISEASES CLASSIFIED ELSEWHERE**
N77.1 **Vaginitis, vulvitis and vulvovaginitis in diseases classified elsewhere**
     Code first underlying disease, such as:
       pinworm (B80)
     Excludes1: candidal vulvovaginitis (B37.3)
       chlamydial vulvovaginitis (A56.02)
       gonococcal vulvovaginitis (A54.02)
       herpesviral [herpes simplex] vulvovaginitis (A60.04)
       trichomonal vulvovaginitis (A59.01)
       tuberculous vulvovaginitis (A18.18)
       vulvovaginitis in early syphilis (A51.0)
       vulvovaginitis in late syphilis (A52.76)

(N80–N98) NONINFLAMMATORY DISORDERS OF FEMALE GENITAL TRACT

N83   **NONINFLAMMATORY DISORDERS OF OVARY, FALLOPIAN**
[4th]   **TUBE AND BROAD LIGAMENT**
Excludes2: hydrosalpinx (N70.1-)
N83.0 **Follicular cyst of ovary**
  [5th]   Cyst of graafian follicle
     Hemorrhagic follicular cyst (of ovary)
     N83.00   **Follicular cyst of ovary, unspecified side**
     N83.01   **Follicular cyst of right ovary**
     N83.02   **Follicular cyst of left ovary**
N83.1 **Corpus luteum cyst**
  [5th]   Hemorrhagic corpus luteum cyst
     N83.10   **Corpus luteum cyst of ovary, unspecified side**
     N83.11   **Corpus luteum cyst of right ovary**
     N83.12   **Corpus luteum cyst of left ovary**
N83.2 **Other and unspecified ovarian cysts**
  [5th]   *Excludes1:* developmental ovarian cyst (Q50.1)
     neoplastic ovarian cyst (D27.-)
     polycystic ovarian syndrome (E28.2)
     Stein-Leventhal syndrome (E28.2)
     N83.20   **Unspecified ovarian cysts**
      [6th]   N83.201   **Unspecified ovarian cyst, right side**
         N83.202   **Unspecified ovarian cyst, left side**
         N83.209   **Unspecified ovarian cyst, unspecified side**
     N83.29   **Other ovarian cysts**
      [6th]   Retention cyst of ovary
       Simple cyst of ovary
         N83.291   **Other ovarian cyst, right side**
         N83.292   **Other ovarian cyst, left side**
         N83.299   **Other ovarian cyst, unspecified side**
N83.4 **Prolapse and hernia of ovary and fallopian tube**
  [5th]

N83.40 Prolapse and hernia of ovary and fallopian tube, unspecified side
Prolapse and hernia of ovary and fallopian tube, NOS

N83.41 Prolapse and hernia of right ovary and fallopian tube

N83.42 Prolapse and hernia of left ovary and fallopian tube

N83.5 [5th] Torsion of ovary, ovarian pedicle and fallopian tube
Torsion of accessory tube

    N83.51 Torsion of ovary and ovarian pedicle

    [6th] N83.511 Torsion of right ovary and ovarian pedicle

    N83.512 Torsion of left ovary and ovarian pedicle

    N83.519 Torsion of ovary and ovarian pedicle, unspecified side
    Torsion of ovary and ovarian pedicle, NOS

    N83.53 Torsion of ovary, ovarian pedicle and fallopian tube

N83.8 Other noninflammatory disorders of ovary, fallopian tube and broad ligament
Broad ligament laceration syndrome [Allen-Masters]

N85 [4th] OTHER NONINFLAMMATORY DISORDERS OF UTERUS, EXCEPT CERVIX

Excludes1: endometriosis (N80.-)
inflammatory diseases of uterus (N71.-)
noninflammatory disorders of cervix, except malposition (N86–N88)
polyp of corpus uteri (N84.0)
uterine prolapse (N81.-)

N85.0 Endometrial hyperplasia

    [5th] N85.00 Endometrial hyperplasia, unspecified
    Hyperplasia (adenomatous) (cystic) (glandular) of endometrium
    Hyperplastic endometritis

N85.8 Other specified noninflammatory disorders of uterus
Atrophy of uterus, acquired
Fibrosis of uterus NOS

N86 [✓] EROSION AND ECTROPION OF CERVIX UTERI

Decubitus (trophic) ulcer of cervix
Eversion of cervix
Excludes1: erosion and ectropion of cervix with cervicitis (N72)

N88 [4th] OTHER NONINFLAMMATORY DISORDERS OF CERVIX UTERI

Excludes2: inflammatory disease of cervix (N72)
polyp of cervix (N84.1)

N88.1 Old laceration of cervix uteri
Adhesions of cervix
Excludes1: current obstetric trauma (O71.3)

N88.2 Stricture and stenosis of cervix uteri
Excludes1: stricture and stenosis of cervix uteri complicating labor (O65.5)

N89 [4th] OTHER NONINFLAMMATORY DISORDERS OF VAGINA

Excludes1: abnormal results from vaginal cytologic examination without histologic confirmation (R87.62-)
carcinoma in situ of vagina (D07.2)
HGSIL of vagina (R87.623)
inflammation of vagina (N76.-)
senile (atrophic) vaginitis (N95.2)
severe dysplasia of vagina (D07.2)
trichomonal leukorrhea (A59.00)
vaginal intraepithelial neoplasia [VAIN], grade III (D07.2)

N89.5 Stricture and atresia of vagina
Vaginal adhesions
Vaginal stenosis
Excludes1: congenital atresia or stricture (Q52.4)
postprocedural adhesions of vagina (N99.2)

N89.6 Tight hymenal ring
Rigid hymen
Tight introitus
Excludes1: imperforate hymen (Q52.3)

N89.7 Hematocolpos
Hematocolpos with hematometra or hematosalpinx

N89.8 Other specified noninflammatory disorders of vagina
Leukorrhea NOS
Old vaginal laceration
Pessary ulcer of vagina
Excludes1: current obstetric trauma (O70.-, O71.4, O71.7–O71.8)
old laceration involving muscles of pelvic floor (N81.8)

N89.9 Noninflammatory disorder of vagina, unspecified

N90 [4th] OTHER NONINFLAMMATORY DISORDERS OF VULVA AND PERINEUM

Excludes1: anogenital (venereal) warts (A63.0)
carcinoma in situ of vulva (D07.1)
condyloma acuminatum (A63.0)
current obstetric trauma (O70.-, O71.7–O71.8)
inflammation of vulva (N76.-)
severe dysplasia of vulva (D07.1)
vulvar intraepithelial neoplasm III [VIN III] (D07.1)

N90.0 Mild vulvar dysplasia
Vulvar intraepithelial neoplasia [VIN], grade I

N90.1 Moderate vulvar dysplasia
Vulvar intraepithelial neoplasia [VIN], grade II

N90.3 Dysplasia of vulva, unspecified

N90.4 Leukoplakia of vulva
Dystrophy of vulva
Kraurosis of vulva
Lichen sclerosus of external female genital organs

N90.5 Atrophy of vulva
Stenosis of vulva

N90.6 Hypertrophy of vulva

    [5th] N90.60 Unspecified hypertrophy of vulva
    Unspecified hypertrophy of labia

    N90.61 Childhood asymmetric labium majus enlargement CALME

    N90.69 Other specified hypertrophy of vulva
    Other specified hypertrophy of labia

N90.7 Vulvar cyst

N90.8 [5th] Other specified noninflammatory disorders of vulva and perineum

    N90.81 [6th] Female genital mutilation status
    Female genital cutting status

      N90.810 Female genital mutilation status, unspecified
      Female genital cutting status, unspecified
      Female genital mutilation status NOS

      N90.811 Female genital mutilation Type I status
      Clitorectomy status
      Female genital cutting Type I status

      N90.812 Female genital mutilation Type II status
      Clitorectomy with excision of labia minora status

      N90.813 Female genital mutilation Type III status
      Female genital cutting Type III status
      Infibulation status

      N90.818 Other female genital mutilation status
      Female genital cutting or mutilation Type IV status
      Other female genital cutting status

    N90.89 Other specified noninflammatory disorders of vulva and perineum
    Adhesions of vulva
    Hypertrophy of clitoris

N90.9 Noninflammatory disorder of vulva and perineum, unspecified

N91 [4th] ABSENT, SCANTY AND RARE MENSTRUATION

Excludes1: ovarian dysfunction (E28.-)

N91.0 Primary amenorrhea

N91.1 Secondary amenorrhea

N91.2 Amenorrhea, unspecified

N92 [4th] EXCESSIVE, FREQUENT AND IRREGULAR MENSTRUATION

Excludes1: postmenopausal bleeding (N95.0)
precocious puberty (menstruation) (E30.1)

  Additional Character Required   3-character code   •=New Code   ▲=Revised Code   *Excludes1*—Not coded here, do not use together   *Excludes2*—Not included here

N92.0   **Excessive and frequent menstruation with regular cycle**
Heavy periods NOS
Menorrhagia NOS
Polymenorrhea

N92.1   **Excessive and frequent menstruation with irregular cycle**
Irregular intermenstrual bleeding
Irregular, shortened intervals between menstrual bleeding
Menometrorrhagia
Metrorrhagia

N92.2   **Excessive menstruation at puberty**
Excessive bleeding associated with onset of menstrual periods
Pubertal menorrhagia
Puberty bleeding

N92.3   **Ovulation bleeding**
Regular intermenstrual bleeding

N92.5   **Other specified irregular menstruation**

N92.6   **Irregular menstruation, unspecified**
Irregular bleeding NOS
Irregular periods NOS
Excludes1: irregular menstruation with:
    lengthened intervals or scanty bleeding (N91.3–N91.5)
    shortened intervals or excessive bleeding (N92.1)

N93 **4th**   **OTHER ABNORMAL UTERINE AND VAGINAL BLEEDING**
Excludes1: neonatal vaginal hemorrhage (P54.6)
    precocious puberty (menstruation) (E30.1)
    pseudomenses (P54.6)

N93.1   **Pre-pubertal vaginal bleeding**

N93.8   **Other specified abnormal uterine and vaginal bleeding**
Dysfunctional or functional uterine or vaginal bleeding NOS

N93.9   **Abnormal uterine and vaginal bleeding, unspecified**

N94 **4th**   **PAIN AND OTHER CONDITIONS ASSOCIATED WITH FEMALE GENITAL ORGANS AND MENSTRUAL CYCLE**

N94.0   **Mittelschmerz**

N94.1 **5th**   **Dyspareunia**
Excludes1: psychogenic dyspareunia (F52.6)
    N94.10   **Unspecified dyspareunia**
    N94.11   **Superficial (introital) dyspareunia**
    N94.12   **Deep dyspareunia**
    N94.19   **Other specified dyspareunia**

N94.2   **Vaginismus**
Excludes1: psychogenic vaginismus (F52.5)

N94.3   **Premenstrual tension syndrome**
Excludes 1: premenstrual dysphoric disorder (F32.81)
Code also associated menstrual migraine (G43.82-, G43.83-)

N94.4   **Primary dysmenorrhea**

N94.5   **Secondary dysmenorrhea**

N94.6   **Dysmenorrhea, unspecified**
Excludes1: psychogenic dysmenorrhea (F45.8)

N94.8 **5th**   **Other specified conditions associated with female genital organs and menstrual cycle**
    N94.81 **6th**   **Vulvodynia**
       N94.810   **Vulvar vestibulitis**
       N94.818   **Other vulvodynia**
       N94.819   **Vulvodynia, unspecified**
          Vulvodynia NOS
    N94.89   **Other specified conditions associated with female genital organs and menstrual cycle**

N94.9   **Unspecified condition associated with female genital organs and menstrual cycle**

N97 **4th**   **FEMALE INFERTILITY**
Includes: inability to achieve a pregnancy
    sterility, female NOS
Excludes1: female infertility associated with:
    hypopituitarism (E23.0)
    Stein-Leventhal syndrome (E28.2)
Excludes2: incompetence of cervix uteri (N88.3)

N97.0   **Female infertility associated with anovulation**

N97.1   **Female infertility of tubal origin**
Female infertility associated with congenital anomaly of tube
Female infertility due to tubal block
Female infertility due to tubal occlusion
Female infertility due to tubal stenosis

N97.9   **Female infertility, unspecified**

(N99) INTRAOPERATIVE AND POSTPROCEDURAL COMPLICATIONS AND DISORDERS OF GENITOURINARY SYSTEM, NEC

N99 **4th**   **INTRAOPERATIVE AND POSTPROCEDURAL COMPLICATIONS AND DISORDERS OF GENITOURINARY SYSTEM, NEC**
Excludes2: irradiation cystitis (N30.4-)
    postoophorectomy osteoporosis with current pathological fracture (M80.8-)
    postoophorectomy osteoporosis without current pathological fracture (M81.8)

N99.0   **Postprocedural (acute) (chronic) kidney failure**
Use additional code to type of kidney disease

N99.1 **5th**   **Postprocedural urethral stricture**
Postcatheterization urethral stricture
    N99.11 **6th**   **Postprocedural urethral stricture, male**
       N99.110   **Postprocedural urethral stricture, male, meatal**
       N99.111   **Postprocedural bulbous urethral stricture, male**
       N99.112   **Postprocedural membranous urethral stricture, male**
       N99.113   **Postprocedural anterior bulbous urethral stricture, male**
       N99.114   **Postprocedural urethral stricture, male, unspecified**
       N99.115   **Postprocedural fossa navicularis urethral stricture**
       N99.116   **Postprocedural urethral stricture, male, overlapping sites**
    N99.12   **Postprocedural urethral stricture, female**

N99.2   **Postprocedural adhesions of vagina**

N99.3   **Prolapse of vaginal vault after hysterectomy**

N99.4   **Postprocedural pelvic peritoneal adhesions**
Excludes2: pelvic peritoneal adhesions NOS (N73.6)
    postinfective pelvic peritoneal adhesions (N73.6)

N99.5 **5th**   **Complications of stoma of urinary tract**
Excludes2: mechanical complication of urinary catheter (T83.0-)
    N99.51 **6th**   **Complication of cystostomy**
       N99.510   **Cystostomy hemorrhage**
       N99.511   **Cystostomy infection**
       N99.512   **Cystostomy malfunction**
       N99.518   **Other cystostomy complication**
    N99.52 **6th**   **Complication of incontinent external stoma of urinary tract**
       N99.520   **Hemorrhage of incontinent external stoma of urinary tract**
       N99.521   **Infection of incontinent external stoma of urinary tract**
       N99.522   **Malfunction of incontinent external stoma of urinary tract**
       N99.523   **Herniation of incontinent stoma of urinary tract**
       N99.524   **Stenosis of incontinent stoma of urinary tract**
       N99.528   **Other complication of incontinent external stoma of urinary tract**
    N99.53 **6th**   **Complication of continent stoma of urinary tract**
       N99.530   **Hemorrhage of continent stoma of urinary tract**
       N99.531   **Infection of continent stoma of urinary tract**
       N99.532   **Malfunction of continent stoma of urinary tract**
       N99.533   **Herniation of continent stoma of urinary tract**
       N99.534   **Stenosis of continent stoma of urinary tract**
       N99.538   **Other complication of continent stoma of urinary tract**

CHAPTER 14. DISEASES OF THE GENITOURINARY SYSTEM (N92.0–N99.538)

4th **5th** **6th** **7th**   Additional Character Required   ✔   3-character code

•=New Code
▲=Revised Code

Excludes1—Not coded here, do not use together
Excludes2—Not included here

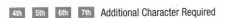

N99.8   **Other intraoperative and postprocedural complications and disorders of GI system**
5th

     N99.81   Other intraoperative complications of GI system

     N99.82   **Postprocedural hemorrhage of a GI system organ or structure following a procedure**
6th

         N99.820   Postprocedural hemorrhage of a GI system organ or structure following a GI system procedure

         N99.821   Postprocedural hemorrhage of a GI system organ or structure following other procedure

     N99.83   Residual ovary syndrome

     N99.84   **Postprocedural hematoma and seroma of a GI system organ or structure following a procedure**
6th

         N99.840   Postprocedural hematoma of a GI system organ or structure following a GI system procedure

         N99.841   Postprocedural hematoma of a GI system organ or structure following other procedure

         N99.842   Postprocedural seroma of a GI system organ or structure following a GI system procedure

         N99.843   Postprocedural seroma of a GI system organ or structure following other procedure

     N99.89   Other postprocedural complications and disorders of GI system

CHAPTER 14. DISEASES OF THE GENITOURINARY SYSTEM   (N99.8–N99.89)

4th   5th   6th   7th   Additional Character Required   ✓   3-character code   •=New Code   ▲=Revised Code   *Excludes1*—Not coded here, do not use together   *Excludes2*—Not included here

278   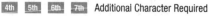PEDIATRIC ICD-10-CM 2021: A MANUAL FOR PROVIDER-BASED CODING

Chapter 15. Pregnancy, childbirth and the puerperium (O00–O9A)

GUIDELINES

General Rules for Obstetric Cases

CODES FROM CHAPTER 15 AND SEQUENCING PRIORITY
Obstetric cases require codes from Chapter 15, codes in the range O00–O9A, Pregnancy, Childbirth, and the Puerperium. Chapter 15 codes have sequencing priority over codes from other chapters. Additional codes from other chapters may be used in conjunction with Chapter 15 codes to further specify conditions. Should the provider document that the pregnancy is incidental to the encounter, then code Z33.1, Pregnant state, incidental, should be used in place of any Chapter 15 codes. It is the provider's responsibility to state that the condition being treated is not affecting the pregnancy.

CHAPTER 15 CODES USED ONLY ON THE MATERNAL RECORD
Chapter 15 codes are to be used only on the maternal record, never on the record of the newborn.

FINAL CHARACTER FOR TRIMESTER
The majority of codes in Chapter 15 have a final character indicating the trimester of pregnancy. The timeframes for the trimesters are indicated at the beginning of the chapter.

Assignment of the final character for trimester should be based on the provider's documentation of the trimester (or number of weeks) for the current admission/encounter. This applies to the assignment of trimester for pre-existing conditions as well as those that develop during or are due to the pregnancy. The provider's documentation of the number of weeks may be used to assign the appropriate code identifying the trimester.

Refer to the *ICD-10-CM* manual for complete guidelines.

SELECTION OF TRIMESTER FOR INPATIENT ADMISSIONS THAT ENCOMPASS MORE THAN ONE TRIMESTER
In instances when a patient is admitted to a hospital for complications of pregnancy during one trimester and remains in the hospital into a subsequent trimester, the trimester character for the antepartum complication code should be assigned on the basis of the trimester when the complication developed, not the trimester of the discharge. If the condition developed prior to the current admission/encounter or represents a pre-existing condition, the trimester character for the trimester at the time of the admission/encounter should be assigned.

UNSPECIFIED TRIMESTER
The "unspecified trimester" code should rarely be used, such as when the documentation in the record is insufficient to determine the trimester and it is not possible to obtain clarification.

7TH CHARACTER FOR FETUS IDENTIFICATION
Refer to categories O31, O35, O36, O40, and O41.

Selection of OB Principal or First-listed Diagnosis

ROUTINE OUTPATIENT PRENATAL VISITS
Refer to the *ICD-10-CM* manual for complete guidelines.

PRENATAL OUTPATIENT VISITS FOR HIGH-RISK PATIENTS
For routine prenatal outpatient visits for patients with high-risk pregnancies, a code from category O09, Supervision of high-risk pregnancy, should be used as the first-listed diagnosis. Secondary Chapter 15 codes may be used in conjunction with these codes if appropriate.

EPISODES WHEN NO DELIVERY OCCURS
Refer to the *ICD-10-CM* manual for complete guidelines.

WHEN A DELIVERY OCCURS
Refer to the *ICD-10-CM* manual for complete guidelines.

OUTCOME OF DELIVERY
A code from category Z37, Outcome of delivery, should be included on every maternal record when a delivery has occurred. These codes are not to be used on subsequent records or on the newborn record.

Pre-existing conditions versus conditions due to the pregnancy
Certain categories in Chapter 15 distinguish between conditions of the mother that existed prior to pregnancy (pre-existing) and those that are a direct result of pregnancy. When assigning codes from Chapter 15, it is important to assess if a condition was pre-existing prior to pregnancy or developed during or due to the pregnancy in order to assign the correct code.

Categories that do not distinguish between pre-existing and pregnancy-related conditions may be used for either. It is acceptable to use codes specifically for the puerperium with codes complicating pregnancy and childbirth if a condition arises postpartum during the delivery encounter.

Pre-existing hypertension in pregnancy
Refer to category O10.
Refer to Chapter 9, Hypertension.

Fetal Conditions Affecting the Management of the Mother

CODES FROM CATEGORIES O35 AND O36
Refer to categories O35 and O36.

IN UTERO SURGERY
Refer to category O35.

No code from Chapter 16, the perinatal codes, should be used on the mother's record to identify fetal conditions. Surgery performed in utero on a fetus is still to be coded as an obstetric encounter.

HIV Infection in Pregnancy, Childbirth and the Puerperium
During pregnancy, childbirth or the puerperium, a patient admitted because of an HIV-related illness should receive a principal diagnosis from subcategory O98.7-, HIV disease complicating pregnancy, childbirth and the puerperium, followed by the code(s) for the HIV-related illness(es).

Patients with asymptomatic HIV infection status admitted during pregnancy, childbirth, or the puerperium should receive codes of O98.7- and Z21, Asymptomatic HIV infection status.

DM in pregnancy
Diabetes mellitus is a significant complicating factor in pregnancy. Pregnant women who are diabetic should be assigned a code from category O24, DM in pregnancy, childbirth, and the puerperium, first, followed by the appropriate diabetes code(s) (E08–E13) from Chapter 4.

Long-term use of insulin
Code Z79.4, Long-term (current) use of insulin, should also be assigned if the DM is being treated with insulin.

Gestational (pregnancy induced) diabetes
Gestational (pregnancy induced) diabetes can occur during the second and third trimester of pregnancy in women who were not diabetic prior to pregnancy. Gestational diabetes can cause complications in the pregnancy similar to those of pre-existing DM. It also puts the woman at greater risk of developing diabetes after the pregnancy. Codes for gestational diabetes are in subcategory O24.4, Gestational DM. No other code from category O24, DM in pregnancy, childbirth, and the puerperium, should be used with a code from O24.4.

The codes under subcategory O24.4 include diet controlled and insulin controlled. *If a patient with gestational diabetes is treated with both diet and insulin, only the code for insulin-controlled is required.*

Refer to the *ICD-10-CM* manual for complete guidelines.

Refer to the *ICD-10-CM* manual for guidelines for normal delivery (O80); peripartum and postpartum periods; sequela of complication of pregnancy, childbirth, and the puerperium (O94); sepsis and septic shock complicating abortion, pregnancy, childbirth and the puerperium; puerperal sepsis; termination of pregnancy and spontaneous abortion and alcohol, tobacco *and drug* use during pregnancy, childbirth and the puerperium.

4th **5th** **6th** **7th** Additional Character Required   ✔ 3-character code

•=New Code
▲=Revised Code

Excludes1—Not coded here, do not use together
Excludes2—Not included here

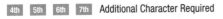

Abuse in a pregnant patient

Refer to the *ICD-10-CM* manual for complete guidelines.
Refer to Chapter 19. Adult and child abuse, neglect and other maltreatment.

Note: CODES FROM THIS CHAPTER ARE FOR USE ONLY ON MATERNAL RECORDS, NEVER ON NEWBORN RECORDS.

Codes from this chapter are for use for conditions related to or aggravated by the pregnancy, childbirth, or by the puerperium (maternal causes or obstetric causes).

Use additional code from category Z3A, Weeks of gestation, to identify the specific week of the pregnancy, if known

Excludes1: supervision of normal pregnancy (Z34.-)

Excludes2: mental and behavioral disorders associated with the puerperium (F53)
obstetrical tetanus (A34)
postpartum necrosis of pituitary gland (E23.0)
puerperal osteomalacia (M83.0)

> Trimesters are counted from the first day of the last menstrual period. They are defined as follows:
> 1st trimester — less than 14 weeks 0 days
> 2nd trimester — 14 weeks 0 days to less than 28 weeks 0 days
> 3rd trimester — 28 weeks 0 days until delivery

(O00–O08) PREGNANCY WITH ABORTIVE OUTCOME

O00 **ECTOPIC PREGNANCY**
[4th]
Includes: ruptured ectopic pregnancy
Use additional code from category O08 to identify any associated complication

O00.0 Abdominal pregnancy
[5th] *Excludes1:* maternal care for viable fetus in abdominal pregnancy (O36.7-)

O00.00 Abdominal pregnancy without intrauterine pregnancy
O00.01 Abdominal pregnancy with intrauterine pregnancy

O00.1 Tubal pregnancy
[5th] Fallopian pregnancy
Rupture of (fallopian) tube due to pregnancy
Tubal abortion

O00.10 Tubal pregnancy without intrauterine pregnancy
[6th] **O00.101** Right tubal pregnancy without intrauterine pregnancy
O00.102 Left tubal pregnancy without intrauterine pregnancy
O00.109 Unspecified tubal pregnancy without intrauterine pregnancy

O00.11 Tubal pregnancy with intrauterine pregnancy
[6th] **O00.111** Right tubal pregnancy with intrauterine pregnancy
O00.112 Left tubal pregnancy with intrauterine pregnancy
O00.119 Unspecified tubal pregnancy with intrauterine pregnancy

O00.2 Ovarian pregnancy
[5th] **O00.20** Ovarian pregnancy without intrauterine pregnancy
[6th] **O00.201** Right ovarian pregnancy without intrauterine pregnancy
O00.202 Left ovarian pregnancy without intrauterine pregnancy
O00.209 Unspecified ovarian pregnancy without intrauterine pregnancy

O00.21 Ovarian pregnancy with intrauterine pregnancy
[6th] **O00.211** Right ovarian pregnancy with intrauterine pregnancy
O00.212 Left ovarian pregnancy without intrauterine pregnancy
O00.219 Unspecified ovarian pregnancy with intrauterine pregnancy

O00.8 Other ectopic pregnancy
[5th] Cervical pregnancy
Cornual pregnancy
Intraligamentous pregnancy
Mural pregnancy
O00.80 Other ectopic pregnancy without intrauterine pregnancy
O00.81 Other ectopic pregnancy with intrauterine pregnancy

O00.9 Ectopic pregnancy, unspecified
[5th] **O00.90** Unspecified ectopic pregnancy without intrauterine pregnancy
O00.91 Unspecified ectopic pregnancy with intrauterine pregnancy

O02 **OTHER ABNORMAL PRODUCTS OF CONCEPTION**
[4th]
Use additional code from category O08 to identify any associated complication.
Excludes1: papyraceous fetus (O31.0-)
O02.1 Missed abortion
Early fetal death, before completion of 20 weeks of gestation, with retention of dead fetus
Excludes1: failed induced abortion (O07.-)
fetal death (intrauterine) (late) (O36.4)
missed abortion with blighted ovum (O02.0)
missed abortion with hydatidiform mole (O01.-)
missed abortion with nonhydatidiform (O02.0)
missed abortion with other abnormal products of conception (O02.8-)
missed delivery (O36.4)
stillbirth (P95)

O03 **SPONTANEOUS ABORTION**
[4th]
Note: Incomplete abortion includes retained products of conception following spontaneous abortion
Includes: miscarriage
O03.4 Incomplete spontaneous abortion without complication
O03.9 Complete or unspecified spontaneous abortion without complication
Miscarriage NOS
Spontaneous abortion NOS

(O09) SUPERVISION OF HIGH RISK PREGNANCY

O09 **SUPERVISION OF HIGH RISK PREGNANCY**
[4th]
O09.6 Supervision of young primigravida and multigravida
[5th] Supervision of pregnancy for a female <16 years old at expected date of delivery
O09.61 Supervision of young primigravida
[6th]
O09.62 Supervision of young multigravida
[6th]

> Requires 6th character to identify trimester
> 1 first trimester
> 2 second trimester
> 3 third trimester
> 9 unspecified trimester

(O10–O16) EDEMA, PROTEINURIA AND HYPERTENSIVE DISORDERS IN PREGNANCY, CHILDBIRTH AND THE PUERPERIUM

Category O10, Pre-existing hypertension complicating pregnancy, childbirth and the puerperium, includes codes for hypertensive heart and hypertensive CKD. When assigning one of the O10 codes that includes hypertensive heart disease or hypertensive CKD, it is necessary to add a secondary code from the appropriate hypertension category to specify the type of heart failure or CKD.

O10 **PRE-EXISTING HYPERTENSION COMPLICATING PREGNANCY, CHILDBIRTH AND THE PUERPERIUM**
[4th]
Includes: pre-existing hypertension with pre-existing proteinuria complicating pregnancy, childbirth and the puerperium
Excludes2: pre-existing hypertension with superimposed pre-eclampsia complicating pregnancy, childbirth and the puerperium (O11.-)
O10.0 Pre-existing essential hypertension complicating pregnancy, childbirth and the puerperium
[5th] Any condition in I10 specified as a reason for obstetric care during pregnancy, childbirth or the puerperium

> Requires 6th character to identify trimester
> 1 first trimester
> 2 second trimester
> 3 third trimester
> 9 unspecified trimester

O10.01 Pre-existing essential hypertension complicating pregnancy
[6th]
O10.02 Pre-existing essential hypertension complicating childbirth
[6th]
O10.03 Pre-existing essential hypertension complicating the puerperium

---

[4th] [5th] [6th] [7th] Additional Character Required ✔ 3-character code
•=New Code *Excludes1*—Not coded here, do not use together
▲=Revised Code *Excludes2*—Not included here

O10.1 **5th** **Pre-existing hypertensive heart disease complicating pregnancy, childbirth and the puerperium**

Any condition in I11 specified as a reason for obstetric care during pregnancy, childbirth or the puerperium

Use additional code from I11 to identify the type of hypertensive heart disease

O10.11 **6th** **Pre-existing hypertensive heart disease complicating pregnancy**

Requires 6th character to identify trimester
1 first trimester
2 second trimester
3 third trimester
9 unspecified trimester

O10.4 **5th** **Pre-existing secondary hypertension complicating pregnancy, childbirth and the puerperium**

Any condition in I15 specified as a reason for obstetric care during pregnancy, childbirth or the puerperium

Use additional code from I15 to identify the type of secondary hypertension

O10.41 **6th** **Pre-existing secondary hypertension complicating pregnancy**

O11 **4th** **PRE-EXISTING HYPERTENSION WITH PRE-ECLAMPSIA**

Includes: conditions in O10 complicated by pre-eclampsia
pre-eclampsia superimposed pre-existing hypertension

Use additional code from O10 to identify the type of hypertension

O11.1 Pre-existing hypertension with pre-eclampsia, first trimester

O11.2 Pre-existing hypertension with pre-eclampsia, second trimester

O11.3 Pre-existing hypertension with pre-eclampsia, third trimester

O14 **4th** **PRE-ECLAMPSIA**

Excludes1: pre-existing hypertension with pre-eclampsia (O11)

O14.0 **5th** **Mild to moderate pre-eclampsia**

O14.1 **5th** **Severe pre-eclampsia**

Excludes1: HELLP syndrome (O14.2-)

O14 requires 5th character
4 complicating childbirth
5 complicating the puerperium

O14.2 **5th** **HELLP syndrome**

Severe pre-eclampsia with hemolysis, elevated liver enzymes and low platelet count (HELLP)

O14.9 **5th** **Unspecified pre-eclampsia**

(O20–O29) OTHER MATERNAL DISORDERS PREDOMINANTLY RELATED TO PREGNANCY

Excludes2: maternal care related to the fetus and amniotic cavity and possible delivery problems (O30–O48)
maternal diseases classifiable elsewhere but complicating pregnancy, labor and delivery, and the puerperium (O98–O99)

O20 **4th** **HEMORRHAGE IN EARLY PREGNANCY**

Includes: hemorrhage before completion of 20 weeks gestation
Excludes1: pregnancy with abortive outcome (O00–O08)

O20.0 Threatened abortion

Hemorrhage specified as due to threatened abortion

O20.8 Other hemorrhage in early pregnancy

O20.9 Hemorrhage in early pregnancy, unspecified

O24 **4th** **DM IN PREGNANCY, CHILDBIRTH, AND THE PUERPERIUM**

O24.0 **5th** **Pre-existing type 1 DM**

Juvenile onset DM, in pregnancy, childbirth and the puerperium
Ketosis-prone DM in pregnancy, childbirth and the puerperium

Use additional code from category E10 to further identify any manifestations

O24.01 **6th** **Pre-existing type 1 DM, in pregnancy**

O24.01 and O24.11 require 6th character to identify trimester
1 first trimester
2 second trimester
3 third trimester
9 unspecified trimester

O24.1 **5th** **Pre-existing type 2 DM**

Insulin-resistant DM

Use additional code (for): from category E11 to further identify any manifestations long-term (current) use of insulin (Z79.4)

O24.11 **6th** **Pre-existing type 2 DM, in pregnancy**

O24.4 **5th** **Gestational DM**

DM arising in pregnancy
Gestational diabetes mellitus NOS

O24.41 **6th** **Gestational DM in pregnancy**

O24.410 Gestational DM in pregnancy, diet controlled

O24.414 Gestational DM in pregnancy, insulin controlled

O24.415 Gestational DM in pregnancy, controlled by oral hypoglycemic drugs

Gestational diabetes mellitus in pregnancy, controlled by oral antidiabetic drugs

O28 **4th** **ABNORMAL FINDINGS ON ANTENATAL SCREENING OF MOTHER**

Excludes1: diagnostic findings classified elsewhere—**see Alphabetical Index**

O28.0 Abnormal hematological finding on antenatal screening of mother

O28.1 Abnormal biochemical finding on antenatal screening of mother

O28.2 Abnormal cytological finding on antenatal screening of mother

O28.3 Abnormal ultrasonic finding on antenatal screening of mother

O28.4 Abnormal radiological finding on antenatal screening of mother

O28.5 Abnormal chromosomal and genetic finding on antenatal screening of mother

O28.8 Other abnormal findings on antenatal screening of mother

O28.9 Unspecified abnormal findings on antenatal screening of mother

(O30–O48) MATERNAL CARE RELATED TO THE FETUS AND AMNIOTIC CAVITY AND POSSIBLE DELIVERY PROBLEMS

O30 **4th** **MULTIPLE GESTATION**

Code also any complications specific to multiple gestation

O30.0 **5th** **Twin pregnancy**

O30.00 **6th** **Twin pregnancy, unspecified number of placenta and unspecified number of amniotic sacs**

O30.01 **6th** **Twin pregnancy, monochorionic/monoamniotic**

Twin pregnancy, one placenta, one amniotic sac
Excludes1: conjoined twins (O30.02-)

O30.02 **6th** **Conjoined twin pregnancy**

O30.03 **6th** **Twin pregnancy, monochorionic/diamniotic**

Twin pregnancy, one placenta, two amniotic sacs

O30.04 **6th** **Twin pregnancy, dichorionic/diamniotic**

Twin pregnancy, two placentae, two amniotic sacs

O30.09 **6th** **Twin pregnancy, unable to determine number of placenta and number of amniotic sacs**

O30.1 **5th** **Triplet pregnancy**

O30.10 **6th** **Triplet pregnancy, unspecified number of placenta and unspecified number of amniotic sacs**

O30.11 **6th** **Triplet pregnancy with two or more monochorionic fetuses**

O30.12 **6th** **Triplet pregnancy with two or more monoamniotic fetuses**

O30 requires 6th character to identify trimester
1 first trimester
2 second trimester
3 third trimester
9 unspecified trimester

O30.13 **6th** **Triplet pregnancy, trichorionic/triamniotic**

O30.19 **6th** **Triplet pregnancy, unable to determine number of placenta and number of amniotic sacs**

O30.2 **5th** **Quadruplet pregnancy**

O30.20 **6th** **Quadruplet pregnancy, unspecified number of placenta**

O30.21 **6th** **Quadruplet pregnancy with two or more monochorionic fetuses**

O30.22 **6th** **Quadruplet pregnancy with two or more monoamniotic fetuses**

O30.23 **6th** **Quadruplet pregnancy, quadrachorionic/quadra-amniotic**

O30.29 **6th** **Quadruplet pregnancy, unable to determine number of placenta and number of amniotic sacs**

4th **5th** **6th** **7th** Additional Character Required   3-character code

•=New Code
▲=Revised Code

Excludes1—Not coded here, do not use together
Excludes2—Not included here

CHAPTER 15. PREGNANCY, CHILDBIRTH AND THE PUERPERIUM   (O30.8–O35.8XX)

O30.8 **Other specified multiple gestation**
[5th] Multiple gestation pregnancy greater then quadruplets

    O30.80 **Other specified multiple gestation, unspecified number of placenta and unspecified number of amniotic sacs**
[6th]

    O30.81 **Other specified multiple gestation with two or more monochorionic fetuses**
[6th]

    O30.82 **Other specified multiple gestation with two or more monoamniotic fetuses**
[6th]

> O30 requires 6th character to identify trimester
> 1 first trimester
> 2 second trimester
> 3 third trimester
> 9 unspecified trimester

    O30.83 **Other specified multiple gestation, number of chorions and amnions are both equal to the number of fetuses**
[6th]
         Pentachorionic, penta-amniotic pregnancy (quintuplets)
         Hexachorionic, hexa-amniotic pregnancy (sextuplets)
         Heptachorionic, hepta-amniotic pregnancy (septuplets)

    O30.89 **Other specified multiple gestation, unable to determine number of placenta and number ofamniotic sacs**
[6th]

O31 **COMPLICATIONS SPECIFIC TO MULTIPLE GESTATION**
[4th] Assign a 7th character to identify the fetus for which the complication code applies.

Assign 7th character "0" for either a single gestation or when the documentation is insufficient to determine the fetus affected and it is not possible to obtain clarification or when it is not possible to clinically determine which fetus is affected.

> Requires 7th character to identify affected fetus
> 0 not applicable (ie, only one fetus) or unspecified
> 1 fetus 1
> 2 fetus 2
> 3 fetus 3
> 4 fetus 4
> 5 fetus 5
> 9 other fetus

Excludes2: delayed delivery of second twin, triplet, etc. (O63.2)
     malpresentation of one fetus or more (O32.9)
     placental transfusion syndromes (O43.0-)

Code also the appropriate code from category O30, Multiple gestation, when assigning a code from category O31 that has a 7th character of 1 through 9.

O31.1 **Continuing pregnancy after spontaneous abortion of one fetus or more**
[5th]

    O31.10 **Continuing pregnancy after spontaneous abortion of one fetus or more, unspecified trimester**

    O31.11 **Continuing pregnancy after spontaneous abortion of one fetus or more, first trimester**

    O31.12 **Continuing pregnancy after spontaneous abortion of one fetus or more, second trimester**

    O31.13 **Continuing pregnancy after spontaneous abortion of one fetus or more, third trimester**

O31.2 **Continuing pregnancy after intrauterine death of one fetus or more**
[5th]

    O31.20 **Continuing pregnancy after intrauterine death of one fetus or more, unspecified trimester**

    O31.21 **Continuing pregnancy after intrauterine death of one fetus or more, first trimester**

    O31.22 **Continuing pregnancy after intrauterine death of one fetus or more, second trimester**

    O31.23 **Continuing pregnancy after intrauterine death of one fetus or more, third trimester**

O31.8 **Other complications specific to multiple gestation**
[5th]   **O31.8X** **Other complications specific to multiple gestation**
[6th]
    O31.8X1 **Other complications specific to multiple gestation, first trimester**
[7th]
    O31.8X2 **Other complications specific to multiple gestation, second trimester**
[7th]
    O31.8X3 **Other complications specific to multiple gestation, third trimester**
[7th]

O35 **MATERNAL CARE FOR KNOWN OR SUSPECTED FETAL ABNORMALITY AND DAMAGE**
[4th] Assign only when the fetal condition is actually responsible for modifying the management of the mother, ie, by requiring diagnostic studies, additional observation, special care, or termination of pregnancy. The fact that the fetal condition exists does not justify assigning a code from this series to the mother's record.

In cases when surgery is performed on the fetus, a diagnosis code from category O35, Maternal care for known or suspected fetal abnormality and damage, should be assigned identifying the fetal condition. Assign the appropriate procedure code for the procedure performed.

No code from Chapter 16, the perinatal codes, should be used on the mother's record to identify fetal conditions. Surgery performed in utero on a fetus is still to be coded as an obstetric encounter.

Assign a 7th character to identify the fetus for which the complication code applies.

Assign 7th character "0" for either a single gestation or when the documentation is insufficient to determine the fetus affected and it is not possible to obtain clarification or when it is not possible to clinically determine which fetus is affected.

Includes: the listed conditions in the fetus as a reason for hospitalization or other obstetric care to the mother, or for termination of pregnancy

> Requires 7th character to identify affected fetus
> 0 not applicable (ie, single gestation) or unspecified
> 1 fetus 1
> 2 fetus 2
> 3 fetus 3
> 4 fetus 4
> 5 fetus 5
> 9 other fetus

Code also any associated maternal condition
Excludes1: encounter for suspected maternal and fetal conditions ruled out (Z03.7-)
Code also the appropriate code from category O30, Multiple gestation, when assigning a code from category O35 that has a 7th character of 1 through 9.
Use placeholder X to complete the full code

O35.0XX **Maternal care for (suspected) central nervous system malformation in fetus**
[7th]
     Maternal care for fetal anencephaly
     Maternal care for fetal hydrocephalus
     Maternal care for fetal spina bifida
     Excludes2: chromosomal abnormality in fetus (O35.1)

O35.1XX **Maternal care for (suspected) chromosomal abnormality in fetus**
[7th]

O35.2XX **Maternal care for (suspected) hereditary disease in fetus**
[7th]
     Excludes2: chromosomal abnormality in fetus (O35.1)

O35.3XX **Maternal care for (suspected) damage to fetus from viral disease in mother**
[7th]
     Maternal care for damage to fetus from maternal cytomegalovirus infection
     Maternal care for damage to fetus from maternal rubella

O35.4XX **Maternal care for (suspected) damage to fetus from alcohol**
[7th]

O35.5XX **Maternal care for (suspected) damage to fetus by drugs**
[7th]
     Maternal care for damage to fetus from drug addiction

O35.6XX **Maternal care for (suspected) damage to fetus by radiation**
[7th]

O35.7XX **Maternal care for (suspected) damage to fetus by other medical procedures**
[7th]
     Maternal care for damage to fetus by amniocentesis
     Maternal care for damage to fetus by biopsy procedures
     Maternal care for damage to fetus by hematological investigation
     Maternal care for damage to fetus by intrauterine contraceptive device
     Maternal care for damage to fetus by intrauterine surgery

O35.8XX **Maternal care for other (suspected) fetal abnormality and damage**
[7th]
     Maternal care for other (suspected) fetal abnormality and damage
     Maternal care for damage to fetus from maternal listeriosis

---

[4th] [5th] [6th] [7th] Additional Character Required   [✓] 3-character code   •=New Code   ▲=Revised Code   *Excludes1*—Not coded here, do not use together   *Excludes2*—Not included here

Maternal care for damage to fetus from maternal toxoplasmosis

O35.9XX **Maternal care for (suspected) fetal abnormality and damage, unspecified**
7th

O36 **MATERNAL CARE FOR OTHER FETAL PROBLEMS**
4th

Assign only when the fetal condition is actually responsible for modifying the management of the mother, ie, by requiring diagnostic studies, additional observation, special care, or termination of pregnancy. The fact that the fetal condition exists does not justify assigning a code from this series to the mother's record.

No code from Chapter 16, the perinatal codes, should be used on the mother's record to identify fetal conditions. Surgery performed in utero on a fetus is still to be coded as an obstetric encounter.

Assign a 7th character to identify the fetus for which the complication code applies.

Assign 7th character "0" for either a single gestation or when the documentation is insufficient to determine the fetus affected and it is not possible to obtain clarification or when it is not possible to clinically determine which fetus is affected.

Includes: the listed conditions in the fetus as a reason for hospitalization or other obstetric care of the mother, or for termination of pregnancy

> Requires 7th character to identify affected fetus
> 0 not applicable (ie, only one fetus) or unspecified
> 1 fetus 1
> 2 fetus 2
> 3 fetus 3
> 4 fetus 4
> 5 fetus 5
> 9 other fetus

Excludes1: encounter for suspected maternal and fetal conditions ruled out (Z03.7-)
placental transfusion syndromes (O43.0-)
Excludes2: labor and delivery complicated by fetal stress (O77.-)
Code also the appropriate code from category O30, Multiple gestation, when assigning a code from category O36 that has a 7th character of 1 through 9.

O36.0 **Maternal care for rhesus isoimmunization**
5th
Maternal care for Rh incompatibility (with hydrops fetalis)

O36.01 **Maternal care for anti-D [Rh] antibodies**
6th

O36.011 **Maternal care for anti-D [Rh] antibodies, first trimester**
7th

O36.012 **Maternal care for anti-D [Rh] antibodies, second trimester**
7th

O36.013 **Maternal care for anti-D [Rh] antibodies, third trimester**
7th

O36.09 **Maternal care for other rhesus isoimmunization**
6th

O36.091 **Maternal care for other rhesus isoimmunization, first trimester**
7th

O36.092 **Maternal care for other rhesus isoimmunization, second trimester**
7th

O36.093 **Maternal care for other rhesus isoimmunization, third trimester**
7th

O36.1 **Maternal care for other isoimmunization**
5th
Maternal care for ABO isoimmunization

O36.11 **Maternal care for Anti-A sensitization**
6th
Maternal care for isoimmunization NOS (with hydrops fetalis)

O36.111 **Maternal care for Anti-A sensitization, first trimester**
7th

O36.112 **Maternal care for Anti-A sensitization, second trimester**
7th

O36.113 **Maternal care for Anti-A sensitization, third trimester**
7th

O36.19 **Maternal care for other isoimmunization**
6th
Maternal care for Anti-B sensitization

O36.191 **Maternal care for other isoimmunization, first trimester**
7th

O36.192 **Maternal care for other isoimmunization, second trimester**
7th

O36.193 **Maternal care for other isoimmunization, third trimester**
7th

O36.2 **Maternal care for hydrops fetalis**
5th
Maternal care for hydrops fetalis NOS
Maternal care for hydrops fetalis not associated with isoimmunization
Excludes1: hydrops fetalis associated with ABO isoimmunization (O36.1-)
hydrops fetalis associated with rhesus isoimmunization (O36.0-)

O36.21X **Maternal care for hydrops fetalis, first trimester**
7th

O36.22X **Maternal care for hydrops fetalis, second trimester**
7th

O36.23X **Maternal care for hydrops fetalis, third trimester**
7th

O36.4XX **Maternal care for intrauterine death**
7th
Maternal care for intrauterine fetal death NOS
Maternal care for intrauterine fetal death after completion of 20 weeks of gestation
Maternal care for late fetal death
Maternal care for missed delivery
Excludes1: missed abortion (O02.1)
stillbirth (P95)

O36.5 **Maternal care for known or suspected poor fetal growth**
5th

O36.51 **Maternal care for known or suspected placental insufficiency**
6th

O36.511 **Maternal care for known or suspected placental insufficiency, first trimester**
7th

O36.512 **Maternal care for known or suspected placental insufficiency, second trimester**
7th

O36.513 **Maternal care for known or suspected placental insufficiency, third trimester**
7th

O36.59 **Maternal care for other known or suspected poor fetal growth**
6th
Maternal care for known or suspected light-for-dates NOS
Maternal care for known or suspected small-for-dates NOS

O36.591 **Maternal care for other known or suspected poor fetal growth, first trimester**
7th

O36.592 **Maternal care for other known or suspected poor fetal growth, second trimester**
7th

O36.593 **Maternal care for other known or suspected poor fetal growth, third trimester**
7th

O36.6 **Maternal care for excessive fetal growth**
5th
Maternal care for known or suspected large-for-dates

O36.61X **Maternal care for excessive fetal growth, first trimester**
7th

O36.62X **Maternal care for excessive fetal growth, second trimester**
7th

O36.63X **Maternal care for excessive fetal growth, third trimester**
7th

O36.7 **Maternal care for viable fetus in abdominal pregnancy**
5th

O36.71X **Maternal care for viable fetus in abdominal pregnancy, first trimester**
7th

O36.72X **Maternal care for viable fetus in abdominal pregnancy, second trimester**
7th

O36.73X **Maternal care for viable fetus in abdominal pregnancy, third trimester**
7th

O36.8 **Maternal care for other specified fetal problems**
5th

O36.80 **Pregnancy with inconclusive fetal viability**
Encounter to determine fetal viability of pregnancy

O36.81 **Decreased fetal movements**
6th

O36.812 **Decreased fetal movements, second trimester**

O36.813 **Decreased fetal movements, third trimester**
7th

O36.82 **Fetal anemia and thrombocytopenia**
6th

O36.821 **Fetal anemia and thrombocytopenia, first trimester**
7th

O36.822 **Fetal anemia and thrombocytopenia, second trimester**
7th

4th 5th 6th 7th Additional Character Required ✔ 3-character code

• =New Code
▲ =Revised Code

Excludes1—Not coded here, do not use together
Excludes2—Not included here

CHAPTER 15. PREGNANCY, CHILDBIRTH AND THE PUERPERIUM   (O36.823–O42.92)

O36.823 **Fetal anemia and thrombocytopenia, third trimester**
[7th]

Requires 7th character to identify affected fetus	
0	not applicable (ie, only one fetus) or unspecified
1	fetus 1
2	fetus 2
3	fetus 3
4	fetus 4
5	fetus 5
9	other fetus

O36.83 **Maternal care for abnormalities of the fetal heart rate or rhythm**
[6th]
   Maternal care for depressed fetal heart rate tones
   Maternal care for fetal bradycardia
   Maternal care for fetal heart rate abnormal variability
   Maternal care for fetal heart rate decelerations
   Maternal care for fetal heart rate irregularity
   Maternal care for fetal tachycardia
   Maternal care for non-reassuring fetal heart rate or rhythm

   O36.831 **Maternal care for abnormalities of the fetal heart rate or rhythm, first trimester**
   [7th]
   O36.832 **Maternal care for abnormalities of the fetal heart rate or rhythm, second trimester**
   [7th]
   O36.833 **Maternal care for abnormalities of the fetal heart rate or rhythm, third trimester**
   [7th]
   O36.839 **Maternal care for abnormalities of the fetal heart rate or rhythm, unspecified trimester**
   [7th]

O36.89 **Maternal care for other specified fetal problems**
[6th]
   O36.891 **Maternal care for other specified fetal problems, first trimester**
   [7th]
   O36.892 **Maternal care for other specified fetal problems, second trimester**
   [7th]
   O36.893 **Maternal care for other specified fetal problems, third trimester**
   [7th]

O40 **POLYHYDRAMNIOS**
[4th]
Assign a 7th character to identify the fetus for which the complication code applies.

Assign 7th character "0" for either a single gestation or when the documentation is insufficient to determine the fetus affected and it is not possible to obtain clarification or when it is not possible to clinically determine which fetus is affected.

Requires 7th character to identify affected fetus	
0	not applicable (ie, only one fetus) or unspecified
1	fetus 1
2	fetus 2
3	fetus 3
4	fetus 4
5	fetus 5
9	other fetus

Includes: hydramnios
Excludes1: encounter for suspected maternal and fetal conditions ruled out (Z03.7-)

O40.1XX **Polyhydramnios, first trimester**
[7th]
O40.2XX **Polyhydramnios, second trimester**
[7th]
O40.3XX **Polyhydramnios, third trimester**
[7th]
O40.9XX **Polyhydramnios, unspecified trimester**
[7th]

O41 **OTHER DISORDERS OF AMNIOTIC FLUID AND MEMBRANES**
[4th]
Assign a 7th character to identify the fetus for which the complication code applies.

Assign 7th character "0" for either a single gestation or when the documentation is insufficient to determine the fetus affected and it is not possible to obtain clarification or when it is not possible to clinically determine which fetus is affected.

Requires 7th character to identify affected fetus	
0	not applicable (ie, only one fetus) or unspecified
1	fetus 1
2	fetus 2
3	fetus 3
4	fetus 4
5	fetus 5
9	other fetus

Excludes1: encounter for suspected maternal and fetal conditions ruled out (Z03.7-)

Code also the appropriate code from category O30, Multiple gestation, when assigning a code from category O41 that has a 7th character of 1 through 9.

O41.01X **Oligohydramnios, first trimester, not applicable or unspecified**
[7th]
O41.02X **Oligohydramnios, second trimester, not applicable or unspecified**
[7th]
O41.03X **Oligohydramnios, third trimester, not applicable or unspecified**
[7th]

O42 **PREMATURE RUPTURE OF MEMBRANES**
[4th]
   O42.00 **Premature rupture of membranes, onset of labor within 24 hours of rupture, unspecified weeks of gestation**
   O42.01 **Preterm premature rupture of membranes, onset of labor within 24 hours of rupture**
   [6th]
     Premature rupture of membranes before 37 completed weeks of gestation
     O42.011 **Preterm premature rupture of membranes, onset of labor within 24 hours of rupture, first trimester**
     O42.012 **second trimester**
     O42.013 **third trimester**
     O42.019 **unspecified trimester**
   O42.02 **Full-term premature rupture of membranes, onset of labor within 24 hours of rupture**
     Premature rupture of membranes at or after 37 completed weeks of gestation, onset of labor within 24hours of rupture

O42.1 **Premature rupture of membranes, onset of labor more than 24 hours following rupture**
[5th]
   O42.10 **Premature rupture of membranes, onset of labor more than 24 hours following rupture, unspecified weeks of gestation**
   O42.11 **Preterm premature rupture of membranes, onset of labor more than 24 hours following rupture**
   [6th]
     Premature rupture of membranes before 37 completed weeks of gestation
     O42.111 **Preterm premature rupture of membranes, onset of labor more than 24 hours following rupture, first trimester**
     O42.112 **second trimester**
     O42.113 **third trimester**
     O42.119 **unspecified trimester**
   O42.12 **Full-term premature rupture of membranes, onset of labor more than 24 hours following rupture**
     Premature rupture of membranes at or after 37 completed weeks of gestation, onset of labor more than 24 hours following rupture

O42.9 **Premature rupture of membranes, unspecified as to length of time between rupture and onset of labor**
   O42.90 **Premature rupture of membranes, unspecified as to length of time between rupture and onset of labor, unspecified weeks of gestation**
   O42.91 **Preterm premature rupture of membranes, unspecified as to length of time between rupture and onset of labor**
   [6th]
     Premature rupture of membranes before 37 completed weeks of gestation
     O42.911 **Preterm premature rupture of membranes, unspecified as to length of time between rupture and onset of labor; first trimester**
     O42.912 **second trimester**
     O42.913 **third trimester**
   O42.92 **Full-term premature rupture of membranes, unspecified as to length of time between rupture and onset of labor**
     Premature rupture of membranes at or after 37 completed weeks of gestation, unspecified as to length of time between rupture and onset of labor

---

[4th] [5th] [6th] [7th]   Additional Character Required   ✓ 3-character code   •=New Code   ▲=Revised Code   *Excludes1*—Not coded here, do not use together   *Excludes2*—Not included here

O43 **PLACENTAL DISORDERS**
`4th`
    Excludes2: maternal care for poor fetal growth due to placental
        insufficiency (O36.5-)
        placenta previa (O44.-)
        placental polyp (O90.89)
        placentitis (O41.14-)
        premature separation of placenta [abruptio placentae] (O45.-)
    O43.0 **Placental transfusion syndromes**
    `5th`   **O43.01** **Fetomaternal placental transfusion syndrome**
        `6th`   Maternofetal placental transfusion syndrome
            O43.011 **Fetomaternal placental transfusion**
                syndrome; first trimester
            O43.012 **second trimester**
            O43.013 **third trimester**
        O43.02 **Fetus-to-fetus placental transfusion syndrome**
        `6th`   **O43.021** **Fetus-to-fetus placental transfusion**
                syndrome; first trimester
            O43.022 **second trimester**
            O43.023 **third trimester**

(O60–O77) COMPLICATIONS OF LABOR AND DELIVERY

O60 **PRETERM LABOR**
`4th`
    Includes: onset (spontaneous) of labor before 37 completed weeks of
    gestation
    Excludes1: false labor (O47.0-)
        threatened labor NOS (O47.0-)
    O60.0 **Preterm labor without delivery**
    `5th`   **O60.02** **Preterm labor without delivery, second trimester**
        O60.03 **Preterm labor without delivery, third trimester**

O75 **OTHER COMPLICATIONS OF LABOR AND DELIVERY, NOT**
`4th` **ELSEWHERE CLASSIFIED**
    Excludes2: puerperal (postpartum) infection (O86.-)
        puerperal (postpartum) sepsis (O85)
    O75.0 **Maternal distress during labor and delivery**
    O75.1 **Shock during or following labor and delivery**
        Obstetric shock following labor and delivery
    O75.2 **Pyrexia during labor, not elsewhere classified**
    O75.3 **Other infection during labor**
        Sepsis during labor
        Use additional code (B95–B97), to identify infectious agent
    O75.4 **Other complications of obstetric surgery and procedures**
        Cardiac arrest following obstetric surgery or procedures
        Cardiac failure following obstetric surgery or procedures
        Cerebral anoxia following obstetric surgery or procedures
        Pulmonary edema following obstetric surgery or procedures
        Use additional code to identify specific complication
        Excludes2: complications of anesthesia during labor and delivery
            (O74.-)
            disruption of obstetrical (surgical) wound (O90.0–O90.1)
            hematoma of obstetrical (surgical) wound (O90.2)
            infection of obstetrical (surgical) wound (O86.0-)
    O75.5 **Delayed delivery after artificial rupture of membranes**
    O75.8 **Other specified complications of labor and delivery**
    `5th`   **O75.81** **Maternal exhaustion complicating labor and delivery**
        O75.82 **Onset (spontaneous) of labor after 37 completed**
                weeks of gestation but before 39 completed weeks
                gestation, with delivery by (planned) cesarean
                section
                Delivery by (planned) cesarean section occurring after
                    37 completed weeks of gestation but before 39
                    completed weeks gestation due to (spontaneous)
                    onset of labor
                Code first to specify reason for planned cesarean
                    section such as:
                    cephalopelvic disproportion (normally formed fetus)
                    (O33.9)
                    previous cesarean delivery (O34.21)
        O75.89 **Other specified complications of labor and delivery**
    O75.9 **Complication of labor and delivery, unspecified**

(O80–O82) ENCOUNTER FOR DELIVERY

(O85–O92) COMPLICATIONS PREDOMINANTLY RELATED TO THE PUERPERIUM

O92 **OTHER DISORDERS OF BREAST AND DISORDERS OF**
`4th` **LACTATION ASSOCIATED WITH PREGNANCY AND THE**
PUERPERIUM
    O92.0 **Retracted nipple associated with pregnancy, the puerperium,**
    `5th` **and lactation**
        O92.02 **Retracted nipple associated with the puerperium**
        O92.03 **Retracted nipple associated with lactation**
    O92.1 **Cracked nipple associated with pregnancy, the puerperium,**
    `5th` **and lactation**
        Fissure of nipple, gestational or puerperal
        O92.12 **Cracked nipple associated with the puerperium**
        O92.13 **Cracked nipple associated with lactation**
    O92.2 **Other and unspecified disorders of breast associated with**
    `5th` **pregnancy and the puerperium**
        O92.20 **Unspecified disorder of breast associated with**
                pregnancy and the puerperium
        O92.29 **Other disorders of breast associated with pregnancy**
                and the puerperium
    O92.3 **Agalactia**
        Primary agalactia
        Excludes1: Elective agalactia (O92.5)
        Secondary agalactia (O92.5)
        Therapeutic agalactia (O92.5)
    O92.4 **Hypogalactia**
    O92.5 **Suppressed lactation**
        Elective agalactia
        Secondary agalactia
        Therapeutic agalactia
        Excludes1: primary agalactia (O92.3)
    O92.6 **Galactorrhea**
    O92.7 **Other and unspecified disorders of lactation**
    `5th`   **O92.70** **Unspecified disorders of lactation**
        O92.79 **Other disorders of lactation**
                Puerperal galactocele

(O94–O9A) OTHER OBSTETRIC CONDITIONS, NOT ELSEWHERE CLASSIFIED

`4th` `5th` `6th` `7th` Additional Character Required   ✔ 3-character code   • =New Code   *Excludes1*—Not coded here, do not use together
    ▲ =Revised Code   *Excludes2*—Not included here

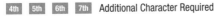

Chapter 16. Certain conditions originating in the perinatal period (P00–P96)

GUIDELINES

For coding and reporting purposes the perinatal period is defined as before birth through the 28th day following birth. The following guidelines are provided for reporting purposes

General Perinatal Rules

Codes in this chapter are never for use on the maternal record. Codes from Chapter 15, the obstetric chapter, are never permitted on the newborn record. Chapter 16 codes may be used throughout the life of the patient if the condition is still present.

PRINCIPAL DIAGNOSIS FOR BIRTH RECORD

When coding the birth episode in a newborn record, assign a code from category Z38, Liveborn infants according to place of birth and type of delivery, as the principal diagnosis. Refer to code Z38 for further guidelines.

A code from category Z38 is used only on the newborn record, not on the mother's record.

USE OF CODES FROM OTHER CHAPTERS WITH CODES FROM CHAPTER 16

Codes from other chapters may be used with codes from Chapter 16 if the codes from the other chapters provide more specific detail. Codes for signs and symptoms may be assigned when a definitive diagnosis has not been established. If the reason for the encounter is a perinatal condition, the code from Chapter 16 should be sequenced first.

USE OF CHAPTER 16 CODES AFTER THE PERINATAL PERIOD

Should a condition originate in the perinatal period, and continue throughout the life of the patient, the perinatal code should continue to be used regardless of the patient's age.

BIRTH PROCESS OR COMMUNITY ACQUIRED CONDITIONS

If a newborn has a condition that may be either due to the birth process or community acquired and the documentation does not indicate which it is, the default is due to the birth process and the code from Chapter 16 should be used. If the condition is community-acquired, a code from Chapter 16 should not be assigned.

CODE ALL CLINICALLY SIGNIFICANT CONDITIONS

All clinically significant conditions noted on routine newborn examination should be coded. A condition is clinically significant if it requires:
- clinical evaluation; or
- therapeutic treatment; or
- diagnostic procedures; or
- extended length of hospital stay; or
- increased nursing care and/or monitoring; or
- has implications for future health care needs

Note: The perinatal guidelines listed above are the same as the general coding guidelines for "additional diagnoses," except for the final point regarding implications for future health care needs. Codes should be assigned for conditions that have been specified by the provider as having implications for future health care needs.

Observation and Evaluation of Newborns for Suspected Condition not Found

See category Z05.

Coding Additional Perinatal Diagnoses

ASSIGNING CODES FOR CONDITIONS THAT REQUIRE TREATMENT

Assign codes for conditions that require treatment or further investigation, prolong the length of stay, or require resource utilization.

CODES FOR CONDITIONS SPECIFIED AS HAVING IMPLICATIONS FOR FUTURE HEALTH CARE NEEDS

Assign codes for conditions that have been specified by the provider as having implications for future health care needs.

Prematurity and Fetal Growth Retardation

Refer to categories P05–P07 for guidelines for prematurity and fetal growth retardation.

LBW and immaturity status

Refer to category P07, Disorders of newborn related to short gestation and LBW, not elsewhere classified, for associated guidelines.

Bacterial Sepsis of Newborn

Refer to category P36, Bacterial sepsis of newborn for guidelines for reporting newborn bacterial sepsis.

Stillbirth

Refer to code P95 for guidelines.

COVID-19 Infection in Newborn

For a newborn that tests positive for COVID-19, assign code U07.1, COVID-19, and the appropriate codes for associated manifestation(s) in neonates/newborns in the absence of documentation indicating a specific type of transmission. For a newborn that tests positive for COVID-19 and the provider documents the condition was contracted in utero or during the birth process, assign codes P35.8, Other congenital viral diseases, and U07.1, COVID-19. When coding the birth episode in a newborn record, the appropriate code from category Z38, Liveborn infants according to place of birth and type of delivery, should be assigned as the principal diagnosis.

Note: Codes from this chapter are for use on newborn records only, never on maternal records

Includes: conditions that have their origin in the fetal or perinatal period (before birth through the first 28 days after birth) even if morbidity occurs later

Excludes2: congenital malformations, deformations and chromosomal abnormalities (Q00–Q99)
endocrine, nutritional and metabolic diseases (E00–E88)
injury, poisoning and certain other consequences of external causes (S00–T88)
neoplasms (C00–D49)
tetanus neonatorum (A33)

(P00–P04) NEWBORN AFFECTED BY MATERNAL FACTORS AND BY COMPLICATIONS OF PREGNANCY, LABOR, AND DELIVERY

Note: These codes are for use when the listed maternal conditions are specified as the cause of confirmed morbidity or potential morbidity which have their origin in the perinatal period (before birth through the first 28 days after birth). Codes from these categories are also for use for newborns who are suspected of having an abnormal condition resulting from exposure from the mother or the birth process.

P00 **NEWBORN AFFECTED BY MATERNAL CONDITIONS THAT**
4th **MAY BE UNRELATED TO PRESENT PREGNANCY**
Code first any current condition in newborn
Excludes2: encounter for observation and evaluation of newborn for suspected diseases and conditions ruled out (Z05.-)
newborn affected by maternal complications of pregnancy (P01.-)
newborn affected by maternal endocrine and metabolic disorders (P70–P74)
newborn affected by noxious substances transmitted via placenta or breast milk (P04.-)
P00.0 **Newborn affected by maternal hypertensive disorders**
Newborn affected by maternal conditions classifiable to O10–O11, O13–O16
P00.1 **Newborn affected by maternal renal and urinary tract diseases**
Newborn affected by maternal conditions classifiable to N00–N39
P00.2 **Newborn affected by maternal infectious and parasitic diseases**
Newborn affected by maternal infectious disease classifiable to A00–B99, J09 and J10
Excludes2: infections specific to the perinatal period (P35–P39)
maternal genital tract or other localized infections (P00.8)

4th **5th** **6th** **7th** Additional Character Required   ✓ 3-character code   •=New Code   *Excludes1*—Not coded here, do not use together
▲=Revised Code   *Excludes2*—Not included here

PEDIATRIC ICD-10-CM 2021: A MANUAL FOR PROVIDER-BASED CODING   287

CHAPTER 16. CERTAIN CONDITIONS ORIGINATING IN THE PERINATAL PERIOD   (P00.3–P03.811)

P00.3 Newborn affected by other maternal circulatory and respiratory diseases
Newborn affected by maternal conditions classifiable to I00–I99, J00–J99, Q20–Q34 and not included in P00.0, P00.2

P00.4 Newborn affected by maternal nutritional disorders
Newborn affected by maternal disorders classifiable to E40–E64
Maternal malnutrition NOS

P00.5 Newborn affected by maternal injury
Newborn affected by maternal conditions classifiable to O9A.2-

P00.6 Newborn affected by surgical procedure on mother
Newborn affected by amniocentesis
Excludes1: cesarean delivery for present delivery (P03.4)
   damage to placenta from amniocentesis, cesarean delivery or surgical induction (P02.1)
   previous surgery to uterus or pelvic organs (P03.89)
Excludes2: newborn affected by complication of (fetal) intrauterine procedure (P96.5)

P00.7 Newborn affected by other medical procedures on mother, NEC
Newborn affected by radiation to mother
Excludes1: damage to placenta from amniocentesis, cesarean delivery or surgical induction (P02.1)
   newborn affected by other complications of labor and delivery (P03.-)

P00.8 Newborn affected by other maternal conditions
5th   **P00.81 Newborn affected by periodontal disease in mother**
P00.89 Newborn affected by other maternal conditions
Newborn affected by conditions classifiable to T80–T88
Newborn affected by maternal genital tract or other localized infections
Newborn affected by maternal SLE
Use additional code to identify infectious agent, if known

P00.9 Newborn affected by unspecified maternal condition

P01   **NEWBORN AFFECTED BY MATERNAL COMPLICATIONS OF PREGNANCY**
4th
Code first any current condition in newborn
Excludes2: encounter for observation of newborn for suspected diseases and conditions ruled out (Z05.-)
P01.0 Newborn affected by incompetent cervix
P01.1 Newborn affected by premature rupture of membranes
P01.2 Newborn affected by oligohydramnios
Excludes1: oligohydramnios due to premature rupture of membranes (P01.1)
P01.3 Newborn affected by polyhydramnios
Newborn affected by hydramnios
P01.4 Newborn affected by ectopic pregnancy
Newborn affected by abdominal pregnancy
P01.5 Newborn affected by multiple pregnancy
Newborn affected by triplet (pregnancy)
Newborn affected by twin (pregnancy)
P01.6 Newborn affected by maternal death
P01.7 Newborn affected by malpresentation before labor
Newborn affected by breech presentation before labor
Newborn affected by external version before labor
Newborn affected by face presentation before labor
Newborn affected by transverse lie before labor
Newborn affected by unstable lie before labor
P01.8 Newborn affected by other maternal complications of pregnancy
P01.9 Newborn affected by maternal complication of pregnancy, unspecified

P02   **NEWBORN AFFECTED BY COMPLICATIONS OF PLACENTA, CORD AND MEMBRANES**
4th
Code first any current condition in newborn
Excludes2: encounter for observation of newborn for suspected diseases and conditions ruled out (Z05.-)
P02.0 Newborn affected by placenta previa
P02.1 Newborn affected by other forms of placental separation and hemorrhage
Newborn affected by abruptio placenta
Newborn affected by accidental hemorrhage
Newborn affected by antepartum hemorrhage

Newborn affected by damage to placenta from amniocentesis, cesarean delivery or surgical induction
Newborn affected by maternal blood loss
Newborn affected by premature separation of placenta

P02.2 Newborn affected by other and unspecified morphological and functional abnormalities of placenta
5th
P02.20 Newborn affected by unspecified morphological and functional abnormalities of placenta
P02.29 Newborn affected by other morphological and functional abnormalities of placenta
Newborn affected by placental dysfunction
Newborn affected by placental infarction
Newborn affected by placental insufficiency

P02.3 Newborn affected by placental transfusion syndromes
Newborn affected by placental and cord abnormalities resulting in twin-to-twin or other transplacental transfusion

P02.4 Newborn affected by prolapsed cord
P02.5 Newborn affected by other compression of umbilical cord
Newborn affected by umbilical cord (tightly) around neck
Newborn affected by entanglement of umbilical cord
Newborn affected by knot in umbilical cord

P02.6 Newborn affected by other and unspecified conditions of umbilical cord
5th
P02.60 Newborn affected by unspecified conditions of umbilical cord
P02.69 Newborn affected by other conditions of umbilical cord
Newborn affected by short umbilical cord
Newborn affected by vasa previa
Excludes1: newborn affected by single umbilical artery (Q27.0)

P02.7 Newborn affected by chorioamnionitis
5th
P02.70 Newborn affected by fetal inflammatory response syndrome
P02.78 Newborn affected by other conditions from chorioamnionitis
Newborn affected by amnionitis
Newborn affected by membranitis
Newborn affected by placentitis

P02.8 Newborn affected by other abnormalities of membranes
P02.9 Newborn affected by abnormality of membranes, unspecified

P03   **NEWBORN AFFECTED BY OTHER COMPLICATIONS OF LABOR AND DELIVERY**
4th
Code first any current condition in newborn
Excludes2: encounter for observation of newborn for suspected diseases and conditions ruled out (Z05.-)
P03.0 Newborn affected by breech delivery and extraction
P03.1 Newborn affected by other malpresentation, malposition and disproportion during labor and delivery
Newborn affected by contracted pelvis
Newborn affected by conditions classifiable to O64–O66
Newborn affected by persistent occipitoposterior
Newborn affected by transverse lie
P03.2 Newborn affected by forceps delivery
P03.3 Newborn affected by delivery by vacuum extractor [ventouse]
P03.4 Newborn affected by cesarean delivery
P03.5 Newborn affected by precipitate delivery
Newborn affected by rapid second stage
P03.6 Newborn affected by abnormal uterine contractions
Newborn affected by conditions classifiable to O62.-, except O62.3
Newborn affected by hypertonic labor
Newborn affected by uterine inertia
P03.8 Newborn affected by other specified complications of labor and delivery
5th
P03.81 Newborn affected by abnormality in fetal (intrauterine) heart rate or rhythm
6th
Excludes1: neonatal cardiac dysrhythmia (P29.1-)
P03.810 Newborn affected by abnormality in fetal (intrauterine) heart rate or rhythm before the onset of labor
P03.811 Newborn affected by abnormality in fetal (intrauterine) heart rate or rhythm during labor

---

4th **5th** **6th** **7th**   Additional Character Required   3-character code   •=New Code   *Excludes1*—Not coded here, do not use together
     ▲=Revised Code   *Excludes2*—Not included here

P03.819 Newborn affected by abnormality in fetal (intrauterine) heart rate or rhythm, unspecified as to time of onset

P03.82 Meconium passage during delivery
Excludes1: meconium aspiration (P24.00, P24.01)
meconium staining (P96.83)

P03.89 Newborn affected by other specified complications of labor and delivery
Newborn affected by abnormality of maternal soft tissues
Newborn affected by conditions classifiable to O60–O75 and by procedures used in labor and delivery not included in P02.- and P03.0–P03.6
Newborn affected by induction of labor

P03.9 Newborn affected by complication of labor and delivery, unspecified

P04 NEWBORN AFFECTED BY NOXIOUS SUBSTANCES `4th` TRANSMITTED VIA PLACENTA OR BREAST MILK
Includes: nonteratogenic effects of substances transmitted via placenta
Excludes2: congenital malformations (Q00–Q99)
encounter for observation of newborn for suspected diseases and conditions ruled out (Z05.-)
neonatal jaundice from excessive hemolysis due to drugs or toxins transmitted from mother (P58.4)
newborn in contact with and (suspected) exposures hazardous to health not transmitted via placenta or breast milk (Z77.-)

P04.0 Newborn affected by maternal anesthesia and analgesia in pregnancy, labor and delivery
Newborn affected by reactions and intoxications from maternal opiates and tranquilizers administered for procedures during pregnancy or labor and delivery
Excludes2: newborn affected by other maternal medication (P04.1-)

P04.1 Newborn affected by other maternal medication
`5th` **Code first** withdrawal symptoms from maternal use of drugs of addiction, if applicable (P96.1)
Excludes1: dysmorphism due to warfarin (Q86.2)
fetal hydantoin syndrome (Q86.1)
Excludes2: maternal anesthesia and analgesia in pregnancy, labor and delivery (P04.0)
maternal use of drugs of addiction (P04.4-)

P04.11 Newborn affected by maternal antineoplastic chemotherapy
P04.12 Newborn affected by maternal cytotoxic drugs
P04.13 Newborn affected by maternal use of anticonvulsants
P04.14 Newborn affected by maternal use of opiates
P04.15 Newborn affected by maternal use of antidepressants
P04.16 Newborn affected by maternal use of amphetamines
P04.17 Newborn affected by maternal use of sedative-hypnotics
P04.18 Newborn affected by other maternal medication
P04.19 Newborn affected by maternal use of unspecified medication
P04.1A Newborn affected by maternal use of anxiolytics

P04.2 Newborn affected by maternal use of tobacco
Newborn affected by exposure in utero to tobacco smoke
Excludes2: newborn exposure to environmental tobacco smoke (P96.81)

P04.3 Newborn affected by maternal use of alcohol
Excludes1: fetal alcohol syndrome (Q86.0)

P04.4 Newborn affected by maternal use of drugs of addiction
`5th` **P04.40** Newborn affected by maternal use of unspecified drugs of addiction
P04.41 Newborn affected by maternal use of cocaine
P04.42 Newborn affected by maternal use of hallucinogens
Excludes2: newborn affected by other maternal medication (P04.1-)
P04.49 Newborn affected by maternal use of other drugs of addiction
Excludes2: newborn affected by maternal anesthesia and analgesia (P04.0)

withdrawal symptoms from maternal use of drugs of addiction (P96.1)

P04.5 Newborn affected by maternal use of nutritional chemical substances
P04.6 Newborn affected by maternal exposure to environmental chemical substances
P04.8 Newborn affected by other maternal noxious substances
`5th` **P04.81** Newborn affected by maternal use of cannabis
P04.89 Newborn affected by other maternal noxious substances
P04.9 Newborn affected by maternal noxious substance, unspecified

(P05–P08) DISORDERS OF NEWBORN RELATED TO LENGTH OF GESTATION AND FETAL GROWTH

Providers utilize different criteria in determining prematurity. A code for prematurity should not be assigned unless it is documented. Assignment of codes in categories P05, Disorders of newborn related to slow fetal growth and fetal malnutrition, and P07, Disorders of newborn related to short gestation and LBW, not elsewhere classified, should be based on the recorded birth weight and estimated gestational age. Codes from category P05 should not be assigned with codes from category P07.

P05 DISORDERS OF NEWBORN RELATED TO SLOW FETAL `4th` GROWTH AND FETAL MALNUTRITION
P05.0 Newborn light for gestational age
`5th` *Light-for-dates newborns are those who are smaller in size than normal for the gestational age, most commonly defined as weight below the 10th percentile but length above the 10th percentile for gestational age.*
Newborn light-for-dates

P05.00 Newborn light for gestational age, unspecified weight
P05.01 Newborn light for gestational age, less than 500 g
P05.02 Newborn light for gestational age, 500–749 g
P05.03 Newborn light for gestational age, 750–999 g
P05.04 Newborn light for gestational age, 1000–1249 g
P05.05 Newborn light for gestational age, 1250–1499 g
P05.06 Newborn light for gestational age, 1500–1749 g
P05.07 Newborn light for gestational age, 1750–1999 g
P05.08 Newborn light for gestational age, 2000–2499 g
P05.09 Newborn light for gestational age, 2500 g and over

P05.1 Newborn small for gestational age
`5th` *Small for gestational age newborns are those who are smaller in size than normal for the gestational age, most commonly defined as weight below the 10th percentile and length below 10th percentile for the gestational age.*
Newborn small-and-light-for-dates
Newborn small-for-dates

P05.10 Newborn small for gestational age, unspecified weight
P05.11 Newborn small for gestational age, less than 500 g
P05.12 Newborn small for gestational age, 500–749 g
P05.13 Newborn small for gestational age, 750–999 g
P05.14 Newborn small for gestational age, 1000–1249 g
P05.15 Newborn small for gestational age, 1250–1499 g
P05.16 Newborn small for gestational age, 1500–1749 g
P05.17 Newborn small for gestational age, 1750–1999 g
P05.18 Newborn small for gestational age, 2000–2499 g
P05.19 Newborn small for gestational age, other
Newborn small for gestational age, 2500 g and over

P05.2 Newborn affected by fetal (intrauterine) malnutrition not light or small for gestational age
Infant, not light or small for gestational age, showing signs of fetal malnutrition, such as dry, peeling skin and loss of subcutaneous tissue
Excludes1: newborn affected by fetal malnutrition with light for gestational age (P05.0-)
newborn affected by fetal malnutrition with small for gestational age (P05.1-)

P05.9 Newborn affected by slow intrauterine growth, unspecified
Newborn affected by fetal growth retardation NOS

`4th` `5th` `6th` `7th` Additional Character Required ✔ 3-character code •=New Code ▲=Revised Code *Excludes1*—Not coded here, do not use together *Excludes2*—Not included here

PEDIATRIC ICD-10-CM 2021: A MANUAL FOR PROVIDER-BASED CODING 289

P07 **DISORDERS OF NEWBORN RELATED TO SHORT**
4th **GESTATION AND LBW, NEC**

Note: When both birth weight and gestational age of the newborn are available, both should be coded with birth weight sequenced before gestational age

Includes: the listed conditions, without further specification, as the cause of morbidity or additional care, in newborn

P07.0 **Extremely LBW newborn**
5th   Newborn birth weight 999 g or less
   Excludes1: LBW due to slow fetal growth and fetal malnutrition (P05.-)

     P07.00   **Extremely LBW newborn, unspecified weight**
     P07.01   **Extremely LBW newborn, less than 500 g**
     P07.02   **Extremely LBW newborn, 500–749 g**
     P07.03   **Extremely LBW newborn, 750–999 g**

P07.1 **Other LBW newborn**
5th   Newborn birth weight 1000–2499 g.
   Excludes1: LBW due to slow fetal growth and fetal malnutrition (P05.-)

     P07.10   **Other LBW newborn, unspecified weight**
     P07.14   **Other LBW newborn, 1000–1249 g**
     P07.15   **Other LBW newborn, 1250–1499 g**
     P07.16   **Other LBW newborn, 1500–1749 g**
     P07.17   **Other LBW newborn, 1750–1999 g**
     P07.18   **Other LBW newborn, 2000–2499 g**

P07.2 **Extreme immaturity of newborn**
5th   Less than 28 completed weeks (less than 196 completed days) of gestation.

     P07.20   **Extreme immaturity of newborn; unspecified weeks of gestation**
        Gestational age less than 28 completed weeks NOS
     P07.21   **gestational age less than 23 completed weeks**
        gestational age less than 23 weeks, 0 days
     P07.22   **gestational age 23 completed weeks**
        gestational age 23 weeks, 0 days through 23 weeks, 6 days
     P07.23   **gestational age 24 completed weeks**
        gestational age 24 weeks, 0 days through 24 weeks, 6 days
     P07.24   **gestational age 25 completed weeks**
        gestational age 25 weeks, 0 days through 25 weeks, 6 days
     P07.25   **gestational age 26 completed weeks**
        gestational age 26 weeks, 0 days through 26 weeks, 6 days
     P07.26   **gestational age 27 completed weeks**
        gestational age 27 weeks, 0 days through 27 weeks, 6 days

P07.3 **Preterm [premature] newborn [other]**
5th   28 completed weeks or more but less than 37 completed weeks (196 completed days but less than 259 completed days) of gestation.
   Prematurity NOS

     P07.30   **Preterm newborn, unspecified weeks of gestation**
     P07.31   **Preterm newborn, gestational age 28 completed weeks**
        Preterm newborn, gestational age 28 weeks, 0 days through 28 weeks, 6 days
     P07.32   **Preterm newborn, gestational age 29 completed weeks**
        Preterm newborn, gestational age 29 weeks, 0 days through 29 weeks, 6 days
     P07.33   **Preterm newborn, gestational age 30 completed weeks**
        Preterm newborn, gestational age 30 weeks, 0 days through 30 weeks, 6 days
     P07.34   **Preterm newborn, gestational age 31 completed weeks**
        Preterm newborn, gestational age 31 weeks, 0 days through 31 weeks, 6 days
     P07.35   **Preterm newborn, gestational age 32 completed**

weeks
        Preterm newborn, gestational age 32 weeks, 0 days through 32 weeks, 6 days
     P07.36   **Preterm newborn, gestational age 33 completed weeks**
        Preterm newborn, gestational age 33 weeks, 0 days through 33 weeks, 6 days
     P07.37   **Preterm newborn, gestational age 34 completed weeks**
        Preterm newborn, gestational age 34 weeks, 0 days through 34 weeks, 6 days
     P07.38   **Preterm newborn, gestational age 35 completed weeks**
        Preterm newborn, gestational age 35 weeks, 0 days through 35 weeks, 6 days
     P07.39   **Preterm newborn, gestational age 36 completed weeks**
        Preterm newborn, gestational age 36 weeks, 0 days through 36 weeks, 6 days

P08 **DISORDERS OF NEWBORN RELATED TO LONG**
4th **GESTATION AND HIGH BIRTH WEIGHT**

Note: When both birth weight and gestational age of the newborn are available, priority of assignment should be given to birth weight

Includes: the listed conditions, without further specification, as causes of morbidity or additional care, in newborn

P08.0 **Exceptionally large newborn baby**
   Usually implies a birth weight of 4500 g. or more
   Excludes1: syndrome of infant of diabetic mother (P70.1)
       syndrome of infant of mother with gestational diabetes (P70.0)

P08.1 **Other heavy for gestational age newborn**
   Other newborn heavy- or large-for-dates regardless of period of gestation
   Usually implies a birth weight of 4000 g. to 4499 g.
   Excludes1: newborn with a birth weight of 4500 or more (P08.0)
       syndrome of infant of diabetic mother (P70.1)
       syndrome of infant of mother with gestational diabetes (P70.0).

P08.2 **Late newborn, not heavy for gestational age**
5th   **P08.21**   **Post-term newborn**
        Newborn with gestation period over 40 completed weeks to 42 completed weeks
     P08.22   **Prolonged gestation of newborn**
        Newborn with gestation period over 42 completed weeks (294 days or more), not heavy- or large-for-dates.
        Postmaturity NOS

(P09) ABNORMAL FINDINGS ON NEONATAL SCREENING

P09 **ABNORMAL FINDINGS ON NEONATAL SCREENING**
✓ **Use additional code** to identify signs, symptoms and conditions associated with the screening
   Excludes2: nonspecific serologic evidence of HIV (R75)

(P10–P15) BIRTH TRAUMA

P10 **INTRACRANIAL LACERATION AND HEMORRHAGE DUE**
4th **TO BIRTH INJURY**
   Excludes1: intracranial hemorrhage of newborn NOS (P52.9)
       intracranial hemorrhage of newborn due to anoxia or hypoxia (P52.-)
       nontraumatic intracranial hemorrhage of newborn (P52.-)

P10.0 **Subdural hemorrhage due to birth injury**
   Subdural hematoma (localized) due to birth injury
P10.1 **Cerebral hemorrhage due to birth injury**
P10.2 **Intraventricular hemorrhage due to birth injury**
P10.3 **Subarachnoid hemorrhage due to birth injury**
P10.4 **Tentorial tear due to birth injury**
P10.8 **Other intracranial lacerations and hemorrhages due to birth injury**
P10.9 **Unspecified intracranial laceration and hemorrhage due to birth injury**
   Excludes1: subdural hemorrhage accompanying tentorial tear (P10.4)

P11 **OTHER BIRTH INJURIES TO CENTRAL NERVOUS SYSTEM**
4th **P11.0** **Cerebral edema due to birth injury**

4th **5th** **6th** **7th**   Additional Character Required   **✓**   3-character code

•=New Code   *Excludes1*—Not coded here, do not use together
▲=Revised Code   *Excludes2*—Not included here

P11.1 Other specified brain damage due to birth injury

P11.2 Unspecified brain damage due to birth injury

P11.3 Birth injury to facial nerve
Facial palsy due to birth injury

P11.4 Birth injury to other cranial nerves

P11.5 Birth injury to spine and spinal cord
Fracture of spine due to birth injury

P11.9 Birth injury to central nervous system, unspecified

P12 BIRTH INJURY TO SCALP

`4th`

P12.0 Cephalhematoma due to birth injury

P12.1 Chignon (from vacuum extraction) due to birth injury

P12.2 Epicranial subaponeurotic hemorrhage due to birth injury
Subgaleal hemorrhage

P12.3 Bruising of scalp due to birth injury

P12.4 Injury of scalp of newborn due to monitoring equipment
Sampling incision of scalp of newborn
Scalp clip (electrode) injury of newborn

P12.8 Other birth injuries to scalp

`5th` **P12.81 Caput succedaneum**

P12.89 Other birth injuries to scalp

P12.9 Birth injury to scalp, unspecified

P13 BIRTH INJURY TO SKELETON

`4th`

Excludes2: birth injury to spine (P11.5)

P13.0 Fracture of skull due to birth injury

P13.1 Other birth injuries to skull
Excludes1: cephalhematoma (P12.0)

P13.2 Birth injury to femur

P13.3 Birth injury to other long bones

P13.4 Fracture of clavicle due to birth injury

P13.8 Birth injuries to other parts of skeleton

P13.9 Birth injury to skeleton, unspecified

P14 BIRTH INJURY TO PERIPHERAL NERVOUS SYSTEM

`4th`

P14.0 Erb's paralysis due to birth injury

P14.1 Klumpke's paralysis due to birth injury

P14.2 Phrenic nerve paralysis due to birth injury

P14.3 Other brachial plexus birth injuries

P14.8 Birth injuries to other parts of peripheral nervous system

P14.9 Birth injury to peripheral nervous system, unspecified

P15 OTHER BIRTH INJURIES

`4th`

P15.0 Birth injury to liver
Rupture of liver due to birth injury

P15.1 Birth injury to spleen
Rupture of spleen due to birth injury

P15.2 Sternomastoid injury due to birth injury

P15.3 Birth injury to eye
Subconjunctival hemorrhage due to birth injury
Traumatic glaucoma due to birth injury

P15.4 Birth injury to face
Facial congestion due to birth injury

P15.5 Birth injury to external genitalia

P15.6 Subcutaneous fat necrosis due to birth injury

P15.8 Other specified birth injuries

P15.9 Birth injury, unspecified

(P19–P29) RESPIRATORY AND CARDIOVASCULAR DISORDERS SPECIFIC TO THE PERINATAL PERIOD

P19 METABOLIC ACIDEMIA IN NEWBORN

`4th`

Includes: metabolic acidemia in newborn

P19.0 Metabolic acidemia in newborn first noted before onset of labor

P19.1 Metabolic acidemia in newborn first noted during labor

P19.2 Metabolic acidemia noted at birth

P19.9 Metabolic acidemia, unspecified

P22 RESPIRATORY DISTRESS OF NEWBORN

`4th`

P22.0 Respiratory distress syndrome of newborn
Cardiorespiratory distress syndrome of newborn
Hyaline membrane disease
Idiopathic respiratory distress syndrome [IRDS or RDS] of newborn
Pulmonary hypoperfusion syndrome

Respiratory distress syndrome, type I
Excludes2: respiratory arrest of newborn (P28.81)
respiratory failure of newborn NOS (P28.5)

P22.1 Transient tachypnea of newborn
Idiopathic tachypnea of newborn
Respiratory distress syndrome, type II
Wet lung syndrome

P22.8 Other respiratory distress of newborn
Excludes1: respiratory arrest of newborn (P28.81)
respiratory failure of newborn NOS (P28.5)

P22.9 Respiratory distress of newborn, unspecified
Excludes1: respiratory arrest of newborn (P28.81)
respiratory failure of newborn NOS (P28.5)

P23 CONGENITAL PNEUMONIA

`4th`

Includes: infective pneumonia acquired in utero or during birth
Excludes1: neonatal pneumonia resulting from aspiration (P24.-)

P23.0 Congenital pneumonia; due to viral agent
Use additional code (B97) to identify organism
Excludes1: congenital rubella pneumonitis (P35.0)

P23.1 due to Chlamydia

P23.2 due to Staphylococcus

P23.3 due to Streptococcus, group B

P23.4 due to E. coli

P23.5 due to Pseudomonas

P23.6 due to other bacterial agents
due to H. influenzae
due to K. pneumoniae
due to Mycoplasma
due to Streptococcus, except group B
Use additional code (B95–B96) to identify organism

P23.8 due to other organisms

P23.9 unspecified

P24 NEONATAL ASPIRATION

`4th`

Includes: aspiration in utero and during delivery

P24.0 Meconium aspiration

`5th` ***Excludes1:*** meconium passage (without aspiration) during delivery (P03.82)
meconium staining (P96.83)

P24.00 Meconium aspiration without respiratory symptoms
Meconium aspiration NOS

P24.01 Meconium aspiration with respiratory symptoms
Meconium aspiration pneumonia
Meconium aspiration pneumonitis
Meconium aspiration syndrome NOS
Use additional code to identify any secondary pulmonary hypertension, if applicable (I27.2-)

P24.1 Neonatal aspiration of (clear) amniotic fluid and mucus

`5th` Neonatal aspiration of liquor (amnii)

P24.10 Neonatal aspiration of (clear) amniotic fluid and mucus; without respiratory symptoms
Neonatal aspiration of amniotic fluid and mucus NOS

P24.11 with respiratory symptoms
with pneumonia
with pneumonitis
Use additional code to identify any secondary pulmonary hypertension, if applicable (I27.2-)

P24.2 Neonatal aspiration of blood;

`5th` **P24.20 without respiratory symptoms**
Neonatal aspiration of blood NOS

P24.21 with respiratory symptoms
with pneumonia
with pneumonitis
Use additional code to identify any secondary pulmonary hypertension, if applicable (I27.2-)

P24.3 Neonatal aspiration of milk and regurgitated food

`5th` Neonatal aspiration of stomach contents

P24.30 Neonatal aspiration of milk and regurgitated food; without respiratory symptoms
Neonatal aspiration of milk and regurgitated food NOS

P24.31 with respiratory symptoms
Use additional code to identify any secondary pulmonary hypertension, if applicable (I27.2-)

CHAPTER 16. CERTAIN CONDITIONS ORIGINATING IN THE PERINATAL PERIOD (P11.1–P24.31)

`4th` `5th` `6th` `7th` Additional Character Required	✓ 3-character code	•=New Code ▲=Revised Code	***Excludes1***—Not coded here, do not use together ***Excludes2***—Not included here

P24.8 Other neonatal aspiration;
5th   **P24.80**   **without respiratory symptoms**
     Neonatal aspiration NEC
   P24.81   **with respiratory symptoms**
     Neonatal aspiration pneumonia NEC
     Neonatal aspiration with pneumonitis NEC
     Neonatal aspiration with pneumonia NOS
     Neonatal aspiration with pneumonitis NOS
     Use additional code to identify any secondary pulmonary hypertension, if applicable (I27.2-)
P24.9 Neonatal aspiration, unspecified

P25 INTERSTITIAL EMPHYSEMA AND RELATED CONDITIONS ORIGINATING IN THE PERINATAL PERIOD
4th
Do not report codes from P25 that do not originate in the perinatal period.
P25.0 Interstitial emphysema originating in the perinatal period
P25.1 Pneumothorax originating in the perinatal period
P25.2 Pneumomediastinum originating in the perinatal period
P25.3 Pneumopericardium originating in the perinatal period
P25.8 Other conditions related to interstitial emphysema originating in the perinatal period

P26 PULMONARY HEMORRHAGE ORIGINATING IN THE PERINATAL PERIOD
4th
Do not report codes from P26 that do not originate in the perinatal period
Excludes1: acute idiopathic hemorrhage in infants over 28 days old (R04.81)
P26.0 Tracheobronchial hemorrhage
P26.1 Massive pulmonary hemorrhage
P26.8 Other pulmonary hemorrhages
P26.9 Unspecified pulmonary hemorrhage

P27 CHRONIC RESPIRATORY DISEASE ORIGINATING IN THE PERINATAL PERIOD
4th
Do not report codes from P27 that do not originate in the perinatal period
Excludes2: respiratory distress of newborn (P22.0–P22.9)
P27.0 Wilson-Mikity syndrome
   Pulmonary dysmaturity
P27.1 Bronchopulmonary dysplasia
P27.8 Other chronic respiratory diseases
   Congenital pulmonary fibrosis
   Ventilator lung in newborn
P27.9 Unspecified chronic respiratory disease

P28 OTHER RESPIRATORY CONDITIONS ORIGINATING IN THE PERINATAL PERIOD
4th
Excludes1: congenital malformations of the respiratory system (Q30–Q34)
P28.0 Primary atelectasis of newborn
   Primary failure to expand terminal respiratory units
   Pulmonary hypoplasia associated with short gestation
   Pulmonary immaturity NOS
P28.1 Other and unspecified atelectasis of newborn
5th   **P28.10**   **Unspecified atelectasis of newborn**
     Atelectasis of newborn NOS
   P28.11   **Resorption atelectasis without respiratory distress syndrome**
     Excludes1: resorption atelectasis with respiratory distress syndrome (P22.0)
   P28.19   **Other atelectasis of newborn**
     Partial atelectasis of newborn
     Secondary atelectasis of newborn
P28.2 Cyanotic attacks of newborn
   Excludes1: apnea of newborn (P28.3–P28.4)
P28.3 Primary sleep apnea of newborn
   Central sleep apnea of newborn
   Obstructive sleep apnea of newborn
   Sleep apnea of newborn NOS
P28.4 Other apnea of newborn
   Apnea of prematurity
   Obstructive apnea of newborn
   Excludes1: obstructive sleep apnea of newborn (P28.3)
P28.5 Respiratory failure of newborn
   Excludes1: respiratory arrest of newborn (P28.81)
     respiratory distress of newborn (P22.0-)
P28.8 Other specified respiratory conditions of newborn
5th   **P28.81**   **Respiratory arrest of newborn**

   P28.89   **Other specified respiratory conditions of newborn**
     Congenital laryngeal stridor
     Sniffles in newborn
     Snuffles in newborn
     Excludes1: early congenital syphilitic rhinitis (A50.05)
P28.9 Respiratory condition of newborn, unspecified
   Respiratory depression in newborn

P29 CARDIOVASCULAR DISORDERS ORIGINATING IN THE PERINATAL PERIOD
4th
Excludes1: congenital malformations of the circulatory system (Q20–Q28)
P29.0 Neonatal cardiac failure
P29.1 Neonatal cardiac dysrhythmia
5th   **P29.11**   **Neonatal tachycardia**
   P29.12   **Neonatal bradycardia**
P29.2 Neonatal hypertension
P29.3 Persistent fetal circulation
5th   **P29.30**   **Pulmonary hypertension of newborn**
     Persistent pulmonary hypertension of newborn
   P29.38   **Other persistent fetal circulation**
     Delayed closure of ductus arteriosus
P29.4 Transient myocardial ischemia in newborn
P29.8 Other cardiovascular disorders originating in the perinatal period
5th
   P29.81   **Cardiac arrest of newborn**
   P29.89   **Other cardiovascular disorders originating in the perinatal period**
P29.9 Cardiovascular disorder originating in the perinatal period, unspecified

(P35–P39) INFECTIONS SPECIFIC TO THE PERINATAL PERIOD

Infections acquired in utero, during birth via the umbilicus, or during the first 28 days after birth
Excludes2: asymptomatic HIV infection status (Z21)
   congenital gonococcal infection (A54.-)
   congenital pneumonia (P23.-)
   congenital syphilis (A50.-)
   HIV disease (B20)
   infant botulism (A48.51)
   infectious diseases not specific to the perinatal period (A00–B99, J09, J10.-)
   intestinal infectious disease (A00–A09)
   laboratory evidence of HIV (R75)
   tetanus neonatorum (A33)

P35 CONGENITAL VIRAL DISEASES
4th
Includes: infections acquired in utero or during birth
P35.0 Congenital rubella syndrome
   Congenital rubella pneumonitis
P35.1 Congenital cytomegalovirus infection
P35.2 Congenital herpesviral [herpes simplex] infection
P35.3 Congenital viral hepatitis
P35.4 Congenital Zika virus disease
   Use additional code to identify manifestations of congenital Zika virus disease
P35.8 Other congenital viral diseases
   Congenital varicella [chickenpox]
P35.9 Congenital viral disease, unspecified

P36 BACTERIAL SEPSIS OF NEWBORN
4th
   GUIDELINES

Category P36, Bacterial sepsis of newborn, includes congenital sepsis. If a perinate is documented as having sepsis without documentation of congenital or community acquired, the default is congenital and a code from category P36 should be assigned. If the P36 code includes the causal organism, an additional code from category B95, Streptococcus, Staphylococcus, and Enterococcus as the cause of diseases classified elsewhere, or B96, Other bacterial agents as the cause of diseases classified elsewhere, should not be assigned. If the P36 code does not include the causal organism, assign an additional code from category B96. If applicable, use additional codes to identify severe sepsis (R65.2-) and any associated acute organ dysfunction.
Includes: congenital sepsis
Use additional code(s), if applicable, to identify severe sepsis (R65.2-) and associated acute organ dysfunction(s)

4th   **5th**   **6th**   **7th**   Additional Character Required   ✔   3-character code   •=New Code   ***Excludes1***—Not coded here, do not use together
                                               ▲=Revised Code   ***Excludes2***—Not included here

P36.0 **Sepsis of newborn due to Streptococcus, group B**
P36.1 **Sepsis of newborn due to other and unspecified streptococci**
> 5th P36.10 **Sepsis of newborn due to unspecified streptococci**
P36.19 **Sepsis of newborn due to other streptococci**
P36.2 **Sepsis of newborn due to Staphylococcus aureus**
P36.3 **Sepsis of newborn due to other and unspecified staphylococci**
> 5th P36.30 **Sepsis of newborn due to unspecified staphylococci**
P36.39 **Sepsis of newborn due to other staphylococci**
P36.4 **Sepsis of newborn due to E. coli**
P36.5 **Sepsis of newborn due to anaerobes**
P36.8 **Other bacterial sepsis of newborn**
Use additional code from category B96 to identify organism
P36.9 **Bacterial sepsis of newborn, unspecified**

P37 4th **OTHER CONGENITAL INFECTIOUS AND PARASITIC DISEASES**
Excludes2: congenital syphilis (A50.-)
infectious neonatal diarrhea (A00–A09)
necrotizing enterocolitis in newborn (P77.-)
noninfectious neonatal diarrhea (P78.3)
ophthalmia neonatorum due to gonococcus (A54.31)
tetanus neonatorum (A33)
P37.0 **Congenital tuberculosis**
P37.1 **Congenital toxoplasmosis**
Hydrocephalus due to congenital toxoplasmosis
P37.2 **Neonatal (disseminated) listeriosis**
P37.3 **Congenital falciparum malaria**
P37.4 **Other congenital malaria**
P37.5 **Neonatal candidiasis**
P37.8 **Other specified congenital infectious and parasitic diseases**
P37.9 **Congenital infectious or parasitic disease, unspecified**

P38 4th **OMPHALITIS OF NEWBORN**
Excludes1: omphalitis not of newborn (L08.82)
tetanus omphalitis (A33)
umbilical hemorrhage of newborn (P51.-)
P38.1 **Omphalitis with mild hemorrhage**
P38.9 **Omphalitis without hemorrhage**
Omphalitis of newborn NOS

P39 4th **OTHER INFECTIONS SPECIFIC TO THE PERINATAL PERIOD**
Use additional code to identify organism or specific infection
P39.0 **Neonatal infective mastitis**
Excludes1: breast engorgement of newborn (P83.4)
noninfective mastitis of newborn (P83.4)
P39.1 **Neonatal conjunctivitis and dacryocystitis**
Neonatal chlamydial conjunctivitis
Ophthalmia neonatorum NOS
Excludes1: gonococcal conjunctivitis (A54.31)
P39.2 **Intra-amniotic infection affecting newborn, NEC**
P39.3 **Neonatal urinary tract infection**
P39.4 **Neonatal skin infection**
Neonatal pyoderma
Excludes1: pemphigus neonatorum (L00)
staphylococcal scalded skin syndrome (L00)
P39.8 **Other specified infections specific to the perinatal period**
P39.9 **Infection specific to the perinatal period, unspecified**

(P50–P61) HEMORRHAGIC AND HEMATOLOGICAL DISORDERS OF NEWBORN

Excludes1: congenital stenosis and stricture of bile ducts (Q44.3)
Crigler-Najjar syndrome (E80.5)
Dubin-Johnson syndrome (E80.6)
Gilbert syndrome (E80.4)
hereditary hemolytic anemias (D55–D58)

P50 4th **NEWBORN AFFECTED BY INTRAUTERINE (FETAL) BLOOD LOSS**
Excludes1: congenital anemia from intrauterine (fetal) blood loss (P61.3)
P50.0 **Newborn affected by intrauterine (fetal) blood loss from vasa previa**
P50.1 **Newborn affected by intrauterine (fetal) blood loss from ruptured cord**

P50.2 **Newborn affected by intrauterine (fetal) blood loss from placenta**
P50.3 **Newborn affected by hemorrhage into co-twin**
P50.4 **Newborn affected by hemorrhage into maternal circulation**
P50.5 **Newborn affected by intrauterine (fetal) blood loss from cut end of co-twin's cord**
P50.8 **Newborn affected by other intrauterine (fetal) blood loss**
P50.9 **Newborn affected by intrauterine (fetal) blood loss, unspecified**
Newborn affected by fetal hemorrhage NOS

P51 4th **UMBILICAL HEMORRHAGE OF NEWBORN**
Excludes1: omphalitis with mild hemorrhage (P38.1)
umbilical hemorrhage from cut end of co-twins cord (P50.5)
P51.0 **Massive umbilical hemorrhage of newborn**
P51.8 **Other umbilical hemorrhages of newborn**
Slipped umbilical ligature NOS
P51.9 **Umbilical hemorrhage of newborn, unspecified**

P52 4th **INTRACRANIAL NONTRAUMATIC HEMORRHAGE OF NEWBORN**
Includes: intracranial hemorrhage due to anoxia or hypoxia
Excludes1: intracranial hemorrhage due to birth injury (P10.-)
intracranial hemorrhage due to other injury (S06.-)
P52.0 **Intraventricular (nontraumatic) hemorrhage, grade 1, of newborn**
Subependymal hemorrhage (without intraventricular extension)
Bleeding into germinal matrix
P52.1 **Intraventricular (nontraumatic) hemorrhage, grade 2, of newborn**
Subependymal hemorrhage with intraventricular extension
Bleeding into ventricle
P52.2 **Intraventricular (nontraumatic) hemorrhage, grade 3 and**
> 5th **grade 4, of newborn**
P52.21 **Intraventricular (nontraumatic) hemorrhage, grade 3, of newborn**
Subependymal hemorrhage with intraventricular extension with enlargement of ventricle
P52.22 **Intraventricular (nontraumatic) hemorrhage, grade 4, of newborn**
Bleeding into cerebral cortex
Subependymal hemorrhage with intracerebral extension
P52.3 **Unspecified intraventricular (nontraumatic) hemorrhage of newborn**
P52.4 **Intracerebral (nontraumatic) hemorrhage of newborn**
P52.5 **Subarachnoid (nontraumatic) hemorrhage of newborn**
P52.6 **Cerebellar (nontraumatic) and posterior fossa hemorrhage of newborn**
P52.8 **Other intracranial (nontraumatic) hemorrhages of newborn**
P52.9 **Intracranial (nontraumatic) hemorrhage of newborn, unspecified**

P53 ✔ **HEMORRHAGIC DISEASE OF NEWBORN**
Vitamin K deficiency of newborn

P54 4th **OTHER NEONATAL HEMORRHAGES**
Excludes1: newborn affected by (intrauterine) blood loss (P50.-)
pulmonary hemorrhage originating in the perinatal period (P26.-)
P54.0 **Neonatal hematemesis**
Excludes1: neonatal hematemesis due to swallowed maternal blood (P78.2)
P54.1 **Neonatal melena**
Excludes1: neonatal melena due to swallowed maternal blood (P78.2)
P54.2 **Neonatal rectal hemorrhage**
P54.3 **Other neonatal gastrointestinal hemorrhage**
P54.4 **Neonatal adrenal hemorrhage**
P54.5 **Neonatal cutaneous hemorrhage**
Neonatal bruising
Neonatal ecchymoses
Neonatal petechiae
Neonatal superficial hematomata
Excludes2: bruising of scalp due to birth injury (P12.3)
cephalhematoma due to birth injury (P12.0)
P54.6 **Neonatal vaginal hemorrhage**
Neonatal pseudomenses

4th	5th	6th	7th	Additional Character Required	✔ 3-character code

•=New Code
▲=Revised Code

Excludes1—Not coded here, do not use together
Excludes2—Not included here

CHAPTER 16. CERTAIN CONDITIONS ORIGINATING IN THE PERINATAL PERIOD   (P54.8–P74.9)

P54.8   Other specified neonatal hemorrhages

P54.9   Neonatal hemorrhage, unspecified

P55   HEMOLYTIC DISEASE OF NEWBORN

`4th`

P55.0   Rh isoimmunization of newborn

P55.1   ABO isoimmunization of newborn

P55.8   Other hemolytic diseases of newborn

P55.9   Hemolytic disease of newborn, unspecified

P56   HYDROPS FETALIS DUE TO HEMOLYTIC DISEASE

`4th`

Excludes1: hydrops fetalis NOS (P83.2)

P56.0   Hydrops fetalis due to isoimmunization

P56.9   Hydrops fetalis due to other and unspecified hemolytic disease

    `5th`   P56.90   Hydrops fetalis due to unspecified hemolytic disease

        P56.99   Hydrops fetalis due to other hemolytic disease

P57   KERNICTERUS

`4th`

P57.0   Kernicterus due to isoimmunization

P57.8   Other specified kernicterus

     Excludes1: Crigler-Najjar syndrome (E80.5)

P57.9   Kernicterus, unspecified

P59   NEONATAL JAUNDICE FROM OTHER AND UNSPECIFIED CAUSES

`4th`

Excludes1: jaundice due to inborn errors of metabolism (E70–E88)

    kernicterus (P57.-)

P59.0   Neonatal jaundice associated with preterm delivery

    Hyperbilirubinemia of prematurity

    Jaundice due to delayed conjugation associated with preterm delivery

P59.1   Inspissated bile syndrome

P59.2   Neonatal jaundice from other and unspecified hepatocellular damage

`5th`

     Excludes1: congenital viral hepatitis (P35.3)

    P59.20   Neonatal jaundice from unspecified hepatocellular damage

    P59.29   Neonatal jaundice from other hepatocellular damage

        Neonatal giant cell hepatitis

        Neonatal (idiopathic) hepatitis

P59.3   Neonatal jaundice from breast milk inhibitor

P59.8   Neonatal jaundice from other specified causes

P59.9   Neonatal jaundice, unspecified

    Neonatal physiological jaundice (intense)(prolonged) NOS

P60   DISSEMINATED INTRAVASCULAR COAGULATION OF NEWBORN

✔

Defibrination syndrome of newborn

P61   OTHER PERINATAL HEMATOLOGICAL DISORDERS

`4th`

Excludes1: transient hypogammaglobulinemia of infancy (D80.7)

P61.0   Transient neonatal thrombocytopenia

    Neonatal thrombocytopenia due to exchange transfusion

    Neonatal thrombocytopenia due to idiopathic maternal thrombocytopenia

    Neonatal thrombocytopenia due to isoimmunization

P61.1   Polycythemia neonatorum

P61.2   Anemia of prematurity

P61.3   Congenital anemia from fetal blood loss

P61.4   Other congenital anemias, NEC

    Congenital anemia NOS

P61.5   Transient neonatal neutropenia

     Excludes1: congenital neutropenia (nontransient) (D70.0)

P61.6   Other transient neonatal disorders of coagulation

P61.8   Other specified perinatal hematological disorders

P61.9   Perinatal hematological disorder, unspecified

(P70–P74) TRANSITORY ENDOCRINE AND METABOLIC DISORDERS SPECIFIC TO NEWBORN

Includes: transitory endocrine and metabolic disturbances caused by the infant's response to maternal endocrine and metabolic factors, or its adjustment to extrauterine environment

P70   TRANSITORY DISORDERS OF CARBOHYDRATE METABOLISM SPECIFIC TO NEWBORN

`4th`

P70.0   Syndrome of infant of mother with gestational diabetes

    Newborn (with hypoglycemia) affected by maternal gestational diabetes

     Excludes1: newborn (with hypoglycemia) affected by maternal (pre-existing) DM (P70.1)

    syndrome of infant of a diabetic mother (P70.1)

P70.1   Syndrome of infant of a diabetic mother

    Newborn (with hypoglycemia) affected by maternal (pre-existing) DM

     Excludes1: newborn (with hypoglycemia) affected by maternal gestational diabetes (P70.0)

    syndrome of infant of mother with gestational diabetes (P70.0)

P70.2   Neonatal DM

P70.3   Iatrogenic neonatal hypoglycemia

P70.4   Other neonatal hypoglycemia

    Transitory neonatal hypoglycemia

P70.8   Other transitory disorders of carbohydrate metabolism of newborn

P71   TRANSITORY NEONATAL DISORDERS OF CALCIUM AND MAGNESIUM METABOLISM

`4th`

P71.0   Cow's milk hypocalcemia in newborn

P71.1   Other neonatal hypocalcemia

     Excludes1: neonatal hypoparathyroidism (P71.4)

P71.3   Neonatal tetany without calcium or magnesium deficiency

    Neonatal tetany NOS

P71.4   Transitory neonatal hypoparathyroidism

P71.8   Other transitory neonatal disorders of calcium and magnesium metabolism

P71.9   Transitory neonatal disorder of calcium and magnesium metabolism, unspecified

P72   OTHER TRANSITORY NEONATAL ENDOCRINE DISORDERS

`4th`

Excludes1: congenital hypothyroidism with or without goiter (E03.0-E03.1)

    dyshormogenetic goiter (E07.1)

    Pendred's syndrome (E07.1)

P72.0   Neonatal goiter, not elsewhere classified

    Transitory congenital goiter with normal functioning

P72.1   Transitory neonatal hyperthyroidism

    Neonatal thyrotoxicosis

P72.2   Other transitory neonatal disorders of thyroid function, not elsewhere classified

    Transitory neonatal hypothyroidism

P72.8   Other specified transitory neonatal endocrine disorders

P72.9   Transitory neonatal endocrine disorder, unspecified

P74   OTHER TRANSITORY NEONATAL ELECTROLYTE AND METABOLIC DISTURBANCES

`4th`

P74.0   Late metabolic acidosis of newborn

     Excludes1: (fetal) metabolic acidosis of newborn (P19)

P74.1   Dehydration of newborn

P74.2   Disturbances of sodium balance of newborn

    `5th`   P74.21   Hypernatremia of newborn

        P74.22   Hyponatremia of newborn

P74.3   Disturbances of potassium balance of newborn

    `5th`   P74.31   Hyperkalemia of newborn

        P74.32   Hypokalemia of newborn

P74.4   Other transitory electrolyte disturbances of newborn

    `5th`   P74.41   Alkalosis of newborn

        P74.42   Disturbances of chlorine balance of newborn

       `6th`   P74.421   Hyperchloremia of newborn

           Hyperchloremic metabolic acidosis

           Excludes2: late metabolic acidosis of the newborn (P47.0)

         P74.422   Hypochloremia of newborn

        P74.49   Other transitory electrolyte disturbance of newborn

P74.5   Transitory tyrosinemia of newborn

P74.6   Transitory hyperammonemia of newborn

P74.8   Other transitory metabolic disturbances of newborn

    Amino-acid metabolic disorders described as transitory

P74.9   Transitory metabolic disturbance of newborn, unspecified

---

`4th` `5th` `6th` `7th`   Additional Character Required   ✔   3-character code

•=New Code   *Excludes1*—Not coded here, do not use together

▲=Revised Code   *Excludes2*—Not included here

(P76–P78) DIGESTIVE SYSTEM DISORDERS OF NEWBORN

P76   **OTHER INTESTINAL OBSTRUCTION OF NEWBORN**
`4th`
    P76.0   **Meconium plug syndrome**
        Meconium ileus NOS
        Excludes1: meconium ileus in cystic fibrosis (E84.11)
    P76.1   **Transitory ileus of newborn**
        Excludes1: Hirschsprung's disease (Q43.1)
    P76.2   **Intestinal obstruction due to inspissated milk**
    P76.8   **Other specified intestinal obstruction of newborn**
        Excludes1: intestinal obstruction classifiable to K56.-
    P76.9   **Intestinal obstruction of newborn, unspecified**

P77   **NECROTIZING ENTEROCOLITIS OF NEWBORN**
`4th`
    P77.1   **Stage 1 necrotizing enterocolitis in newborn**
        Necrotizing enterocolitis without
        pneumatosis, without perforation
    P77.2   **Stage 2 necrotizing enterocolitis in newborn**
        Necrotizing enterocolitis with
        pneumatosis, without perforation
    P77.3   **Stage 3 necrotizing enterocolitis in newborn**
        Necrotizing enterocolitis with perforation
        Necrotizing enterocolitis with pneumatosis and perforation
    P77.9   **Necrotizing enterocolitis in newborn, unspecified**
        Necrotizing enterocolitis in newborn, NOS

> For necrotizing enterocolitis that begins after the 28th day, see the alphabetic index for the appropriate reference (eg, necrotizing enterocolitis due to C. difficile A04.7).

P78   **OTHER PERINATAL DIGESTIVE SYSTEM DISORDERS**
`4th`
    Excludes1: cystic fibrosis (E84.0–E84.9)
        neonatal gastrointestinal hemorrhages (P54.0–P54.3)
    P78.0   **Perinatal intestinal perforation**
        Meconium peritonitis
    P78.1   **Other neonatal peritonitis**
        Neonatal peritonitis NOS
    P78.2   **Neonatal hematemesis and melena due to swallowed maternal blood**
    P78.3   **Noninfective neonatal diarrhea**
        Neonatal diarrhea NOS
    P78.8   **Other specified perinatal digestive system disorders**
      `5th`   **P78.81**   **Congenital cirrhosis (of liver)**
           P78.82   **Peptic ulcer of newborn**
           P78.83   **Newborn esophageal reflux**
               Neonatal esophageal reflux
           P78.84   **Gestational alloimmune liver disease**
               GALD
               Neonatal hemochromatosis
               Excludes 1: hemochromatosis (E83.11-)
           P78.89   **Other specified perinatal digestive system disorders**
    P78.9   **Perinatal digestive system disorder, unspecified**

(P80–P83) CONDITIONS INVOLVING THE INTEGUMENT AND TEMPERATURE REGULATION OF NEWBORN

P80   **HYPOTHERMIA OF NEWBORN**
`4th`
    P80.0   **Cold injury syndrome**
        Severe and usually chronic hypothermia associated with a pink
        flushed appearance, edema and neurological and biochemical
        abnormalities.
        Excludes1: mild hypothermia of newborn (P80.8)
    P80.8   **Other hypothermia of newborn**
        Mild hypothermia of newborn
    P80.9   **Hypothermia of newborn, unspecified**

P81   **OTHER DISTURBANCES OF TEMPERATURE REGULATION OF NEWBORN**
`4th`
    P81.0   **Environmental hyperthermia of newborn**
    P81.8   **Other specified disturbances of temperature regulation of newborn**
    P81.9   **Disturbance of temperature regulation of newborn, unspecified**
        Fever of newborn NOS

P83   **OTHER CONDITIONS OF INTEGUMENT SPECIFIC TO NEWBORN**
`4th`
    Excludes1: congenital malformations of skin and integument (Q80–Q84)
        hydrops fetalis due to hemolytic disease (P56.-)
        neonatal skin infection (P39.4)
        staphylococcal scalded skin syndrome (L00)
    Excludes2: cradle cap (L21.0)
        diaper [napkin] dermatitis (L22)
    P83.0   **Sclerema neonatorum**
    P83.1   **Neonatal erythema toxicum**
    P83.2   **Hydrops fetalis not due to hemolytic disease**
        Hydrops fetalis NOS
    P83.3   **Other and unspecified edema specific to newborn**
        P83.30   **Unspecified edema specific to newborn**
        P83.39   **Other edema specific to newborn**
    P83.4   **Breast engorgement of newborn**
        Noninfective mastitis of newborn
    P83.5   **Congenital hydrocele**
    P83.6   **Umbilical polyp of newborn**
    P83.8   **Other specified conditions of integument specific to newborn**
      `5th`   **P83.81**   **Umbilical granuloma**
               Excludes2: Granulomatous disorder of the skin and
                   subcutaneous tissue, unspecified (L92.9)
           P83.88   **Other specified conditions of integument specific to newborn**
               Bronze baby syndrome
               Neonatal scleroderma
               Urticaria neonatorum
    P83.9   **Condition of the integument specific to newborn, unspecified**

(P84) OTHER PROBLEMS WITH NEWBORN

P84   **OTHER PROBLEMS WITH NEWBORN**
`✔`
    Acidemia of newborn
    Acidosis of newborn
    Anoxia of newborn NOS
    Asphyxia of newborn NOS
    Hypercapnia of newborn
    Hypoxemia of newborn
    Hypoxia of newborn NOS
    Mixed metabolic and respiratory acidosis of newborn
    Excludes1: intracranial hemorrhage due to anoxia or hypoxia (P52.-)
        hypoxic ischemic encephalopathy [HIE] (P91.6-)
        late metabolic acidosis of newborn (P74.0)

(P90–P96) OTHER DISORDERS ORIGINATING IN THE PERINATAL PERIOD

P90   **CONVULSIONS OF NEWBORN**
`✔`
    Excludes1: benign myoclonic epilepsy in infancy (G40.3-)
        benign neonatal convulsions (familial) (G40.3-)

P91   **OTHER DISTURBANCES OF CEREBRAL STATUS OF NEWBORN**
`4th`
    P91.0   **Neonatal cerebral ischemia**
        Excludes1: Neonatal cerebral infarction (P91.82-)
    P91.1   **Acquired periventricular cysts of newborn**
    P91.2   **Neonatal cerebral leukomalacia**
        Periventricular leukomalacia
    P91.3   **Neonatal cerebral irritability**
    P91.4   **Neonatal cerebral depression**
    P91.5   **Neonatal coma**
    P91.6   **Hypoxic ischemic encephalopathy [HIE]**
      `5th`   *Excludes1:* Neonatal cerebral depression (P91.4)
        Neonatal cerebral irritability (P91.3)
        Neonatal coma (P91.5)
        P91.60   **HIE, unspecified**
        P91.61   **Mild HIE**
        P91.62   **Moderate HIE**
        P91.63   **Severe HIE**
    P91.8   **Other specified disturbances of cerebral status of newborn**
      `5th`

`4th` `5th` `6th` `7th`   Additional Character Required   `✔`   3-character code

● =New Code
▲ =Revised Code

Excludes1—Not coded here, do not use together
Excludes2—Not included here

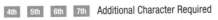

P91.81 Neonatal encephalopathy

6th   P91.811 Neonatal encephalopathy in diseases classified elsewhere
    Code first underlying condition, if known, such as:
        congenital cirrhosis (of liver) (P78.81)
        intracranial nontraumatic hemorrhage of newborn (P52.-)
        kernicterus (P57.-)

   P91.819 Neonatal encephalopathy, unspecified

•P91.82 Neonatal cerebral infarction
6th
   Neonatal stroke
   Perinatal arterial ischemic stroke
   Perinatal cerebral infarction
   Excludes1: cerebral infarction (I63.-)
   Excludes2: intracranial hemorrhage of newborn (P52.-)

   •P91.821 Neonatal cerebral infarction, right side of brain
   •P91.822 Neonatal cerebral infarction, left side of brain
   •P91.823 Neonatal cerebral infarction, bilateral
   •P91.829 Neonatal cerebral infarction, unspecified side

P91.88 Other specified disturbances of cerebral status of newborn

P91.9 Disturbance of cerebral status of newborn, unspecified

P92 FEEDING PROBLEMS OF NEWBORN
4th
Excludes1: eating disorders (F50.-)
   feeding problems in child over 28 days old (R63.3)

> Note: Report a code from P92 after 28 days of life if the feeding problem began within the first 28 days of life

P92.0 Vomiting of newborn
5th
Excludes1: vomiting of child over 28 days old (R11.-)

   P92.01 Bilious vomiting of newborn
      Excludes1: bilious vomiting in child over 28 days old (R11.14)

   P92.09 Other vomiting of newborn
      Excludes1: regurgitation of food in newborn (P92.1)

P92.1 Regurgitation and rumination of newborn
P92.2 Slow feeding of newborn
P92.3 Underfeeding of newborn
P92.4 Overfeeding of newborn
P92.5 Neonatal difficulty in feeding at breast
P92.6 Failure to thrive in newborn
   Excludes1: failure to thrive in child over 28 days old (R62.51)
P92.8 Other feeding problems of newborn
P92.9 Feeding problem of newborn, unspecified

P93 REACTIONS AND INTOXICATIONS DUE TO DRUGS ADMINISTERED TO NEWBORN
4th
Includes: reactions and intoxications due to drugs administered to fetus affecting newborn
Excludes1: jaundice due to drugs or toxins transmitted from mother or given to newborn (P58.4-)
   reactions and intoxications from maternal opiates, tranquilizers and other medication (P04.0-P04.1, P04.4-)
   withdrawal symptoms from maternal use of drugs of addiction (P96.1)
   withdrawal symptoms from therapeutic use of drugs in newborn (P96.2)

P93.0 Grey baby syndrome
P93.8 Other reactions and intoxications due to drugs administered to newborn
   Use additional code for adverse effect, if applicable, to identify drug (T36-T50 with fifth or sixth character 5)

P94 DISORDERS OF MUSCLE TONE OF NEWBORN
4th
P94.0 Transient neonatal myasthenia gravis
   myasthenia gravis (G70.0)
P94.1 Congenital hypertonia
P94.2 Congenital hypotonia
   Floppy baby syndrome, unspecified
P94.8 Other disorders of muscle tone of newborn
P94.9 Disorder of muscle tone of newborn, unspecified

P95 STILLBIRTH
✔
Deadborn fetus NOS
Fetal death of unspecified cause
Stillbirth NOS
Excludes1: maternal care for intrauterine death (O36.4)
   missed abortion (O02.1)
   outcome of delivery, stillbirth (Z37.1, Z37.3, Z37.4, Z37.7)
Code P95, Stillbirth, is only for use in institutions that maintain separate records for stillbirths. No other code should be used with P95. Code P95 should not be used on the mother's record.

P96 OTHER CONDITIONS ORIGINATING IN THE PERINATAL PERIOD
4th
P96.0 Congenital renal failure
   Uremia of newborn
P96.1 Neonatal withdrawal symptoms from maternal use of drugs of addiction
   Drug withdrawal syndrome in infant of dependent mother
   Neonatal abstinence syndrome
   Excludes1: reactions and intoxications from maternal opiates and tranquilizers administered during labor and delivery (P04.0)
P96.2 Withdrawal symptoms from therapeutic use of drugs in newborn
P96.3 Wide cranial sutures of newborn
   Neonatal craniotabes
P96.5 Complication to newborn due to (fetal) intrauterine procedure
   newborn affected by amniocentesis (P00.6)
P96.8 Other specified conditions originating in the perinatal period
5th   P96.81 Exposure to (parental) (environmental) tobacco smoke in the perinatal period
      Excludes2: newborn affected by in utero exposure to tobacco (P04.2)
        exposure to environmental tobacco smoke after the perinatal period (Z77.22)
   P96.82 Delayed separation of umbilical cord
   P96.83 Meconium staining
      Excludes1: meconium aspiration (P24.00, P24.01)
        meconium passage during delivery (P03.82)
   P96.89 Other specified conditions originating in the perinatal period
      Use additional code to specify condition
P96.9 Condition originating in the perinatal period, unspecified
   Congenital debility NOS

4th **5th** **6th** **7th** Additional Character Required   ✔ 3-character code   •=New Code   *Excludes1*—Not coded here, do not use together
    ▲=Revised Code   *Excludes2*—Not included here

296   PEDIATRIC ICD-10-CM 2021: A MANUAL FOR PROVIDER-BASED CODING

Chapter 17. Congenital malformations, deformations and chromosomal abnormalities (Q00–Q99)

GUIDELINES

Assign an appropriate code(s) from categories Q00–Q99, Congenital malformations, deformations, and chromosomal abnormalities when a malformation/deformation or chromosomal abnormality is documented. A malformation/deformation or chromosomal abnormality may be the principal/first-listed diagnosis on a record or a secondary diagnosis.

When a malformation/deformation or chromosomal abnormality does not have a unique code assignment, assign additional code(s) for any manifestations that may be present.

When the code assignment specifically identifies the malformation/deformation or chromosomal abnormality, manifestations that are an inherent component of the anomaly should not be coded separately. Additional codes should be assigned for manifestations that are not an inherent component.

Codes from Chapter 17 may be used throughout the life of the patient. If a congenital malformation or deformity has been corrected, a personal history code should be used to identify the history of the malformation or deformity. Although present at birth, a malformation/deformation or chromosomal abnormality may not be identified until later in life. Whenever the condition is diagnosed by the provider, it is appropriate to assign a code from codes Q00–Q99. For the birth admission, the appropriate code from category Z38, Liveborn infants, according to place of birth and type of delivery, should be sequenced as the principal diagnosis, followed by any congenital anomaly codes, Q00–Q99.

Note: Codes from this chapter are not for use on maternal records
Excludes2: inborn errors of metabolism (E70–E88)

(Q00–Q07) CONGENITAL MALFORMATIONS OF THE NERVOUS SYSTEM

Q00 ANENCEPHALY AND SIMILAR MALFORMATIONS
`4th`
- **Q00.0 Anencephaly**
  Acephaly
  Acrania
  Amyelencephaly
  Hemianencephaly
  Hemicephaly
- **Q00.1 Craniorachischisis**
- **Q00.2 Iniencephaly**

Q01 ENCEPHALOCELE
`4th`
Includes: Arnold-Chiari syndrome, type III
  encephalocystocele
  encephalomyelocele
  hydroencephalocele
  hydromeningocele, cranial
  meningocele, cerebral
  meningoencephalocele
Excludes1: Meckel-Gruber syndrome (Q61.9)
- **Q01.0 Frontal encephalocele**
- **Q01.1 Nasofrontal encephalocele**
- **Q01.2 Occipital encephalocele**
- **Q01.8 Encephalocele of other sites**
- **Q01.9 Encephalocele, unspecified**

Q02 MICROCEPHALY
`✓`
Includes: hydromicrocephaly
  micrencephalon
Code first, if applicable, to identify congenital Zika virus disease
Excludes1: Meckel-Gruber syndrome (Q61.9)

Q03 CONGENITAL HYDROCEPHALUS
`4th`
Includes: hydrocephalus in newborn
Excludes1: Arnold-Chiari syndrome, type II (Q07.0-)
  acquired hydrocephalus (G91.-)
  hydrocephalus due to congenital toxoplasmosis (P37.1)
  hydrocephalus with spina bifida (Q05.0–Q05.4)
- **Q03.0 Malformations of aqueduct of Sylvius**
  Anomaly of aqueduct of Sylvius
  Obstruction of aqueduct of Sylvius, congenital
  Stenosis of aqueduct of Sylvius
- **Q03.1 Atresia of foramina of Magendie and Luschka**
  Dandy-Walker syndrome
- **Q03.8 Other congenital hydrocephalus**
- **Q03.9 Congenital hydrocephalus, unspecified**

Q04 OTHER CONGENITAL MALFORMATIONS OF BRAIN
`4th`
Excludes1: cyclopia (Q87.0)
  macrocephaly (Q75.3)
- **Q04.0 Congenital malformations of corpus callosum**
  Agenesis of corpus callosum
- **Q04.3 Other reduction deformities of brain**
  Absence of part of brain
  Agenesis of part of brain
  Agyria
  Aplasia of part of brain
  Hydranencephaly
  Hypoplasia of part of brain
  Lissencephaly
  Microgyria
  Pachygyria
  Excludes1: congenital malformations of corpus callosum (Q04.0)
- **Q04.6 Congenital cerebral cysts**
  Porencephaly
  Schizencephaly
  Excludes1: acquired porencephalic cyst (G93.0)
- **Q04.8 Other specified congenital malformations of brain**
  Arnold-Chiari syndrome, type IV
  Macrogyria
- **Q04.9 Congenital malformation of brain, unspecified**
  Congenital anomaly NOS of brain
  Congenital deformity NOS of brain
  Congenital disease or lesion NOS of brain
  Multiple anomalies NOS of brain, congenital

Q05 SPINA BIFIDA
`4th`
Includes: hydromeningocele (spinal)
  meningocele (spinal)
  meningomyelocele
  myelocele
  myelomeningocele
  rachischisis
  spina bifida (aperta) (cystica)
  syringomyelocele

> Lipomeningocele in spina bifida is also included in category Q05.

Use additional code for any associated paraplegia (paraparesis) (G82.2-)
Excludes1: Arnold-Chiari syndrome, type II (Q07.0-)
  spina bifida occulta (Q76.0)
- **Q05.0 Cervical spina bifida with hydrocephalus**
- **Q05.1 Thoracic spina bifida with hydrocephalus**
  Dorsal spina bifida with hydrocephalus
  Thoracolumbar spina bifida with hydrocephalus
- **Q05.2 Lumbar spina bifida with hydrocephalus**
  Lumbosacral spina bifida with hydrocephalus
- **Q05.3 Sacral spina bifida with hydrocephalus**
- **Q05.4 Unspecified spina bifida with hydrocephalus**
- **Q05.5 Cervical spina bifida without hydrocephalus**
- **Q05.6 Thoracic spina bifida without hydrocephalus**
  Dorsal spina bifida NOS
  Thoracolumbar spina bifida NOS
- **Q05.7 Lumbar spina bifida without hydrocephalus**
  Lumbosacral spina bifida NOS
- **Q05.8 Sacral spina bifida without hydrocephalus**
- **Q05.9 Spina bifida, unspecified**

Q06 OTHER CONGENITAL MALFORMATIONS OF SPINAL CORD
`4th`
- **Q06.0 Amyelia**
- **Q06.1 Hypoplasia and dysplasia of spinal cord**
  Atelomyelia
  Myelatelia
  Myelodysplasia of spinal cord
- **Q06.2 Diastematomyelia**
- **Q06.3 Other congenital cauda equina malformations**
- **Q06.4 Hydromyelia**
  Hydrorachis
- **Q06.8 Other specified congenital malformations of spinal cord**

`4th` `5th` `6th` `7th` Additional Character Required   `✓` 3-character code

•=New Code
▲=Revised Code

Excludes1—Not coded here, do not use together
Excludes2—Not included here

CHAPTER 17. CONGENITAL MALFORMATIONS, DEFORMATIONS AND CHROMOSOMAL ABNORMALITIES   (Q06.9–Q15.9)

Q06.9 Congenital malformation of spinal cord, unspecified
Congenital anomaly NOS of spinal cord
Congenital deformity NOS of spinal cord
Congenital disease or lesion NOS of spinal cord

Q07   OTHER CONGENITAL MALFORMATIONS OF NERVOUS SYSTEM
[4th]
Excludes2: congenital central alveolar hypoventilation syndrome (G47.35)
familial dysautonomia [Riley-Day] (G90.1)
neurofibromatosis (nonmalignant) (Q85.0-)

Q07.0 Arnold-Chiari syndrome
[5th] Arnold-Chiari syndrome, type II
Excludes1: Arnold-Chiari syndrome, type III (Q01.-)
Arnold-Chiari syndrome, type IV (Q04.8)
Q07.00   without spina bifida or hydrocephalus
Q07.01   with spina bifida
Q07.02   with hydrocephalus
Q07.03   with spina bifida and hydrocephalus
Q07.8 Other specified congenital malformations of nervous system
Agenesis of nerve
Displacement of brachial plexus
Jaw-winking syndrome
Marcus Gunn's syndrome
Q07.9 Congenital malformation of nervous system, unspecified
Congenital anomaly NOS of nervous system
Congenital deformity NOS of nervous system
Congenital disease or lesion NOS of nervous system

(Q10–Q18) CONGENITAL MALFORMATIONS OF EYE, EAR, FACE AND NECK

Excludes2: cleft lip and cleft palate (Q35–Q37)
congenital malformation of cervical spine (Q05.0, Q05.5, Q67.5, Q76.0–Q76.4)
congenital malformation of larynx (Q31.-)
congenital malformation of lip NEC (Q38.0)
congenital malformation of nose (Q30.-)
congenital malformation of parathyroid gland (Q89.2)
congenital malformation of thyroid gland (Q89.2)

Q10   CONGENITAL MALFORMATIONS OF EYELID, LACRIMAL APPARATUS AND ORBIT
[4th]
Excludes1: cryptophthalmos NOS (Q11.2)
cryptophthalmos syndrome (Q87.0)
Q10.0 Congenital ptosis
Q10.1 Congenital ectropion
Q10.2 Congenital entropion
Q10.3 Other congenital malformations of eyelid
Ablepharon
Blepharophimosis, congenital
Coloboma of eyelid
Congenital absence or agenesis of cilia
Congenital absence or agenesis of eyelid
Congenital accessory eyelid
Congenital accessory eye muscle
Congenital malformation of eyelid NOS
Q10.4 Absence and agenesis of lacrimal apparatus
Congenital absence of punctum lacrimale
Q10.5 Congenital stenosis and stricture of lacrimal duct
Q10.6 Other congenital malformations of lacrimal apparatus
Congenital malformation of lacrimal apparatus NOS
Q10.7 Congenital malformation of orbit

Q11   ANOPHTHALMOS, MICROPHTHALMOS AND MACROPHTHALMOS
[4th]
Q11.0 Cystic eyeball
Q11.1 Other anophthalmos
Anophthalmos NOS
Agenesis of eye
Aplasia of eye
Q11.2 Microphthalmos
Cryptophthalmos NOS
Dysplasia of eye
Hypoplasia of eye
Rudimentary eye
Excludes1: cryptophthalmos syndrome (Q87.0)

Q11.3 Macrophthalmos
Excludes1: macrophthalmos in congenital glaucoma (Q15.0)

Q12   CONGENITAL LENS MALFORMATIONS
[4th]
Q12.0 Congenital cataract
Q12.1 Congenital displaced lens
Q12.2 Coloboma of lens
Q12.3 Congenital aphakia
Q12.4 Spherophakia
Q12.8 Other congenital lens malformations
Microphakia
Q12.9 Congenital lens malformation, unspecified

Q13   CONGENITAL MALFORMATIONS OF ANTERIOR SEGMENT OF EYE
[4th]
Q13.0 Coloboma of iris
Coloboma NOS
Q13.1 Absence of iris
Aniridia
Use additional code for associated glaucoma (H42)
Q13.2 Other congenital malformations of iris
Anisocoria, congenital
Atresia of pupil
Congenital malformation of iris NOS
Corectopia
Q13.3 Congenital corneal opacity
Q13.4 Other congenital corneal malformations
Congenital malformation of cornea NOS
Microcornea
Peter's anomaly
Q13.5 Blue sclera
Q13.8 Other congenital malformations of anterior segment of eye
[5th] **Q13.81   Rieger's anomaly**
Use additional code for associated glaucoma (H42)
Q13.89   Other congenital malformations of anterior segment of eye
Q13.9 Congenital malformation of anterior segment of eye, unspecified

Q14   CONGENITAL MALFORMATIONS OF POSTERIOR SEGMENT OF EYE
[4th]
Excludes2: optic nerve hypoplasia (H47.03-)
Q14.0 Congenital malformation of vitreous humor
Congenital vitreous opacity
Q14.1 Congenital malformation of retina
Congenital retinal aneurysm
Q14.2 Congenital malformation of optic disc
Coloboma of optic disc
Q14.3 Congenital malformation of choroid
Q14.8 Other congenital malformations of posterior segment of eye
Coloboma of the fundus
Q14.9 Congenital malformation of posterior segment of eye, unspecified

Q15   OTHER CONGENITAL MALFORMATIONS OF EYE
[4th]
Excludes1: congenital nystagmus (H55.01)
ocular albinism (E70.31-)
optic nerve hypoplasia (H47.03-)
retinitis pigmentosa (H35.52)
Q15.0 Congenital glaucoma
Axenfeld's anomaly
Buphthalmos
Glaucoma of childhood
Glaucoma of newborn
Hydrophthalmos
Keratoglobus, congenital, with glaucoma
Macrocornea with glaucoma
Macrophthalmos in congenital glaucoma
Megalocornea with glaucoma
Q15.8 Other specified congenital malformations of eye
Q15.9 Congenital malformation of eye, unspecified
Congenital anomaly of eye
Congenital deformity of eye

[4th] [5th] [6th] [7th]   Additional Character Required   ☑   3-character code   •=New Code   ▲=Revised Code   *Excludes1*—Not coded here, do not use together   *Excludes2*—Not included here

Q16 CONGENITAL MALFORMATIONS OF EAR CAUSING IMPAIRMENT OF HEARING
`4th`

Excludes1: congenital deafness (H90.-)

Q16.0 Congenital absence of (ear) auricle

Q16.1 Congenital absence, atresia and stricture of auditory canal (external)
Congenital atresia or stricture of osseous meatus

Q16.2 Absence of eustachian tube

Q16.3 Congenital malformation of ear ossicles
Congenital fusion of ear ossicles

Q16.4 Other congenital malformations of middle ear
Congenital malformation of middle ear NOS

Q16.5 Congenital malformation of inner ear
Congenital anomaly of membranous labyrinth
Congenital anomaly of organ of Corti

Q16.9 Congenital malformation of ear causing impairment of hearing, unspecified
Congenital absence of ear NOS

Q17 OTHER CONGENITAL MALFORMATIONS OF EAR
`4th`

*Excludes*1: congenital malformations of ear with impairment of hearing (Q16.0–Q16.9)
preauricular sinus (Q18.1)

Q17.0 Accessory auricle
Accessory tragus
Polyotia
Preauricular appendage or tag
Supernumerary ear
Supernumerary lobule

Q17.1 Macrotia

Q17.2 Microtia

Q17.3 Other misshapen ear
Pointed ear

Q17.4 Misplaced ear
Low-set ears
Excludes1: cervical auricle (Q18.2)

Q17.5 Prominent ear
Bat ear

Q17.8 Other specified congenital malformations of ear
Congenital absence of lobe of ear

Q17.9 Congenital malformation of ear, unspecified
Congenital anomaly of ear NOS

Q18 OTHER CONGENITAL MALFORMATIONS OF FACE AND NECK
`4th`

Excludes1: cleft lip and cleft palate (Q35-Q37)
conditions classified to Q67.0-Q67.4
congenital malformations of skull and face bones (Q75.-)
cyclopia (Q87.0)
dentofacial anomalies [including malocclusion] (M26.-)
malformation syndromes affecting facial appearance (Q87.0)
persistent thyroglossal duct (Q89.2)

Q18.0 Sinus, fistula and cyst of branchial cleft
Branchial vestige

Q18.1 Preauricular sinus and cyst
Fistula of auricle, congenital
Cervicoaural fistula

Q18.2 Other branchial cleft malformations
Branchial cleft malformation NOS
Cervical auricle
Otocephaly

Q18.6 Macrocheilia
Hypertrophy of lip, congenital

Q18.8 Other specified congenital malformations of face and neck
Medial cyst of face and neck
Medial fistula of face and neck
Medial sinus of face and neck

Q18.9 Congenital malformation of face and neck, unspecified
Congenital anomaly NOS of face and neck

(Q20–Q28) CONGENITAL MALFORMATIONS OF THE CIRCULATORY SYSTEM

Q20 CONGENITAL MALFORMATIONS OF CARDIAC CHAMBERS AND CONNECTIONS
`4th`

Excludes1: dextrocardia with situs inversus (Q89.3)
mirror-image atrial arrangement with situs inversus (Q89.3)

Q20.0 Common arterial trunk
Persistent truncus arteriosus
Excludes1: aortic septal defect (Q21.4)

Q20.3 Discordant ventriculoarterial connection
Dextrotransposition of aorta
Transposition of great vessels (complete)

Q20.8 Other congenital malformations of cardiac chambers and connections
Cor binoculare

Q21 CONGENITAL MALFORMATIONS OF CARDIAC SEPTA
`4th`

Excludes1: acquired cardiac septal defect (I51.0)

Q21.0 Ventricular septal defect
Roger's disease

Q21.1 Atrial septal defect
Coronary sinus defect
Patent or persistent foramen ovale
Patent or persistent ostium secundum defect (type II)
Patent or persistent sinus venosus defect

Q21.2 Atrioventricular septal defect
Common atrioventricular canal
Endocardial cushion defect
Ostium primum atrial septal defect (type I)

Q21.3 Tetralogy of Fallot
Ventricular septal defect with pulmonary stenosis or atresia, dextroposition of aorta and hypertrophy of right ventricle

Q21.8 Other congenital malformations of cardiac septa
Eisenmenger's defect
Pentalogy of Fallot
Code also Eisenmenger's complex or syndrome (I27.83)

Q21.9 Congenital malformation of cardiac septum, unspecified
Septal (heart) defect NOS

Q22 CONGENITAL MALFORMATIONS OF PULMONARY AND TRICUSPID VALVES
`4th`

Q22.0 Pulmonary valve atresia

Q22.1 Congenital pulmonary valve stenosis

Q22.2 Congenital pulmonary valve insufficiency
Congenital pulmonary valve regurgitation

Q22.3 Other congenital malformations of pulmonary valve
Congenital malformation of pulmonary valve NOS
Supernumerary cusps of pulmonary valve

Q22.4 Congenital tricuspid stenosis
Congenital tricuspid atresia

Q22.5 Ebstein's anomaly

Q22.6 Hypoplastic right heart syndrome

Q22.8 Other congenital malformations of tricuspid valve

Q22.9 Congenital malformation of tricuspid valve, unspecified

Q23 CONGENITAL MALFORMATIONS OF AORTIC AND MITRAL VALVES
`4th`

Q23.0 Congenital stenosis of aortic valve
Congenital aortic atresia
Congenital aortic stenosis NOS
Excludes1: congenital stenosis of aortic valve in hypoplastic left heart syndrome (Q23.4)
congenital subaortic stenosis (Q24.4)
supravalvular aortic stenosis (congenital) (Q25.3)

Q23.1 Congenital insufficiency of aortic valve
Bicuspid aortic valve
Congenital aortic insufficiency

Q23.2 Congenital mitral stenosis
Congenital mitral atresia

Q23.3 Congenital mitral insufficiency

Q23.4 Hypoplastic left heart syndrome

Q23.8 Other congenital malformations of aortic and mitral valves

---

`4th` `5th` `6th` `7th` Additional Character Required	3-character code	• =New Code	*Excludes1*—Not coded here, do not use together
		▲=Revised Code	*Excludes2*—Not included here

CHAPTER 17. CONGENITAL MALFORMATIONS, DEFORMATIONS AND CHROMOSOMAL ABNORMALITIES   (Q23.9–Q28.8)

Q23.9   **Congenital malformation of aortic and mitral valves, unspecified**

Q24   **OTHER CONGENITAL MALFORMATIONS OF HEART**
> `4th`   *Excludes1:* endocardial fibroelastosis (I42.4)

Q24.0   **Dextrocardia**
Excludes1: dextrocardia with situs inversus (Q89.3)
     isomerism of atrial appendages (with asplenia or polysplenia) (Q20.6)
     mirror-image atrial arrangement with situs inversus (Q89.3)

Q24.1   **Levocardia**

Q24.3   **Pulmonary infundibular stenosis**
Subvalvular pulmonic stenosis

Q24.4   **Congenital subaortic stenosis**

Q24.6   **Congenital heart block**

Q24.8   **Other specified congenital malformations of heart**
Congenital diverticulum of left ventricle
Congenital malformation of myocardium
Congenital malformation of pericardium
Malposition of heart
Uhl's disease

Q24.9   **Congenital malformation of heart, unspecified**
Congenital anomaly of heart
Congenital disease of heart

Q25   **CONGENITAL MALFORMATIONS OF GREAT ARTERIES**
> `4th`   **Q25.0**   **Patent ductus arteriosus**
Patent ductus Botallo
Persistent ductus arteriosus

Q25.1   **Coarctation of aorta**
Coarctation of aorta (preductal) (postductal)
Stenosis of aorta

Q25.2   **Atresia of aorta**
> `5th`   **Q25.21**   **Interruption of aortic arch**
Atresia of aortic arch
Q25.29   **Other atresia of aorta**
Atresia of aorta

Q25.3   **Supravalvular aortic stenosis**
Excludes1: congenital aortic stenosis NOS (Q23.0)
     congenital stenosis of aortic valve (Q23.0)

Q25.4   **Other congenital malformations of aorta**
> `5th`   **Q25.40**   **Congenital malformation of aorta unspecified**
Q25.41   **Absence and aplasia of aorta**
Q25.42   **Hypoplasia of aorta**
Q25.43   **Congenital aneurysm of aorta**
Congenital aneurysm of aortic root
Congenital aneurysm of aortic sinus
Q25.44   **Congenital dilation of aorta**
Q25.45   **Double aortic arch**
Vascular ring of aorta
Q25.46   **Tortuous aortic arch**
Persistent convolutions of aortic arch
Q25.47   **Right aortic arch**
Persistent right aortic arch
Q25.48   **Anomalous origin of subclavian artery**
Q25.49   **Other congenital malformations of aorta**
Aortic arch
Bovine arch

Q25.5   **Atresia of pulmonary artery**

Q25.6   **Stenosis of pulmonary artery**
Supravalvular pulmonary stenosis

Q25.7   **Other congenital malformations of pulmonary artery**
> `5th`   **Q25.71**   **Coarctation of pulmonary artery**
Q25.72   **Congenital pulmonary arteriovenous malformation**
Congenital pulmonary arteriovenous aneurysm
Q25.79   **Other congenital malformations of pulmonary artery**
Aberrant pulmonary artery
Agenesis of pulmonary artery
Congenital aneurysm of pulmonary artery
Congenital anomaly of pulmonary artery
Hypoplasia of pulmonary artery

Q25.9   **Congenital malformation of great arteries, unspecified**

Q26   **CONGENITAL MALFORMATIONS OF GREAT VEINS**
> `4th`   **Q26.2**   **Total anomalous pulmonary venous connection**
TAPVR, subdiaphragmatic
TAPVR, supradiaphragmatic

Q26.3   **Partial anomalous pulmonary venous connection**
Partial anomalous pulmonary venous return

Q26.4   **Anomalous pulmonary venous connection, unspecified**

Q26.8   **Other congenital malformations of great veins**
Absence of vena cava (inferior) (superior)
Azygos continuation of inferior vena cava
Persistent left posterior cardinal vein
Scimitar syndrome

Q26.9   **Congenital malformation of great vein, unspecified**
Congenital anomaly of vena cava (inferior) (superior) NOS

Q27   **OTHER CONGENITAL MALFORMATIONS OF PERIPHERAL VASCULAR SYSTEM**
> `4th`   *Excludes2:* anomalies of cerebral and precerebral vessels (Q28.0–Q28.3)
     anomalies of coronary vessels (Q24.5)
     anomalies of pulmonary artery (Q25.5–Q25.7)
     congenital retinal aneurysm (Q14.1)
     hemangioma and lymphangioma (D18.-)

Q27.0   **Congenital absence and hypoplasia of umbilical artery**
Single umbilical artery

Q27.3   **Arteriovenous malformation (peripheral)**
> `5th`   Arteriovenous aneurysm
Excludes1: acquired arteriovenous aneurysm (I77.0)
Excludes2: arteriovenous malformation of cerebral vessels (Q28.2)
     arteriovenous malformation of precerebral vessels (Q28.0)
Q27.30   **Arteriovenous malformation, site unspecified**
Q27.31   **Arteriovenous malformation of vessel of upper limb**
Q27.32   **Arteriovenous malformation of vessel of lower limb**
Q27.33   **Arteriovenous malformation of digestive system vessel**
Q27.34   **Arteriovenous malformation of renal vessel**
Q27.39   **Arteriovenous malformation, other site**

Q27.8   **Other specified congenital malformations of peripheral vascular system**
Absence of peripheral vascular system
Atresia of peripheral vascular system
Congenital aneurysm (peripheral)
Congenital stricture, artery
Congenital varix
Excludes 1: arteriovenous malformation (Q27.3-)

Q27.9   **Congenital malformation of peripheral vascular system, unspecified**
Anomaly of artery or vein NOS

Q28   **OTHER CONGENITAL MALFORMATIONS OF CIRCULATORY SYSTEM**
> `4th`   *Excludes1:* congenital aneurysm NOS (Q27.8)
     congenital coronary aneurysm (Q24.5)
     ruptured cerebral arteriovenous malformation (I60.8)
     ruptured malformation of precerebral vessels (I72.0)
Excludes2: congenital peripheral aneurysm (Q27.8)
     congenital pulmonary aneurysm (Q25.79)
     congenital retinal aneurysm (Q14.1)

Q28.2   **Arteriovenous malformation of cerebral vessels**
Arteriovenous malformation of brain NOS
Congenital arteriovenous cerebral aneurysm (nonruptured)

Q28.3   **Other malformations of cerebral vessels**
Congenital cerebral aneurysm (nonruptured)
Congenital malformation of cerebral vessels NOS
Developmental venous anomaly

Q28.8   **Other specified congenital malformations of circulatory system**
Congenital aneurysm, specified site NEC
Spinal vessel anomaly

`4th` `5th` `6th` `7th`   Additional Character Required   ✔   3-character code

•=New Code   *Excludes1*—Not coded here, do not use together
▲=Revised Code   *Excludes2*—Not included here

(Q30–Q34) CONGENITAL MALFORMATIONS OF THE RESPIRATORY SYSTEM

Q30 **CONGENITAL MALFORMATIONS OF NOSE**
`4th`
  Excludes1: congenital deviation of nasal septum (Q67.4)
  Q30.0 **Choanal atresia**
    Atresia of nares (anterior) (posterior)
    Congenital stenosis of nares (anterior) (posterior)
  Q30.3 **Congenital perforated nasal septum**
  Q30.8 **Other congenital malformations of nose**
    Accessory nose
    Congenital anomaly of nasal sinus wall
  Q30.9 **Congenital malformation of nose, unspecified**

Q31 **CONGENITAL MALFORMATIONS OF LARYNX**
`4th`
  Excludes1: congenital laryngeal stridor NOS (P28.89)
  Q31.2 **Laryngeal hypoplasia**
  Q31.5 **Congenital laryngomalacia**
  Q31.8 **Other congenital malformations of larynx**
    Absence of larynx
    Agenesis of larynx
    Atresia of larynx
    Congenital cleft thyroid cartilage
    Congenital fissure of epiglottis
    Congenital stenosis of larynx NEC
    Posterior cleft of cricoid cartilage

Q32 **CONGENITAL MALFORMATIONS OF TRACHEA AND BRONCHUS**
`4th`
  Excludes1: congenital bronchiectasis (Q33.4)

> For congenital tracheoesophageal fistula, see category Q39.

  Q32.0 **Congenital tracheomalacia**
  Q32.4 **Other congenital malformations of bronchus**
    Absence of bronchus
    Agenesis of bronchus
    Atresia of bronchus
    Congenital diverticulum of bronchus
    Congenital malformation of bronchus NOS

Q33 **CONGENITAL MALFORMATIONS OF LUNG**
`4th`
  Excludes1: pulmonary hypoplasia associated with short gestation (P28.0)
  Q33.6 **Congenital hypoplasia and dysplasia of lung**
  Q33.9 **Congenital malformation of lung, unspecified**

Q34 **OTHER CONGENITAL MALFORMATIONS OF RESPIRATORY SYSTEM**
`4th`
  Excludes2: congenital central alveolar hypoventilation syndrome (G47.35)
  Q34.8 **Other specified congenital malformations of respiratory system**
    Atresia of nasopharynx
  Q34.9 **Congenital malformation of respiratory system, unspecified**
    Congenital absence of respiratory system
    Congenital anomaly of respiratory system NOS

(Q35–Q37) CLEFT LIP AND CLEFT PALATE

Use additional code to identify associated malformation of the nose (Q30.2)
Excludes2: Robin's syndrome (Q87.0)

Q35 **CLEFT PALATE**
`4th`
  Includes: fissure of palate
    palatoschisis
  Excludes1: cleft palate with cleft lip (Q37.-)
  Q35.1 **Cleft hard palate**
  Q35.3 **Cleft soft palate**
  Q35.5 **Cleft hard palate with cleft soft palate**
  Q35.7 **Cleft uvula**
  Q35.9 **Cleft palate, unspecified**
    Cleft palate NOS

Q36 **CLEFT LIP**
`4th`
  Includes: cheiloschisis
    congenital fissure of lip
    harelip
    labium leporinum
  Excludes1: cleft lip with cleft palate (Q37.-)

Q36.0 **Cleft lip, bilateral**
Q36.1 **Cleft lip, median**
Q36.9 **Cleft lip, unilateral**
  Cleft lip NOS

Q37 **CLEFT PALATE WITH CLEFT LIP**
`4th`
  Includes: cheilopalatoschisis
  Q37.0 **Cleft hard palate with bilateral cleft lip**
  Q37.1 **Cleft hard palate with unilateral cleft lip**
    Cleft hard palate with cleft lip NOS
  Q37.2 **Cleft soft palate with bilateral cleft lip**
  Q37.3 **Cleft soft palate with unilateral cleft lip**
    Cleft soft palate with cleft lip NOS
  Q37.4 **Cleft hard and soft palate with bilateral cleft lip**
  Q37.5 **Cleft hard and soft palate with unilateral cleft lip**
    Cleft hard and soft palate with cleft lip NOS
  Q37.8 **Unspecified cleft palate with bilateral cleft lip**
  Q37.9 **Unspecified cleft palate with unilateral cleft lip**

(Q38–Q45) OTHER CONGENITAL MALFORMATIONS OF THE DIGESTIVE SYSTEM

Q38 **OTHER CONGENITAL MALFORMATIONS OF TONGUE, MOUTH AND PHARYNX**
`4th`
  Excludes1: dentofacial anomalies (M26.-)
    macrostomia (Q18.4)
    microstomia (Q18.5)
  Q38.0 **Congenital malformations of lips, not elsewhere classified**
    Congenital fistula of lip
    Congenital malformation of lip NOS
    Van der Woude's syndrome
    Excludes1: cleft lip (Q36.-)
      cleft lip with cleft palate (Q37.-)
      macrocheilia (Q18.6)
      microcheilia (Q18.7)
  Q38.1 **Ankyloglossia**
    Tongue tie
  Q38.2 **Macroglossia**
    Congenital hypertrophy of tongue
  Q38.3 **Other congenital malformations of tongue**
    Aglossia
    Bifid tongue
    Congenital adhesion of tongue
    Congenital fissure of tongue
    Congenital malformation of tongue NOS
    Double tongue
    Hypoglossia
    Hypoplasia of tongue
    Microglossia
  Q38.5 **Congenital malformations of palate, not elsewhere classified**
    Congenital absence of uvula
    Congenital malformation of palate NOS
    Congenital high arched palate
    Excludes1: cleft palate (Q35.-)
      cleft palate with cleft lip (Q37.-)
  Q38.6 **Other congenital malformations of mouth**
    Congenital malformation of mouth NOS
  Q38.8 **Other congenital malformations of pharynx**
    Congenital malformation of pharynx NOS
    Imperforate pharynx

Q39 **CONGENITAL MALFORMATIONS OF ESOPHAGUS**
`4th`
  Q39.0 **Atresia of esophagus without fistula**
    Atresia of esophagus NOS

> Code Q39.1 may be used to report congenital tracheo-esophageal fistula with atresia of esophagus.

  Q39.1 **Atresia of esophagus with tracheo-esophageal fistula**
    Atresia of esophagus with broncho-esophageal fistula
  Q39.2 **Congenital tracheo-esophageal fistula without atresia**
    Congenital tracheo-esophageal fistula NOS
  Q39.5 **Congenital dilatation of esophagus**
    Congenital cardiospasm

`4th` `5th` `6th` `7th` Additional Character Required   ✓ 3-character code

•=New Code
▲=Revised Code

Excludes1—Not coded here, do not use together
Excludes2—Not included here

CHAPTER 17. CONGENITAL MALFORMATIONS, DEFORMATIONS AND CHROMOSOMAL ABNORMALITIES (Q40–Q50.32)

Q40 OTHER CONGENITAL MALFORMATIONS OF UPPER ALIMENTARY TRACT
[4th]

Q40.0 Congenital hypertrophic pyloric stenosis
Congenital or infantile constriction or hypertrophy or spasm
Congenital or infantile stenosis
Congenital or infantile stricture or stricture

Q40.1 Congenital hiatus hernia
Congenital displacement of cardia through esophageal hiatus
Excludes1: congenital diaphragmatic hernia (Q79.0)

Q40.2 Other specified congenital malformations of stomach
Congenital displacement of stomach
Congenital diverticulum of stomach
Congenital hourglass stomach
Congenital duplication of stomach
Megalogastria
Microgastria

Q40.8 Other specified congenital malformations of upper alimentary tract

Q40.9 Congenital malformation of upper alimentary tract, unspecified
Congenital anomaly of upper alimentary tract
Congenital deformity of upper alimentary tract

Q41 CONGENITAL ABSENCE, ATRESIA AND STENOSIS OF SMALL INTESTINE
[4th]

Includes: congenital obstruction, occlusion or stricture of small intestine or intestine NOS
Excludes1: cystic fibrosis with intestinal manifestation (E84.11)
meconium ileus NOS (without cystic fibrosis) (P76.0)

Q41.0 Congenital absence, atresia and stenosis of duodenum

Q41.1 Congenital absence, atresia and stenosis of jejunum
Apple peel syndrome
Imperforate jejunum

Q41.2 Congenital absence, atresia and stenosis of ileum

Q41.8 Congenital absence, atresia and stenosis of other specified parts of small intestine

Q41.9 Congenital absence, atresia and stenosis of small intestine, part unspecified
Congenital absence, atresia and stenosis of intestine NOS

Q42 CONGENITAL ABSENCE, ATRESIA AND STENOSIS OF LARGE INTESTINE
[4th]

Includes: congenital obstruction, occlusion and stricture of large intestine

Q42.0 Congenital absence, atresia and stenosis of rectum with fistula

Q42.1 Congenital absence, atresia and stenosis of rectum without fistula
Imperforate rectum

Q42.2 Congenital absence, atresia and stenosis of anus with fistula

Q42.3 Congenital absence, atresia and stenosis of anus without fistula
Imperforate anus

Q42.8 Congenital absence, atresia and stenosis of other parts of large intestine

Q42.9 Congenital absence, atresia and stenosis of large intestine, part unspecified

Q43 OTHER CONGENITAL MALFORMATIONS OF INTESTINE
[4th]

Q43.0 Meckel's diverticulum (displaced) (hypertrophic)
Persistent omphalomesenteric duct
Persistent vitelline duct

Q43.1 Hirschsprung's disease
Aganglionosis
Congenital (aganglionic) megacolon

Q43.2 Other congenital functional disorders of colon
Congenital dilatation of colon

Q43.3 Congenital malformations of intestinal fixation
Congenital omental, anomalous adhesions [bands]
Congenital peritoneal adhesions [bands]
Incomplete rotation of cecum and colon
Insufficient rotation of cecum and colon
Jackson's membrane
Malrotation of colon
Rotation failure of cecum and colon
Universal mesentery

Q43.6 Congenital fistula of rectum and anus
Excludes1: congenital fistula of anus with absence, atresia and stenosis (Q42.2)
congenital fistula of rectum with absence, atresia and stenosis (Q42.0)
congenital rectovaginal fistula (Q52.2)
congenital urethrorectal fistula (Q64.73)
pilonidal fistula or sinus (L05.-)

Q43.8 Other specified congenital malformations of intestine
Congenital blind loop syndrome
Congenital diverticulitis, colon
Congenital diverticulum, intestine
Dolichocolon
Megaloappendix
Megaloduodenum
Microcolon
Transposition of appendix
Transposition of colon
Transposition of intestine

Q43.9 Congenital malformation of intestine, unspecified

Q44 CONGENITAL MALFORMATIONS OF GALLBLADDER, BILE DUCTS AND LIVER
[4th]

Q44.0 Agenesis, aplasia and hypoplasia of gallbladder
Congenital absence of gallbladder

Q44.1 Other congenital malformations of gallbladder
Congenital malformation of gallbladder NOS
Intrahepatic gallbladder

Q44.2 Atresia of bile ducts

Q44.3 Congenital stenosis and stricture of bile ducts

Q44.4 Choledochal cyst

Q44.5 Other congenital malformations of bile ducts
Accessory hepatic duct
Biliary duct duplication
Congenital malformation of bile duct NOS
Cystic duct duplication

Q44.7 Other congenital malformations of liver
Accessory liver
Alagille's syndrome
Congenital absence of liver
Congenital hepatomegaly
Congenital malformation of liver NOS

Q45 OTHER CONGENITAL MALFORMATIONS OF DIGESTIVE SYSTEM
[4th]

Excludes2: congenital diaphragmatic hernia (Q79.0)
congenital hiatus hernia (Q40.1)

Q45.8 Other specified congenital malformations of digestive system
Absence (complete) (partial) of alimentary tract NOS
Duplication of digestive system
Malposition, congenital of digestive system

Q45.9 Congenital malformation of digestive system, unspecified
Congenital anomaly of digestive system
Congenital deformity of digestive system

(Q50–Q56) CONGENITAL MALFORMATIONS OF GENITAL ORGANS

Excludes1: androgen insensitivity syndrome (E34.5-)
syndromes associated with anomalies in the number and form of chromosomes (Q90–Q99)

Q50 CONGENITAL MALFORMATIONS OF OVARIES, FALLOPIAN TUBES AND BROAD LIGAMENTS
[4th]

Q50.0 Congenital absence of ovary
[5th] *Excludes1:* Turner's syndrome (Q96.-)

Q50.01 Congenital absence of ovary, unilateral
Q50.02 Congenital absence of ovary, bilateral

Q50.1 Developmental ovarian cyst

Q50.2 Congenital torsion of ovary

Q50.3 Other congenital malformations of ovary
[5th] **Q50.31 Accessory ovary**
Q50.32 Ovarian streak
46, XX with streak gonads

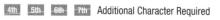 Additional Character Required

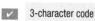 3-character code

•=New Code
▲=Revised Code

Excludes1—Not coded here, do not use together
Excludes2—Not included here

Q50.39   **Other congenital malformation of ovary**
Congenital malformation of ovary NOS

Q50.4   **Embryonic cyst of fallopian tube**
Fimbrial cyst

Q50.5   **Embryonic cyst of broad ligament**
Epoophoron cyst
Parovarian cyst

Q50.6   **Other congenital malformations of fallopian tube and broad ligament**
Absence of fallopian tube and broad ligament
Accessory fallopian tube and broad ligament
Atresia of fallopian tube and broad ligament
Congenital malformation of fallopian tube or broad ligament NOS

Q51   **CONGENITAL MALFORMATIONS OF UTERUS AND CERVIX**
`4th`

Q51.0   **Agenesis and aplasia of uterus**
Congenital absence of uterus

Q51.1   **Doubling of uterus with doubling of cervix and vagina**
`5th`   **Q51.10**   **Doubling of uterus with doubling of cervix and vagina without obstruction**
Doubling of uterus with doubling of cervix and vagina NOS

    Q51.11   **Doubling of uterus with doubling of cervix and vagina with obstruction**

Q51.2   **Other doubling of uterus**
`5th`   Doubling of uterus NOS
Septate uterus

    Q51.21   **Complete doubling of uterus**
Complete septate uterus

    Q51.22   **Partial doubling of uterus**
Partial septate uterus

    Q51.28   **Other and unspecified doubling of uterus**
Septate uterus NOS

Q51.3   **Bicornate uterus**
Bicornate uterus, complete or partial

Q51.4   **Unicornate uterus**
Unicornate uterus with or without a separate uterine horn
Uterus with only one functioning horn

Q51.5   **Agenesis and aplasia of cervix**
Congenital absence of cervix

Q51.6   **Embryonic cyst of cervix**

Q51.7   **Congenital fistulae between uterus and digestive and urinary tracts**

Q51.8   **Other congenital malformations of uterus and cervix**
`5th`   **Q51.81**   **Other congenital malformations of uterus**
`6th`   **Q51.810**   **Arcuate uterus**
Arcuatus uterus

      Q51.811   **Hypoplasia of uterus**

      Q51.818   **Other congenital malformations of uterus**
Müllerian anomaly of uterus NEC

    Q51.82   **Other congenital malformations of cervix**
`6th`   **Q51.820**   **Cervical duplication**

      Q51.821   **Hypoplasia of cervix**

      Q51.828   **Other congenital malformations of cervix**

Q51.9   **Congenital malformation of uterus and cervix, unspecified**

Q52   **OTHER CONGENITAL MALFORMATIONS OF FEMALE GENITALIA**
`4th`

Q52.0   **Congenital absence of vagina**
Vaginal agenesis, total or partial

Q52.1   **Doubling of vagina**
`5th`   *Excludes1*: doubling of vagina with doubling of uterus and cervix (Q51.1-)

    Q52.10   **Doubling of vagina, unspecified**
Septate vagina NOS

    Q52.11   **Transverse vaginal septum**

    Q52.12   **Longitudinal vaginal septum**
`6th`   **Q52.120**   **Longitudinal vaginal septum, nonobstructing**

      Q52.121   **Longitudinal vaginal septum, obstructing, right side**

      Q52.122   **Longitudinal vaginal septum, obstructing, left side**

      Q52.123   **Longitudinal vaginal septum, microperforate, right side**

      Q52.124   **Longitudinal vaginal septum, microperforate, left side**

      Q52.129   **Other and unspecified longitudinal vaginal septum**

Q52.2   **Congenital rectovaginal fistula**
Excludes1: cloaca (Q43.7)

Q52.4   **Other congenital malformations of vagina**
Canal of Nuck cyst, congenital
Congenital malformation of vagina NOS
Embryonic vaginal cyst
Gartner's duct cyst

Q52.5   **Fusion of labia**

Q52.6   **Congenital malformation of clitoris**

Q52.7   **Other and unspecified congenital malformations of vulva**
`5th`   **Q52.70**   **Unspecified congenital malformations of vulva**
Congenital malformation of vulva NOS

    Q52.71   **Congenital absence of vulva**

    Q52.79   **Other congenital malformations of vulva**
Congenital cyst of vulva

Q52.3   **Imperforate hymen**

Q52.8   **Other specified congenital malformations of female genitalia**

Q52.9   **Congenital malformation of female genitalia, unspecified**

Q53   **UNDESCENDED AND ECTOPIC TESTICLE**
`4th`

Q53.0   **Ectopic testis**
`5th`   **Q53.00**   **Ectopic testis, unspecified**

    Q53.01   **Ectopic testis, unilateral**

    Q53.02   **Ectopic testes, bilateral**

Q53.1   **Undescended testicle, unilateral**
`5th`   **Q53.10**   **Unspecified undescended testicle, unilateral**

    Q53.11   **Abdominal testis, unilateral**
`6th`   **Q53.111**   **Unilateral intraabdominal testis**

      Q53.112   **Unilateral inguinal testis**

    Q53.12   **Ectopic perineal testis, unilateral**

    Q53.13   **Unilateral high scrotal testis**

Q53.2   **Undescended testicle, bilateral**
`5th`   **Q53.20**   **Undescended testicle, unspecified, bilateral**

    Q53.21   **Abdominal testis, bilateral**
`6th`   **Q53.211**   **Bilateral intraabdominal testes**

      Q53.212   **Bilateral inguinal testes**

    Q53.22   **Ectopic perineal testis, bilateral**

    Q53.23   **Bilateral high scrotal testes**

Q53.9   **Undescended testicle, unspecified**
Cryptorchism NOS

Q54   **HYPOSPADIAS**
`4th`   *Excludes1:* epispadias (Q64.0)

Q54.0   **Hypospadias, balanic**
Hypospadias, coronal
Hypospadias, glandular

Q54.1   **Hypospadias, penile**

Q54.2   **Hypospadias, penoscrotal**

Q54.3   **Hypospadias, perineal**

Q54.4   **Congenital chordee**
Chordee without hypospadias

Q54.8   **Other hypospadias**
Hypospadias with intersex state

Q54.9   **Hypospadias, unspecified**

Q55   **OTHER CONGENITAL MALFORMATIONS OF MALE GENITAL ORGANS**
`4th`   *Excludes1:* congenital hydrocele (P83.5)
    hypospadias (Q54.-)

Q55.0   **Absence and aplasia of testis**
Monorchism

Q55.1   **Hypoplasia of testis and scrotum**
Fusion of testes

Q55.2   **Other and unspecified congenital malformations of testis and scrotum**
`5th`   **Q55.20**   **Unspecified congenital malformations of testis and scrotum**
Congenital malformation of testis or scrotum NOS

`4th` `5th` `6th` `7th` Additional Character Required   ✔ 3-character code

•=New Code
▲=Revised Code

Excludes1—Not coded here, do not use together
Excludes2—Not included here

CHAPTER 17. CONGENITAL MALFORMATIONS, DEFORMATIONS AND CHROMOSOMAL ABNORMALITIES   (Q55.21–Q64.6)

Q55.21 **Polyorchism**
Q55.22 **Retractile testis**
Q55.23 **Scrotal transposition**
Q55.29 **Other congenital malformations of testis and scrotum**
Q55.4 **Other congenital malformations of vas deferens, epididymis, seminal vesicles and prostate**
Absence or aplasia of prostate
Absence or aplasia of spermatic cord
Congenital malformation of vas deferens, epididymis, seminal vesicles or prostate NOS
Q55.5 **Congenital absence and aplasia of penis**
Q55.6 **Other congenital malformations of penis**
`5th` Q55.61 **Curvature of penis (lateral)**
Q55.62 **Hypoplasia of penis**
Micropenis
Q55.63 **Congenital torsion of penis**
Excludes1: acquired torsion of penis (N48.82)
Q55.64 **Hidden penis**
Buried penis
Concealed penis
Excludes1: acquired buried penis (N48.83)
Q55.69 **Other congenital malformation of penis**
Congenital malformation of penis NOS
Q55.8 **Other specified congenital malformations of male genital organs**
Q55.9 **Congenital malformation of male genital organ, unspecified**
Congenital anomaly of male genital organ
Congenital deformity of male genital organ

Q56 **INDETERMINATE SEX AND PSEUDOHERMAPHRODITISM**
`4th` *Excludes1:* 46, XX true hermaphrodite (Q99.1)
androgen insensitivity syndrome (E34.5-)
chimera 46, XX/46, XY true hermaphrodite (Q99.0)
female pseudohermaphroditism with adrenocortical disorder (E25.-)
pseudohermaphroditism with specified chromosomal anomaly (Q96–Q99)
pure gonadal dysgenesis (Q99.1)
Q56.1 **Male pseudohermaphroditism, not elsewhere classified**
46, XY with streak gonads
Male pseudohermaphroditism NOS
Q56.2 **Female pseudohermaphroditism, not elsewhere classified**
Female pseudohermaphroditism NOS
Q56.3 **Pseudohermaphroditism, unspecified**
Q56.4 **Indeterminate sex, unspecified**
Ambiguous genitalia

(Q60–Q64) CONGENITAL MALFORMATIONS OF THE URINARY SYSTEM

Q60 **RENAL AGENESIS AND OTHER REDUCTION DEFECTS OF KIDNEY**
`4th` *Includes:* congenital absence of kidney
congenital atrophy of kidney
infantile atrophy of kidney
Q60.0 **Renal agenesis, unilateral**
Q60.1 **Renal agenesis, bilateral**
Q60.3 **Renal hypoplasia, unilateral**
Q60.4 **Renal hypoplasia, bilateral**
Q60.6 **Potter's syndrome**

Q61 **CYSTIC KIDNEY DISEASE**
`4th` *Excludes1:* acquired cyst of kidney (N28.1)
Potter's syndrome (Q60.6)
Q61.0 **Congenital renal cyst**
`5th` Q61.00 **Congenital renal cyst, unspecified**
Cyst of kidney NOS (congenital)
Q61.01 **Congenital single renal cyst**
Q61.02 **Congenital multiple renal cysts**
Q61.1 **Polycystic kidney, infantile type**
`5th` Polycystic kidney, autosomal recessive
Q61.11 **Cystic dilatation of collecting ducts**
Q61.19 **Other polycystic kidney, infantile type**

Q61.2 **Polycystic kidney, adult type**
Polycystic kidney, autosomal dominant
Q61.3 **Polycystic kidney, unspecified**
Q61.4 **Renal dysplasia**
Multicystic dysplastic kidney
Multicystic kidney (development)
Multicystic kidney disease
Multicystic renal dysplasia
Excludes1: polycystic kidney disease (Q61.11–Q61.3)
Q61.5 **Medullary cystic kidney**
Nephronopthisis
Sponge kidney NOS
Q61.8 **Other cystic kidney diseases**
Fibrocystic kidney
Fibrocystic renal degeneration or disease
Q61.9 **Cystic kidney disease, unspecified**
Meckel-Gruber syndrome

Q62 **CONGENITAL OBSTRUCTIVE DEFECTS OF RENAL PELVIS**
`4th` **AND CONGENITAL MALFORMATIONS OF URETER**
Q62.0 **Congenital hydronephrosis**
Q62.1 **Congenital occlusion of ureter**
`5th` Atresia and stenosis of ureter
Q62.10 **Congenital occlusion of ureter, unspecified**
Q62.11 **Congenital occlusion of ureteropelvic junction**
Q62.12 **Congenital occlusion of ureterovesical orifice**
Q62.3 **Other obstructive defects of renal pelvis and ureter**
`5th` Q62.31 **Congenital ureterocele, orthotopic**
Q62.32 **Cecoureterocele**
Ectopic ureterocele
Q62.39 **Other obstructive defects of renal pelvis and ureter**
Ureteropelvic junction obstruction NOS
Q62.8 **Other congenital malformations of ureter**
Anomaly of ureter NOS

Q63 **OTHER CONGENITAL MALFORMATIONS OF KIDNEY**
`4th` *Excludes1:* congenital nephrotic syndrome (N04.-)
Q63.0 **Accessory kidney**
Q63.1 **Lobulated, fused and horseshoe kidney**
Q63.2 **Ectopic kidney**
Congenital displaced kidney
Malrotation of kidney
Q63.3 **Hyperplastic and giant kidney**
Compensatory hypertrophy of kidney
Q63.8 **Other specified congenital malformations of kidney**
Congenital renal calculi
Q63.9 **Congenital malformation of kidney, unspecified**

Q64 **OTHER CONGENITAL MALFORMATIONS OF**
`4th` **URINARY SYSTEM**
Q64.0 **Epispadias**
Excludes1: hypospadias (Q54.-)
Q64.1 **Exstrophy of urinary bladder**
`5th` Q64.10 **Exstrophy of urinary bladder, unspecified**
Ectopia vesicae
Q64.11 **Supravesical fissure of urinary bladder**
Q64.12 **Cloacal exstrophy of urinary bladder**
Q64.19 **Other exstrophy of urinary bladder**
Extroversion of bladder
Q64.2 **Congenital posterior urethral valves**
Q64.3 **Other atresia and stenosis of urethra and bladder neck**
`5th` Q64.31 **Congenital bladder neck obstruction**
Congenital obstruction of vesicourethral orifice
Q64.39 **Other atresia and stenosis of urethra and bladder neck**
Atresia and stenosis of urethra and bladder neck NOS
Q64.4 **Malformation of urachus**
Cyst of urachus
Patent urachus
Prolapse of urachus
Q64.5 **Congenital absence of bladder and urethra**
Q64.6 **Congenital diverticulum of bladder**

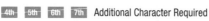 Additional Character Required   ✔ 3-character code

•=New Code   *Excludes1*—Not coded here, do not use together
▲=Revised Code   *Excludes2*—Not included here

Q64.7 Other and unspecified congenital malformations of bladder and urethra
5th
> *Excludes1:* congenital prolapse of bladder (mucosa) (Q79.4)
>
> **Q64.70** Unspecified congenital malformation of bladder and urethra
> Malformation of bladder or urethra NOS
>
> **Q64.79** Other congenital malformations of bladder and urethra

Q64.9 Congenital malformation of urinary system, unspecified
Congenital anomaly NOS of urinary system
Congenital deformity NOS of urinary system

(Q65–Q79) CONGENITAL MALFORMATIONS AND DEFORMATIONS OF THE MUSCULOSKELETAL SYSTEM

Q65 CONGENITAL DEFORMITIES OF HIP
4th
Excludes1: clicking hip (R29.4)

Q65.0 Congenital dislocation of hip, unilateral
5th
> **Q65.00** Congenital dislocation of unspecified hip, unilateral
> **Q65.01** Congenital dislocation of right hip, unilateral
> **Q65.02** Congenital dislocation of left hip, unilateral

Q65.1 Congenital dislocation of hip, bilateral
Q65.2 Congenital dislocation of hip, unspecified
Q65.3 Congenital partial dislocation of hip, unilateral
5th
> **Q65.30** Congenital partial dislocation of unspecified hip, unilateral
> **Q65.31** Congenital partial dislocation of right hip, unilateral
> **Q65.32** Congenital partial dislocation of left hip, unilateral

Q65.4 Congenital partial dislocation of hip, bilateral
Q65.5 Congenital partial dislocation of hip, unspecified
Q65.6 Congenital unstable hip
Congenital dislocatable hip
Q65.8 Other congenital deformities of hip
5th
> **Q65.81** Congenital coxa valga
> **Q65.82** Congenital coxa vara
> **Q65.89** Other specified congenital deformities of hip
> Anteversion of femoral neck
> Congenital acetabular dysplasia

Q66 CONGENITAL DEFORMITIES OF FEET
4th
Excludes1: reduction defects of feet (Q72.-)
valgus deformities (acquired) (M21.0-)
varus deformities (acquired) (M21.1-)

Q66.0 Congenital talipes equinovarus
5th
> **Q66.01** Congenital talipes equinovarus, right foot
> **Q66.02** Congenital talipes equinovarus, left foot

Q66.1 Congenital talipes calcaneovarus
5th
> **Q66.11** Congenital talipes calcaneovarus, right foot
> **Q66.12** Congenital talipes calcaneovarus, left foot

Q66.2 Congenital metatarsus deformities
5th
> **Q66.21** Congenital metatarsus primus varus
> *6th*
> > **Q66.211** Congenital metatarsus primus varus, right foot
> > **Q66.212** Congenital metatarsus primus varus, left foot
>
> **Q66.22** Congenital metatarsus adductus
> *6th*
> Congenital metatarsus varus
> > **Q66.221** Congenital metatarsus adductus, right foot
> > **Q66.222** Congenital metatarsus adductus, left foot

Q66.3 Other congenital varus deformities of feet
5th
Hallux varus, congenital
> **Q66.31** Other congenital varus deformities of feet, right foot
> **Q66.32** Other congenital varus deformities of feet, left foot

Q66.4 Congenital talipes calcaneovalgus
5th
> **Q66.41** Congenital talipes calcaneovalgus, right foot
> **Q66.42** Congenital talipes calcaneovalgus, left foot

Q66.5 Congenital pes planus
5th
Congenital flat foot
Congenital rigid flat foot
Congenital spastic (everted) flat foot
Excludes1: pes planus, acquired (M21.4)
> **Q66.50** Congenital pes planus, unspecified foot
> **Q66.51** Congenital pes planus, right foot

Q66.52 Congenital pes planus, left foot
Q66.6 Other congenital valgus deformities of feet
Congenital metatarsus valgus
Q66.7 Congenital pes cavus
5th
> **Q66.71** Congenital pes cavus, right foot
> **Q66.72** Congenital pes cavus, left foot

Q66.8 Other congenital deformities of feet
5th
> **Q66.80** Congenital vertical talus deformity, unspecified foot
> **Q66.81** Congenital vertical talus deformity, right foot
> **Q66.82** Congenital vertical talus deformity, left foot
> **Q66.89** Other specified congenital deformities of feet
> Congenital asymmetric talipes
> Congenital clubfoot NOS
> Congenital talipes NOS
> Congenital tarsal coalition
> Hammer toe, congenital

Q66.9 Congenital deformity of feet, unspecified
5th
> **Q66.91** Congenital deformity of feet, unspecified, right foot
> **Q66.92** Congenital deformity of feet, unspecified, left foot

Q67 CONGENITAL MUSCULOSKELETAL DEFORMITIES OF HEAD, FACE, SPINE AND CHEST
4th
Excludes1: congenital malformation syndromes classified to Q87.- Potter's syndrome (Q60.6)

Q67.0 Congenital facial asymmetry
Q67.1 Congenital compression facies
Q67.2 Dolichocephaly
Q67.3 Plagiocephaly
Q67.4 Other congenital deformities of skull, face and jaw
Congenital depressions in skull
Congenital hemifacial atrophy or hypertrophy
Deviation of nasal septum, congenital
Squashed or bent nose, congenital
Excludes1: dentofacial anomalies [including malocclusion] (M26.-)
syphilitic saddle nose (A50.5)
Q67.5 Congenital deformity of spine
Congenital postural scoliosis
Congenital scoliosis NOS
Excludes1: infantile idiopathic scoliosis (M41.0)
scoliosis due to congenital bony malformation (Q76.3)
Q67.6 Pectus excavatum
Congenital funnel chest
Q67.7 Pectus carinatum
Congenital pigeon chest
Q67.8 Other congenital deformities of chest
Congenital deformity of chest wall NOS

Q68 OTHER CONGENITAL MUSCULOSKELETAL DEFORMITIES
4th
Excludes1: reduction defects of limb(s) (Q71-Q73)
Excludes2: congenital myotonic chondrodystrophy (G71.13)
Q68.0 Congenital deformity of sternocleidomastoid muscle
Congenital contracture of sternocleidomastoid (muscle)
Congenital (sternomastoid) torticollis
Sternomastoid tumor (congenital)
Q68.1 Congenital deformity of finger(s) and hand
Congenital clubfinger
Spade-like hand (congenital)
Q68.2 Congenital deformity of knee
Congenital dislocation of knee
Congenital genu recurvatum
Q68.5 Congenital bowing of long bones of leg, unspecified
Q68.8 Other specified congenital musculoskeletal deformities
Congenital deformity of clavicle or scapula
Congenital deformity of elbow or forearm or wrist
Congenital dislocation of elbow or shoulder or wrist

Q69 POLYDACTYLY
4th
Q69.0 Accessory finger(s)
Q69.1 Accessory thumb(s)
Q69.2 Accessory toe(s)
Accessory hallux
Q69.9 Polydactyly, unspecified
Supernumerary digit(s) NOS

4th *5th* *6th* *7th* Additional Character Required | ✔ 3-character code

•=New Code
▲=Revised Code

Excludes1—Not coded here, do not use together
Excludes2—Not included here

CHAPTER 17. CONGENITAL MALFORMATIONS, DEFORMATIONS AND CHROMOSOMAL ABNORMALITIES (Q64.7–Q69.9)

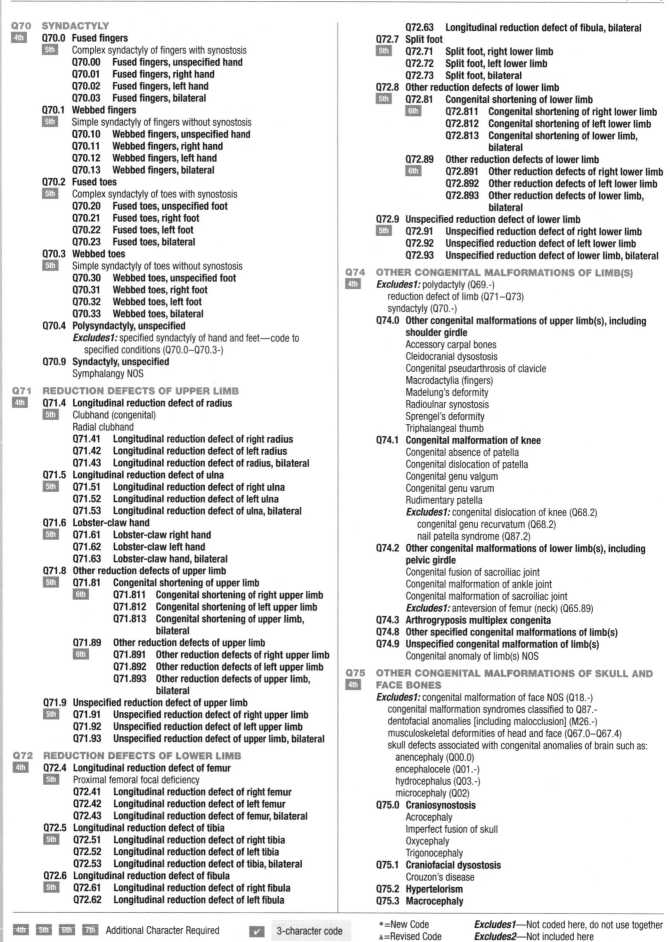

CHAPTER 17. CONGENITAL MALFORMATIONS, DEFORMATIONS AND CHROMOSOMAL ABNORMALITIES (Q70–Q75.3)

Q70   **SYNDACTYLY**
`4th`

Q70.0 Fused fingers
   `5th` Complex syndactyly of fingers with synostosis
- **Q70.00**   **Fused fingers, unspecified hand**
- **Q70.01**   **Fused fingers, right hand**
- **Q70.02**   **Fused fingers, left hand**
- **Q70.03**   **Fused fingers, bilateral**

Q70.1 Webbed fingers
   `5th` Simple syndactyly of fingers without synostosis
- **Q70.10**   **Webbed fingers, unspecified hand**
- **Q70.11**   **Webbed fingers, right hand**
- **Q70.12**   **Webbed fingers, left hand**
- **Q70.13**   **Webbed fingers, bilateral**

Q70.2 Fused toes
   `5th` Complex syndactyly of toes with synostosis
- **Q70.20**   **Fused toes, unspecified foot**
- **Q70.21**   **Fused toes, right foot**
- **Q70.22**   **Fused toes, left foot**
- **Q70.23**   **Fused toes, bilateral**

Q70.3 Webbed toes
   `5th` Simple syndactyly of toes without synostosis
- **Q70.30**   **Webbed toes, unspecified foot**
- **Q70.31**   **Webbed toes, right foot**
- **Q70.32**   **Webbed toes, left foot**
- **Q70.33**   **Webbed toes, bilateral**

Q70.4 Polysyndactyly, unspecified
   Excludes1: specified syndactyly of hand and feet—code to specified conditions (Q70.0–Q70.3-)

Q70.9 Syndactyly, unspecified
   Symphalangy NOS

Q71   **REDUCTION DEFECTS OF UPPER LIMB**
`4th`

Q71.4 Longitudinal reduction defect of radius
   `5th` Clubhand (congenital)
   Radial clubhand
- **Q71.41**   **Longitudinal reduction defect of right radius**
- **Q71.42**   **Longitudinal reduction defect of left radius**
- **Q71.43**   **Longitudinal reduction defect of radius, bilateral**

Q71.5 Longitudinal reduction defect of ulna
   `5th`
- **Q71.51**   **Longitudinal reduction defect of right ulna**
- **Q71.52**   **Longitudinal reduction defect of left ulna**
- **Q71.53**   **Longitudinal reduction defect of ulna, bilateral**

Q71.6 Lobster-claw hand
   `5th`
- **Q71.61**   **Lobster-claw right hand**
- **Q71.62**   **Lobster-claw left hand**
- **Q71.63**   **Lobster-claw hand, bilateral**

Q71.8 Other reduction defects of upper limb
   `5th` **Q71.81**   **Congenital shortening of upper limb**
     `6th`
- **Q71.811**   **Congenital shortening of right upper limb**
- **Q71.812**   **Congenital shortening of left upper limb**
- **Q71.813**   **Congenital shortening of upper limb, bilateral**

   Q71.89   **Other reduction defects of upper limb**
     `6th`
- **Q71.891**   **Other reduction defects of right upper limb**
- **Q71.892**   **Other reduction defects of left upper limb**
- **Q71.893**   **Other reduction defects of upper limb, bilateral**

Q71.9 Unspecified reduction defect of upper limb
   `5th`
- **Q71.91**   **Unspecified reduction defect of right upper limb**
- **Q71.92**   **Unspecified reduction defect of left upper limb**
- **Q71.93**   **Unspecified reduction defect of upper limb, bilateral**

Q72   **REDUCTION DEFECTS OF LOWER LIMB**
`4th`

Q72.4 Longitudinal reduction defect of femur
   `5th` Proximal femoral focal deficiency
- **Q72.41**   **Longitudinal reduction defect of right femur**
- **Q72.42**   **Longitudinal reduction defect of left femur**
- **Q72.43**   **Longitudinal reduction defect of femur, bilateral**

Q72.5 Longitudinal reduction defect of tibia
   `5th`
- **Q72.51**   **Longitudinal reduction defect of right tibia**
- **Q72.52**   **Longitudinal reduction defect of left tibia**
- **Q72.53**   **Longitudinal reduction defect of tibia, bilateral**

Q72.6 Longitudinal reduction defect of fibula
   `5th`
- **Q72.61**   **Longitudinal reduction defect of right fibula**
- **Q72.62**   **Longitudinal reduction defect of left fibula**

   Q72.63   **Longitudinal reduction defect of fibula, bilateral**

Q72.7 Split foot
   `5th`
- **Q72.71**   **Split foot, right lower limb**
- **Q72.72**   **Split foot, left lower limb**
- **Q72.73**   **Split foot, bilateral**

Q72.8 Other reduction defects of lower limb
   `5th` **Q72.81**   **Congenital shortening of lower limb**
     `6th`
- **Q72.811**   **Congenital shortening of right lower limb**
- **Q72.812**   **Congenital shortening of left lower limb**
- **Q72.813**   **Congenital shortening of lower limb, bilateral**

   Q72.89   **Other reduction defects of lower limb**
     `6th`
- **Q72.891**   **Other reduction defects of right lower limb**
- **Q72.892**   **Other reduction defects of left lower limb**
- **Q72.893**   **Other reduction defects of lower limb, bilateral**

Q72.9 Unspecified reduction defect of lower limb
   `5th`
- **Q72.91**   **Unspecified reduction defect of right lower limb**
- **Q72.92**   **Unspecified reduction defect of left lower limb**
- **Q72.93**   **Unspecified reduction defect of lower limb, bilateral**

Q74   **OTHER CONGENITAL MALFORMATIONS OF LIMB(S)**
`4th`
   Excludes1: polydactyly (Q69.-)
   reduction defect of limb (Q71–Q73)
   syndactyly (Q70.-)

Q74.0 Other congenital malformations of upper limb(s), including shoulder girdle
   Accessory carpal bones
   Cleidocranial dysostosis
   Congenital pseudarthrosis of clavicle
   Macrodactylia (fingers)
   Madelung's deformity
   Radioulnar synostosis
   Sprengel's deformity
   Triphalangeal thumb

Q74.1 Congenital malformation of knee
   Congenital absence of patella
   Congenital dislocation of patella
   Congenital genu valgum
   Congenital genu varum
   Rudimentary patella
   Excludes1: congenital dislocation of knee (Q68.2)
     congenital genu recurvatum (Q68.2)
     nail patella syndrome (Q87.2)

Q74.2 Other congenital malformations of lower limb(s), including pelvic girdle
   Congenital fusion of sacroiliac joint
   Congenital malformation of ankle joint
   Congenital malformation of sacroiliac joint
   Excludes1: anteversion of femur (neck) (Q65.89)

Q74.3 Arthrogryposis multiplex congenita

Q74.8 Other specified congenital malformations of limb(s)

Q74.9 Unspecified congenital malformation of limb(s)
   Congenital anomaly of limb(s) NOS

Q75   **OTHER CONGENITAL MALFORMATIONS OF SKULL AND FACE BONES**
`4th`
   Excludes1: congenital malformation of face NOS (Q18.-)
   congenital malformation syndromes classified to Q87.-
   dentofacial anomalies [including malocclusion] (M26.-)
   musculoskeletal deformities of head and face (Q67.0–Q67.4)
   skull defects associated with congenital anomalies of brain such as:
     anencephaly (Q00.0)
     encephalocele (Q01.-)
     hydrocephalus (Q03.-)
     microcephaly (Q02)

Q75.0 Craniosynostosis
   Acrocephaly
   Imperfect fusion of skull
   Oxycephaly
   Trigonocephaly

Q75.1 Craniofacial dysostosis
   Crouzon's disease

Q75.2 Hypertelorism

Q75.3 Macrocephaly

`4th` `5th` `6th` `7th`   Additional Character Required   ✔ 3-character code   •=New Code   ▲=Revised Code   ***Excludes1***—Not coded here, do not use together   ***Excludes2***—Not included here

Q75.4 **Mandibulofacial dysostosis**
Franceschetti syndrome
Treacher Collins syndrome

Q75.5 **Oculomandibular dysostosis**

Q75.8 **Other specified congenital malformations of skull and face bones**
Absence of skull bone, congenital
Congenital deformity of forehead
Platybasia

Q75.9 **Congenital malformation of skull and face bones, unspecified**
Congenital anomaly of face bones NOS
Congenital anomaly of skull NOS

Q76 **CONGENITAL MALFORMATIONS OF SPINE AND BONY THORAX** `4th`
Excludes1: congenital musculoskeletal deformities of spine and chest (Q67.5–Q67.8)

Q76.0 **Spina bifida occulta**
Excludes1: meningocele (spinal) (Q05.-)
spina bifida (aperta) (cystica) (Q05.-)

Q76.2 **Congenital spondylolisthesis**
Congenital spondylolysis
Excludes1: spondylolisthesis (acquired) (M43.1-)
spondylolysis (acquired) (M43.0-)

Q76.3 **Congenital scoliosis due to congenital bony malformation**
Hemivertebra fusion or failure of segmentation with scoliosis

Q76.4 **Other congenital malformations of spine, not associated with scoliosis** `5th`
Q76.42 **Congenital lordosis** `6th`
Q76.425 **Congenital lordosis, thoracolumbar region**
Q76.426 **Congenital lordosis, lumbar region**
Q76.427 **Congenital lordosis, lumbosacral region**
Q76.428 **Congenital lordosis, sacral and sacrococcygeal region**
Q76.429 **Congenital lordosis, unspecified region**
Q76.49 **Other congenital malformations of spine, not associated with scoliosis**
Congenital absence of vertebra NOS
Congenital fusion of spine NOS
Congenital malformation of lumbosacral (joint) (region) NOS
Congenital malformation of spine NOS
Hemivertebra NOS
Malformation of spine NOS
Platyspondylisis NOS
Supernumerary vertebra NOS

Q77 **OSTEOCHONDRODYSPLASIA WITH DEFECTS OF GROWTH OF TUBULAR BONES AND SPINE** `4th`
Excludes1: mucopolysaccharidosis (E76.0-E76.3)
Excludes2: congenital myotonic chondrodystrophy (G71.13)

Q77.0 **Achondrogenesis**
Hypochondrogenesis

Q77.1 **Thanatophoric short stature**

Q77.2 **Short rib syndrome**
Asphyxiating thoracic dysplasia [Jeune]

Q77.3 **Chondrodysplasia punctata**
Excludes1: Rhizomelic chondrodysplasia punctata (E71.43)

Q77.4 **Achondroplasia**
Hypochondroplasia
Osteosclerosis congenita

Q77.5 **Diastrophic dysplasia**

Q77.6 **Chondroectodermal dysplasia**
Ellis-van Creveld syndrome

Q77.7 **Spondyloepiphyseal dysplasia**

Q77.8 **Other osteochondrodysplasia with defects of growth of tubular bones and spine**

Q77.9 **Osteochondrodysplasia with defects of growth of tubular bones and spine, unspecified**

Q78 **OTHER OSTEOCHONDRODYSPLASIAS** `4th`
Excludes2: congenital myotonic chondrodystrophy (G71.13)

Q78.0 **Osteogenesis imperfecta**
Fragilitas ossium
Osteopsathyrosis

Q78.2 **Osteopetrosis**
Albers-Schönberg syndrome
Osteosclerosis NOS

Q78.4 **Enchondromatosis**
Maffucci's syndrome
Ollier's disease

Q78.8 **Other specified osteochondrodysplasias**
Osteopoikilosis

Q78.9 **Osteochondrodysplasia, unspecified**
Chondrodystrophy NOS
Osteodystrophy NOS

Q79 **CONGENITAL MALFORMATIONS OF MUSCULOSKELETAL SYSTEM, NEC** `4th`
Excludes2: congenital (sternomastoid) torticollis (Q68.0)

Q79.0 **Congenital diaphragmatic hernia**
Excludes1: congenital hiatus hernia (Q40.1)

Q79.1 **Other congenital malformations of diaphragm**
Absence of diaphragm
Congenital malformation of diaphragm NOS
Eventration of diaphragm

Q79.2 **Exomphalos**
Omphalocele
Excludes1: umbilical hernia (K42.-)

Q79.3 **Gastroschisis**

Q79.4 **Prune belly syndrome**
Congenital prolapse of bladder mucosa
Eagle-Barrett syndrome

Q79.5 **Other congenital malformations of abdominal wall** `5th`
Excludes1: umbilical hernia (K42.-)
Q79.51 **Congenital hernia of bladder**
Q79.59 **Other congenital malformations of abdominal wall**

Q79.6 **Ehlers-Danlos syndromes** `5th`
Q79.60 **Ehlers-Danlos syndrome, unspecified**
Q79.61 **Classical Ehlers-Danlos syndrome**
Classical EDS (cEDS)
Q79.62 **Hypermobile Ehlers-Danlos syndrome**
Hypermobile EDS (hEDS)
Q79.63 **Vascular Ehlers-Danlos syndrome**
Vascular EDS (vEDS)
Q79.69 **Other Ehlers-Danlos syndromes**

Q79.8 **Other congenital malformations of musculoskeletal system**
Absence of muscle
Absence of tendon
Accessory muscle
Amyotrophia congenita
Congenital constricting bands
Congenital shortening of tendon
Poland syndrome

Q79.9 **Congenital malformation of musculoskeletal system, unspecified**
Congenital anomaly of musculoskeletal system NOS
Congenital deformity of musculoskeletal system NOS

(Q80–Q89) OTHER CONGENITAL MALFORMATIONS

Q80 **CONGENITAL ICHTHYOSIS** `4th`
Excludes1: Refsum's disease (G60.1)

Q80.0 **Ichthyosis vulgaris**

Q80.1 **X-linked ichthyosis**

Q80.2 **Lamellar ichthyosis**
Collodion baby

Q80.3 **Congenital bullous ichthyosiform erythroderma**

Q80.4 **Harlequin fetus**

Q80.8 **Other congenital ichthyosis**

Q80.9 **Congenital ichthyosis, unspecified**

Q81 **EPIDERMOLYSIS BULLOSA** `4th`
Q81.0 **Epidermolysis bullosa simplex**
Excludes1: Cockayne's syndrome (Q87.19)

Q81.1 **Epidermolysis bullosa letalis**
Herlitz' syndrome

Q81.2 **Epidermolysis bullosa dystrophica**

Q81.8 **Other epidermolysis bullosa**

Q81.9 **Epidermolysis bullosa, unspecified**

`4th` `5th` `6th` `7th` Additional Character Required   ✔ 3-character code

•=New Code   *Excludes1*—Not coded here, do not use together
▲=Revised Code   *Excludes2*—Not included here

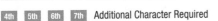

CHAPTER 17. CONGENITAL MALFORMATIONS, DEFORMATIONS AND CHROMOSOMAL ABNORMALITIES (Q82–Q87.2)

Q82 4th **OTHER CONGENITAL MALFORMATIONS OF SKIN**

Excludes1: acrodermatitis enteropathica (E83.2)
congenital erythropoietic porphyria (E80.0)
pilonidal cyst or sinus (L05.-)
Sturge-Weber (-Dimitri) syndrome (Q85.8)

Q82.0 Hereditary lymphedema

Q82.1 Xeroderma pigmentosum

Q82.2 Congenital cutaneous mastocytosis
Congenital diffuse cutaneous mastocytosis
Congenital maculopapular cutaneous mastocytosis
Congenital urticaria pigmentosa
Excludes1: cutaneous mastocytosis NOS (D47.01)
diffuse cutaneous mastocytosis (with onset after newborn period) (D47.01)
malignant mastocytosis (C96.2-)
systemic mastocytosis (D47.02)
urticaria pigmentosa (non-congenital) (with onset after newborn period) (D47.01)

Q82.3 Incontinentia pigmenti

Q82.4 Ectodermal dysplasia (anhidrotic)
Excludes1: Ellis-van Creveld syndrome (Q77.6)

Q82.5 Congenital non-neoplastic nevus
Birthmark NOS
Flammeus nevus
Portwine nevus
Sanguineous nevus
Strawberry nevus
Vascular nevus NOS
Verrucous nevus
Excludes2: Café au lait spots (L81.3)
lentigo (L81.4)
nevus NOS (D22.-)
araneus nevus (I78.1)
melanocytic nevus (D22.-)
pigmented nevus (D22.-)
spider nevus (I78.1)
stellar nevus (I78.1)

Q82.6 Congenital sacral dimple
Parasacral dimple
Excludes2: pilonidal cyst with abscess (L05.01)
pilonidal cyst without abscess (L05.91)

Q82.8 Other specified congenital malformations of skin
Abnormal palmar creases
Accessory skin tags
Benign familial pemphigus [Hailey-Hailey]
Congenital poikiloderma
Cutis laxa (hyperelastica)
Dermatoglyphic anomalies
Inherited keratosis palmaris et plantaris
Keratosis follicularis *[Darier-White]*
Excludes1: Ehlers-Danlos syndromes (Q79.6-).

Q82.9 Congenital malformation of skin, unspecified

Q83 4th **CONGENITAL MALFORMATIONS OF BREAST**

Excludes2: absence of pectoral muscle (Q79.8)
hypoplasia of breast (N64.82)
micromastia (N64.82)

Q83.0 Congenital absence of breast with absent nipple

Q83.3 Accessory nipple
Supernumerary nipple

Q83.8 Other congenital malformations of breast

Q84 4th **OTHER CONGENITAL MALFORMATIONS OF INTEGUMENT**

Q84.2 Other congenital malformations of hair
Congenital hypertrichosis
Congenital malformation of hair NOS
Persistent lanugo

Q84.3 Anonychia
Excludes1: nail patella syndrome (Q87.2)

Q84.4 Congenital leukonychia

Q84.6 Other congenital malformations of nails
Congenital clubnail
Congenital koilonychia
Congenital malformation of nail NOS

Q84.8 Other specified congenital malformations of integument
Aplasia cutis congenita

Q84.9 Congenital malformation of integument, unspecified
Congenital anomaly of integument NOS
Congenital deformity of integument NOS

Q85 4th **PHAKOMATOSES, NES**

Excludes1: ataxia telangiectasia [Louis-Bar] (G11.3)
familial dysautonomia [Riley-Day] (G90.1)

Q85.0 Neurofibromatosis (nonmalignant)
5th **Q85.00 Neurofibromatosis, unspecified**
Q85.01 Neurofibromatosis, type 1
Von Recklinghausen disease
Q85.02 Neurofibromatosis, type 2
Acoustic neurofibromatosis
Q85.03 Schwannomatosis
Q85.09 Other neurofibromatosis

Q85.1 Tuberous sclerosis
Bourneville's disease
Epiloia

Q85.8 Other phakomatoses, NEC
Peutz-Jeghers syndrome
Sturge-Weber (-Dimitri) syndrome
von Hippel-Lindau syndrome
Excludes1: Meckel-Gruber syndrome (Q61.9)

Q85.9 Phakomatosis, unspecified
Hamartosis NOS

Q86 4th **CONGENITAL MALFORMATION SYNDROMES DUE TO KNOWN EXOGENOUS CAUSES, NEC**

Excludes2: iodine-deficiency-related hypothyroidism (E00–E02)
nonteratogenic effects of substances transmitted via placenta or breast milk (P04.-)

Q86.0 Fetal alcohol syndrome (dysmorphic)

Q87 4th **OTHER SPECIFIED CONGENITAL MALFORMATION SYNDROMES AFFECTING MULTIPLE SYSTEMS**

Use additional code(s) to identify all associated manifestations

Q87.0 Congenital malformation syndromes predominantly affecting facial appearance
Acrocephalopolysyndactyly
Acrocephalosyndactyly [Apert]
Cryptophthalmos syndrome
Cyclopia
Goldenhar syndrome
Moebius syndrome
Oro-facial-digital syndrome
Robin syndrome
Whistling face
Production note-replace text with Insert 17E:

Q87.1 5th **Congenital malformation syndromes predominantly associated with short stature**
Excludes1: Ellis-van Creveld syndrome (Q77.6)
Smith-Lemli-Opitz syndrome (E78.72)
Q87.11 Prader-Willi syndrome
Q87.19 Other congenital malformation syndromes predominantly associated with short stature
Aarskog syndrome
Cockayne syndrome
De Lange syndrome
Dubowitz syndrome
Noonan syndrome
Robinow-Silverman-Smith syndrome
Russell-Silver syndrome
Seckel syndrome

Q87.2 Congenital malformation syndromes predominantly involving limbs
Holt-Oram syndrome
Klippel-Trenaunay-Weber syndrome
Nail patella syndrome
Rubinstein-Taybi syndrome
Sirenomelia syndrome
TAR syndrome
VATER syndrome

  Additional Character Required   3-character code

•=New Code   *Excludes1*—Not coded here, do not use together
▲=Revised Code   *Excludes2*—Not included here

Q87.3 **Congenital malformation syndromes involving early overgrowth**
Beckwith-Wiedemann syndrome
Sotos syndrome
Weaver syndrome

Q87.4 **Marfan's syndrome**
  `5th` Q87.40 **Marfan's syndrome, unspecified**
     Q87.41 **Marfan's syndrome with cardiovascular manifestations**
      `6th`
       Q87.410 **Marfan's syndrome with aortic dilation**
       Q87.418 **Marfan's syndrome with other cardiovascular manifestations**
     Q87.42 **Marfan's syndrome with ocular manifestations**
     Q87.43 **Marfan's syndrome with skeletal manifestation**

Q87.8 **Other specified congenital malformation syndromes, NEC**
  `5th` *Excludes1:* Zellweger syndrome (E71.510)
     Q87.81 **Alport syndrome**
       Use additional code to identify stage of CKD (N18.1–N18.6)
     Q87.82 **Arterial tortuosity syndrome**
     Q87.89 **Other specified congenital malformation syndromes, NEC**
       Laurence-Moon (-Bardet)-Biedl syndrome

Q89 `4th` **OTHER CONGENITAL MALFORMATIONS, NEC**

Q89.0 **Congenital absence and malformations of spleen**
  `5th` *Excludes1:* isomerism of atrial appendages (with asplenia or polysplenia) (Q20.6)
     Q89.01 **Asplenia (congenital)**
     Q89.09 **Congenital malformations of spleen**
       Congenital splenomegaly

Q89.1 **Congenital malformations of adrenal gland**
Excludes1: adrenogenital disorders (E25.-)
  congenital adrenal hyperplasia (E25.0)

Q89.2 **Congenital malformations of other endocrine glands**
Congenital malformation of parathyroid or thyroid gland
Persistent thyroglossal duct
Thyroglossal cyst
Excludes1: congenital goiter (E03.0)
  congenital hypothyroidism (E03.1)

Q89.3 **Situs inversus**
Dextrocardia with situs inversus
Mirror-image atrial arrangement with situs inversus
Situs inversus or transversus abdominalis
Situs inversus or transversus thoracis
Transposition of abdominal viscera
Transposition of thoracic viscera
Excludes1: dextrocardia NOS (Q24.0)

Q89.7 **Multiple congenital malformations, NEC**
Multiple congenital anomalies NOS
Multiple congenital deformities NOS
Excludes1: congenital malformation syndromes affecting multiple systems (Q87.-)

Q89.8 **Other specified congenital malformations**
Use additional code(s) to identify all associated manifestations

Q89.9 **Congenital malformation, unspecified**
Congenital anomaly NOS
Congenital deformity NOS

(Q90–Q99) CHROMOSOMAL ABNORMALITIES, NEC

Excludes2: mitochondrial metabolic disorders (E88.4-)

Q90 `4th` **DOWN SYNDROME**
Use additional code(s) to identify any associated physical conditions and degree of intellectual disabilities (F70–F79)

Q90.0 **Trisomy 21, nonmosaicism (meiotic nondisjunction)**
Q90.1 **Trisomy 21, mosaicism (mitotic nondisjunction)**
Q90.2 **Trisomy 21, translocation**
Q90.9 **Down syndrome, unspecified**
  Trisomy 21 NOS

Q91 `4th` **TRISOMY 18 AND TRISOMY 13**
Q91.0 **Trisomy 18, nonmosaicism (meiotic nondisjunction)**
Q91.1 **Trisomy 18, mosaicism (mitotic nondisjunction)**
Q91.2 **Trisomy 18, translocation**

Q91.3 **Trisomy 18, unspecified**
Q91.4 **Trisomy 13, nonmosaicism (meiotic nondisjunction)**
Q91.5 **Trisomy 13, mosaicism (mitotic nondisjunction)**
Q91.6 **Trisomy 13, translocation**
Q91.7 **Trisomy 13, unspecified**

Q92 `4th` **OTHER TRISOMIES AND PARTIAL TRISOMIES OF THE AUTOSOMES, NOT ELSEWHERE CLASSIFIED**
Includes: unbalanced translocations and insertions
Excludes1: trisomies of chromosomes 13, 18, 21 (Q90-Q91)
Q92.9 **Trisomy and partial trisomy of autosomes, unspecified**

Q93 `4th` **MONOSOMIES AND DELETIONS FROM THE AUTOSOMES, NEC**
Q93.0 **Whole chromosome monosomy, nonmosaicism (meiotic nondisjunction)**
Q93.1 **Whole chromosome monosomy, mosaicism (mitotic nondisjunction)**
Q93.2 **Chromosome replaced with ring, dicentric or isochromosome**
Q93.3 **Deletion of short arm of chromosome 4**
  Wolff-Hirschorn syndrome
Q93.4 **Deletion of short arm of chromosome 5**
  Cri-du-chat syndrome
Q93.5 **Other deletions of part of a chromosome**
  `5th` Q93.51 **Angelman syndrome**
     Q93.59 **Other deletions of part of a chromosome**
Q93.7 **Deletions with other complex rearrangements**
  Deletions due to unbalanced translocations, inversions and insertions
  Code also any associated duplications due to unbalanced translocations, inversions and insertions (Q92.5)
Q93.8 **Other deletions from the autosomes**
  `5th` Q93.81 **Velo-cardio-facial syndrome**
     Deletion 22q11.2
     Q93.82 **Williams syndrome**
     Q93.88 **Other microdeletions**
       Miller-Dieker syndrome
       Smith-Magenis syndrome
     Q93.89 **Other deletions from the autosomes**
       Deletions identified by fluorescence in situ hybridization (FISH)
       Deletions identified by in situ hybridization (ISH)
       Deletions seen only at prometaphase
Q93.9 **Deletion from autosomes, unspecified**

Q95 `4th` **BALANCED REARRANGEMENTS AND STRUCTURAL MARKERS, NOT ELSEWHERE CLASSIFIED**
Includes: Robertsonian and balanced reciprocal translocations and insertions
Q95.0 **Balanced translocation and insertion in normal individual**
Q95.9 **Balanced rearrangement and structural marker, unspecified**

Q96 `4th` **TURNER'S SYNDROME**
Excludes1: Noonan syndrome (Q87.19)
Q96.0 **Karyotype 45, X**
Q96.1 **Karyotype 46, X iso (Xq)**
  Karyotype 46, isochromosome Xq
Q96.2 **Karyotype 46, X with abnormal sex chromosome, except iso (Xq)**
  Karyotype 46, X with abnormal sex chromosome, except isochromosome Xq
Q96.3 **Mosaicism, 45, X/46, XX or XY**
Q96.4 **Mosaicism, 45, X/other cell line(s) with abnormal sex chromosome**
Q96.8 **Other variants of Turner's syndrome**
Q96.9 **Turner's syndrome, unspecified**

Q97 `4th` **OTHER SEX CHROMOSOME ABNORMALITIES, FEMALE PHENOTYPE, NEC**
Excludes1: Turner's syndrome (Q96.-)
Q97.0 **Karyotype 47, XXX**
Q97.2 **Mosaicism, lines with various numbers of X chromosomes**
Q97.8 **Other specified sex chromosome abnormalities, female phenotype**
Q97.9 **Sex chromosome abnormality, female phenotype, unspecified**

`4th` `5th` `6th` `7th` Additional Character Required   ✓ 3-character code

•=New Code
▲=Revised Code

Excludes1—Not coded here, do not use together
Excludes2—Not included here

Q98 **OTHER SEX CHROMOSOME ABNORMALITIES, MALE**
4th   **PHENOTYPE, NEC**
    Q98.3 **Other male with 46, XX karyotype**
    Q98.4 **Klinefelter syndrome, unspecified**
    Q98.5 **Karyotype 47, XYY**
    Q98.7 **Male with sex chromosome mosaicism**
    Q98.9 **Sex chromosome abnormality, male phenotype, unspecified**

Q99 **OTHER CHROMOSOME ABNORMALITIES, NEC**
4th   **Q99.1** **46, XX true hermaphrodite**
       46, XX with streak gonads
       46, XY with streak gonads
       Pure gonadal dysgenesis
    Q99.2 **Fragile X chromosome**
       Fragile X syndrome
    Q99.8 **Other specified chromosome abnormalities**
    Q99.9 **Chromosomal abnormality, unspecified**

4th   5th   6th   7th   Additional Character Required   ✔ 3-character code   •=New Code   *Excludes1*—Not coded here, do not use together
                                                       ▲=Revised Code   *Excludes2*—Not included here

Chapter 18. Symptoms, signs, and abnormal clinical and laboratory findings, not elsewhere classified (R00–R99)

GUIDELINES

Chapter 18 includes symptoms, signs, abnormal results of clinical or other investigative procedures, and ill-defined conditions regarding which no diagnosis classifiable elsewhere is recorded. Signs and symptoms that point to a specific diagnosis have been assigned to a category in other chapters of the classification.

Use of symptom codes

Codes that describe symptoms and signs are acceptable for reporting purposes when a related definitive diagnosis has not been established (confirmed) by the provider.

Use of a symptom code with a definitive diagnosis code

Codes for signs and symptoms may be reported in addition to a related definitive diagnosis when the sign or symptom is not routinely associated with that diagnosis, such as the various signs and symptoms associated with complex syndromes. The definitive diagnosis code should be sequenced before the symptom code.

Signs or symptoms that are associated routinely with a disease process should not be assigned as additional codes, unless otherwise instructed by the classification.

Combination codes that include symptoms

ICD-10-CM contains a number of combination codes that identify both the definitive diagnosis and common symptoms of that diagnosis. When using one of these combination codes, an additional code should not be assigned for the symptom.

Repeated falls

Refer to the ICD-10-CM manual.

Coma scale

Refer to subcategory R40.2 for guidelines.

SIRS due to Non-Infectious Process

Refer to codes R65.10-R65.11.

Death NOS

Refer to code R99.

Note: This chapter includes symptoms, signs, abnormal results of clinical or other investigative procedures, and ill-defined conditions regarding which no diagnosis classifiable elsewhere is recorded.

Signs and symptoms that point rather definitely to a given diagnosis have been assigned to a category in other chapters of the classification. In general, categories in this chapter include the less well-defined conditions and symptoms that, without the necessary study of the case to establish a final diagnosis, point perhaps equally to two or more diseases or to two or more systems of the body. Practically all categories in the chapter could be designated 'not otherwise specified,' 'unknown etiology' or 'transient'. The Alphabetical Index should be consulted to determine which symptoms and signs are to be allocated here and which to other chapters. The residual subcategories, numbered .8, are generally provided for other relevant symptoms that cannot be allocated elsewhere in the classification.

The conditions and signs or symptoms included in categories R00–R94 consist of:
a) cases for which no more specific diagnosis can be made even after all the facts bearing on the case have been investigated;
b) signs or symptoms existing at the time of initial encounter that proved to be transient and whose causes could not be determined;
c) provisional diagnosis in a patient who failed to return for further investigation or care;
d) cases referred elsewhere for investigation or treatment before the diagnosis was made;
e) cases in which a more precise diagnosis was not available for any other reason;
f) certain symptoms, for which supplementary information is provided, that represent important problems in medical care in their own right.

Excludes2: abnormal findings on antenatal screening of mother (O28.-)
   certain conditions originating in the perinatal period (P04–P96)
   signs and symptoms classified in the body system chapters signs and
      symptoms of breast (N63, N64.5)

(R00–R09) SYMPTOMS AND SIGNS INVOLVING THE CIRCULATORY AND RESPIRATORY SYSTEMS

R00 **ABNORMALITIES OF HEART BEAT**
`4th` *Excludes1:* abnormalities originating in the perinatal period (P29.1-)
Excludes 2: specified arrhythmias (I47–I49)
  R00.0 **Tachycardia, unspecified**
    Rapid heart beat
    Sinoauricular tachycardia NOS
    Sinus [sinusal] tachycardia NOS
    Excludes1: neonatal tachycardia (P29.11)
      paroxysmal tachycardia (I47.-)
  R00.1 **Bradycardia, unspecified**
    Sinoatrial bradycardia
    Sinus bradycardia
    Slow heart beat
    Vagal bradycardia
    Use additional code for adverse effect, if applicable, to identify
      drug (T36–T50 with fifth or sixth character 5)
    Excludes1: neonatal bradycardia (P29.12)
  R00.2 **Palpitations**
    Awareness of heart beat
  R00.8 **Other abnormalities of heart beat**
  R00.9 **Unspecified abnormalities of heart beat**

R01 **CARDIAC MURMURS AND OTHER CARDIAC SOUNDS**
`4th` *Excludes1:* cardiac murmurs and sounds originating in the perinatal period
  (P29.8)
  R01.0 **Benign and innocent cardiac murmurs**
    Functional cardiac murmur
  R01.1 **Cardiac murmur, unspecified**
    Cardiac bruit NOS
    Heart murmur NOS
    Systolic murmur NOS
  R01.2 **Other cardiac sounds**
    Cardiac dullness, increased or decreased
    Precordial friction

R03 **ABNORMAL BLOOD-PRESSURE READING, WITHOUT**
`4th` **DIAGNOSIS**
  R03.0 **Elevated blood-pressure reading, without diagnosis of**
    hypertension
    Note: This category is to be used to record an episode of elevated
      blood pressure in a patient in whom no formal diagnosis of
      hypertension has been made, or as an isolated incidental finding.
  R03.1 **Nonspecific low blood-pressure reading**
    Excludes1: hypotension (I95.-)
      maternal hypotension syndrome (O26.5-)
      neurogenic orthostatic hypotension (G90.3)

R04 **HEMORRHAGE FROM RESPIRATORY PASSAGES**
`4th`   **R04.0** **Epistaxis**
    Hemorrhage from nose
    Nosebleed
  R04.2 **Hemoptysis**
    Blood-stained sputum
    Cough with hemorrhage
  R04.8 **Hemorrhage from other sites in respiratory passages**
  `5th` **R04.81** **Acute idiopathic pulmonary hemorrhage in infants**
      AIPHI
      Acute idiopathic hemorrhage in infants over 28 days old
      Excludes1: perinatal pulmonary hemorrhage (P26.-)
        von Willebrand's disease (D68.0)
    R04.89 **Hemorrhage from other sites in respiratory passages**
      Pulmonary hemorrhage NOS
  R04.9 **Hemorrhage from respiratory passages, unspecified**

`4th` `5th` `6th` `7th` Additional Character Required   ☑ 3-character code

•=New Code
▲=Revised Code

Excludes1—Not coded here, do not use together
Excludes2—Not included here

CHAPTER 18. SYMPTOMS, SIGNS, AND ABNORMAL CLINICAL AND LABORATORY FINDINGS, NOT ELSEWHERE CLASSIFIED   (R05–R10.2)

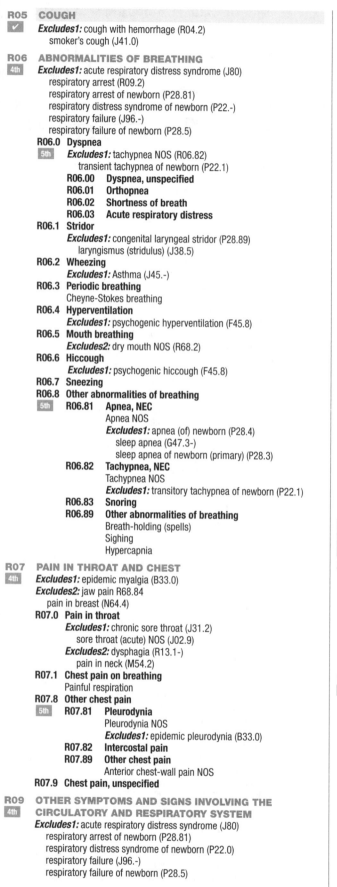

R05   COUGH
☑
Excludes1: cough with hemorrhage (R04.2)
   smoker's cough (J41.0)

R06   ABNORMALITIES OF BREATHING
4th
Excludes1: acute respiratory distress syndrome (J80)
   respiratory arrest (R09.2)
   respiratory arrest of newborn (P28.81)
   respiratory distress syndrome of newborn (P22.-)
   respiratory failure (J96.-)
   respiratory failure of newborn (P28.5)

R06.0   Dyspnea
5th
Excludes1: tachypnea NOS (R06.82)
   transient tachypnea of newborn (P22.1)

R06.00   Dyspnea, unspecified
R06.01   Orthopnea
R06.02   Shortness of breath
R06.03   Acute respiratory distress

R06.1   Stridor
Excludes1: congenital laryngeal stridor (P28.89)
   laryngismus (stridulus) (J38.5)

R06.2   Wheezing
Excludes1: Asthma (J45.-)

R06.3   Periodic breathing
Cheyne-Stokes breathing

R06.4   Hyperventilation
Excludes1: psychogenic hyperventilation (F45.8)

R06.5   Mouth breathing
Excludes2: dry mouth NOS (R68.2)

R06.6   Hiccough
Excludes1: psychogenic hiccough (F45.8)

R06.7   Sneezing

R06.8   Other abnormalities of breathing
5th
R06.81   Apnea, NEC
Apnea NOS
Excludes1: apnea (of) newborn (P28.4)
   sleep apnea (G47.3-)
   sleep apnea of newborn (primary) (P28.3)

R06.82   Tachypnea, NEC
Tachypnea NOS
Excludes1: transitory tachypnea of newborn (P22.1)

R06.83   Snoring
R06.89   Other abnormalities of breathing
Breath-holding (spells)
Sighing
Hypercapnia

R07   PAIN IN THROAT AND CHEST
4th
Excludes1: epidemic myalgia (B33.0)
Excludes2: jaw pain R68.84
   pain in breast (N64.4)

R07.0   Pain in throat
Excludes1: chronic sore throat (J31.2)
   sore throat (acute) NOS (J02.9)
Excludes2: dysphagia (R13.1-)
   pain in neck (M54.2)

R07.1   Chest pain on breathing
Painful respiration

R07.8   Other chest pain
5th
R07.81   Pleurodynia
Pleurodynia NOS
Excludes1: epidemic pleurodynia (B33.0)

R07.82   Intercostal pain
R07.89   Other chest pain
Anterior chest-wall pain NOS

R07.9   Chest pain, unspecified

R09   OTHER SYMPTOMS AND SIGNS INVOLVING THE CIRCULATORY AND RESPIRATORY SYSTEM
4th
Excludes1: acute respiratory distress syndrome (J80)
   respiratory arrest of newborn (P28.81)
   respiratory distress syndrome of newborn (P22.0)
   respiratory failure (J96.-)
   respiratory failure of newborn (P28.5)

R09.0   Asphyxia and hypoxemia
5th
Excludes1: asphyxia due to carbon monoxide (T58.-)
   asphyxia due to FB in respiratory tract (T17.-)
   birth (intrauterine) asphyxia (P84)
   hyperventilation (R06.4)
   traumatic asphyxia (T71.-)
Excludes 2: hypercapnia (R06.89)

R09.01   Asphyxia
R09.02   Hypoxemia

R09.1   Pleurisy
Excludes1: pleurisy with effusion (J90)

R09.2   Respiratory arrest
Cardiorespiratory failure
Excludes1: cardiac arrest (I46.-)
   respiratory arrest of newborn (P28.81)
   respiratory distress of newborn (P22.0)
   respiratory failure (J96.-)
   respiratory failure of newborn (P28.5)
   respiratory insufficiency (R06.89)
   respiratory insufficiency of newborn (P28.5)

R09.3   Abnormal sputum
Abnormal amount of sputum
Abnormal color of sputum
Abnormal odor of sputum
Excessive sputum
Excludes1: blood-stained sputum (R04.2)

R09.8   Other specified symptoms and signs involving the circulatory and respiratory systems
5th
R09.81   Nasal congestion
R09.82   Postnasal drip
R09.89   Other specified symptoms and signs involving the circulatory and respiratory systems
Bruit (arterial)
Abnormal chest percussion
Feeling of FB in throat
Friction sounds in chest
Chest tympany
Choking sensation
Rales
Weak pulse
Excludes2: FB in throat (T17.2-)
   wheezing (R06.2)

(R10–R19) SYMPTOMS AND SIGNS INVOLVING THE DIGESTIVE SYSTEM AND ABDOMEN

Excludes2: congenital or infantile pylorospasm (Q40.0)
   gastrointestinal hemorrhage (K92.0–K92.2)
   intestinal obstruction (K56.-)
   newborn gastrointestinal hemorrhage (P54.0–P54.3)
   newborn intestinal obstruction (P76.-)
   pylorospasm (K31.3)
   signs and symptoms involving the urinary system (R30–R39)
   symptoms referable to female genital organs (N94.-)
   symptoms referable to male genital organs male (N48–N50)

R10   ABDOMINAL AND PELVIC PAIN
4th
Excludes1: renal colic (N23)
Excludes2: dorsalgia (M54.-)
   flatulence and related conditions (R14.-)

R10.0   Acute abdomen
Severe abdominal pain (generalized) (with abdominal rigidity)
Excludes1: abdominal rigidity NOS (R19.3)
   generalized abdominal pain NOS (R10.84)
   localized abdominal pain (R10.1-R10.3-)

R10.1   Pain localized to upper abdomen
5th
R10.10   Upper abdominal pain, unspecified
R10.11   RUQ pain
R10.12   LUQ pain
R10.13   Epigastric pain
Dyspepsia
Excludes1: functional dyspepsia (K30)

R10.2   Pelvic and perineal pain
Excludes1: vulvodynia (N94.81)

4th	5th	6th	7th	Additional Character Required		☑	3-character code	•=New Code	*Excludes1*—Not coded here, do not use together
								▲=Revised Code	*Excludes2*—Not included here

R10.3 **Pain localized to other parts of lower abdomen**
- **5th** R10.30 **Lower abdominal pain, unspecified**
- R10.31 **RLQ pain**
- R10.32 **LLQ pain**
- R10.33 **Periumbilical pain**

R10.8 **Other abdominal pain**
- **5th** R10.81 **Abdominal tenderness**
  - **6th** Abdominal tenderness NOS
  - R10.811 **RUQ abdominal tenderness**
  - R10.812 **LUQ abdominal tenderness**
  - R10.813 **RLQ abdominal tenderness**
  - R10.814 **LLQ abdominal tenderness**
  - R10.815 **Periumbilic abdominal tenderness**
  - R10.816 **Epigastric abdominal tenderness**
  - R10.817 **Generalized abdominal tenderness**
  - R10.819 **Abdominal tenderness, unspecified site**
- R10.82 **Rebound abdominal tenderness**
  - **6th** R10.821 **RUQ rebound abdominal tenderness**
  - R10.822 **LUQ rebound abdominal tenderness**
  - R10.823 **RLQ rebound abdominal tenderness**
  - R10.824 **LLQ rebound abdominal tenderness**
  - R10.825 **Periumbilic rebound abdominal tenderness**
  - R10.826 **Epigastric rebound abdominal tenderness**
  - R10.827 **Generalized rebound abdominal tenderness**
  - R10.829 **Rebound abdominal tenderness, unspecified site**
- R10.83 **Colic**
  - Colic NOS
  - Infantile colic
  - *Excludes1:* colic in adult and child over 12 months old (R10.84)
- R10.84 **Generalized abdominal pain**
  - *Excludes1:* generalized abdominal pain associated with acute abdomen (R10.0)

R10.9 **Unspecified abdominal pain**

R11 **NAUSEA AND VOMITING**
- **4th** *Excludes1:* cyclical vomiting associated with migraine (G43.A-)
  - excessive vomiting in pregnancy (O21.-)
  - hematemesis (K92.0)
  - neonatal hematemesis (P54.0)
  - newborn vomiting (P92.0-)
  - psychogenic vomiting (F50.89)
  - vomiting associated with bulimia nervosa (F50.2)
  - vomiting following gastrointestinal surgery (K91.0)
- R11.0 **Nausea**
  - Nausea NOS
  - Nausea without vomiting
- R11.1 **Vomiting**
  - **5th** R11.10 **Vomiting, unspecified**
    - Vomiting NOS
  - R11.11 **Vomiting without nausea**
  - R11.12 **Projectile vomiting**
  - R11.13 **Vomiting of fecal matter**
  - R11.14 **Bilious vomiting**
    - Bilious emesis
  - R11.15 **Cyclical vomiting syndrome unrelated to migraine**
    - Cyclic vomiting syndrome NOS
    - Persistent vomiting
    - *Excludes1:* cyclical vomiting in migraine (G43.A-)
    - *Excludes2:* bulimia nervosa (F50.2)
      - diabetes mellitus due to underlying condition (E08.-)
- R11.2 **Nausea with vomiting, unspecified**
  - Persistent nausea with vomiting NOS

R12 **HEARTBURN**
- ✔ *Excludes1:* dyspepsia NOS (R10.13)
  - functional dyspepsia (K30)

R13 **APHAGIA AND DYSPHAGIA**
- **4th** R13.0 **Aphagia**
  - Inability to swallow
  - *Excludes1:* psychogenic aphagia (F50.9)

R13.1 **Dysphagia**
- **5th** **Code first**, if applicable, dysphagia following cerebrovascular disease (I69. with final characters -91)
  - *Excludes1:* psychogenic dysphagia (F45.8)
  - R13.10 **Dysphagia, unspecified**
    - Difficulty in swallowing NOS
  - R13.11 **Dysphagia, oral phase**
  - R13.12 **Dysphagia, oropharyngeal phase**
  - R13.13 **Dysphagia, pharyngeal phase**
  - R13.14 **Dysphagia, pharyngoesophageal phase**
  - R13.19 **Other dysphagia**
    - Cervical dysphagia
    - Neurogenic dysphagia

R14 **FLATULENCE AND RELATED CONDITIONS**
- **4th** *Excludes1:* psychogenic aerophagy (F45.8)
- R14.0 **Abdominal distension (gaseous)**
  - Bloating
  - Tympanites (abdominal) (intestinal)
- R14.1 **Gas pain**
- R14.2 **Eructation**
- R14.3 **Flatulence**

R15 **FECAL INCONTINENCE**
- **4th** *Includes:* encopresis NOS
- *Excludes1:* fecal incontinence of nonorganic origin (F98.1)
- R15.0 **Incomplete defecation**
  - *Excludes1:* constipation (K59.0-)
    - fecal impaction (K56.41)
- R15.1 **Fecal smearing**
  - Fecal soiling
- R15.2 **Fecal urgency**
- R15.9 **Full incontinence of feces**
  - Fecal incontinence NOS

R16 **HEPATOMEGALY AND SPLENOMEGALY, NEC**
- **4th** R16.0 **Hepatomegaly, NEC**
  - Hepatomegaly NOS
- R16.1 **Splenomegaly, NEC**
  - Splenomegaly NOS
- R16.2 **Hepatomegaly with splenomegaly, NEC**
  - Hepatosplenomegaly NOS

R17 **UNSPECIFIED JAUNDICE**
- ✔ *Excludes1:* neonatal jaundice (P55, P57–P59)

R18 **ASCITES**
- **4th** *Includes:* fluid in peritoneal cavity
- *Excludes1:* ascites in alcoholic cirrhosis (K70.31)
  - ascites in alcoholic hepatitis (K70.11)
  - ascites in toxic liver disease with chronic active hepatitis (K71.51)
- R18.0 **Malignant ascites**
  - **Code first** malignancy, such as: malignant neoplasm of ovary (C56.-)
    - secondary malignant neoplasm of retroperitoneum and peritoneum (C78.6)
- R18.8 **Other ascites**
  - Ascites NOS
  - Peritoneal effusion (chronic)

R19 **OTHER SYMPTOMS AND SIGNS INVOLVING THE DIGESTIVE SYSTEM AND ABDOMEN**
- **4th** *Excludes1:* acute abdomen (R10.0)
- R19.0 **Intra-abdominal and pelvic swelling, mass and lump**
  - **5th** *Excludes1:* abdominal distension (gaseous) (R14.-)
    - ascites (R18.-)
  - R19.00 **Intra-abdominal and pelvic swelling, mass and lump, unspecified site**
  - R19.01 **RUQ abdominal swelling, mass and lump**
  - R19.02 **LUQ abdominal swelling, mass and lump**
  - R19.03 **RLQ abdominal swelling, mass and lump**
  - R19.04 **LLQ abdominal swelling, mass and lump**
  - R19.05 **Periumbilic swelling, mass or lump**
    - Diffuse or generalized umbilical swelling or mass
  - R19.06 **Epigastric swelling, mass or lump**

4th **5th** **6th** **7th** Additional Character Required	✔ 3-character code	•=New Code ▲=Revised Code	***Excludes1***—Not coded here, do not use together ***Excludes2***—Not included here

R19.07 **Generalized intra-abdominal and pelvic swelling, mass and lump**
Diffuse or generalized intra-abdominal swelling or mass NOS
Diffuse or generalized pelvic swelling or mass NOS

R19.09 **Other intra-abdominal and pelvic swelling, mass and lump**

R19.1 **Abnormal bowel sounds**
`5th` R19.11 **Absent bowel sounds**
R19.12 **Hyperactive bowel sounds**
R19.15 **Other abnormal bowel sounds**
Abnormal bowel sounds NOS

R19.2 **Visible peristalsis**
Hyperperistalsis

R19.3 **Abdominal rigidity**
`5th` *Excludes1:* abdominal rigidity with severe abdominal pain (R10.0)
R19.30 **Abdominal rigidity, unspecified site**
R19.31 **RUQ abdominal rigidity**
R19.32 **LUQ abdominal rigidity**
R19.33 **RLQ abdominal rigidity**
R19.34 **LLQ abdominal rigidity**
R19.35 **Periumbilic abdominal rigidity**
R19.36 **Epigastric abdominal rigidity**
R19.37 **Generalized abdominal rigidity**

R19.4 **Change in bowel habit**
Excludes1: constipation (K59.0-)
functional diarrhea (K59.1)

R19.5 **Other fecal abnormalities**
Abnormal stool color
Bulky stools
Mucus in stools
Occult blood in feces
Occult blood in stools
Excludes1: melena (K92.1)
neonatal melena (P54.1)

R19.6 **Halitosis**
R19.7 **Diarrhea, unspecified**
Diarrhea NOS
Excludes1: functional diarrhea (K59.1)
neonatal diarrhea (P78.3)
psychogenic diarrhea (F45.8)

R19.8 **Other specified symptoms and signs involving the digestive system and abdomen**

(R20–R23) SYMPTOMS AND SIGNS INVOLVING THE SKIN AND SUBCUTANEOUS TISSUE

Excludes2: symptoms relating to breast (N64.4–N64.5)

R20 DISTURBANCES OF SKIN SENSATION
`4th` *Excludes1:* dissociative anesthesia and sensory loss (F44.6)
psychogenic disturbances (F45.8)
R20.0 **Anesthesia of skin**
R20.1 **Hypoesthesia of skin**
R20.2 **Paresthesia of skin**
Formication
Pins and needles
Tingling skin
Excludes1: acroparesthesia (I73.8)
R20.3 **Hyperesthesia**
R20.8 **Other disturbances of skin sensation**
R20.9 **Unspecified disturbances of skin sensation**

R21 RASH AND OTHER NONSPECIFIC SKIN ERUPTION
☑ *Includes:* rash NOS
Excludes1: specified type of rash — code to condition
vesicular eruption (R23.8)

R22 LOCALIZED SWELLING, MASS AND LUMP OF SKIN AND SUBCUTANEOUS TISSUE
`4th`
Includes: subcutaneous nodules (localized)(superficial)
Excludes1: abnormal findings on diagnostic imaging (R90–R93)
edema (R60.-)
enlarged lymph nodes (R59.-)
localized adiposity (E65)
swelling of joint (M25.4-)
R22.0 **Localized swelling, mass and lump; head**
R22.1 **neck**
R22.2 **trunk**
Excludes1: intra-abdominal or pelvic mass and lump (R19.0-)
intra-abdominal or pelvic swelling (R19.0-)
Excludes2: breast mass and lump (N63)
R22.3 **Localized swelling, mass and lump, upper limb**
`5th` R22.31 **Localized swelling, mass and lump; right upper limb**
R22.32 **left upper limb**
R22.33 **upper limb, bilateral**
R22.4 **Localized swelling, mass and lump, lower limb**
`5th` R22.41 **Localized swelling, mass and lump; right lower limb**
R22.42 **left lower limb**
R22.43 **lower limb, bilateral**
R22.9 **Localized swelling, mass and lump, unspecified**

R23 OTHER SKIN CHANGES
`4th` R23.0 **Cyanosis**
Excludes1: acrocyanosis (I73.8)
cyanotic attacks of newborn (P28.2)
R23.1 **Pallor**
Clammy skin
R23.2 **Flushing**
Excessive blushing
Code first, if applicable, menopausal and female climacteric states (N95.1)
R23.3 **Spontaneous ecchymoses**
Petechiae
Excludes1: ecchymoses of newborn (P54.5)
purpura (D69.-)
R23.8 **Other skin changes**
R23.9 **Unspecified skin changes**

(R25–R29) SYMPTOMS AND SIGNS INVOLVING THE NERVOUS AND MUSCULOSKELETAL SYSTEMS

R25 ABNORMAL INVOLUNTARY MOVEMENTS
`4th` *Excludes1:* specific movement disorders (G20–G26)
stereotyped movement disorders (F98.4)
tic disorders (F95.-)
R25.1 **Tremor, unspecified**
Excludes1: chorea NOS (G25.5)
essential tremor (G25.0)
hysterical tremor (F44.4)
intention tremor (G25.2)
R25.2 **Cramp and spasm**
Excludes2: carpopedal spasm (R29.0)
charley-horse (M62.831)
infantile spasms (G40.4-)
muscle spasm of back (M62.830)
muscle spasm of calf (M62.831)
R25.8 **Other abnormal involuntary movements**
R25.9 **Unspecified abnormal involuntary movements**

R26 ABNORMALITIES OF GAIT AND MOBILITY
`4th` *Excludes1:* ataxia NOS (R27.0)
hereditary ataxia (G11.-)
locomotor (syphilitic) ataxia (A52.11)
immobility syndrome (paraplegic) (M62.3)
R26.0 **Ataxic gait**
Staggering gait
R26.1 **Paralytic gait**
Spastic gait
R26.2 **Difficulty in walking, NEC**
Excludes1: falling (R29.6)
unsteadiness on feet (R26.81)

`4th` `5th` `6th` `7th` Additional Character Required   ☑ 3-character code

●=New Code   *Excludes1*—Not coded here, do not use together
▲=Revised Code   *Excludes2*—Not included here

R26.8 Other abnormalities of gait and mobility
> **5th** **R26.81 Unsteadiness on feet**
> **R26.89 Other abnormalities of gait and mobility**

R26.9 Unspecified abnormalities of gait and mobility

R27 OTHER LACK OF COORDINATION
4th *Excludes1:* ataxic gait (R26.0)
> hereditary ataxia (G11.-)
> vertigo NOS (R42)

R27.0 Ataxia, unspecified
> *Excludes1:* ataxia following cerebrovascular disease (I69. with final characters -93)

R27.8 Other lack of coordination
R27.9 Unspecified lack of coordination

R29 OTHER SYMPTOMS AND SIGNS INVOLVING THE
4th **NERVOUS AND MUSCULOSKELETAL SYSTEMS**

R29.0 Tetany
> Carpopedal spasm
> *Excludes1:* hysterical tetany (F44.5)
> neonatal tetany (P71.3)
> parathyroid tetany (E20.9)
> post-thyroidectomy tetany (E89.2)

R29.1 Meningismus
R29.2 Abnormal reflex
> *Excludes2:* abnormal pupillary reflex (H57.0)
> hyperactive gag reflex (J39.2)
> vasovagal reaction or syncope (R55)

R29.3 Abnormal posture
R29.4 Clicking hip
> *Excludes1:* congenital deformities of hip (Q65.-)

R29.8 Other symptoms and signs involving the nervous and
5th **musculoskeletal systems**
> **R29.81 Other symptoms and signs involving the nervous**
> **6th** **system**
>> **R29.810 Facial weakness**
>> Facial droop
>> **R29.818 Other symptoms and signs involving the nervous system**

> **R29.89 Other symptoms and signs involving the**
> **6th** **musculoskeletal system**
>> *Excludes2:* pain in limb (M79.6-)
>> **R29.891 Ocular torticollis**
>>> *Excludes1:* congenital (sternomastoid) torticollis Q68.0
>>> psychogenic torticollis (F45.8)
>>> spasmodic torticollis (G24.3)
>>> torticollis due to birth injury (P15.8)
>>> torticollis NOS M43.6
>> **R29.898 Other symptoms and signs involving the musculoskeletal system**

R29.9 Unspecified symptoms and signs involving the; nervous and
5th **musculoskeletal systems**
> **R29.90 Nervous system**
> **R29.91 Musculoskeletal system**

(R30–R39) SYMPTOMS AND SIGNS INVOLVING THE GENITOURINARY SYSTEM

R30 PAIN ASSOCIATED WITH MICTURITION
4th *Excludes1:* psychogenic pain associated with micturition (F45.8)

R30.0 Dysuria
> Strangury

R30.9 Painful micturition, unspecified
> Painful urination NOS

R31 HEMATURIA
4th *Excludes1:* hematuria included with underlying conditions, such as:
> acute cystitis with hematuria (N30.01)
> recurrent and persistent hematuria in glomerular diseases (N02.-)

R31.0 Gross hematuria
R31.1 Benign essential microscopic hematuria
R31.2 Other microscopic hematuria
> **5th** **R31.21 Asymptomatic microscopic hematuria**

> **R31.29 Other microscopic hematuria**

R31.9 Hematuria, unspecified

R32 UNSPECIFIED URINARY INCONTINENCE
✔ Enuresis NOS
Excludes1: functional urinary incontinence (R39.81)
> nonorganic enuresis (F98.0)
> stress incontinence and other specified urinary incontinence (N39.3–N39.4-)
> urinary incontinence associated with cognitive impairment (R39.81)

R33 RETENTION OF URINE
4th *Excludes1:* psychogenic retention of urine (F45.8)

R33.8 Other retention of urine
> **Code first**, if applicable, any causal condition, such as: enlarged prostate (N40.1)

R33.9 Retention of urine, unspecified

R34 ANURIA AND OLIGURIA
✔ *Excludes1:* anuria and oliguria complicating abortion or ectopic or molar pregnancy (O00–O07, O08.4)
> anuria and oliguria complicating pregnancy (O26.83–)

R35 POLYURIA
4th **Code first,** if applicable, any causal condition, such as: enlarged prostate (N40.1)
Excludes1: psychogenic polyuria (F45.8)

R35.0 Frequency of micturition
R35.1 Nocturia
R35.8 Other polyuria
> Polyuria NOS

R36 URETHRAL DISCHARGE
4th **R36.0 Urethral discharge without blood**
R36.1 Hematospermia
R36.9 Urethral discharge, unspecified
> Penile discharge NOS
> Urethrorrhea

R37 SEXUAL DYSFUNCTION, UNSPECIFIED
✔

R39 OTHER AND UNSPECIFIED SYMPTOMS AND SIGNS
4th **INVOLVING THE GENITOURINARY SYSTEM**

R39.0 Extravasation of urine
R39.1 Other difficulties with micturition
> **5th** **Code first**, if applicable, any causal condition, such as: enlarged prostate (N40.1)
> **R39.11 Hesitancy of micturition**
> **R39.12 Poor urinary stream**
>> Weak urinary steam
> **R39.13 Splitting of urinary stream**
> **R39.14 Feeling of incomplete bladder emptying**
> **R39.15 Urgency of urination**
>> *Excludes1:* urge incontinence (N39.41, N39.46)
> **R39.16 Straining to void**
> **R39.19 Other difficulties with micturition**
>> **6th** **R39.191 Need to immediately re-void**
>> **R39.192 Position dependent micturition**
>> **R39.198 Other difficulties with micturition**

R39.8 Other symptoms and signs involving the genitourinary system
> **5th** **R39.81 Functional urinary incontinence**
> **R39.82 Chronic bladder pain**
> **R39.83 Unilateral non-palpable testicle**
> **R39.84 Bilateral non-palpable testicles**
> **R39.89 Other symptoms and signs involving the genitourinary system**

R39.9 Unspecified symptoms and signs involving the genitourinary system

(R40–R46) SYMPTOMS AND SIGNS INVOLVING COGNITION, PERCEPTION, EMOTIONAL STATE AND BEHAVIOR

Excludes2: symptoms and signs constituting part of a pattern of mental disorder (F01–F99)

| **4th** | **5th** | **6th** | **7th** | Additional Character Required | ✔ 3-character code |

• =New Code   *Excludes1*—Not coded here, do not use together
▲ =Revised Code   *Excludes2*—Not included here

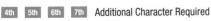

CHAPTER 18. SYMPTOMS, SIGNS, AND ABNORMAL CLINICAL AND LABORATORY FINDINGS, NOT ELSEWHERE CLASSIFIED   (R40–R41)

R40 SOMNOLENCE, STUPOR AND COMA
[4th]

Excludes1: neonatal coma (P91.5)
somnolence, stupor and coma in diabetes (E08–E13)
somnolence, stupor and coma in hepatic failure (K72.-)
somnolence, stupor and coma in hypoglycemia (nondiabetic) (E15)

R40.0 Somnolence
Drowsiness
Excludes1: coma (R40.2-)

R40.1 Stupor
Catatonic stupor
Semicoma
Excludes1: catatonic schizophrenia (F20.2)
    coma (R40.2-)
    depressive stupor (F31–F33)
    dissociative stupor (F44.2)
    manic stupor (F30.2)

R40.2 Coma
[5th]

GUIDELINES

The coma scale codes (R40.2-) can be used in conjunction with traumatic brain injury codes, acute cerebrovascular disease or sequelae of cerebrovascular disease codes. These codes are primarily for use by trauma registries, but they may be used in any setting where this information is collected. The coma scale codes should be sequenced after the diagnosis code(s).

These codes, one from each subcategory, are needed to complete the scale. The 7th character indicates when the scale was recorded. The 7th character should match for all three codes.

At a minimum, report the initial score documented on presentation at your facility. This may be a score from the emergency medicine technician (EMT) or in the emergency department. If desired, a facility may choose to capture multiple coma scale scores.

Assign code R40.24, Glasgow coma scale, total score, when only the total score is documented in the medical record and not the individual score(s). **Do not report codes for individual or total Glasgow coma scale scores for a patient with a medically induced coma or a sedated patient.**

See Section I.B.14 for coma scale documentation by clinicians other than patient's provider.
Code first any associated: fracture of skull (S02.-)
    intracranial injury (S06.-)
Note: One code from each subcategory R40.21–R40.23 is required to complete the coma scale

R40.20 Unspecified coma
Coma NOS
Unconsciousness NOS

R40.21 Coma scale, eyes open
[6th]

R40.211 Coma scale, eyes open, never
Coma scale eye opening score of 1

R40.212 Coma scale, eyes open, to pain
[7th]
Coma scale eye opening score of 2

> 7th character is to be added to subcategory R40.21- or R40.22-
> 0–unspecified time
> 1–in the field [EMT/ambulance]
> 2–at arrival to ED
> 3–at hospital admission
> 4–24 hours or more after hospital admission

R40.213 Coma scale, eyes open, to sound
[7th]
Coma scale eye opening score of 3

R40.214 Coma scale, eyes open, spontaneous
[7th]
Coma scale eye opening score of 4

R40.22 Coma scale, best verbal response
[6th]

R40.221 Coma scale, best verbal response, none
[7th]
Coma scale verbal score of 1

R40.222 Coma scale, best verbal response, incomprehensible words
[7th]
Coma scale verbal score of 2
Incomprehensible sounds (2–5 years of age)
Moans/grunts to pain; restless (<2 years old)

R40.223 Coma scale, best verbal response, inappropriate words
[7th]
Coma scale verbal score of 3
Inappropriate crying or screaming (< 2 years of age)
Screaming (2–5 years of age)

R40.224 Coma scale, best verbal response, confused conversation
[7th]
Coma scale verbal score of 4
Inappropriate words (2–5 years of age)
Irritable cries (< 2 years of age)

R40.225 Coma scale, best verbal response, oriented
[7th]
Coma scale verbal score of 5
Cooing or babbling or crying appropriately (< 2 years of age)
Uses appropriate words (2–5 years of age)

R40.23 Coma scale, best motor response
[6th]

R40.231 Coma scale, best motor response, none
[7th]
Coma scale motor score of 1

> 7th character is to be added to subcategory R40.23- or R40.24-
> 0–unspecified time
> 1–in the field [EMT/ambulance]
> 2–at arrival to ED
> 3–at hospital admission
> 4–24 hours or more after hospital admission

R40.232 Coma scale, best motor response, extension
[7th]
Coma scale motor score of 2
Abnormal extensor posturing to pain or noxious stimuli (< 2 years of age)
Extensor posturing to pain or noxious stimuli (2–5 years of age)

R40.233 Coma scale, best motor response, abnormal
[7th]
Coma scale motor score of 3
Abnormal flexure posturing to pain or noxious stimuli (0–5 years of age)
Flexion/decorticate posturing (< 2 years of age)

R40.234 Coma scale, best motor response, flexion withdrawal
[7th]
Coma scale motor score of 4
Withdraws from pain or noxious stimuli (0–5 years of age)

R40.235 Coma scale, best motor response, localizes pain
[7th]
Coma scale motor score of 5
Localizes pain (2-5 years of age)
Withdraws to touch (< 2 years of age)

R40.236 Coma scale, best motor response, obeys commands
[7th]
Coma scale motor score of 6
Normal or spontaneous movement (< 2 years of age)
Obeys commands (2-5 years of age)

R40.24 Glasgow coma scale, total score
[6th]
Note: Assign a code from subcategory R40.24, when only the total coma score is documented

R40.241 Glasgow coma scale score 13–15
[7th]

R40.242 Glasgow coma scale score 9–12
[7th]

R40.243 Glasgow coma scale score 3–8
[7th]

R40.244 Other coma, without documented Glasgow coma scale score, or with partial score reported
[7th]

R40.3 Persistent vegetative state

R41 OTHER SYMPTOMS AND SIGNS INVOLVING COGNITIVE FUNCTIONS AND AWARENESS
[4th]

Excludes1: dissociative [conversion] disorders (F44.-)
    mild cognitive impairment, so stated (G31.84)

[4th] [5th] [6th] [7th] Additional Character Required   ✔ 3-character code   •=New Code   **Excludes1**—Not coded here, do not use together
▲=Revised Code   **Excludes2**—Not included here

R41.0 Disorientation, unspecified
Confusion NOS
Delirium NOS

R41.8 [5th] Other symptoms and signs involving cognitive functions and awareness

    R41.82 Altered mental status, unspecified
    Change in mental status NOS
    Excludes1: altered level of consciousness (R40.-)
      altered mental status due to known condition—code to condition
      delirium NOS (R41.0)

    R41.83 Borderline intellectual functioning
    IQ level 71 to 84
    Excludes1: intellectual disabilities (F70–F79)

    R41.84 [6th] Other specified cognitive deficit
    Excludes1: cognitive deficits as sequelae of cerebrovascular disease (I69.01-, I69.11-, I69.21-, I69.31-, I69.81-, I69.91-)

      R41.840 Attention and concentration deficit
      Excludes1: attention-deficit hyperactivity disorders (F90.-)

      R41.841 Cognitive communication deficit
      R41.842 Visuospatial deficit
      R41.843 Psychomotor deficit
      R41.844 Frontal lobe and executive function deficit

    R41.89 Other symptoms and signs involving cognitive functions and awareness
    Anosognosia

R41.9 Unspecified symptoms and signs involving cognitive functions and awareness
Unspecified neurocognitive disorder

R42 ✔ DIZZINESS AND GIDDINESS
Light-headedness
Vertigo NOS
Excludes1: vertiginous syndromes (H81.-)
  vertigo from infrasound (T75.23)

R43 [4th] DISTURBANCES OF SMELL AND TASTE
R43.0 Anosmia
R43.1 Parosmia
R43.2 Parageusia
R43.8 Other disturbances of smell and taste
Mixed disturbance of smell and taste
R43.9 Unspecified disturbances of smell and taste

R44 [4th] OTHER SYMPTOMS AND SIGNS INVOLVING GENERAL SENSATIONS AND PERCEPTIONS
Excludes1: alcoholic hallucinations (F10.151, F10.251, F10.951)
  hallucinations in drug psychosis (F11-F19 with fifth to sixth characters 51)
  hallucinations in mood disorders with psychotic symptoms (F30.2, F31.5, F32.3, F33.3)
  hallucinations in schizophrenia, schizotypal and delusional disorders (F20–F29)
Excludes2: disturbances of skin sensation (R20.-)
R44.0 Auditory hallucinations
R44.1 Visual hallucinations
R44.2 Other hallucinations
R44.3 Hallucinations, unspecified
R44.8 Other symptoms and signs involving general sensations and perceptions
R44.9 Unspecified symptoms and signs involving general sensations and perceptions

R45 [4th] SYMPTOMS AND SIGNS INVOLVING EMOTIONAL STATE
R45.0 Nervousness
Nervous tension
R45.1 Restlessness and agitation
R45.2 Unhappiness
R45.3 Demoralization and apathy
Excludes1: anhedonia (R45.84)
R45.4 Irritability and anger
R45.5 Hostility
R45.6 Violent behavior

R45.7 State of emotional shock and stress, unspecified
R45.8 [5th] Other symptoms and signs involving emotional state
  R45.81 Low self-esteem
  R45.82 Worries
  R45.83 Excessive crying of child, adolescent or adult
  Excludes1: excessive crying of infant (baby) R68.11
  R45.84 Anhedonia
  R45.85 [6th] Homicidal and suicidal ideations
  Excludes1: suicide attempt (T14.91)
    R45.850 Homicidal ideations
    R45.851 Suicidal ideations
  R45.86 Emotional lability
  R45.87 Impulsiveness
  R45.89 Other symptoms and signs involving emotional state

R46 [4th] SYMPTOMS AND SIGNS INVOLVING APPEARANCE AND BEHAVIOR
Excludes1: appearance and behavior in schizophrenia, schizotypal and delusional disorders (F20–F29)
  mental and behavioral disorders (F01– F99)
R46.0 Very low level of personal hygiene
R46.1 Bizarre personal appearance
R46.2 Strange and inexplicable behavior
R46.3 Overactivity
R46.4 Slowness and poor responsiveness
Excludes 1: stupor (R40.1)
R46.5 Suspiciousness and marked evasiveness
R46.6 Undue concern and preoccupation with stressful events
R46.7 Verbosity and circumstantial detail obscuring reason for contact
R46.8 [5th] Other symptoms and signs involving appearance and behavior
  R46.81 Obsessive-compulsive behavior
  obsessive-compulsive disorder (F42.-)
  R46.89 Other symptoms and signs involving appearance and behavior

(R47–R49) SYMPTOMS AND SIGNS INVOLVING SPEECH AND VOICE

R47 [4th] SPEECH DISTURBANCES, NEC
Excludes1: autism (F84.0)
  cluttering (F80.81)
  specific developmental disorders of speech and language (F80.-)
  stuttering (F80.81)
R47.1 Dysarthria and anarthria
Excludes1: dysarthria following cerebrovascular disease (I69. with final characters -22)
R47.8 [5th] Other speech disturbances
Excludes1: dysarthria following cerebrovascular disease (I69. with final characters -28)
  R47.81 Slurred speech
  R47.82 Fluency disorder in conditions classified elsewhere
  Stuttering in conditions classified elsewhere
  Code first underlying disease or condition, such as:
    Parkinson's disease (G20)
  Excludes1: adult onset fluency disorder (F98.5)
    childhood onset fluency disorder (F80.81)
    fluency disorder (stuttering) following cerebrovascular disease (I69. with final characters -23)
  R47.89 Other speech disturbances
R47.9 Unspecified speech disturbances

R48 [4th] DYSLEXIA AND OTHER SYMBOLIC DYSFUNCTIONS, NEC
Excludes1: specific developmental disorders of scholastic skills (F81.-)
R48.0 Dyslexia and alexia
R48.1 Agnosia
Astereognosia (astereognosis)
Autotopagnosia
Excludes1: visual object agnosia (R48.3)
R48.8 Other symbolic dysfunctions
Acalculia
Agraphia
R48.9 Unspecified symbolic dysfunctions

[4th] [5th] [6th] [7th] Additional Character Required   ✔ 3-character code

•=New Code
▲=Revised Code

Excludes1—Not coded here, do not use together
Excludes2—Not included here

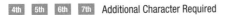

R49 VOICE AND RESONANCE DISORDERS
[4th] *Excludes1:* psychogenic voice and resonance disorders (F44.4)
- **R49.0 Dysphonia**
  Hoarseness
- **R49.1 Aphonia**
  Loss of voice
- **R49.2 Hypernasality and hyponasality**
  - **[5th] R49.21 Hypernasality**
  - **R49.22 Hyponasality**
- **R49.8 Other voice and resonance disorders**
- **R49.9 Unspecified voice and resonance disorder**
  Change in voice NOS
  Resonance disorder NOS

(R50–R69) GENERAL SYMPTOMS AND SIGNS

R50 FEVER OF OTHER AND UNKNOWN ORIGIN
[4th] *Excludes1:* chills without fever (R68.83)
- febrile convulsions (R56.0-)
- fever of unknown origin during labor (O75.2)
- fever of unknown origin in newborn (P81.9)
- hypothermia due to illness (R68.0)
- malignant hyperthermia due to anesthesia (T88.3)
- puerperal pyrexia NOS (O86.4)
- **R50.2 Drug-induced fever**
  Use additional code for adverse effect, if applicable, to identify drug (T36–T50 with fifth or sixth character 5)
  Excludes1: postvaccination (postimmunization) fever (R50.83)
- **R50.8 Other specified fever**
  - **[5th] R50.81 Fever presenting with conditions classified elsewhere**
    Code first underlying condition when associated fever is present, such as with: leukemia (C91–C95)
    neutropenia (D70.-)
    sickle-cell disease
    (D57.-)
    | Do not use R50.81 with acute conditions |
  - **R50.82 Postprocedural fever**
    Excludes1:
    postprocedural infection (T81.4-)
    posttransfusion fever (R50.84)
    postvaccination (postimmunization) fever (R50.83)
  - **R50.83 Postvaccination fever**
    Postimmunization fever
  - **R50.84 Febrile nonhemolytic transfusion reaction**
    FNHTR
    Posttransfusion fever
- **R50.9 Fever, unspecified**
  Fever NOS
  Fever of unknown origin [FUO]
  Fever with chills
  Fever with rigors
  Hyperpyrexia NOS
  Persistent fever

R51 HEADACHE
[4th] *Excludes2:* atypical face pain (G50.1)
- migraine and other headache syndromes (G43–G44)
- trigeminal neuralgia (G50.0)
- •**R51.0 Headache with orthostatic component, NEC**
  Headache with positional component, NEC
- •**R51.9 Headache, unspecified**
  Facial pain NOS

R52 PAIN, UNSPECIFIED
[✔]
Acute pain NOS
Generalized pain NOS
Pain NOS
Excludes1: acute and chronic pain, NEC (G89.-)
localized pain, unspecified type — code to pain by site, such as:
abdomen pain (R10.-)
back pain (M54.9)
breast pain (N64.4)
chest pain (R07.1–R07.9)
ear pain (H92.0-)
eye pain (H57.1)
headache (R51.9)

joint pain (M25.5-)
limb pain (M79.6-)
lumbar region pain (M54.5)
pelvic and perineal pain (R10.2)
shoulder pain (M25.51-)
spine pain (M54.-)
throat pain (R07.0)
tongue pain (K14.6)
tooth pain (K08.8)
renal colic (N23)
pain disorders exclusively related to psychological factors (F45.41)

R53 MALAISE AND FATIGUE
[4th]
- **R53.1 Weakness**
  Asthenia NOS
  Excludes1: muscle weakness (M62.81)
  sarcopenia (M62.84)
- **R53.8 Other malaise and fatigue**
  - **[5th]** *Excludes1:* combat exhaustion and fatigue (F43.0)
    congenital debility (P96.9)
    exhaustion and fatigue due to excessive exertion (T73.3)
    exhaustion and fatigue due to exposure (T73.2)
    exhaustion and fatigue due to heat (T67.-)
    exhaustion and fatigue due to recurrent depressive episode (F33)
  - **R53.81 Other malaise**
    Chronic debility
    Debility NOS
    General physical deterioration
    Malaise NOS
    Nervous debility
    Excludes1: age-related physical debility (R54)
  - **R53.82 Chronic fatigue, unspecified**
    Chronic fatigue syndrome NOS
    Excludes1: postviral fatigue syndrome (G93.3)
  - **R53.83 Other fatigue**
    Fatigue NOS
    Lack of energy
    Lethargy
    Tiredness
    Excludes 2: exhaustion and fatigue due to depressive episode (F32.-)

R55 SYNCOPE AND COLLAPSE
[✔]
Blackout
Fainting
Vasovagal attack
Excludes1: cardiogenic shock (R57.0)
carotid sinus syncope (G90.01)
heat syncope (T67.1)
neurocirculatory asthenia (F45.8)
neurogenic orthostatic hypotension (G90.3)
orthostatic hypotension (I95.1)
postprocedural shock (T81.1-)
psychogenic syncope (F48.8)
shock NOS (R57.9)
shock complicating or following abortion or ectopic or molar pregnancy (O00–O07, O08.3)
Stokes-Adams attack (I45.9)
unconsciousness NOS (R40.2-)

R56 CONVULSIONS, NEC
[4th] *Excludes1:* dissociative convulsions and seizures (F44.5)
epileptic convulsions and seizures (G40.-)
newborn convulsions and seizures (P90)
- **R56.0 Febrile convulsions**
  - **[5th] R56.00 Simple febrile convulsions**
    Febrile convulsion NOS
    Febrile seizure NOS
  - **R56.01 Complex febrile convulsions**
    Atypical febrile seizure
    Complex febrile seizure
    Complicated febrile seizure
    Excludes1: status epilepticus (G40.901)
- **R56.1 Post traumatic seizures**
  Excludes1: post traumatic epilepsy (G40.-)

[4th] [5th] [6th] [7th] Additional Character Required   **[✔]** 3-character code

•=New Code   *Excludes1*—Not coded here, do not use together
▲=Revised Code   *Excludes2*—Not included here

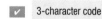

R56.9   Unspecified convulsions
Convulsion disorder
Fit NOS
Recurrent convulsions
Seizure(s) (convulsive) NOS

R57   SHOCK, NEC
`4th`

Excludes1: anaphylactic shock NOS (T78.2)
anaphylactic reaction or shock due to adverse food reaction (T78.0-)
anaphylactic shock due to adverse effect of correct drug or medicament properly administered (T88.6)
anaphylactic shock due to serum (T80.5-)
anesthetic shock (T88.3)
electric shock (T75.4)
obstetric shock (O75.1)
postprocedural shock (T81.1-)
psychic shock (F43.0)
shock complicating or following ectopic or molar pregnancy (O00–O07, O08.3)
shock due to lightning (T75.01)
traumatic shock (T79.4)
toxic shock syndrome (A48.3)

R57.0   Cardiogenic shock
Excludes 2: septic shock (R65.21)

R57.1   Hypovolemic shock

R57.8   Other shock

R57.9   Shock, unspecified
Failure of peripheral circulation NOS

R58   HEMORRHAGE, NEC
✔

Hemorrhage NOS
Excludes1: hemorrhage included with underlying conditions, such as:
acute duodenal ulcer with hemorrhage (K26.0)
acute gastritis with bleeding (K29.01)
ulcerative enterocolitis with rectal bleeding (K51.01)

R59   ENLARGED LYMPH NODES
`4th`

Includes: swollen glands
Excludes1: lymphadenitis NOS (I88.9)
acute lymphadenitis (L04.-)
chronic lymphadenitis (I88.1)
mesenteric (acute) (chronic) lymphadenitis (I88.0)

R59.0   Localized enlarged lymph nodes

R59.1   Generalized enlarged lymph nodes
Lymphadenopathy NOS

R59.9   Enlarged lymph nodes, unspecified

R60   EDEMA, NEC
`4th`

Excludes1: angioneurotic edema (T78.3)
ascites (R18.-)
cerebral edema (G93.6)
cerebral edema due to birth injury (P11.0)
edema of larynx (J38.4)
edema of nasopharynx (J39.2)
edema of pharynx (J39.2)
gestational edema (O12.0-)
hereditary edema (Q82.0)
hydrops fetalis NOS (P83.2)
hydrothorax (J94.8)
hydrops fetalis NOS (P83.2)
newborn edema (P83.3)
pulmonary edema (J81.-)

R60.0   Localized edema

R60.1   Generalized edema
Excludes 2: nutritional edema (E40–E46)

R60.9   Edema, unspecified
Fluid retention NOS

R61   GENERALIZED HYPERHIDROSIS
✔

Excessive sweating
Night sweats
Secondary hyperhidrosis
Code first, if applicable, menopausal and female climacteric states (N95.1)
Excludes1: focal (primary) (secondary) hyperhidrosis (L74.5-)
Frey's syndrome (L74.52)
localized (primary) (secondary) hyperhidrosis (L74.5-)

R62   LACK OF EXPECTED NORMAL PHYSIOLOGICAL DEVELOPMENT IN CHILDHOOD AND ADULTS
`4th`

Excludes1: delayed puberty (E30.0)
gonadal dysgenesis (Q99.1)
hypopituitarism (E23.0)

R62.0   Delayed milestone in childhood
Delayed attainment of expected physiological developmental stage
Late talker
Late walker

R62.5   Other and unspecified lack of expected normal physiological development in childhood
`5th`
Excludes1: HIV disease resulting in failure to thrive (B20)
physical retardation due to malnutrition (E45)

R62.50   Unspecified lack of expected normal physiological development in childhood
Infantilism NOS

R62.51   Failure to thrive (child)
Failure to gain weight
Excludes1: failure to thrive in child under 28 days old (P92.6)

R62.52   Short stature (child)
Lack of growth
Physical retardation
Short stature NOS
Excludes1: short stature due to endocrine disorder (E34.3)

R62.59   Other lack of expected normal physiological development in childhood

R63   SYMPTOMS AND SIGNS CONCERNING FOOD AND FLUID INTAKE
`4th`

Excludes1: bulimia NOS (F50.2)

R63.0   Anorexia
Loss of appetite
Excludes1: anorexia nervosa (F50.0-)
loss of appetite of nonorganic origin (F50.89)

R63.1   Polydipsia
Excessive thirst

R63.2   Polyphagia
Excessive eating
Hyperalimentation NOS

R63.3   Feeding difficulties
Feeding problem (elderly) (infant) NOS
Picky eater
Excludes1: eating disorders (F50.-)
feeding problems of newborn (P92.-)
infant feeding disorder of nonorganic origin (F98.2-)

R63.4   Abnormal weight loss

R63.5   Abnormal weight gain
Excludes1: excessive weight gain in pregnancy (O26.0-)
obesity (E66.-)

R63.6   Underweight
Use additional code to identify body mass index (BMI), if known (Z68.-)
Excludes1: abnormal weight loss (R63.4)
anorexia nervosa (F50.0-)
malnutrition (E40–E46)

R63.8   Other symptoms and signs concerning food and fluid intake

R64   CACHEXIA
✔

Wasting syndrome
Code first underlying condition, if known
Excludes1: abnormal weight loss (R63.4)
nutritional marasmus (E41)

R65   SYMPTOMS AND SIGNS SPECIFICALLY ASSOCIATED WITH SYSTEMIC INFLAMMATION AND INFECTION
`4th`

R65.1   SIRS of non-infectious origin
`5th`

> **GUIDELINE**
>
> The SIRS can develop as a result of certain non-infectious disease processes, such as trauma, malignant neoplasm, or pancreatitis. When SIRS is documented with a noninfectious condition, and no subsequent infection is documented, the code for the underlying condition, such as an injury, should be assigned, followed by code R65.10 or code R65.11. If an associated acute organ dysfunction is documented, the appropriate code(s) for the specific type

---

`4th` `5th` `6th` `7th`   Additional Character Required   ✔   3-character code

•=New Code
▲=Revised Code

Excludes1—Not coded here, do not use together
Excludes2—Not included here

CHAPTER 18. SYMPTOMS, SIGNS, AND ABNORMAL CLINICAL AND LABORATORY FINDINGS, NOT ELSEWHERE CLASSIFIED   (R65.10–R73.0)

of organ dysfunction(s) should be assigned in addition to code R65.11. If acute organ dysfunction is documented, but it cannot be determined if the acute organ dysfunction is associated with SIRS or due to another condition (e.g., directly due to the trauma), the provider should be queried.

Code first underlying condition, such as: heatstroke (T67.0-)
  injury and trauma (S00–T88)
Excludes1: sepsis- code to infection
  severe sepsis (R65.2)

R65.10   SIRS of non-infectious origin without acute organ dysfunction
  SIRS NOS

R65.11   SIRS of non-infectious origin with acute organ dysfunction
  Use additional code to identify specific acute organ
    dysfunction, such as:
    acute kidney failure (N17.-)
    cute respiratory failure (J96.0-)
    critical illness myopathy (G72.81)
    critical illness polyneuropathy (G62.81)
    disseminated intravascular coagulopathy [DIC] (D65)
    encephalopathy (metabolic) (septic) (G93.41)
    hepatic failure (K72.0-)

R65.2   Severe sepsis
5th
  Infection with associated acute organ dysfunction
  Sepsis with acute organ dysfunction
  Sepsis with multiple organ dysfunction
  SIRS due to infectious process with acute organ dysfunction
  Code first underlying infection, such as: infection following a
    procedure (T81.4-)
    infections following infusion, transfusion and therapeutic
      injection (T80.2-)
    puerperal sepsis (O85)
    sepsis following complete or unspecified spontaneous abortion
      (O03.87)
    sepsis following ectopic and molar pregnancy (O08.82)
    sepsis following incomplete spontaneous abortion (O03.37)
    sepsis following (induced) termination of pregnancy (O04.87)
    sepsis NOS (A41.9)
  Use additional code to identify specific acute organ dysfunction,
    such as:
    acute kidney failure (N17.-)
    acute respiratory failure (J96.0-)
    critical illness myopathy (G72.81)
    critical illness polyneuropathy (G62.81)
    disseminated intravascular coagulopathy [DIC] (D65)
    encephalopathy (metabolic) (septic) (G93.41)
    hepatic failure (K72.0-)

R65.20   Severe sepsis without septic shock
  Severe sepsis NOS

R65.21   Severe sepsis with septic shock

R68   OTHER GENERAL SYMPTOMS AND SIGNS
4th
R68.0   Hypothermia, not associated with low environmental temperature
  Excludes1: hypothermia NOS (accidental) (T68)
    hypothermia due to anesthesia (T88.51)
    hypothermia due to low environmental temperature (T68)
    newborn hypothermia (P80.-)

R68.1   Nonspecific symptoms peculiar to infancy
5th
  Excludes1: colic, infantile (R10.83)
    neonatal cerebral irritability (P91.3)
    teething syndrome (K00.7)

R68.11   Excessive crying of infant (baby)
  Excludes1: excessive crying of child, adolescent, or
    adult (R45.83)

R68.12   Fussy infant (baby)
  Irritable infant

R68.13   Apparent life threatening event in infant (ALTE)
  Apparent life threatening event in newborn
  Brief resolved unexplained event (BRUE)
  Code first confirmed diagnosis, if known
  Use additional code(s) for associated signs and

symptoms if no confirmed diagnosis established, or if signs and symptoms are not associated routinely with confirmed diagnosis, or provide additional information for cause of ALTE

R68.19   Other nonspecific symptoms peculiar to infancy

R68.2   Dry mouth, unspecified
  Excludes1: dry mouth due to dehydration (E86.0)
    dry mouth due to sicca syndrome [Sjögren] (M35.0-)
    salivary gland hyposecretion (K11.7)

R68.3   Clubbing of fingers
  Clubbing of nails
  Excludes1: congenital club finger (Q68.1)

R68.8   Other general symptoms and signs
5th
R68.81   Early satiety
R68.83   Chills (without fever)
  Chills NOS
  Excludes1: chills with fever (R50.9)

R68.84   Jaw pain
  Mandibular pain
  Maxilla pain
  Excludes1: temporomandibular joint arthralgia (M26.62-)

R68.89   Other general symptoms and signs

R69   ILLNESS, UNSPECIFIED
✔
  Unknown and unspecified cases of morbidity

(R70–R79) ABNORMAL FINDINGS ON EXAMINATION OF BLOOD, WITHOUT DIAGNOSIS

Excludes2: abnormalities (of) (on):
  abnormal findings on antenatal screening of mother (O28.-)
  coagulation hemorrhagic disorders (D65–D68)
  lipids (E78.-)
  platelets and thrombocytes (D69.-)
  white blood cells classified elsewhere (D70–D72)
  diagnostic abnormal findings classified elsewhere—see Alphabetical Index
  hemorrhagic and hematological disorders of newborn (P50–P61)

R70   ELEVATED ERYTHROCYTE SEDIMENTATION RATE AND
4th   ABNORMALITY OF PLASMA VISCOSITY
R70.0   Elevated erythrocyte sedimentation rate
R70.1   Abnormal plasma viscosity

R71   ABNORMALITY OF RED BLOOD CELLS
4th
  Excludes1: anemias (D50–D64)
    anemia of premature infant (P61.2)
    benign (familial) polycythemia (D75.0)
    congenital anemias (P61.2–P61.4)
    newborn anemia due to isoimmunization (P55.-)
    polycythemia neonatorum (P61.1)
    polycythemia NOS (D75.1)
    polycythemia vera (D45)
    secondary polycythemia (D75.1)

R71.0   Precipitous drop in hematocrit
  Drop (precipitous) in hemoglobin
  Drop in hematocrit

R71.8   Other abnormality of red blood cells
  Abnormal red-cell morphology NOS
  Abnormal red-cell volume NOS
  Anisocytosis
  Poikilocytosis

R73   ELEVATED BLOOD GLUCOSE LEVEL
4th
  Excludes1: DM (E08–E13)
    DM in pregnancy, childbirth and the puerperium (O24.-)
    neonatal disorders (P70.0–P70.2)
    postsurgical hypoinsulinemia (E89.1)

R73.0   Abnormal glucose
5th
  Excludes1: abnormal glucose in pregnancy (O99.81-)
    DM (E08–E13)
    dysmetabolic syndrome X (E88.81)
    gestational diabetes (O24.4-)
    glycosuria (R81)
    hypoglycemia (E16.2)

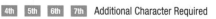

4th	5th	6th	7th	Additional Character Required		✔ 3-character code

•=New Code   *Excludes1*—Not coded here, do not use together
▲=Revised Code   *Excludes2*—Not included here

R73.01 **Impaired fasting glucose**
Elevated fasting glucose

R73.02 **Impaired glucose tolerance (oral)**
Elevated glucose tolerance

R73.03 **Prediabetes**
Latent diabetes

R73.09 **Other abnormal glucose** [Do not report for hyperglycemia caused by DM]
Abnormal glucose NOS
Abnormal non-fasting glucose tolerance

R73.9 **Hyperglycemia, unspecified**

R74 **ABNORMAL SERUM ENZYME LEVELS**
4th ▲R74.0 **Nonspecific elevation of levels of transaminase and lactic acid dehydrogenase [LDH]**
5th
• R74.01 **Elevation of levels of liver transaminase levels**
Elevation of levels of alanine transaminase (ALT)
Elevation of levels of aspartate transaminase (AST)
• R74.02 **Elevation of levels of lactic acid dehydrogenase [LDH]**

R74.8 **Abnormal levels of other serum enzymes**
Abnormal level of acid phosphatase
Abnormal level of alkaline phosphatase
Abnormal level of amylase
Abnormal level of lipase [triacylglycerol lipase]

R74.9 **Abnormal serum enzyme level, unspecified**

R75 **INCONCLUSIVE LABORATORY EVIDENCE OF HIV**
✓

GUIDELINES

Patients with inconclusive HIV serology, but no definitive diagnosis or manifestations of the illness, may be assigned code R75, Inconclusive laboratory evidence of HIV.
Nonconclusive HIV-test finding in infants
Excludes1: asymptomatic HIV infection status (Z21)
HIV disease (B20)

R76 **OTHER ABNORMAL IMMUNOLOGICAL FINDINGS IN SERUM**
4th
R76.0 **Raised antibody titer**
Excludes1: isoimmunization in pregnancy (O36.0–O36.1)
isoimmunization affecting newborn (P55.-)

R76.1 **Nonspecific reaction to test for tuberculosis**
5th R76.11 **Nonspecific reaction to tuberculin skin test without active tuberculosis**
Abnormal result of Mantoux test
PPD positive
Tuberculin (skin test) positive
Tuberculin (skin test) reactor
Excludes1: nonspecific reaction to cell mediated immunity measurement of gamma interferon antigen response without active tuberculosis (R76.12)

R76.12 **Nonspecific reaction to cell mediated immunity measurement of gamma interferon antigen response without active tuberculosis**
Nonspecific reaction to QFT without active tuberculosis
Excludes1: nonspecific reaction to tuberculin skin test without active tuberculosis (R76.11)
positive tuberculin skin test (R76.11)

R76.8 **Other specified abnormal immunological findings in serum**
Raised level of immunoglobulins NOS

R76.9 **Abnormal immunological finding in serum, unspecified**

R77 **OTHER ABNORMALITIES OF PLASMA PROTEINS**
4th *Excludes1:* disorders of plasma-protein metabolism (E88.0-)
R77.1 **Abnormality of globulin**
Hyperglobulinemia NOS
R77.8 **Other specified abnormalities of plasma proteins**
R77.9 **Abnormality of plasma protein, unspecified**

R78 **FINDINGS OF DRUGS AND OTHER SUBSTANCES, NOT NORMALLY FOUND IN BLOOD**
4th **Use additional code** to identify the any retained FB, if applicable (Z18.-)
Excludes1: mental or behavioral disorders due to psychoactive substance use (F10–F19)

R78.0 **Finding of alcohol in blood**
Use additional external cause code (Y90.-), for detail regarding alcohol level

R78.1 **Finding of opiate drug in blood**

R78.2 **Finding of cocaine in blood**

R78.3 **Finding of hallucinogen in blood**

R78.4 **Finding of other drugs of addictive potential in blood**

R78.5 **Finding of other psychotropic drug in blood**

R78.6 **Finding of steroid agent in blood**

R78.7 **Finding of abnormal level of heavy metals in blood**
5th R78.71 **Abnormal lead level in blood**
Excludes1: lead poisoning (T56.0-)
R78.79 **Finding of abnormal level of heavy metals in blood**

R78.8 **Finding of other specified substances, not normally found in blood**
5th
R78.81 **Bacteremia**
Excludes1: sepsis-code to specified infection
R78.89 **Finding of other specified substances, not normally found in blood**
Finding of abnormal level of lithium in blood

R78.9 **Finding of unspecified substance, not normally found in blood**

R79 **OTHER ABNORMAL FINDINGS OF BLOOD CHEMISTRY**
4th **Use additional code** to identify any retained FB, if applicable (Z18.-)
Excludes1: asymptomatic hyperuricemia (E79.0)
hyperglycemia NOS (R73.9)
hypoglycemia NOS (E16.2)
neonatal hypoglycemia (P70.3–P70.4)
specific findings indicating disorder of amino-acid metabolism (E70–E72)
specific findings indicating disorder of carbohydrate metabolism (E73–E74)
specific findings indicating disorder of lipid metabolism (E75.-)

R79.1 **Abnormal coagulation profile**
Abnormal or prolonged bleeding time
Abnormal or prolonged coagulation time
Abnormal or prolonged partial thromboplastin time [PTT]
Abnormal or prolonged prothrombin time [PT]
Excludes1: coagulation defects (D68.-)
Excludes2: abnormality of fluid, electrolyte or acid-base balance (E86–E87)

R79.8 **Other specified abnormal findings of blood chemistry**
5th R79.81 **Abnormal blood-gas level**
R79.82 **Elevated C-reactive protein (CRP)**
R79.89 **Other specified abnormal findings of blood chemistry**
R79.9 **Abnormal finding of blood chemistry, unspecified**

(R80–R82) ABNORMAL FINDINGS ON EXAMINATION OF URINE, WITHOUT DIAGNOSIS

Excludes1: abnormal findings on antenatal screening of mother (O28.-)
diagnostic abnormal findings classified elsewhere—see Alphabetical Index
specific findings indicating disorder of amino-acid metabolism (E70–E72)
specific findings indicating disorder of carbohydrate metabolism (E73–E74)

R80 **PROTEINURIA**
4th *Excludes1:* gestational proteinuria (O12.1-)
R80.0 **Isolated proteinuria**
Idiopathic proteinuria
Excludes1: isolated proteinuria with specific morphological lesion (N06.-)

R80.1 **Persistent proteinuria, unspecified**

R80.2 **Orthostatic proteinuria, unspecified**
Postural proteinuria

R80.3 **Bence Jones proteinuria**

R80.8 **Other proteinuria**

R80.9 **Proteinuria, unspecified**
Albuminuria NOS

R81 **GLYCOSURIA**
✓ *Excludes1:* renal glycosuria (E74.818)

4th 5th 6th 7th Additional Character Required ✓ 3-character code

• =New Code
▲ =Revised Code

Excludes1—Not coded here, do not use together
Excludes2—Not included here

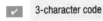

321

CHAPTER 18. SYMPTOMS, SIGNS, AND ABNORMAL CLINICAL AND LABORATORY FINDINGS, NOT ELSEWHERE CLASSIFIED (R82–R93.0)

R82 **OTHER AND UNSPECIFIED ABNORMAL FINDINGS IN URINE**
[4th]
Includes: chromoabnormalities in urine
Use additional code to identify any retained FB, if applicable (Z18.-)
Excludes2: hematuria (R31.-)
R82.0 Chyluria
    Excludes1: filarial chyluria (B74.-)
R82.1 Myoglobinuria
R82.2 Biliuria
R82.3 Hemoglobinuria
    Excludes1: hemoglobinuria due to hemolysis from external causes NEC (D59.6)
    hemoglobinuria due to paroxysmal nocturnal [Marchiafava-Micheli] (D59.5)
R82.7 Abnormal findings on microbiological examination of urine
[5th]
    Excludes1: colonization status (Z22.-)
    R82.71 Bacteriuria
    R82.79 Other abnormal findings on microbiological examination of urine
R82.8 Abnormal findings on cytological and histological examination of urine
[5th]
    R82.81 Pyuria
        sterile pyuria
    R82.89 Other abnormal findings on cytological and histological examination of urine
R82.9 Other and unspecified abnormal findings in urine
[5th]
    R82.90 Unspecified abnormal findings in urine
    R82.91 Other chromoabnormalities of urine
        Chromoconversion (dipstick)
        Idiopathic dipstick converts positive for blood with no cellular forms in sediment
        Excludes1: hemoglobinuria (R82.3)
        myoglobinuria (R82.1)
    R82.99 Other abnormal findings in urine
    [6th]
        R82.991 Hypocitraturia
        R82.992 Hyperoxaluria
            Excludes1: primary hyperoxaluria (E72.53)
        R82.993 Hyperuricosuria
        R82.994 Hypercalciuria
            Idiopathic hypercalciuria
        R82.998 Other abnormal findings in urine
            Cells and casts in urine
            Crystalluria
            Melanuria

(R83–R89) ABNORMAL FINDINGS ON EXAMINATION OF OTHER BODY FLUIDS, SUBSTANCES AND TISSUES, WITHOUT DIAGNOSIS

Excludes1: abnormal findings on antenatal screening of mother (O28.-)
diagnostic abnormal findings classified elsewhere — see Alphabetical Index
Excludes2: abnormal findings on examination of blood, without diagnosis (R70–R79)
abnormal findings on examination of urine, without diagnosis (R80–R82)
abnormal tumor markers (R97.-)

R83 **ABNORMAL FINDINGS IN CEREBROSPINAL FLUID**
[4th]
    R83.3 Abnormal level of substances chiefly nonmedicinal as to source in cerebrospinal fluid
    R83.4 Abnormal immunological findings in cerebrospinal fluid
    R83.5 Abnormal microbiological findings in cerebrospinal fluid
        Positive culture findings in cerebrospinal fluid
        Excludes1: colonization status (Z22.-)
    R83.6 Abnormal cytological findings in cerebrospinal fluid
    R83.8 Other abnormal findings in cerebrospinal fluid
        Abnormal chromosomal findings in cerebrospinal fluid
    R83.9 Unspecified abnormal finding in cerebrospinal fluid

R84 **ABNORMAL FINDINGS IN SPECIMENS FROM RESPIRATORY ORGANS AND THORAX**
[4th]
Includes: abnormal findings in bronchial washings
abnormal findings in nasal secretions
abnormal findings in pleural fluid
abnormal findings in sputum
abnormal findings in throat scrapings
Excludes1: blood-stained sputum (R04.2)
R84.3 Abnormal level of substances chiefly nonmedicinal as to source in specimens from respiratory organs and thorax
R84.4 Abnormal immunological findings in specimens from respiratory organs and thorax
R84.5 Abnormal microbiological findings in specimens from respiratory organs and thorax
    Positive culture findings in specimens from respiratory organs and thorax
    Excludes1: colonization status (Z22.-)
R84.6 Abnormal cytological findings in specimens from respiratory organs and thorax

R89 **ABNORMAL FINDINGS IN SPECIMENS FROM OTHER ORGANS, SYSTEMS AND TISSUES**
[4th]
Includes: abnormal findings in nipple discharge
abnormal findings in synovial fluid
abnormal findings in wound secretions
R89.0 Abnormal level of enzymes in specimens from other organs, systems and tissues
R89.1 Abnormal level of hormones in specimens from other organs, systems and tissues
R89.2 Abnormal level of other drugs, medicaments and biological substances in specimens from other organs, systems and tissues
R89.3 Abnormal level of substances chiefly nonmedicinal as to source in specimens from other organs, systems and tissues
R89.4 Abnormal immunological findings in specimens from other organs, systems and tissues
R89.5 Abnormal microbiological findings in specimens from other organs, systems and tissues
    Positive culture findings in specimens from other organs, systems and tissues
    Excludes1: colonization status (Z22.-)
R89.6 Abnormal cytological findings in specimens from other organs, systems and tissues
R89.7 Abnormal histological findings in specimens from other organs, systems and tissues
R89.8 Other abnormal findings in specimens from other organs, systems and tissues
    Abnormal chromosomal findings in specimens from other organs, systems and tissues
R89.9 Unspecified abnormal finding in specimens from other organs, systems and tissues

(R90–R94) ABNORMAL FINDINGS ON DIAGNOSTIC IMAGING AND IN FUNCTION STUDIES, WITHOUT DIAGNOSIS

Includes: nonspecific abnormal findings on diagnostic imaging by CAT scan
nonspecific abnormal findings on diagnostic imaging by MRI [NMR] or PET scan
nonspecific abnormal findings on diagnostic imaging by thermography
nonspecific abnormal findings on diagnostic imaging by ultrasound [echogram]
nonspecific abnormal findings on diagnostic imaging by X-ray examination
Excludes1: abnormal findings on antenatal screening of mother (O28.-)
diagnostic abnormal findings classified elsewhere — **see Alphabetical Index**

R91 **ABNORMAL FINDINGS ON DIAGNOSTIC IMAGING OF LUNG**
[4th]
    R91.1 Solitary pulmonary nodule
        Coin lesion lung
        Solitary pulmonary nodule, subsegmental branch of the bronchial tree
    R91.8 Other nonspecific abnormal finding of lung field
        Lung mass NOS found on diagnostic imaging of lung
        Pulmonary infiltrate NOS
        Shadow, lung

R93 **ABNORMAL FINDINGS ON DIAGNOSTIC IMAGING OF OTHER BODY STRUCTURES**
[4th]
    R93.0 Abnormal findings on diagnostic imaging of skull and head, NEC
        Excludes1: intracranial space-occupying lesion found on diagnostic imaging (R90.0)

[4th] [5th] [6th] [7th] Additional Character Required   ✔ 3-character code   ●=New Code   *Excludes1*—Not coded here, do not use together
▲=Revised Code   *Excludes2*—Not included here

R93.1 Abnormal findings on diagnostic imaging of heart and coronary circulation
Abnormal echocardiogram NOS
Abnormal heart shadow

R93.2 Abnormal findings on diagnostic imaging of liver and biliary tract
Nonvisualization of gallbladder

R93.3 Abnormal findings on diagnostic imaging of other parts of digestive tract

R93.4 Abnormal findings on diagnostic imaging of urinary organs
   5th *Excludes2:* hypertrophy of kidney (N28.81)

   R93.41 Abnormal radiologic findings on diagnostic imaging of renal pelvis, ureter, or bladder
     Filling defect of bladder found on diagnostic imaging
     Filling defect of renal pelvis found on diagnostic imaging
     Filling defect of ureter found on diagnostic imaging

   R93.42 Abnormal radiologic findings on diagnostic imaging of kidney
     6th
     R93.421 right kidney
     R93.422 left kidney
     R93.429 unspecified kidney

   R93.49 Abnormal radiologic findings on diagnostic imaging of other urinary organs

R93.5 Abnormal findings on diagnostic imaging of other abdominal regions, including retroperitoneum

R93.6 Abnormal findings on diagnostic imaging of limbs
   Excludes2: abnormal finding in skin and subcutaneous tissue (R93.8-)

R93.7 Abnormal findings on diagnostic imaging of other parts of musculoskeletal system
   Excludes2: abnormal findings on diagnostic imaging of skull (R93.0)

R93.8 Abnormal findings on diagnostic imaging of other specified body structures
   5th

   R93.81 Abnormal radiologic findings on diagnostic imaging of testicles
     6th
     R93.811 Abnormal radiologic findings on diagnostic imaging of right testicle
     R93.812 Abnormal radiologic findings on diagnostic imaging of left testicle
     R93.813 Abnormal radiologic findings on diagnostic imaging of testicles, bilateral
     R93.819 Abnormal radiologic findings on diagnostic imaging of unspecified testicle

   R93.89 Abnormal findings on diagnostic imaging of other specified body structures
     Abnormal finding by radioisotope localization of placenta
     Abnormal radiological finding in skin and subcutaneous tissue
     Mediastinal shift

R94 ABNORMAL RESULTS OF FUNCTION STUDIES
   4th *Includes:* abnormal results of radionuclide [radioisotope] uptake studies
     abnormal results of scintigraphy

R94.0 Abnormal results of function studies of central nervous system
   5th **R94.01 Abnormal electroencephalogram [EEG]**
     R94.02 Abnormal brain scan
     R94.09 Abnormal results of other function studies of central nervous system

R94.1 Abnormal results of function studies of peripheral nervous system and special senses
   5th
   R94.11 Abnormal results of function studies of eye
     6th
     R94.110 Abnormal electro-oculogram [EOG]
     R94.111 Abnormal electroretinogram[ERG]
       Abnormal retinal function study

     R94.112 Abnormal visually evoked potential [VEP]
     R94.113 Abnormal oculomotor study
     R94.118 Abnormal results of other function studies of eye

   R94.12 Abnormal results of function studies of ear and other special senses
     6th
     R94.120 Abnormal auditory function study
     R94.121 Abnormal vestibular function study
     R94.128 Abnormal results of other function studies of ear and other special senses

   R94.13 Abnormal results of function studies of peripheral nervous system
     6th
     R94.130 Abnormal response to nerve stimulation, unspecified
     R94.131 Abnormal electromyogram [EMG]
       Excludes1: electromyogram of eye (R94.113)
     R94.138 Abnormal results of other function studies of peripheral nervous system

R94.2 Abnormal results of pulmonary function studies
Reduced ventilatory capacity
Reduced vital capacity

R94.3 Abnormal results of cardiovascular function studies
   5th **R94.30 Abnormal result of cardiovascular function study, unspecified**
     R94.31 Abnormal electrocardiogram [ECG] [EKG]
       Excludes1: long QT syndrome (I45.81)
     R94.39 Abnormal result of other cardiovascular function study
       Abnormal electrophysiological intracardiac studies
       Abnormal phonocardiogram
       Abnormal vectorcardiogram

R94.4 Abnormal results of kidney function studies
Abnormal renal function test

R94.5 Abnormal results of liver function studies

R94.6 Abnormal results of thyroid function studies

R94.7 Abnormal results of other endocrine function studies
   Excludes2: abnormal glucose (R73.0-)

R94.8 Abnormal results of function studies of other organs and systems
Abnormal basal metabolic rate [BMR]
Abnormal bladder function test
Abnormal splenic function test

(R97) ABNORMAL TUMOR MARKERS

R97 ABNORMAL TUMOR MARKERS
   4th Elevated tumor associated antigens [TAA]
     Elevated tumor specific antigens [TSA]
   R97.0 Elevated carcinoembryonic antigen [CEA]
   R97.1 Elevated cancer antigen 125 [CA 125]
   R97.8 Other abnormal tumor markers

(R99) ILL-DEFINED AND UNKNOWN CAUSE OF MORTALITY

R99 ILL-DEFINED AND UNKNOWN CAUSE OF MORTALITY
   ✔ Code R99, Ill-defined and unknown cause of mortality, is only for use in the very limited circumstance when a patient who has already died is brought into an emergency department or other healthcare facility and is pronounced dead upon arrival. It does not represent the discharge disposition of death.
     Death (unexplained) NOS
     Unspecified cause of mortality

4th **5th** **6th** **7th** Additional Character Required   ✔ 3-character code

•=New Code
▲=Revised Code

Excludes1—Not coded here, do not use together
Excludes2—Not included here

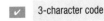

Chapter 19. Injury, poisoning and certain other consequences of external causes (S00–T88)

GUIDELINES

Application of 7th Characters in Chapter 19

Most categories in Chapter 19 have a 7th character requirement for each applicable code. Most categories in this chapter have three 7th character values (with the exception of fractures): A, initial encounter, D, subsequent encounter and S, sequela. Categories for traumatic fractures have additional 7th character values. While the patient may be seen by a new or different provider over the course of treatment for an injury, assignment of the 7th character is based on whether the patient is undergoing active treatment and not whether the provider is seeing the patient for the first time.

For complication codes, active treatment refers to treatment for the condition described by the code, even though it may be related to an earlier precipitating problem. For example, code T84.50XA, Infection and inflammatory reaction due to unspecified internal joint prosthesis, initial encounter, is used when active treatment is provided for the infection, even though the condition relates to the prosthetic device, implant or graft that was placed at a previous encounter.

7th character "A," initial encounter, is used while the patient is receiving active treatment for the condition. Examples of active treatment are: surgical treatment, emergency department encounter, and evaluation and continuing treatment by the same or a different physician.

7th character "D," subsequent encounter, is used for encounters after the patient has received active treatment of the condition and is receiving routine care for the condition during the healing or recovery phase. Examples of subsequent care are: cast change or removal, an x-ray to check healing status of fracture, removal of external or internal fixation device, medication adjustment, other aftercare and follow up visits following treatment of the injury or condition.

The aftercare Z codes should not be used for aftercare for conditions such as injuries or poisonings, where 7th characters are provided to identify subsequent care. For example, for aftercare of an injury, assign the acute injury code with the 7th character "D" (subsequent encounter).

7th character "S," sequela, is for use for complications or conditions that arise as a direct result of a condition, such as scar formation after a burn. The scars are sequelae of the burn. When using 7th character "S," it is necessary to use both the injury code that precipitated the sequela and the code for the sequela itself. The "S" is added only to the injury code, not the sequela code. The 7th character "S" identifies the injury responsible for the sequela. The specific type of sequela (eg, scar) is sequenced first, followed by the injury code.

An "X" may be listed at the end of the code to indicate a placeholder digit(s). The X will be required in order to get to the 7th character, which indicates the type of encounter. Be sure to use all indicated placeholder digits prior to the appropriate 7th character digit.

Coding of Injuries

When coding injuries, assign separate codes for each injury unless a combination code is provided, in which case the combination code is assigned. Codes from category T07, Unspecified multiple injuries should not be assigned in the inpatient setting unless information for a more specific code is not available. Traumatic injury codes (S00–T14.9) are not to be used for normal, healing surgical wounds or to identify complications of surgical wounds.

The code for the most serious injury, as determined by the provider and the focus of treatment, is sequenced first.

SUPERFICIAL INJURIES

Superficial injuries such as abrasions or contusions are not coded when associated with more severe injuries of the same site.

PRIMARY INJURY WITH DAMAGE TO NERVES/BLOOD VESSELS

When a primary injury results in minor damage to peripheral nerves or blood vessels, the primary injury is sequenced first with additional code(s) for injuries to nerves and spinal cord (such as category S04), and/or injury to blood vessels (such as category S15). When the primary injury is to the blood vessels or nerves, that injury should be sequenced first.

IATROGENIC INJURIES

Injury codes from Chapter 19 should not be assigned for injuries that occur during, or as a result of, a medical intervention. Assign the appropriate complication code(s).

Coding of Traumatic Fractures

The principles of multiple coding of injuries should be followed in coding fractures. Fractures of specified sites are coded individually by site in accordance with both the provisions within categories S02, S12, S22, S32, S42, S49, S52, S59, S62, S72, S79, S82, S89, S92 and the level of detail furnished by medical record content.

A fracture not indicated as open or closed should be coded to closed. A fracture not indicated whether displaced or not displaced should be coded to displaced.

More specific guidelines are as follows:

INITIAL VS. SUBSEQUENT ENCOUNTER FOR FRACTURES

Traumatic fractures are coded using the appropriate 7th character for initial encounter (A, B, C) while the patient is receiving active treatment for the fracture. Examples of active treatment are: surgical treatment, emergency department encounter, and evaluation and continuing (ongoing) treatment by the same or different physician. The appropriate 7th character for initial encounter should also be assigned for a patient who delayed seeking treatment for the fracture or nonunion. Fractures are coded using the appropriate 7th character for subsequent care for encounters after the patient has completed active treatment of the fracture and is receiving routine care for the fracture during the healing or recovery phase. Examples of fracture aftercare are: cast change or removal, an x-ray to check healing status of fracture, removal of external or internal fixation device, medication adjustment, and follow-up visits following fracture treatment.

Care for complications of surgical treatment for fracture repairs during the healing or recovery phase should be coded with the appropriate complication codes.

Care of complications of fractures, such as malunion and nonunion, should be reported with the appropriate 7th character for subsequent care with nonunion (K, M, N,) or subsequent care with malunion (P, Q, R).

Malunion/nonunion: The appropriate 7th character for initial encounter should also be assigned for a patient who delayed seeking treatment for the fracture or nonunion.

A code from category M80, not a traumatic fracture code, should be used for any patient with known osteoporosis who suffers a fracture, even if the patient had a minor fall or trauma, if that fall or trauma would not usually break a normal, healthy bone.

The aftercare Z codes should not be used for aftercare for traumatic fractures. For aftercare of a traumatic fracture, assign the acute fracture code with the appropriate 7th character.

MULTIPLE FRACTURES SEQUENCING

Multiple fractures are sequenced in accordance with the severity of the fracture.

PHYSEAL FRACTURES

For physeal fractures, assign only the code identifying the type of physeal fracture. Do not assign a separate code to identify the specific bone that is fractured.

Coding of Burns and Corrosions

Refer to category T20 for guidelines.

Adverse Effects, Poisoning, Underdosing and Toxic Effects

Refer to category T36 for guidelines.

Adult and Child Abuse, Neglect and Other Maltreatment

Refer to category T74 for guidelines.

Complications of care

GENERAL GUIDELINES FOR COMPLICATIONS OF CARE

See Section I.B.16 (page XVIII) for information on documentation of complications of care.

PAIN DUE TO MEDICAL DEVICES

Pain associated with devices, implants or grafts left in a surgical site (for example painful hip prosthesis) is assigned to the appropriate code(s) found in Chapter 19, Injury, poisoning, and certain other consequences of external causes. Specific codes for pain due to medical devices are found in the T code section of the *ICD-10-CM*. **Use additional code(s)** from category G89 to identify acute or chronic pain due to presence of the device, implant or graft (G89.18 or G89.28).

TRANSPLANT COMPLICATIONS

Transplant complications other than kidney

| 4th | 5th | 6th | 7th | Additional Character Required | ✔ | 3-character code | Unspecified laterality codes were excluded here. | • =New Code
▲ =Revised Code
☐ =Social determinants of health | ***Excludes1***—Not coded here, do not use together
Excludes2—Not included here |

CHAPTER 19. INJURY, POISONING AND CERTAIN OTHER CONSEQUENCES OF EXTERNAL CAUSES   (S00–S00.37X)

Please see category T86 for guidelines for complications of transplanted organs and tissue other than kidney.

Kidney transplant complications
Refer to code T86.1 for guidelines for complications of kidney transplant.

COMPLICATION CODES THAT INCLUDE THE EXTERNAL CAUSE
As with certain other T codes, some of the complications of care codes have the external cause included in the code. The code includes the nature of the complication as well as the type of procedure that caused the complication. No external cause code indicating the type of procedure is necessary for these codes.

COMPLICATIONS OF CARE CODES WITHIN THE BODY SYSTEM CHAPTERS
Intraoperative and postprocedural complication codes are found within the body system chapters with codes specific to the organs and structures of that body system. These codes should be sequenced first, followed by a code(s) for the specific complication, if applicable.

Note: Use secondary code(s) from Chapter 20, External causes of morbidity, to indicate cause of injury. Codes within the T-section that include the external cause do not require an additional external cause code
    Use additional code to identify any retained FB, if applicable (Z18.-)
Excludes1: birth trauma (P10–P15)
    obstetric trauma (O70–O71)

Note: The chapter uses the S-section for coding different types of injuries related to single body regions and the T-section to cover injuries to unspecified body regions as well as poisoning and certain other consequences of external causes.
    Most codes in Chapter 19 require the addition of 7th characters to form complete codes. Descriptors for 7th characters are provided in text boxes throughout the chapter.

(S00–S09) INJURIES TO THE HEAD

Includes: Injuries of ear
    injuries of eye
    injuries of face [any part]
    injuries of gum
    injuries of jaw
    injuries of oral cavity
    injuries of palate
    injuries of periocular area
    injuries of scalp
    injuries of temporomandibular joint area
    injuries of tongue
    injuries of tooth

> **7th characters for category S00**
> A—initial encounter
> D—subsequent encounter
> S—sequela

Code also for any associated infection
Excludes2: burns and corrosions (T20–T32)
    effects of FB in ear (T16)
    effects of FB in larynx (T17.3)
    effects of FB in mouth NOS (T18.0)
    effects of FB in nose (T17.0–T17.1)
    effects of FB in pharynx (T17.2)
    effects of FB on external eye (T15.-)
    frostbite (T33–T34)
    insect bite or sting, venomous (T63.4)

S00   **SUPERFICIAL INJURY OF HEAD**
[4th]   ***Excludes1:*** diffuse cerebral contusion (S06.2-)
    focal cerebral contusion (S06.3-)
    injury of eye and orbit (S05.-)
    open wound of head (S01.-)

    S00.0   **Superficial injury of scalp**
    [5th]   **S00.00X**   Unspecified superficial injury of scalp
        [7th]
        S00.01X   Abrasion of scalp
        [7th]
        S00.02X   Blister (nonthermal) of scalp
        [7th]
        S00.03X   Contusion of scalp
        [7th]   Bruise of scalp
             Hematoma of scalp
        S00.04X   External constriction of part of scalp
        [7th]
        S00.05X   Superficial FB of scalp
        [7th]   Splinter in the scalp

        S00.06X   Insect bite (nonvenomous) of scalp
        [7th]
        S00.07X   Other superficial bite of scalp
        [7th]   ***Excludes1:*** open bite of scalp (S01.05)

    S00.1   **Contusion of eyelid and periocular area**
    [5th]   Black eye
         Excludes2: contusion of eyeball and orbital tissues (S05.1)
        S00.10X   Contusion of unspecified eyelid and periocular area
        [7th]
        S00.11X   Contusion of right eyelid and periocular area
        [7th]
        S00.12X   Contusion of left eyelid and periocular area
        [7th]

    S00.2   **Other and unspecified superficial injuries of eyelid and periocular area**
    [5th]
         Excludes2: superficial injury of conjunctiva and cornea (S05.0-)
        S00.20   Unspecified superficial injury of eyelid and periocular area
        [6th]
            S00.201   Unspecified superficial injury of right eyelid and periocular area
            [7th]
            S00.202   Unspecified superficial injury of left eyelid and periocular area
            [7th]
         S00.21   Abrasion of eyelid and periocular area
         [6th]
            S00.211   Abrasion of right eyelid and periocular area
            [7th]
            S00.212   Abrasion of left eyelid and periocular area
            [7th]
         S00.22   Blister (nonthermal) of eyelid and periocular area
         [6th]
            S00.221   Blister (nonthermal) of right eyelid and periocular area
            [7th]
            S00.222   Blister (nonthermal) of left eyelid and periocular area
            [7th]
         S00.24   External constriction of eyelid and periocular area
         [6th]
            S00.241   External constriction of right eyelid and periocular area
            [7th]
            S00.242   External constriction of left eyelid and periocular area
            [7th]
         S00.25   Superficial FB of eyelid and periocular area
         [6th]   Splinter of eyelid and periocular area
             Excludes2: retained FB in eyelid (H02.81-)
            S00.251   Superficial FB of right eyelid and periocular area
            [7th]
            S00.252   Superficial FB of left eyelid and periocular area
            [7th]
         S00.26   Insect bite (nonvenomous) of eyelid and periocular area
         [6th]
            S00.261   Insect bite (nonvenomous) of right eyelid and periocular area
            [7th]
            S00.262   Insect bite (nonvenomous) of left eyelid and periocular area
            [7th]
         S00.27   Other superficial bite of eyelid and periocular area
         [6th]   ***Excludes1:*** open bite of eyelid and periocular area (S01.15)
            S00.271   Other superficial bite of right eyelid and periocular area
            [7th]
            S00.272   Other superficial bite of left eyelid and periocular area
            [7th]

    S00.3   **Superficial injury of nose**
    [5th]   **S00.30X**   Unspecified superficial injury of nose
        S00.31X   Abrasion of nose
        [7th]
        S00.32X   Blister (nonthermal) of nose
        [7th]
        S00.33X   Contusion of nose
        [7th]   Bruise of nose
             Hematoma of nose
        S00.34X   External constriction of nose
        [7th]
        S00.35X   Superficial FB of nose
        [7th]   Splinter in the nose
        S00.36X   Insect bite (nonvenomous) of nose
        [7th]
        S00.37X   Other superficial bite of nose
        [7th]   ***Excludes1:*** open bite of nose (S01.25)

[4th]   [5th]   [6th]   [7th]   Additional Character Required   ✓   3-character code   Unspecified laterality codes were excluded here.   • =New Code   ▲ =Revised Code   ¤ =Social determinants of health   ***Excludes1***—Not coded here, do not use together   ***Excludes2***—Not included here

S00.4   **Superficial injury of ear**
- `5th` **S00.40**   **Unspecified superficial injury of ear**
  - `6th` **S00.401**   **Unspecified superficial injury of right ear**
    - `7th`
  - **S00.402**   **Unspecified superficial injury of left ear**
    - `7th`
- **S00.41**   **Abrasion of ear**
  - `6th`
  - **S00.411**   **Abrasion of right ear**
    - `7th`
  - **S00.412**   **Abrasion of left ear**
    - `7th`

> **7th characters for category S00**
> A—initial encounter
> D—subsequent encounter
> S—sequela

- **S00.42**   **Blister (nonthermal) of ear**
  - `6th`
  - **S00.421**   **Blister (nonthermal) of right ear**
    - `7th`
  - **S00.422**   **Blister (nonthermal) of left ear**
    - `7th`
- **S00.43**   **Contusion of ear**
  - `6th`   Bruise of ear
  - Hematoma of ear
  - **S00.431**   **Contusion of right ear**
    - `7th`
  - **S00.432**   **Contusion of left ear**
    - `7th`
- **S00.44**   **External constriction of ear**
  - `6th`
  - **S00.441**   **External constriction of right ear**
    - `7th`
  - **S00.442**   **External constriction of left ear**
    - `7th`
- **S00.45**   **Superficial FB of ear**
  - `6th`   Splinter in the ear
  - **S00.451**   **Superficial FB of right ear**
    - `7th`
  - **S00.452**   **Superficial FB of left ear**
    - `7th`
- **S00.46**   **Insect bite (nonvenomous) of ear**
  - `6th`
  - **S00.461**   **Insect bite (nonvenomous) of right ear**
    - `7th`
  - **S00.462**   **Insect bite (nonvenomous) of left ear**
    - `7th`
- **S00.47**   **Other superficial bite of ear**
  - `6th`   *Excludes1:* open bite of ear (S01.35)
  - **S00.471**   **Other superficial bite of right ear**
    - `7th`
  - **S00.472**   **Other superficial bite of left ear**
    - `7th`

S00.5   **Superficial injury of lip and oral cavity**
- `5th` **S00.50**   **Unspecified superficial injury of lip and oral cavity**
  - `6th` **S00.501**   **Unspecified superficial injury of lip**
    - `7th`
  - **S00.502**   **Unspecified superficial injury of oral cavity**
    - `7th`
- **S00.51**   **Abrasion of lip and oral cavity**
  - `6th` **S00.511**   **Abrasion of lip**
    - `7th`
  - **S00.512**   **Abrasion of oral cavity**
    - `7th`
- **S00.52**   **Blister (nonthermal) of lip and oral cavity**
  - `6th` **S00.521**   **Blister (nonthermal) of lip**
    - `7th`
  - **S00.522**   **Blister (nonthermal) of oral cavity**
    - `7th`
- **S00.53**   **Contusion of lip and oral cavity**
  - `6th` **S00.531**   **Contusion of lip**
    - `7th`   Bruise of lip
    - Hematoma of lip
  - **S00.532**   **Contusion of oral cavity**
    - `7th`   Bruise of oral cavity
    - Hematoma of oral cavity
- **S00.54**   **External constriction of lip and oral cavity**
  - `6th` **S00.541**   **External constriction of lip**
    - `7th`
  - **S00.542**   **External constriction of oral cavity**
    - `7th`

S00.55   **Superficial FB of lip and oral cavity**
- `6th` **S00.551**   **Superficial FB of lip**
  - `7th`   Splinter of lip and oral cavity
- **S00.552**   **Superficial FB of oral cavity**
  - `7th`   Splinter of lip and oral cavity

S00.56   **Insect bite (nonvenomous) of lip and oral cavity**
- `6th` **S00.561**   **Insect bite (nonvenomous) of lip**
  - `7th`
- **S00.562**   **Insect bite (nonvenomous) of oral cavity**
  - `7th`

S00.57   **Other superficial bite of lip and oral cavity**
- `6th` **S00.571**   **Other superficial bite of lip**
  - `7th`   *Excludes1:* open bite of lip (S01.551)
- **S00.572**   **Other superficial bite of oral cavity**
  - `7th`   *Excludes1:* open bite of oral cavity (S01.552)

S00.8   **Superficial injury of other parts of head**
- `5th`   Superficial injuries of face [any part]
- **S00.80X**   **Unspecified superficial injury of other part of head**
  - `7th`
- **S00.81X**   **Abrasion of other part of head**
  - `7th`
- **S00.82X**   **Blister (nonthermal) of other part of head**
  - `7th`
- **S00.83X**   **Contusion of other part of head**
  - `7th`   Bruise of other part of head
  - Hematoma of other part of head
- **S00.84X**   **External constriction of other part of head**
  - `7th`
- **S00.85X**   **Superficial FB of other part of head**
  - `7th`   *Splinter in other part of head*
- **S00.86X**   **Insect bite (nonvenomous) of other part of head**
  - `7th`
- **S00.87X**   **Other superficial bite of other part of head**
  - `7th`   *Excludes1:* open bite of other part of head (S01.85)

S00.9   **Superficial injury of unspecified part of head**
- `5th` **S00.90X**   **Unspecified superficial injury of unspecified part of head**
  - `7th`
- **S00.91X**   **Abrasion of unspecified part of head**
  - `7th`
- **S00.92X**   **Blister (nonthermal) of unspecified part of head**
  - `7th`
- **S00.93X**   **Contusion of unspecified part of head**
  - `7th`   Bruise of head
  - Hematoma of head
- **S00.94X**   **External constriction of unspecified part of head**
  - `7th`
- **S00.95X**   **Superficial FB of unspecified part of head**
  - `7th`   Splinter of head
- **S00.96X**   **Insect bite (nonvenomous) of unspecified part of head**
  - `7th`
- **S00.97X**   **Other superficial bite of unspecified part of head**
  - `7th`   *Excludes1:* open bite of head (S01.95)

S01   **OPEN WOUND OF HEAD**
- `4th` **Code also** any associated:
  - injury of cranial nerve (S04.-)
  - injury of muscle and tendon of head (S09.1-)
  - intracranial injury (S06.-)
  - wound infection

> **7th characters for category S01**
> A—initial encounter
> D—subsequent encounter
> S—sequela

Excludes1: open skull fracture (S02.- with 7th character)
Excludes2: injury of eye and orbit (S05.-)
traumatic amputation of part of head (S08.-)

S01.0   **Open wound of scalp**
- `5th`   *Excludes1:* avulsion of scalp (S08.0)
- **S01.01X**   **Laceration without FB of scalp**
  - `7th`
- **S01.02X**   **Laceration with FB of scalp**
  - `7th`
- **S01.03X**   **Puncture wound without FB of scalp**
  - `7th`
- **S01.04X**   **Puncture wound with FB of scalp**
  - `7th`

`4th` `5th` `6th` `7th`   Additional Character Required   ✓   3-character code   Unspecified laterality codes were excluded here.

- • =New Code
- ▲ =Revised Code
- � =Social determinants of health

Excludes1—Not coded here, do not use together
Excludes2—Not included here

CHAPTER 19. INJURY, POISONING AND CERTAIN OTHER CONSEQUENCES OF EXTERNAL CAUSES   (S01.05X–S01.81X)

S01.05X   **Open bite of scalp**
[7th]   Bite of scalp NOS
    Excludes1: superficial bite of scalp (S00.06, S00.07-)

S01.1   **Open wound of eyelid and periocular area**
[5th]   Open wound of eyelid and periocular area with or without involvement of lacrimal passages

   S01.11   **Laceration without FB of eyelid and periocular area**
[6th]
     S01.111   **Laceration without FB of right eyelid and periocular area**
[7th]

> 7th characters for category S01
> A—initial encounter
> D—subsequent encounter
> S—sequela

     S01.112   **Laceration without FB of left eyelid and periocular area**
[7th]

   S01.12   **Laceration with FB of eyelid and periocular area**
[6th]
     S01.121   **Laceration with FB of right eyelid and periocular area**
[7th]
     S01.122   **Laceration with FB of left eyelid and periocular area**
[7th]

   S01.13   **Puncture wound without FB of eyelid and periocular area**
[6th]
     S01.131   **Puncture wound without FB of right eyelid and periocular area**
[7th]
     S01.132   **Puncture wound without FB of left eyelid and periocular area**
[7th]

   S01.14   **Puncture wound with FB of eyelid and periocular area**
[6th]
     S01.141   **Puncture wound with FB of right eyelid and periocular area**
[7th]
     S01.142   **Puncture wound with FB of left eyelid and periocular area**
[7th]

   S01.15   **Open bite of eyelid and periocular area**
[6th]
     Bite of eyelid and periocular area NOS
     Excludes1: superficial bite of eyelid and periocular area (S00.26, S00.27)
     S01.151   **Open bite of right eyelid and periocular area**
[7th]
     S01.152   **Open bite of left eyelid and periocular area**
[7th]

S01.2   **Open wound of nose**
[5th]
   S01.21X   **Laceration without FB of nose**
[7th]
   S01.22X   **Laceration with FB of nose**
[7th]
   S01.23X   **Puncture wound without FB of nose**
[7th]
   S01.24X   **Puncture wound with FB of nose**
[7th]
   S01.25X   **Open bite of nose**
[7th]
     Bite of nose NOS
     Excludes1: superficial bite of nose (S00.36, S00.37)

S01.3   **Open wound of ear**
[5th]
   S01.31   **Laceration without FB of ear**
[6th]
     S01.311   **Laceration without FB of right ear**
[7th]
     S01.312   **Laceration without FB of left ear**
[7th]
   S01.32   **Laceration with FB of ear**
[6th]
     S01.321   **Laceration with FB of right ear**
[7th]
     S01.322   **Laceration with FB of left ear**
[7th]
   S01.33   **Puncture wound without FB of ear**
[6th]
     S01.331   **Puncture wound without FB of right ear**
[7th]
     S01.332   **Puncture wound without FB of left ear**
[7th]
   S01.34   **Puncture wound with FB of ear**
[6th]
     S01.341   **Puncture wound with FB of right ear**
[7th]
     S01.342   **Puncture wound with FB of left ear**
[7th]

S01.35   **Open bite of ear**
[6th]
   Bite of ear NOS
   Excludes1: superficial bite of ear (S00.46, S00.47)
   S01.351   **Open bite of right ear**
[7th]
   S01.352   **Open bite of left ear**
[7th]

S01.4   **Open wound of cheek and temporomandibular area**
[5th]
   S01.41   **Laceration without FB of cheek and temporomandibular area**
[6th]
     S01.411   **Laceration without FB of right cheek and temporomandibular area**
[7th]
     S01.412   **Laceration without FB of left cheek and temporomandibular area**
[7th]
   S01.42   **Laceration with FB of cheek and temporomandibular area**
[6th]
     S01.421   **Laceration with FB of right cheek and temporomandibular area**
[7th]
     S01.422   **Laceration with FB of left cheek and temporomandibular area**
[7th]
   S01.43   **Puncture wound without FB of cheek and temporomandibular area**
[6th]
     S01.431   **Puncture wound without FB of right cheek and temporomandibular area**
[7th]
     S01.432   **Puncture wound without FB of left cheek and temporomandibular area**
[7th]
   S01.44   **Puncture wound with FB of cheek and temporomandibular area**
[6th]
     S01.441   **Puncture wound with FB of right cheek and temporomandibular area**
[7th]
     S01.442   **Puncture wound with FB of left cheek and temporomandibular area**
[7th]
   S01.45   **Open bite of cheek and temporomandibular area**
[6th]
     Bite of cheek and temporomandibular area NOS
     Excludes2: superficial bite of cheek and temporomandibular area (S00.86, S00.87)
     S01.451   **Open bite of right cheek and temporomandibular area**
[7th]
     S01.452   **Open bite of left cheek and temporomandibular area**
[7th]

S01.5   **Open wound of lip and oral cavity**
[5th]
   Excludes2: tooth dislocation (S03.2)
     tooth fracture (S02.5)
   S01.51   **Laceration of lip and oral cavity without FB**
[6th]
     S01.511   **Laceration without FB of lip**
[7th]
     S01.512   **Laceration without FB of oral cavity**
[7th]
   S01.52   **Laceration of lip and oral cavity with FB**
[6th]
     S01.521   **Laceration with FB of lip**
[7th]
     S01.522   **Laceration with FB of oral cavity**
[7th]
   S01.53   **Puncture wound of lip and oral cavity without FB**
[6th]
     S01.531   **Puncture wound without FB of lip**
[7th]
     S01.532   **Puncture wound without FB of oral cavity**
[7th]
   S01.54   **Puncture wound of lip and oral cavity with FB**
[6th]
     S01.541   **Puncture wound with FB of lip**
[7th]
     S01.542   **Puncture wound with FB of oral cavity**
[7th]
   S01.55   **Open bite of lip and oral cavity**
[6th]
     S01.551   **Open bite of lip**
[7th]
      Bite of lip NOS
      Excludes1: superficial bite of lip (S00.571)
     S01.552   **Open bite of oral cavity**
[7th]
      Bite of oral cavity NOS
      Excludes1: superficial bite of oral cavity (S00.572)

S01.8   **Open wound of other parts of head**
[5th]
   S01.81X   **Laceration without FB of other part of head**
[7th]

[4th] [5th] [6th] [7th]   Additional Character Required   [✔]   3-character code   Unspecified laterality codes were excluded here.

•=New Code
▲=Revised Code
�=Social determinants of health

Excludes1—Not coded here, do not use together
Excludes2—Not included here

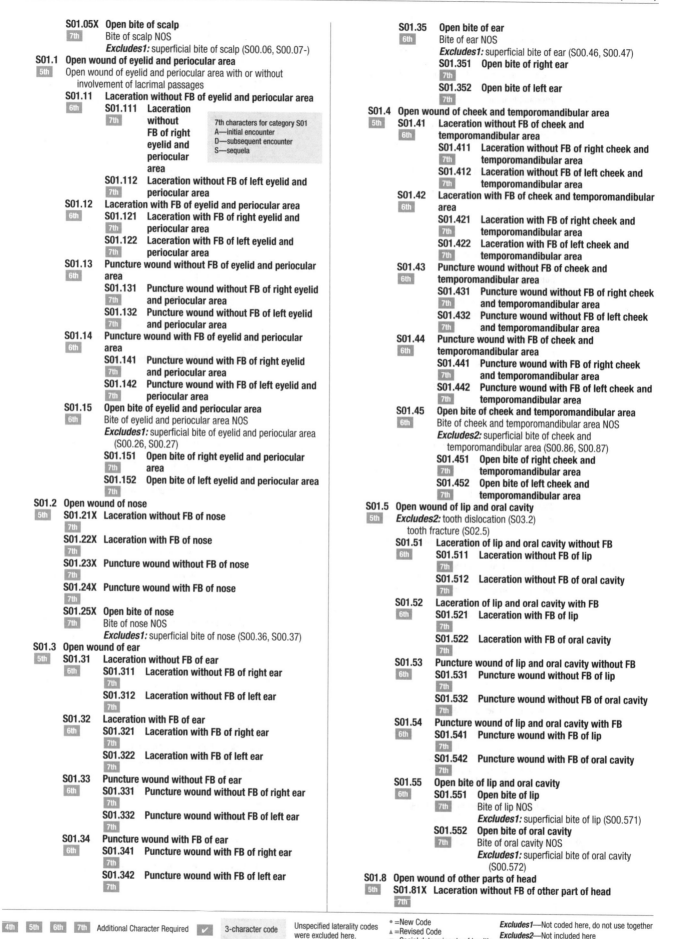

S01.82X Laceration with FB of other part of head
[7th]

S01.83X Puncture wound without FB of other part of head
[7th]

S01.84X Puncture wound with FB of other part of head
[7th]

S01.85X Open bite of other part of head
[7th]
Bite of other part of head NOS
Excludes1: superficial bite of other part of head (S00.87)

> 7th characters for category S01
> A—initial encounter
> D—subsequent encounter
> S—sequela

S01.9 Open wound of unspecified part of head
[5th]

S01.90X Unspecified open wound of unspecified part of head
[7th]

S01.91X Laceration without FB of unspecified part of head
[7th]

S01.92X Laceration with FB of unspecified part of head
[7th]

S01.93X Puncture wound without FB of unspecified part of head
[7th]

S01.94X Puncture wound with FB of unspecified part of head
[7th]

S01.95X Open bite of unspecified part of head
[7th]
Bite of head NOS
Excludes1: superficial bite of head NOS (S00.97)

S02 **FRACTURE OF SKULL AND FACIAL BONES**
[4th]
Note: A fracture not indicated as open or closed should be coded to closed
Code also any associated intracranial injury (S06.-)

S02.0 Fracture of vault of skull
Fracture of frontal bone
Fracture of parietal bone

S02.1 Fracture of base of skull
[5th]
Excludes2: lateral orbital wall (S02.84-)
medial orbital wall (S02.83-)
orbital floor (S02.3-)

> 7th characters for category S02
> A—initial encounter for closed fracture
> B—initial encounter for open fracture
> D—subsequent encounter for fracture with routine healing
> G—subsequent encounter for fracture with delayed healing
> K—subsequent encounter for fracture with nonunion
> S—sequela

S02.101 Fracture of base of skull, right side
[7th]

S02.102 Fracture of base of skull, left side
[7th]

S02.109 Fracture of base of skull, unspecified side
[7th]

S02.11 Fracture of occiput
[6th]

S02.111 Type II occipital condyle fracture, unspecified side
[7th]

S02.112 Type III occipital condyle fracture, unspecified side
[7th]

S02.113 Unspecified occipital condyle fracture
[7th]

S02.118 Other fracture of occiput, unspecified side
[7th]

S02.119 Unspecified fracture of occiput
[7th]

S02.11A Type I occipital condyle fracture, right side
[7th]

S02.11B Type I occipital condyle fracture, left side
[7th]

S02.11C Type II occipital condyle fracture, right side
[7th]

S02.11D Type II occipital condyle fracture, left side
[7th]

S02.11E Type III occipital condyle fracture, right side
[7th]

S02.11F Type III occipital condyle fracture, left side
[7th]

S02.11G Other fracture of occiput, right side
[7th]

S02.11H Other fracture of occiput, left side
[7th]

S02.12 Fracture of orbital roof

S02.121 Fracture of orbital roof, right side, closed fracture
[7th]

S02.122 Fracture of orbital roof, left side, closed fracture
[7th]

S02.129 Fracture of orbital roof, unspecified side, closed fracture
[7th]

S02.19X Other fracture of base of skull
[7th]
Fracture of anterior fossa of base of skull
Fracture of ethmoid or frontal sinus
Fracture of middle fossa of base of skull
Fracture of orbital roof
Fracture of posterior fossa of base of skull
Fracture of sphenoid
Fracture of temporal bone

S02.2XX Fracture of nasal bones
[7th]

S02.3 Fracture of orbital floor
[5th]
Fracture of inferior orbital wall
Excludes1: orbit NOS (S02.85)
Excludes2: lateral orbital wall (S02.84-)
medial orbital wall (S02.83-)
orbital roof (S02.1-)

S02.30X Fracture of orbital floor, unspecified side
[7th]
Excludes1: orbit NOS (S02.85)
Excludes2: orbital roof (S02.1-)

S02.31X Fracture of orbital floor, right side
[7th]
Excludes1: orbit NOS (S02.8)
Excludes2: orbital roof (S02.1-)

S02.32X Fracture of orbital floor, left side
[7th]
Excludes1: orbit NOS (S02.8)
Excludes2: orbital roof (S02.1-)

S02.4 Fracture of malar, maxillary and zygoma bones
[5th]
Fracture of superior maxilla
Fracture of upper jaw (bone)
Fracture of zygomatic process of temporal bone

S02.40 Fracture of malar, maxillary and zygoma bones, unspecified
[6th]

S02.400 Malar fracture, unspecified side
[7th]

S02.401 Maxillary fracture, unspecified side
[7th]

S02.402 Zygomatic fracture, unspecified side
[7th]

S02.40A Malar fracture, right side
[7th]

S02.40B Malar fracture, left side
[7th]

S02.40C Maxillary fracture, right side
[7th]

S02.40D Maxillary fracture, left side
[7th]

S02.40E Zygomatic fracture, right side
[7th]

S02.40F Zygomatic fracture, left side
[7th]

S02.5XX Fracture of tooth (traumatic)
[7th]
Broken tooth
Excludes1: cracked tooth (nontraumatic) (K03.81)

S02.6 Fracture of mandible
[5th]
Fracture of lower jaw (bone)

S02.60 Fracture of mandible, unspecified
[6th]

S02.600 Fracture of unspecified part of body of mandible, unspecified side
[7th]

S02.601 Fracture of unspecified part of body of right mandible
[7th]

S02.602 Fracture of unspecified part of body of left mandible
[7th]

S02.609 Fracture of mandible, unspecified
[7th]

S02.61 Fracture of condylar process of mandible
[6th]

S02.610 Fracture of condylar process of mandible, unspecified side
[7th]

[4th] [5th] [6th] [7th] Additional Character Required | ✓ 3-character code | Unspecified laterality codes were excluded here.

• =New Code
▲ =Revised Code
▫ =Social determinants of health

Excludes1—Not coded here, do not use together
Excludes2—Not included here

PEDIATRIC ICD-10-CM 2021: A MANUAL FOR PROVIDER-BASED CODING

329

CHAPTER 19. INJURY, POISONING AND CERTAIN OTHER CONSEQUENCES OF EXTERNAL CAUSES (S01.82X–S02.610)

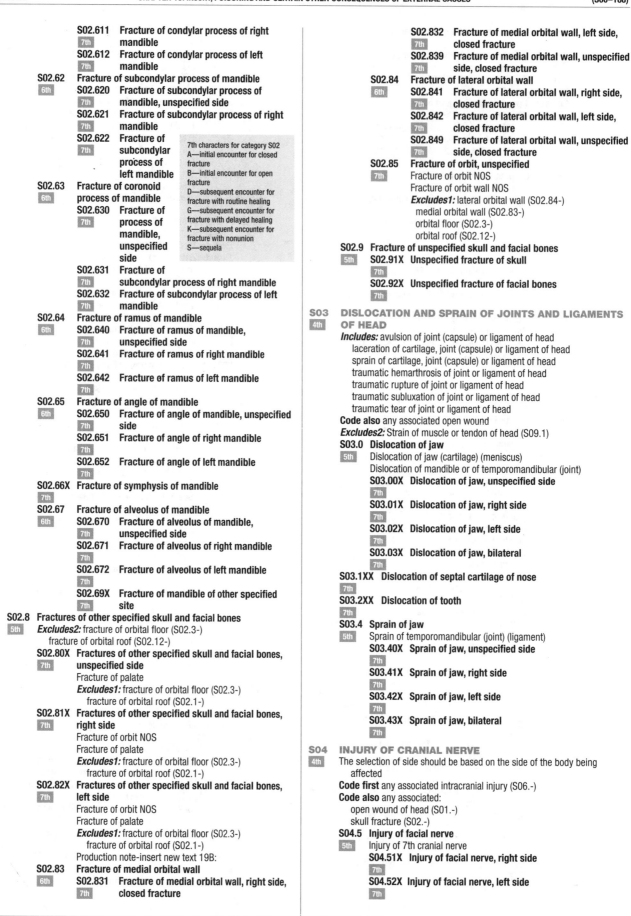

S02.611 [7th] **Fracture of condylar process of right mandible**

S02.612 [7th] **Fracture of condylar process of left mandible**

S02.62 [6th] **Fracture of subcondylar process of mandible**

S02.620 [7th] **Fracture of subcondylar process of mandible, unspecified side**

S02.621 [7th] **Fracture of subcondylar process of right mandible**

S02.622 [7th] **Fracture of subcondylar process of left mandible**

> 7th characters for category S02
> A—initial encounter for closed fracture
> B—initial encounter for open fracture
> D—subsequent encounter for fracture with routine healing
> G—subsequent encounter for fracture with delayed healing
> K—subsequent encounter for fracture with nonunion
> S—sequela

S02.63 [6th] **Fracture of coronoid process of mandible**

S02.630 [7th] **Fracture of process of mandible, unspecified side**

S02.631 [7th] **Fracture of subcondylar process of right mandible**

S02.632 [7th] **Fracture of subcondylar process of left mandible**

S02.64 [6th] **Fracture of ramus of mandible**

S02.640 [7th] **Fracture of ramus of mandible, unspecified side**

S02.641 [7th] **Fracture of ramus of right mandible**

S02.642 [7th] **Fracture of ramus of left mandible**

S02.65 [6th] **Fracture of angle of mandible**

S02.650 [7th] **Fracture of angle of mandible, unspecified side**

S02.651 [7th] **Fracture of angle of right mandible**

S02.652 [7th] **Fracture of angle of left mandible**

S02.66X [7th] **Fracture of symphysis of mandible**

S02.67 [6th] **Fracture of alveolus of mandible**

S02.670 [7th] **Fracture of alveolus of mandible, unspecified side**

S02.671 [7th] **Fracture of alveolus of right mandible**

S02.672 [7th] **Fracture of alveolus of left mandible**

S02.69X [7th] **Fracture of mandible of other specified site**

S02.8 [5th] **Fractures of other specified skull and facial bones**

Excludes2: fracture of orbital floor (S02.3-)
fracture of orbital roof (S02.12-)

S02.80X [7th] **Fractures of other specified skull and facial bones, unspecified side**
Fracture of palate
Excludes1: fracture of orbital floor (S02.3-)
fracture of orbital roof (S02.1-)

S02.81X [7th] **Fractures of other specified skull and facial bones, right side**
Fracture of orbit NOS
Fracture of palate
Excludes1: fracture of orbital floor (S02.3-)
fracture of orbital roof (S02.1-)

S02.82X [7th] **Fractures of other specified skull and facial bones, left side**
Fracture of orbit NOS
Fracture of palate
Excludes1: fracture of orbital floor (S02.3-)
fracture of orbital roof (S02.1-)
Production note-insert new text 19B:

S02.83 [6th] **Fracture of medial orbital wall**

S02.831 [7th] **Fracture of medial orbital wall, right side, closed fracture**

S02.832 [7th] **Fracture of medial orbital wall, left side, closed fracture**

S02.839 [7th] **Fracture of medial orbital wall, unspecified side, closed fracture**

S02.84 [6th] **Fracture of lateral orbital wall**

S02.841 [7th] **Fracture of lateral orbital wall, right side, closed fracture**

S02.842 [7th] **Fracture of lateral orbital wall, left side, closed fracture**

S02.849 [7th] **Fracture of lateral orbital wall, unspecified side, closed fracture**

S02.85 [7th] **Fracture of orbit, unspecified**
Fracture of orbit NOS
Fracture of orbit wall NOS
Excludes1: lateral orbital wall (S02.84-)
medial orbital wall (S02.83-)
orbital floor (S02.3-)
orbital roof (S02.12-)

S02.9 **Fracture of unspecified skull and facial bones**

S02.91X [5th] [7th] **Unspecified fracture of skull**

S02.92X [7th] **Unspecified fracture of facial bones**

S03 [4th] **DISLOCATION AND SPRAIN OF JOINTS AND LIGAMENTS OF HEAD**
Includes: avulsion of joint (capsule) or ligament of head
laceration of cartilage, joint (capsule) or ligament of head
sprain of cartilage, joint (capsule) or ligament of head
traumatic hemarthrosis of joint or ligament of head
traumatic rupture of joint or ligament of head
traumatic subluxation of joint or ligament of head
traumatic tear of joint or ligament of head
Code also any associated open wound
Excludes2: Strain of muscle or tendon of head (S09.1)

S03.0 [5th] **Dislocation of jaw**
Dislocation of jaw (cartilage) (meniscus)
Dislocation of mandible or of temporomandibular (joint)

S03.00X [7th] **Dislocation of jaw, unspecified side**

S03.01X [7th] **Dislocation of jaw, right side**

S03.02X [7th] **Dislocation of jaw, left side**

S03.03X [7th] **Dislocation of jaw, bilateral**

S03.1XX [7th] **Dislocation of septal cartilage of nose**

S03.2XX [7th] **Dislocation of tooth**

S03.4 [5th] **Sprain of jaw**
Sprain of temporomandibular (joint) (ligament)

S03.40X [7th] **Sprain of jaw, unspecified side**

S03.41X [7th] **Sprain of jaw, right side**

S03.42X [7th] **Sprain of jaw, left side**

S03.43X [7th] **Sprain of jaw, bilateral**

S04 [4th] **INJURY OF CRANIAL NERVE**
The selection of side should be based on the side of the body being affected
Code first any associated intracranial injury (S06.-)
Code also any associated:
open wound of head (S01.-)
skull fracture (S02.-)

S04.5 [5th] **Injury of facial nerve**
Injury of 7th cranial nerve

S04.51X [7th] **Injury of facial nerve, right side**

S04.52X [7th] **Injury of facial nerve, left side**

| [4th] | [5th] | [6th] | [7th] | Additional Character Required | ✓ | 3-character code | Unspecified laterality codes were excluded here. | • =New Code ▲ =Revised Code ▢ =Social determinants of health | *Excludes1*—Not coded here, do not use together *Excludes2*—Not included here |

S05   INJURY OF EYE AND ORBIT
4th

Includes: open wound of eye and orbit
Excludes2: 2nd cranial [optic] nerve injury
    (S04.0-)
    3rd cranial [oculomotor] nerve injury
    (S04.1-)
    open wound of eyelid and periocular
    area (S01.1-)
    orbital bone fracture (S02.1-, S02.3-, S02.8-)
    superficial injury of eyelid (S00.1–S00.2)

7th characters for categories
S05 & S06
A—initial encounter
D—subsequent encounter
S—sequela

S05.0   Injury of conjunctiva and corneal abrasion without FB
5th
Excludes1: FB in conjunctival sac
    (T15.1)
    FB in cornea (T15.0)

S05.01X Injury of conjunctiva and corneal abrasion without
7th   FB, right eye

S05.02X Injury of conjunctiva and corneal abrasion without
7th   FB, left eye

S05.1   Contusion of eyeball and orbital tissues
5th
Traumatic hyphema
Excludes2: black eye NOS (S00.1)
    contusion of eyelid and periocular area (S00.1)

S05.11X Contusion of eyeball and orbital tissues, right eye
7th

S05.12X Contusion of eyeball and orbital tissues, left eye
7th

S05.8   Other injuries of eye and orbit
5th
Lacrimal duct injury

S05.8X   Other injuries of eye and orbit
6th
    S05.8X1   Other injuries of right eye and orbit
    7th

    S05.8X2   Other injuries of left eye and orbit
    7th

S05.9   Unspecified injury of eye and orbit
5th
Injury of eye NOS

S05.91X Unspecified injury of right eye and orbit
7th

S05.92X Unspecified injury of left eye and orbit
7th

S06   INTRACRANIAL INJURY
4th

Includes: traumatic brain injury
Code also any associated:
    open wound of head (S01.-)
    skull fracture (S02.-)
Excludes1: head injury NOS (S09.90)

7th characters for categories
S05 & S06
A—initial encounter
D—subsequent encounter
S—sequela

S06.0   Concussion
5th
Commotio cerebri
Excludes1: concussion with other intracranial injuries classified in
    subcategories S06.1- to S06.6-, S06.81- and S06.82- code to
    specified intracranial injury

S06.0X   Concussion
6th
    S06.0X0   Concussion without LOC
    7th

    S06.0X1   Concussion with LOC of 30 min or less
    7th

    S06.0X9   Concussion with LOC unspecified duration
    7th   Concussion NOS

S06.3   Focal traumatic brain injury
5th
Excludes1: any condition classifiable to S06.4–S06.6
Excludes2: focal cerebral edema (S06.1)

S06.30   Unspecified focal traumatic brain injury
    S06.300   Unspecified focal traumatic brain injury
    7th   without LOC
    S06.301   Unspecified focal traumatic brain injury
    7th   with LOC of; 30 min or less
    S06.302   31 min to
    7th   59 min
    S06.303   1 hour to
    7th   5 h 59 min
    S06.304   6 h to 24 h
    7th
    S06.305   greater than 24 h with return to pre-
    7th   existing conscious level

S06.306   greater than 24 h without return to pre-
7th   existing conscious level with patient
    surviving
S06.307A   any duration with death due to brain
    injury prior to regaining consciousness
S06.308A   any duration with death due to other
    cause prior to regaining consciousness
S06.309   unspecified duration
7th   Unspecified focal traumatic brain injury NOS

S06.31   Contusion and laceration of right cerebrum
6th
    S06.310   Contusion and laceration of right
    7th   cerebrum without loss of consciousness
    S06.311   Contusion and laceration of right
    7th   cerebrum with LOC of; 30 min or less
    S06.312   31 min to 59 min
    7th
    S06.313   1 hour to 5 h 59 min
    7th
    S06.314   6 h to 24 h
    7th
    S06.315   greater than 24 h with return to pre-
    7th   existing conscious level
    S06.316   greater than 24 h without return to pre-
    7th   existing conscious level with patient
    surviving
    S06.317A   any duration with death
        due to brain injury prior to
        regaining consciousness
    S06.318A   any duration with death
        due to other cause prior to
        regaining consciousness
    S06.319   unspecified duration
    7th   Contusion and laceration of right cerebrum
        NOS

S06.32   Contusion and laceration of left cerebrum
6th
    S06.320   Contusion and laceration of left cerebrum
    7th   without loss of consciousness
    S06.321   Contusion and laceration of left cerebrum
    7th   with LOC of; 30 min or less
    S06.322   31 min to 59 min
    7th
    S06.323   1 hour to 5 h 59 min
    7th
    S06.324   6 h to 24 h
    7th
    S06.325   greater than 24 h with return to pre-
    7th   existing conscious level
    S06.326   greater than 24 h without return to pre-
    7th   existing conscious level with patient
    surviving
    S06.327A   any duration with death due to brain
        injury prior to regaining consciousness
    S06.328A   any duration with death due to other
        cause prior to regaining consciousness
    S06.329   unspecified duration
    7th   Contusion and laceration of left cerebrum
        NOS

S06.34   Traumatic hemorrhage of right cerebrum
6th
Traumatic intracerebral hemorrhage and hematoma of
right cerebrum
    S06.340   Traumatic hemorrhage of right cerebrum
    7th   without LOC
    S06.341   Traumatic hemorrhage of right cerebrum
    7th   with LOC of; 30 min or less
    S06.342   31 min to 59 min
    7th
    S06.343   1 h to 5 h 59 min
    7th
    S06.344   6 h to 24 h
    7th
    S06.345   greater than 24 h with return to pre-
    7th   existing conscious level

4th	**5th**	**6th**	**7th**	Additional Character Required	✔	3-character code

Unspecified laterality codes
were excluded here.

• =New Code
▲ =Revised Code
▢ =Social determinants of health

Excludes1—Not coded here, do not use together
Excludes2—Not included here

S06.346 greater than 24 h without return to pre-existing conscious level with patient surviving
[7th]

S06.347A any duration with death due to brain injury prior to regaining consciousness

> 7th characters for categories S06
> A—initial encounter
> D—subsequent encounter
> S—sequela

S06.348A any duration with death due to other cause prior to regaining consciousness

S06.349 unspecified duration
[7th] Traumatic hemorrhage of right cerebrum NOS

S06.35 Traumatic hemorrhage of left cerebrum
[6th] Traumatic intracerebral hemorrhage and hematoma of left cerebrum

S06.350 Traumatic hemorrhage of left cerebrum without LOC
[7th]

S06.351 Traumatic hemorrhage of left cerebrum with LOC of; 30 min or less
[7th]

S06.352 31 min to 59 min
[7th]

S06.353 1 h to 5 h 59 min
[7th]

S06.354 6 h to 24 h
[7th]

S06.355 greater than 24 h with return to pre-existing conscious level
[7th]

S06.356 greater than 24 h without return to pre-existing conscious level with patient surviving
[7th]

S06.357A any duration with death due to brain injury prior to regaining consciousness

S06.358A any duration with death due to other cause prior to regaining consciousness

S06.359 unspecified duration
[7th] Traumatic hemorrhage of left cerebrum NOS

S06.37 Contusion, laceration, and hemorrhage of cerebellum
[6th]

S06.370 Contusion, laceration, and hemorrhage of cerebellum without LOC
[7th]

S06.371 Contusion, laceration, and hemorrhage of cerebellum with LOC of; 30 min or less
[7th]

S06.372 31 min to 59 min
[7th]

S06.373 1 hour to 5 h 59 min
[7th]

S06.374 6 h to 24 h
[7th]

S06.375 greater than 24 h with return to pre-existing conscious level
[7th]

S06.376 greater than 24 h without return to pre-existing conscious level with patient surviving
[7th]

S06.377A any duration with death due to brain injury prior to regaining consciousness

S06.378A any duration with death due to other cause prior to regaining consciousness

S06.379 unspecified duration
[7th] Contusion, laceration, and hemorrhage of cerebellum NOS

S06.38 Contusion, laceration, and hemorrhage of brainstem
[6th]

S06.380 Contusion, laceration, and hemorrhage of brainstem without LOC
[7th]

S06.381 Contusion, laceration, and hemorrhage of brainstem with LOC of; 30 min or less
[7th]

S06.382 31 min to 59 min
[7th]

S06.383 1 hour to 5 h 59 min
[7th]

S06.384 6 h to 24 h
[7th]

S06.385 greater than 24 h with return to pre-existing conscious level
[7th]

S06.386 greater than 24 h without return to pre-existing conscious level with patient surviving
[7th]

S06.387A any duration with death due to brain injury prior to regaining consciousness

S06.388A any duration with death due to other cause prior to regaining consciousness

S06.389 unspecified duration
[7th] Contusion, laceration, and hemorrhage of brainstem NOS

S06.4 Epidural hemorrhage
[5th] Extradural hemorrhage NOS
Extradural hemorrhage (traumatic)

S06.4X Epidural hemorrhage
[6th]

S06.4X0 Epidural hemorrhage without loss of consciousness
[7th]

S06.4X1 Epidural hemorrhage with loss of consciousness of 30 minutes or less
[7th]

S06.4X2 Epidural hemorrhage with loss of consciousness of 31 minutes to 59 minutes
[7th]

S06.4X3 Epidural hemorrhage with loss of consciousness of 1 hour to 5 hours 59 minutes
[7th]

S06.4X4 Epidural hemorrhage with loss of consciousness of 6 hours to 24 hours
[7th]

S06.4X5 Epidural hemorrhage with loss of consciousness greater than 24 hours with return to pre-existing conscious level
[7th]

S06.4X6 Epidural hemorrhage with loss of consciousness greater than 24 hours without return to pre-existing conscious level with patient surviving
[7th]

S06.4X7A Epidural hemorrhage with loss of consciousness of any duration with death due to brain injury prior to regaining consciousness

S06.4X8A Epidural hemorrhage with loss of consciousness of any duration with death due to other causes prior to regaining consciousness

S06.4X9 Epidural hemorrhage with loss of consciousness of unspecified duration
[7th] Epidural hemorrhage NOS

S06.5 Traumatic subdural hemorrhage
[5th]

S06.5X Traumatic subdural hemorrhage
[6th]

S06.5X0 Traumatic subdural hemorrhage without LOC
[7th]

S06.5X1 Traumatic subdural hemorrhage with LOC of; 30 min or less
[7th]

S06.5X2 31 min to 59 min
[7th]

S06.5X3 1 hour to 5 h 59 min
[7th]

S06.5X4 6 h to 24 h
[7th]

S06.5X5 greater than 24 h with return to pre-existing conscious level
[7th]

S06.5X6 greater than 24 h without return to pre-existing conscious level with patient surviving
[7th]

S06.5X7A any duration with death due to brain injury before regaining consciousness

S06.5X8A any duration with death due to other cause before regaining consciousness

S06.5X9 unspecified duration
[7th] Traumatic subdural hemorrhage NOS

S06.6 Traumatic subarachnoid hemorrhage
[5th]

S06.6X Traumatic subarachnoid hemorrhage
[6th]

S06.6X0 Traumatic subarachnoid hemorrhage without LOC
[7th]

S06.6X1 Traumatic subarachnoid hemorrhage with LOC of; 30 min or less
[7th]

[4th] [5th] [6th] [7th] Additional Character Required   ✔ 3-character code   Unspecified laterality codes were excluded here.

• =New Code
▲ =Revised Code
▫ =Social determinants of health

Excludes1—Not coded here, do not use together
Excludes2—Not included here

S06.6X2 31 min to 59 min
<small>7th</small>

S06.6X3 1 hour to 5 h 59 min
<small>7th</small>

S06.6X4 6 h to 24 h
<small>7th</small>

S06.6X5	greater	7th characters for categories S06
<small>7th</small>	than 24 h	A—initial encounter
	with return	D—subsequent encounter
	to pre-existing conscious level	S—sequela

S06.6X6 greater than 24 h without return to pre-
<small>7th</small>   existing conscious level with patient
          surviving

S06.6X7A any duration with death due to brain
          injury prior to regaining consciousness

S06.6X8A any duration with death due to other
          cause prior to regaining consciousness

S06.6X9 unspecified duration
<small>7th</small>   Traumatic subarachnoid hemorrhage NOS

S06.8 **Other specified intracranial injuries**
<small>5th</small>
      S06.89 **Other specified intracranial injury**
<small>6th</small>
          Excludes1: concussion (S06.0X-)
          S06.890 **Other specified intracranial injury without**
<small>7th</small>   **LOC**
          S06.891 **Other specified intracranial injury with**
<small>7th</small>   **LOC of 30 min or less**
          S06.892 **Other specified intracranial injury with**
<small>7th</small>   **LOC of; 31 min to 59 min**
          S06.893 **1 hour to 5 h 59 min**
<small>7th</small>

          S06.894 **6 h to 24 h**
<small>7th</small>

          S06.895 **greater than 24 h with return to pre-**
<small>7th</small>   **existing conscious level**
          S06.896 **greater than 24 h without return to pre-**
<small>7th</small>   **existing conscious level with patient**
              surviving
          S06.897A **any duration with death due to brain**
              injury prior to regaining consciousness
          S06.898A **any duration with death due to other**
              cause prior to regaining consciousness
          S06.899 **unspecified duration**
<small>7th</small>

S06.9 **Unspecified intracranial injury**
<small>5th</small>
      Brain injury NOS
      Head injury NOS with LOC
      Traumatic brain injury NOS
      Excludes1: conditions classifiable to S06.0- to S06.8- code to
          specified intracranial injury
        head injury NOS (S09.90)
      S06.9X **Unspecified intracranial injury**
<small>6th</small>
          S06.9X0 **Unspecified intracranial injury without**
<small>7th</small>   **LOC**
          S06.9X1 **Unspecified intracranial injury with LOC**
<small>7th</small>   **of; 30 min or less**
          S06.9X2 **31 min to 59 min**
<small>7th</small>

          S06.9X3 **1 hour to 5 h 59 min**
<small>7th</small>

          S06.9X4 **6 h to 24 h**
<small>7th</small>

          S06.9X5 **greater than 24 h with return to pre-**
<small>7th</small>   **existing conscious level**
          S06.9X6 **greater than 24 h without return to pre-**
<small>7th</small>   **existing conscious level with patient**
              surviving
          S06.9X7A **any duration with death due to brain**
              injury prior to regaining consciousness
          S06.9X8A **any duration with death due to other**
              cause prior to regaining consciousness
          S06.9X9 **unspecified duration**
<small>7th</small>

S09 **OTHER AND UNSPECIFIED INJURIES OF HEAD**
<small>4th</small>
      S09.0 **Injury of blood vessels of head, NEC**
          Excludes1: injury of cerebral blood
              vessels (S06.-)
            injury of precerebral blood
              vessels (S15.-)

	7th characters for categories S09
	A—initial encounter
	D—subsequent encounter
	S—sequela

      S09.1 **Injury of muscle and tendon**
<small>5th</small>   **of head**
          Code also any associated open wound (S01.-)
          Excludes2: sprain to joints and ligament of head (S03.9)
          S09.10X **Unspecified injury of muscle and tendon of head**
<small>7th</small>   Injury of muscle and tendon of head NOS
          S09.11X **Strain of muscle and tendon of head**
<small>7th</small>

          S09.12X **Laceration of muscle and tendon of head**
<small>7th</small>

          S09.19X **Other specified injury of muscle and tendon of head**
<small>7th</small>

      S09.2 **Traumatic rupture of ear drum**
<small>5th</small>
          Excludes1: traumatic rupture of ear drum due to blast injury
              (S09.31-)
          S09.21X **Traumatic rupture of right ear drum**
<small>7th</small>

          S09.22X **Traumatic rupture of left ear drum**
<small>7th</small>

      S09.8 **Other specified injuries of head**
<small>5th</small>

      S09.9 **Unspecified injury of face and head**
          S09.90X **Unspecified injury of head**
<small>7th</small>   Head injury NOS
                Excludes1: brain injury NOS (S06.9-)
                    head injury NOS with LOC (S06.9-)
                    intracranial injury NOS (S06.9-)
          S09.91X **Unspecified injury of ear**
<small>7th</small>   Injury of ear NOS
          S09.92X **Unspecified injury of nose**
<small>7th</small>   Injury of nose NOS
          S09.93X **Unspecified injury of face**
<small>7th</small>   Injury of face NOS
                Injuries to the neck (S10–S19)
                Includes: injuries of nape
                    injuries of supraclavicular region
                    injuries of throat
                Excludes2: burns and corrosions (T20–T32)
                    effects of FB in esophagus (T18.1)
                    effects of FB in larynx (T17.3)
                    effects of FB in pharynx (T17.2)
                    effects of FB in trachea (T17.4)
                    frostbite (T33–T34)
                    insect bite or sting, venomous (T63.4)

(S10–S19) INJURIES TO THE NECK

Includes: injuries of nape
    injuries of supraclavicular region
    injuries of throat
Excludes2: burns and corrosions (T20–T32)
    effects of FB in esophagus (T18.1)
    effects of FB in larynx (T17.3)
    effects of FB in pharynx (T17.2)
    effects of FB in trachea (T17.4)
    frostbite (T33–T34)
    insect bite or sting, venomous (T63.4)

S10 **SUPERFICIAL INJURY OF NECK**
<small>4th</small>
      S10.0XX **Contusion of throat**
<small>7th</small>   Contusion of cervical esophagus
          Contusion of larynx
          Contusion of pharynx
          Contusion of trachea

	7th characters for category S10
	& S11
	A—initial encounter
	D—subsequent encounter
	S—sequela

      S10.1 **Other and unspecified superficial**
<small>5th</small>   **injuries of throat**
          S10.10X **Unspecified superficial injuries of throat**
<small>7th</small>

<small>4th</small> <small>5th</small> <small>6th</small> <small>7th</small> Additional Character Required ✓ 3-character code	Unspecified laterality codes were excluded here.	• =New Code ▲ =Revised Code ▫ =Social determinants of health	*Excludes1*—Not coded here, do not use together *Excludes2*—Not included here

CHAPTER 19. INJURY, POISONING AND CERTAIN OTHER CONSEQUENCES OF EXTERNAL CAUSES   (S10.11X–S12.600)

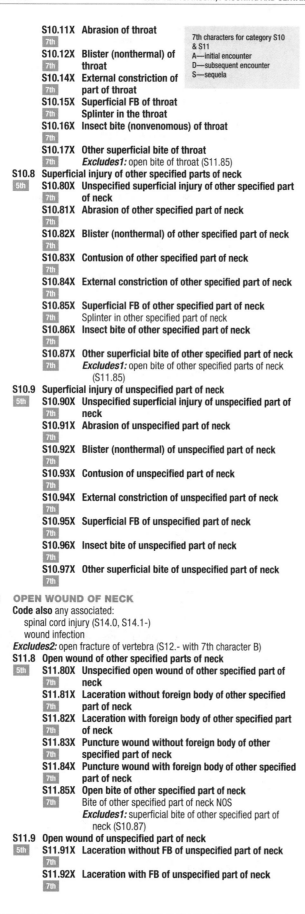

S10.11X   Abrasion of throat
7th

S10.12X   Blister (nonthermal) of throat
7th

S10.14X   External constriction of part of throat
7th

S10.15X   Superficial FB of throat
7th   Splinter in the throat

S10.16X   Insect bite (nonvenomous) of throat
7th

S10.17X   Other superficial bite of throat
7th   *Excludes1:* open bite of throat (S11.85)

S10.8   Superficial injury of other specified parts of neck
5th

    S10.80X   Unspecified superficial injury of other specified part of neck
    7th

    S10.81X   Abrasion of other specified part of neck
    7th

    S10.82X   Blister (nonthermal) of other specified part of neck
    7th

    S10.83X   Contusion of other specified part of neck
    7th

    S10.84X   External constriction of other specified part of neck
    7th

    S10.85X   Superficial FB of other specified part of neck
    7th   Splinter in other specified part of neck

    S10.86X   Insect bite of other specified part of neck
    7th

    S10.87X   Other superficial bite of other specified part of neck
    7th   *Excludes1:* open bite of other specified parts of neck (S11.85)

S10.9   Superficial injury of unspecified part of neck
5th

    S10.90X   Unspecified superficial injury of unspecified part of neck
    7th

    S10.91X   Abrasion of unspecified part of neck
    7th

    S10.92X   Blister (nonthermal) of unspecified part of neck
    7th

    S10.93X   Contusion of unspecified part of neck
    7th

    S10.94X   External constriction of unspecified part of neck
    7th

    S10.95X   Superficial FB of unspecified part of neck
    7th

    S10.96X   Insect bite of unspecified part of neck
    7th

    S10.97X   Other superficial bite of unspecified part of neck
    7th

S11   **OPEN WOUND OF NECK**
4th

Code also any associated:
   spinal cord injury (S14.0, S14.1-)
   wound infection

Excludes2: open fracture of vertebra (S12.- with 7th character B)

S11.8   Open wound of other specified parts of neck
5th

    S11.80X   Unspecified open wound of other specified part of neck
    7th

    S11.81X   Laceration without foreign body of other specified part of neck
    7th

    S11.82X   Laceration with foreign body of other specified part of neck
    7th

    S11.83X   Puncture wound without foreign body of other specified part of neck
    7th

    S11.84X   Puncture wound with foreign body of other specified part of neck
    7th

    S11.85X   Open bite of other specified part of neck
    7th   Bite of other specified part of neck NOS
      Excludes1: superficial bite of other specified part of neck (S10.87)

S11.9   Open wound of unspecified part of neck
5th

    S11.91X   Laceration without FB of unspecified part of neck
    7th

    S11.92X   Laceration with FB of unspecified part of neck
    7th

> 7th characters for category S10 & S11
> A—initial encounter
> D—subsequent encounter
> S—sequela

S11.93X   Puncture wound without FB of unspecified part of neck
7th

S11.94X   Puncture wound with FB of unspecified part of neck
7th

S11.95X   Open bite of unspecified part of neck
7th   Bite of neck NOS
    Excludes1: superficial bite of neck (S10.97)

S12   **FRACTURE OF CERVICAL VERTEBRA AND OTHER PARTS OF NECK**
4th

Note: A fracture not indicated as displaced or nondisplaced should be coded to displaced

A fracture not indicated as open or closed should be coded to closed

Includes: fracture of cervical neural arch
    fracture of cervical spine
    fracture of cervical spinous process
    fracture of cervical transverse process
    fracture of cervical vertebral arch
    fracture of neck

Code first any associated cervical spinal cord injury (S14.0, S14.1-)

S12.0   Fracture of first cervical vertebra
5th   Atlas

    S12.00   Unspecified fracture of first cervical vertebra
    6th

       S12.000   Unspecified displaced fracture of first cervical vertebra
       7th

       S12.001   Unspecified nondisplaced fracture of first cervical vertebra
       7th

    S12.03   Posterior arch fracture of first cervical vertebra
    6th

       S12.030   Displaced posterior arch fracture of first cervical vertebra
       7th

       S12.031   Nondisplaced posterior arch fracture of first cervical vertebra
       7th

S12.1   Fracture of second cervical vertebra
5th   Axis

    S12.10   Unspecified fracture of second cervical vertebra
    6th

       S12.100   Unspecified displaced fracture of second cervical vertebra
       7th

       S12.101   Unspecified nondisplaced fracture of second cervical vertebra
       7th

S12.2   Fracture of third cervical vertebra
5th

    S12.20   Unspecified fracture of third cervical vertebra
    6th

       S12.200   Unspecified displaced fracture of third cervical vertebra
       7th

       S12.201   Unspecified nondisplaced fracture of third cervical vertebra
       7th

S12.3   Fracture of fourth cervical vertebra
5th

    S12.30   Unspecified fracture of fourth cervical vertebra
    6th

       S12.300   Unspecified displaced fracture of fourth cervical vertebra
       7th

       S12.301   Unspecified nondisplaced fracture of fourth cervical vertebra
       7th

S12.4   Fracture of fifth cervical vertebra
5th

    S12.40   Unspecified fracture of fifth cervical vertebra
    6th

       S12.400   Unspecified displaced fracture of fifth cervical vertebra
       7th

       S12.401   Unspecified nondisplaced fracture of fifth cervical vertebra
       7th

S12.5   Fracture of sixth cervical vertebra
5th

    S12.50   Unspecified fracture of sixth cervical vertebra
    6th

       S12.500   Unspecified displaced fracture of sixth cervical vertebra
       7th

       S12.501   Unspecified nondisplaced fracture of sixth cervical vertebra
       7th

S12.6   Fracture of seventh cervical vertebra
5th

    S12.60   Unspecified fracture of seventh cervical vertebra
    6th

       S12.600   Unspecified displaced fracture of seventh cervical vertebra
       7th

> 7th characters for category S12.0–12.6
> A—initial encounter for closed fracture
> B—initial encounter for open fracture
> D—subsequent encounter for fracture with routine healing
> G—subsequent encounter for fracture with delayed healing
> K—subsequent encounter for fracture with nonunion
> S—sequela

4th   5th   6th   7th   Additional Character Required   ✔   3-character code   Unspecified laterality codes were excluded here.   • =New Code   ▲ =Revised Code   ¤ =Social determinants of health   *Excludes1*—Not coded here, do not use together   *Excludes2*—Not included here

334   PEDIATRIC ICD-10-CM 2021: A MANUAL FOR PROVIDER-BASED CODING

S12.601 **Unspecified nondisplaced fracture of seventh cervical vertebra**
`7th`

S12.8XX **Fracture of other parts of neck**
Hyoid bone
Larynx
Thyroid cartilage
Trachea

> 7th characters for category S12.8 & S12.9
> A—initial encounter
> D—subsequent encounter
> S—sequela

S12.9XX **Fracture of neck, unspecified**
`7th`
Fracture of neck NOS
Fracture of cervical spine NOS
Fracture of cervical vertebra NOS

S13 **DISLOCATION AND SPRAIN OF JOINTS AND LIGAMENTS AT NECK LEVEL**
`4th`
Includes: avulsion of joint or ligament at neck level
laceration of cartilage, joint or ligament at neck level
sprain of cartilage, joint or ligament at neck level
traumatic hemarthrosis of joint or ligament at neck level
traumatic rupture of joint or ligament at neck level
traumatic subluxation of joint or ligament at neck level
traumatic tear of joint or ligament at neck level

> 7th characters for category S13
> A—initial encounter
> D—subsequent encounter
> S—sequela

Code also any associated open wound
Excludes2: strain of muscle or tendon at neck level (S16.1)

S13.4XX **Sprain of ligaments of cervical spine**
`7th`
Sprain of anterior longitudinal (ligament), cervical
Sprain of atlanto-axial (joints)
Sprain of atlanto-occipital (joints)
Whiplash injury of cervical spine

S13.8XX **Sprain of joints and ligaments of other parts of neck**
`7th`

S13.9XX **Sprain of joints and ligaments of unspecified parts of neck**
`7th`

S14 **INJURY OF NERVES AND SPINAL CORD AT NECK LEVEL**
`4th`
Note: Code to highest level of cervical cord injury
Code also any associated:
fracture of cervical vertebra (S12.0–S12.6.-)
open wound of neck (S11.-)
transient paralysis (R29.5)

> 7th characters for category S14
> A—initial encounter
> D—subsequent encounter
> S—sequela

S14.0XX **Concussion and edema of cervical spinal cord**
`7th`

S14.1 **Other and unspecified injuries of cervical spinal cord**
`5th`
    S14.10 **Unspecified injury of cervical spinal cord**
`6th`
       S14.101 **Unspecified injury at; C1 level of cervical spinal cord**
`7th`
       S14.102 **C2 level of cervical spinal cord**
`7th`
       S14.103 **C3 level of cervical spinal cord**
`7th`
       S14.104 **C4 level of cervical spinal cord**
`7th`
       S14.105 **C5 level of cervical spinal cord**
`7th`
       S14.106 **C6 level of cervical spinal cord**
`7th`
       S14.107 **C7 level of cervical spinal cord**
`7th`
       S14.108 **C8 level of cervical spinal cord**
`7th`
       S14.109 **unspecified level of cervical spinal cord**
`7th`
       Injury of cervical spinal cord NOS

S14.2XX **Injury of nerve root of cervical spine**
`7th`

S14.3XX **Injury of brachial plexus**
`7th`

S14.4XX **Injury of peripheral nerves of neck**
`7th`

S14.5XX **Injury of cervical sympathetic nerves**
`7th`

S14.8XX **Injury of other specified nerves of neck**
`7th`

S14.9XX **Injury of unspecified nerves of neck**
`7th`

S15 **INJURY OF BLOOD VESSELS AT NECK LEVEL**
`4th`
Code also any associated open wound (S11.-)

S15.8XX **Injury of other specified blood vessels at neck level**
`7th`

S15.9XX **Injury of unspecified blood vessel at neck level**
`7th`

S16 **INJURY OF MUSCLE, FASCIA AND TENDON AT NECK LEVEL**
`4th`
Code also any associated open wound (S11.-)
Excludes2: sprain of joint or ligament at neck level (S13.9)

S16.1XX **Strain of muscle, fascia and tendon at neck level**
`7th`

S16.2XX **Laceration of muscle, fascia and tendon at neck level**
`7th`

S16.8XX **Other specified injury of muscle, fascia and tendon at neck level**
`7th`

S16.9XX **Unspecified injury of muscle, fascia and tendon at neck level**
`7th`
Injuries to the thorax (S20–S29)
Includes: injuries of breast
injuries of chest (wall)
injuries of interscapular area
Excludes2: burns and corrosions (T20–T32)
effects of FB in bronchus (T17.5)
effects of FB in esophagus (T18.1)
effects of FB in lung (T17.8)
effects of FB in trachea (T17.4)
frostbite (T33–T34)
injuries of axilla
injuries of clavicle
injuries of scapular region
injuries of shoulder
insect bite or sting, venomous (T63.4)

(S20–S29) INJURIES TO THE THORAX

Includes: injuries of breast
injuries of chest (wall)
injuries of interscapular area
Excludes2: burns and corrosions (T20–T32)
effects of FB in bronchus (T17.5)
effects of FB in esophagus (T18.1)
effects of FB in lung (T17.8)
effects of FB in trachea (T17.4)
frostbite (T33–T34)
injuries of axilla
injuries of clavicle
injuries of scapular region
injuries of shoulder
insect bite or sting, venomous (T63.4)

> 7th characters for category S20
> A—initial encounter
> D—subsequent encounter
> S—sequela

S20 **SUPERFICIAL INJURY OF THORAX**
`4th`
    S20.0 **Contusion of breast**
`5th`
       S20.00X **Contusion of breast, unspecified breast**
`7th`
       S20.01X **Contusion of right breast**
`7th`
       S20.02X **Contusion of left breast**
`7th`
    S20.1 **Other and unspecified superficial injuries of breast**
`5th`
       S20.11 **Abrasion of breast**
`6th`
          S20.111 **Abrasion of breast, right breast**
`7th`
          S20.112 **Abrasion of breast, left breast**
`7th`
          S20.119 **Abrasion of breast, unspecified breast**
`7th`
       S20.12 **Blister (nonthermal) of breast**
`6th`
          S20.121 **Blister (nonthermal) of breast, right breast**
`7th`
          S20.122 **Blister (nonthermal) of breast, left breast**
`7th`

`4th` `5th` `6th` `7th`   Additional Character Required   ✓   3-character code | Unspecified laterality codes were excluded here.   • =New Code   ▲ =Revised Code   ▫ =Social determinants of health   *Excludes1*—Not coded here, do not use together   *Excludes2*—Not included here

CHAPTER 19. INJURY, POISONING AND CERTAIN OTHER CONSEQUENCES OF EXTERNAL CAUSES   (S20.129–S20.411)

S20.129   7th   Blister (nonthermal) of breast, unspecified breast

S20.14   6th   External constriction of part of breast

> 7th characters for category S20
> A—initial encounter
> D—subsequent encounter
> S—sequela

S20.141   7th   External constriction of part of breast, right breast

S20.142   7th   External constriction of part of breast, left breast

S20.15   6th   Superficial FB of breast
Splinter in the breast

S20.151   7th   Superficial FB of breast, right breast

S20.152   7th   Superficial FB of breast, left breast

S20.16   6th   Insect bite (nonvenomous) of breast

S20.161   7th   Insect bite (nonvenomous) of breast, right breast

S20.162   7th   Insect bite (nonvenomous) of breast, left breast

S20.17   6th   Other superficial bite of breast
Excludes1: open bite of breast (S21.05-)

S20.171   7th   Other superficial bite of breast, right breast

S20.172   7th   Other superficial bite of breast, left breast

S20.2   5th   Contusion of thorax

S20.20X   7th   Contusion of thorax, unspecified

S20.21   6th   Contusion of front wall of thorax

S20.211   7th   Contusion of right front wall of thorax

S20.212   7th   Contusion of left front wall of thorax

•**S20.213**   7th   Contusion of bilateral front wall of thorax

•**S20.214**   7th   Contusion of middle front wall of thorax

S20.219   7th   Contusion of unspecified front wall of thorax

S20.22   6th   Contusion of back wall of thorax

S20.221   7th   Contusion of right back wall of thorax

S20.222   7th   Contusion of left back wall of thorax

•**S20.223**   7th   Contusion of bilateral back wall of thorax

•**S20.224**   7th   Contusion of middle back wall of thorax

S20.229   7th   Contusion of unspecified back wall of thorax
Interscapular contusion

S20.3   5th   Other and unspecified superficial injuries of front wall of thorax

S20.30   6th   Unspecified superficial injuries of front wall of thorax

S20.301   7th   Unspecified superficial injuries of right front wall of thorax

S20.302   7th   Unspecified superficial injuries of left front wall of thorax

•**S20.303**   7th   Unspecified superficial injuries of bilateral front wall of thorax

•**S20.304**   7th   Unspecified superficial injuries of middle front wall of thorax

S20.309   7th   Unspecified superficial injuries of unspecified front wall of thorax

S20.31   6th   Abrasion of front wall of thorax

S20.311   7th   Abrasion of right front wall of thorax

S20.312   7th   Abrasion of left front wall of thorax

•**S20.313**   7th   Abrasion of bilateral front wall of thorax

•**S20.314**   7th   Abrasion of middle front wall of thorax

S20.319   7th   Abrasion of unspecified front wall of thorax

S20.32   6th   Blister (nonthermal) of front wall of thorax

S20.321   7th   Blister (nonthermal) of right front wall of thorax

S20.322   7th   Blister (nonthermal) of left front wall of thorax

•**S20.323**   7th   Blister (nonthermal) of bilateral front wall of thorax

•**S20.324**   7th   Blister (nonthermal) of middle front wall of thorax

S20.329   7th   Blister (nonthermal) of unspecified front wall of thorax

S20.34   6th   External constriction of front wall of thorax

S20.341   7th   External constriction of right front wall of thorax

S20.342   7th   External constriction of left front wall of thorax

•**S20.343**   7th   External constriction of bilateral front wall of thorax

•**S20.344**   7th   External constriction of middle front wall of thorax

S20.349   7th   External constriction of unspecified front wall of thorax

S20.35   6th   Superficial foreign body of front wall of thorax
Splinter in front wall of thorax

S20.351   7th   Superficial foreign body of right front wall of thorax

S20.352   7th   Superficial foreign body of left front wall of thorax

•**S20.353**   7th   Superficial foreign body of bilateral front wall of thorax

•**S20.354**   7th   Superficial foreign body of middle front wall of thorax

S20.359   7th   Superficial foreign body of unspecified front wall of thorax

S20.36   6th   Insect bite (nonvenomous) of front wall of thorax

S20.361   7th   Insect bite (nonvenomous) of right front wall of thorax

S20.362   7th   Insect bite (nonvenomous) of left front wall of thorax

•**S20.363**   7th   Insect bite (nonvenomous) of bilateral front wall of thorax

•**S20.364**   7th   Insect bite (nonvenomous) of middle front wall of thorax

S20.369   7th   Insect bite (nonvenomous) of unspecified front wall of thorax

S20.37   6th   Other superficial bite of front wall of thorax
Excludes1: open bite of front wall of thorax (S21.14)

S20.371   7th   Other superficial bite of right front wall of thorax

S20.372   7th   Other superficial bite of left front wall of thorax

•**S20.373**   7th   Other superficial bite of bilateral front wall of thorax

•**S20.374**   7th   Other superficial bite of middle front wall of thorax

S20.379   7th   Other superficial bite of unspecified front wall of thorax

S20.4   5th   Other and unspecified superficial injuries of back wall of thorax

S20.40   6th   Unspecified superficial injuries of back wall of thorax

S20.401   7th   Unspecified superficial injuries of right back wall of thorax

S20.402   7th   Unspecified superficial injuries of left back wall of thorax

S20.409   7th   Unspecified superficial injuries of unspecified back wall of thorax

S20.41   6th   Abrasion of back wall of thorax

S20.411   7th   Abrasion of right back wall of thorax

4th   5th   6th   7th   Additional Character Required   ✓   3-character code   Unspecified laterality codes were excluded here.   • =New Code   ▲ =Revised Code   ¤ =Social determinants of health   *Excludes1*—Not coded here, do not use together   *Excludes2*—Not included here

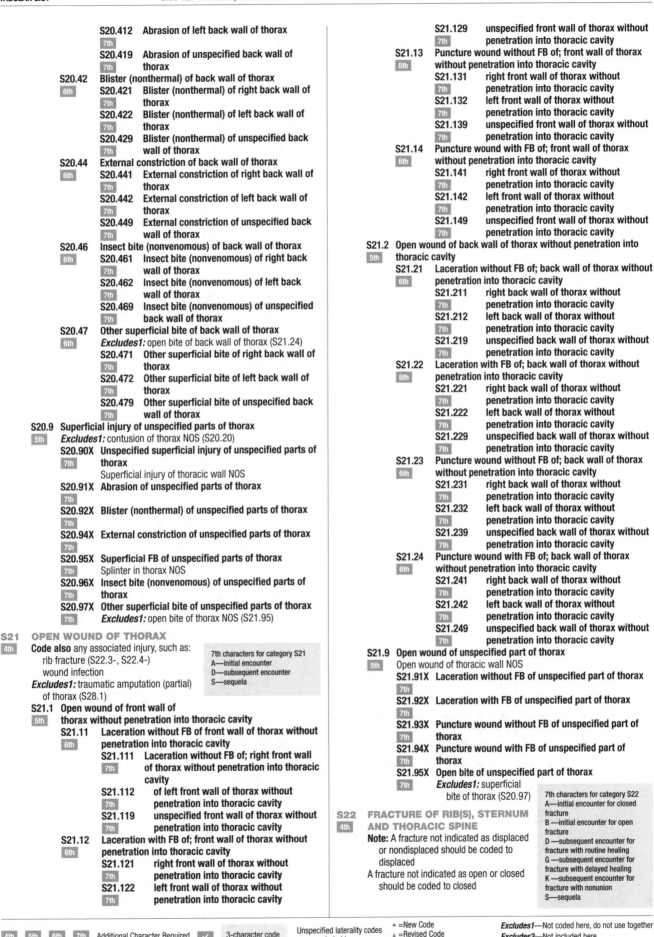

S20.412 Abrasion of left back wall of thorax
7th

S20.419 Abrasion of unspecified back wall of thorax
7th

S20.42 Blister (nonthermal) of back wall of thorax
6th

    S20.421 Blister (nonthermal) of right back wall of thorax
7th

    S20.422 Blister (nonthermal) of left back wall of thorax
7th

    S20.429 Blister (nonthermal) of unspecified back wall of thorax
7th

S20.44 External constriction of back wall of thorax
6th

    S20.441 External constriction of right back wall of thorax
7th

    S20.442 External constriction of left back wall of thorax
7th

    S20.449 External constriction of unspecified back wall of thorax
7th

S20.46 Insect bite (nonvenomous) of back wall of thorax
6th

    S20.461 Insect bite (nonvenomous) of right back wall of thorax
7th

    S20.462 Insect bite (nonvenomous) of left back wall of thorax
7th

    S20.469 Insect bite (nonvenomous) of unspecified back wall of thorax
7th

S20.47 Other superficial bite of back wall of thorax
6th

    Excludes1: open bite of back wall of thorax (S21.24)

    S20.471 Other superficial bite of right back wall of thorax
7th

    S20.472 Other superficial bite of left back wall of thorax
7th

    S20.479 Other superficial bite of unspecified back wall of thorax
7th

S20.9 Superficial injury of unspecified parts of thorax
5th

    Excludes1: contusion of thorax NOS (S20.20)

S20.90X Unspecified superficial injury of unspecified parts of thorax
7th

    Superficial injury of thoracic wall NOS

S20.91X Abrasion of unspecified parts of thorax
7th

S20.92X Blister (nonthermal) of unspecified parts of thorax
7th

S20.94X External constriction of unspecified parts of thorax
7th

S20.95X Superficial FB of unspecified parts of thorax
7th

    Splinter in thorax NOS

S20.96X Insect bite (nonvenomous) of unspecified parts of thorax
7th

S20.97X Other superficial bite of unspecified parts of thorax
7th

    Excludes1: open bite of thorax NOS (S21.95)

S21   **OPEN WOUND OF THORAX**
4th

Code also any associated injury, such as:
    rib fracture (S22.3-, S22.4-)
    wound infection
Excludes1: traumatic amputation (partial) of thorax (S28.1)

7th characters for category S21
A—initial encounter
D—subsequent encounter
S—sequela

S21.1 Open wound of front wall of thorax without penetration into thoracic cavity
5th

    S21.11 Laceration without FB of front wall of thorax without penetration into thoracic cavity
6th

        S21.111 Laceration without FB of; right front wall of thorax without penetration into thoracic cavity
7th

        S21.112 of left front wall of thorax without penetration into thoracic cavity
7th

        S21.119 unspecified front wall of thorax without penetration into thoracic cavity
7th

    S21.12 Laceration with FB of; front wall of thorax without penetration into thoracic cavity
6th

        S21.121 right front wall of thorax without penetration into thoracic cavity
7th

        S21.122 left front wall of thorax without penetration into thoracic cavity
7th

        S21.129 unspecified front wall of thorax without penetration into thoracic cavity
7th

    S21.13 Puncture wound without FB of; front wall of thorax without penetration into thoracic cavity
6th

        S21.131 right front wall of thorax without penetration into thoracic cavity
7th

        S21.132 left front wall of thorax without penetration into thoracic cavity
7th

        S21.139 unspecified front wall of thorax without penetration into thoracic cavity
7th

    S21.14 Puncture wound with FB of; front wall of thorax without penetration into thoracic cavity
6th

        S21.141 right front wall of thorax without penetration into thoracic cavity
7th

        S21.142 left front wall of thorax without penetration into thoracic cavity
7th

        S21.149 unspecified front wall of thorax without penetration into thoracic cavity
7th

S21.2 Open wound of back wall of thorax without penetration into thoracic cavity
5th

    S21.21 Laceration without FB of; back wall of thorax without penetration into thoracic cavity
6th

        S21.211 right back wall of thorax without penetration into thoracic cavity
7th

        S21.212 left back wall of thorax without penetration into thoracic cavity
7th

        S21.219 unspecified back wall of thorax without penetration into thoracic cavity
7th

    S21.22 Laceration with FB of; back wall of thorax without penetration into thoracic cavity
6th

        S21.221 right back wall of thorax without penetration into thoracic cavity
7th

        S21.222 left back wall of thorax without penetration into thoracic cavity
7th

        S21.229 unspecified back wall of thorax without penetration into thoracic cavity
7th

    S21.23 Puncture wound without FB of; back wall of thorax without penetration into thoracic cavity
6th

        S21.231 right back wall of thorax without penetration into thoracic cavity
7th

        S21.232 left back wall of thorax without penetration into thoracic cavity
7th

        S21.239 unspecified back wall of thorax without penetration into thoracic cavity
7th

    S21.24 Puncture wound with FB of; back wall of thorax without penetration into thoracic cavity
6th

        S21.241 right back wall of thorax without penetration into thoracic cavity
7th

        S21.242 left back wall of thorax without penetration into thoracic cavity
7th

        S21.249 unspecified back wall of thorax without penetration into thoracic cavity
7th

S21.9 Open wound of unspecified part of thorax
5th

    Open wound of thoracic wall NOS

S21.91X Laceration without FB of unspecified part of thorax
7th

S21.92X Laceration with FB of unspecified part of thorax
7th

S21.93X Puncture wound without FB of unspecified part of thorax
7th

S21.94X Puncture wound with FB of unspecified part of thorax
7th

S21.95X Open bite of unspecified part of thorax
7th

    Excludes1: superficial bite of thorax (S20.97)

S22   **FRACTURE OF RIB(S), STERNUM AND THORACIC SPINE**
4th

Note: A fracture not indicated as displaced or nondisplaced should be coded to displaced

A fracture not indicated as open or closed should be coded to closed

7th characters for category S22
A—initial encounter for closed fracture
B —initial encounter for open fracture
D —subsequent encounter for fracture with routine healing
G —subsequent encounter for fracture with delayed healing
K —subsequent encounter for fracture with nonunion
S—sequela

| 4th | 5th | 6th | 7th | Additional Character Required | ✓ | 3-character code |

Unspecified laterality codes were excluded here.

• =New Code
▲ =Revised Code
⌑ =Social determinants of health

Excludes1—Not coded here, do not use together
Excludes2—Not included here

Includes: fracture of thoracic neural arch
fracture of thoracic spinous process
fracture of thoracic transverse process
fracture of thoracic vertebra or of
thoracic vertebral arch
Code first any associated:
injury of intrathoracic organ (S27.-)
spinal cord injury (S24.0-, S24.1-)
Excludes1: transection of thorax (S28.1)
Excludes2: fracture of clavicle (S42.0-)
fracture of scapula (S42.1-)

> 7th characters for category S22
> A—initial encounter for closed fracture
> B—initial encounter for open fracture
> D—subsequent encounter for fracture with routine healing
> G—subsequent encounter for fracture with delayed healing
> K—subsequent encounter for fracture with nonunion
> S—sequela

S22.2 Fracture of sternum
  5th **S22.20X** Unspecified fracture of sternum
    7th

    S22.21X Fracture of manubrium
    7th

    S22.22X Fracture of body of sternum
    7th

    S22.23X Sternal manubrial dissociation
    7th

    S22.24X Fracture of xiphoid process
    7th

S22.3 Fracture of one rib
  5th **S22.31X** Fracture of one rib, right side
    7th

    S22.32X Fracture of one rib, left side
    7th

    S22.39X Fracture of one rib, unspecified side
    7th

S22.4 Multiple fractures of ribs
  5th Fractures of two or more ribs
    Excludes1: flail chest (S22.5-)
    S22.41X Multiple fractures of ribs, right side
    7th

    S22.42X Multiple fractures of
    7th   ribs, left side
    S22.43X Multiple fractures of ribs, bilateral
    7th

    S22.49X Multiple fractures of ribs, unspecified side
    7th

S22.5XX Flail chest
  7th

S22.9XX Fracture of bony thorax, part unspecified
  7th

S24   **INJURY OF NERVES AND SPINAL CORD AT THORAX**
4th   **LEVEL**
Note: Code to highest level of thoracic spinal cord injury
Injuries to the spinal cord (S24.0 and S24.1) refer to the cord level and not bone level injury, and can affect nerve roots at and below the level given.
Code also any associated:
fracture of thoracic vertebra (S22.0-)
open wound of thorax (S21.-)
transient paralysis (R29.5)

> 7th characters for category S24
> A—initial encounter
> D—subsequent encounter
> S—sequela

Excludes2: injury of brachial plexus (S14.3)
S24.0XX Concussion and edema of thoracic spinal cord
  7th

S24.1 Other and unspecified injuries of thoracic spinal cord
  5th **S24.10** Unspecified injury of thoracic spinal cord
    6th **S24.101** Unspecified injury at; T1 level of thoracic
      7th   spinal cord
      S24.102 T2–T6 level of thoracic spinal cord
      7th
      S24.103 T7–T10 level of thoracic spinal cord
      7th
      S24.104 T11–T12 level of thoracic spinal cord
      7th
      S24.109 unspecified level of thoracic spinal cord
      7th   Injury of thoracic spinal cord NOS

S27   **INJURY OF OTHER AND UNSPECIFIED INTRATHORACIC**
4th   **ORGANS**
Code also any associated open wound of thorax (S21.-)
Excludes2: injury of cervical esophagus (S10–S19)
injury of trachea (cervical) (S10–S19)

> 7th characters for category S27
> A—initial encounter
> D—subsequent encounter
> S—sequela

S27.0XX Traumatic pneumothorax
  7th   *Excludes1:* spontaneous pneumothorax (J93.-)

S27.3 Other and unspecified injuries of lung
  5th **S27.30** Unspecified injury of lung
    6th **S27.301** Unspecified injury of lung, unilateral
      7th
      S27.302 Unspecified injury of lung, bilateral
      7th

    S27.32 Contusion of lung
    6th **S27.321** Contusion of lung, unilateral
      7th
      S27.322 Contusion of lung, bilateral
      7th
      S27.329 Contusion of lung, unspecified
      7th

(S30–S39) INJURIES TO THE ABDOMEN, LOWER BACK, LUMBAR SPINE, PELVIS AND EXTERNAL GENITALS

Includes: injuries to the abdominal wall
injuries to the anus
injuries to the buttock
injuries to the external genitalia
injuries to the flank
injuries to the groin
Excludes2: burns and corrosions (T20–T32)
effects of FB in anus and rectum (T18.5)
effects of FB in genitourinary tract (T19.-)
effects of FB in stomach, small intestine and colon (T18.2–T18.4)
frostbite (T33–T34)
insect bite or sting, venomous (T63.4)

S30   **SUPERFICIAL INJURY OF ABDOMEN, LOWER BACK,**
4th   **PELVIS AND EXTERNAL GENITALS**
  Excludes2: superficial injury of hip (S70.-)
  S30.0XX Contusion of lower back and
  7th   pelvis
      Contusion of buttock

> 7th characters for category S30
> A—initial encounter
> D—subsequent encounter
> S—sequela

  S30.1XX Contusion of abdominal wall
  7th   Contusion of flank
      Contusion of groin

S30.2 Contusion of external genital organs
  5th **S30.20** Contusion of unspecified external genital organ
    6th **S30.201** Contusion of unspecified external genital
      7th   organ, male
      S30.202 Contusion of unspecified external genital
      7th   organ, female
    S30.21X Contusion of penis
    7th

    S30.22X Contusion of scrotum and testes
    7th

    S30.23X Contusion of vagina and vulva
    7th

S30.3XX Contusion of anus
  7th

S30.8 Other superficial injuries of abdomen, lower back, pelvis and
  5th **external genitals**
    S30.81 Abrasion of abdomen, lower back, pelvis and
    6th   external genitals
      S30.810 Abrasion of lower back and pelvis
      7th
      S30.811 Abrasion of abdominal wall
      7th
      S30.812 Abrasion of penis
      7th
      S30.813 Abrasion of scrotum and testes
      7th

4th   *5th*   *6th*   *7th*   Additional Character Required   ✔   3-character code   Unspecified laterality codes were excluded here.   • =New Code   ▲ =Revised Code   ¤ =Social determinants of health   *Excludes1*—Not coded here, do not use together   *Excludes2*—Not included here

S30.814   **Abrasion of vagina and vulva**
`7th`

S30.815   **Abrasion of unspecified external genital organs, male**
`7th`

> 7th characters for category S30
> A—initial encounter
> D—subsequent encounter
> S—sequela

S30.816   **Abrasion of unspecified external genital organs, female**
`7th`

S30.817   **Abrasion of anus**
`7th`

S30.82   **Blister (nonthermal) of abdomen, lower back, pelvis and external genitals**
`6th`

S30.820   **Blister (non-thermal) of lower back and pelvis**
`7th`

S30.821   **Blister (nonthermal) of abdominal wall**
`7th`

S30.822   **Blister (nonthermal) of penis**
`7th`

S30.823   **Blister (nonthermal) of scrotum and testes**
`7th`

S30.824   **Blister (nonthermal) of vagina and vulva**
`7th`

S30.825   **Blister (nonthermal) of unspecified external genital organs, male**
`7th`

S30.826   **Blister (nonthermal) of unspecified external genital organs, female**
`7th`

S30.827   **Blister (nonthermal) of anus**
`7th`

S30.84   **External constriction of abdomen, lower back, pelvis and external genitals**
`6th`

S30.840   **External constriction of lower back and pelvis**
`7th`

S30.841   **External constriction of abdominal wall**
`7th`

S30.842   **External constriction of penis**
`7th`
Hair tourniquet syndrome of penis
Use additional cause code to identify the constricting item (W49.0-)

S30.843   **External constriction of scrotum and testes**
`7th`

S30.844   **External constriction of vagina and vulva**
`7th`

S30.845   **External constriction of unspecified external genital organs, male**
`7th`

S30.846   **External constriction of unspecified external genital organs, female**
`7th`

S30.85   **Superficial FB of abdomen, lower back, pelvis and external genitals**
`6th`
Splinter in the abdomen, lower back, pelvis and external genitals

S30.850   **Superficial FB of; lower back and pelvis**
`7th`

S30.851   **abdominal wall**
`7th`

S30.852   **penis**
`7th`

S30.853   **scrotum and testes**
`7th`

S30.854   **vagina and vulva**
`7th`

S30.855   **unspecified external genital organs, male**
`7th`

S30.856   **unspecified external genital organs, female**
`7th`

S30.857   **anus**
`7th`

S30.86   **Insect bite (nonvenomous) of abdomen, lower back, pelvis and external genitals**
`6th`

S30.860   **Insect bite (nonvenomous) of; lower back and pelvis**
`7th`

S30.861   **abdominal wall**
`7th`

S30.862   **penis**
`7th`

S30.863   **scrotum and testes**
`7th`

S30.864   **vagina and vulva**
`7th`

S30.865   **unspecified external genital organs, male**
`7th`

S30.866   **unspecified external genital organs, female**
`7th`

S30.867   **anus**
`7th`

S30.87   **Other superficial bite of abdomen, lower back, pelvis and external genitals**
`6th`
Excludes1: open bite of abdomen, lower back, pelvis and external genitals (S31.05, S31.15, S31.25, S31.35, S31.45, S31.55)

S30.870   **Other superficial bite of; lower back and pelvis**
`7th`

S30.871   **abdominal wall**
`7th`

S30.872   **penis**
`7th`

S30.873   **scrotum and testes**
`7th`

S30.874   **vagina and vulva**
`7th`

S30.875   **unspecified external genital organs, male**
`7th`

S30.876   **unspecified external genital organs, female**
`7th`

S30.877   **anus**
`7th`

S30.9   **Unspecified superficial injury of abdomen, lower back, pelvis and external genitals**
`5th`

S30.91X   **Unspecified superficial injury of; lower back and pelvis**
`7th`

S30.92X   **abdominal wall**
`7th`

S30.93X   **penis**
`7th`

S30.94X   **scrotum and testes**
`7th`

S30.95X   **vagina and vulva**
`7th`

S30.96X   **unspecified external genital organs, male**
`7th`

S30.97X   **unspecified external genital organs, female**
`7th`

S30.98X   **anus**
`7th`

S31   **OPEN WOUND OF ABDOMEN, LOWER BACK, PELVIS AND EXTERNAL GENITALS**
`4th`
Code also any associated:
   spinal cord injury (S24.0, S24.1-, S34.0-, S34.1-)
   wound infection

> 7th characters for categories S31
> A—initial encounter
> D—subsequent encounter
> S—sequela

Excludes1: traumatic amputation of part of abdomen, lower back and pelvis (S38.2-, S38.3)
Excludes2: open wound of hip (S71.00–S71.02)
   open fracture of pelvis (S32.1–S32.9 with 7th character B)

S31.0   **Open wound of lower back and pelvis**
`5th`

S31.01   **Laceration without FB of lower back and pelvis;**
`6th`

> For subcategory S31.0, use 6th character of 1 for penetration into the retroperitoneum, along with the appropriate 7th character.

S31.010   **without penetration into retroperitoneum**
`7th`
Laceration without FB of lower back and pelvis NOS

S31.02   **Laceration with FB of lower back and pelvis;**
`6th`

`4th` `5th` `6th` `7th`   Additional Character Required   ✓   3-character code   Unspecified laterality codes were excluded here.

• =New Code
▲ =Revised Code
▣ =Social determinants of health

Excludes1—Not coded here, do not use together
Excludes2—Not included here

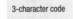

S31.020 `7th` **without penetration into retroperitoneum**
Laceration with FB of lower back and pelvis NOS

7th characters for category S31
A—initial encounter
D—subsequent encounter
S—sequela

S31.03 `6th` **Puncture wound without FB of lower back and pelvis**

S31.030 `7th` **Puncture wound without FB of lower back and pelvis without penetration into retroperitoneum**
Puncture wound without FB of lower back and pelvis NOS

S31.04 `6th` **Puncture wound with FB of lower back and pelvis**

S31.040 `7th` **Puncture wound with FB of lower back and pelvis; without penetration into retroperitoneum**
Puncture wound with FB of lower back and pelvis NOS

S31.05 `6th` **Open bite of lower back and pelvis**
Bite of lower back and pelvis NOS
Excludes1: superficial bite of lower back and pelvis (S30.860, S30.870)

S31.050 `7th` **Open bite of lower back and pelvis without penetration into retroperitoneum**
Open bite of lower back and pelvis NOS

S31.1 `5th` **Open wound of abdominal wall without penetration into peritoneal cavity**
Open wound of abdominal wall NOS
Excludes2: open wound of abdominal wall with penetration into peritoneal cavity (S31.6-)

S31.11 `6th` **Laceration without FB of abdominal wall without penetration into peritoneal cavity**

S31.110 `7th` **Laceration without FB of abdominal wall; RUQ without penetration into peritoneal cavity**

S31.111 `7th` **LUQ without penetration into peritoneal cavity**

S31.112 `7th` **epigastric region without penetration into peritoneal cavity**

S31.113 `7th` **RLQ without penetration into peritoneal cavity**

S31.114 `7th` **LLQ without penetration into peritoneal cavity**

S31.115 `7th` **periumbilic region without penetration into peritoneal cavity**

S31.119 `7th` **unspecified quadrant without penetration into peritoneal cavity**

S31.12 `6th` **Laceration with FB of abdominal wall without penetration into peritoneal cavity**

S31.120 `7th` **Laceration of abdominal wall with FB; RUQ without penetration into peritoneal cavity**

S31.121 `7th` **LUQ without penetration into peritoneal cavity**

S31.122 `7th` **epigastric region without penetration into peritoneal cavity**

S31.123 `7th` **RLQ without penetration into peritoneal cavity**

S31.124 `7th` **LLQ without penetration into peritoneal cavity**

S31.125 `7th` **periumbilic region without penetration into peritoneal cavity**

S31.129 `7th` **unspecified quadrant without penetration into peritoneal cavity**

S31.13 `6th` **Puncture wound of abdominal wall without FB without penetration into peritoneal cavity**

S31.130 `7th` **Puncture wound of abdominal wall without FB; RUQ without penetration into peritoneal cavity**

S31.131 `7th` **LUQ without penetration into peritoneal cavity**

S31.132 `7th` **epigastric region without penetration into peritoneal cavity**

S31.133 `7th` **RLQ without penetration into peritoneal cavity**

S31.134 `7th` **LLQ without penetration into peritoneal cavity**

S31.135 `7th` **periumbilic region without penetration into peritoneal cavity**

S31.139 `7th` **unspecified quadrant without penetration into peritoneal cavity**

S31.14 `6th` **Puncture wound of abdominal wall with FB without penetration into peritoneal cavity**

S31.140 `7th` **Puncture wound of abdominal wall with FB; RUQ without penetration into peritoneal cavity**

S31.141 `7th` **LUQ without penetration into peritoneal cavity**

S31.142 `7th` **epigastric region without penetration into peritoneal cavity**

S31.143 `7th` **RLQ without penetration into peritoneal cavity**

S31.144 `7th` **LLQ without penetration into peritoneal cavity**

S31.145 `7th` **periumbilic region without penetration into peritoneal cavity**

S31.149 `7th` **unspecified quadrant without penetration into peritoneal cavity**

S31.15 `6th` **Open bite of abdominal wall without penetration into peritoneal cavity**
Bite of abdominal wall NOS
Excludes1: superficial bite of abdominal wall (S30.871)

S31.150 `7th` **Open bite of abdominal wall; RUQ without penetration into peritoneal cavity**

S31.151 `7th` **LUQ without penetration into peritoneal cavity**

S31.152 `7th` **epigastric region without penetration into peritoneal cavity**

S31.153 `7th` **RLQ without penetration into peritoneal cavity**

S31.154 `7th` **LLQ without penetration into peritoneal cavity**

S31.155 `7th` **periumbilic region without penetration into peritoneal cavity**

S31.159 `7th` **unspecified quadrant without penetration into peritoneal cavity**

S31.2 `5th` **Open wound of penis**

S31.21X `7th` **Laceration without FB of penis**

S31.23X `7th` **Puncture wound without foreign body of penis**

S31.24X `7th` **Puncture wound with foreign body of penis**

S31.25X `7th` **Open bite of penis**
Bite of penis NOS
Excludes1: superficial bite of penis (S30.862, S30.872)

S31.3 `5th` **Open wound of scrotum and testes**

S31.31X `7th` **Laceration without FB of scrotum and testes**

S31.33X `7th` **Puncture wound without foreign body of scrotum and testes**

S31.34X `7th` **Puncture wound with foreign body of scrotum and testes**

S31.35X `7th` **Open bite of scrotum and testes**
Bite of scrotum and testes NOS
Excludes1: superficial bite of scrotum and testes (S30.863, S30.873)

S31.4 `5th` **Open wound of vagina and vulva**
Excludes1: injury to vagina and vulva during delivery (O70.-, O71.4)

S31.41X `7th` **Laceration without FB of vagina and vulva**

S31.42X `7th` **Laceration with FB of vagina and vulva**

S31.43X `7th` **Puncture wound without FB of vagina and vulva**

`4th` `5th` `6th` `7th` Additional Character Required   ✔   3-character code

Unspecified laterality codes were excluded here.

• =New Code
▲ =Revised Code
✍ =Social determinants of health

Excludes1—Not coded here, do not use together
Excludes2—Not included here

S31.44X **Puncture wound with FB of vagina and vulva**
`7th`

S31.45X **Open bite of vagina and vulva**
`7th`
Bite of vagina and vulva NOS

> 7th characters for category S31
> A—initial encounter
> D—subsequent encounter
> S—sequela

Excludes1: superficial bite of vagina and vulva (S30.864, S30.874)

S31.8 **Open wound of other parts of abdomen, lower back and pelvis**
`5th`
 S31.81 **Open wound of right buttock**
 `6th`
  S31.811 **Laceration without FB of right buttock**
  `7th`
  S31.812 **Laceration with FB of right buttock**
  `7th`
  S31.813 **Puncture wound without FB of right buttock**
  `7th`
  S31.814 **Puncture wound with FB of right buttock**
  `7th`
  S31.815 **Open bite of right buttock**
  `7th`
   Bite of right buttock NOS
   Excludes1: superficial bite of buttock (S30.870)

 S31.82 **Open wound of left buttock**
 `6th`
  S31.821 **Laceration without FB of left buttock**
  `7th`
  S31.822 **Laceration with FB of left buttock**
  `7th`
  S31.823 **Puncture wound without FB of left buttock**
  `7th`
  S31.824 **Puncture wound with FB of left buttock**
  `7th`
  S31.825 **Open bite of left buttock**
  `7th`
   Bite of left buttock NOS
   Excludes1: superficial bite of buttock (S30.870)

 S31.83 **Open wound of anus**
 `6th`
  S31.831 **Laceration without FB of anus**
  `7th`
  S31.832 **Laceration with FB of anus**
  `7th`
  S31.833 **Puncture wound without FB of anus**
  `7th`
  S31.834 **Puncture wound with FB of anus**
  `7th`
  S31.835 **Open bite of anus**
  `7th`
   Bite of anus NOS
   Excludes1: superficial bite of anus (S30.877)

S32 **FRACTURE OF LUMBAR SPINE AND PELVIS**
`4th`
Note: A fracture not indicated as displaced or nondisplaced should be coded to displaced
A fracture not indicated as opened or closed should be coded to closed
Includes: fracture of lumbosacral neural arch
fracture of lumbosacral spinous process
fracture of lumbosacral transverse process
fracture of lumbosacral vertebra or of lumbosacral vertebral arch

> 7th characters for category S32
> A—initial encounter for closed fracture
> B—initial encounter for open fracture
> D—subsequent encounter for fracture with routine healing
> G—subsequent encounter for fracture with delayed healing
> K—subsequent encounter for fracture with nonunion
> S—sequela

Code first any associated spinal cord and spinal nerve injury (S34.-)
Excludes1: transection of abdomen (S38.3)
Excludes2: fracture of hip NOS (S72.0-)

S32.1 **Fracture of sacrum**
`5th`
For vertical fractures, code to most medial fracture extension
Use two codes if both a vertical and transverse fracture are present
Code also any associated fracture of pelvic ring (S32.8-)
 S32.10X **Unspecified fracture of sacrum**
 `7th`
 S32.11 **Zone I fracture of sacrum**
 `6th`
  Vertical sacral ala fracture of sacrum

S32.110 **Nondisplaced Zone I fracture of sacrum**
`7th`
S32.111 **Minimally displaced Zone I fracture of sacrum**
`7th`
S32.112 **Severely displaced Zone I fracture of sacrum**
`7th`
S32.119 **Unspecified Zone I fracture of sacrum**

S32.12 **Zone II fracture of sacrum**
`6th`
Vertical foraminal region fracture of sacrum
 S32.120 **Nondisplaced Zone II fracture of sacrum**
 `7th`
 S32.121 **Minimally displaced Zone II fracture of sacrum**
 `7th`
 S32.122 **Severely displaced Zone II fracture of sacrum**
 `7th`
 S32.129 **Unspecified Zone II fracture of sacrum**
 `7th`

S32.13 **Zone III fracture of sacrum**
`6th`
Vertical fracture into spinal canal region of sacrum
 S32.130 **Nondisplaced Zone III fracture of sacrum**
 `7th`
 S32.131 **Minimally displaced Zone III fracture of sacrum**
 `7th`
 S32.132 **Severely displaced Zone III fracture of sacrum**
 `7th`
 S32.139 **Unspecified Zone III fracture of sacrum**
 `7th`

S32.14X **Type 1 fracture of sacrum**
`7th`
Transverse flexion fracture of sacrum without displacement
S32.15X **Type 2 fracture of sacrum**
`7th`
Transverse flexion fracture of sacrum with posterior displacement
S32.16X **Type 3 fracture of sacrum**
`7th`
Transverse extension fracture of sacrum with anterior displacement
S32.17X **Type 4 fracture of sacrum**
`7th`
Transverse segmental comminution of upper sacrum
S32.19X **Other fracture of sacrum**
`7th`

S32.2XX **Fracture of coccyx**
`7th`

S32.3 **Fracture of ilium**
`5th`
Excludes1: fracture of ilium with associated disruption of pelvic ring (S32.8-)
 S32.30 **Unspecified fracture of ilium**
 `6th`
  S32.301 **Unspecified fracture of right ilium**
  `7th`
  S32.302 **Unspecified fracture of left ilium**
  `7th`
  S32.309 **Unspecified fracture of unspecified ilium**
  `7th`

 S32.31 **Avulsion fracture of ilium**
 `6th`
  S32.311 **Displaced avulsion fracture of right ilium**
  `7th`
  S32.312 **Displaced avulsion fracture of left ilium**
  `7th`
  S32.313 **Displaced avulsion fracture of unspecified ilium**
  `7th`
  S32.314 **Nondisplaced avulsion fracture of right ilium**
  `7th`
  S32.315 **Nondisplaced avulsion fracture of left ilium**
  `7th`
  S32.316 **Nondisplaced avulsion fracture of unspecified ilium**
  `7th`

 S32.39 **Other fracture of ilium**
 `6th`
  S32.391 **Other fracture of right ilium**
  `7th`
  S32.392 **Other fracture of left ilium**
  `7th`
  S32.399 **Other fracture of unspecified ilium**
  `7th`

S32.4 **Fracture of acetabulum**
`5th`
Code also any associated fracture of pelvic ring (S32.8-)

`4th` `5th` `6th` `7th` Additional Character Required   ✔ 3-character code   Unspecified laterality codes were excluded here.

• =New Code
▲ =Revised Code
▫ =Social determinants of health

Excludes1—Not coded here, do not use together
Excludes2—Not included here

S32.40 `6th` **Unspecified fracture of acetabulum**

  S32.401 `7th` **Unspecified fracture of right acetabulum**

  S32.402 `7th` **Unspecified fracture of left acetabulum**

> 7th characters for category S32
> A—initial encounter for closed fracture
> B—initial encounter for open fracture
> D—subsequent encounter for fracture with routine healing
> G—subsequent encounter for fracture with delayed healing
> K—subsequent encounter for fracture with nonunion
> S—sequela

S32.41 `6th` **Fracture of anterior wall of acetabulum**

  S32.411 `7th` **Displaced fracture of anterior wall of right acetabulum**

  S32.412 `7th` **Displaced fracture of anterior wall of left acetabulum**

  S32.414 `7th` **Nondisplaced fracture of anterior wall of right acetabulum**

  S32.415 `7th` **Nondisplaced fracture of anterior wall of left acetabulum**

S32.42 `6th` **Fracture of posterior wall of acetabulum**

  S32.421 `7th` **Displaced fracture of posterior wall of right acetabulum**

  S32.422 `7th` **Displaced fracture of posterior wall of left acetabulum**

  S32.424 `7th` **Nondisplaced fracture of posterior wall of right acetabulum**

  S32.425 `7th` **Nondisplaced fracture of posterior wall of left acetabulum**

S32.43 `6th` **Fracture of anterior column [iliopubic] of acetabulum**

  S32.431 `7th` **Displaced fracture of anterior column [iliopubic] of right acetabulum**

  S32.432 `7th` **Displaced fracture of anterior column [iliopubic] of left acetabulum**

  S32.434 `7th` **Nondisplaced fracture of anterior column [iliopubic] of right aceta-bulum**

  S32.435 `7th` **Nondisplaced fracture of anterior column [iliopubic] of left aceta-bulum**

S32.44 `6th` **Fracture of posterior column [ilioischial] of acetabulum**

  S32.441 `7th` **Displaced fracture of posterior column [ilioischial] of right acetabulum**

  S32.442 `7th` **Displaced fracture of posterior column [ilioischial] of left acetabulum**

  S32.444 `7th` **Nondisplaced fracture of posterior column [ilioischial] of right acetabulum**

  S32.445 `7th` **Nondisplaced fracture of posterior column [ilioischial] of left acetabulum**

S32.45 `6th` **Transverse fracture of acetabulum**

  S32.451 `7th` **Displaced transverse fracture of right acetabulum**

  S32.452 `7th` **Displaced transverse fracture of left acetabulum**

  S32.454 `7th` **Nondisplaced transverse fracture of right acetabulum**

  S32.455 `7th` **Nondisplaced transverse fracture of left acetabulum**

  S32.456 `7th` **Nondisplaced transverse fracture of unspecified acetabulum**

S32.46 `6th` **Associated transverse-posterior fracture of acetabulum**

  S32.461 `7th` **Displaced associated transverse-posterior fracture of right acetabulum**

  S32.462 `7th` **Displaced associated transverse-posterior fracture of left acetabulum**

  S32.464 `7th` **Nondisplaced associated transverse-posterior fracture of right acetabulum**

  S32.465 `7th` **Nondisplaced associated transverse-posterior fracture of left acetabulum**

S32.47 `6th` **Fracture of medial wall of acetabulum**

  S32.471 `7th` **Displaced fracture of medial wall of right acetabulum**

  S32.472 `7th` **Displaced fracture of medial wall of left acetabulum**

  S32.474 `7th` **Nondisplaced fracture of medial wall of right acetabulum**

  S32.475 `7th` **Nondisplaced fracture of medial wall of left acetabulum**

S32.48 `6th` **Dome fracture of acetabulum**

  S32.481 `7th` **Displaced dome fracture of right acetabulum**

  S32.482 `7th` **Displaced dome fracture of left acetabulum**

  S32.484 `7th` **Nondisplaced dome fracture of right acetabulum**

  S32.485 `7th` **Nondisplaced dome fracture of left acetabulum**

S32.49 `6th` **Other specified fracture of acetabulum**

  S32.491 `7th` **Other specified fracture of right acetabulum**

  S32.492 `7th` **Other specified fracture of left acetabulum**

S32.5 `5th` **Fracture of pubis**

  Excludes1: fracture of pubis with associated disruption of pelvic ring (S32.8-)

  S32.50 `6th` **Unspecified fracture of pubis**

    S32.501 `7th` **Unspecified fracture of right pubis**

    S32.502 `7th` **Unspecified fracture of left pubis**

  S32.51 `6th` **Fracture of superior rim of pubis**

    S32.511 `7th` **Fracture of superior rim of right pubis**

    S32.512 `7th` **Fracture of superior rim of left pubis**

  S32.59 `6th` **Other specified fracture of pubis**

    S32.591 `7th` **Other specified fracture of right pubis**

    S32.592 `7th` **Other specified fracture of left pubis**

S32.6 `5th` **Fracture of ischium**

  Excludes1: fracture of ischium with associated disruption of pelvic ring (S32.8-)

  S32.60 `6th` **Unspecified fracture of ischium**

    S32.601 `7th` **Unspecified fracture of right ischium**

    S32.602 `7th` **Unspecified fracture of left ischium**

  S32.61 `6th` **Avulsion fracture of ischium**

    S32.611 `7th` **Displaced avulsion fracture of right ischium**

    S32.612 `7th` **Displaced avulsion fracture of left ischium**

    S32.614 `7th` **Nondisplaced avulsion fracture of right ischium**

    S32.615 `7th` **Nondisplaced avulsion fracture of left ischium**

  S32.69 `6th` **Other specified fracture of ischium**

    S32.691 `7th` **Other specified fracture of right ischium**

    S32.692 `7th` **Other specified fracture of left ischium**

S32.8 `5th` **Fracture of other parts of pelvis**

  Code also any associated: fracture of acetabulum (S32.4-)
    sacral fracture (S32.1-)

  S32.81 `6th` **Multiple fractures of pelvis with disruption of pelvic ring**

  Multiple pelvic fractures with disruption of pelvic circle

    S32.810 `7th` **Multiple fractures of pelvis with stable disruption of pelvic ring**

    S32.811 `7th` **Multiple fractures of pelvis with unstable disruption of pelvic ring**

`4th` `5th` `6th` `7th` Additional Character Required ✔ `3-character code` Unspecified laterality codes were excluded here.

∗ =New Code
▲ =Revised Code
◻ =Social determinants of health

Excludes1—Not coded here, do not use together
Excludes2—Not included here

S32.82X **Multiple fractures of pelvis without disruption of pelvic ring**
7th
Multiple pelvic fractures without disruption of pelvic circle

S32.89X **Fracture of other parts of pelvis**
7th

S32.9XX **Fracture of unspecified parts of lumbosacral spine and pelvis**
7th
Fracture of lumbosacral spine NOS
Fracture of pelvis NOS

S33 **DISLOCATION AND SPRAIN OF JOINTS AND LIGAMENTS OF LUMBAR SPINE AND PELVIS**
4th

Includes: avulsion of joint or ligament of lumbar spine and pelvis
laceration of cartilage, joint or ligament of lumbar spine and pelvis
sprain of cartilage, joint or ligament of lumbar spine and pelvis
traumatic hemarthrosis of joint or ligament of lumbar spine and pelvis
traumatic rupture of joint or ligament of lumbar spine and pelvis
traumatic subluxation of joint or ligament of lumbar spine and pelvis
traumatic tear of joint or ligament of lumbar spine and pelvis

7th characters for category S33
A—initial encounter
D—subsequent encounter
S—sequela

Code also any associated open wound
Excludes1: nontraumatic rupture or displacement of lumbar intervertebral disc NOS (M51.-)
obstetric damage to pelvic joints and ligaments (O71.6)
Excludes2: dislocation and sprain of joints and ligaments of hip (S73.-)
strain of muscle of lower back and pelvis (S39.01-)

S33.2XX **Dislocation of sacroiliac and sacrococcygeal joint**
7th

S33.5XX **Sprain of ligaments of lumbar spine**
7th

S33.6XX **Sprain of sacroiliac joint**
7th

S33.8XX **Sprain of other parts of lumbar spine and pelvis**
7th

S33.9XX **Sprain of unspecified parts of lumbar spine and pelvis**
7th

S34 **INJURY OF LUMBAR AND SACRAL SPINAL CORD AND NERVES AT ABDOMEN, LOWER BACK AND PELVIS LEVEL**
4th

Note: Code to highest level of lumbar cord injury
Injuries to the spinal cord (S34.0 and S34.1) refer to the cord level and not bone level injury, and can affect nerve roots at and below the level given.

7th characters for category S34
A—initial encounter
D—subsequent encounter
S—sequela

Code also any associated: fracture of vertebra (S22.0-, S32.0-)
open wound of abdomen, lower back and pelvis (S31.-)
transient paralysis (R29.5)

S34.0 **Concussion and edema of lumbar and sacral spinal cord**
5th   **S34.01X** **Concussion and edema of lumbar spinal cord**
7th

     S34.02X **Concussion and edema of sacral spinal cord**
7th
Concussion and edema of conus medullaris

S34.1 **Other and unspecified injury of lumbar and sacral spinal cord**
5th   **S34.10** **Unspecified injury to lumbar spinal cord (level)**
6th   **S34.101** **Unspecified injury to; L1 level of lumbar spinal cord**
7th
     S34.102 **L2 level of lumbar spinal cord**
7th
     S34.103 **L3 level of lumbar spinal cord**
7th
     S34.104 **L4 level of lumbar spinal cord**
7th
     S34.105 **L5 level of lumbar spinal cord**
7th
     S34.109 **unspecified level of lumbar spinal cord**
7th

   S34.12 **Incomplete lesion of lumbar spinal cord (level)**
6th   **S34.121** **Incomplete lesion of; L1 level of lumbar spinal cord**
7th
     S34.123 **L3 level of lumbar spinal cord**
7th

S34.124 **L4 level of lumbar spinal cord**
7th

S34.125 **L5 level of lumbar spinal cord**
7th

S34.129 **unspecified level of lumbar spinal cord**
7th

S34.13 **Other and unspecified injury to sacral spinal cord**
6th
Other injury to conus medullaris
   S34.131 **Complete lesion of sacral spinal cord**
7th
Complete lesion of conus medullaris
   S34.132 **Incomplete lesion of sacral spinal cord**
7th
Incomplete lesion of conus medullaris
   S34.139 **Unspecified injury to sacral spinal cord**
7th
Unspecified injury of conus medullaris

S34.2 **Injury of nerve root of lumbar and sacral spine**
5th   **S34.21X** **Injury of nerve root of lumbar spine**
7th

     S34.22X **Injury of nerve root of sacral spine**
7th

     S34.3XX **Injury of cauda equina**
7th

     S34.4XX **Injury of lumbosacral plexus**
7th

     S34.5XX **Injury of lumbar, sacral and pelvic sympathetic nerves**
7th
Injury of celiac ganglion or plexus
Injury of hypogastric plexus
Injury of mesenteric plexus (inferior) (superior)
Injury of splanchnic nerve

     S34.6XX **Injury of peripheral nerve(s) at abdomen, lower back and pelvis level**
7th
     S34.8XX **Injury of other nerves at abdomen, lower back and pelvis level**
7th
     S34.9XX **Injury of unspecified nerves at abdomen, lower back and pelvis level**
7th

S36 **INJURY OF INTRA-ABDOMINAL ORGANS**
4th
Code also any associated open wound (S31.-)

S36.0 **Injury of spleen**
5th   **S36.02** **Contusion of spleen**
6th   **S36.020** **Minor contusion of spleen**
7th
Contusion of spleen less than 2 cm
     S36.021 **Major contusion of spleen**
7th
Contusion of spleen greater than 2 cm
   S36.03 **Laceration of spleen**
6th   **S36.030** **Superficial (capsular) laceration of spleen**
7th

7th characters for category S36
A—initial encounter
D—subsequent encounter
S—sequela

Laceration of spleen less than 1 cm
Minor laceration of spleen
     S36.032 **Major laceration of spleen**
7th
Avulsion of spleen
Laceration of spleen greater than 3 cm
Massive laceration of spleen
Multiple moderate lacerations of spleen
Stellate laceration of spleen

S36.3 **Injury of stomach**
5th   **S36.30** **Unspecified injury of stomach**
   S36.32 **Contusion of stomach**

S36.6 **Injury of rectum**
5th   **S36.60X** **Unspecified injury of rectum**
7th

     S36.62X **Contusion of rectum**
7th

     S36.63X **Laceration of rectum**
7th

S36.9 **Injury of unspecified intra-abdominal organ**
5th   **S36.90X** **Unspecified injury of unspecified intra-abdominal organ**
7th
     S36.92X **Contusion of unspecified intra-abdominal organ**
7th

4th	5th	6th	7th	Additional Character Required	✓	3-character code

Unspecified laterality codes were excluded here.

• =New Code
▲ =Revised Code
▣ =Social determinants of health

Excludes1—Not coded here, do not use together
Excludes2—Not included here

CHAPTER 19. INJURY, POISONING AND CERTAIN OTHER CONSEQUENCES OF EXTERNAL CAUSES (S36.93X–S40.87)

S36.93X   Laceration of unspecified intra-abdominal organ
7th

S36.99X   Other injury of unspecified intra-abdominal organ
7th

S37   **INJURY OF URINARY AND PELVIC ORGANS**
4th
Code also any associated open wound (S31.-)
Excludes1: obstetric trauma to pelvic organs (O71.-)
Excludes2: injury of peritoneum (S36.81)
   injury of retroperitoneum (S36.89-)

S37.0   **Injury of kidney**
5th
   Excludes2: acute kidney injury
      (nontraumatic) (N17.9)

> 7th characters for category S37
> A—initial encounter
> D—subsequent encounter
> S—sequela

   S37.01   **Minor contusion of**
   6th   **kidney**
     Contusion of kidney less
      than 2 cm
     Contusion of kidney NOS
     S37.011   **Minor contusion of right kidney**
     7th

     S37.012   **Minor contusion of left kidney**
     7th

   S37.02   **Major contusion of kidney**
   6th
     Contusion of kidney greater than 2 cm
     S37.021   **Major contusion of right kidney**
     7th

     S37.022   **Major contusion of left kidney**
     7th

S39   **OTHER AND UNSPECIFIED INJURIES OF ABDOMEN, LOWER BACK, PELVIS AND EXTERNAL GENITALS**
4th
Code also any associated open wound (S31.-)
Excludes2: sprain of joints and ligaments of lumbar spine and pelvis
   (S33.-)

S39.0   **Injury of muscle, fascia and tendon of abdomen, lower back and pelvis**
5th
   S39.01   **Strain of muscle,**
   6th   **fascia and tendon of**
     abdomen, lower back
     and pelvis

> 7th characters for category S39
> A—initial encounter
> D—subsequent encounter
> S—sequela

     S39.011   **Strain of**
     7th   **muscle, fascia and tendon of abdomen**
     S39.012   **Strain of muscle, fascia and tendon of**
     7th   **lower back**

S39.8   **Other specified injuries of abdomen, lower back, pelvis and external genitals**
5th
   S39.83X   **Other specified injuries of pelvis**
   7th

   S39.84   **Other specified injuries of external genitals**
   6th   **S39.848**   **Other specified injuries of external**
     7th   **genitals**

S39.9   **Unspecified injury of abdomen, lower back, pelvis and external genitals**
5th
   S39.91   **Unspecified injury of abdomen**
   7th

   S39.92   **Unspecified injury of lower back**
   7th

   S39.93   **Unspecified injury of pelvis**
   7th

   S39.94   **Unspecified injury of external genitals**
   7th

(S40–S49) INJURIES TO THE SHOULDER AND UPPER ARM

Includes: injuries of axilla
   injuries of scapular region
Excludes2: burns and corrosions (T20–T32)
   frostbite (T33–T34)
   injuries of elbow (S50–S59)
   insect bite or sting, venomous (T63.4)

S40   **SUPERFICIAL INJURY OF**
4th   **SHOULDER AND UPPER ARM**

> 7th characters for category S40
> A—initial encounter
> D—subsequent encounter
> S—sequela

   S40.0   **Contusion of shoulder and upper**
   5th   **arm**

     S40.01   **Contusion of shoulder**
     6th   **S40.011**   **Contusion of right shoulder**
       7th

       S40.012   **Contusion of left shoulder**
       7th

     S40.02   **Contusion of upper arm**
     6th   **S40.021**   **Contusion of right upper arm**
       7th

       S40.022   **Contusion of left upper arm**
       7th

S40.2   **Other superficial injuries of shoulder**
5th
   S40.21   **Abrasion of shoulder**
   6th   **S40.211**   **Abrasion of right shoulder**
     7th

     S40.212   **Abrasion of left shoulder**
     7th

   S40.22   **Blister (nonthermal) of shoulder**
   6th   **S40.221**   **Blister (nonthermal) of right shoulder**
     7th

     S40.222   **Blister (nonthermal) of left shoulder**
     7th

   S40.24   **External constriction of shoulder**
   6th   **S40.241**   **External constriction of right shoulder**
     7th

     S40.242   **External constriction of left shoulder**
     7th

   S40.25   **Superficial FB of shoulder**
   6th   Splinter in the shoulder
     S40.251   **Superficial FB of right shoulder**
     7th

     S40.252   **Superficial FB of left shoulder**
     7th

   S40.26   **Insect bite (nonvenomous) of shoulder**
   6th   **S40.261**   **Insect bite (nonvenomous) of right**
     7th   **shoulder**
     S40.262   **Insect bite (nonvenomous) of left shoulder**
     7th

   S40.27   **Other superficial bite of shoulder**
   6th   ***Excludes1:*** open bite of shoulder (S41.05)
     S40.271   **Other superficial bite of right shoulder**
     7th

     S40.272   **Other superficial bite of left shoulder**
     7th

S40.8   **Other superficial injuries of upper arm**
5th
   S40.81   **Abrasion of upper arm**
   6th   **S40.811**   **Abrasion of right upper arm**
     7th

     S40.812   **Abrasion of left upper arm**
     7th

   S40.82   **Blister (nonthermal) of upper arm**
   6th   **S40.821**   **Blister (nonthermal) of right upper arm**
     7th

     S40.822   **Blister (nonthermal) of left upper arm**
     7th

   S40.84   **External constriction of upper arm**
   6th   **S40.841**   **External constriction of right upper arm**
     7th

     S40.842   **External constriction of left upper arm**
     7th

   S40.85   **Superficial FB of upper arm**
   6th   Splinter in the upper arm
     S40.851   **Superficial FB of right upper arm**
     7th

     S40.852   **Superficial FB of left upper arm**
     7th

   S40.86   **Insect bite (nonvenomous) of upper arm**
   6th   **S40.861**   **Insect bite (nonvenomous) of right upper**
     7th   **arm**
     S40.862   **Insect bite (nonvenomous) of left upper**
     7th   **arm**

   S40.87   **Other superficial bite of upper arm**
   6th   ***Excludes1:*** open bite of upper arm (S41.14)
     Excludes2: other superficial bite of shoulder (S40.27-)

4th *5th* *6th* *7th*   Additional Character Required   ✔   3-character code   Unspecified laterality codes were excluded here.   ✱ =New Code   ▲ =Revised Code   ◻ =Social determinants of health   ***Excludes1***—Not coded here, do not use together   ***Excludes2***—Not included here

S40.871 **Other superficial bite of right upper arm**
7th

S40.872 **Other superficial bite of left upper arm**
7th

S40.9 **Unspecified superficial injury of shoulder and upper arm**
5th

    S40.91 **Unspecified superficial injury of shoulder**
6th

       S40.911 **Unspecified superficial injury of right shoulder**
7th

       S40.912 **Unspecified superficial injury of left shoulder**
7th

    S40.92 **Unspecified superficial injury of upper arm**
6th

       S40.921 **Unspecified superficial injury of right upper arm**
7th

       S40.922 **Unspecified superficial injury of left upper arm**
7th

> 7th characters for categories S40 & S41
> A—initial encounter
> D—subsequent encounter
> S—sequela

S41   OPEN WOUND OF SHOULDER AND UPPER ARM
4th

Code also any associated wound infection
Excludes1: traumatic amputation of shoulder and upper arm (S48.-)
Excludes2: open fracture of shoulder and upper arm (S42.- with 7th character B or C)

S41.0 **Open wound of shoulder**
5th

    S41.01 **Laceration without FB of shoulder**
6th

       S41.011 **Laceration without FB of right shoulder**
7th

       S41.012 **Laceration without FB of left shoulder**
7th

    S41.02 **Laceration with FB of shoulder**
6th

       S41.021 **Laceration with FB of right shoulder**
7th

       S41.022 **Laceration with FB of left shoulder**
7th

    S41.03 **Puncture wound without FB of shoulder**
6th

       S41.031 **Puncture wound without FB of right shoulder**
7th

       S41.032 **Puncture wound without FB of left shoulder**
7th

    S41.04 **Puncture wound with FB of shoulder**
6th

       S41.041 **Puncture wound with FB of right shoulder**
7th

       S41.042 **Puncture wound with FB of left shoulder**
7th

    S41.05 **Open bite of shoulder**
6th

       Bite of shoulder NOS
       Excludes1: superficial bite of shoulder (S40.27)

       S41.051 **Open bite of right shoulder**
7th

       S41.052 **Open bite of left shoulder**
7th

S41.1 **Open wound of upper arm**
5th

    S41.11 **Laceration without FB of upper arm**
6th

       S41.111 **Laceration without FB of right upper arm**
7th

       S41.112 **Laceration without FB of left upper arm**
7th

    S41.12 **Laceration with FB of upper arm**
6th

       S41.121 **Laceration with FB of right upper arm**
7th

       S41.122 **Laceration with FB of left upper arm**
7th

    S41.13 **Puncture wound without FB of upper arm**
6th

       S41.131 **Puncture wound without FB of right upper arm**
7th

       S41.132 **Puncture wound without FB of left upper arm**
7th

    S41.14 **Puncture wound with FB of upper arm**
6th

       S41.141 **Puncture wound with FB of right upper arm**
7th

       S41.142 **Puncture wound with FB of left upper arm**
7th

    S41.15 **Open bite of upper arm**
6th

       Bite of upper arm NOS
       Excludes1: superficial bite of upper arm (S40.87)

       S41.151 **Open bite of right upper arm**
7th

       S41.152 **Open bite of left upper arm**
7th

S42   FRACTURE OF SHOULDER AND UPPER ARM
4th

Note: A fracture not indicated as displaced or nondisplaced should be coded to displaced

A fracture not indicated as open or closed should be coded to closed

Excludes1: traumatic amputation of shoulder and upper arm (S48.-)

> 7th characters for category S42
> A—initial encounter for closed fracture
> B—initial encounter for open fracture
> D—subsequent encounter for fracture with routine healing
> G—subsequent encounter for fracture with delayed healing
> K—subsequent encounter for fracture with nonunion
> P—subsequent encounter for fracture with malunion
> S—sequela

S42.0 **Fracture of clavicle**
5th

    S42.00 **Fracture of unspecified part of clavicle**
6th

       S42.001 **Fracture of unspecified part of right clavicle**
7th

       S42.002 **Fracture of unspecified part of left clavicle**
7th

    S42.01 **Fracture of sternal end of clavicle**
6th

       S42.011 **Anterior displaced fracture of sternal end of right clavicle**
7th

       S42.012 **Anterior displaced fracture of sternal end of left clavicle**
7th

       S42.014 **Posterior displaced fracture of sternal end of right clavicle**
7th

       S42.015 **Posterior displaced fracture of sternal end of left clavicle**
7th

       S42.017 **Nondisplaced fracture of sternal end of right clavicle**
7th

       S42.018 **Nondisplaced fracture of sternal end of left clavicle**
7th

    S42.02 **Fracture of shaft of clavicle**
6th

       S42.021 **Displaced fracture of shaft of right clavicle**
7th

       S42.022 **Displaced fracture of shaft of left clavicle**
7th

       S42.024 **Nondisplaced fracture of shaft of right clavicle**
7th

       S42.025 **Nondisplaced fracture of shaft of left clavicle**
7th

    S42.03 **Fracture of lateral end of clavicle**
6th

       Fracture of acromial end of clavicle

       S42.031 **Displaced fracture of lateral end of right clavicle**
7th

       S42.032 **Displaced fracture of lateral end of left clavicle**
7th

       S42.034 **Nondisplaced fracture of lateral end of right clavicle**
7th

       S42.035 **Nondisplaced fracture of lateral end of left clavicle**
7th

S42.2 **Fracture of upper end of humerus**
5th

    Fracture of proximal end of humerus
    Excludes2: fracture of shaft of humerus (S42.3-)
       physeal fracture of upper end of humerus (S49.0-)

    S42.20 **Unspecified fracture of upper end of; humerus**
6th

       S42.201   **right humerus**
7th

       S42.202   **left humerus**
7th

    S42.21 **Unspecified fracture of surgical neck of humerus**
6th

       Fracture of neck of humerus NOS

       S42.211 **Unspecified displaced fracture of surgical neck of right humerus**
7th

       S42.212 **Unspecified displaced fracture of surgical neck of left humerus**
7th

       S42.214 **Unspecified nondisplaced fracture of surgical neck of right humerus**
7th

• =New Code   ***Excludes1***—Not coded here, do not use together
▲ =Revised Code   ***Excludes2***—Not included here
□ =Social determinants of health

| 4th | 5th | 6th | 7th | Additional Character Required | ✔ | 3-character code |

Unspecified laterality codes were excluded here.

CHAPTER 19. INJURY, POISONING AND CERTAIN OTHER CONSEQUENCES OF EXTERNAL CAUSES   (S42.215–S42.411)

S42.215 Unspecified nondisplaced fracture of [7th] surgical neck of left humerus

S42.22 2-part fracture of surgical neck of humerus
[6th]
    S42.221 2-part displaced fracture of surgical neck [7th] of right humerus
    S42.222 2-part dis-[7th] placed fracture of surgical neck of left humerus
    S42.224 2-part [7th] nondisplaced fracture of surgical neck of right humerus
    S42.225 2-part [7th] nondisplaced fracture of surgical neck of left humerus

> 7th characters for category S42
> A—initial encounter for closed fracture
> B—initial encounter for open fracture
> D—subsequent encounter for fracture with routine healing
> G—subsequent encounter for fracture with delayed healing
> K—subsequent encounter for fracture with nonunion
> P—subsequent encounter for fracture with malunion
> S—sequela

S42.23 3-part fracture of surgical neck of humerus
[6th]
    S42.231 3-part fracture of surgical neck of right [7th] humerus
    S42.232 3-part fracture of surgical neck of left [7th] humerus

S42.24 4-part fracture of surgical neck of humerus
[6th]
    S42.241 4-part fracture of surgical neck of right [7th] humerus
    S42.242 4-part fracture of surgical neck of left [7th] humerus

S42.25 Fracture of greater tuberosity of humerus
[6th]
    S42.251 Displaced fracture of greater tuberosity of [7th] right humerus
    S42.252 Displaced fracture of greater tuberosity of [7th] left humerus
    S42.254 Nondisplaced fracture of greater [7th] tuberosity of right humerus
    S42.255 Nondisplaced fracture of greater [7th] tuberosity of left humerus

S42.26 Fracture of lesser tuberosity of humerus
[6th]
    S42.261 Displaced fracture of lesser tuberosity of [7th] right humerus
    S42.262 Displaced fracture of lesser tuberosity of [7th] left humerus
    S42.264 Nondisplaced fracture of lesser tuberosity [7th] of right humerus
    S42.265 Nondisplaced fracture of lesser tuberosity [7th] of left humerus

S42.27 Torus fracture of upper end of humerus
[6th]
    S42.271 Torus fracture of upper end of right [7th] humerus
    S42.272 Torus fracture of upper end of left [7th] humerus

S42.29 Other fracture of upper end of humerus
[6th]
    Fracture of anatomical neck of humerus
    Fracture of articular head of humerus
    S42.291 Other displaced fracture of upper end of [7th] right humerus
    S42.292 Other displaced fracture of upper end of [7th] left humerus
    S42.293 Other displaced fracture of upper end of [7th] unspecified humerus
    S42.294 Other nondisplaced fracture of upper end [7th] of right humerus
    S42.295 Other nondisplaced fracture of upper end [7th] of left humerus

S42.3 Fracture of shaft of humerus
[5th]
    Fracture of humerus NOS
    Fracture of upper arm NOS
    Excludes2: physeal fractures of upper end of humerus (S49.0-)
    physeal fractures of lower end of humerus (S49.1-)
    S42.30 Unspecified fracture of shaft of humerus
    [6th]
        S42.301 Unspecified fracture of shaft of humerus, [7th] right arm

S42.302 Unspecified fracture of shaft of humerus, [7th] left arm

S42.31 Greenstick fracture of shaft of humerus
[6th]
    S42.311 Greenstick fracture of shaft of humerus, [7th] right arm
    S42.312 Greenstick fracture of shaft of humerus, [7th] left arm

S42.32 Transverse fracture of shaft of humerus
[6th]
    S42.321 Displaced transverse fracture of shaft of [7th] humerus, right arm
    S42.322 Displaced transverse fracture of shaft of [7th] humerus, left arm
    S42.324 Nondisplaced transverse fracture of shaft [7th] of humerus, right arm
    S42.325 Nondisplaced transverse fracture of shaft [7th] of humerus, left arm

S42.33 Oblique fracture of shaft of humerus
[6th]
    S42.331 Displaced oblique fracture of shaft of [7th] humerus, right arm
    S42.332 Displaced oblique fracture of shaft of [7th] humerus, left arm
    S42.334 Nondisplaced oblique fracture of shaft of [7th] humerus, right arm
    S42.335 Nondisplaced oblique fracture of shaft of [7th] humerus, left arm

S42.34 Spiral fracture of shaft of humerus
[6th]
    S42.341 Displaced spiral fracture of shaft of [7th] humerus, right arm
    S42.342 Displaced spiral fracture of shaft of [7th] humerus, left arm
    S42.343 Displaced spiral fracture of shaft of [7th] humerus, unspecified arm
    S42.344 Nondisplaced spiral fracture of shaft of [7th] humerus, right arm
    S42.345 Nondisplaced spiral fracture of shaft of [7th] humerus, left arm

S42.35 Comminuted fracture of shaft of humerus
[6th]
    S42.351 Displaced comminuted fracture of shaft of [7th] humerus, right arm
    S42.352 Displaced comminuted fracture of shaft of [7th] humerus, left arm
    S42.354 Nondisplaced comminuted fracture of [7th] shaft of humerus, right arm
    S42.355 Nondisplaced comminuted fracture of [7th] shaft of humerus, left arm

S42.36 Segmental fracture of shaft of humerus
[6th]
    S42.361 Displaced segmental fracture of shaft of [7th] humerus, right arm
    S42.362 Displaced segmental fracture of shaft of [7th] humerus, left arm
    S42.364 Nondisplaced segmental fracture of shaft [7th] of humerus, right arm
    S42.365 Nondisplaced segmental fracture of shaft [7th] of humerus, left arm

S42.39 Other fracture of shaft of humerus
[6th]
    S42.391 Other fracture of shaft of right humerus [7th]
    S42.392 Other fracture of shaft of left humerus [7th]

S42.4 Fracture of lower end of humerus
[5th]
    Fracture of distal end of humerus
    Excludes2: fracture of shaft of humerus (S42.3-)
    physeal fracture of lower end of humerus (S49.1-)
    S42.40 Unspecified fracture of lower end of humerus
    [6th]
    Fracture of elbow NOS
        S42.401 Unspecified fracture of lower end of right [7th] humerus
        S42.402 Unspecified fracture of lower end of left [7th] humerus
    S42.41 Simple supracondylar fracture without intercondylar
    [6th] fracture of humerus
        S42.411 Displaced simple supracondylar fracture [7th] without intercondylar fracture of right humerus

[4th] [5th] [6th] [7th] Additional Character Required   ✓   3-character code   Unspecified laterality codes were excluded here.   •=New Code   ▲=Revised Code   ▭=Social determinants of health   *Excludes1*—Not coded here, do not use together   *Excludes2*—Not included here

346   **PEDIATRIC ICD-10-CM 2021: A MANUAL FOR PROVIDER-BASED CODING**

S42.412 Displaced simple supracondylar fracture without intercondylar fracture of left humerus
7th

S42.414 Nondisplaced simple supracondylar fracture without intercondylar fracture of right humerus
7th

> 7th characters for category S42
> A—initial encounter for closed fracture
> B—initial encounter for open fracture
> D—subsequent encounter for fracture with routine healing
> G—subsequent encounter for fracture with delayed healing
> K—subsequent encounter for fracture with nonunion
> P—subsequent encounter for fracture with malunion
> S—sequela

S42.415 Nondisplaced simple supracondylar fracture without intercondylar fracture of left humerus
7th

S42.42 Comminuted supracondylar fracture without intercondylar fracture of humerus
6th

S42.421 Displaced comminuted supracondylar fracture without intercondylar fracture of right humerus
7th

S42.422 Displaced comminuted supracondylar fracture without intercondylar fracture of left humerus
7th

S42.424 Nondisplaced comminuted supracondylar fracture without intercondylar fracture of right humerus
7th

S42.425 Nondisplaced comminuted supracondylar fracture without intercondylar fracture of left humerus
7th

S42.43 Fracture (avulsion) of lateral epicondyle of humerus
6th

S42.431 Displaced fracture (avulsion) of lateral epicondyle of right humerus
7th

S42.432 Displaced fracture (avulsion) of lateral epicondyle of left humerus
7th

S42.434 Nondisplaced fracture (avulsion) of lateral epicondyle of right humerus
7th

S42.435 Nondisplaced fracture (avulsion) of lateral epicondyle of left humerus
7th

S42.44 Fracture (avulsion) of medial epicondyle of humerus
6th

S42.441 Displaced fracture (avulsion) of medial epicondyle of right humerus
7th

S42.442 Displaced fracture (avulsion) of medial epicondyle of left humerus
7th

S42.444 Nondisplaced fracture (avulsion) of medial epicondyle of right humerus
7th

S42.445 Nondisplaced fracture (avulsion) of medial epicondyle of left humerus
7th

S42.447 Incarcerated fracture (avulsion) of medial epicondyle of right humerus
7th

S42.448 Incarcerated fracture (avulsion) of medial epicondyle of left humerus
7th

S42.45 Fracture of lateral condyle of humerus
6th
Fracture of capitellum of humerus

S42.451 Displaced fracture of lateral condyle of right humerus
7th

S42.452 Displaced fracture of lateral condyle of left humerus
7th

S42.454 Nondisplaced fracture of lateral condyle of right humerus
7th

S42.455 Nondisplaced fracture of lateral condyle of left humerus
7th

S42.46 Fracture of medial condyle of humerus
6th
Trochlea fracture of humerus

S42.461 Displaced fracture of medial condyle of right humerus
7th

S42.462 Displaced fracture of medial condyle of left humerus
7th

S42.464 Nondisplaced fracture of medial condyle of right humerus
7th

S42.465 Nondisplaced fracture of medial condyle of left humerus
7th

S42.47 Transcondylar fracture of humerus
6th

S42.471 Displaced transcondylar fracture of right humerus
7th

S42.472 Displaced transcondylar fracture of left humerus
7th

S42.474 Nondisplaced transcondylar fracture of right humerus
7th

S42.475 Nondisplaced transcondylar fracture of left humerus
7th

S42.48 Torus fracture of lower end of humerus
6th

S42.481 Torus fracture of lower end of right humerus
7th

S42.482 Torus fracture of lower end of left humerus
7th

S42.49 Other fracture of lower end of humerus
6th

S42.491 Other displaced fracture of lower end of right humerus
7th

S42.492 Other displaced fracture of lower end of left humerus
7th

S42.494 Other nondisplaced fracture of lower end of right humerus
7th

S42.495 Other nondisplaced fracture of lower end of left humerus
7th

S42.9 Fracture of shoulder girdle, part unspecified
5th
Fracture of shoulder NOS

S42.91X Fracture of right shoulder girdle, part unspecified
7th

S42.92X Fracture of left shoulder girdle, part unspecified
7th

S43 **DISLOCATION AND SPRAIN OF JOINTS AND LIGAMENTS OF SHOULDER GIRDLE**
4th

Includes: avulsion of joint or ligament of shoulder girdle

laceration of cartilage, joint or ligament of shoulder girdle

sprain of cartilage, joint or ligament of shoulder girdle

traumatic hemarthrosis of joint or ligament of shoulder girdle

traumatic rupture of joint or ligament of shoulder girdle

traumatic subluxation of joint or ligament of shoulder girdle

traumatic tear of joint or ligament of shoulder girdle

> 7th characters for category S43
> A—initial encounter
> D—subsequent encounter
> S—sequela

Code also any associated open wound

Excludes2: strain of muscle, fascia and tendon of shoulder and upper arm (S46.-)

S43.0 Subluxation and dislocation of shoulder joint
5th
Dislocation of glenohumeral joint
Subluxation of glenohumeral joint

S43.00 Unspecified subluxation and dislocation of shoulder joint
6th
Dislocation of humerus NOS
Subluxation of humerus NOS

S43.001 Unspecified subluxation of right shoulder joint
7th

S43.002 Unspecified subluxation of left shoulder joint
7th

S43.004 Unspecified dislocation of right shoulder joint
7th

S43.005 Unspecified dislocation of left shoulder joint
7th

S43.01 Anterior subluxation and dislocation of humerus
6th

S43.011 Anterior subluxation of right humerus
7th

S43.012 Anterior subluxation of left humerus
7th

S43.014 Anterior dislocation of right humerus
7th

S43.015 Anterior dislocation of left humerus
7th

S43.02 Posterior subluxation and dislocation of humerus
6th

S43.021 Posterior subluxation of right humerus
7th

S43.022 Posterior subluxation of left humerus
7th

4th	5th	6th	7th	Additional Character Required	✓	3-character code

Unspecified laterality codes were excluded here.

• =New Code
▲ =Revised Code
▫ =Social determinants of health

Excludes1—Not coded here, do not use together
Excludes2—Not included here

CHAPTER 19. INJURY, POISONING AND CERTAIN OTHER CONSEQUENCES OF EXTERNAL CAUSES   (S43.024–S43.491)

S43.024 Posterior dislocation of right humerus
7th

S43.025 Posterior dislocation of left humerus
7th

7th characters for category S43
A—initial encounter
D—subsequent encounter
S—sequela

S43.03 Inferior subluxation and dislocation of humerus
6th

S43.031 Inferior subluxation of right humerus
7th

S43.032 Inferior subluxation of left humerus
7th

S43.034 Inferior dislocation of right humerus
7th

S43.035 Inferior dislocation of left humerus
7th

S43.08 Other subluxation and dislocation of shoulder joint
6th

S43.081 Other subluxation of right shoulder joint
7th

S43.082 Other subluxation of left shoulder joint
7th

S43.084 Other dislocation of right shoulder joint
7th

S43.085 Other dislocation of left shoulder joint
7th

S43.1 Subluxation and dislocation of acromioclavicular joint
5th

S43.10 Unspecified dislocation of acromioclavicular joint
6th

S43.101 Unspecified dislocation of right acromioclavicular joint
7th

S43.102 Unspecified dislocation of left acromioclavicular joint
7th

S43.11 Subluxation of acromioclavicular joint
6th

S43.111 Subluxation of right acromioclavicular joint
7th

S43.112 Subluxation of left acromioclavicular joint
7th

S43.12 Dislocation of acromioclavicular joint, 100%–200% displacement
6th

S43.121 Dislocation of right acromioclavicular joint, 100%–200% displacement
7th

S43.122 Dislocation of left acromioclavicular joint, 100%–200% displacement
7th

S43.13 Dislocation of acromioclavicular joint, greater than 200% displacement
6th

S43.131 Dislocation of right acromioclavicular joint, greater than 200% displacement
7th

S43.132 Dislocation of left acromioclavicular joint, greater than 200% displacement
7th

S43.14 Inferior dislocation of acromioclavicular joint
6th

S43.141 Inferior dislocation of right acromioclavicular joint
7th

S43.142 Inferior dislocation of left acromioclavicular joint
7th

S43.15 Posterior dislocation of acromioclavicular joint
6th

S43.151 Posterior dislocation of right acromioclavicular joint
7th

S43.152 Posterior dislocation of left acromioclavicular joint
7th

S43.2 Subluxation and dislocation of sternoclavicular joint
5th

S43.20 Unspecified subluxation and dislocation of sternoclavicular joint

S43.201 Unspecified subluxation of right sternoclavicular joint
7th

S43.202 Unspecified subluxation of left sternoclavicular joint
7th

S43.204 Unspecified dislocation of right sternoclavicular joint
7th

S43.205 Unspecified dislocation of left sternoclavicular joint
7th

S43.21 Anterior subluxation and dislocation of sternoclavicular joint
6th

S43.211 Anterior subluxation of right sternoclavicular joint
7th

S43.212 Anterior subluxation of left sternoclavicular joint
7th

S43.214 Anterior dislocation of right sternoclavicular joint
7th

S43.215 Anterior dislocation of left sternoclavicular joint
7th

S43.22 Posterior subluxation and dislocation of sternoclavicular joint
6th

S43.221 Posterior subluxation of right sternoclavicular joint
7th

S43.222 Posterior subluxation of left sternoclavicular joint
7th

S43.224 Posterior dislocation of right sternoclavicular joint
7th

S43.225 Posterior dislocation of left sternoclavicular joint
7th

S43.3 Subluxation and dislocation of other and unspecified parts of shoulder girdle
5th

S43.30 Subluxation and dislocation of unspecified parts of shoulder girdle
6th

Dislocation/subluxation of shoulder girdle NOS

S43.301 Subluxation of unspecified parts of right shoulder girdle
7th

S43.302 Subluxation of unspecified parts of left shoulder girdle
7th

S43.304 Dislocation of unspecified parts of right shoulder girdle
7th

S43.305 Dislocation of unspecified parts of left shoulder girdle
7th

S43.31 Subluxation and dislocation of scapula
6th

S43.311 Subluxation of right scapula
7th

S43.312 Subluxation of left scapula
7th

S43.314 Dislocation of right scapula
7th

S43.315 Dislocation of left scapula
7th

S43.39 Subluxation and dislocation of other parts of shoulder girdle
6th

S43.391 Subluxation of other parts of right shoulder girdle
7th

S43.392 Subluxation of other parts of left shoulder girdle
7th

S43.394 Dislocation of other parts of right shoulder girdle
7th

S43.395 Dislocation of other parts of left shoulder girdle
7th

S43.4 Sprain of shoulder joint
5th

S43.40 Unspecified sprain of shoulder joint
6th

S43.401 Unspecified sprain of right shoulder joint
7th

S43.402 Unspecified sprain of left shoulder joint
7th

S43.41 Sprain of coracohumeral (ligament)
6th

S43.411 Sprain of right coracohumeral (ligament)
7th

S43.412 Sprain of left coracohumeral (ligament)
7th

S43.42 Sprain of rotator cuff capsule
6th

Excludes1: rotator cuff syndrome (complete) (incomplete), not specified as traumatic (M75.1-)

Excludes2: injury of tendon of rotator cuff (S46.0-)

S43.421 Sprain of right rotator cuff capsule
7th

S43.422 Sprain of left rotator cuff capsule
7th

S43.43 Superior glenoid labrum lesion
6th

SLAP lesion

S43.431 Superior glenoid labrum lesion of right shoulder
7th

S43.432 Superior glenoid labrum lesion of left shoulder
7th

S43.49 Other sprain of shoulder joint
6th

S43.491 Other sprain of right shoulder joint
7th

4th	5th	6th	7th	Additional Character Required	✓	3-character code	Unspecified laterality codes were excluded here.	•=New Code ▲=Revised Code ▢=Social determinants of health	*Excludes1*—Not coded here, do not use together *Excludes2*—Not included here

S43.492   Other sprain of left shoulder joint
> 7th

S43.5   Sprain of acromioclavicular joint
> 5th

Sprain of acromioclavicular ligament

S43.51X   Sprain of right acromioclavicular joint
> 7th

S43.52X   Sprain of left acromioclavicular joint
> 7th

S43.6   Sprain of sternoclavicular joint
> 5th

S43.61X   Sprain of right sternoclavicular joint
> 7th

S43.62X   Sprain of left sternoclavicular joint
> 7th

S43.8   Sprain of other specified parts of shoulder girdle
> 5th

S43.81X   Sprain of other specified parts of right shoulder girdle
> 7th

S43.82X   Sprain of other specified parts of left shoulder girdle
> 7th

> 7th characters for categories S43 & S46
> A—initial encounter
> D—subsequent encounter
> S—sequela

S46   **INJURY OF MUSCLE, FASCIA AND TENDON AT SHOULDER AND UPPER ARM LEVEL**
> 4th

Code also any associated open wound (S41.-)

Excludes2: injury of muscle, fascia and tendon at elbow (S56.-)

sprain of joints and ligaments of shoulder girdle (S43.9)

S46.0   Injury of muscle(s) and tendon(s) of the rotator cuff of shoulder
> 5th

S46.00   Unspecified injury of muscle(s) and tendon(s) of the rotator cuff of shoulder
> 6th

S46.001   Unspecified injury of muscle(s) and tendon(s) of the rotator cuff of right shoulder
> 7th

S46.002   Unspecified injury of muscle(s) and tendon(s) of the rotator cuff of left shoulder
> 7th

S46.01   Strain of muscle(s) and tendon(s) of the rotator cuff of shoulder
> 6th

S46.011   Strain of muscle(s) and tendon(s) of the rotator cuff of right shoulder
> 7th

S46.012   Strain of muscle(s) and tendon(s) of the rotator cuff of left shoulder
> 7th

S46.02   Laceration of muscle(s) and tendon(s) of the rotator cuff of shoulder
> 6th

S46.021   Laceration of muscle(s) and tendon(s) of the rotator cuff of right shoulder
> 7th

S46.022   Laceration of muscle(s) and tendon(s) of the rotator cuff of left shoulder
> 7th

S46.09   Other injury of muscle(s) and tendon(s) of the rotator cuff of shoulder
> 6th

S46.091   Other injury of muscle(s) and tendon(s) of the rotator cuff of right shoulder
> 7th

S46.092   Other injury of muscle(s) and tendon(s) of the rotator cuff of left shoulder
> 7th

S46.91   Strain of unspecified muscle, fascia and tendon at shoulder and upper arm level
> 6th

S46.911   Strain of unspecified muscle, fascia and tendon at shoulder and upper arm level, right arm
> 7th

S46.912   Strain of unspecified muscle, fascia and tendon at shoulder and upper arm level, left arm
> 7th

S46.92   Laceration of unspecified muscle, fascia and tendon at shoulder and upper arm level
> 6th

S46.921   Laceration of unspecified muscle, fascia and tendon at shoulder and upper arm level, right arm
> 7th

S46.922   Laceration of unspecified muscle, fascia and tendon at shoulder and upper arm level, left arm
> 7th

S46.99   Other injury of unspecified muscle, fascia and tendon at shoulder and upper arm level
> 6th

S46.991   Other injury of unspecified muscle, fascia and tendon at shoulder and upper arm level, right arm
> 7th

S46.992   Other injury of unspecified muscle, fascia and tendon at shoulder and upper arm level, left arm
> 7th

S49   **OTHER AND UNSPECIFIED INJURIES OF SHOULDER AND UPPER ARM**
> 4th

S49.0   Physeal fracture of upper end of humerus
> 5th

S49.00   Unspecified physeal fracture of upper end of humerus
> 6th

S49.001   Unspecified physeal fracture of upper end of humerus, right arm
> 7th

> 7th characters for category S49
> A—initial encounter for closed fracture
> D—subsequent encounter for fracture with routine healing
> G—subsequent encounter for fracture with delayed healing
> K—subsequent encounter for fracture with nonunion
> P—subsequent encounter for fracture with malunion
> S—sequela

S49.002   Unspecified physeal fracture of upper end of humerus, left arm
> 7th

S49.01   Salter-Harris Type I physeal fracture of upper end of humerus
> 6th

S49.011   Salter-Harris Type I physeal fractureof upper end of humerus, right arm
> 7th

S49.012   Salter-Harris Type I physeal fracture of upper end of humerus, left arm
> 7th

S49.02   Salter-Harris Type II physeal fracture of upper end of humerus
> 6th

S49.021   Salter-Harris Type II physeal fracture of upper end of humerus, right arm
> 7th

S49.022   Salter-Harris Type II physeal fracture of upper end of humerus, left arm
> 7th

S49.03   Salter-Harris Type III physeal fracture of upper end of humerus
> 6th

S49.031   Salter-Harris Type III physeal fracture of upper end of humerus, right arm
> 7th

S49.032   Salter-Harris Type III physeal fracture of upper end of humerus, left arm
> 7th

S49.04   Salter-Harris Type IV physeal fracture of upper end of humerus
> 6th

S49.041   Salter-Harris Type IV physeal fracture of upper end of humerus, right arm
> 7th

S49.042   Salter-Harris Type IV physeal fracture of upper end of humerus, left arm
> 7th

S49.09   Other physeal fracture of upper end of humerus
> 6th

S49.091   Other physeal fracture of upper end of humerus, right arm
> 7th

S49.092   Other physeal fracture of upper end of humerus, left arm
> 7th

S49.1   Physeal fracture of lower end of humerus
> 5th

S49.10   Unspecified physeal fracture of lower end of humerus
> 6th

S49.101   Unspecified physeal fracture of lower end of humerus, right arm
> 7th

S49.102   Unspecified physeal fracture of lower end of humerus, left arm
> 7th

S49.11   Salter-Harris Type I physeal fracture of lower end of humerus
> 6th

S49.111   Salter-Harris Type I physeal fracture of lower end of humerus, right arm
> 7th

S49.112   Salter-Harris Type I physeal fracture of lower end of humerus, left arm
> 7th

S49.12   Salter-Harris Type II physeal fracture of lower end of humerus
> 6th

S49.121   Salter-Harris Type II physeal fracture of lower end of humerus, right arm
> 7th

S49.122   Salter-Harris Type II physeal fracture of lower end of humerus, left arm
> 7th

S49.13   Salter-Harris Type III physeal fracture of lower end of humerus
> 6th

| 4th | 5th | 6th | 7th | Additional Character Required   ✓   3-character code |

Unspecified laterality codes were excluded here.

• =New Code
▲ =Revised Code
▫ =Social determinants of health

Excludes1—Not coded here, do not use together
Excludes2—Not included here

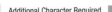

CHAPTER 19. INJURY, POISONING AND CERTAIN OTHER CONSEQUENCES OF EXTERNAL CAUSES   (S49.131–S51.82)

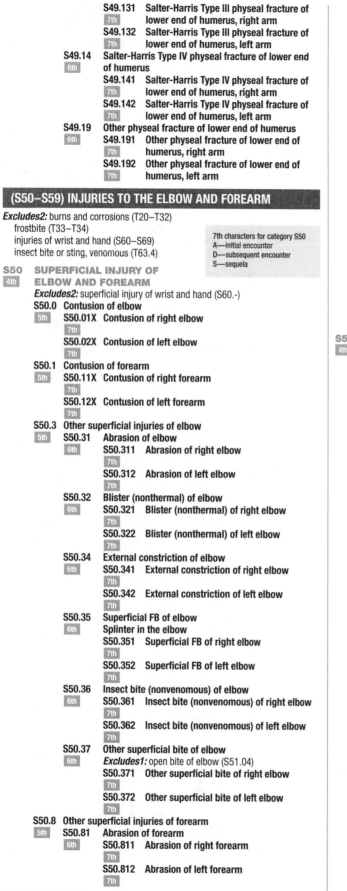

S49.131 [7th] Salter-Harris Type III physeal fracture of lower end of humerus, right arm
S49.132 [7th] Salter-Harris Type III physeal fracture of lower end of humerus, left arm
S49.14 [6th] Salter-Harris Type IV physeal fracture of lower end of humerus
S49.141 [7th] Salter-Harris Type IV physeal fracture of lower end of humerus, right arm
S49.142 [7th] Salter-Harris Type IV physeal fracture of lower end of humerus, left arm
S49.19 [6th] Other physeal fracture of lower end of humerus
S49.191 [7th] Other physeal fracture of lower end of humerus, right arm
S49.192 [7th] Other physeal fracture of lower end of humerus, left arm

(S50–S59) INJURIES TO THE ELBOW AND FOREARM

Excludes2: burns and corrosions (T20–T32)
    frostbite (T33–T34)
    injuries of wrist and hand (S60–S69)
    insect bite or sting, venomous (T63.4)

> 7th characters for category S50
> A—initial encounter
> D—subsequent encounter
> S—sequela

S50 [4th] **SUPERFICIAL INJURY OF ELBOW AND FOREARM**
Excludes2: superficial injury of wrist and hand (S60.-)
S50.0 Contusion of elbow
[5th] **S50.01X** [7th] Contusion of right elbow
S50.02X [7th] Contusion of left elbow
S50.1 Contusion of forearm
[5th] **S50.11X** [7th] Contusion of right forearm
S50.12X [7th] Contusion of left forearm
S50.3 Other superficial injuries of elbow
[5th] **S50.31** [6th] Abrasion of elbow
S50.311 [7th] Abrasion of right elbow
S50.312 [7th] Abrasion of left elbow
S50.32 [6th] Blister (nonthermal) of elbow
S50.321 [7th] Blister (nonthermal) of right elbow
S50.322 [7th] Blister (nonthermal) of left elbow
S50.34 [6th] External constriction of elbow
S50.341 [7th] External constriction of right elbow
S50.342 [7th] External constriction of left elbow
S50.35 [6th] Superficial FB of elbow
Splinter in the elbow
S50.351 [7th] Superficial FB of right elbow
S50.352 [7th] Superficial FB of left elbow
S50.36 [6th] Insect bite (nonvenomous) of elbow
S50.361 [7th] Insect bite (nonvenomous) of right elbow
S50.362 [7th] Insect bite (nonvenomous) of left elbow
S50.37 [6th] Other superficial bite of elbow
Excludes1: open bite of elbow (S51.04)
S50.371 [7th] Other superficial bite of right elbow
S50.372 [7th] Other superficial bite of left elbow
S50.8 Other superficial injuries of forearm
[5th] **S50.81** [6th] Abrasion of forearm
S50.811 [7th] Abrasion of right forearm
S50.812 [7th] Abrasion of left forearm

S50.82 [6th] Blister (nonthermal) of forearm
S50.821 [7th] Blister (nonthermal) of right forearm
S50.822 [7th] Blister (nonthermal) of left forearm
S50.84 [6th] External constriction of forearm
S50.841 [7th] External constriction of right forearm
S50.842 [7th] External constriction of left forearm
S50.85 [6th] Superficial FB of forearm
Splinter in the forearm
S50.851 [7th] Superficial FB of right forearm
S50.852 [7th] Superficial FB of left forearm
S50.86 [6th] Insect bite (nonvenomous) of forearm
S50.861 [7th] Insect bite (nonvenomous) of right forearm
S50.862 [7th] Insect bite (nonvenomous) of left forearm
S50.87 [6th] Other superficial bite of forearm
Excludes1: open bite of forearm (S51.84)
S50.871 [7th] Other superficial bite of right forearm
S50.872 [7th] Other superficial bite of left forearm

S51 [4th] **OPEN WOUND OF ELBOW AND FOREARM**
Code also any associated wound infection
Excludes1: open fracture of elbow and forearm (S52.- with open fracture 7th character)
    traumatic amputation of elbow and forearm (S58.-)
Excludes2: open wound of wrist and hand (S61.-)

> 7th characters for category S51
> A—initial encounter
> D—subsequent encounter
> S—sequela

S51.0 Open wound of elbow
[5th] **S51.01** [6th] Laceration without FB of elbow
S51.011 [7th] Laceration without FB of right elbow
S51.012 [7th] Laceration without FB of left elbow
S51.02 [6th] Laceration with FB of elbow
S51.021 [7th] Laceration with FB of right elbow
S51.022 [7th] Laceration with FB of left elbow
S51.03 [6th] Puncture wound without FB of elbow
S51.031 [7th] Puncture wound without FB of right elbow
S51.032 [7th] Puncture wound without FB of left elbow
S51.04 [6th] Puncture wound with FB of elbow
S51.041 [7th] Puncture wound with FB of right elbow
S51.042 [7th] Puncture wound with FB of left elbow
S51.05 [6th] Open bite of elbow
Bite of elbow NOS
Excludes1: superficial bite of elbow (S50.36, S50.37)
S51.051 [7th] Open bite, right elbow
S51.052 [7th] Open bite, left elbow
S51.8 Open wound of forearm
[5th] ***Excludes2:*** open wound of elbow (S51.0-)
S51.81 [6th] Laceration without FB of forearm
S51.811 [7th] Laceration without FB of right forearm
S51.812 [7th] Laceration without FB of left forearm
S51.82 [6th] Laceration with FB of forearm

[4th] [5th] [6th] [7th] Additional Character Required ☑ 3-character code Unspecified laterality codes were excluded here.

● =New Code
▲ =Revised Code
⊡ =Social determinants of health

Excludes1—Not coded here, do not use together
Excludes2—Not included here

S51.821 **Laceration with FB of right forearm**
`7th`

S51.822 **Laceration with FB of left forearm**
`7th`

S51.83 **Puncture wound without FB of forearm**
`6th`
    S51.831 **Puncture wound without FB of right forearm**
    `7th`
    S51.832 **Puncture wound without FB of left forearm**
    `7th`

S51.84 **Puncture wound with FB of forearm**
`6th`
    S51.841 **Puncture wound with FB of right forearm**
    `7th`
    S51.842 **Puncture wound with FB of left forearm**
    `7th`

S51.85 **Open bite of forearm**
`6th`
Bite of forearm NOS
Excludes1: superficial bite of forearm (S50.86, S50.87)
    S51.851 **Open bite of right forearm**
    `7th`
    S51.852 **Open bite of left forearm**
    `7th`

S52 FRACTURE OF FOREARM
`4th`
Note: A fracture not indicated as displaced or nondisplaced should be coded to displaced
A fracture not indicated as open or closed should be coded to closed
The open fracture designations are based on the Gustilo open fracture classification
Excludes1: traumatic amputation of forearm (S58.-)
Excludes2: fracture at wrist and hand level (S62.-)

S52.0 **Fracture of upper end of ulna**
`5th`
Fracture of proximal end of ulna
Excludes2: fracture of elbow NOS (S42.40-)
    fractures of shaft of ulna (S52.2-)

    S52.00 **Unspecified fracture of upper end of ulna**
    `6th`
        S52.001 **Unspecified fracture of upper end of right ulna**
        `7th`
        S52.002 **Unspecified fracture of upper end of left ulna**
        `7th`

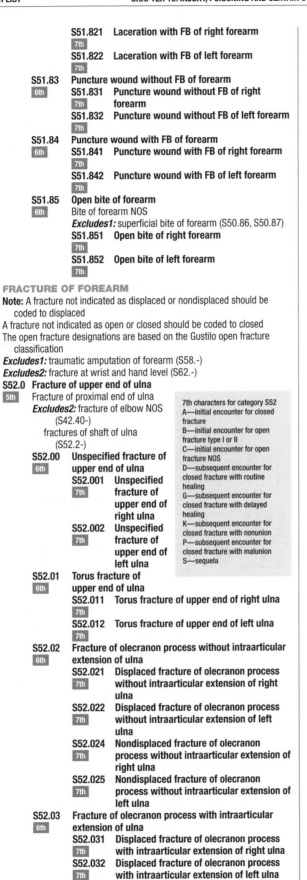

7th characters for category S52
A—initial encounter for closed fracture
B—initial encounter for open fracture type I or II
C—initial encounter for open fracture NOS
D—subsequent encounter for closed fracture with routine healing
G—subsequent encounter for closed fracture with delayed healing
K—subsequent encounter for closed fracture with nonunion
P—subsequent encounter for closed fracture with malunion
S—sequela

    S52.01 **Torus fracture of upper end of ulna**
    `6th`
        S52.011 **Torus fracture of upper end of right ulna**
        `7th`
        S52.012 **Torus fracture of upper end of left ulna**
        `7th`

    S52.02 **Fracture of olecranon process without intraarticular extension of ulna**
    `6th`
        S52.021 **Displaced fracture of olecranon process without intraarticular extension of right ulna**
        `7th`
        S52.022 **Displaced fracture of olecranon process without intraarticular extension of left ulna**
        `7th`
        S52.024 **Nondisplaced fracture of olecranon process without intraarticular extension of right ulna**
        `7th`
        S52.025 **Nondisplaced fracture of olecranon process without intraarticular extension of left ulna**
        `7th`

    S52.03 **Fracture of olecranon process with intraarticular extension of ulna**
    `6th`
        S52.031 **Displaced fracture of olecranon process with intraarticular extension of right ulna**
        `7th`
        S52.032 **Displaced fracture of olecranon process with intraarticular extension of left ulna**
        `7th`

S52.034 **Nondisplaced fracture of olecranon process with intraarticular extension of right ulna**
`7th`
S52.035 **Nondisplaced fracture of olecranon process with intraarticular extension of left ulna**
`7th`

S52.04 **Fracture of coronoid process of ulna**
`6th`
    S52.041 **Displaced fracture of coronoid process of right ulna**
    `7th`
    S52.042 **Displaced fracture of coronoid process of left ulna**
    `7th`
    S52.044 **Nondisplaced fracture of coronoid process of right ulna**
    `7th`
    S52.045 **Nondisplaced fracture of coronoid process of left ulna**
    `7th`

S52.09 **Other fracture of upper end of ulna**
`6th`
    S52.091 **Other fracture of upper end of right ulna**
    `7th`
    S52.092 **Other fracture of upper end of left ulna**
    `7th`

S52.1 **Fracture of upper end of radius**
`5th`
Fracture of proximal end of radius
Excludes2: physeal fractures of upper end of radius (S59.2-) fracture of shaft of radius (S52.3-)

    S52.10 **Unspecified fracture of upper end of radius**
    `6th`
        S52.101 **Unspecified fracture of upper end of right radius**
        `7th`
        S52.102 **Unspecified fracture of upper end of left radius**
        `7th`

    S52.11 **Torus fracture of upper end of radius**
    `6th`
        S52.111 **Torus fracture of upper end of right radius**
        `7th`
        S52.112 **Torus fracture of upper end of left radius**
        `7th`

    S52.12 **Fracture of head of radius**
    `6th`
        S52.121 **Displaced fracture of head of right radius**
        `7th`
        S52.122 **Displaced fracture of head of left radius**
        `7th`
        S52.124 **Nondis-placed fracture of head of right radius**
        `7th`
        S52.125 **Nondisplaced fracture of head of left radius**
        `7th`

    S52.13 **Fracture of neck of radius**
    `6th`
        S52.131 **Displaced fracture of neck of right radius**
        `7th`
        S52.132 **Displaced fracture of neck of eft radius**
        `7th`
        S52.134 **Nondisplaced fracture of neck of right radius**
        `7th`
        S52.135 **Nondisplaced fracture of neck of left radius**
        `7th`

    S52.18 **Other fracture of upper end of radius**
    `6th`
        S52.181 **Other fracture of upper end of right radius**
        `7th`
        S52.182 **Other fracture of upper end of left radius**
        `7th`

S52.2 **Fracture of shaft of ulna**
`5th`
    S52.20 **Unspecified fracture of shaft of ulna**
    `6th`
    Fracture of ulna NOS
        S52.201 **Unspecified fracture of shaft of right ulna**
        `7th`
        S52.202 **Unspecified fracture of shaft of left ulna**
        `7th`

    S52.21 **Greenstick fracture of shaft of ulna**
    `6th`
        S52.211 **Greenstick fracture of shaft of right ulna**
        `7th`
        S52.212 **Greenstick fracture of shaft of left ulna**
        `7th`

    S52.22 **Transverse fracture of shaft of ulna**
    `6th`
        S52.221 **Displaced transverse fracture of shaft of right ulna**
        `7th`

`4th` `5th` `6th` `7th` Additional Character Required ✔ `3-character code` Unspecified laterality codes were excluded here.

• =New Code
▲ =Revised Code
▫ =Social determinants of health

Excludes1—Not coded here, do not use together
Excludes2—Not included here

PEDIATRIC ICD-10-CM 2021: A MANUAL FOR PROVIDER-BASED CODING   351

S52.222 Displaced transverse fracture of shaft of left ulna
`7th`

S52.224 Nondisplaced transverse fracture of shaft of right ulna
`7th`

S52.225 Nondisplaced transverse fracture of shaft of left ulna
`7th`

S52.23 Oblique fracture of shaft of ulna
`6th`

S52.231 Displaced oblique fracture of shaft of right ulna
`7th`

S52.232 Displaced oblique fracture of shaft of left ulna
`7th`

S52.234 Nondisplaced oblique fracture of shaft of right ulna
`7th`

S52.235 Nondisplaced oblique fracture of shaft of left ulna
`7th`

> 7th characters for category S52
> A—initial encounter for closed fracture
> B—initial encounter for open fracture type I or II
> C—initial encounter for open fracture NOS
> D—subsequent encounter for closed fracture with routine healing
> G—subsequent encounter for closed fracture with delayed healing
> K—subsequent encounter for closed fracture with nonunion
> P—subsequent encounter for closed fracture with malunion
> S—sequela

S52.24 Spiral fracture of shaft of ulna
`6th`

S52.241 Displaced spiral fracture of shaft of ulna, right arm
`7th`

S52.242 Displaced spiral fracture of shaft of ulna, left arm
`7th`

S52.244 Nondisplaced spiral fracture of shaft of ulna, right arm
`7th`

S52.245 Nondisplaced spiral fracture of shaft of ulna, left arm
`7th`

S52.25 Comminuted fracture of shaft of ulna
`6th`

S52.251 Displaced comminuted fracture of shaft of ulna, right arm
`7th`

S52.252 Displaced comminuted fracture of shaft of ulna, left arm
`7th`

S52.254 Nondisplaced comminuted fracture of shaft of ulna, right arm
`7th`

S52.255 Nondisplaced comminuted fracture of shaft of ulna, left arm
`7th`

S52.26 Segmental fracture of shaft of ulna
`6th`

S52.261 Displaced segmental fracture of shaft of ulna, right arm
`7th`

S52.262 Displaced segmental fracture of shaft of ulna, left arm
`7th`

S52.264 Nondisplaced segmental fracture of shaft of ulna, right arm
`7th`

S52.265 Nondisplaced segmental fracture of shaft of ulna, left arm
`7th`

S52.27 Monteggia's fracture of ulna
`6th`
Fracture of upper shaft of ulna with dislocation of radial head

S52.271 Monteggia's fracture of right ulna
`7th`

S52.272 Monteggia's fracture of left ulna
`7th`

S52.28 Bent bone of ulna
`6th`

S52.281 Bent bone of right ulna
`7th`

S52.282 Bent bone of left ulna
`7th`

S52.29 Other fracture of shaft of ulna
`6th`

S52.291 Other fracture of shaft of right ulna
`7th`

S52.292 Other fracture of shaft of left ulna
`7th`

S52.3 Fracture of shaft of radius
`5th`

S52.30 Unspecified fracture of shaft of radius
`6th`

S52.301 Unspecified fracture of shaft of right radius
`7th`

S52.302 Unspecified fracture of shaft of left radius
`7th`

S52.31 Greenstick fracture of shaft of radius
`6th`

S52.311 Greenstick fracture of shaft of radius, right arm
`7th`

S52.312 Greenstick fracture of shaft of radius, left arm
`7th`

S52.32 Transverse fracture of shaft of radius
`6th`

S52.321 Displaced transverse fracture of shaft of right radius
`7th`

S52.322 Displaced transverse fracture of shaft of left radius
`7th`

S52.324 Nondisplaced transverse fracture of shaft of right radius
`7th`

S52.325 Nondisplaced transverse fracture of shaft of left radius
`7th`

S52.33 Oblique fracture of shaft of radius
`6th`

S52.331 Displaced oblique fracture of shaft of right radius
`7th`

S52.332 Displaced oblique fracture of shaft of left radius
`7th`

S52.334 Nondisplaced oblique fracture of shaft of right radius
`7th`

S52.335 Nondisplaced oblique fracture of shaft of left radius
`7th`

S52.34 Spiral fracture of shaft of radius
`6th`

S52.341 Displaced spiral fracture of shaft of radius, right arm
`7th`

S52.342 Displaced spiral fracture of shaft of radius, left arm
`7th`

S52.344 Nondisplaced spiral fracture of shaft of radius, right arm
`7th`

S52.345 Nondisplaced spiral fracture of shaft of radius, left arm
`7th`

S52.35 Comminuted fracture of shaft of radius
`6th`

S52.351 Displaced comminuted fracture of shaft of radius, right arm
`7th`

S52.352 Displaced comminuted fracture of shaft of radius, left arm
`7th`

S52.354 Nondisplaced comminuted fracture of shaft of radius, right arm
`7th`

S52.355 Nondisplaced comminuted fracture of shaft of radius, left arm
`7th`

S52.36 Segmental fracture of shaft of radius
`6th`

S52.361 Displaced segmental fracture of shaft of radius, right arm
`7th`

S52.362 Displaced segmental fracture of shaft of radius, left arm
`7th`

S52.364 Nondisplaced segmental fracture of shaft of radius, right arm
`7th`

S52.365 Nondisplaced segmental fracture of shaft of radius, left arm
`7th`

S52.37 Galeazzi's fracture
`6th`
Fracture of lower shaft of radius with radioulnar joint dislocation

S52.371 Galeazzi's fracture of right radius
`7th`

S52.372 Galeazzi's fracture of left radius
`7th`

S52.38 Bent bone of radius
`6th`

S52.381 Bent bone of right radius
`7th`

S52.382 Bent bone of left radius
`7th`

S52.39 Other fracture of shaft of radius
`6th`

S52.391 Other fracture of shaft of radius, right arm
`7th`

S52.392 Other fracture of shaft of radius, left arm
`7th`

S52.5 Fracture of lower end of radius
`5th`
Fracture of distal end of radius
Excludes: physeal fractures of lower end of radius (S59.2-)

S52.50 Unspecified fracture of the lower end of radius
`6th`

`4th` `5th` `6th` `7th`   Additional Character Required   ✔   3-character code

Unspecified laterality codes were excluded here.

• =New Code
▲ =Revised Code
⌑ =Social determinants of health

Excludes1—Not coded here, do not use together
Excludes2—Not included here

S52.501   **7th**   Unspecified fracture of the lower end of right radius

S52.502   **7th**   Unspecified fracture of the lower end of left radius

S52.51   **6th**   Fracture of radial styloid process

S52.511   **7th**   Displaced fracture of right radial styloid process

S52.512   **7th**   Displaced fracture of left radial styloid process

S52.514   **7th**   Nondisplaced fracture of right radial styloid process

S52.515   **7th**   Nondisplaced fracture of left radial styloid process

> 7th characters for category S52
> A—initial encounter for closed fracture
> B—initial encounter for open fracture type I or II
> C—initial encounter for open fracture NOS
> D—subsequent encounter for closed fracture with routine healing
> G—subsequent encounter for closed fracture with delayed healing
> K—subsequent encounter for closed fracture with nonunion
> P—subsequent encounter for closed fracture with malunion
> S—sequela

S52.52   **6th**   Torus fracture of lower end of radius

S52.521   **7th**   Torus fracture of lower end of right radius

S52.522   **7th**   Torus fracture of lower end of left radius

S52.53   **6th**   Colles' fracture

S52.531   **7th**   Colles' fracture of right radius

S52.532   **7th**   Colles' fracture of left radius

S52.54   **6th**   Smith's fracture

S52.541   **7th**   Smith's fracture of right radius

S52.542   **7th**   Smith's fracture of left radius

S52.55   **6th**   Other extraarticular fracture of lower end of radius

S52.551   **7th**   Other extra-articular fracture of lower end of right radius

S52.552   **7th**   Other extra-articular fracture of lower end of left radius

S52.56   **6th**   Barton's fracture

S52.561   **7th**   Barton's fracture of right radius

S52.562   **7th**   Barton's fracture of left radius

S52.57   **6th**   Other intraarticular fracture of lower end of radius

S52.571   **7th**   Other intraarticular fracture of lower end of right radius

S52.572   **7th**   Other intraarticular fracture of lower end of left radius

S52.59   **6th**   Other fractures of lower end of radius

S52.591   **7th**   Other fractures of lower end of right radius

S52.592   **7th**   Other fractures of lower end of left radius

S52.6   **5th**   Fracture of lower end of ulna

S52.60   **6th**   Unspecified fracture of lower end of ulna

S52.601   **7th**   Unspecified fracture of lower end of right ulna

S52.602   **7th**   Unspecified fracture of lower end of left ulna

S52.61   **6th**   Fracture of ulna styloid process

S52.611   **7th**   Displaced fracture of right ulna styloid process

S52.612   **7th**   Displaced fracture of left ulna styloid process

S52.614   **7th**   Nondisplaced fracture of right ulna styloid process

S52.615   **7th**   Nondisplaced fracture of left ulna styloid process

S52.62   **6th**   Torus fracture of lower end of ulna

S52.621   **7th**   Torus fracture of lower end of right ulna

S52.622   **7th**   Torus fracture of lower end of left ulna

S52.69   **6th**   Other fracture of lower end of ulna

S52.691   **7th**   Other fracture of lower end of right ulna

S52.692   **7th**   Other fracture of lower end of left ulna

S52.9   **5th**   Unspecified fracture of forearm

S52.91X   **7th**   Unspecified fracture of right forearm

S52.92X   **7th**   Unspecified fracture of left forearm

S53   **4th**   DISLOCATION AND SPRAIN OF JOINTS AND LIGAMENTS OF ELBOW

Includes: avulsion of joint or ligament of elbow

laceration of cartilage, joint or ligament of elbow

sprain of cartilage, joint or ligament of elbow

traumatic hemarthrosis of joint or ligament of elbow

traumatic rupture of joint or ligament of elbow

traumatic subluxation of joint or ligament of elbow

traumatic tear of joint or ligament of elbow

Code also any associated open wound

Excludes2: strain of muscle, fascia and tendon at forearm level (S56.-)

> 7th characters for category S53
> A—initial encounter
> D—subsequent encounter
> S—sequela

S53.0   **5th**   Subluxation and dislocation of radial head

Dislocation of radiohumeral joint

Subluxation of radiohumeral joint

Excludes1: Monteggia's fracture-dislocation (S52.27-)

S53.00   **6th**   Unspecified subluxation and dislocation of radial head

S53.001   **7th**   Unspecified subluxation of right radial head

S53.002   **7th**   Unspecified subluxation of left radial head

S53.004   **7th**   Unspecified dislocation of right radial head

S53.005   **7th**   Unspecified dislocation of left radial head

S53.02   **6th**   Posterior subluxation and dislocation of radial head

Posteriolateral subluxation and dislocation of radial head

S53.021   **7th**   Posterior subluxation of right radial head

S53.022   **7th**   Posterior subluxation of left radial head

S53.024   **7th**   Posterior dislocation of right radial head

S53.025   **7th**   Posterior dislocation of left radial head

S53.03   **6th**   Nursemaid's elbow

S53.031   **7th**   Nursemaid's elbow, right elbow

S53.032   **7th**   Nursemaid's elbow, left elbow

S53.09   **6th**   Other subluxation and dislocation of radial head

S53.091   **7th**   Other subluxation of right radial head

S53.092   **7th**   Other subluxation of left radial head

S53.094   **7th**   Other dislocation of right radial head

S53.095   **7th**   Other dislocation of left radial head

S53.4   **5th**   Sprain of elbow

Excludes2: traumatic rupture of radial collateral ligament (S53.2-)

traumatic rupture of ulnar collateral ligament (S53.3-)

S53.40   **6th**   Unspecified sprain of elbow

S53.401   **7th**   Unspecified sprain of right elbow

| **4th** **5th** **6th** **7th**   Additional Character Required | ✓   3-character code | Unspecified laterality codes were excluded here. | • =New Code
▲ =Revised Code
▣ =Social determinants of health | ***Excludes1***—Not coded here, do not use together
Excludes2—Not included here |

S53.402   Unspecified sprain of left elbow
[7th]

S53.41   Radiohumeral (joint) sprain
[6th]
   S53.411   Radiohumeral (joint) sprain of right elbow
   [7th]
   S53.412   Radiohumeral (joint) sprain of left elbow
   [7th]

S53.42   Ulnohumeral (joint) sprain
[6th]
   S53.421   Ulnohumeral (joint) sprain of right elbow
   [7th]
   S53.422   Ulnohumeral (joint) sprain of left elbow
   [7th]

S53.43   Radial collateral ligament sprain
[6th]
   S53.431   Radial collateral ligament sprain of right elbow
   [7th]
   S53.432   Radial collateral ligament sprain of left elbow
   [7th]

S53.44   Ulnar collateral ligament sprain
[6th]
   S53.441   Ulnar collateral ligament sprain of right elbow
   [7th]
   S53.442   Ulnar collateral ligament sprain of left elbow
   [7th]

S53.49   Other sprain of elbow
[6th]
   S53.491   Other sprain of right elbow
   [7th]
   S53.492   Other sprain of left elbow
   [7th]

S56 INJURY OF MUSCLE, FASCIA AND TENDON AT FOREARM LEVEL
[4th]

Code also any associated open wound (S51.-)

Excludes2: injury of muscle, fascia and tendon at or below wrist (S66.-)
sprain of joints and ligaments of elbow (S53.4-)

> 7th characters for category S56
> A—initial encounter
> D—subsequent encounter
> S—sequela

S56.0   Injury of flexor muscle, fascia and tendon of thumb at forearm level
[5th]
   S56.01   Strain of flexor muscle, fascia and tendon of thumb at forearm level
   [6th]
     S56.011   Strain of flexor muscle, fascia and tendon of right thumb at forearm level
     [7th]
     S56.012   Strain of flexor muscle, fascia and tendon of left thumb at forearm level
     [7th]
   S56.02   Laceration of flexor muscle, fascia and tendon of thumb at forearm level
   [6th]
     S56.021   Laceration of flexor muscle, fascia and tendon of right thumb at forearm level
     [7th]
     S56.022   Laceration of flexor muscle, fascia and tendon of left thumb at forearm level
     [7th]

S56.1   Injury of flexor muscle, fascia and tendon of other and unspecified finger at forearm level
[5th]
   S56.11   Strain of flexor muscle, fascia and tendon of other and unspecified finger at forearm level
   [6th]
     S56.111   Strain of flexor muscle, fascia and tendon of right index finger at forearm level
     [7th]
     S56.112   Strain of flexor muscle, fascia and tendon of left index finger at forearm level
     [7th]
     S56.113   Strain of flexor muscle, fascia and tendon of right middle finger at forearm level
     [7th]
     S56.114   Strain of flexor muscle, fascia and tendon of left middle finger at forearm level
     [7th]
     S56.115   Strain of flexor muscle, fascia and tendon of right ring finger at forearm level
     [7th]
     S56.116   Strain of flexor muscle, fascia and tendon of left ring finger at forearm level
     [7th]
     S56.117   Strain of flexor muscle, fascia and tendon of right little finger at forearm level
     [7th]
     S56.118   Strain of flexor muscle, fascia and tendon of left little finger at forearm level
     [7th]
   S56.12   Laceration of flexor muscle, fascia and tendon of other and unspecified finger at forearm level
   [6th]
     S56.121   Laceration of flexor muscle, fascia and tendon of right index finger at forearm level
     [7th]
     S56.122   Laceration of flexor muscle, fascia and tendon of left index finger at forearm level
     [7th]
     S56.123   Laceration of flexor muscle, fascia and tendon of right middle finger at forearm level
     [7th]
     S56.124   Laceration of flexor muscle, fascia and tendon of left middle finger at forearm level
     [7th]
     S56.125   Laceration of flexor muscle, fascia and tendon of right ring finger at forearm level
     [7th]
     S56.126   Laceration of flexor muscle, fascia and tendon of left ring finger at forearm level
     [7th]
     S56.127   Laceration of flexor muscle, fascia and tendon of right little finger at forearm level
     [7th]
     S56.128   Laceration of flexor muscle, fascia and tendon of left little finger at forearm level
     [7th]

S56.2   Injury of other flexor muscle, fascia and tendon at forearm level
[5th]
   S56.21   Strain of other flexor muscle, fascia and tendon at forearm level
   [6th]
     S56.211   Strain of other flexor muscle, fascia and tendon at forearm level, right arm
     [7th]
     S56.212   Strain of other flexor muscle, fascia and tendon at forearm level, left arm
     [7th]
   S56.22   Laceration of other flexor muscle, fascia and tendon at forearm level
   [6th]
     S56.221   Laceration of other flexor muscle, fascia and tendon at forearm level, right arm
     [7th]
     S56.222   Laceration of other flexor muscle, fascia and tendon at forearm level, left arm
     [7th]

S56.3   Injury of extensor or abductor muscles, fascia and tendons of thumb at forearm level
[5th]
   S56.31   Strain of extensor or abductor muscles, fascia and tendons of thumb at forearm level
   [6th]
     S56.311   Strain of extensor or abductor muscles, fascia and tendons of right thumb at forearm level
     [7th]
     S56.312   Strain of extensor or abductor muscles, fascia and tendons of left thumb at forearm level
     [7th]
   S56.32   Laceration of extensor or abductor muscles, fascia and tendons of thumb at forearm level
   [6th]
     S56.321   Laceration of extensor or abductor muscles, fascia and tendons of right thumb at forearm level
     [7th]
     S56.322   Laceration of extensor or abductor muscles, fascia and tendons of left thumb at forearm level
     [7th]
   S56.39   Other injury of extensor or abductor muscles, fascia and tendons of thumb at forearm level
   [6th]
     S56.391   Other injury of extensor or abductor muscles, fascia and tendons of right thumb at forearm level
     [7th]
     S56.392   Other injury of extensor or abductor muscles, fascia and tendons of left thumb at forearm level
     [7th]

S56.4   Injury of extensor muscle, fascia and tendon of other and unspecified finger at forearm level
[5th]
   S56.41   Strain of extensor muscle, fascia and tendon of other and unspecified finger at forearm level
   [6th]
     S56.411   Strain of extensor muscle, fascia and tendon of right index finger at forearm level
     [7th]
     S56.412   Strain of extensor muscle, fascia and tendon of left index finger at forearm level
     [7th]
     S56.413   Strain of extensor muscle, fascia and tendon of right middle finger at forearm level
     [7th]
     S56.414   Strain of extensor muscle, fascia and tendon of left middle finger at forearm level
     [7th]
     S56.415   Strain of extensor muscle, fascia and tendon of right ring finger at forearm level
     [7th]

[4th] [5th] [6th] [7th] Additional Character Required   ✔ 3-character code   Unspecified laterality codes were excluded here.   • =New Code   ▲ =Revised Code   ¤ =Social determinants of health   *Excludes1*—Not coded here, do not use together   *Excludes2*—Not included here

354   PEDIATRIC ICD-10-CM 2021: A MANUAL FOR PROVIDER-BASED CODING

S56.416   Strain of extensor muscle, fascia and
[7th]   tendon of left ring finger at forearm level

S56.417   Strain of extensor muscle, fascia and
[7th]   tendon of right little finger at forearm level

S56.418   Strain of extensor muscle, fascia and
[7th]   tendon of left little finger at forearm level

S56.42   Laceration of extensor
[6th]   muscle, fascia and
tendon of other and
unspecified finger at
forearm level

> 7th characters for category S56
> A—initial encounter
> D—subsequent encounter
> S—sequela

S56.421   Laceration
[7th]   of extensor muscle, fascia and tendon of
right index finger at forearm level

S56.422   Laceration of extensor muscle, fascia and
[7th]   tendon of left index finger at forearm level

S56.423   Laceration of extensor muscle, fascia and
[7th]   tendon of right middle finger at forearm
level

S56.424   Laceration of extensor muscle, fascia and
[7th]   tendon of left middle finger at forearm
level

S56.425   Laceration of extensor muscle, fascia and
[7th]   tendon of right ring finger at forearm level

S56.426   Laceration of extensor muscle, fascia and
[7th]   tendon of left ring finger at forearm level

S56.427   Laceration of extensor muscle, fascia and
[7th]   tendon of right little finger at forearm level

S56.428   Laceration of extensor muscle, fascia and
[7th]   tendon of left little finger at forearm level

S56.5   Injury of other extensor muscle, fascia and tendon at forearm
[5th]   level

S56.51   Strain of other extensor muscle, fascia and tendon at
[6th]   forearm level

S56.511   Strain of other extensor muscle, fascia and
[7th]   tendon at forearm level, right arm

S56.512   Strain of other extensor muscle, fascia and
[7th]   tendon at forearm level, left arm

S56.52   Laceration of other extensor muscle, fascia and
[6th]   tendon at forearm level

S56.521   Laceration of other extensor muscle,
[7th]   fascia and tendon at forearm level, right
arm

S56.522   Laceration of other extensor muscle,
[7th]   fascia and tendon at forearm level, left
arm

S56.8   Injury of other muscles, fascia and tendons at forearm level
[5th]

S56.81   Strain of other muscles, fascia and tendons at
[6th]   forearm level

S56.811   Strain of other muscles, fascia and
[7th]   tendons at forearm level, right arm

S56.812   Strain of other muscles, fascia and
[7th]   tendons at forearm level, left arm

S56.82   Laceration of other muscles, fascia and tendons at
[6th]   forearm level

S56.821   Laceration of other muscles, fascia and
[7th]   tendons at forearm level, right arm

S56.822   Laceration of other muscles, fascia and
[7th]   tendons at forearm level, left arm

S56.9   Injury of unspecified muscles, fascia and tendons at forearm
[5th]   level

S56.90   Unspecified injury of unspecified muscles, fascia and
[6th]   tendons at forearm level

S56.901   Unspecified injury of unspecified muscles,
[7th]   fascia and tendons at forearm level, right
arm

S56.902   Unspecified injury of unspecified muscles,
[7th]   fascia and tendons at forearm level, left
arm

S56.91   Strain of unspecified muscles, fascia and tendons at
[6th]   forearm level

S56.911   Strain of unspecified muscles, fascia and
[7th]   tendons at forearm level, right arm

S56.912   Strain of unspecified muscles, fascia and
[7th]   tendons at forearm level, left arm

S56.92   Laceration of unspecified muscles, fascia and
[6th]   tendons at forearm level

S56.921   Laceration of unspecified muscles, fascia
[7th]   and tendons at forearm level, right arm

S56.922   Laceration of unspecified muscles, fascia
[7th]   and tendons at forearm level, left arm

S59   **OTHER AND UNSPECIFIED INJURIES OF ELBOW**
[4th]   **AND FOREARM**

Excludes2: other and unspecified injuries
[2nd]   of wrist and hand (S69.-)

S59.0   Physeal fracture of lower end
[5th]   of ulna

> 7th characters for category S59
> A—initial encounter for closed fracture
> D—subsequent encounter for fracture with routine healing
> G—subsequent encounter for fracture with delayed healing
> K—subsequent encounter for fracture with nonunion

S59.00   Unspecified physeal
[6th]   fracture of lower end
of ulna

S59.001   Unspecified
[7th]   physeal
fracture of
lower end of
ulna, right
arm

> 7th characters for category S59
> A—initial encounter for closed fracture
> D—subsequent encounter for fracture with routine healing
> G—subsequent encounter for fracture with delayed healing
> K—subsequent encounter for fracture with nonunion
> P—subsequent encounter for fracture with malunion
> S—sequela

S59.002   Unspecified
[7th]   physeal
fracture of
lower end
of ulna,
left arm

S59.01   Salter-Harris Type I physeal fracture of lower end
[6th]   of ulna

S59.011   Salter-Harris Type I physeal fracture of
[7th]   lower end of ulna, right arm

S59.012   Salter-Harris Type I physeal fracture of
[7th]   lower end of ulna, left arm

S59.02   Salter-Harris Type II physeal fracture of lower end of
[6th]   ulna

S59.021   Salter-Harris Type II physeal fracture of
[7th]   lower end of ulna, right arm

S59.022   Salter-Harris Type II physeal fracture of
[7th]   lower end of ulna, left arm

S59.03   Salter-Harris Type III physeal fracture of lower end of
[6th]   ulna

S59.031   Salter-Harris Type III physeal fracture of
[7th]   lower end of ulna, right arm

S59.032   Salter-Harris Type III physeal fracture of
[7th]   lower end of ulna, left arm

S59.04   Salter-Harris Type IV physeal fracture of lower end of
[6th]   ulna

S59.041   Salter-Harris Type IV physeal fracture of
[7th]   lower end of ulna, right arm

S59.042   Salter-Harris Type IV physeal fracture of
[7th]   lower end of ulna, left arm

S59.09   Other physeal fracture of lower end of ulna
[6th]

S59.091   Other physeal fracture of lower end of
[7th]   ulna, right arm

S59.092   Other physeal fracture of lower end of
[7th]   ulna, left arm

S59.1   Physeal fracture of upper end of radius
[5th]

S59.10   Unspecified physeal fracture of upper end of radius
[6th]

S59.101   Unspecified physeal fracture of upper end
[7th]   of radius, right arm

S59.102   Unspecified physeal fracture of upper end
[7th]   of radius, left arm

S59.11   Salter-Harris Type I physeal fracture of upper end of
[6th]   radius

S59.111   Salter-Harris Type I physeal fracture of
[7th]   upper end of radius, right arm

S59.112   Salter-Harris Type I physeal fracture of
[7th]   upper end of radius, left arm

S59.12   Salter-Harris Type II physeal fracture of upper end of
[6th]   radius

| [4th] | [5th] | [6th] | [7th] | Additional Character Required | ✔ | 3-character code | Unspecified laterality codes were excluded here. | • =New Code   ▲ =Revised Code   ▭ =Social determinants of health | *Excludes1*—Not coded here, do not use together   *Excludes2*—Not included here |

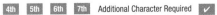

S59.121 [7th] Salter-Harris Type II physeal fracture of upper end of radius, right arm

S59.122 [7th] Salter-Harris Type II physeal fracture of upper end of radius, left arm

S59.13 [6th] Salter-Harris Type III physeal fracture of upper end of radius

S59.131 [7th] Salter-Harris Type III physeal fracture of upper end of radius, right arm

S59.132 [7th] Salter-Harris Type III physeal fracture of upper end of radius, left arm

> 7th characters for category S59
> A—initial encounter for closed fracture
> D—subsequent encounter for fracture with routine healing
> G—subsequent encounter for fracture with delayed healing
> K—subsequent encounter for fracture with nonunion
> P—subsequent encounter for fracture with malunion
> S—sequela

S59.14 [6th] Salter-Harris Type IV physeal fracture of upper end of radius

S59.141 [7th] Salter-Harris Type IV physeal fracture of upper end of radius, right arm

S59.142 [7th] Salter-Harris Type IV physeal fracture of upper end of radius, left arm

S59.19 [6th] Other physeal fracture of upper end of radius

S59.191 [7th] Other physeal fracture of upper end of radius, right arm

S59.192 [7th] Other physeal fracture of upper end of radius, left arm

S59.2 [5th] Physeal fracture of lower end of radius

S59.20 [6th] Unspecified physeal fracture of lower end of radius

S59.201 [7th] Unspecified physeal fracture of lower end of radius, right arm

S59.202 [7th] Unspecified physeal fracture of lower end of radius, left arm

S59.21 [6th] Salter-Harris Type I physeal fracture of lower end of radius

S59.211 [7th] Salter-Harris Type I physeal fracture of lower end of radius, right arm

S59.212 [7th] Salter-Harris Type I physeal fracture of lower end of radius, left arm

S59.22 [6th] Salter-Harris Type II physeal fracture of lower end of radius

S59.221 [7th] Salter-Harris Type II physeal fracture of lower end of radius, right arm

S59.222 [7th] Salter-Harris Type II physeal fracture of lower end of radius, left arm

S59.23 [6th] Salter-Harris Type III physeal fracture of lower end of radius

S59.231 [7th] Salter-Harris Type III physeal fracture of lower end of radius, right arm

S59.232 [7th] Salter-Harris Type III physeal fracture of lower end of radius, left arm

S59.24 [6th] Salter-Harris Type IV physeal fracture of lower end of radius

S59.241 [7th] Salter-Harris Type IV physeal fracture of lower end of radius, right arm

S59.242 [7th] Salter-Harris Type IV physeal fracture of lower end of radius, left arm

S59.29 [6th] Other physeal fracture of lower end of radius

S59.291 [7th] Other physeal fracture of lower end of radius, right arm

S59.292 [7th] Other physeal fracture of lower end of radius, left arm

S59.8 [5th] Other specified injuries of elbow and forearm

S59.80 [6th] Other specified injuries of elbow

S59.801 [7th] Other specified injuries of right elbow

> 7th characters for subcategory S59.8
> A—initial encounter
> D—subsequent encounter
> S—sequela

S59.802 [7th] Other specified injuries of left elbow

S59.81 [6th] Other specified injuries of forearm

S59.811 [7th] Other specified injuries right forearm

S59.812 [7th] Other specified injuries left forearm

(S60–S69) INJURIES TO THE WRIST, HAND AND FINGERS

Excludes2: burns and corrosions (T20–T32)
frostbite (T33–T34)
insect bite or sting, venomous (T63.4)

S60   **SUPERFICIAL INJURY OF WRIST, HAND AND FINGERS** [4th]

S60.0 [5th] Contusion of finger without damage to nail

Excludes1: contusion involving nail (matrix) (S60.1)

> 7th characters for category S60
> A—initial encounter
> D—subsequent encounter
> S—sequela

S60.00X [7th] Contusion of unspecified finger without damage to nail
Contusion of finger(s) NOS

S60.01 [6th] Contusion of thumb without damage to nail

S60.011 [7th] Contusion of right thumb without damage to nail

S60.02 [6th] Contusion of index finger without damage to nail

S60.021 [7th] Contusion of right index finger without damage to nail

S60.022 [7th] Contusion of left index finger without damage to nail

S60.03 [6th] Contusion of middle finger without damage to nail

S60.031 [7th] Contusion of right middle finger without damage to nail

S60.032 [7th] Contusion of left middle finger without damage to nail

S60.04 [6th] Contusion of ring finger without damage to nail

S60.041 [7th] Contusion of right ring finger without damage to nail

S60.042 [7th] Contusion of left ring finger without damage to nail

S60.05 [6th] Contusion of little finger without damage to nail

S60.051 [7th] Contusion of right little finger without damage to nail

S60.052 [7th] Contusion of left little finger without damage to nail

S60.1 [5th] Contusion of finger with damage to nail

S60.11 [6th] Contusion of thumb with damage to nail

S60.111 [7th] Contusion of right thumb with damage to nail

S60.112 [7th] Contusion of left thumb with damage to nail

S60.12 [6th] Contusion of index finger with damage to nail

S60.121 [7th] Contusion of right index finger with damage to nail

S60.122 [7th] Contusion of left index finger with damage to nail

S60.13 [6th] Contusion of middle finger with damage to nail

S60.131 [7th] Contusion of right middle finger with damage to nail

S60.132 [7th] Contusion of left middle finger with damage to nail

S60.14 [6th] Contusion of ring finger with damage to nail

S60.141 [7th] Contusion of right ring finger with damage to nail

S60.142 [7th] Contusion of left ring finger with damage to nail

S60.15 [6th] Contusion of little finger with damage to nail

S60.151 [7th] Contusion of right little finger with damage to nail

S60.152 [7th] Contusion of left little finger with damage to nail

S60.2 [5th] Contusion of wrist and hand

Excludes2: contusion of fingers (S60.0-, S60.1-)

[4th] [5th] [6th] [7th] Additional Character Required   ✓ 3-character code   Unspecified laterality codes were excluded here.

• =New Code
▲ =Revised Code
☐ =Social determinants of health

Excludes1—Not coded here, do not use together
Excludes2—Not included here

S60.21 **Contusion of wrist**
    `6th`
      S60.211 **Contusion of right wrist**
        `7th`
      S60.212 **Contusion of left wrist**
        `7th`

S60.22 **Contusion of hand**
    `6th`
      S60.221 **Contusion of right hand**
        `7th`
      S60.222 **Contusion of left hand**
        `7th`

> **7th characters for category S60**
> A—initial encounter
> D—subsequent encounter
> S—sequela

S60.3 **Other superficial injuries of thumb**
   `5th`
    S60.31 **Abrasion of thumb**
     `6th`
       S60.311 **Abrasion of right thumb**
         `7th`
       S60.312 **Abrasion of left thumb**
         `7th`

    S60.32 **Blister (nonthermal) of thumb**
     `6th`
       S60.321 **Blister (nonthermal) of right thumb**
         `7th`
       S60.322 **Blister (nonthermal) of left thumb**
         `7th`

    S60.34 **External constriction of thumb**
     `6th`
     Hair tourniquet syndrome of thumb
     Use additional cause code to identify the constricting item (W49.0-)
       S60.341 **External constriction of right thumb**
         `7th`
       S60.342 **External constriction of left thumb**
         `7th`

    S60.35 **Superficial FB of thumb**
     `6th`
     Splinter in the thumb
       S60.351 **Superficial FB of right thumb**
         `7th`
       S60.352 **Superficial FB of left thumb**
         `7th`

    S60.36 **Insect bite (nonvenomous) of thumb**
     `6th`
       S60.361 **Insect bite (nonvenomous) of right thumb**
         `7th`
       S60.362 **Insect bite (nonvenomous) of left thumb**
         `7th`

    S60.37 **Other superficial bite of thumb**
     `6th`
     Excludes1: open bite of thumb (S61.05-, S61.15-)
       S60.371 **Other superficial bite of right thumb**
         `7th`
       S60.372 **Other superficial bite of left thumb**
         `7th`

S60.4 **Other superficial injuries of other fingers**
   `5th`
    S60.41 **Abrasion of fingers**
     `6th`
       S60.410 **Abrasion of right index finger**
         `7th`
       S60.411 **Abrasion of left index finger**
         `7th`
       S60.412 **Abrasion of right middle finger**
         `7th`
       S60.413 **Abrasion of left middle finger**
         `7th`
       S60.414 **Abrasion of right ring finger**
         `7th`
       S60.415 **Abrasion of left ring finger**
         `7th`
       S60.416 **Abrasion of right little finger**
         `7th`
       S60.417 **Abrasion of left little finger**
         `7th`

    S60.42 **Blister (nonthermal) of fingers**
     `6th`
       S60.420 **Blister (nonthermal) of right index finger**
         `7th`
       S60.421 **Blister (nonthermal) of left index finger**
         `7th`
       S60.422 **Blister (nonthermal) of right middle finger**
         `7th`
       S60.423 **Blister (nonthermal) of left middle finger**
         `7th`

       S60.424 **Blister (nonthermal) of right ring finger**
         `7th`
       S60.425 **Blister (nonthermal) of left ring finger**
         `7th`
       S60.426 **Blister (nonthermal) of right little finger**
         `7th`
       S60.427 **Blister (nonthermal) of left little finger**
         `7th`

S60.44 **External constriction of fingers**
   `6th`
    Hair tourniquet syndrome of finger
    Use additional cause code to identify the constricting item (W49.0-)
      S60.440 **External constriction of right index finger**
        `7th`
      S60.441 **External constriction of left index finger**
        `7th`
      S60.442 **External constriction of right middle finger**
        `7th`
      S60.443 **External constriction of left middle finger**
        `7th`
      S60.444 **External constriction of right ring finger**
        `7th`
      S60.445 **External constriction of left ring finger**
        `7th`
      S60.446 **External constriction of right little finger**
        `7th`
      S60.447 **External constriction of left little finger**
        `7th`

S60.45 **Superficial FB of fingers**
   `6th`
    Splinter in the finger(s)
      S60.450 **Superficial FB of right index finger**
        `7th`
      S60.451 **Superficial FB of left index finger**
        `7th`
      S60.452 **Superficial FB of right middle finger**
        `7th`
      S60.453 **Superficial FB of left middle finger**
        `7th`
      S60.454 **Superficial FB of right ring finger**
        `7th`
      S60.455 **Superficial FB of left ring finger**
        `7th`
      S60.456 **Superficial FB of right little finger**
        `7th`
      S60.457 **Superficial FB of left little finger**
        `7th`

S60.46 **Insect bite (nonvenomous) of fingers**
   `6th`
      S60.460 **Insect bite (nonvenomous) of right index finger**
        `7th`
      S60.461 **Insect bite (nonvenomous) of left index finger**
        `7th`
      S60.462 **Insect bite (nonvenomous) of right middle finger**
        `7th`
      S60.463 **Insect bite (nonvenomous) of left middle finger**
        `7th`
      S60.464 **Insect bite (nonvenomous) of right ring finger**
        `7th`
      S60.465 **Insect bite (nonvenomous) of left ring finger**
        `7th`
      S60.466 **Insect bite (nonvenomous) of right little finger**
        `7th`
      S60.467 **Insect bite (nonvenomous) of left little finger**
        `7th`

S60.47 **Other superficial bite of fingers**
   `6th`
    Excludes1: open bite of fingers (S61.25-, S61.35-)
      S60.470 **Other superficial bite of right index finger**
        `7th`
      S60.471 **Other superficial bite of left index finger**
        `7th`
      S60.472 **Other superficial bite of right middle finger**
        `7th`
      S60.473 **Other superficial bite of left middle finger**
        `7th`

`4th` `5th` `6th` `7th` Additional Character Required   ✔   3-character code   Unspecified laterality codes were excluded here.

• =New Code
▲ =Revised Code
▣ =Social determinants of health

Excludes1—Not coded here, do not use together
Excludes2—Not included here

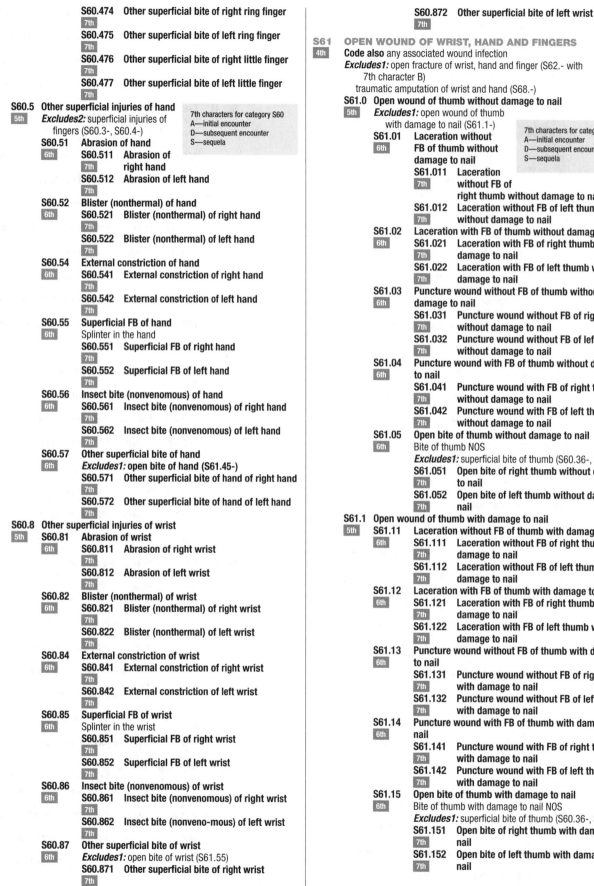

S60.474 Other superficial bite of right ring finger
> 7th

S60.475 Other superficial bite of left ring finger
> 7th

S60.476 Other superficial bite of right little finger
> 7th

S60.477 Other superficial bite of left little finger
> 7th

S60.5 Other superficial injuries of hand
> 5th
>
> *Excludes2:* superficial injuries of fingers (S60.3-, S60.4-)

7th characters for category S60
A—initial encounter
D—subsequent encounter
S—sequela

    S60.51 Abrasion of hand
> 6th
>
> **S60.511** Abrasion of right hand
> > 7th
>
> **S60.512** Abrasion of left hand
> > 7th

    S60.52 Blister (nonthermal) of hand
> 6th
>
> **S60.521** Blister (nonthermal) of right hand
> > 7th
>
> **S60.522** Blister (nonthermal) of left hand
> > 7th

    S60.54 External constriction of hand
> 6th
>
> **S60.541** External constriction of right hand
> > 7th
>
> **S60.542** External constriction of left hand
> > 7th

    S60.55 Superficial FB of hand
> 6th
>
> Splinter in the hand
>
> **S60.551** Superficial FB of right hand
> > 7th
>
> **S60.552** Superficial FB of left hand
> > 7th

    S60.56 Insect bite (nonvenomous) of hand
> 6th
>
> **S60.561** Insect bite (nonvenomous) of right hand
> > 7th
>
> **S60.562** Insect bite (nonvenomous) of left hand
> > 7th

    S60.57 Other superficial bite of hand
> 6th
>
> *Excludes1:* open bite of hand (S61.45-)
>
> **S60.571** Other superficial bite of hand of right hand
> > 7th
>
> **S60.572** Other superficial bite of hand of left hand
> > 7th

S60.8 Other superficial injuries of wrist
> 5th

    S60.81 Abrasion of wrist
> 6th
>
> **S60.811** Abrasion of right wrist
> > 7th
>
> **S60.812** Abrasion of left wrist
> > 7th

    S60.82 Blister (nonthermal) of wrist
> 6th
>
> **S60.821** Blister (nonthermal) of right wrist
> > 7th
>
> **S60.822** Blister (nonthermal) of left wrist
> > 7th

    S60.84 External constriction of wrist
> 6th
>
> **S60.841** External constriction of right wrist
> > 7th
>
> **S60.842** External constriction of left wrist
> > 7th

    S60.85 Superficial FB of wrist
> 6th
>
> Splinter in the wrist
>
> **S60.851** Superficial FB of right wrist
> > 7th
>
> **S60.852** Superficial FB of left wrist
> > 7th

    S60.86 Insect bite (nonvenomous) of wrist
> 6th
>
> **S60.861** Insect bite (nonvenomous) of right wrist
> > 7th
>
> **S60.862** Insect bite (nonveno-mous) of left wrist
> > 7th

    S60.87 Other superficial bite of wrist
> 6th
>
> *Excludes1:* open bite of wrist (S61.55)
>
> **S60.871** Other superficial bite of right wrist
> > 7th

S60.872 Other superficial bite of left wrist
> 7th

S61 **OPEN WOUND OF WRIST, HAND AND FINGERS**
> 4th
>
> **Code also** any associated wound infection
> *Excludes1:* open fracture of wrist, hand and finger (S62.- with 7th character B)
> traumatic amputation of wrist and hand (S68.-)

S61.0 Open wound of thumb without damage to nail
> 5th
>
> *Excludes1:* open wound of thumb with damage to nail (S61.1-)

7th characters for category S61
A—initial encounter
D—subsequent encounter
S—sequela

    S61.01 Laceration without FB of thumb without damage to nail
> 6th
>
> **S61.011** Laceration without FB of right thumb without damage to nail
> > 7th
>
> **S61.012** Laceration without FB of left thumb without damage to nail
> > 7th

    S61.02 Laceration with FB of thumb without damage to nail
> 6th
>
> **S61.021** Laceration with FB of right thumb without damage to nail
> > 7th
>
> **S61.022** Laceration with FB of left thumb without damage to nail
> > 7th

    S61.03 Puncture wound without FB of thumb without damage to nail
> 6th
>
> **S61.031** Puncture wound without FB of right thumb without damage to nail
> > 7th
>
> **S61.032** Puncture wound without FB of left thumb without damage to nail
> > 7th

    S61.04 Puncture wound with FB of thumb without damage to nail
> 6th
>
> **S61.041** Puncture wound with FB of right thumb without damage to nail
> > 7th
>
> **S61.042** Puncture wound with FB of left thumb without damage to nail
> > 7th

    S61.05 Open bite of thumb without damage to nail
> 6th
>
> Bite of thumb NOS
>
> *Excludes1:* superficial bite of thumb (S60.36-, S60.37-)
>
> **S61.051** Open bite of right thumb without damage to nail
> > 7th
>
> **S61.052** Open bite of left thumb without damage to nail
> > 7th

S61.1 Open wound of thumb with damage to nail
> 5th

    S61.11 Laceration without FB of thumb with damage to nail
> 6th
>
> **S61.111** Laceration without FB of right thumb with damage to nail
> > 7th
>
> **S61.112** Laceration without FB of left thumb with damage to nail
> > 7th

    S61.12 Laceration with FB of thumb with damage to nail
> 6th
>
> **S61.121** Laceration with FB of right thumb with damage to nail
> > 7th
>
> **S61.122** Laceration with FB of left thumb with damage to nail
> > 7th

    S61.13 Puncture wound without FB of thumb with damage to nail
> 6th
>
> **S61.131** Puncture wound without FB of right thumb with damage to nail
> > 7th
>
> **S61.132** Puncture wound without FB of left thumb with damage to nail
> > 7th

    S61.14 Puncture wound with FB of thumb with damage to nail
> 6th
>
> **S61.141** Puncture wound with FB of right thumb with damage to nail
> > 7th
>
> **S61.142** Puncture wound with FB of left thumb with damage to nail
> > 7th

    S61.15 Open bite of thumb with damage to nail
> 6th
>
> Bite of thumb with damage to nail NOS
>
> *Excludes1:* superficial bite of thumb (S60.36-, S60.37-)
>
> **S61.151** Open bite of right thumb with damage to nail
> > 7th
>
> **S61.152** Open bite of left thumb with damage to nail
> > 7th

CHAPTER 19. INJURY, POISONING AND CERTAIN OTHER CONSEQUENCES OF EXTERNAL CAUSES   (S60.474–S61.152)

4th	5th	6th	7th	Additional Character Required	✔	3-character code	Unspecified laterality codes were excluded here.	• =New Code	*Excludes1*—Not coded here, do not use together

▲ =Revised Code
▫ =Social determinants of health

Excludes2—Not included here

S61.2 **Open wound of other finger without damage to nail**
[5th] *Excludes1:* open wound of finger involving nail (matrix) (S61.3-)
Excludes2: open wound of thumb without damage to nail (S61.0-)

S61.21 **Laceration without FB of finger without damage to nail**
[6th]

> 7th characters for category S61
> A—initial encounter
> D—subsequent encounter
> S—sequela

S61.210 Laceration without FB of right index finger without damage to nail
[7th]

S61.211 Laceration without FB of left index finger without damage to nail
[7th]

S61.212 Laceration without FB of right middle finger without damage to nail
[7th]

S61.213 Laceration without FB of left middle finger without damage to nail
[7th]

S61.214 Laceration without FB of right ring finger without damage to nail
[7th]

S61.215 Laceration without FB of left ring finger without damage to nail
[7th]

S61.216 Laceration without FB of right little finger without damage to nail
[7th]

S61.217 Laceration without FB of left little finger without damage to nail
[7th]

S61.22 **Laceration with FB of finger without damage to nail**
[6th]

S61.220 Laceration with FB of right index finger without damage to nail
[7th]

S61.221 Laceration with FB of left index finger without damage to nail
[7th]

S61.222 Laceration with FB of right middle finger without damage to nail
[7th]

S61.223 Laceration with FB of left middle finger without damage to nail
[7th]

S61.224 Laceration with FB of right ring finger without damage to nail
[7th]

S61.225 Laceration with FB of left ring finger without damage to nail
[7th]

S61.226 Laceration with FB of right little finger without damage to nail
[7th]

S61.227 Laceration with FB of left little finger without damage to nail
[7th]

S61.23 **Puncture wound without FB of finger without damage to nail**
[6th]

S61.230 Puncture wound without FB of right index finger without damage to nail
[7th]

S61.231 Puncture wound without FB of left index finger without damage to nail
[7th]

S61.232 Puncture wound without FB of right middle finger without damage to nail
[7th]

S61.233 Puncture wound without FB of left middle finger without damage to nail
[7th]

S61.234 Puncture wound without FB of right ring finger without damage to nail
[7th]

S61.235 Puncture wound without FB of left ring finger without damage to nail
[7th]

S61.236 Puncture wound without FB of right little finger without damage to nail
[7th]

S61.237 Puncture wound without FB of left little finger without damage to nail
[7th]

S61.24 **Puncture wound with FB of finger without damage to nail**
[6th]

S61.240 Puncture wound with FB of right index finger with-out damage to nail
[7th]

S61.241 Puncture wound with FB of left index finger without damage to nail
[7th]

S61.242 Puncture wound with FB of right middle finger without damage to nail
[7th]

S61.243 Puncture wound with FB of left middle finger without damage to nail
[7th]

S61.244 Puncture wound with FB of right ring finger without damage to nail
[7th]

S61.245 Puncture wound with FB of left ring finger without damage to nail
[7th]

S61.246 Puncture wound with FB of right little finger without damage to nail
[7th]

S61.247 Puncture wound with FB of left little finger without damage to nail
[7th]

S61.25 **Open bite of finger without damage to nail**
[6th] Bite of finger without damage to nail NOS
Excludes1: superficial bite of finger (S60.46-, S60.47-)

S61.250 Open bite of right index finger without damage to nail
[7th]

S61.251 Open bite of left index finger without damage to nail
[7th]

S61.252 Open bite of right middle finger without damage to nail
[7th]

S61.253 Open bite of left middle finger without damage to nail
[7th]

S61.254 Open bite of right ring finger without damage to nail
[7th]

S61.255 Open bite of left ring finger without damage to nail
[7th]

S61.256 Open bite of right little finger without damage to nail
[7th]

S61.257 Open bite of left little finger without damage to nail
[7th]

S61.3 **Open wound of other finger with damage to nail**
[5th]

S61.31 **Laceration without FB of finger with damage to nail**
[6th]

S61.310 Laceration without FB of right index finger with damage to nail
[7th]

S61.311 Laceration without FB of left index finger with damage to nail
[7th]

S61.312 Laceration without FB of right middle finger with damage to nail
[7th]

S61.313 Laceration without FB of left middle finger with damage to nail
[7th]

S61.314 Laceration without FB of right ring finger with damage to nail
[7th]

S61.315 Laceration without FB of left ring finger with damage to nail
[7th]

S61.316 Laceration without FB of right little finger with damage to nail
[7th]

S61.317 Laceration without FB of left little finger with damage to nail
[7th]

S61.32 **Laceration with FB of finger with damage to nail**
[6th]

S61.320 Laceration with FB of right index finger with damage to nail
[7th]

S61.321 Laceration with FB of left index finger with damage to nail
[7th]

S61.322 Laceration with FB of right middle finger with damage to nail
[7th]

S61.323 Laceration with FB of left middle finger with damage to nail
[7th]

S61.324 Laceration with FB of right ring finger with damage to nail
[7th]

S61.325 Laceration with FB of left ring finger with damage to nail
[7th]

S61.326 Laceration with FB of right little finger with damage to nail
[7th]

S61.327 Laceration with FB of left little finger with damage to nail
[7th]

S61.33 **Puncture wound without FB of finger with damage to nail**
[6th]

S61.330 Puncture wound without FB of right index finger with damage to nail
[7th]

S61.331 Puncture wound without FB of left index finger with damage to nail
[7th]

S61.332 Puncture wound without FB of right middle finger with damage to nail
[7th]

S61.333 Puncture wound without FB of left middle finger with damage to nail
[7th]

S61.334 Puncture wound without FB of right ring finger with damage to nail
[7th]

S61.335 Puncture wound without FB of left ring finger with damage to nail
[7th]

S61.336 Puncture wound without FB of right little finger with damage to nail
[7th]

[4th] [5th] [6th] [7th] Additional Character Required   ✓   3-character code   Unspecified laterality codes were excluded here.   • =New Code   ▲ =Revised Code   ▪ =Social determinants of health   *Excludes1*—Not coded here, do not use together   *Excludes2*—Not included here

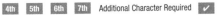

S61.337   Puncture wound without FB of left little finger with damage to nail   7th

S61.34   6th   Puncture wound with FB of finger with damage to nail

S61.340   7th   Puncture wound with FB of right index finger with damage to nail

> 7th characters for category S61
> A—initial encounter
> D—subsequent encounter
> S—sequela

S61.341   7th   Puncture wound with FB of left index finger with damage to nail

S61.342   7th   Puncture wound with FB of right middle finger with damage to nail

S61.343   7th   Puncture wound with FB of left middle finger with damage to nail

S61.344   7th   Puncture wound with FB of right ring finger with damage to nail

S61.345   7th   Puncture wound with FB of left ring finger with damage to nail

S61.346   7th   Puncture wound with FB of right little finger with damage to nail

S61.347   7th   Puncture wound with FB of left little finger with damage to nail

S61.35   6th   Open bite of finger with damage to nail

Bite of finger with damage to nail NOS

Excludes1: superficial bite of finger (S60.46-, S60.47-)

S61.350   7th   Open bite of right index finger with damage to nail

S61.351   7th   Open bite of left index finger with damage to nail

S61.352   7th   Open bite of right middle finger with damage to nail

S61.353   7th   Open bite of left middle finger with damage to nail

S61.354   7th   Open bite of right ring finger with damage to nail

S61.355   7th   Open bite of left ring finger with damage to nail

S61.356   7th   Open bite of right little finger with damage to nail

S61.357   7th   Open bite of left little finger with damage to nail

S61.4   5th   Open wound of hand

S61.41   6th   Laceration without FB of hand

S61.411   7th   Laceration without FB of right hand

S61.412   7th   Laceration without FB of left hand

S61.42   6th   Laceration with FB of hand

S61.421   7th   Laceration with FB of right hand

S61.422   7th   Laceration with FB of left hand

S61.43   6th   Puncture wound without FB of hand

S61.431   7th   Puncture wound without FB of right hand

S61.432   7th   Puncture wound without FB of left hand

S61.44   6th   Puncture wound with FB of hand

S61.441   7th   Puncture wound with FB of right hand

S61.442   7th   Puncture wound with FB of left hand

S61.45   6th   Open bite of hand

Bite of hand NOS

Excludes1: superficial bite of hand (S60.56-, S60.57-)

S61.451   7th   Open bite of right hand

S61.452   7th   Open bite of left hand

S61.5   5th   Open wound of wrist

S61.51   6th   Laceration without FB of wrist

S61.511   7th   Laceration without FB of right wrist

S61.512   7th   Laceration without FB of left wrist

S61.52   6th   Laceration with FB of wrist

S61.521   7th   Laceration with FB of right wrist

S61.522   7th   Laceration with FB of left wrist

S61.53   6th   Puncture wound without FB of wrist

S61.531   7th   Puncture wound without FB of right wrist

S61.532   7th   Puncture wound without FB of left wrist

S61.54   6th   Puncture wound with FB of wrist

S61.541   7th   Puncture wound with FB of right wrist

S61.542   7th   Puncture wound with FB of left wrist

S61.55   6th   Open bite of wrist

Bite of wrist NOS

Excludes1: superficial bite of wrist (S60.86-, S60.87-)

S61.551   7th   Open bite of right wrist

S61.552   7th   Open bite of left wrist

S62   4th   **FRACTURE AT WRIST AND HAND LEVEL**

Note: A fracture not indicated as displaced or nondisplaced should be coded to displaced

A fracture not indicated as open or closed should be coded to closed

Excludes1: traumatic amputation of wrist and hand (S68.-)

Excludes2: fracture of distal parts of ulna and radius (S52.-)

> 7th characters for category S62
> A—initial encounter for closed fracture
> B—initial encounter for open fracture
> D—subsequent encounter for fracture with routine healing
> G—subsequent encounter for fracture with delayed healing
> K—subsequent encounter for fracture with nonunion
> P—subsequent encounter for fracture with malunion
> S—sequela

S62.0   5th   Fracture of navicular [scaphoid] bone of wrist

S62.00   6th   Unspecified fracture of navicular [scaphoid] bone of wrist

S62.001   7th   Unspecified fracture of navicular [scaphoid] bone of right wrist

S62.002   7th   Unspecified fracture of navicular [scaphoid] bone of left wrist

S62.01   6th   Fracture of distal pole of navicular [scaphoid] bone of wrist

Fracture of volar tuberosity of navicular [scaphoid] bone of wrist

S62.011   7th   Displaced fracture of distal pole of navicular [scaphoid] bone of right wrist

S62.012   7th   Displaced fracture of distal pole of navicular [scaphoid] bone of left wrist

S62.014   7th   Nondisplaced fracture of distal pole of navicular [scaphoid] bone of right wrist

S62.015   7th   Nondisplaced fracture of distal pole of navicular [scaphoid] bone of left wrist

S62.02   6th   Fracture of middle third of navicular [scaphoid] bone of wrist

S62.021   7th   Displaced fracture of middle third of navicular [scaphoid] bone of right wrist

S62.022   7th   Displaced fracture of middle third of navicular [scaphoid] bone of left wrist

S62.024   7th   Nondisplaced fracture of middle third of navicular [scaphoid] bone of right wrist

S62.025   7th   Nondisplaced fracture of middle third of navicular [scaphoid] bone of left wrist

S62.03   6th   Fracture of proximal third of navicular [scaphoid] bone of wrist

S62.031   7th   Displaced fracture of proximal third of navicular [scaphoid] bone of right wrist

S62.032   7th   Displaced fracture of proximal third of navicular [scaphoid] bone of left wrist

---

4th   5th   6th   7th   Additional Character Required   ✓   3-character code

Unspecified laterality codes were excluded here.

• =New Code
▲ =Revised Code
▫ =Social determinants of health

Excludes1—Not coded here, do not use together
Excludes2—Not included here

360   PEDIATRIC ICD-10-CM 2021: A MANUAL FOR PROVIDER-BASED CODING

S62.034 `7th` Nondisplaced fracture of proximal third of navicular [scaphoid] bone of right wrist

S62.035 `7th` Nondisplaced fracture of proximal third of navicular [scaphoid] bone of left wrist

S62.1 `5th` **Fracture of other and unspecified carpal bone(s)**

Excludes2: fracture of scaphoid of wrist (S62.0-)

S62.10 `6th` **Fracture of unspecified carpal bone**

Fracture of wrist NOS

S62.101 `7th` Fracture of unspecified carpal bone, right wrist

S62.102 `7th` Fracture of unspecified carpal bone, left wrist

> 7th characters for category S62
> A—initial encounter for closed fracture
> B—initial encounter for open fracture
> D—subsequent encounter for fracture with routine healing
> G—subsequent encounter for fracture with delayed healing
> K—subsequent encounter for fracture with nonunion
> P—subsequent encounter for fracture with malunion
> S—sequela

S62.11 `6th` **Fracture of triquetrum [cuneiform] bone of wrist**

S62.111 `7th` Displaced fracture of triquetrum [cuneiform] bone, right wrist

S62.112 `7th` Displaced fracture of triquetrum [cuneiform] bone, left wrist

S62.114 `7th` Nondisplaced fracture of triquetrum [cuneiform] bone, right wrist

S62.115 `7th` Nondisplaced fracture of triquetrum [cuneiform] bone, left wrist

S62.12 `6th` **Fracture of lunate [semilunar]**

S62.121 `7th` Displaced fracture of lunate [semilunar], right wrist

S62.122 `7th` Displaced fracture of lunate [semilunar], left wrist

S62.124 `7th` Nondisplaced fracture of lunate [semilunar], right wrist

S62.125 `7th` Nondisplaced fracture of lunate [semilunar], left wrist

S62.13 `6th` **Fracture of capitate [os magnum] bone**

S62.131 `7th` Displaced fracture of capitate [os magnum] bone, right wrist

S62.132 `7th` Displaced fracture of capitate [os magnum] bone, left wrist

S62.134 `7th` Nondisplaced fracture of capitate [os magnum] bone, right wrist

S62.135 `7th` Nondisplaced fracture of capitate [os magnum] bone, left wrist

S62.14 `6th` **Fracture of body of hamate [unciform] bone**

Fracture of hamate [unciform] bone NOS

S62.141 `7th` Displaced fracture of body of hamate [unciform] bone, right wrist

S62.142 `7th` Displaced fracture of body of hamate [unciform] bone, left wrist

S62.144 `7th` Nondisplaced fracture of body of hamate [unciform] bone, right wrist

S62.145 `7th` Nondisplaced fracture of body of hamate [unciform] bone, left wrist

S62.15 `6th` **Fracture of hook process of hamate [unciform] bone**

Fracture of unciform process of hamate [unciform] bone

S62.151 `7th` Displaced fracture of hook process of hamate [unciform] bone, right wrist

S62.152 `7th` Displaced fracture of hook process of hamate [unciform] bone, left wrist

S62.154 `7th` Nondisplaced fracture of hook process of hamate [unciform] bone, right wrist

S62.155 `7th` Nondisplaced fracture of hook process of hamate [unciform] bone, left wrist

S62.16 `6th` **Fracture of pisiform**

S62.161 `7th` Displaced fracture of pisiform, right wrist

S62.162 `7th` Displaced fracture of pisiform, left wrist

S62.164 `7th` Nondisplaced fracture of pisiform, right wrist

S62.165 `7th` Nondisplaced fracture of pisiform, left wrist

S62.17 `6th` **Fracture of trapezium [larger multangular]**

S62.171 `7th` Displaced fracture of trapezium [larger multangular], right wrist

S62.172 `7th` Displaced fracture of trapezium [larger multangular], left wrist

S62.174 `7th` Nondisplaced fracture of trapezium [larger multangular], right wrist

S62.175 `7th` Nondisplaced fracture of trapezium [larger multangular], left wrist

S62.18 `6th` **Fracture of trapezoid [smaller multangular]**

S62.181 `7th` Displaced fracture of trapezoid [smaller multangular], right wrist

S62.182 `7th` Displaced fracture of trapezoid [smaller multangular], left wrist

S62.184 `7th` Nondisplaced fracture of trapezoid [smaller multangular], right wrist

S62.185 `7th` Nondisplaced fracture of trapezoid [smaller multangular], left wrist

S62.2 `5th` **Fracture of first metacarpal bone**

S62.20 `6th` **Unspecified fracture of first metacarpal bone**

S62.201 `7th` Unspecified fracture of first metacarpal bone, right hand

S62.202 `7th` Unspecified fracture of first metacarpal bone, left hand

S62.21 `6th` **Bennett's fracture**

S62.211 `7th` Bennett's fracture, right hand

S62.212 `7th` Bennett's fracture, left hand

S62.22 `6th` **Rolando's fracture**

S62.221 `7th` Displaced Rolando's fracture, right hand

S62.222 `7th` Displaced Rolando's fracture, left hand

S62.224 `7th` Nondisplaced Rolando's fracture, right hand

S62.225 `7th` Nondisplaced Rolando's fracture, left hand

S62.23 `6th` **Other fracture of base of first metacarpal bone**

S62.231 `7th` Other displaced fracture of base of first metacarpal bone, right hand

S62.232 `7th` Other displaced fracture of base of first metacarpal bone, left hand

S62.234 `7th` Other nondisplaced fracture of base of first metacarpal bone, right hand

S62.235 `7th` Other nondisplaced fracture of base of first metacarpal bone, left hand

S62.24 `6th` **Fracture of shaft of first metacarpal bone**

S62.241 `7th` Displaced fracture of shaft of first metacarpal bone, right hand

S62.242 `7th` Displaced fracture of shaft of first metacarpal bone, left hand

S62.244 `7th` Nondisplaced fracture of shaft of first metacarpal bone, right hand

S62.245 `7th` Nondisplaced fracture of shaft of first metacarpal bone, left hand

S62.25 `6th` **Fracture of neck of first metacarpal bone**

S62.251 `7th` Displaced fracture of neck of first metacarpal bone, right hand

S62.252 `7th` Displaced fracture of neck of first metacarpal bone, left hand

S62.254 `7th` Nondisplaced fracture of neck of first metacarpal bone, right hand

S62.255 `7th` Nondisplaced fracture of neck of first metacarpal bone, left hand

S62.29 `6th` **Other fracture of first metacarpal bone**

S62.291 `7th` Other fracture of first metacarpal bone, right hand

S62.292 `7th` Other fracture of first metacarpal bone, left hand

S62.3 `5th` **Fracture of other and unspecified metacarpal bone**

Excludes2: fracture of first metacarpal bone (S62.2-)

`4th` `5th` `6th` `7th`   Additional Character Required   ✔ `3-character code`   Unspecified laterality codes were excluded here.

• =New Code
▲ =Revised Code
▯ =Social determinants of health

Excludes1—Not coded here, do not use together
Excludes2—Not included here

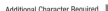

CHAPTER 19. INJURY, POISONING AND CERTAIN OTHER CONSEQUENCES OF EXTERNAL CAUSES   (S62.30–S62.395)

S62.30 `6th` **Unspecified fracture of other metacarpal bone**
- **S62.300** `7th` **Unspecified fracture of second metacarpal bone, right hand**
- **S62.301** `7th` **Unspecified fracture of second metacarpal bone, left hand**
- **S62.302** `7th` **Unspecified fracture of third metacarpal bone, right hand**
- **S62.303** `7th` **Unspecified fracture of third metacarpal bone, left hand**
- **S62.304** `7th` **Unspecified fracture of fourth metacarpal bone, right hand**
- **S62.305** `7th` **Unspecified fracture of fourth metacarpal bone, left hand**
- **S62.306** `7th` **Unspecified fracture of fifth metacarpal bone, right hand**
- **S62.307** `7th` **Unspecified fracture of fifth metacarpal bone, left hand**

> 7th characters for category S62
> A—initial encounter for closed fracture
> B—initial encounter for open fracture
> D—subsequent encounter for fracture with routine healing
> G—subsequent encounter for fracture with delayed healing
> K—subsequent encounter for fracture with nonunion
> P—subsequent encounter for fracture with malunion
> S—sequela

S62.31 `6th` **Displaced fracture of base of other metacarpal bone**
- **S62.310** `7th` **Displaced fracture of base of second metacarpal bone, right hand**
- **S62.311** `7th` **Displaced fracture of base of second metacarpal bone, left hand**
- **S62.312** `7th` **Displaced fracture of base of third metacarpal bone, right hand**
- **S62.313** `7th` **Displaced fracture of base of third metacarpal bone, left hand**
- **S62.314** `7th` **Displaced fracture of base of fourth metacarpal bone, right hand**
- **S62.315** `7th` **Displaced fracture of base of fourth metacarpal bone, left hand**
- **S62.316** `7th` **Displaced fracture of base of fifth metacarpal bone, right hand**
- **S62.317** `7th` **Displaced fracture of base of fifth metacarpal bone, left hand**

S62.32 `6th` **Displaced fracture of shaft of other metacarpal bone**
- **S62.320** `7th` **Displaced fracture of shaft of second metacarpal bone, right hand**
- **S62.321** `7th` **Displaced fracture of shaft of second metacarpal bone, left hand**
- **S62.322** `7th` **Displaced fracture of shaft of third metacarpal bone, right hand**
- **S62.323** `7th` **Displaced fracture of shaft of third metacarpal bone, left hand**
- **S62.324** `7th` **Displaced fracture of shaft of fourth metacarpal bone, right hand**
- **S62.325** `7th` **Displaced fracture of shaft of fourth metacarpal bone, left hand**
- **S62.326** `7th` **Displaced fracture of shaft of fifth metacarpal bone, right hand**
- **S62.327** `7th` **Displaced fracture of shaft of fifth metacarpal bone, left hand**

S62.33 `6th` **Displaced fracture of neck of other metacarpal bone**
- **S62.330** `7th` **Displaced fracture of neck of second metacarpal bone, right hand**
- **S62.331** `7th` **Displaced fracture of neck of second metacarpal bone, left hand**
- **S62.332** `7th` **Displaced fracture of neck of third metacarpal bone, right hand**
- **S62.333** `7th` **Displaced fracture of neck of third metacarpal bone, left hand**
- **S62.334** `7th` **Displaced fracture of neck of fourth metacarpal bone, right hand**
- **S62.335** `7th` **Displaced fracture of neck of fourth metacarpal bone, left hand**
- **S62.336** `7th` **Displaced fracture of neck of fifth metacarpal bone, right hand**
- **S62.337** `7th` **Displaced fracture of neck of fifth metacarpal bone, left hand**

S62.34 `6th` **Nondisplaced fracture of base of other metacarpal bone**
- **S62.340** `7th` **Nondisplaced fracture of base of second metacarpal bone, right hand**
- **S62.341** `7th` **Nondisplaced fracture of base of second metacarpal bone left hand**
- **S62.342** `7th` **Nondisplaced fracture of base of third metacarpal bone, right hand**
- **S62.343** `7th` **Nondisplaced fracture of base of third metacarpal bone, left hand**
- **S62.344** `7th` **Nondisplaced fracture of base of fourth metacarpal bone, right hand**
- **S62.345** `7th` **Nondisplaced fracture of base of fourth metacarpal bone, left hand**
- **S62.346** `7th` **Nondisplaced fracture of base of fifth metacarpal bone, right hand**
- **S62.347** `7th` **Nondisplaced fracture of base of fifth metacarpal bone, left hand**

S62.35 `6th` **Nondisplaced fracture of shaft of other metacarpal bone**
- **S62.350** `7th` **Nondisplaced fracture of shaft of second metacarpal bone, right hand**
- **S62.351** `7th` **Nondisplaced fracture of shaft of second metacarpal bone, left hand**
- **S62.352** `7th` **Nondisplaced fracture of shaft of third metacarpal bone, right hand**
- **S62.353** `7th` **Nondisplaced fracture of shaft of third metacarpal bone, left hand**
- **S62.354** `7th` **Nondisplaced fracture of shaft of fourth metacarpal bone, right hand**
- **S62.355** `7th` **Nondisplaced fracture of shaft of fourth metacarpal bone, left hand**
- **S62.356** `7th` **Nondisplaced fracture of shaft of fifth metacarpal bone, right hand**
- **S62.357** `7th` **Nondisplaced fracture of shaft of fifth metacarpal bone, left hand**

S62.36 `6th` **Nondisplaced fracture of neck of other metacarpal bone**
- **S62.360** `7th` **Nondisplaced fracture of neck of second metacarpal bone, right hand**
- **S62.361** `7th` **Nondisplaced fracture of neck of second metacarpal bone, left hand**
- **S62.362** `7th` **Nondisplaced fracture of neck of third metacarpal bone, right hand**
- **S62.363** `7th` **Nondisplaced fracture of neck of third metacarpal bone, left hand**
- **S62.364** `7th` **Nondisplaced fracture of neck of fourth metacarpal bone, right hand**
- **S62.365** `7th` **Nondisplaced fracture of neck of fourth metacarpal bone, left hand**
- **S62.366** `7th` **Nondisplaced fracture of neck of fifth metacarpal bone, right hand**
- **S62.367** `7th` **Nondisplaced fracture of neck of fifth metacarpal bone, left hand**

S62.39 `6th` **Other fracture of other metacarpal bone**
- **S62.390** `7th` **Other fracture of second metacarpal bone, right hand**
- **S62.391** `7th` **Other fracture of second metacarpal bone, left hand**
- **S62.392** `7th` **Other fracture of third metacarpal bone, right hand**
- **S62.393** `7th` **Other fracture of third metacarpal bone, left hand**
- **S62.394** `7th` **Other fracture of fourth metacarpal bone, right hand**
- **S62.395** `7th` **Other fracture of fourth metacarpal bone, left hand**

`4th` `5th` `6th` `7th` Additional Character Required   ✓ 3-character code   Unspecified laterality codes were excluded here.   • =New Code   ▲ =Revised Code   ▫ =Social determinants of health   **Excludes1**—Not coded here, do not use together   **Excludes2**—Not included here

S62.396 **7th** Other fracture of fifth metacarpal bone, right hand

S62.397 **7th** Other fracture of fifth metacarpal bone, left hand

S62.5 5th Fracture of thumb

S62.50 6th Fracture of unspecified phalanx of thumb

S62.501 **7th** Fracture of unspecified phalanx of right thumb

S62.502 **7th** Fracture of unspecified phalanx of left thumb

> 7th characters for category S62
> A—initial encounter for closed fracture
> B—initial encounter for open fracture
> D—subsequent encounter for fracture with routine healing
> G—subsequent encounter for fracture with delayed healing
> K—subsequent encounter for fracture with nonunion
> P—subsequent encounter for fracture with malunion
> S—sequela

S62.51 6th Fracture of proximal phalanx of thumb

S62.511 **7th** Displaced fracture of proximal phalanx of right thumb

S62.512 **7th** Displaced fracture of proximal phalanx of left thumb

S62.514 **7th** Nondisplaced fracture of proximal phalanx of right thumb

S62.515 **7th** Nondisplaced fracture of proximal phalanx of left thumb

S62.52 6th Fracture of distal phalanx of thumb

S62.521 **7th** Displaced fracture of distal phalanx of right thumb

S62.522 **7th** Displaced fracture of distal phalanx of left thumb

S62.524 **7th** Nondisplaced fracture of distal phalanx of right thumb

S62.525 **7th** Nondisplaced fracture of distal phalanx of left thumb

S62.6 5th Fracture of other and unspecified finger(s)

Excludes2: fracture of thumb (S62.5-)

S62.61 6th Displaced fracture of proximal phalanx of finger

S62.610 **7th** Displaced fracture of proximal phalanx of right index finger

S62.611 **7th** Displaced fracture of proximal phalanx of left index finger

S62.612 **7th** Displaced fracture of proximal phalanx of right middle finger

S62.613 **7th** Displaced fracture of proximal phalanx of left middle finger

S62.614 **7th** Displaced fracture of proximal phalanx of right ring finger

S62.615 **7th** Displaced fracture of proximal phalanx of left ring finger

S62.616 **7th** Displaced fracture of proximal phalanx of right little finger

S62.617 **7th** Displaced fracture of proximal phalanx of left little finger

S62.62 6th Displaced fracture of middle phalanx of finger

S62.620 **7th** Displaced fracture of middle phalanx of right index finger

S62.621 **7th** Displaced fracture of middle phalanx of left index finger

S62.622 **7th** Displaced fracture of middle phalanx of right middle finger

S62.623 **7th** Displaced fracture of middle phalanx of left middle finger

S62.624 **7th** Displaced fracture of middle phalanx of right ring finger

S62.625 **7th** Displaced fracture of middle phalanx of left ring finger

S62.626 **7th** Displaced fracture of middle phalanx of right little finger

S62.627 **7th** Displaced fracture of middle phalanx of left little finger

S62.63 6th Displaced fracture of distal phalanx of finger

S62.630 **7th** Displaced fracture of distal phalanx of right index finger

S62.631 **7th** Displaced fracture of distal phalanx of left index finger

S62.632 **7th** Displaced fracture of distal phalanx of right middle finger

S62.633 **7th** Displaced fracture of distal phalanx of left middle finger

S62.634 **7th** Displaced fracture of distal phalanx of right ring finger

S62.635 **7th** Displaced fracture of distal phalanx of left ring finger

S62.636 **7th** Displaced fracture of distal phalanx of right little finger

S62.637 **7th** Displaced fracture of distal phalanx of left little finger

S62.64 6th Nondisplaced fracture of proximal phalanx of finger

S62.640 **7th** Nondisplaced fracture of proximal phalanx of right index finger

S62.641 **7th** Nondisplaced fracture of proximal phalanx of left index finger

S62.642 **7th** Nondisplaced fracture of proximal phalanx of right middle finger

S62.643 **7th** Nondisplaced fracture of proximal phalanx of left middle finger

S62.644 **7th** Nondisplaced fracture of proximal phalanx of right ring finger

S62.645 **7th** Nondisplaced fracture of proximal phalanx of left ring finger

S62.646 **7th** Nondisplaced fracture of proximal phalanx of right little finger

S62.647 **7th** Nondisplaced fracture of proximal phalanx of left little finger

S62.65 6th Nondisplaced fracture of medial phalanx of finger

S62.650 **7th** Nondisplaced fracture of middle phalanx of right index finger

S62.651 **7th** Nondisplaced fracture of middle phalanx of left index finger

S62.652 **7th** Nondisplaced fracture of middle phalanx of right middle finger

S62.653 **7th** Nondisplaced fracture of middle phalanx of left middle finger

S62.654 **7th** Nondisplaced fracture of middle phalanx of right ring finger

S62.655 **7th** Nondisplaced fracture of middle phalanx of left ring finger

S62.656 **7th** Nondisplaced fracture of middle phalanx of right little finger

S62.657 **7th** Nondisplaced fracture of middle phalanx of left little finger

S62.66 6th Nondisplaced fracture of distal phalanx of finger

S62.660 **7th** Nondisplaced fracture of distal phalanx of right index finger

S62.661 **7th** Nondisplaced fracture of distal phalanx of left index finger

S62.662 **7th** Nondisplaced fracture of distal phalanx of right middle finger

S62.663 **7th** Nondisplaced fracture of distal phalanx of left middle finger

S62.664 **7th** Nondisplaced fracture of distal phalanx of right ring finger

S62.665 **7th** Nondisplaced fracture of distal phalanx of left ring finger

S62.666 **7th** Nondisplaced fracture of distal phalanx of right little finger

S62.667 **7th** Nondisplaced fracture of distal phalanx of left little finger

S63 4th DISLOCATION AND SPRAIN OF JOINTS AND LIGAMENTS AT WRIST AND HAND LEVEL

Includes: avulsion of joint or ligament at wrist and hand level

laceration of cartilage, joint or ligament at wrist and hand level

sprain of cartilage, joint or ligament at wrist and hand level

> 7th characters for category S63
> A—initial encounter
> D—subsequent encounter
> S—sequela

4th **5th** **6th** **7th** Additional Character Required ✓ 3-character code

Unspecified laterality codes were excluded here.

• =New Code
▲ =Revised Code
⊡ =Social determinants of health

Excludes1—Not coded here, do not use together
Excludes2—Not included here

PEDIATRIC ICD-10-CM 2021: A MANUAL FOR PROVIDER-BASED CODING

363

traumatic hemarthrosis of joint or ligament at wrist and hand level

traumatic rupture of joint or ligament at wrist and hand level

traumatic subluxation of joint or ligament at wrist and hand level

traumatic tear of joint or ligament at wrist and hand level

Code also any associated open wound

Excludes2: strain of muscle, fascia and tendon of wrist and hand (S66.-)

S63.0 **[5th]** **Subluxation and dislocation of wrist and hand joints**

7th characters for category S63
A—initial encounter
D—subsequent encounter
S—sequela

S63.06 **[6th]** **Subluxation and dislocation of metacarpal (bone), proximal end**

S63.061 **[7th]** Subluxation of metacarpal (bone), proximal end of right hand

S63.062 **[7th]** Subluxation of metacarpal (bone), proximal end of left hand

S63.063 **[7th]** Subluxation of metacarpal (bone), proximal end of unspecified hand

S63.064 **[7th]** Dislocation of metacarpal (bone), proximal end of right hand

S63.065 **[7th]** Dislocation of metacarpal (bone), proximal end of left hand

S63.1 **[5th]** **Subluxation and dislocation of thumb**

S63.10 **[6th]** **Unspecified subluxation and dislocation of thumb**

S63.101 **[7th]** Unspecified subluxation of right thumb

S63.102 **[7th]** Unspecified subluxation of left thumb

S63.104 **[7th]** Unspecified dislocation of right thumb

S63.105 **[7th]** Unspecified dislocation of left thumb

S63.11 **[6th]** **Subluxation and dislocation of metacarpophalangeal joint of thumb**

S63.111 **[7th]** Subluxation of metacarpophalangeal joint of right thumb

S63.112 **[7th]** Subluxation of metacarpophalangeal joint of left thumb

S63.114 **[7th]** Dislocation of metacarpophalangeal joint of right thumb

S63.115 **[7th]** Dislocation of metacarpophalangeal joint of left thumb

S63.12 **[6th]** **Subluxation and dislocation of interphalangeal joint of thumb**

S63.121 **[7th]** Subluxation of interphalangeal joint of right thumb

S63.122 **[7th]** Subluxation of interphalangeal joint of left thumb

S63.124 **[7th]** Dislocation of interphalangeal joint of right thumb

S63.125 **[7th]** Dislocation of interphalangeal joint of left thumb

S63.2 **[5th]** **Subluxation and dislocation of other finger(s)**

Excludes2: subluxation and dislocation of thumb (S63.1-)

S63.20 **[6th]** **Unspecified subluxation of other finger**

S63.200 **[7th]** Unspecified subluxation of right index finger

S63.201 **[7th]** Unspecified subluxation of left index finger

S63.202 **[7th]** Unspecified subluxation of right middle finger

S63.203 **[7th]** Unspecified subluxation of left middle finger

S63.204 **[7th]** Unspecified subluxation of right ring finger

S63.205 **[7th]** Unspecified subluxation of left ring finger

S63.206 **[7th]** Unspecified subluxation of right little finger

S63.207 **[7th]** Unspecified subluxation of left little finge

S63.21 **[6th]** **Subluxation of metacarpophalangeal joint of finger**

S63.210 **[7th]** Subluxation of metacarpophalangeal joint of right index finger

S63.211 **[7th]** Subluxation of metacar-pophalan-geal joint of left index finger

S63.212 **[7th]** Subluxation of metacarpophalangeal joint of right middle finger

S63.213 **[7th]** Subluxation of metacarpophalangeal joint of left middle finger

S63.214 **[7th]** Subluxation of metacarpophalangeal joint of right ring finger

S63.215 **[7th]** Subluxation of metacarpophalangeal joint of left ring finger

S63.216 **[7th]** Subluxation of metacarpophalangeal joint of right little finger

S63.217 **[7th]** Subluxation of metacarpophalangeal joint of left little finger

S63.23 **[6th]** **Subluxation of proximal interphalangeal joint of finger**

S63.230 **[7th]** Subluxation of proximal interphalangeal joint of right index finger

S63.231 **[7th]** Subluxation of proximal interphalangeal joint of left index finger

S63.232 **[7th]** Subluxation of proximal interphalangeal joint of right middle finger

S63.233 **[7th]** Subluxation of proximal interphalangeal joint of left middle finger

S63.234 **[7th]** Subluxation of proximal interphalangeal joint of right ring finger

S63.235 **[7th]** Subluxation of proximal interphalangeal joint of left ring finger

S63.236 **[7th]** Subluxation of proximal interphalangeal joint of right little finger

S63.237 **[7th]** Subluxation of proximal interphalangeal joint of left little finger

S63.24 **[6th]** **Subluxation of distal interphalangeal joint of finger**

S63.240 **[7th]** Subluxation of distal interphalangeal joint of right index finger

S63.241 **[7th]** Subluxation of distal interphalangeal joint of left index finger

S63.242 **[7th]** Subluxation of distal interphalangeal joint of right middle finger

S63.243 **[7th]** Subluxation of distal interphalangeal joint of left middle finger

S63.244 **[7th]** Subluxation of distal interphalangeal joint of right ring finger

S63.245 **[7th]** Subluxation of distal interphalangeal joint of left ring finger

S63.246 **[7th]** Subluxation of distal interphalangeal joint of right little finger

S63.247 **[7th]** Subluxation of distal interphalangeal joint of left little finger

S63.26 **[6th]** **Dislocation of metacarpophalangeal joint of finger**

S63.260 **[7th]** Dislocation of metacarpophalangeal joint of right index finger

S63.261 **[7th]** Dislocation of metacarpophalangeal joint of left index finger

S63.262 **[7th]** Dislocation of metacarpophalangeal joint of right middle finger

S63.263 **[7th]** Dislocation of metacarpophalangeal joint of left middle finger

S63.264 **[7th]** Dislocation of metacarpophalangeal joint of right ring finger

S63.265 **[7th]** Dislocation of metacarpophalangeal joint of left ring finger

S63.266 **[7th]** Dislocation of metacarpophalangeal joint of right little finger

S63.267 **[7th]** Dislocation of metacarpophalangeal joint of left little finger

S63.28 **[6th]** **Dislocation of proximal interphalangeal joint of finger**

S63.280 **[7th]** Dislocation of proximal interphalangeal joint of right index finger

S63.281 **[7th]** Dislocation of proximal interphalangeal joint of left index finger

S63.282 **[7th]** Dislocation of proximal interphalan-geal joint of right middle finger

---

| **[4th]** **[5th]** **[6th]** **[7th]** Additional Character Required | ✔ 3-character code | Unspecified laterality codes were excluded here. | • =New Code
▲ =Revised Code
☐ =Social determinants of health | ***Excludes1***—Not coded here, do not use together
Excludes2—Not included here |

S63.283 7th Dislocation of proximal interphalangeal joint of left middle finger

S63.284 7th Dislocation of proximal interphalangeal joint of right ring finger

S63.285 7th Dislocation of proximal interphalangeal joint of left ring finger

S63.286 7th Dislocation of proximal interphalangeal joint of right little finger

> 7th characters for category S63
> A—initial encounter
> D—subsequent encounter
> S—sequela

S63.287 7th Dislocation of proximal interphalangeal joint of left little finger

S63.29 6th Dislocation of distal interphalangeal joint of finger

S63.290 7th Dislocation of distal interphalangeal joint of right index finger

S63.291 7th Dislocation of distal interphalangeal joint of left index finger

S63.292 7th Dislocation of distal interphalangeal joint of right middle finger

S63.293 7th Dislocation of distal interphalangeal joint of left middle finger

S63.294 7th Dislocation of distal interphalangeal joint of right ring finger

S63.295 7th Dislocation of distal interphalangeal joint of left ring finger

S63.296 7th Dislocation of distal interphalangeal joint of right little finger

S63.297 7th Dislocation of distal inter-phalangeal joint of left little finger

S63.5 5th Other and unspecified sprain of wrist

S63.50 6th Unspecified sprain of wrist

S63.501 7th Unspecified sprain of right wrist

S63.502 7th Unspecified sprain of left wrist

S63.51 6th Sprain of carpal (joint)

S63.511 7th Sprain of carpal joint of right wrist

S63.512 7th Sprain of carpal joint of left wrist

S63.52 6th Sprain of radiocarpal joint

Excludes1: traumatic rupture of radiocarpal ligament (S63.32-)

S63.521 7th Sprain of radiocarpal joint of right wrist

S63.522 7th Sprain of radiocarpal joint of left wrist

S63.59 6th Other specified sprain of wrist

S63.591 7th Other specified sprain of right wrist

S63.592 7th Other specified sprain of left wrist

S63.6 5th Other and unspecified sprain of finger(s)

Excludes1: traumatic rupture of ligament of finger at metacarpophalangeal and interphalangeal joint(s) (S63.4-)

S63.60 6th Unspecified sprain of thumb

S63.601 7th Unspecified sprain of right thumb

S63.602 7th Unspecified sprain of left thumb

S63.61 6th Unspecified sprain of other and unspecified finger(s)

S63.610 7th Unspecified sprain of right index finger

S63.611 7th Unspecified sprain of left index finger

S63.612 7th Unspecified sprain of right middle finger

S63.613 7th Unspecified sprain of left middle finger

S63.614 7th Unspecified sprain of right ring finger

S63.615 7th Unspecified sprain of left ring finger

S63.616 7th Unspecified sprain of right little finger

S63.617 7th Unspecified sprain of left little finger

S63.62 6th Sprain of interphalangeal joint of thumb

S63.621 7th Sprain of interphalangeal joint of right thumb

S63.622 7th Sprain of interphalangeal joint of left thumb

S63.63 6th Sprain of interphalangeal joint of other and unspecified finger(s)

S63.630 7th Sprain of interphalangeal joint of right index finger

S63.631 7th Sprain of interphalangeal joint of left index finger

S63.632 7th Sprain of interphalangeal joint of right middle finger

S63.633 7th Sprain of interphalangeal joint of left middle finger

S63.634 7th Sprain of interphalangeal joint of right ring finger

S63.635 7th Sprain of interphalangeal joint of left ring finger

S63.636 7th Sprain of interphalangeal joint of right little finger

S63.637 7th Sprain of interphalangeal joint of left little finger

S63.64 6th Sprain of metacarpophalangeal joint of thumb

S63.641 7th Sprain of metacarpophalangeal joint of right thumb

S63.642 7th Sprain of metacarpophalangeal joint of left thumb

S63.65 6th Sprain of metacarpophalangeal joint of other and unspecified finger(s)

S63.650 7th Sprain of metacarpophalangeal joint of right index finger

S63.651 7th Sprain of metacarpophalangeal joint of left index finger

S63.652 7th Sprain of metacarpophalangeal joint of right middle finger

S63.653 7th Sprain of metacarpophalangeal joint of left middle finger

S63.654 7th Sprain of metacarpophalangeal joint of right ring finger

S63.655 7th Sprain of metacarpophalangeal joint of left ring finger

S63.656 7th Sprain of metacarpophalangeal joint of right little finger

S63.657 7th Sprain of metacarpophalangeal joint of left little finger

S63.68 6th Other sprain of thumb

S63.681 7th Other sprain of right thumb

S63.682 7th Other sprain of left thumb

S63.69 6th Other sprain of other and unspecified finger(s)

S63.690 7th Other sprain of right index finger

S63.691 7th Other sprain of left index finger

S63.692 7th Other sprain of right middle finger

S63.693 7th Other sprain of left middle finger

S63.694 7th Other sprain of right ring finger

S63.695 7th Other sprain of left ring finger

S63.696 7th Other sprain of right little finger

S63.697 7th Other sprain of left little finger

CHAPTER 19. INJURY, POISONING AND CERTAIN OTHER CONSEQUENCES OF EXTERNAL CAUSES (S63.283–S63.697)

4th 5th 6th 7th Additional Character Required ✔ 3-character code

Unspecified laterality codes were excluded here.

• =New Code
▲ =Revised Code
▣ =Social determinants of health

Excludes1—Not coded here, do not use together
Excludes2—Not included here

CHAPTER 19. INJURY, POISONING AND CERTAIN OTHER CONSEQUENCES OF EXTERNAL CAUSES   (S63.8–S66.51)

S63.8 Sprain of other part of wrist and hand
- **5th** **S63.8X** Sprain of other part of wrist and hand
  - **6th** **S63.8X1** Sprain of other part of right wrist and **7th** hand
  - **S63.8X2** Sprain of other part of left wrist and hand **7th**

S63.9 Sprain of unspecified part of wrist and hand
- **5th** **S63.91X** Sprain of unspecified part of right wrist and hand **7th**
- **S63.92X** Sprain of unspecified part of left wrist and hand **7th**

S65   **INJURY OF BLOOD VESSELS AT WRIST AND HAND LEVEL**
4th   **Code also** any associated open wound (S61.-)

> 7th characters for category S63 & S65
> A—initial encounter
> D—subsequent encounter
> S—sequela

S65.2 Injury of superficial palmar arch
- **5th** **S65.21** Laceration of superficial palmar arch
  - **6th**
    - **S65.211** Laceration of superficial palmar arch of right hand **7th**
    - **S65.212** Laceration of superficial palmar arch of left hand **7th**
- **S65.29** Other specified injury of superficial palmar arch
  - **6th**
    - **S65.291** Other specified injury of superficial palmar arch of right hand **7th**
    - **S65.292** Other specified injury of superficial palmar arch of left hand **7th**

S65.3 Injury of deep palmar arch
- **5th** **S65.30** Unspecified injury of deep palmar arch
  - **6th**
    - **S65.301** Unspecified injury of deep palmar arch of right hand **7th**
    - **S65.302** Unspecified injury of deep palmar arch of left hand **7th**
- **S65.31** Laceration of deep palmar arch
  - **6th**
    - **S65.311** Laceration of deep palmar arch of right hand **7th**
    - **S65.312** Laceration of deep palmar arch of left hand **7th**
- **S65.39** Other specified injury of deep palmar arch
  - **6th**
    - **S65.391** Other specified injury of deep palmar arch of right hand **7th**
    - **S65.392** Other specified injury of deep palmar arch of left hand **7th**

S65.9 Injury of unspecified blood vessel at wrist and hand level
- **5th** **S65.91** Laceration of unspecified blood vessel at wrist and hand level
  - **6th**
    - **S65.911** Laceration of unspecified blood vessel at wrist and hand level of right arm **7th**
    - **S65.912** Laceration of unspecified blood vessel at wrist and hand level of left arm **7th**
- **S65.99** Other specified injury of unspecified blood vessel at wrist and hand level
  - **6th**
    - **S65.991** Other specified injury of unspecified blood vessel at wrist and hand of right arm **7th**
    - **S65.992** Other specified injury of unspecified blood vessel at wrist and hand of left arm **7th**

S66   **INJURY OF MUSCLE, FASCIA AND TENDON AT WRIST AND HAND LEVEL**
4th   **Code also** any associated open wound (S61.-)

> 7th characters for categories S65 & S66
> A—initial encounter
> D—subsequent encounter
> S—sequela

Excludes2: sprain of joints and ligaments of wrist and hand (S63.-)

S66.0 Injury of long flexor muscle, fascia, and tendon of thumb at wrist and hand level
- **5th** **S66.01** Strain of long flexor muscle, fascia and tendon of thumb at wrist and hand level
  - **6th**
    - **S66.011** Strain of long flexor muscle, fascia and tendon of right thumb at wrist and hand level **7th**
    - **S66.012** Strain of long flexor muscle, fascia and tendon of left thumb at wrist and hand level **7th**

S66.02 Laceration of long flexor muscle, fascia and tendon of thumb at wrist and hand level
- **6th**
  - **S66.021** Laceration of long flexor muscle, fascia and tendon of right thumb at wrist and hand level **7th**
  - **S66.022** Laceration of long flexor muscle, fascia and tendon of left thumb at wrist and hand level **7th**

S66.11 Strain of flexor muscle, fascia and tendon of other and unspecified finger at wrist and hand level
- **6th**
  - **S66.110** Strain of flexor muscle, fascia and tendon of right index finger at wrist and hand level **7th**
  - **S66.111** Strain of flexor muscle, fascia and tendon of left index finger at wrist and hand level **7th**
  - **S66.112** Strain of flexor muscle, fascia and tendon of right middle finger at wrist and hand level **7th**
  - **S66.113** Strain of flexor muscle, fascia and tendon of left middle finger at wrist and hand level **7th**
  - **S66.114** Strain of flexor muscle, fascia and tendon of right ring finger at wrist and hand level **7th**
  - **S66.115** Strain of flexor muscle, fascia and tendon of left ring finger at wrist and hand level **7th**
  - **S66.116** Strain of flexor muscle, fascia and tendon of right little finger at wrist and hand level **7th**
  - **S66.117** Strain of flexor muscle, fascia and tendon of left little finger at wrist and hand level **7th**

S66.21 Strain of extensor muscle, fascia and tendon of thumb at wrist and hand level
- **6th**
  - **S66.211** Strain of extensor muscle, fascia and tendon of right thumb at wrist and hand level **7th**
  - **S66.212** Strain of extensor muscle, fascia and tendon of left thumb at wrist and hand level **7th**

S66.31 Strain of extensor muscle, fascia and tendon of other and unspecified finger at wrist and hand level
- **6th**
  - **S66.310** Strain of extensor muscle, fascia and tendon of right index finger at wrist and hand level **7th**
  - **S66.311** Strain of extensor muscle, fascia and tendon of left index finger at wrist and hand level **7th**
  - **S66.312** Strain of extensor muscle, fascia and tendon of right middle finger at wrist and hand level **7th**
  - **S66.313** Strain of extensor muscle, fascia and tendon of left middle finger at wrist and hand level **7th**
  - **S66.314** Strain of extensor muscle, fascia and tendon of right ring finger at wrist and hand level **7th**
  - **S66.315** Strain of extensor muscle, fascia and tendon of left ring finger at wrist and hand level **7th**
  - **S66.316** Strain of extensor muscle, fascia and tendon of right little finger at wrist and hand level **7th**
  - **S66.317** Strain of extensor muscle, fascia and tendon of left little finger at wrist and hand level **7th**

S66.41 Strain of intrinsic muscle, fascia and tendon of thumb at wrist and hand level
- **6th**
  - **S66.411** Strain of intrinsic muscle, fascia and tendon of right thumb at wrist and hand level **7th**
  - **S66.412** Strain of intrinsic muscle, fascia and tendon of left thumb at wrist and hand level **7th**

S66.51 Strain of intrinsic muscle, fascia and tendon of other and unspecified finger at wrist and hand level
- **6th**

4th **5th** **6th** **7th** Additional Character Required   ✔ 3-character code   Unspecified laterality codes were excluded here.   • =New Code   ▲ =Revised Code   ▫ =Social determinants of health   **Excludes1**—Not coded here, do not use together   **Excludes2**—Not included here

S66.510 `7th` Strain of intrinsic muscle, fascia and tendon of right index finger at wrist and hand level

S66.511 `7th` Strain of intrinsic muscle, fascia and tendon of left index finger at wrist and hand level

S66.512 `7th` Strain of intrinsic muscle, fascia and tendon of right middle finger at wrist and hand level

7th characters for category S66
A—initial encounter
D—subsequent encounter
S—sequela

S66.513 `7th` Strain of intrinsic muscle, fascia and tendon of left middle finger at wrist and hand level

S66.514 `7th` Strain of intrinsic muscle, fascia and tendon of right ring finger at wrist and hand level

S66.515 `7th` Strain of intrinsic muscle, fascia and tendon of left ring finger at wrist and hand level

S66.516 `7th` Strain of intrinsic muscle, fascia and tendon of right little finger at wrist and hand level

S66.517 `7th` Strain of intrinsic muscle, fascia and tendon of left little finger at wrist and hand level

S66.91 `6th` Strain of unspecified muscle, fascia and tendon at wrist and hand level

S66.911 `7th` Strain of unspecified muscle, fascia and tendon at wrist and hand level, right hand

S66.912 `7th` Strain of unspecified muscle, fascia and tendon at wrist and hand level, left hand

S67 `4th` **CRUSHING INJURY OF WRIST, HAND AND FINGERS**

Use additional code for all associated injuries, such as: fracture of wrist and hand (S62.-)
open wound of wrist and hand (S61.-)

7th characters for category S67
A—initial encounter
D—subsequent encounter
S—sequela

S67.0 `5th` Crushing injury of thumb

S67.01X `7th` Crushing injury of right thumb

S67.02X `7th` Crushing injury of left thumb

S67.1 `5th` Crushing injury of other and unspecified finger(s)

Excludes2: crushing injury of thumb (S67.0-)

S67.19 `6th` Crushing injury of other finger(s)

S67.190 `7th` Crushing injury of right index finger

S67.191 `7th` Crushing injury of left index finger

S67.192 `7th` Crushing injury of right middle finger

S67.193 `7th` Crushing injury of left middle finger

S67.194 `7th` Crushing injury of right ring finger

S67.195 `7th` Crushing injury of left ring finger

S67.196 `7th` Crushing injury of right little finger

S67.197 `7th` Crushing injury of left little finger, initial encounter

S67.198 `7th` Crushing injury of other finger-
Crushing injury of specified finger with unspecified laterality

S67.2 `5th` Crushing injury of hand

Excludes2: crushing injury of fingers (S67.1-)
crushing injury of thumb (S67.0-)

S67.21X `7th` Crushing injury of right hand

S67.22X `7th` Crushing injury of left hand

S67.3 Crushing injury of wrist

S67.31X `7th` Crushing injury of right wrist

S67.32X `7th` Crushing injury of left wrist

S67.4 `5th` Crushing injury of wrist and hand

Excludes1: crushing injury of hand alone (S67.2-)
crushing injury of wrist alone (S67.3-)

Excludes2: crushing injury of fingers (S67.1-)
crushing injury of thumb (S67.0-)

S67.41X `7th` Crushing injury of right wrist and hand

S67.42X `7th` Crushing injury of left wrist and hand

(S70–S79) INJURIES TO THE HIP AND THIGH

Excludes2: burns and corrosions (T20–T32)
frostbite (T33–T34)
snake bite (T63.0-)
venomous insect bite or sting (T63.4-)

7th characters for category S70
A—initial encounter
D—subsequent encounter
S—sequela

S70 `4th` **SUPERFICIAL INJURY OF HIP AND THIGH**

S70.0 `5th` Contusion of hip

S70.01X `7th` Contusion of right hip

S70.02X `7th` Contusion of left hip

S70.1 `5th` Contusion of thigh

S70.11X `7th` Contusion of right thigh

S70.12X `7th` Contusion of left thigh

S70.2 `5th` Other superficial injuries of hip

S70.21 `6th` Abrasion of hip

S70.211 `7th` Abrasion, right hip

S70.212 `7th` Abrasion, left hip

S70.22 `6th` Blister (nonthermal) of hip

S70.221 `7th` Blister (nonthermal), right hip

S70.222 `7th` Blister (nonthermal), left hip

S70.24 `6th` External constriction of hip

S70.241 `7th` External constriction, right hip

S70.242 `7th` External constriction, left hip

S70.25 `6th` Superficial FB of hip
Splinter in the hip

S70.251 `7th` Superficial FB, right hip

S70.252 `7th` Superficial FB, left hip

S70.26 `6th` Insect bite (nonvenomous) of hip

S70.261 `7th` Insect bite (nonvenomous), right hip

S70.262 `7th` Insect bite (nonvenomous), left hip

S70.27 `6th` Other superficial bite of hip

Excludes1: open bite of hip (S71.05-)

S70.271 `7th` Other superficial bite of hip, right hip

S70.272 `7th` Other superficial bite of hip, left hip

S70.3 `5th` Other superficial injuries of thigh

S70.31 `6th` Abrasion of thigh

S70.311 `7th` Abrasion, right thigh

S70.312 `7th` Abrasion, left thigh

S70.32 `6th` Blister (nonthermal) of thigh

| `4th` `5th` `6th` `7th` Additional Character Required | ✔ 3-character code | Unspecified laterality codes were excluded here. | • =New Code
▲ =Revised Code
⌂ =Social determinants of health | *Excludes1*—Not coded here, do not use together
Excludes2—Not included here |

CHAPTER 19. INJURY, POISONING AND CERTAIN OTHER CONSEQUENCES OF EXTERNAL CAUSES   (S70.321–S72.025)

S70.321 **Blister (nonthermal), right thigh**
`7th`

S70.322 **Blister (nonthermal), left thigh**
`7th`

S70.34 **External constriction of thigh**
`6th`
S70.341 **External constriction, right thigh**
`7th`
S70.342 **External constriction, left thigh**
`7th`

S70.35 **Superficial FB of thigh**
`6th`
Splinter in the thigh
S70.351 **Superficial FB, right thigh**
`7th`
S70.352 **Superficial FB, left thigh**
`7th`

S70.36 **Insect bite (nonvenomous) of thigh**
`6th`
S70.361 **Insect bite (nonvenomous), right thigh**
`7th`
S70.362 **Insect bite (nonvenomous), left thigh**
`7th`

S70.37 **Other superficial bite of thigh**
`6th`
Excludes1: open bite of thigh (S71.15)
S70.371 **Other superficial bite of right thigh**
`7th`
S70.372 **Other superficial bite of left thigh**
`7th`

> 7th characters for categories S70 & S71
> A—initial encounter
> D—subsequent encounter
> S—sequela

S71 OPEN WOUND OF HIP AND THIGH
`4th`

Code also any associated wound infection
Excludes1: open fracture of hip and thigh (S72.-)
traumatic amputation of hip and thigh (S78.-)
Excludes2: bite of venomous animal (T63.-)
open wound of ankle, foot and toes (S91.-)
open wound of knee and lower leg (S81.-)

S71.0 **Open wound of hip**
`5th`
S71.01 **Laceration without FB of hip**
`6th`
S71.011 **Laceration without FB, right hip**
`7th`
S71.012 **Laceration without FB, left hip**
`7th`

S71.02 **Laceration with FB of hip**
`6th`
S71.021 **Laceration with FB, right hip**
`7th`
S71.022 **Laceration with FB, left hip**
`7th`

S71.03 **Puncture wound without FB of hip**
`6th`
S71.031 **Puncture wound without FB, right hip**
`7th`
S71.032 **Puncture wound without FB, left hip**
`7th`

S71.04 **Puncture wound with FB of hip**
`6th`
S71.041 **Puncture wound with FB, right hip**
`7th`
S71.042 **Puncture wound with FB, left hip**
`7th`

S71.05 **Open bite of hip**
`6th`
Bite of hip NOS
Excludes1: superficial bite of hip (S70.26, S70.27)
S71.051 **Open bite, right hip**
`7th`
S71.052 **Open bite, left hip**
`7th`

S71.1 **Open wound of thigh**
`5th`
S71.11 **Laceration without FB of thigh**
`6th`
S71.111 **Laceration without FB, right thigh**
`7th`
S71.112 **Laceration without FB, left thigh**
`7th`

S71.12 **Laceration with FB of thigh**
`6th`
S71.121 **Laceration with FB, right thigh**
`7th`

S71.122 **Laceration with FB, left thigh**
`7th`

S71.13 **Puncture wound without FB of thigh**
`6th`
S71.131 **Puncture wound without FB, right thigh**
`7th`
S71.132 **Puncture wound without FB, left thigh**
`7th`

S71.14 **Puncture wound with FB of thigh**
`6th`
S71.141 **Puncture wound with FB, right thigh**
`7th`
S71.142 **Puncture wound with FB, left thigh**
`7th`

S71.15 **Open bite of thigh**
`6th`
Bite of thigh NOS
Excludes1: superficial bite of thigh (S70.37-)
S71.151 **Open bite, right thigh**
`7th`
S71.152 **Open bite, left thigh**
`7th`

S72 FRACTURE OF FEMUR
`4th`

Please see full *ICD-10-CM* manual for seventh characters applicable to open fracture types IIIA, IIIB, or IIIC.
Note: A fracture not indicated as displaced or nondisplaced should be coded to displaced
A fracture not indicated as open or closed should be coded to closed
The open fracture designations are based on the Gustilo open fracture classification
Excludes1: traumatic amputation of hip and thigh (S78.-)
Excludes2: fracture of lower leg and ankle (S82.-)
fracture of foot (S92.-)
periprosthetic fracture of prosthetic implant of hip (M97.0-)

S72.0 **Fracture of head and neck of femur**
`5th`
Excludes2: physeal fracture of upper end of femur (S79.0-)
S72.00 **Fracture of unspecified part of neck of femur**
`6th`
Fracture of hip NOS
Fracture of neck of femur NOS
S72.001 **Fracture of unspecified part of neck of right femur**
`7th`
S72.002 **Fracture of unspecified part of neck of left femur**
`7th`

S72.01 **Unspecified intracapsular fracture of femur**
`6th`
Subcapital fracture of femur
S72.011 **Unspecified intracapsular fracture of right femur**
`7th`
S72.012 **Unspecified intracapsular fracture of left femur**
`7th`

S72.02 **Fracture of epiphysis (separation) (upper) of femur**
`6th`
Transepiphyseal fracture of femur
Excludes1: capital femoral epiphyseal fracture (pediatric) of femur (S79.01-)
Salter-Harris Type I physeal fracture of upper end of femur (S79.01-)
S72.021 **Displaced fracture of epiphysis (separation) (upper) of right femur**
`7th`
S72.022 **Displaced fracture of epiphysis (separation) (upper) of left femur**
`7th`
S72.023 **Displaced fracture of epiphysis (separation) (upper) of unspecified femur**
`7th`
S72.024 **Nondisplaced fracture of epiphysis (separation) (upper) of right femur**
`7th`
S72.025 **Nondisplaced fracture of epiphysis (separation) (upper) of left femur**
`7th`

> 7th characters for category S72 except S72.47-
> A—initial encounter for closed fracture
> B—initial encounter for open fracture type I or II initial encounter for open fracture NOS
> D—subsequent encounter for closed fracture with routine healing
> E—subsequent encounter for open fracture type I or II with routine healing
> G—subsequent encounter for closed fracture with delayed healing
> H—subsequent encounter for open fracture type I or II with delayed healing
> K—subsequent encounter for closed fracture with nonunion
> M—subsequent encounter for open fracture type I or II with nonunion
> P—subsequent encounter for closed fracture with malunion
> Q—subsequent encounter for open fracture type I or II with malunion
> S—sequela

`4th` `5th` `6th` `7th`   Additional Character Required   ✔   3-character code   Unspecified laterality codes were excluded here.   • =New Code   ▲ =Revised Code   ▢ =Social determinants of health   *Excludes1*—Not coded here, do not use together   *Excludes2*—Not included here

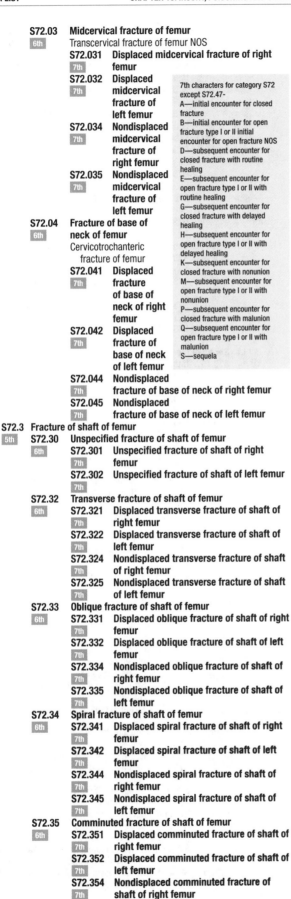

S72.03 **6th** **Midcervical fracture of femur**
Transcervical fracture of femur NOS

S72.031 **7th** Displaced midcervical fracture of right femur

S72.032 **7th** Displaced midcervical fracture of left femur

S72.034 **7th** Nondisplaced midcervical fracture of right femur

S72.035 **7th** Nondisplaced midcervical fracture of left femur

S72.04 **6th** **Fracture of base of neck of femur**
Cervicotrochanteric fracture of femur

S72.041 **7th** Displaced fracture of base of neck of right femur

S72.042 **7th** Displaced fracture of base of neck of left femur

S72.044 **7th** Nondisplaced fracture of base of neck of right femur

S72.045 **7th** Nondisplaced fracture of base of neck of left femur

S72.3 **5th** **Fracture of shaft of femur**

S72.30 **6th** **Unspecified fracture of shaft of femur**

S72.301 **7th** Unspecified fracture of shaft of right femur

S72.302 **7th** Unspecified fracture of shaft of left femur

S72.32 **6th** **Transverse fracture of shaft of femur**

S72.321 **7th** Displaced transverse fracture of shaft of right femur

S72.322 **7th** Displaced transverse fracture of shaft of left femur

S72.324 **7th** Nondisplaced transverse fracture of shaft of right femur

S72.325 **7th** Nondisplaced transverse fracture of shaft of left femur

S72.33 **6th** **Oblique fracture of shaft of femur**

S72.331 **7th** Displaced oblique fracture of shaft of right femur

S72.332 **7th** Displaced oblique fracture of shaft of left femur

S72.334 **7th** Nondisplaced oblique fracture of shaft of right femur

S72.335 **7th** Nondisplaced oblique fracture of shaft of left femur

S72.34 **6th** **Spiral fracture of shaft of femur**

S72.341 **7th** Displaced spiral fracture of shaft of right femur

S72.342 **7th** Displaced spiral fracture of shaft of left femur

S72.344 **7th** Nondisplaced spiral fracture of shaft of right femur

S72.345 **7th** Nondisplaced spiral fracture of shaft of left femur

S72.35 **6th** **Comminuted fracture of shaft of femur**

S72.351 **7th** Displaced comminuted fracture of shaft of right femur

S72.352 **7th** Displaced comminuted fracture of shaft of left femur

S72.354 **7th** Nondisplaced comminuted fracture of shaft of right femur

7th characters for category S72 except S72.47-
A—initial encounter for closed fracture
B—initial encounter for open fracture type I or II initial encounter for open fracture NOS
D—subsequent encounter for closed fracture with routine healing
E—subsequent encounter for open fracture type I or II with routine healing
G—subsequent encounter for closed fracture with delayed healing
H—subsequent encounter for open fracture type I or II with delayed healing
K—subsequent encounter for closed fracture with nonunion
M—subsequent encounter for open fracture type I or II with nonunion
P—subsequent encounter for closed fracture with malunion
Q—subsequent encounter for open fracture type I or II with malunion
S—sequela

S72.355 **7th** Nondisplaced comminuted fracture of shaft of left femur

S72.36 **6th** **Segmental fracture of shaft of femur**

S72.361 **7th** Displaced segmental fracture of shaft of right femur

S72.362 **7th** Displaced segmental fracture of shaft of left femur

S72.364 **7th** Nondisplaced segmental fracture of shaft of right femur

S72.365 **7th** Nondisplaced segmental fracture of shaft of left femur

S72.39 **6th** **Other fracture of shaft of femur**

S72.391 **7th** Other fracture of shaft of right femur

S72.392 **7th** Other fracture of shaft of left femur

S72.4 **5th** **Fracture of lower end of femur**
Fracture of distal end of femur
Excludes2: fracture of shaft of femur (S72.3-)
physeal fracture of lower end of femur (S79.1-)

S72.40 **6th** **Unspecified fracture of lower end of femur**

S72.401 **7th** Unspecified fracture of lower end of right femur

S72.402 **7th** Unspecified fracture of lower end of left femur

S72.41 **6th** **Unspecified condyle fracture of lower end of femur**
Condyle fracture of femur NOS

S72.411 **7th** Displaced unspecified condyle fracture of lower end of right femur

S72.412 **7th** Displaced unspecified condyle fracture of lower end of left femur

S72.414 **7th** Nondisplaced unspecified condyle fracture of lower end of right femur

S72.415 **7th** Nondisplaced unspecified condyle fracture of lower end of left femur

S72.42 **6th** **Fracture of lateral condyle of femur**

S72.421 **7th** Displaced fracture of lateral condyle of right femur

S72.422 **7th** Displaced fracture of lateral condyle of left femur

S72.424 **7th** Nondisplaced fracture of lateral condyle of right femur

S72.425 **7th** Nondisplaced fracture of lateral condyle of left femur

S72.43 **6th** **Fracture of medial condyle of femur**

S72.431 **7th** Displaced fracture of medial condyle of right femur

S72.432 **7th** Displaced fracture of medial condyle of left femur

S72.434 **7th** Nondisplaced fracture of medial condyle of right femur

S72.435 **7th** Nondisplaced fracture of medial condyle of left femur

S72.44 **6th** **Fracture of lower epiphysis (separation) of femur**
Excludes1: Salter-Harris Type I physeal fracture of lower end of femur (S79.11-)

S72.441 **7th** Displaced fracture of lower epiphysis (separation) of right femur

S72.442 **7th** Displaced fracture of lower epiphysis (separation) of left femur

S72.444 **7th** Nondisplaced fracture of lower epiphysis (separation) of right femur

S72.445 **7th** Nondisplaced fracture of lower epiphysis (separation) of left femur

S72.45 **6th** **Supracondylar fracture without intracondylar extension of lower end of femur**
Supracondylar fracture of lower end of femur NOS
Excludes1: supracondylar fracture with intracondylar extension of lower end of femur (S72.46-)

S72.451 **7th** Displaced supracondylar fracture without intracondylar extension of lower end of right femur

| 4th | 5th | 6th | 7th | Additional Character Required | ✓ | 3-character code | Unspecified laterality codes were excluded here. | • =New Code ▲ =Revised Code ▫ =Social determinants of health | *Excludes1*—Not coded here, do not use together *Excludes2*—Not included here |

CHAPTER 19. INJURY, POISONING AND CERTAIN OTHER CONSEQUENCES OF EXTERNAL CAUSES   (S72.452–S76.31)

S72.452 **Displaced supracondylar fracture without intracondylar extension of lower end of left femur** [7th]

S72.454 **Nondisplaced supracondylar fracture without intracondylar extension of lower end of right femur** [7th]

S72.455 **Nondisplaced supracondylar fracture without intracondylar extension of lower end of left femur** [7th]

S72.46 [6th] **Supracondylar fracture with intracondylar extension of lower end of femur**
Excludes1: supracondylar fracture without intracondylar extension of lower end of femur (S72.45-)

S72.461 **Displaced supracondylar fracture with intracondylar extension of lower end of right femur** [7th]

S72.462 **Displaced supracondylar fracture with intracondylar extension of lower end of left femur** [7th]

S72.464 **Nondisplaced supracondylar fracture with intracondylar extension of lower end of right femur** [7th]

S72.465 **Nondisplaced supracondylar fracture with intracondylar extension of lower end of left femur** [7th]

S72.47 [6th] **Torus fracture of lower end of femur**

S72.471 **Torus fracture of lower end of right femur** [7th]

S72.472 **Torus fracture of lower end of left femur** [7th]

S72.49 [6th] **Other fracture of lower end of femur**

S72.491 **Other fracture of lower end of right femur** [7th]

S72.492 **Other fracture of lower end of left femur** [7th]

S72.8 [5th] **Other fracture of femur**

S72.8X [6th] **Other fracture of femur**

S72.8X1 **Other fracture of right femur** [7th]

S72.8X2 **Other fracture of left femur** [7th]

S72.9 [5th] **Unspecified fracture of femur**
Fracture of thigh NOS
Fracture of upper leg NOS
Excludes1: fracture of hip NOS (S72.00-, S72.01-)

S72.91X **Unspecified fracture of right femur** [7th]

S72.92X **Unspecified fracture of left femur** [7th]

S73 [4th] DISLOCATION AND SPRAIN OF JOINT AND LIGAMENTS OF HIP

Includes: avulsion of joint or ligament of hip
laceration of cartilage, joint or ligament of hip
sprain of cartilage, joint or ligament of hip
traumatic hemarthrosis of joint or ligament of hip
traumatic rupture of joint or ligament of hip
traumatic subluxation of joint or ligament of hip
traumatic tear of joint or ligament of hip

7th characters for category S73
A—initial encounter
D—subsequent encounter
S—sequela

Code also any associated open wound
Excludes2: strain of muscle, fascia and tendon of hip and thigh (S76.-)

S73.0 [5th] **Subluxation and dislocation of hip**

S73.01 [6th] **Posterior subluxation and dislocation of hip**

S73.011 **Posterior subluxation of right hip** [7th]

S73.012 **Posterior subluxation of left hip** [7th]

S73.014 **Posterior dislocation of right hip** [7th]

S73.015 **Posterior dislocation of left hip** [7th]

S73.02 [6th] **Obturator subluxation and dislocation of hip**

S73.021 **Obturator subluxation of right hip** [7th]

S73.022 **Obturator subluxation of left hip** [7th]

S73.024 **Obturator dislocation of right hip** [7th]

S73.025 **Obturator dislocation of left hip** [7th]

S73.03 [6th] **Other anterior subluxation and dislocation of hip**

S73.031 **Other anterior subluxation of right hip** [7th]

S73.032 **Other anterior subluxation of left hip** [7th]

S73.034 **Other anterior dislocation of right hip** [7th]

S73.035 **Other anterior dislocation of left hip** [7th]

S73.04 [6th] **Central subluxation and dislocation of hip**

S73.041 **Central subluxation of right hip** [7th]

S73.042 **Central subluxation of left hip** [7th]

S73.044 **Central dislocation of right hip** [7th]

S73.045 **Central dislocation of left hip** [7th]

S73.1 [5th] **Sprain of hip**

S73.10 [6th] **Unspecified sprain of hip**

S73.101 **Unspecified sprain of right hip** [7th]

S73.102 **Unspecified sprain of left hip** [7th]

S73.11 [6th] **Iliofemoral ligament sprain of hip**

S73.111 **Iliofemoral ligament sprain of right hip** [7th]

S73.112 **Iliofemoral ligament sprain of left hip** [7th]

S73.12 [6th] **Ischiocapsular (ligament) sprain of hip**

S73.121 **Ischiocapsular ligament sprain of right hip** [7th]

S73.122 **Ischiocapsular ligament sprain of left hip** [7th]

S73.19 [6th] **Other sprain of hip**

S73.191 **Other sprain of right hip** [7th]

S73.192 **Other sprain of left hip** [7th]

S76 [4th] INJURY OF MUSCLE, FASCIA AND TENDON AT HIP AND THIGH LEVEL

Code also any associated open wound (S71.-)
Excludes2: injury of muscle, fascia and tendon at lower leg level (S86)
sprain of joint and ligament of hip (S73.1)

S76.0 [5th] **Injury of muscle, fascia and tendon of hip**

S76.01 [6th] **Strain of muscle, fascia and tendon of hip**

S76.011 **Strain of muscle, fascia and tendon of right hip** [7th]

S76.012 **Strain of muscle, fascia and tendon of left hip** [7th]

S76.1 [5th] **Injury of quadriceps muscle, fascia and tendon**
Injury of patellar ligament (tendon)

S76.11 [6th] **Strain of quadriceps muscle, fascia and tendon**

S76.111 **Strain of right quadriceps muscle, fascia and tendon** [7th]

S76.112 **Strain of left quadriceps muscle, fascia and tendon** [7th]

S76.21 [6th] **Strain of adductor muscle, fascia and tendon of thigh**

S76.211 **Strain of adductor muscle, fascia and tendon of right thigh** [7th]

S76.212 **Strain of adductor muscle, fascia and tendon of left thigh** [7th]

S76.31 [6th] **Strain of muscle, fascia and tendon of the posterior muscle group at thigh level**

[4th] [5th] [6th] [7th] Additional Character Required	✔ 3-character code	Unspecified laterality codes were excluded here.	• =New Code ▲ =Revised Code ▫ =Social determinants of health	*Excludes1*—Not coded here, do not use together *Excludes2*—Not included here

S76.311 `7th` Strain of muscle, fascia and tendon of the posterior muscle group at thigh level, right thigh

S76.312 `7th` Strain of muscle, fascia and tendon of the posterior muscle group at thigh level, left thigh

S76.91 `6th` Strain of unspecified muscles, fascia and tendons at thigh level

    S76.911 `7th` Strain of unspecified muscles, fascia and tendons at thigh level, right thigh

    S76.912 `7th` Strain of unspecified muscles, fascia and tendons at thigh level, left thigh

S79 `4th` OTHER AND UNSPECIFIED INJURIES OF HIP AND THIGH

Note: A fracture not indicated as open or closed should be coded to closed

S79.0 `5th` Physeal fracture of upper end of femur

Excludes1: apophyseal fracture of upper end of femur (S72.13-) nontraumatic slipped upper femoral epiphysis (M93.0-)

> 7th characters for subcategories
> S79.0–S79.1
> A—initial encounter for closed fracture
> D—subsequent encounter for fracture with routine healing
> G—subsequent encounter for fracture with delayed healing
> K—subsequent encounter for fracture with nonunion
> P—subsequent encounter for fracture with malunion
> S—sequela

S79.00 `6th` Unspecified physeal fracture of upper end of femur

    S79.001 `7th` Unspecified physeal fracture of upper end of right femur

    S79.002 `7th` Unspecified physeal fracture of upper end of left femur

S79.01 `6th` Salter-Harris Type I physeal fracture of upper end of femur

Acute on chronic slipped capital femoral epiphysis (traumatic)

Acute slipped capital femoral epiphysis (traumatic)

Capital femoral epiphyseal fracture

Excludes1: chronic slipped upper femoral epiphysis (nontraumatic) (M93.02-)

    S79.011 `7th` Salter-Harris Type I physeal fracture of upper end of right femur,

    S79.012 `7th` Salter-Harris Type I physeal fracture of upper end of left femur

S79.09 `6th` Other physeal fracture of upper end of femur

    S79.091 `7th` Other physeal fracture of upper end of right femur

    S79.092 `7th` Other physeal fracture of upper end of left femur

S79.1 `5th` Physeal fracture of lower end of femur

S79.10 `6th` Unspecified physeal fracture of lower end of femur

    S79.101 `7th` Unspecified physeal fracture of lower end of right femur

    S79.102 `7th` Unspecified physeal fracture of lower end of left femur

S79.11 `6th` Salter-Harris Type I physeal fracture of lower end of femur

    S79.111 `7th` Salter-Harris Type I physeal fracture of lower end of right femur

    S79.112 `7th` Salter-Harris Type I physeal fracture of lower end of left femur

S79.12 `6th` Salter-Harris Type II physeal fracture of lower end of femur

    S79.121 `7th` Salter-Harris Type II physeal fracture of lower end of right femur

    S79.122 `7th` Salter-Harris Type II physeal fracture of lower end of left femur

S79.13 `6th` Salter-Harris Type III physeal fracture of lower end of femur

    S79.131 `7th` Salter-Harris Type III physeal fracture of lower end of right femur

    S79.132 `7th` Salter-Harris Type III physeal fracture of lower end of left femur

S79.14 `6th` Salter-Harris Type IV physeal fracture of lower end of femur

S79.141 `7th` Salter-Harris Type IV physeal fracture of lower end of right femur

S79.142 `7th` Salter-Harris Type IV physeal fracture of lower end of left femur

S79.19 `6th` Other physeal fracture of lower end of femur

    S79.191 `7th` Other physeal fracture of lower end of right femur

    S79.192 `7th` Other physeal fracture of lower end of left femur

S79.8 `5th` Other specified injuries of hip and thigh

S79.81 `6th` Other specified injuries of hip

> 7th characters for subcategory
> S79.8
> A—initial encounter
> D—subsequent encounter
> S—sequela

    S79.811 `7th` Other specified injuries of right hip

    S79.812 `7th` Other specified injuries of left hip

S79.82 `6th` Other specified injuries of thigh

    S79.821 `7th` Other specified injuries of right thigh

    S79.822 `7th` Other specified injuries of left thigh

(S80–S89) INJURIES TO THE KNEE AND LOWER LEG

Excludes2: burns and corrosions (T20–T32)
frostbite (T33–T34)
injuries of ankle and foot, except fracture of ankle and malleolus (S90–S99)
insect bite or sting, venomous (T63.4)

S80 `4th` SUPERFICIAL INJURY OF KNEE AND LOWER LEG

Excludes2: superficial injury of ankle and foot (S90.-)

> 7th characters for category S80
> A—initial encounter
> D—subsequent encounter
> S—sequela

S80.0 `5th` Contusion of knee

S80.01X `7th` Contusion of right knee

S80.02X `7th` Contusion of left knee

S80.1 `5th` Contusion of lower leg

S80.11X `7th` Contusion of right lower leg

S80.12X `7th` Contusion of left lower leg

S80.2 `5th` Other superficial injuries of knee

S80.21 `6th` Abrasion of knee

    S80.211 `7th` Abrasion, right knee

    S80.212 `7th` Abrasion, left knee

S80.22 `6th` Blister (nonthermal) of knee

    S80.221 `7th` Blister (nonthermal), right knee

    S80.222 `7th` Blister (nonthermal), left knee

S80.24 `6th` External constriction of knee

    S80.241 `7th` External constriction, right knee

    S80.242 `7th` External constriction, left knee

S80.25 `6th` Superficial FB of knee

Splinter in the knee

    S80.251 `7th` Superficial FB, right knee

    S80.252 `7th` Superficial FB, left knee

S80.26 `6th` Insect bite (nonvenomous) of knee

    S80.261 `7th` Insect bite (nonvenomous), right knee

    S80.262 `7th` Insect bite (nonvenomous), left knee

S80.27 `6th` Other superficial bite of knee

Excludes1: open bite of knee (S81.05-)

`4th` `5th` `6th` `7th` Additional Character Required ✓ 3-character code

Unspecified laterality codes were excluded here.

● =New Code
▲ =Revised Code
⌑ =Social determinants of health

Excludes1—Not coded here, do not use together
Excludes2—Not included here

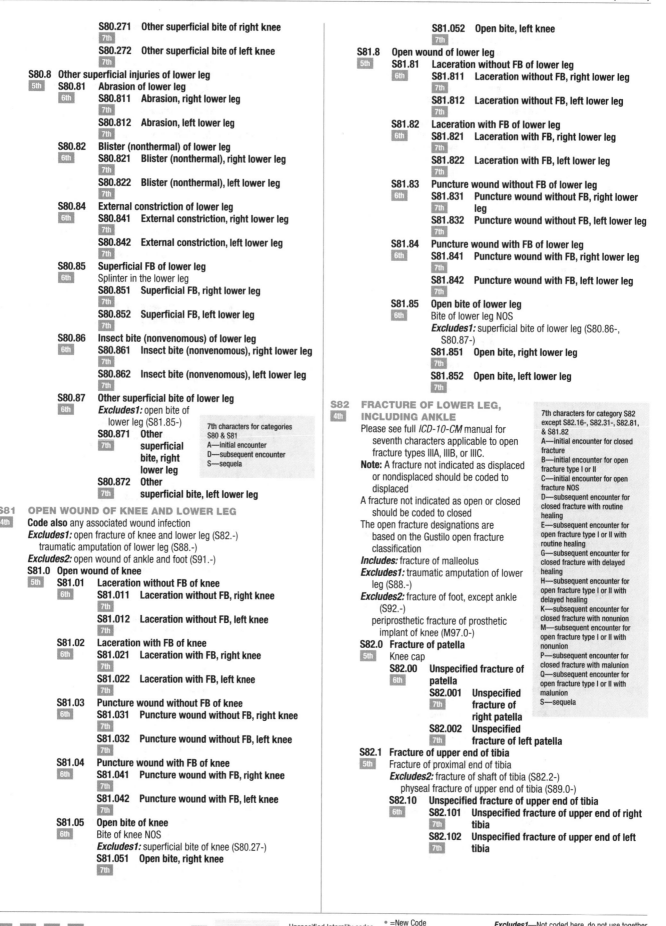

CHAPTER 19. INJURY, POISONING AND CERTAIN OTHER CONSEQUENCES OF EXTERNAL CAUSES   (S80.271–S82.102)

S80.271   Other superficial bite of right knee
7th

S80.272   Other superficial bite of left knee
7th

S80.8   **Other superficial injuries of lower leg**
5th

   S80.81   **Abrasion of lower leg**
    6th

     S80.811   Abrasion, right lower leg
     7th

     S80.812   Abrasion, left lower leg
     7th

   S80.82   **Blister (nonthermal) of lower leg**
    6th

     S80.821   Blister (nonthermal), right lower leg
     7th

     S80.822   Blister (nonthermal), left lower leg
     7th

   S80.84   **External constriction of lower leg**
    6th

     S80.841   External constriction, right lower leg
     7th

     S80.842   External constriction, left lower leg
     7th

   S80.85   **Superficial FB of lower leg**
    6th
    Splinter in the lower leg

     S80.851   Superficial FB, right lower leg
     7th

     S80.852   Superficial FB, left lower leg
     7th

   S80.86   **Insect bite (nonvenomous) of lower leg**
    6th

     S80.861   Insect bite (nonvenomous), right lower leg
     7th

     S80.862   Insect bite (nonvenomous), left lower leg
     7th

   S80.87   **Other superficial bite of lower leg**
    6th
    Excludes1: open bite of lower leg (S81.85-)

	7th characters for categories S80 & S81
	A—initial encounter
	D—subsequent encounter
	S—sequela

     S80.871   Other superficial bite, right lower leg
     7th

     S80.872   Other superficial bite, left lower leg
     7th

S81   **OPEN WOUND OF KNEE AND LOWER LEG**
4th
  Code also any associated wound infection
  Excludes1: open fracture of knee and lower leg (S82.-)
    traumatic amputation of lower leg (S88.-)
  Excludes2: open wound of ankle and foot (S91.-)

S81.0   **Open wound of knee**
5th

   S81.01   **Laceration without FB of knee**
    6th

     S81.011   Laceration without FB, right knee
     7th

     S81.012   Laceration without FB, left knee
     7th

   S81.02   **Laceration with FB of knee**
    6th

     S81.021   Laceration with FB, right knee
     7th

     S81.022   Laceration with FB, left knee
     7th

   S81.03   **Puncture wound without FB of knee**
    6th

     S81.031   Puncture wound without FB, right knee
     7th

     S81.032   Puncture wound without FB, left knee
     7th

   S81.04   **Puncture wound with FB of knee**
    6th

     S81.041   Puncture wound with FB, right knee
     7th

     S81.042   Puncture wound with FB, left knee
     7th

   S81.05   **Open bite of knee**
    6th
    Bite of knee NOS
    Excludes1: superficial bite of knee (S80.27-)

     S81.051   Open bite, right knee
     7th

     S81.052   Open bite, left knee
     7th

S81.8   **Open wound of lower leg**
5th

   S81.81   **Laceration without FB of lower leg**
    6th

     S81.811   Laceration without FB, right lower leg
     7th

     S81.812   Laceration without FB, left lower leg
     7th

   S81.82   **Laceration with FB of lower leg**
    6th

     S81.821   Laceration with FB, right lower leg
     7th

     S81.822   Laceration with FB, left lower leg
     7th

   S81.83   **Puncture wound without FB of lower leg**
    6th

     S81.831   Puncture wound without FB, right lower leg
     7th

     S81.832   Puncture wound without FB, left lower leg
     7th

   S81.84   **Puncture wound with FB of lower leg**
    6th

     S81.841   Puncture wound with FB, right lower leg
     7th

     S81.842   Puncture wound with FB, left lower leg
     7th

   S81.85   **Open bite of lower leg**
    6th
    Bite of lower leg NOS
    Excludes1: superficial bite of lower leg (S80.86-, S80.87-)

     S81.851   Open bite, right lower leg
     7th

     S81.852   Open bite, left lower leg
     7th

S82   **FRACTURE OF LOWER LEG, INCLUDING ANKLE**
4th
  Please see full *ICD-10-CM* manual for seventh characters applicable to open fracture types IIIA, IIIB, or IIIC.
  Note: A fracture not indicated as displaced or nondisplaced should be coded to displaced
  A fracture not indicated as open or closed should be coded to closed
  The open fracture designations are based on the Gustilo open fracture classification
  Includes: fracture of malleolus
  Excludes1: traumatic amputation of lower leg (S88.-)
  Excludes2: fracture of foot, except ankle (S92.-)
    periprosthetic fracture of prosthetic implant of knee (M97.0-)

S82.0   **Fracture of patella**
5th
  Knee cap

   S82.00   **Unspecified fracture of patella**
    6th

     S82.001   Unspecified fracture of right patella
     7th

     S82.002   Unspecified fracture of left patella
     7th

S82.1   **Fracture of upper end of tibia**
5th
  Fracture of proximal end of tibia
  Excludes2: fracture of shaft of tibia (S82.2-)
    physeal fracture of upper end of tibia (S89.0-)

   S82.10   **Unspecified fracture of upper end of tibia**
    6th

     S82.101   Unspecified fracture of upper end of right tibia
     7th

     S82.102   Unspecified fracture of upper end of left tibia
     7th

7th characters for category S82 except S82.16-, S82.31-, S82.81, & S81.82
A—initial encounter for closed fracture
B—initial encounter for open fracture type I or II
C—initial encounter for open fracture NOS
D—subsequent encounter for closed fracture with routine healing
E—subsequent encounter for open fracture type I or II with routine healing
G—subsequent encounter for closed fracture with delayed healing
H—subsequent encounter for open fracture type I or II with delayed healing
K—subsequent encounter for closed fracture with nonunion
M—subsequent encounter for open fracture type I or II with nonunion
P—subsequent encounter for closed fracture with malunion
Q—subsequent encounter for open fracture type I or II with malunion
S—sequela

4th   5th   6th   7th   Additional Character Required   ✓   3-character code   Unspecified laterality codes were excluded here.   • =New Code   ▲ =Revised Code   ▫ =Social determinants of health   *Excludes1*—Not coded here, do not use together   *Excludes2*—Not included here

372   PEDIATRIC ICD-10-CM 2021: A MANUAL FOR PROVIDER-BASED CODING

S82.16 **[6th]** Torus fracture of upper end of tibia

    S82.161 **[7th]** Torus fracture of upper end of right tibia

    S82.162 **[7th]** Torus fracture of upper end of left tibia

7th characters for subcategory S82.16
A—initial encounter for closed fracture
D—subsequent encounter for fracture with routine healing
G—subsequent encounter for fracture with delayed healing
K—subsequent encounter for fracture with nonunion
P—subsequent encounter for fracture with malunion
S—sequela

S82.19 **[6th]** Other fracture of upper end of tibia

    S82.191 **[7th]** Other fracture of upper end of right tibia

    S82.192 **[7th]** Other fracture of upper end of left tibia

7th characters for category S82 except S82.16-, S82.31-, S82.81, & S81.82
A—initial encounter for closed fracture
B—initial encounter for open fracture type I or II
C—initial encounter for open fracture NOS
D—subsequent encounter for closed fracture with routine healing
E—subsequent encounter for open fracture type I or II with routine healing
G—subsequent encounter for closed fracture with delayed healing
H—subsequent encounter for open fracture type I or II with delayed healing
K—subsequent encounter for closed fracture with nonunion
M—subsequent encounter for open fracture type I or II with nonunion
P—subsequent encounter for closed fracture with malunion
Q—subsequent encounter for open fracture type I or II with malunion
S—sequela

S82.2 **[5th]** Fracture of shaft of tibia

    S82.20 **[6th]** Unspecified fracture of shaft of tibia

        Fracture of tibia NOS

    S82.201 **[7th]** Unspecified fracture of shaft of right tibia

    S82.202 **[7th]** Unspecified fracture of shaft of left tibia

    S82.24 **[6th]** Spiral fracture of shaft of tibia

        Toddler fracture

    S82.241 **[7th]** Displaced spiral fracture of shaft of right tibia

    S82.242 **[7th]** Displaced spiral fracture of shaft of left tibia

    S82.244 **[7th]** Nondisplaced spiral fracture of shaft of right tibia

    S82.245 **[7th]** Nondisplaced spiral fracture of shaft of left tibia

S82.3 **[5th]** Fracture of lower end of tibia

    Excludes1: bimalleolar fracture of lower leg (S82.84-)
    fracture of medial malleolus alone (S82.5-)
    Maisonneuve's fracture (S82.86-)
    pilon fracture of distal tibia (S82.87-)
    trimalleolar fractures of lower leg (S82.85-)

    S82.30 **[6th]** Unspecified fracture of lower end of tibia

    S82.301 **[7th]** Unspecified fracture of lower end of right tibia

    S82.302 **[7th]** Unspecified fracture of lower end of left tibia

    S82.31 **[6th]** Torus fracture of lower end of tibia

    S82.311 **[7th]** Torus fracture of lower end of right tibia

    S82.312 **[7th]** Torus fracture of lower end of left tibia

7th characters for subcategory S82.31
A—initial encounter for closed fracture
D—subsequent encounter for fracture with routine healing
G—subsequent encounter for fracture with delayed healing
K—subsequent encounter for fracture with nonunion
P—subsequent encounter for fracture with malunion
S—sequela

    S82.39 **[6th]** Other fracture of lower end of tibia

    S82.391 **[7th]** Other fracture of lower end of right tibia

    S82.392 **[7th]** Other fracture of lower end of left tibia

S82.4 **[5th]** Fracture of shaft of fibula

    Excludes2: fracture of lateral malleolus alone (S82.6-)

    S82.40 **[6th]** Unspecified fracture of shaft of fibula

    S82.401 **[7th]** Unspecified fracture of shaft of right fibula

    S82.402 **[7th]** Unspecified fracture of shaft of left fibula

S82.5 **[5th]** Fracture of medial malleolus

    Excludes1: pilon fracture of distal tibia (S82.87-)
    Salter-Harris type III of lower end of tibia (S89.13-)
    Salter-Harris type IV of lower end of tibia (S89.14-)

    S82.51X **[7th]** Displaced fracture of medial malleolus of right tibia

    S82.52X **[7th]** Displaced fracture of medial malleolus of left tibia

    S82.54X **[7th]** Nondisplaced fracture of medial malleolus of right tibia

    S82.55X **[7th]** Nondisplaced fracture of medial malleolus of left tibia

S82.6 **[5th]** Fracture of lateral malleolus

    Excludes1: pilon fracture of distal tibia (S82.87-)

    S82.61X **[7th]** Displaced fracture of lateral malleolus of right fibula

    S82.62X **[7th]** Displaced fracture of lateral malleolus of left fibula

    S82.64X **[7th]** Nondisplaced fracture of lateral malleolus of right fibula

    S82.65X **[7th]** Nondisplaced fracture of lateral malleolus of left fibula

S82.8 **[5th]** Other fractures of lower leg

    S82.81 **[6th]** Torus fracture of upper end of fibula

    S82.811 **[7th]** Torus fracture of upper end of right fibula

    S82.812 **[7th]** Torus fracture of upper end of left fibula

7th character for subcategories S82.81- & S82.82-
A—initial encounter for closed fracture
D—subsequent encounter for fracture with routine healing
G—subsequent encounter for fracture with delayed healing
K—subsequent encounter for fracture with nonunion
P—subsequent encounter for fracture with malunion
S—sequela

    S82.82 **[6th]** Torus fracture of lower end of fibula

    S82.821 **[7th]** Torus fracture of lower end of right fibula

    S82.822 **[7th]** Torus fracture of lower end of left fibula

    S82.83 **[6th]** Other fracture of upper and lower end of fibula

    S82.831 **[7th]** Other fracture of upper and lower end of right fibula

    S82.832 **[7th]** Other fracture of upper and lower end of left fibula

    S82.84 **[6th]** Bimalleolar fracture of lower leg

    S82.841 **[7th]** Displaced bimalleolar fracture of right lower leg

    S82.842 **[7th]** Displaced bimalleolar fracture of left lower leg

    S82.844 **[7th]** Nondisplaced bimalleolar fracture of right lower leg

    S82.845 **[7th]** Nondisplaced bimalleolar fracture of left lower leg

    S82.85 **[6th]** Trimalleolar fracture of lower leg

    S82.851 **[7th]** Displaced trimalleolar fracture of right lower leg

    S82.852 **[7th]** Displaced trimalleolar fracture of left lower leg

    S82.854 **[7th]** Nondisplaced trimalleolar fracture of right lower leg

    S82.855 **[7th]** Nondisplaced trimalleolar fracture of left lower leg

    S82.86 **[6th]** Maisonneuve's fracture

    S82.861 **[7th]** Displaced Maisonneuve's fracture of right leg

---

[4th] **[5th]** **[6th]** **[7th]** Additional Character Required   ✔   3-character code

Unspecified laterality codes were excluded here.

• =New Code
▲ =Revised Code
▫ =Social determinants of health

Excludes1—Not coded here, do not use together
Excludes2—Not included here

S82.862 7th **Displaced Maisonneuve's fracture of left leg**

S82.864 7th **Nondisplaced Maisonneuve's fracture of right leg**

S82.865 7th **Nondisplaced Maisonneuve's fracture of left leg**

S82.87 6th **Pilon fracture of tibia**

S82.871 7th **Displaced pilon fracture of right tibia**

S82.872 7th **Displaced pilon fracture of left tibia**

S82.874 7th **Nondisplaced pilon fracture of right tibia**

S82.875 7th **Nondisplaced pilon fracture of left tibia**

S82.89 6th **Other fractures of lower leg**
Fracture of ankle NOS

S82.891 7th **Other fracture of right lower leg**

S82.892 7th **Other fracture of left lower leg**

S83 4th **DISLOCATION AND SPRAIN OF JOINTS AND LIGAMENTS OF KNEE**

Includes: avulsion of joint or ligament of knee
     laceration of cartilage, joint or ligament of knee
     sprain of cartilage, joint or ligament of knee
     traumatic hemarthrosis of joint or ligament of knee
     traumatic rupture of joint or ligament of knee
     traumatic subluxation of joint or ligament of knee
     traumatic tear of joint or ligament of knee

> 7th characters for category S83
> A—initial encounter
> D—subsequent encounter
> S—sequela

Code also any associated open wound

Excludes1: derangement of patella (M22.0–M22.3)
     injury of patellar ligament (tendon) (S76.1-)
     internal derangement of knee (M23.-)
     old dislocation of knee (M24.36)
     pathological dislocation of knee (M24.36)
     recurrent dislocation of knee (M22.0)

Excludes2: strain of muscle, fascia and tendon of lower leg (S86.-)

S83.0 5th **Subluxation and dislocation of patella**

S83.00 6th **Unspecified subluxation and dislocation of patella**

S83.001 7th **Unspecified subluxation of right patella**

S83.002 7th **Unspecified subluxation of left patella**

S83.004 7th **Unspecified dislocation of right patella**

S83.005 7th **Unspecified dislocation of left patella**

S83.01 6th **Lateral subluxation and dislocation of patella**

S83.011 7th **Lateral subluxation of right patella**

S83.012 7th **Lateral subluxation of left patella**

S83.014 7th **Lateral dislocation of right patella**

S83.015 7th **Lateral dislocation of left patella**

S83.09 6th **Other subluxation and dislocation of patella**

S83.091 7th **Other subluxation of right patella**

S83.092 7th **Other subluxation of left patella**

S83.094 7th **Other dislocation of right patella**

S83.095 7th **Other dislocation of left patella**

S83.1 5th **Subluxation and dislocation of knee**
Excludes2: instability of knee prosthesis (T84.022, T84.023)

S83.10 6th **Unspecified subluxation and dislocation of knee**

S83.101 7th **Unspecified subluxation of right knee**

S83.102 7th **Unspecified subluxation of left knee**

S83.104 7th **Unspecified dislocation of right knee**

S83.105 7th **Unspecified dislocation of left knee**

S83.11 6th **Anterior subluxation and dislocation of proximal end of tibia**
Posterior subluxation and dislocation of distal end of femur

S83.111 7th **Anterior subluxation of proximal end of tibia, right knee**

S83.112 7th **Anterior subluxation of proximal end of tibia, left knee**

S83.114 7th **Anterior dislocation of proximal end of tibia, right knee**

S83.115 7th **Anterior dislocation of proximal end of tibia, left knee**

S83.12 6th **Posterior subluxation and dislocation of proximal end of tibia**
Anterior dislocation of distal end of femur

S83.121 7th **Posterior subluxation of proximal end of tibia, right knee**

S83.122 7th **Posterior subluxation of proximal end of tibia, left knee**

S83.124 7th **Posterior dislocation of proximal end of tibia, right knee**

S83.125 7th **Posterior dislocation of proximal end of tibia, left knee**

S83.13 6th **Medial subluxation and dislocation of proximal end of tibia**

S83.131 7th **Medial subluxation of proximal end of tibia, right knee**

S83.132 7th **Medial subluxation of proximal end of tibia, left knee**

S83.134 7th **Medial dislocation of proximal end of tibia, right knee**

S83.135 7th **Medial dislocation of proximal end of tibia, left knee**

S83.14 6th **Lateral subluxation and dislocation of proximal end of tibia**

S83.141 7th **Lateral subluxation of proximal end of tibia, right knee**

S83.142 7th **Lateral subluxation of proximal end of tibia, left knee**

S83.144 7th **Lateral dislocation of proximal end of tibia, right knee**

S83.145 7th **Lateral dislocation of proximal end of tibia, left knee**

S83.19 6th **Other subluxation and dislocation of knee**

S83.191 7th **Other subluxation of right knee**

S83.192 7th **Other subluxation of left knee**

S83.194 7th **Other dislocation of right knee**

S83.195 7th **Other dislocation of left knee**

S83.4 **Sprain of collateral ligament of knee**

S83.40 5th **Sprain of unspecified collateral ligament of knee**

S83.401 6th 7th **Sprain of unspecified collateral ligament of right knee**

S83.402 7th **Sprain of unspecified collateral ligament of left knee**

S83.41 6th **Sprain of medial collateral ligament of knee**
Sprain of tibial collateral ligament

S83.411 7th **Sprain of medial collateral ligament of right knee**

S83.412 7th **Sprain of medial collateral ligament of left knee**

S83.42 6th **Sprain of lateral collateral ligament of knee**
Sprain of fibular collateral ligament

4th   5th   6th   7th   Additional Character Required   ✔   3-character code   Unspecified laterality codes were excluded here.

• =New Code
▲ =Revised Code
▫ =Social determinants of health

Excludes1—Not coded here, do not use together
Excludes2—Not included here

S83.421 **7th** Sprain of lateral collateral ligament of right knee

S83.422 **7th** Sprain of lateral collateral ligament of left knee

S83.5 **5th** Sprain of cruciate ligament of knee

S83.50 **6th** Sprain of unspecified cruciate ligament of knee

S83.501 **7th** Sprain of unspecified cruciate ligament of right knee

S83.502 **7th** Sprain of unspecified cruciate ligament of left knee

S83.51 **6th** Sprain of anterior cruciate ligament of knee

S83.511 **7th** Sprain of anterior cruciate ligament of right knee

S83.512 **7th** Sprain of anterior cruciate ligament of left knee

S83.52 **6th** Sprain of posterior cruciate ligament of knee

S83.521 **7th** Sprain of posterior cruciate ligament of right knee

S83.522 **7th** Sprain of posterior cruciate ligament of left knee

S83.6 **5th** Sprain of the superior tibiofibular joint and ligament

S83.60X **7th** Sprain of the superior tibiofibular joint and ligament, unspecified knee

S83.61X **7th** Sprain of the superior tibiofibular joint and ligament, right knee

S83.62X **7th** Sprain of the superior tibiofibular joint and ligament, left knee

S83.8 **5th** Sprain of other specified parts of knee

S83.8X **6th** Sprain of other specified parts of knee

S83.8X1 **7th** Sprain of other specified parts of right knee

S83.8X2 **7th** Sprain of other specified parts of left knee

S83.9 **5th** Sprain of unspecified site of knee

S83.91X **7th** Sprain of unspecified site of right knee

S83.92X **7th** Sprain of unspecified site of left knee

> **7th characters for categories S83 & S86**
> A—initial encounter
> D—subsequent encounter
> S—sequela

S86 **4th** **INJURY OF MUSCLE, FASCIA AND TENDON AT LOWER LEG LEVEL**

Code also any associated open wound (S81.-)

Excludes2: injury of muscle, fascia and tendon at ankle (S96.-)

injury of patellar ligament (tendon) (S76.1-)

sprain of joints and ligaments of knee (S83.-)

S86.0 **5th** Injury of Achilles tendon

S86.00 **6th** Unspecified injury of Achilles tendon

S86.001 **7th** Unspecified injury of right Achilles tendon

S86.002 **7th** Unspecified injury of left Achilles tendon

S86.01 **6th** Strain of Achilles tendon

S86.011 **7th** Strain of right Achilles tendon

S86.012 **7th** Strain of left Achilles tendon

S86.02 **6th** Laceration of Achilles tendon

S86.021 **7th** Laceration of right Achilles tendon

S86.022 **7th** Laceration of left Achilles tendon

S86.09 **6th** Other specified injury of Achilles tendon

S86.091 **7th** Other specified injury of right Achilles tendon

S86.092 **7th** Other specified injury of left Achilles tendon

S86.1 **5th** Injury of other muscle(s) and tendon(s) of posterior muscle group at lower leg level

S86.11 **6th** Strain of other muscle(s) and tendon(s) of posterior muscle group at lower leg level

S86.111 **7th** Strain of other muscle(s) and tendon(s) of posterior muscle group at lower leg level, right leg

S86.112 **7th** Strain of other muscle(s) and tendon(s) of posterior muscle group at lower leg level, left leg

S86.2 **5th** Injury of muscle(s) and tendon(s) of anterior muscle group at lower leg level

S86.21 **6th** Strain of muscle(s) and tendon(s) of anterior muscle group at lower leg level

S86.211 **7th** Strain of muscle(s) and tendon(s) of anterior muscle group at lower leg level, right leg

S86.212 **7th** Strain of muscle(s) and tendon(s) of anterior muscle group at lower leg level, left leg

S86.3 **5th** Injury of muscle(s) and tendon(s) of peroneal muscle group at lower leg level

S86.31 **6th** Strain of muscle(s) and tendon(s) of peroneal muscle group at lower leg level

S86.311 **7th** Strain of muscle(s) and tendon(s) of peroneal muscle group at lower leg level, right leg

S86.312 **7th** Strain of muscle(s) and tendon(s) of peroneal muscle group at lower leg level, left leg

S86.32 **6th** Laceration of muscle(s) and tendon(s) of peroneal muscle group at lower leg level

S86.321 **7th** Laceration of mus-cle(s) and tendon(s) of peroneal muscle group at lower leg level, right leg

S86.322 **7th** Laceration of muscle(s) and tendon(s) of peroneal muscle group at lower leg level, left leg

S86.39 **6th** Other injury of muscle(s) and tendon(s) of peroneal muscle group at lower leg level

S86.391 **7th** Other injury of muscle(s) and tendon(s) of peroneal muscle group at lower leg level, right leg

S86.392 **7th** Other injury of muscle(s) and tendon(s) of peroneal muscle group at lower leg level, left leg

S86.8 **5th** Injury of other muscles and tendons at lower leg level

S86.81 **6th** Strain of other muscles and tendons at lower leg level

S86.811 **7th** Strain of other muscle(s) and tendon(s) at lower leg level, right leg

S86.812 **7th** Strain of other muscle(s) and tendon(s) at lower leg level, left leg

S86.82 **6th** Laceration of other muscles and tendons at lower leg level

S86.821 **7th** Laceration of other muscle(s) and tendon(s) at lower leg level, right leg

S86.822 **7th** Laceration of other muscle(s) and tendon(s) at lower leg level, left leg

S86.89 **6th** Other injury of other muscles and tendons at lower leg level

S86.891 **7th** Other injury of other muscle(s) and tendon(s) at lower leg level, right leg

S86.892 **7th** Other injury of other muscle(s) and tendon(s) at lower leg level, left leg

S86.9 **5th** Injury of unspecified muscle and tendon at lower leg level

S86.91 **6th** Strain of unspecified muscle and tendon at lower leg level

S86.911 **7th** Strain of unspecified muscle(s) and tendon(s) at lower leg level, right leg

S86.912 **7th** Strain of unspecified muscle(s) and tendon(s) at lower leg level, left leg

---

4th **5th** **6th** **7th** Additional Character Required   ✔   3-character code   Unspecified laterality codes were excluded here.

• =New Code
▲ =Revised Code
▫ =Social determinants of health

Excludes1—Not coded here, do not use together
Excludes2—Not included here

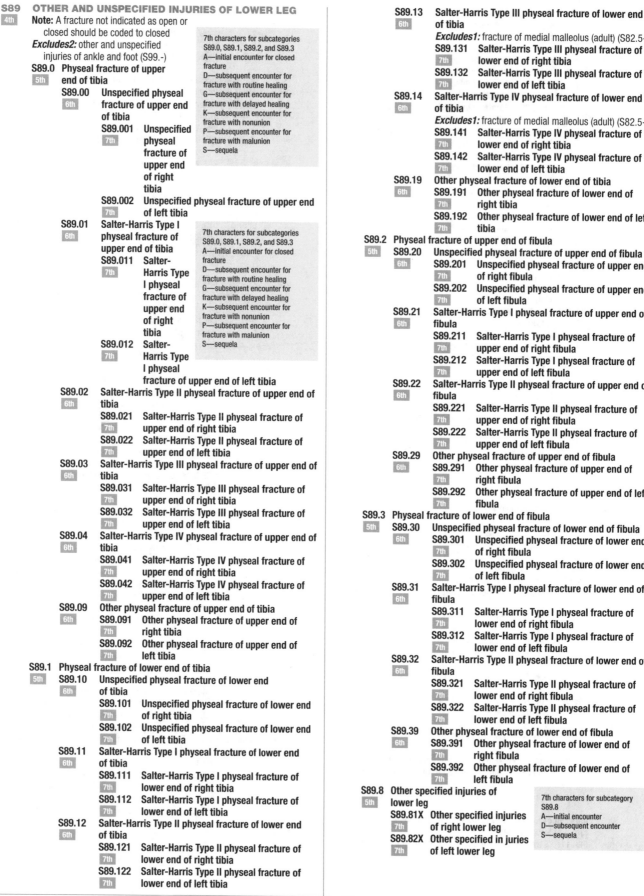

CHAPTER 19. INJURY, POISONING AND CERTAIN OTHER CONSEQUENCES OF EXTERNAL CAUSES   (S89–S89.82X)

S89 **OTHER AND UNSPECIFIED INJURIES OF LOWER LEG**
[4th]
Note: A fracture not indicated as open or closed should be coded to closed
Excludes2: other and unspecified injuries of ankle and foot (S99.-)

S89.0 **Physeal fracture of upper end of tibia**
[5th]

S89.00 Unspecified physeal fracture of upper end of tibia
[6th]

S89.001 Unspecified physeal fracture of upper end of right tibia
[7th]

S89.002 Unspecified physeal fracture of upper end of left tibia
[7th]

7th characters for subcategories S89.0, S89.1, S89.2, and S89.3
A—initial encounter for closed fracture
D—subsequent encounter for fracture with routine healing
G—subsequent encounter for fracture with delayed healing
K—subsequent encounter for fracture with nonunion
P—subsequent encounter for fracture with malunion
S—sequela

S89.01 Salter-Harris Type I physeal fracture of upper end of tibia
[6th]

S89.011 Salter-Harris Type I physeal fracture of upper end of right tibia
[7th]

7th characters for subcategories S89.0, S89.1, S89.2, and S89.3
A—initial encounter for closed fracture
D—subsequent encounter for fracture with routine healing
G—subsequent encounter for fracture with delayed healing
K—subsequent encounter for fracture with nonunion
P—subsequent encounter for fracture with malunion
S—sequela

S89.012 Salter-Harris Type I physeal fracture of upper end of left tibia
[7th]

S89.02 Salter-Harris Type II physeal fracture of upper end of tibia
[6th]

S89.021 Salter-Harris Type II physeal fracture of upper end of right tibia
[7th]

S89.022 Salter-Harris Type II physeal fracture of upper end of left tibia
[7th]

S89.03 Salter-Harris Type III physeal fracture of upper end of tibia
[6th]

S89.031 Salter-Harris Type III physeal fracture of upper end of right tibia
[7th]

S89.032 Salter-Harris Type III physeal fracture of upper end of left tibia
[7th]

S89.04 Salter-Harris Type IV physeal fracture of upper end of tibia
[6th]

S89.041 Salter-Harris Type IV physeal fracture of upper end of right tibia
[7th]

S89.042 Salter-Harris Type IV physeal fracture of upper end of left tibia
[7th]

S89.09 Other physeal fracture of upper end of tibia
[6th]

S89.091 Other physeal fracture of upper end of right tibia
[7th]

S89.092 Other physeal fracture of upper end of left tibia
[7th]

S89.1 **Physeal fracture of lower end of tibia**
[5th]

S89.10 Unspecified physeal fracture of lower end of tibia
[6th]

S89.101 Unspecified physeal fracture of lower end of right tibia
[7th]

S89.102 Unspecified physeal fracture of lower end of left tibia
[7th]

S89.11 Salter-Harris Type I physeal fracture of lower end of tibia
[6th]

S89.111 Salter-Harris Type I physeal fracture of lower end of right tibia
[7th]

S89.112 Salter-Harris Type I physeal fracture of lower end of left tibia
[7th]

S89.12 Salter-Harris Type II physeal fracture of lower end of tibia
[6th]

S89.121 Salter-Harris Type II physeal fracture of lower end of right tibia
[7th]

S89.122 Salter-Harris Type II physeal fracture of lower end of left tibia
[7th]

S89.13 Salter-Harris Type III physeal fracture of lower end of tibia
[6th]

Excludes1: fracture of medial malleolus (adult) (S82.5-)

S89.131 Salter-Harris Type III physeal fracture of lower end of right tibia
[7th]

S89.132 Salter-Harris Type III physeal fracture of lower end of left tibia
[7th]

S89.14 Salter-Harris Type IV physeal fracture of lower end of tibia
[6th]

Excludes1: fracture of medial malleolus (adult) (S82.5-)

S89.141 Salter-Harris Type IV physeal fracture of lower end of right tibia
[7th]

S89.142 Salter-Harris Type IV physeal fracture of lower end of left tibia
[7th]

S89.19 Other physeal fracture of lower end of tibia
[6th]

S89.191 Other physeal fracture of lower end of right tibia
[7th]

S89.192 Other physeal fracture of lower end of left tibia
[7th]

S89.2 **Physeal fracture of upper end of fibula**
[5th]

S89.20 Unspecified physeal fracture of upper end of fibula
[6th]

S89.201 Unspecified physeal fracture of upper end of right fibula
[7th]

S89.202 Unspecified physeal fracture of upper end of left fibula
[7th]

S89.21 Salter-Harris Type I physeal fracture of upper end of fibula
[6th]

S89.211 Salter-Harris Type I physeal fracture of upper end of right fibula
[7th]

S89.212 Salter-Harris Type I physeal fracture of upper end of left fibula
[7th]

S89.22 Salter-Harris Type II physeal fracture of upper end of fibula
[6th]

S89.221 Salter-Harris Type II physeal fracture of upper end of right fibula
[7th]

S89.222 Salter-Harris Type II physeal fracture of upper end of left fibula
[7th]

S89.29 Other physeal fracture of upper end of fibula
[6th]

S89.291 Other physeal fracture of upper end of right fibula
[7th]

S89.292 Other physeal fracture of upper end of left fibula
[7th]

S89.3 **Physeal fracture of lower end of fibula**
[5th]

S89.30 Unspecified physeal fracture of lower end of fibula
[6th]

S89.301 Unspecified physeal fracture of lower end of right fibula
[7th]

S89.302 Unspecified physeal fracture of lower end of left fibula
[7th]

S89.31 Salter-Harris Type I physeal fracture of lower end of fibula
[6th]

S89.311 Salter-Harris Type I physeal fracture of lower end of right fibula
[7th]

S89.312 Salter-Harris Type I physeal fracture of lower end of left fibula
[7th]

S89.32 Salter-Harris Type II physeal fracture of lower end of fibula
[6th]

S89.321 Salter-Harris Type II physeal fracture of lower end of right fibula
[7th]

S89.322 Salter-Harris Type II physeal fracture of lower end of left fibula
[7th]

S89.39 Other physeal fracture of lower end of fibula
[6th]

S89.391 Other physeal fracture of lower end of right fibula
[7th]

S89.392 Other physeal fracture of lower end of left fibula
[7th]

S89.8 **Other specified injuries of lower leg**
[5th]

S89.81X Other specified injuries of right lower leg
[7th]

S89.82X Other specified injuries of left lower leg
[7th]

7th characters for subcategory S89.8
A—initial encounter
D—subsequent encounter
S—sequela

[4th] [5th] [6th] [7th] Additional Character Required   ✔ 3-character code   Unspecified laterality codes were excluded here.

* =New Code
▲ =Revised Code
⌂ =Social determinants of health

Excludes1—Not coded here, do not use together
Excludes2—Not included here

(S90–S99) INJURIES TO THE ANKLE AND FOOT

Excludes2: burns and corrosions (T20–T32)
    fracture of ankle and malleolus (S82.-)
    frostbite (T33–T34)
    insect bite or sting, venomous (T63.4)

> 7th characters for category S90
> A—initial encounter
> D—subsequent encounter
> S—sequela

S90 `4th` **SUPERFICIAL INJURY OF ANKLE, FOOT AND TOES**

S90.0 `5th` **Contusion of ankle**
    S90.01X `7th` **Contusion of right ankle**
    S90.02X `7th` **Contusion of left ankle**

S90.1 `5th` **Contusion of toe without damage to nail**
    S90.11 `6th` **Contusion of great toe without damage to nail**
       S90.111 `7th` **Contusion of right great toe without damage to nail**
       S90.112 `7th` **Contusion of left great toe without damage to nail**

> 7th characters for category S90
> A—initial encounter
> D—subsequent encounter
> S—sequela

    S90.12 `6th` **Contusion of lesser toe without damage to nail**
       S90.121 `7th` **Contusion of right lesser toe(s) without damage to nail**
       S90.122 `7th` **Contusion of left lesser toe(s) without damage to nail**

S90.2 `5th` **Contusion of toe with damage to nail**
    S90.21 `6th` **Contusion of great toe with damage to nail**
       S90.211 `7th` **Contusion of right great toe with damage to nail**
       S90.212 `7th` **Contusion of left great toe with damage to nail**
    S90.22 `6th` **Contusion of lesser toe with damage to nail**
       S90.221 `7th` **Contusion of right lesser toe(s) with damage to nail**
       S90.222 `7th` **Contusion of left lesser toe(s) with damage to nail**

S90.3 `5th` **Contusion of foot**
    Excludes2: contusion of toes (S90.1-, S90.2-)
    S90.31X `7th` **Contusion of right foot**
    S90.32X `7th` **Contusion of left foot**

S90.4 `5th` **Other superficial injuries of toe**
    S90.41 `6th` **Abrasion of toe**
       S90.411 `7th` **Abrasion, right great toe**
       S90.412 `7th` **Abrasion, left great toe**
       S90.414 `7th` **Abrasion, right lesser toe(s)**
       S90.415 `7th` **Abrasion, left lesser toe(s)**
    S90.42 `6th` **Blister (nonthermal) of toe**
       S90.421 `7th` **Blister (nonthermal), right great toe**
       S90.422 `7th` **Blister (nonthermal), left great toe**
       S90.424 `7th` **Blister (nonthermal), right lesser toe(s)**
       S90.425 `7th` **Blister (nonthermal), left lesser toe(s)**
    S90.44 `6th` **External constriction of toe**
       TIP: See category W49 for external cause code (eg, W49.01-, hair causing external constriction).
       Hair tourniquet syndrome of toe
       S90.441 `7th` **External constriction, right great toe**
       S90.442 `7th` **External constriction, left great toe**

       S90.444 `7th` **External constriction, right lesser toe(s)**
       S90.445 `7th` **External constriction, left lesser toe(s)**
    S90.45 `6th` **Superficial FB of toe**
       Splinter in the toe
       S90.451 `7th` **Superficial FB, right great toe**
       S90.452 `7th` **Superficial FB, left great toe**
       S90.454 `7th` **Superficial FB, right lesser toe(s)**
       S90.455 `7th` **Superficial FB, left lesser toe(s)**
    S90.46 `6th` **Insect bite (nonvenomous) of toe**
       S90.461 `7th` **Insect bite (nonvenomous), right great toe**
       S90.462 `7th` **Insect bite (nonvenomous), left great toe**
       S90.464 `7th` **Insect bite (nonvenomous), right lesser toe(s)**
       S90.465 `7th` **Insect bite (nonvenomous), left lesser toe(s)**
    S90.47 `6th` **Other superficial bite of toe**
       Excludes1: open bite of toe (S91.15-, S91.25-)
       S90.471 `7th` **Other superficial bite of right great toe**
       S90.472 `7th` **Other superficial bite of left great toe**
       S90.474 `7th` **Other superficial bite of right lesser toe(s)**
       S90.475 `7th` **Other superficial bite of left lesser toe(s)**

S90.5 `5th` **Other superficial injuries of ankle**
    S90.51 `6th` **Abrasion of ankle**
       S90.511 `7th` **Abrasion, right ankle**
       S90.512 `7th` **Abrasion, left ankle**
    S90.52 `6th` **Blister (nonthermal) of ankle**
       S90.521 `7th` **Blister (nonthermal), right ankle**
       S90.522 `7th` **Blister (nonthermal), left ankle**
    S90.54 `6th` **External constriction of ankle**
       S90.541 `7th` **External constriction, right ankle**
       S90.542 `7th` **External constriction, left ankle**
    S90.55 `6th` **Superficial FB of ankle**
       Splinter in the ankle
       S90.551 `7th` **Superficial FB, right ankle**
       S90.552 `7th` **Superficial FB, left ankle**
    S90.56 `6th` **Insect bite (nonvenomous) of ankle**
       S90.561 `7th` **Insect bite (nonvenomous), right ankle**
       S90.562 `7th` **Insect bite (nonvenomous), left ankle**
    S90.57 `6th` **Other superficial bite of ankle**
       Excludes1: open bite of ankle (S91.05-)
       S90.571 `7th` **Other superficial bite of ankle, right ankle**
       S90.572 `7th` **Other superficial bite of ankle, left ankle**

S90.8 `5th` **Other superficial injuries of foot**
    S90.81 `6th` **Abrasion of foot**
       S90.811 `7th` **Abrasion, right foot**
       S90.812 `7th` **Abrasion, left foot**
    S90.82 `6th` **Blister (nonthermal) of foot**

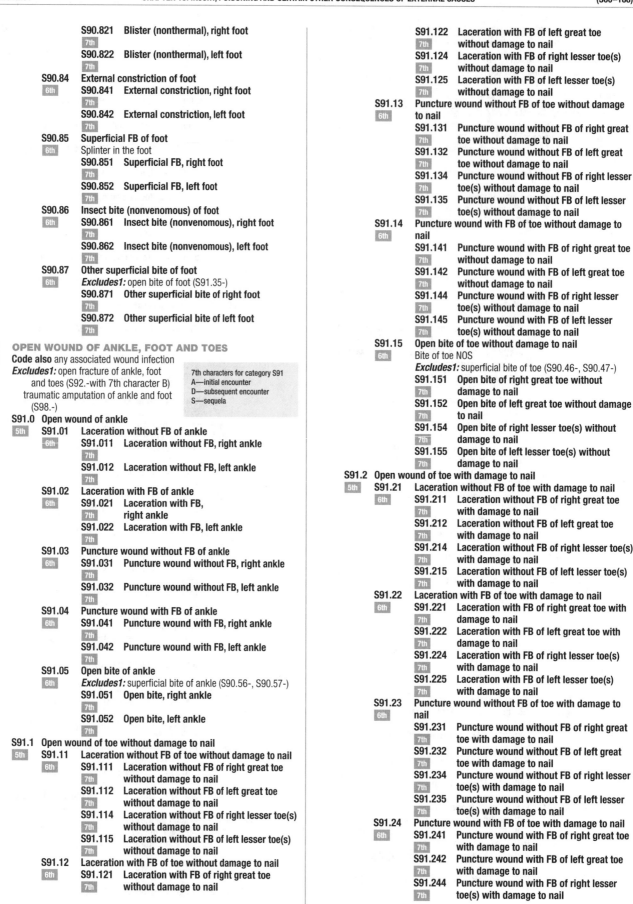

CHAPTER 19. INJURY, POISONING AND CERTAIN OTHER CONSEQUENCES OF EXTERNAL CAUSES   (S90.821–S91.244)

S90.821 **Blister (nonthermal), right foot**
7th

S90.822 **Blister (nonthermal), left foot**
7th

S90.84 **External constriction of foot**
6th
  S90.841 **External constriction, right foot**
  7th

  S90.842 **External constriction, left foot**
  7th

S90.85 **Superficial FB of foot**
6th
Splinter in the foot
  S90.851 **Superficial FB, right foot**
  7th

  S90.852 **Superficial FB, left foot**
  7th

S90.86 **Insect bite (nonvenomous) of foot**
6th
  S90.861 **Insect bite (nonvenomous), right foot**
  7th

  S90.862 **Insect bite (nonvenomous), left foot**
  7th

S90.87 **Other superficial bite of foot**
6th
Excludes1: open bite of foot (S91.35-)
  S90.871 **Other superficial bite of right foot**
  7th

  S90.872 **Other superficial bite of left foot**
  7th

S91 **OPEN WOUND OF ANKLE, FOOT AND TOES**
4th
Code also any associated wound infection
Excludes1: open fracture of ankle, foot
and toes (S92.-with 7th character B)
traumatic amputation of ankle and foot
(S98.-)

7th characters for category S91
A—initial encounter
D—subsequent encounter
S—sequela

S91.0 **Open wound of ankle**
5th
  S91.01 **Laceration without FB of ankle**
  6th
    S91.011 **Laceration without FB, right ankle**
    7th

    S91.012 **Laceration without FB, left ankle**
    7th

  S91.02 **Laceration with FB of ankle**
  6th
    S91.021 **Laceration with FB, right ankle**
    7th
    S91.022 **Laceration with FB, left ankle**
    7th

  S91.03 **Puncture wound without FB of ankle**
  6th
    S91.031 **Puncture wound without FB, right ankle**
    7th

    S91.032 **Puncture wound without FB, left ankle**
    7th

  S91.04 **Puncture wound with FB of ankle**
  6th
    S91.041 **Puncture wound with FB, right ankle**
    7th

    S91.042 **Puncture wound with FB, left ankle**
    7th

  S91.05 **Open bite of ankle**
  6th
  Excludes1: superficial bite of ankle (S90.56-, S90.57-)
    S91.051 **Open bite, right ankle**
    7th

    S91.052 **Open bite, left ankle**
    7th

S91.1 **Open wound of toe without damage to nail**
5th
  S91.11 **Laceration without FB of toe without damage to nail**
  6th
    S91.111 **Laceration without FB of right great toe without damage to nail**
    7th
    S91.112 **Laceration without FB of left great toe without damage to nail**
    7th
    S91.114 **Laceration without FB of right lesser toe(s) without damage to nail**
    7th
    S91.115 **Laceration without FB of left lesser toe(s) without damage to nail**
    7th
  S91.12 **Laceration with FB of toe without damage to nail**
  6th
    S91.121 **Laceration with FB of right great toe without damage to nail**
    7th

    S91.122 **Laceration with FB of left great toe without damage to nail**
    7th
    S91.124 **Laceration with FB of right lesser toe(s) without damage to nail**
    7th
    S91.125 **Laceration with FB of left lesser toe(s) without damage to nail**
    7th

  S91.13 **Puncture wound without FB of toe without damage to nail**
  6th
    S91.131 **Puncture wound without FB of right great toe without damage to nail**
    7th
    S91.132 **Puncture wound without FB of left great toe without damage to nail**
    7th
    S91.134 **Puncture wound without FB of right lesser toe(s) without damage to nail**
    7th
    S91.135 **Puncture wound without FB of left lesser toe(s) without damage to nail**
    7th

  S91.14 **Puncture wound with FB of toe without damage to nail**
  6th
    S91.141 **Puncture wound with FB of right great toe without damage to nail**
    7th
    S91.142 **Puncture wound with FB of left great toe without damage to nail**
    7th
    S91.144 **Puncture wound with FB of right lesser toe(s) without damage to nail**
    7th
    S91.145 **Puncture wound with FB of left lesser toe(s) without damage to nail**
    7th

  S91.15 **Open bite of toe without damage to nail**
  6th
  Bite of toe NOS
  Excludes1: superficial bite of toe (S90.46-, S90.47-)
    S91.151 **Open bite of right great toe without damage to nail**
    7th
    S91.152 **Open bite of left great toe without damage to nail**
    7th
    S91.154 **Open bite of right lesser toe(s) without damage to nail**
    7th
    S91.155 **Open bite of left lesser toe(s) without damage to nail**
    7th

S91.2 **Open wound of toe with damage to nail**
5th
  S91.21 **Laceration without FB of toe with damage to nail**
  6th
    S91.211 **Laceration without FB of right great toe with damage to nail**
    7th
    S91.212 **Laceration without FB of left great toe with damage to nail**
    7th
    S91.214 **Laceration without FB of right lesser toe(s) with damage to nail**
    7th
    S91.215 **Laceration without FB of left lesser toe(s) with damage to nail**
    7th

  S91.22 **Laceration with FB of toe with damage to nail**
  6th
    S91.221 **Laceration with FB of right great toe with damage to nail**
    7th
    S91.222 **Laceration with FB of left great toe with damage to nail**
    7th
    S91.224 **Laceration with FB of right lesser toe(s) with damage to nail**
    7th
    S91.225 **Laceration with FB of left lesser toe(s) with damage to nail**
    7th

  S91.23 **Puncture wound without FB of toe with damage to nail**
  6th
    S91.231 **Puncture wound without FB of right great toe with damage to nail**
    7th
    S91.232 **Puncture wound without FB of left great toe with damage to nail**
    7th
    S91.234 **Puncture wound without FB of right lesser toe(s) with damage to nail**
    7th
    S91.235 **Puncture wound without FB of left lesser toe(s) with damage to nail**
    7th

  S91.24 **Puncture wound with FB of toe with damage to nail**
  6th
    S91.241 **Puncture wound with FB of right great toe with damage to nail**
    7th
    S91.242 **Puncture wound with FB of left great toe with damage to nail**
    7th
    S91.244 **Puncture wound with FB of right lesser toe(s) with damage to nail**
    7th

4th 5th 6th 7th	Additional Character Required	✓ 3-character code	Unspecified laterality codes were excluded here.	• =New Code ▲ =Revised Code ▱ =Social determinants of health	*Excludes1*—Not coded here, do not use together *Excludes2*—Not included here

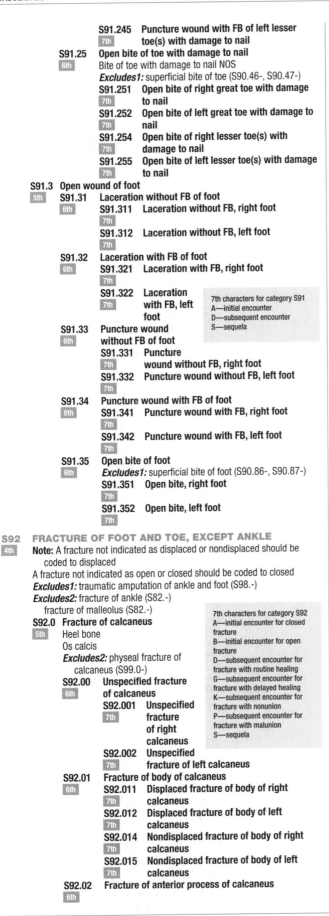

S91.245 Puncture wound with FB of left lesser
[7th] toe(s) with damage to nail

S91.25 Open bite of toe with damage to nail
[6th] Bite of toe with damage to nail NOS
Excludes1: superficial bite of toe (S90.46-, S90.47-)

S91.251 Open bite of right great toe with damage
[7th] to nail

S91.252 Open bite of left great toe with damage to
[7th] nail

S91.254 Open bite of right lesser toe(s) with
[7th] damage to nail

S91.255 Open bite of left lesser toe(s) with damage
[7th] to nail

S91.3 Open wound of foot
[5th]

S91.31 Laceration without FB of foot
[6th]

S91.311 Laceration without FB, right foot
[7th]

S91.312 Laceration without FB, left foot
[7th]

S91.32 Laceration with FB of foot
[6th]

S91.321 Laceration with FB, right foot
[7th]

S91.322 Laceration
[7th] with FB, left
foot

> 7th characters for category S91
> A—initial encounter
> D—subsequent encounter
> S—sequela

S91.33 Puncture wound
[6th] without FB of foot

S91.331 Puncture
[7th] wound without FB, right foot

S91.332 Puncture wound without FB, left foot
[7th]

S91.34 Puncture wound with FB of foot
[6th]

S91.341 Puncture wound with FB, right foot
[7th]

S91.342 Puncture wound with FB, left foot
[7th]

S91.35 Open bite of foot
[6th] *Excludes1:* superficial bite of foot (S90.86-, S90.87-)

S91.351 Open bite, right foot
[7th]

S91.352 Open bite, left foot
[7th]

S92 FRACTURE OF FOOT AND TOE, EXCEPT ANKLE
[4th] **Note:** A fracture not indicated as displaced or nondisplaced should be
coded to displaced
A fracture not indicated as open or closed should be coded to closed
Excludes1: traumatic amputation of ankle and foot (S98.-)
Excludes2: fracture of ankle (S82.-)
fracture of malleolus (S82.-)

S92.0 Fracture of calcaneus
[5th] Heel bone
Os calcis
Excludes2: physeal fracture of
calcaneus (S99.0-)

> 7th characters for category S92
> A—initial encounter for closed fracture
> B—initial encounter for open fracture
> D—subsequent encounter for fracture with routine healing
> G—subsequent encounter for fracture with delayed healing
> K—subsequent encounter for fracture with nonunion
> P—subsequent encounter for fracture with malunion
> S—sequela

S92.00 Unspecified fracture
[6th] of calcaneus

S92.001 Unspecified
[7th] fracture
of right
calcaneus

S92.002 Unspecified
[7th] fracture of left calcaneus

S92.01 Fracture of body of calcaneus
[6th]

S92.011 Displaced fracture of body of right
[7th] calcaneus

S92.012 Displaced fracture of body of left
[7th] calcaneus

S92.014 Nondisplaced fracture of body of right
[7th] calcaneus

S92.015 Nondisplaced fracture of body of left
[7th] calcaneus

S92.02 Fracture of anterior process of calcaneus
[6th]

S92.021 Displaced fracture of anterior process of
[7th] right calcaneus

S92.022 Displaced fracture of anterior process of
[7th] left calcaneus

S92.024 Nondis-placed fracture of anterior process
[7th] of right calcaneus

S92.025 Nondisplaced fracture of anterior process
[7th] of left calcaneus

S92.03 Avulsion fracture of tuberosity of calcaneus
[6th]

S92.031 Displaced avulsion fracture of tuberosity
[7th] of right calcaneus

S92.032 Displaced avulsion fracture of tuberosity
[7th] of left calcaneus

S92.034 Nondisplaced avulsion fracture of
[7th] tuberosity of right calcaneus

S92.035 Nondisplaced avulsion fracture of
[7th] tuberosity of left calcaneus

S92.04 Other fracture of tuberosity of calcaneus
[6th]

S92.041 Displaced other fracture of tuberosity of
[7th] right calcaneus

S92.042 Displaced other fracture of tuberosity of
[7th] left calcaneus

S92.044 Nondisplaced other fracture of tuberosity
[7th] of right calcaneus

S92.045 Nondisplaced other fracture of tuberosity
[7th] of left calcaneus

S92.05 Other extraarticular fracture of calcaneus
[6th]

S92.051 Displaced other extraarticular fracture of
[7th] right calcaneus

S92.052 Displaced other extraarticular fracture of
[7th] left calcaneus

S92.054 Nondisplaced other extraarticular fracture
[7th] of right calcaneus

S92.055 Nondisplaced other extraarticular fracture
[7th] of left calcaneus

S92.06 Intraarticular fracture of calcaneus
[6th]

S92.061 Displaced intraarticular fracture of right
[7th] calcaneus

S92.062 Displaced intraarticular fracture of left
[7th] calcaneus

S92.064 Nondisplaced intraarticular fracture of
[7th] right calcaneus

S92.065 Nondisplaced intraarticular fracture of left
[7th] calcaneus

S92.1 Fracture of talus
[5th] Astragalus

S92.10 Unspecified fracture of talus
[6th]

S92.101 Unspecified fracture of right talus
[7th]

S92.102 Unspecified fracture of left talus
[7th]

S92.11 Fracture of neck of talus
[6th]

S92.111 Displaced fracture of neck of right talus
[7th]

S92.112 Displaced fracture of neck of left talus
[7th]

S92.114 Nondisplaced fracture of neck of right
[7th] talus

S92.115 Nondisplaced fracture of neck of left talus
[7th]

S92.12 Fracture of body of talus
[6th]

S92.121 Displaced fracture of body of right talus
[7th]

S92.122 Displaced fracture of body of left talus
[7th]

S92.124 Nondisplaced fracture of body of right
[7th] talus

S92.125 Nondisplaced fracture of body of left talus
[7th]

S92.13 Fracture of posterior process of talus
[6th]

S92.131 Displaced fracture of posterior process of
[7th] right talus

S92.132 Displaced fracture of posterior process of
[7th] left talus

[4th] [5th] [6th] [7th] Additional Character Required　☑ 3-character code

Unspecified laterality codes
were excluded here.

• =New Code
▲ =Revised Code
▫ =Social determinants of health

Excludes1—Not coded here, do not use together
Excludes2—Not included here

CHAPTER 19. INJURY, POISONING AND CERTAIN OTHER CONSEQUENCES OF EXTERNAL CAUSES (S92.134–S92.415)

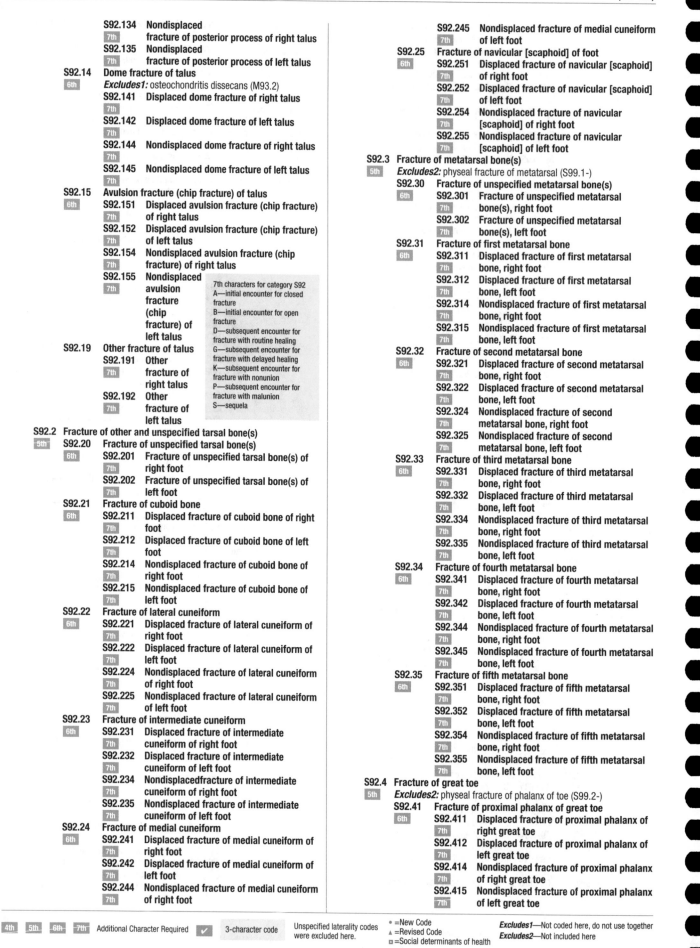

S92.134 **Nondisplaced**
 7th **fracture of posterior process of right talus**

S92.135 **Nondisplaced**
 7th **fracture of posterior process of left talus**

S92.14 **Dome fracture of talus**
 6th *Excludes1:* osteochondritis dissecans (M93.2)

 S92.141 **Displaced dome fracture of right talus**
  7th

 S92.142 **Displaced dome fracture of left talus**
  7th

 S92.144 **Nondisplaced dome fracture of right talus**
  7th

 S92.145 **Nondisplaced dome fracture of left talus**
  7th

S92.15 **Avulsion fracture (chip fracture) of talus**
 6th **S92.151** **Displaced avulsion fracture (chip fracture)**
  7th **of right talus**

 S92.152 **Displaced avulsion fracture (chip fracture)**
  7th **of left talus**

 S92.154 **Nondisplaced avulsion fracture (chip**
  7th **fracture) of right talus**

 S92.155 **Nondisplaced**
  7th **avulsion**
  fracture
  (chip
  fracture) of
  left talus

> 7th characters for category S92
> A—initial encounter for closed fracture
> B—initial encounter for open fracture
> D—subsequent encounter for fracture with routine healing
> G—subsequent encounter for fracture with delayed healing
> K—subsequent encounter for fracture with nonunion
> P—subsequent encounter for fracture with malunion
> S—sequela

S92.19 **Other fracture of talus**
 S92.191 **Other**
  7th **fracture of**
  right talus

 S92.192 **Other**
  7th **fracture of**
  left talus

S92.2 **Fracture of other and unspecified tarsal bone(s)**
 5th **S92.20** **Fracture of unspecified tarsal bone(s)**
  6th **S92.201** **Fracture of unspecified tarsal bone(s) of**
   7th **right foot**

  S92.202 **Fracture of unspecified tarsal bone(s) of**
   7th **left foot**

 S92.21 **Fracture of cuboid bone**
  6th **S92.211** **Displaced fracture of cuboid bone of right**
   7th **foot**

  S92.212 **Displaced fracture of cuboid bone of left**
   7th **foot**

  S92.214 **Nondisplaced fracture of cuboid bone of**
   7th **right foot**

  S92.215 **Nondisplaced fracture of cuboid bone of**
   7th **left foot**

 S92.22 **Fracture of lateral cuneiform**
  6th **S92.221** **Displaced fracture of lateral cuneiform of**
   7th **right foot**

  S92.222 **Displaced fracture of lateral cuneiform of**
   7th **left foot**

  S92.224 **Nondisplaced fracture of lateral cuneiform**
   7th **of right foot**

  S92.225 **Nondisplaced fracture of lateral cuneiform**
   7th **of left foot**

 S92.23 **Fracture of intermediate cuneiform**
  6th **S92.231** **Displaced fracture of intermediate**
   7th **cuneiform of right foot**

  S92.232 **Displaced fracture of intermediate**
   7th **cuneiform of left foot**

  S92.234 **Nondisplacedfracture of intermediate**
   7th **cuneiform of right foot**

  S92.235 **Nondisplaced fracture of intermediate**
   7th **cuneiform of left foot**

 S92.24 **Fracture of medial cuneiform**
  6th **S92.241** **Displaced fracture of medial cuneiform of**
   7th **right foot**

  S92.242 **Displaced fracture of medial cuneiform of**
   7th **left foot**

  S92.244 **Nondisplaced fracture of medial cuneiform**
   7th **of right foot**

  S92.245 **Nondisplaced fracture of medial cuneiform**
   7th **of left foot**

 S92.25 **Fracture of navicular [scaphoid] of foot**
  6th **S92.251** **Displaced fracture of navicular [scaphoid]**
   7th **of right foot**

  S92.252 **Displaced fracture of navicular [scaphoid]**
   7th **of left foot**

  S92.254 **Nondisplaced fracture of navicular**
   7th **[scaphoid] of right foot**

  S92.255 **Nondisplaced fracture of navicular**
   7th **[scaphoid] of left foot**

S92.3 **Fracture of metatarsal bone(s)**
 5th *Excludes2:* physeal fracture of metatarsal (S99.1-)
 S92.30 **Fracture of unspecified metatarsal bone(s)**
  6th **S92.301** **Fracture of unspecified metatarsal**
   7th **bone(s), right foot**

  S92.302 **Fracture of unspecified metatarsal**
   7th **bone(s), left foot**

 S92.31 **Fracture of first metatarsal bone**
  6th **S92.311** **Displaced fracture of first metatarsal**
   7th **bone, right foot**

  S92.312 **Displaced fracture of first metatarsal**
   7th **bone, left foot**

  S92.314 **Nondisplaced fracture of first metatarsal**
   7th **bone, right foot**

  S92.315 **Nondisplaced fracture of first metatarsal**
   7th **bone, left foot**

 S92.32 **Fracture of second metatarsal bone**
  6th **S92.321** **Displaced fracture of second metatarsal**
   7th **bone, right foot**

  S92.322 **Displaced fracture of second metatarsal**
   7th **bone, left foot**

  S92.324 **Nondisplaced fracture of second**
   7th **metatarsal bone, right foot**

  S92.325 **Nondisplaced fracture of second**
   7th **metatarsal bone, left foot**

 S92.33 **Fracture of third metatarsal bone**
  6th **S92.331** **Displaced fracture of third metatarsal**
   7th **bone, right foot**

  S92.332 **Displaced fracture of third metatarsal**
   7th **bone, left foot**

  S92.334 **Nondisplaced fracture of third metatarsal**
   7th **bone, right foot**

  S92.335 **Nondisplaced fracture of third metatarsal**
   7th **bone, left foot**

 S92.34 **Fracture of fourth metatarsal bone**
  6th **S92.341** **Displaced fracture of fourth metatarsal**
   7th **bone, right foot**

  S92.342 **Displaced fracture of fourth metatarsal**
   7th **bone, left foot**

  S92.344 **Nondisplaced fracture of fourth metatarsal**
   7th **bone, right foot**

  S92.345 **Nondisplaced fracture of fourth metatarsal**
   7th **bone, left foot**

 S92.35 **Fracture of fifth metatarsal bone**
  6th **S92.351** **Displaced fracture of fifth metatarsal**
   7th **bone, right foot**

  S92.352 **Displaced fracture of fifth metatarsal**
   7th **bone, left foot**

  S92.354 **Nondisplaced fracture of fifth metatarsal**
   7th **bone, right foot**

  S92.355 **Nondisplaced fracture of fifth metatarsal**
   7th **bone, left foot**

S92.4 **Fracture of great toe**
 5th *Excludes2:* physeal fracture of phalanx of toe (S99.2-)
 S92.41 **Fracture of proximal phalanx of great toe**
  6th **S92.411** **Displaced fracture of proximal phalanx of**
   7th **right great toe**

  S92.412 **Displaced fracture of proximal phalanx of**
   7th **left great toe**

  S92.414 **Nondisplaced fracture of proximal phalanx**
   7th **of right great toe**

  S92.415 **Nondisplaced fracture of proximal phalanx**
   7th **of left great toe**

| 4th | 5th | 6th | 7th | Additional Character Required | ✔ 3-character code | Unspecified laterality codes were excluded here. | • =New Code
▲ =Revised Code
⌂ =Social determinants of health | *Excludes1*—Not coded here, do not use together
Excludes2—Not included here |

S92.42 Fracture of distal phalanx of great toe
- **6th**
  - **S92.421 Displaced fracture of distal phalanx of right great toe** — 7th
  - **S92.422 Displaced fracture of distal phalanx of left great toe** — 7th
  - **S92.424 Nondisplaced fracture of distal phalanx of right great toe** — 7th
  - **S92.425 Nondisplaced fracture of distal phalanx of left great toe** — 7th

S92.49 Other fracture of great toe
- **6th**
  - **S92.491 Other fracture of right great toe** — 7th
  - **S92.492 Other fracture of left great toe** — 7th

S92.5 Fracture of lesser toe(s)
- **5th**
  - *Excludes2:* physeal fracture of toe (S99.2-)

  S92.51 Fracture of proximal phalanx of lesser toe(s)
  - **6th**
    - **S92.511 Displaced fracture of proximal phalanx of right lesser toe(s)** — 7th
    - **S92.512 Displaced fracture of proximal phalanx of left lesser toe(s)** — 7th
    - **S92.514 Nondisplaced fracture of proximal phalanx of right lesser toe(s)** — 7th
    - **S92.515 Nondisplaced fracture of proximal phalanx of left lesser toe(s)** — 7th

  > 7th characters for category S92
  > A—initial encounter for closed fracture
  > B—initial encounter for open fracture
  > D—subsequent encounter for fracture with routine healing
  > G—subsequent encounter for fracture with delayed healing
  > K—subsequent encounter for fracture with nonunion
  > P—subsequent encounter for fracture with malunion
  > S—sequela

  S92.52 Fracture of middle phalanx of lesser toe(s)
  - **6th**
    - **S92.521 Displaced fracture of middle phalanx of right lesser toe(s)** — 7th
    - **S92.522 Displaced fracture of middle phalanx of left lesser toe(s)** — 7th
    - **S92.524 Nondisplaced fracture of middle phalanx of right lesser toe(s)** — 7th
    - **S92.525 Nondisplaced fracture of middle phalanx of left lesser toe(s)** — 7th

  S92.53 Fracture of distal phalanx of lesser toe(s)
  - **6th**
    - **S92.531 Displaced fracture of distal phalanx of right lesser toe(s)** — 7th
    - **S92.532 Displaced fracture of distal phalanx of left lesser toe(s)** — 7th
    - **S92.534 Nondisplaced fracture of distal phalanx of right lesser toe(s)** — 7th
    - **S92.535 Nondisplaced fracture of distal phalanx of left lesser toe(s)** — 7th

  S92.59 Other fracture of lesser toe(s)
  - **6th**
    - **S92.591 Other fracture of right lesser toe(s)** — 7th
    - **S92.592 Other fracture of left lesser toe(s)** — 7th

S92.8 Other fracture of foot
- **5th**
  S92.81 Other fracture of foot
  - **6th**
    - Sesamoid fracture of foot
    - **S92.811 Other fracture of right foot** — 7th
    - **S92.812 Other fracture of left foot** — 7th

S92.9 Unspecified fracture of foot and toe
- **5th**
  S92.90 Unspecified fracture of foot
  - **6th**
    - **S92.901 Unspecified fracture of right foot** — 7th
    - **S92.902 Unspecified fracture of left foot** — 7th

  S92.91 Unspecified fracture of toe
  - **6th**
    - **S92.911 Unspecified fracture of right toe(s)** — 7th

S92.912 Unspecified fracture of left toe(s) — 7th

S93 DISLOCATION AND SPRAIN OF JOINTS AND LIGAMENTS AT ANKLE, FOOT AND TOE LEVEL
- **4th**

  > 7th characters for category S93
  > A—initial encounter
  > D—subsequent encounter
  > S—sequela

  Includes: avulsion of joint or ligament of ankle, foot and toe
  laceration of cartilage, joint or ligament of ankle, foot and toe
  sprain of cartilage, joint or ligament of ankle, foot and toe
  traumatic hemarthrosis of joint or ligament of ankle, foot and toe
  traumatic rupture of joint or ligament of ankle, foot and toe
  traumatic subluxation of joint or ligament of ankle, foot and toe
  traumatic tear of joint or ligament of ankle, foot and toe

  Code also any associated open wound
  Excludes2: strain of muscle and tendon of ankle and foot (S96.-)

  S93.0 Subluxation and dislocation of ankle joint
  - **5th**
    - Subluxation and dislocation of astragalus
    - Subluxation and dislocation of fibula, lower end
    - Subluxation and dislocation of talus or of tibia, lower end
    - **S93.01X Subluxation of right ankle joint** — 7th
    - **S93.02X Subluxation of left ankle joint** — 7th
    - **S93.04X Dislocation of right ankle joint** — 7th
    - **S93.05X Dislocation of left ankle joint** — 7th

  S93.1 Subluxation and dislocation of toe
  - **5th**
    S93.10 Unspecified subluxation and dislocation of toe
    - **6th**
      - Dislocation/subluxation of toe NOS
      - **S93.101 Unspecified subluxation of right toe(s)** — 7th
      - **S93.102 Unspecified subluxation of left toe(s)** — 7th
      - **S93.104 Unspecified dislocation of right toe(s)** — 7th
      - **S93.105 Unspecified dislocation of left toe(s)** — 7th

    S93.11 Dislocation of interphalangeal joint
    - **6th**
      - **S93.111 Dislocation of interphalangeal joint of right great toe** — 7th
      - **S93.112 Dislocation of interphalangeal joint of left great toe** — 7th
      - **S93.114 Dislocation of inter-phalangeal joint of right lesser toe(s)** — 7th
      - **S93.115 Dislocation of interphalangeal joint of left lesser toe(s)** — 7th

    S93.12 Dislocation of metatarsophalangeal joint
    - **6th**
      - **S93.121 Dislocation of metatarsophalangeal joint of right great toe** — 7th
      - **S93.122 Dislocation of metatarsophalangeal joint of left great toe** — 7th
      - **S93.124 Dislocation of metatarsophalangeal joint of right lesser toe(s)** — 7th
      - **S93.125 Dislocation of metatarsophalangeal joint of left lesser toe(s)** — 7th

    S93.13 Subluxation of interphalangeal joint
    - **6th**
      - **S93.131 Subluxation of interphalangeal joint of right great toe** — 7th
      - **S93.132 Subluxation of interphalangeal joint of left great toe** — 7th
      - **S93.134 Subluxation of interphalangeal joint of right lesser toe(s)** — 7th
      - **S93.135 Subluxation of interphalangeal joint of left lesser toe(s)** — 7th

    S93.14 Subluxation of metatarsophalangeal joint
    - **6th**
      - **S93.141 Subluxation of metatarsophalangeal joint of right great toe** — 7th
      - **S93.142 Subluxation of metatarsophalangeal joint of left great toe** — 7th
      - **S93.144 Subluxation of metatarsophalangeal joint of right lesser toe(s)** — 7th

---

4th 5th 6th 7th Additional Character Required   ✓ 3-character code   Unspecified laterality codes were excluded here.

• =New Code
▲ =Revised Code
□ =Social determinants of health

Excludes1—Not coded here, do not use together
Excludes2—Not included here

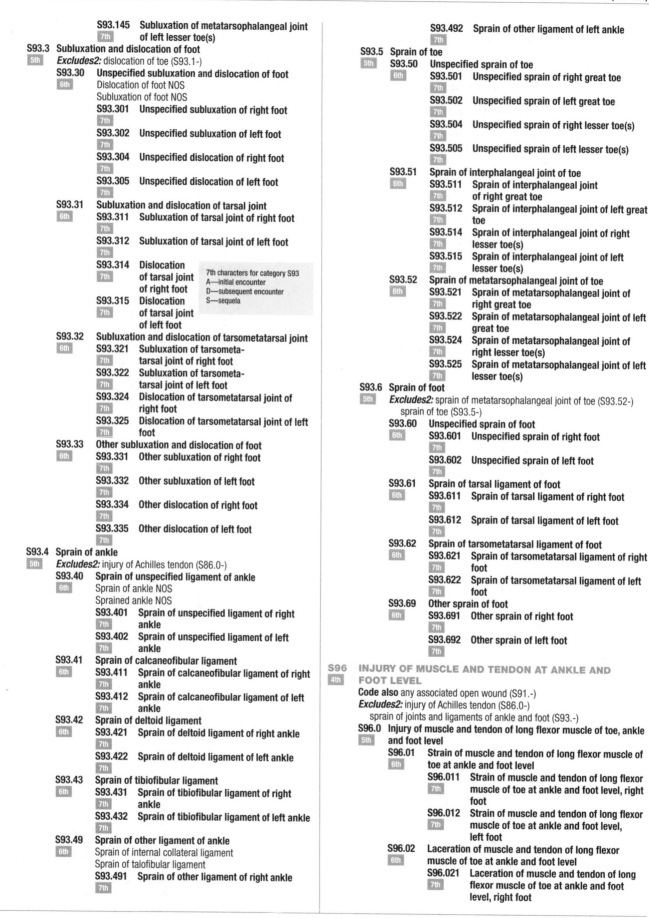

S93.145 Subluxation of metatarsophalangeal joint of left lesser toe(s)
7th

S93.3 Subluxation and dislocation of foot
5th
Excludes2: dislocation of toe (S93.1-)

S93.30 Unspecified subluxation and dislocation of foot
6th
Dislocation of foot NOS
Subluxation of foot NOS

S93.301 Unspecified subluxation of right foot
7th

S93.302 Unspecified subluxation of left foot
7th

S93.304 Unspecified dislocation of right foot
7th

S93.305 Unspecified dislocation of left foot
7th

S93.31 Subluxation and dislocation of tarsal joint
6th
S93.311 Subluxation of tarsal joint of right foot
7th

S93.312 Subluxation of tarsal joint of left foot
7th

S93.314 Dislocation of tarsal joint of right foot
7th

S93.315 Dislocation of tarsal joint of left foot
7th

> 7th characters for category S93
> A—initial encounter
> D—subsequent encounter
> S—sequela

S93.32 Subluxation and dislocation of tarsometatarsal joint
6th
S93.321 Subluxation of tarsometatarsal joint of right foot
7th

S93.322 Subluxation of tarsometatarsal joint of left foot
7th

S93.324 Dislocation of tarsometatarsal joint of right foot
7th

S93.325 Dislocation of tarsometatarsal joint of left foot
7th

S93.33 Other subluxation and dislocation of foot
6th
S93.331 Other subluxation of right foot
7th

S93.332 Other subluxation of left foot
7th

S93.334 Other dislocation of right foot
7th

S93.335 Other dislocation of left foot
7th

S93.4 Sprain of ankle
5th
Excludes2: injury of Achilles tendon (S86.0-)

S93.40 Sprain of unspecified ligament of ankle
6th
Sprain of ankle NOS
Sprained ankle NOS

S93.401 Sprain of unspecified ligament of right ankle
7th

S93.402 Sprain of unspecified ligament of left ankle
7th

S93.41 Sprain of calcaneofibular ligament
6th
S93.411 Sprain of calcaneofibular ligament of right ankle
7th

S93.412 Sprain of calcaneofibular ligament of left ankle
7th

S93.42 Sprain of deltoid ligament
6th
S93.421 Sprain of deltoid ligament of right ankle
7th

S93.422 Sprain of deltoid ligament of left ankle
7th

S93.43 Sprain of tibiofibular ligament
6th
S93.431 Sprain of tibiofibular ligament of right ankle
7th

S93.432 Sprain of tibiofibular ligament of left ankle
7th

S93.49 Sprain of other ligament of ankle
6th
Sprain of internal collateral ligament
Sprain of talofibular ligament
S93.491 Sprain of other ligament of right ankle
7th

S93.492 Sprain of other ligament of left ankle
7th

S93.5 Sprain of toe
5th
S93.50 Unspecified sprain of toe
6th
S93.501 Unspecified sprain of right great toe
7th

S93.502 Unspecified sprain of left great toe
7th

S93.504 Unspecified sprain of right lesser toe(s)
7th

S93.505 Unspecified sprain of left lesser toe(s)
7th

S93.51 Sprain of interphalangeal joint of toe
6th
S93.511 Sprain of interphalangeal joint of right great toe
7th

S93.512 Sprain of interphalangeal joint of left great toe
7th

S93.514 Sprain of interphalangeal joint of right lesser toe(s)
7th

S93.515 Sprain of interphalangeal joint of left lesser toe(s)
7th

S93.52 Sprain of metatarsophalangeal joint of toe
6th
S93.521 Sprain of metatarsophalangeal joint of right great toe
7th

S93.522 Sprain of metatarsophalangeal joint of left great toe
7th

S93.524 Sprain of metatarsophalangeal joint of right lesser toe(s)
7th

S93.525 Sprain of metatarsophalangeal joint of left lesser toe(s)
7th

S93.6 Sprain of foot
5th
Excludes2: sprain of metatarsophalangeal joint of toe (S93.52-)
sprain of toe (S93.5-)

S93.60 Unspecified sprain of foot
6th
S93.601 Unspecified sprain of right foot
7th

S93.602 Unspecified sprain of left foot
7th

S93.61 Sprain of tarsal ligament of foot
6th
S93.611 Sprain of tarsal ligament of right foot
7th

S93.612 Sprain of tarsal ligament of left foot
7th

S93.62 Sprain of tarsometatarsal ligament of foot
6th
S93.621 Sprain of tarsometatarsal ligament of right foot
7th

S93.622 Sprain of tarsometatarsal ligament of left foot
7th

S93.69 Other sprain of foot
6th
S93.691 Other sprain of right foot
7th

S93.692 Other sprain of left foot
7th

S96 INJURY OF MUSCLE AND TENDON AT ANKLE AND FOOT LEVEL
4th
Code also any associated open wound (S91.-)
Excludes2: injury of Achilles tendon (S86.0-)
sprain of joints and ligaments of ankle and foot (S93.-)

S96.0 Injury of muscle and tendon of long flexor muscle of toe, ankle and foot level
5th
S96.01 Strain of muscle and tendon of long flexor muscle of toe at ankle and foot level
6th
S96.011 Strain of muscle and tendon of long flexor muscle of toe at ankle and foot level, right foot
7th

S96.012 Strain of muscle and tendon of long flexor muscle of toe at ankle and foot level, left foot
7th

S96.02 Laceration of muscle and tendon of long flexor muscle of toe at ankle and foot level
6th
S96.021 Laceration of muscle and tendon of long flexor muscle of toe at ankle and foot level, right foot
7th

4th 5th 6th 7th Additional Character Required ✔ 3-character code | Unspecified laterality codes were excluded here. | • =New Code ▲ =Revised Code ▫ =Social determinants of health | *Excludes1*—Not coded here, do not use together *Excludes2*—Not included here

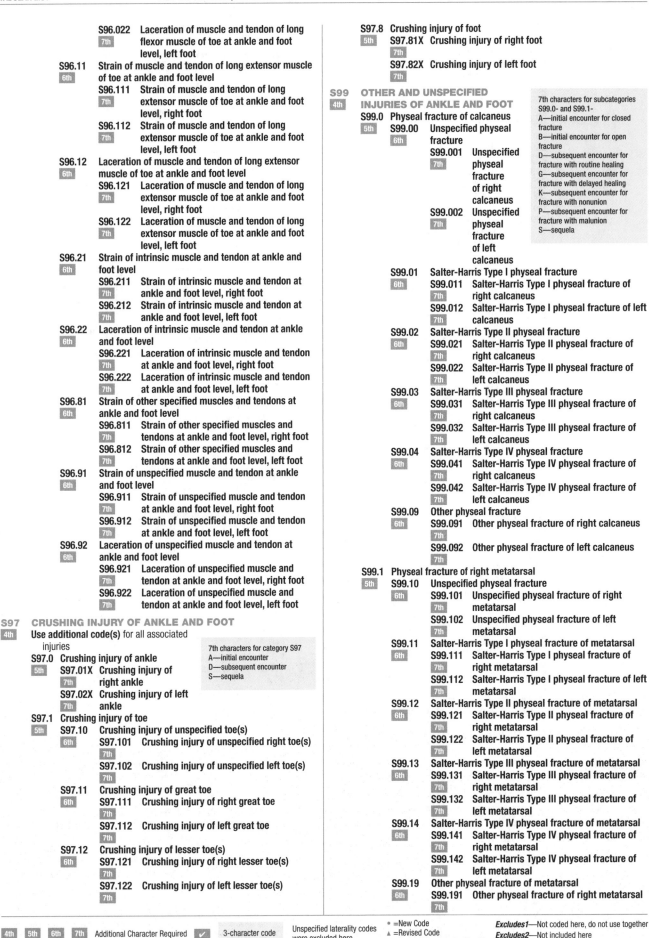

S96.022 Laceration of muscle and tendon of long flexor muscle of toe at ankle and foot level, left foot
— 7th

S96.11 Strain of muscle and tendon of long extensor muscle of toe at ankle and foot level
— 6th
    S96.111 Strain of muscle and tendon of long extensor muscle of toe at ankle and foot level, right foot
    — 7th
    S96.112 Strain of muscle and tendon of long extensor muscle of toe at ankle and foot level, left foot
    — 7th

S96.12 Laceration of muscle and tendon of long extensor muscle of toe at ankle and foot level
— 6th
    S96.121 Laceration of muscle and tendon of long extensor muscle of toe at ankle and foot level, right foot
    — 7th
    S96.122 Laceration of muscle and tendon of long extensor muscle of toe at ankle and foot level, left foot
    — 7th

S96.21 Strain of intrinsic muscle and tendon at ankle and foot level
— 6th
    S96.211 Strain of intrinsic muscle and tendon at ankle and foot level, right foot
    — 7th
    S96.212 Strain of intrinsic muscle and tendon at ankle and foot level, left foot
    — 7th

S96.22 Laceration of intrinsic muscle and tendon at ankle and foot level
— 6th
    S96.221 Laceration of intrinsic muscle and tendon at ankle and foot level, right foot
    — 7th
    S96.222 Laceration of intrinsic muscle and tendon at ankle and foot level, left foot
    — 7th

S96.81 Strain of other specified muscles and tendons at ankle and foot level
— 6th
    S96.811 Strain of other specified muscles and tendons at ankle and foot level, right foot
    — 7th
    S96.812 Strain of other specified muscles and tendons at ankle and foot level, left foot
    — 7th

S96.91 Strain of unspecified muscle and tendon at ankle and foot level
— 6th
    S96.911 Strain of unspecified muscle and tendon at ankle and foot level, right foot
    — 7th
    S96.912 Strain of unspecified muscle and tendon at ankle and foot level, left foot
    — 7th

S96.92 Laceration of unspecified muscle and tendon at ankle and foot level
— 6th
    S96.921 Laceration of unspecified muscle and tendon at ankle and foot level, right foot
    — 7th
    S96.922 Laceration of unspecified muscle and tendon at ankle and foot level, left foot
    — 7th

S97 **CRUSHING INJURY OF ANKLE AND FOOT**
— 4th
  Use additional code(s) for all associated injuries

7th characters for category S97
A—initial encounter
D—subsequent encounter
S—sequela

S97.0 Crushing injury of ankle
— 5th
    S97.01X Crushing injury of right ankle
    — 7th
    S97.02X Crushing injury of left ankle
    — 7th

S97.1 Crushing injury of toe
— 5th
    S97.10 Crushing injury of unspecified toe(s)
    — 6th
        S97.101 Crushing injury of unspecified right toe(s)
        — 7th
        S97.102 Crushing injury of unspecified left toe(s)
        — 7th
    S97.11 Crushing injury of great toe
    — 6th
        S97.111 Crushing injury of right great toe
        — 7th
        S97.112 Crushing injury of left great toe
        — 7th
    S97.12 Crushing injury of lesser toe(s)
    — 6th
        S97.121 Crushing injury of right lesser toe(s)
        — 7th
        S97.122 Crushing injury of left lesser toe(s)
        — 7th

S97.8 Crushing injury of foot
— 5th
    S97.81X Crushing injury of right foot
    — 7th
    S97.82X Crushing injury of left foot
    — 7th

S99 **OTHER AND UNSPECIFIED INJURIES OF ANKLE AND FOOT**
— 4th

7th characters for subcategories S99.0- and S99.1-
A—initial encounter for closed fracture
B—initial encounter for open fracture
D—subsequent encounter for fracture with routine healing
G—subsequent encounter for fracture with delayed healing
K—subsequent encounter for fracture with nonunion
P—subsequent encounter for fracture with malunion
S—sequela

S99.0 Physeal fracture of calcaneus
— 5th
    S99.00 Unspecified physeal fracture
    — 6th
        S99.001 Unspecified physeal fracture of right calcaneus
        — 7th
        S99.002 Unspecified physeal fracture of left calcaneus
        — 7th
    S99.01 Salter-Harris Type I physeal fracture
    — 6th
        S99.011 Salter-Harris Type I physeal fracture of right calcaneus
        — 7th
        S99.012 Salter-Harris Type I physeal fracture of left calcaneus
        — 7th
    S99.02 Salter-Harris Type II physeal fracture
    — 6th
        S99.021 Salter-Harris Type II physeal fracture of right calcaneus
        — 7th
        S99.022 Salter-Harris Type II physeal fracture of left calcaneus
        — 7th
    S99.03 Salter-Harris Type III physeal fracture
    — 6th
        S99.031 Salter-Harris Type III physeal fracture of right calcaneus
        — 7th
        S99.032 Salter-Harris Type III physeal fracture of left calcaneus
        — 7th
    S99.04 Salter-Harris Type IV physeal fracture
    — 6th
        S99.041 Salter-Harris Type IV physeal fracture of right calcaneus
        — 7th
        S99.042 Salter-Harris Type IV physeal fracture of left calcaneus
        — 7th
    S99.09 Other physeal fracture
    — 6th
        S99.091 Other physeal fracture of right calcaneus
        — 7th
        S99.092 Other physeal fracture of left calcaneus
        — 7th

S99.1 Physeal fracture of right metatarsal
— 5th
    S99.10 Unspecified physeal fracture
    — 6th
        S99.101 Unspecified physeal fracture of right metatarsal
        — 7th
        S99.102 Unspecified physeal fracture of left metatarsal
        — 7th
    S99.11 Salter-Harris Type I physeal fracture of metatarsal
    — 6th
        S99.111 Salter-Harris Type I physeal fracture of right metatarsal
        — 7th
        S99.112 Salter-Harris Type I physeal fracture of left metatarsal
        — 7th
    S99.12 Salter-Harris Type II physeal fracture of metatarsal
    — 6th
        S99.121 Salter-Harris Type II physeal fracture of right metatarsal
        — 7th
        S99.122 Salter-Harris Type II physeal fracture of left metatarsal
        — 7th
    S99.13 Salter-Harris Type III physeal fracture of metatarsal
    — 6th
        S99.131 Salter-Harris Type III physeal fracture of right metatarsal
        — 7th
        S99.132 Salter-Harris Type III physeal fracture of left metatarsal
        — 7th
    S99.14 Salter-Harris Type IV physeal fracture of metatarsal
    — 6th
        S99.141 Salter-Harris Type IV physeal fracture of right metatarsal
        — 7th
        S99.142 Salter-Harris Type IV physeal fracture of left metatarsal
        — 7th
    S99.19 Other physeal fracture of metatarsal
    — 6th
        S99.191 Other physeal fracture of right metatarsal
        — 7th

| 4th | 5th | 6th | 7th | Additional Character Required   ✓ 3-character code   Unspecified laterality codes were excluded here.

•=New Code
▲=Revised Code
▫=Social determinants of health

Excludes1—Not coded here, do not use together
Excludes2—Not included here

CHAPTER 19. INJURY, POISONING AND CERTAIN OTHER CONSEQUENCES OF EXTERNAL CAUSES (S96.022–S99.191)

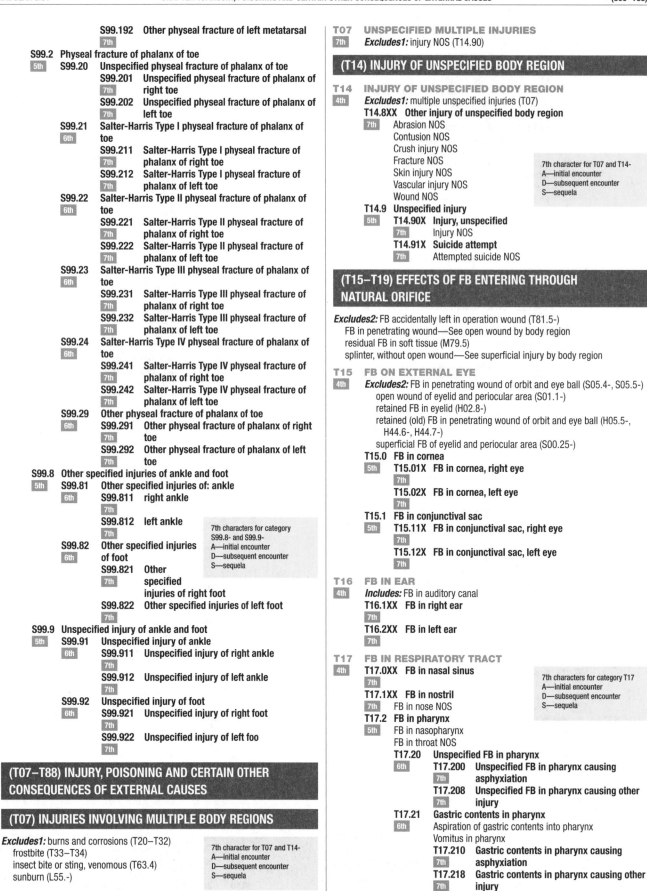

S99.192 Other physeal fracture of left metatarsal
7th

S99.2 Physeal fracture of phalanx of toe
5th
　S99.20 Unspecified physeal fracture of phalanx of toe
　　S99.201 Unspecified physeal fracture of phalanx of right toe
　　7th
　　S99.202 Unspecified physeal fracture of phalanx of left toe
　　7th
　S99.21 Salter-Harris Type I physeal fracture of phalanx of toe
　6th
　　S99.211 Salter-Harris Type I physeal fracture of phalanx of right toe
　　7th
　　S99.212 Salter-Harris Type I physeal fracture of phalanx of left toe
　　7th
　S99.22 Salter-Harris Type II physeal fracture of phalanx of toe
　6th
　　S99.221 Salter-Harris Type II physeal fracture of phalanx of right toe
　　7th
　　S99.222 Salter-Harris Type II physeal fracture of phalanx of left toe
　　7th
　S99.23 Salter-Harris Type III physeal fracture of phalanx of toe
　6th
　　S99.231 Salter-Harris Type III physeal fracture of phalanx of right toe
　　7th
　　S99.232 Salter-Harris Type III physeal fracture of phalanx of left toe
　　7th
　S99.24 Salter-Harris Type IV physeal fracture of phalanx of toe
　6th
　　S99.241 Salter-Harris Type IV physeal fracture of phalanx of right toe
　　7th
　　S99.242 Salter-Harris Type IV physeal fracture of phalanx of left toe
　　7th
　S99.29 Other physeal fracture of phalanx of toe
　6th
　　S99.291 Other physeal fracture of phalanx of right toe
　　7th
　　S99.292 Other physeal fracture of phalanx of left toe
　　7th

S99.8 Other specified injuries of ankle and foot
5th
　S99.81 Other specified injuries of: ankle
　6th
　　S99.811 right ankle
　　7th
　　S99.812 left ankle
　　7th
　S99.82 Other specified injuries of foot
　6th
　　S99.821 Other specified injuries of right foot
　　7th
　　S99.822 Other specified injuries of left foot
　　7th

> 7th characters for category
> S99.8- and S99.9-
> A—initial encounter
> D—subsequent encounter
> S—sequela

S99.9 Unspecified injury of ankle and foot
5th
　S99.91 Unspecified injury of ankle
　6th
　　S99.911 Unspecified injury of right ankle
　　7th
　　S99.912 Unspecified injury of left ankle
　　7th
　S99.92 Unspecified injury of foot
　6th
　　S99.921 Unspecified injury of right foot
　　7th
　　S99.922 Unspecified injury of left foo
　　7th

(T07–T88) INJURY, POISONING AND CERTAIN OTHER CONSEQUENCES OF EXTERNAL CAUSES

(T07) INJURIES INVOLVING MULTIPLE BODY REGIONS

Excludes1: burns and corrosions (T20–T32)
　frostbite (T33–T34)
　insect bite or sting, venomous (T63.4)
　sunburn (L55.-)

> 7th character for T07 and T14-
> A—initial encounter
> D—subsequent encounter
> S—sequela

T07　UNSPECIFIED MULTIPLE INJURIES
7th
　Excludes1: injury NOS (T14.90)

(T14) INJURY OF UNSPECIFIED BODY REGION

T14　INJURY OF UNSPECIFIED BODY REGION
4th
　Excludes1: multiple unspecified injuries (T07)
　T14.8XX Other injury of unspecified body region
　7th
　　Abrasion NOS
　　Contusion NOS
　　Crush injury NOS
　　Fracture NOS
　　Skin injury NOS
　　Vascular injury NOS
　　Wound NOS

> 7th character for T07 and T14-
> A—initial encounter
> D—subsequent encounter
> S—sequela

　T14.9 Unspecified injury
　5th
　　T14.90X Injury, unspecified
　　7th
　　　Injury NOS
　　T14.91X Suicide attempt
　　7th
　　　Attempted suicide NOS

(T15–T19) EFFECTS OF FB ENTERING THROUGH NATURAL ORIFICE

Excludes2: FB accidentally left in operation wound (T81.5-)
　FB in penetrating wound—See open wound by body region
　residual FB in soft tissue (M79.5)
　splinter, without open wound—See superficial injury by body region

T15　FB ON EXTERNAL EYE
4th
　Excludes2: FB in penetrating wound of orbit and eye ball (S05.4-, S05.5-)
　　open wound of eyelid and periocular area (S01.1-)
　　retained FB in eyelid (H02.8-)
　　retained (old) FB in penetrating wound of orbit and eye ball (H05.5-, H44.6-, H44.7-)
　　superficial FB of eyelid and periocular area (S00.25-)
　T15.0 FB in cornea
　5th
　　T15.01X FB in cornea, right eye
　　7th
　　T15.02X FB in cornea, left eye
　　7th
　T15.1 FB in conjunctival sac
　5th
　　T15.11X FB in conjunctival sac, right eye
　　7th
　　T15.12X FB in conjunctival sac, left eye
　　7th

T16　FB IN EAR
4th
　Includes: FB in auditory canal
　T16.1XX FB in right ear
　7th
　T16.2XX FB in left ear
　7th

T17　FB IN RESPIRATORY TRACT
4th
　T17.0XX FB in nasal sinus
　7th
　T17.1XX FB in nostril
　7th
　　FB in nose NOS
　T17.2 FB in pharynx
　5th
　　FB in nasopharynx
　　FB in throat NOS
　　T17.20 Unspecified FB in pharynx
　　6th
　　　T17.200 Unspecified FB in pharynx causing asphyxiation
　　　7th
　　　T17.208 Unspecified FB in pharynx causing other injury
　　　7th
　　T17.21 Gastric contents in pharynx
　　6th
　　　Aspiration of gastric contents into pharynx
　　　Vomitus in pharynx
　　　T17.210 Gastric contents in pharynx causing asphyxiation
　　　7th
　　　T17.218 Gastric contents in pharynx causing other injury
　　　7th

> 7th characters for category T17
> A—initial encounter
> D—subsequent encounter
> S—sequela

4th　5th　6th　7th　Additional Character Required　✓ 3-character code

Unspecified laterality codes were excluded here.

● =New Code
▲ =Revised Code
▱ =Social determinants of health

Excludes1—Not coded here, do not use together
Excludes2—Not included here

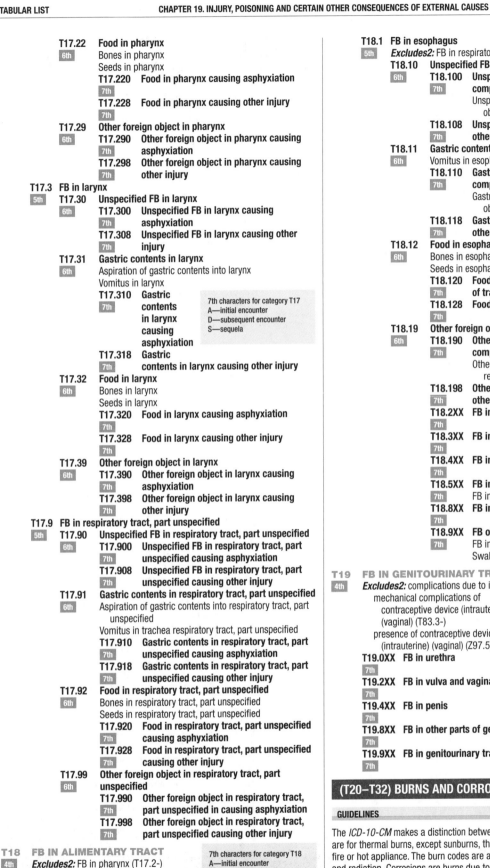

T17.22   **Food in pharynx**
`6th`
    Bones in pharynx
    Seeds in pharynx
      T17.220   **Food in pharynx causing asphyxiation**
      `7th`
      T17.228   **Food in pharynx causing other injury**
      `7th`

T17.29   **Other foreign object in pharynx**
`6th`
      T17.290   **Other foreign object in pharynx causing asphyxiation**
      `7th`
      T17.298   **Other foreign object in pharynx causing other injury**
      `7th`

T17.3   **FB in larynx**
`5th`
    T17.30   **Unspecified FB in larynx**
    `6th`
      T17.300   **Unspecified FB in larynx causing asphyxiation**
      `7th`
      T17.308   **Unspecified FB in larynx causing other injury**
      `7th`

    T17.31   **Gastric contents in larynx**
    `6th`
      Aspiration of gastric contents into larynx
      Vomitus in larynx
      T17.310   **Gastric contents in larynx causing asphyxiation**
      `7th`

> 7th characters for category T17
> A—initial encounter
> D—subsequent encounter
> S—sequela

      T17.318   **Gastric contents in larynx causing other injury**
      `7th`

    T17.32   **Food in larynx**
    `6th`
      Bones in larynx
      Seeds in larynx
      T17.320   **Food in larynx causing asphyxiation**
      `7th`
      T17.328   **Food in larynx causing other injury**
      `7th`

    T17.39   **Other foreign object in larynx**
    `6th`
      T17.390   **Other foreign object in larynx causing asphyxiation**
      `7th`
      T17.398   **Other foreign object in larynx causing other injury**
      `7th`

T17.9   **FB in respiratory tract, part unspecified**
`5th`
    T17.90   **Unspecified FB in respiratory tract, part unspecified**
    `6th`
      T17.900   **Unspecified FB in respiratory tract, part unspecified causing asphyxiation**
      `7th`
      T17.908   **Unspecified FB in respiratory tract, part unspecified causing other injury**
      `7th`

    T17.91   **Gastric contents in respiratory tract, part unspecified**
    `6th`
      Aspiration of gastric contents into respiratory tract, part unspecified
      Vomitus in trachea respiratory tract, part unspecified
      T17.910   **Gastric contents in respiratory tract, part unspecified causing asphyxiation**
      `7th`
      T17.918   **Gastric contents in respiratory tract, part unspecified causing other injury**
      `7th`

    T17.92   **Food in respiratory tract, part unspecified**
    `6th`
      Bones in respiratory tract, part unspecified
      Seeds in respiratory tract, part unspecified
      T17.920   **Food in respiratory tract, part unspecified causing asphyxiation**
      `7th`
      T17.928   **Food in respiratory tract, part unspecified causing other injury**
      `7th`

    T17.99   **Other foreign object in respiratory tract, part unspecified**
    `6th`
      T17.990   **Other foreign object in respiratory tract, part unspecified in causing asphyxiation**
      `7th`
      T17.998   **Other foreign object in respiratory tract, part unspecified causing other injury**
      `7th`

T18   **FB IN ALIMENTARY TRACT**
`4th`
   Excludes2: FB in pharynx (T17.2-)
   T18.0XX   **Foreign body in mouth**
   `7th`

> 7th characters for category T18
> A—initial encounter
> D—subsequent encounter
> S—sequela

T18.1   **FB in esophagus**
`5th`
   Excludes2: FB in respiratory tract (T17.-)
    T18.10   **Unspecified FB in esophagus**
    `6th`
      T18.100   **Unspecified FB in esophagus causing compression of trachea**
      `7th`
       Unspecified FB in esophagus causing obstruction of respiration
      T18.108   **Unspecified FB in esophagus causing other injury**
      `7th`

    T18.11   **Gastric contents in esophagus**
    `6th`
      Vomitus in esophagus
      T18.110   **Gastric contents in esophagus causing compression of trachea**
      `7th`
       Gastric contents in esophagus causing obstruction of respiration
      T18.118   **Gastric contents in esophagus causing other injury**
      `7th`

    T18.12   **Food in esophagus**
    `6th`
      Bones in esophagus
      Seeds in esophagus
      T18.120   **Food in esophagus causing compression of trachea**
      `7th`
      T18.128   **Food in esophagus causing other injury**
      `7th`

    T18.19   **Other foreign object in esophagus**
    `6th`
      T18.190   **Other foreign object in esophagus causing compression of trachea**
      `7th`
       Other FB in esophagus causing obstruction of respiration
      T18.198   **Other foreign object in esophagus causing other injury**
      `7th`

    T18.2XX   **FB in stomach**
    `7th`
    T18.3XX   **FB in small intestine**
    `7th`
    T18.4XX   **FB in colon**
    `7th`
    T18.5XX   **FB in anus and rectum**
    `7th`
      FB in rectosigmoid (junction)
    T18.8XX   **FB in other parts of alimentary tract**
    `7th`
    T18.9XX   **FB of alimentary tract, part unspecified**
    `7th`
      FB in digestive system NOS
      Swallowed FB NOS

T19   **FB IN GENITOURINARY TRACT**
`4th`
   Excludes2: complications due to implanted mesh (T83.7-)
     mechanical complications of contraceptive device (intrauterine) (vaginal) (T83.3-)
     presence of contraceptive device (intrauterine) (vaginal) (Z97.5)

> 7th characters for category T19
> A—initial encounter
> D—subsequent encounter
> S—sequela

   T19.0XX   **FB in urethra**
   `7th`
   T19.2XX   **FB in vulva and vagina**
   `7th`
   T19.4XX   **FB in penis**
   `7th`
   T19.8XX   **FB in other parts of genitourinary tract**
   `7th`
   T19.9XX   **FB in genitourinary tract, part unspecified**
   `7th`

(T20–T32) BURNS AND CORROSIONS

GUIDELINES

The *ICD-10-CM* makes a distinction between burns and corrosions. The burn codes are for thermal burns, except sunburns, that come from a heat source, such as a fire or hot appliance. The burn codes are also for burns resulting from electricity and radiation. Corrosions are burns due to chemicals. The guidelines are the same for burns and corrosions.

    Current burns (T20–T25) are classified by depth, extent and by agent (X code). Burns are classified by depth as first degree (erythema), second degree (blistering),

---

`4th` `5th` `6th` `7th` Additional Character Required	✔ 3-character code	Unspecified laterality codes were excluded here.	• =New Code ▲ =Revised Code ◘ =Social determinants of health	*Excludes1*—Not coded here, do not use together *Excludes2*—Not included here

PEDIATRIC ICD-10-CM 2021: A MANUAL FOR PROVIDER-BASED CODING   385

and third degree (full-thickness involvement). Burns of the eye and internal organs (T26–T28) are classified by site, but not by degree.

Sequencing of burn and related condition codes

Sequence first the code that reflects the highest degree of burn when more than one burn is present.

When the reason for the admission or encounter is for treatment of external multiple burns, sequence first the code that reflects the burn of the highest degree.

When a patient has both internal and external burns, the circumstances of admission govern the selection of the principal diagnosis or first-listed diagnosis.

When a patient is admitted for burn injuries and other related conditions such as smoke inhalation and/or respiratory failure, the circumstances of admission govern the selection of the principal or first-listed diagnosis.

Burns of the same anatomical site

Classify burns of the same **anatomic** site **and on the same side** but of different degrees to the subcategory identifying the highest degree recorded in the diagnosis **(e.g., for second and third degree burns of right thigh, assign only code T24.311-).**

Non-healing burns

Non-healing burns are coded as acute burns.
Necrosis of burned skin should be coded as a non-healed burn.

Infected burn

For any documented infected burn site, use an additional code for the infection.

Assign separate codes for each burn site

When coding burns, assign separate codes for each burn site. Category T30, Burn and corrosion, body region unspecified is extremely vague and should rarely be used.

Codes for burns of "multiple sites" should only be assigned when the medical record documentation does not specify the individual sites.

Burns and corrosions classified according to extent of body surface involved

Refer to category T31 for guidelines.

Encounters for treatment of sequela of burns

Encounters for the treatment of the late effects of burns or corrosions (ie, scars or joint contractures) should be coded with a burn or corrosion code with the 7th character S for sequela.

Sequela with a late effect code and current burn

When appropriate, both a code for a current burn or corrosion with 7th character A or D and a burn or corrosion code with 7th character S may be assigned on the same record (when both a current burn and sequela of an old burn exist). Burns and corrosions do not heal at the same rate and a current healing wound may still exist with sequela of a healed burn or corrosion.

Use of an external cause code with burns and corrosions

An external cause code should be used with burns and corrosions to identify the source and intent of the burn, as well as the place where it occurred.

Includes: burns (thermal) from electrical heating appliances
    burns (thermal) from electricity
    burns (thermal) from flame
    burns (thermal) from friction
    burns (thermal) from hot air and hot gases
    burns (thermal) from hot objects
    burns (thermal) from lightning
    burns (thermal) from radiation
    chemical burn [corrosion] (external) (internal)
    scalds
Excludes2: erythema [dermatitis] ab igne (L59.0)
    radiation-related disorders of the skin and subcutaneous tissue (L55–L59)
    sunburn (L55.-)

(T20–T25) BURNS AND CORROSIONS OF EXTERNAL BODY SURFACE, SPECIFIED BY SITE

Includes: burns and corrosions of first degree [erythema]
    burns and corrosions of second degree [blisters] [epidermal loss]
    burns and corrosions of third degree [deep necrosis of underlying tissue] [full- thickness skin loss]

Use additional code from category T31 or T32 to identify extent of body surface involved

7th characters for categories T20–T25
A—initial encounter
D—subsequent encounter
S—sequela

T20 **BURN AND CORROSION OF**
4th **HEAD, FACE, AND NECK**
    Excludes2: burn and corrosion of ear drum (T28.41, T28.91)
      burn and corrosion of eye and adnexa (T26.-)
      burn and corrosion of mouth and pharynx (T28.0)

  T20.0 **Burn of unspecified degree of head, face, and neck**
  5th **Use additional external cause code** to identify the source, place and intent of the burn (X00–X19, X75–X77, X96–X98, Y92)
    T20.00X **Burn of unspecified degree of head, face, and neck,**
    7th unspecified site
    T20.01 **Burn of unspecified degree of ear [any part, except**
    6th ear drum]
      Excludes2: burn of ear drum (T28.41-)
      T20.011 **Burn of unspecified degree of right ear**
      7th [any part, except ear drum]
      T20.012 **Burn of unspecified degree of left ear [any**
      7th part, except ear drum]
    T20.02X **Burn of unspecified degree of lip(s)**
    7th
    T20.03X **Burn of unspecified degree of chin**
    7th
    T20.04X **Burn of unspecified degree of nose (septum)**
    7th
    T20.05X **Burn of unspecified degree of scalp [any part]**
    7th
    T20.06X **Burn of unspecified degree of forehead and cheek**
    7th
    T20.07X **Burn of unspecified degree of neck, initial encounter**
    7th
    T20.09X **Burn of unspecified degree of multiple sites of head,**
    7th face, and neck

  T20.1 **Burn of first degree of head, face, and neck**
  5th **Use additional external cause code** to identify the source, place and intent of the burn (X00–X19, X75–X77, X96–X98, Y92)
    T20.10X **Burn of first degree of head, face, and neck,**
    7th unspecified site
    T20.11 **Burn of first degree of ear [any part, except ear**
    6th drum]
      Excludes2: burn of ear drum (T28.41-)
      T20.111 **Burn of first degree of right ear [any part,**
      7th except ear drum]
      T20.112 **Burn of first degree of left ear [any part,**
      7th except ear drum]
      T20.119 **Burn of first degree of unspecified ear**
      7th [any part, except ear drum]
    T20.12X **Burn of first degree of lip(s)**
    7th
    T20.13X **Burn of first degree of chin**
    7th
    T20.14X **Burn of first degree of nose (septum)**
    7th
    T20.15X **Burn of first degree of scalp [any part]**
    7th
    T20.16X **Burn of first degree of forehead and cheek**
    7th
    T20.17X **Burn of first degree of neck**
    7th
    T20.19X **Burn of first degree of multiple sites of head, face,**
    7th and neck

  T20.2 **Burn of second degree of head, face, and neck**
  5th **Use additional external cause code** to identify the source, place and intent of the burn (X00–X19, X75–X77, X96–X98, Y92)

   4th **5th** **6th** **7th** Additional Character Required   ✓   3-character code   Unspecified laterality codes were excluded here.   •=New Code   ▲=Revised Code   ▨=Social determinants of health   **Excludes1**—Not coded here, do not use together   **Excludes2**—Not included here

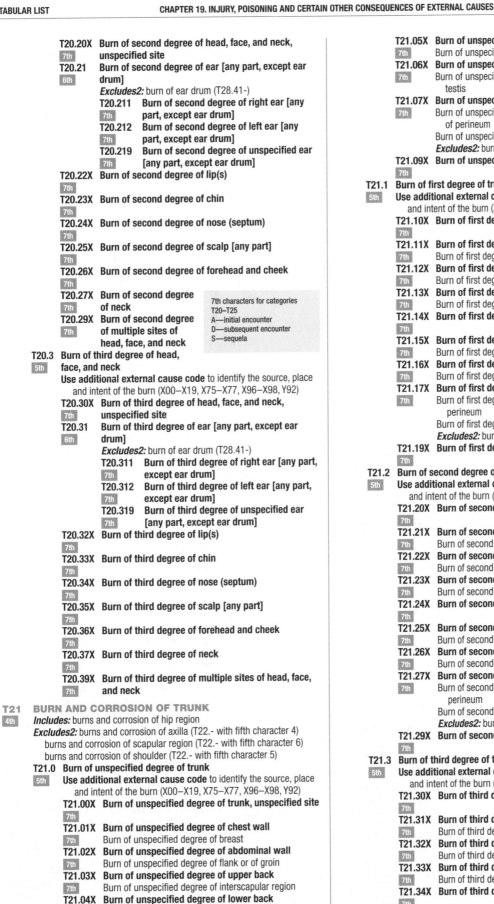

T20.20X [7th] Burn of second degree of head, face, and neck, unspecified site

T20.21 [6th] Burn of second degree of ear [any part, except ear drum]

Excludes2: burn of ear drum (T28.41-)

    T20.211 [7th] Burn of second degree of right ear [any part, except ear drum]

    T20.212 [7th] Burn of second degree of left ear [any part, except ear drum]

    T20.219 [7th] Burn of second degree of unspecified ear [any part, except ear drum]

T20.22X [7th] Burn of second degree of lip(s)

T20.23X [7th] Burn of second degree of chin

T20.24X [7th] Burn of second degree of nose (septum)

T20.25X [7th] Burn of second degree of scalp [any part]

T20.26X [7th] Burn of second degree of forehead and cheek

T20.27X [7th] Burn of second degree of neck

T20.29X [7th] Burn of second degree of multiple sites of head, face, and neck

> 7th characters for categories
> T20–T25
> A—initial encounter
> D—subsequent encounter
> S—sequela

T20.3 [5th] Burn of third degree of head, face, and neck

Use additional external cause code to identify the source, place and intent of the burn (X00–X19, X75–X77, X96–X98, Y92)

T20.30X [7th] Burn of third degree of head, face, and neck, unspecified site

T20.31 [6th] Burn of third degree of ear [any part, except ear drum]

Excludes2: burn of ear drum (T28.41-)

    T20.311 [7th] Burn of third degree of right ear [any part, except ear drum]

    T20.312 [7th] Burn of third degree of left ear [any part, except ear drum]

    T20.319 [7th] Burn of third degree of unspecified ear [any part, except ear drum]

T20.32X [7th] Burn of third degree of lip(s)

T20.33X [7th] Burn of third degree of chin

T20.34X [7th] Burn of third degree of nose (septum)

T20.35X [7th] Burn of third degree of scalp [any part]

T20.36X [7th] Burn of third degree of forehead and cheek

T20.37X [7th] Burn of third degree of neck

T20.39X [7th] Burn of third degree of multiple sites of head, face, and neck

T21 [4th] **BURN AND CORROSION OF TRUNK**

Includes: burns and corrosion of hip region

Excludes2: burns and corrosion of axilla (T22.- with fifth character 4)

burns and corrosion of scapular region (T22.- with fifth character 6)

burns and corrosion of shoulder (T22.- with fifth character 5)

T21.0 [5th] Burn of unspecified degree of trunk

Use additional external cause code to identify the source, place and intent of the burn (X00–X19, X75–X77, X96–X98, Y92)

T21.00X [7th] Burn of unspecified degree of trunk, unspecified site

T21.01X [7th] Burn of unspecified degree of chest wall

Burn of unspecified degree of breast

T21.02X [7th] Burn of unspecified degree of abdominal wall

Burn of unspecified degree of flank or of groin

T21.03X [7th] Burn of unspecified degree of upper back

Burn of unspecified degree of interscapular region

T21.04X [7th] Burn of unspecified degree of lower back

T21.05X [7th] Burn of unspecified degree of buttock

Burn of unspecified degree of anus

T21.06X [7th] Burn of unspecified degree of male genital region

Burn of unspecified degree of penis or of scrotum or of testis

T21.07X [7th] Burn of unspecified degree of female genital region

Burn of unspecified degree of labium (majus) (minus) or of perineum

Burn of unspecified degree of vulva

Excludes2: burn of vagina (T28.3)

T21.09X [7th] Burn of unspecified degree of other site of trunk

T21.1 [5th] Burn of first degree of trunk

Use additional external cause code to identify the source, place and intent of the burn (X00–X19, X75–X77, X96–X98, Y92)

T21.10X [7th] Burn of first degree of trunk, unspecified site

T21.11X [7th] Burn of first degree of chest wall

Burn of first degree of breast

T21.12X [7th] Burn of first degree of abdominal wall

Burn of first degree of flank OR OF GROIN

T21.13X [7th] Burn of first degree of upper back

Burn of first degree of interscapular region

T21.14X [7th] Burn of first degree of lower back

T21.15X [7th] Burn of first degree of buttock

Burn of first degree of anus

T21.16X [7th] Burn of first degree of male genital region

Burn of first degree of penis or of scrotum or of testis

T21.17X [7th] Burn of first degree of female genital region

Burn of first degree of labium (majus) (minus) or of perineum

Burn of first degree of vulva

Excludes2: burn of vagina (T28.3)

T21.19X [7th] Burn of first degree of other site of trunk

T21.2 [5th] Burn of second degree of trunk

Use additional external cause code to identify the source, place and intent of the burn (X00–X19, X75–X77, X96–X98, Y92)

T21.20X [7th] Burn of second degree of trunk, unspecified site

T21.21X [7th] Burn of second degree of chest wall

Burn of second degree of breast

T21.22X [7th] Burn of second degree of abdominal wall

Burn of second degree of flank or of groin

T21.23X [7th] Burn of second degree of upper back

Burn of second degree of interscapular region

T21.24X [7th] Burn of second degree of lower back

T21.25X [7th] Burn of second degree of buttock

Burn of second degree of anus

T21.26X [7th] Burn of second degree of male genital region

Burn of second degree of penis or of scrotum or of testis

T21.27X [7th] Burn of second degree of female genital region

Burn of second degree of labium (majus) (minus) or of perineum

Burn of second degree of vulva

Excludes2: burn of vagina (T28.3)

T21.29X [7th] Burn of second degree of other site of trunk

T21.3 [5th] Burn of third degree of trunk

Use additional external cause code to identify the source, place and intent of the burn (X00–X19, X75–X77, X96–X98, Y92)

T21.30X [7th] Burn of third degree of trunk, unspecified site

T21.31X [7th] Burn of third degree of chest wall

Burn of third degree of breast

T21.32X [7th] Burn of third degree of abdominal wall

Burn of third degree of flank OR GROIN

T21.33X [7th] Burn of third degree of upper back

Burn of third degree of interscapular region

T21.34X [7th] Burn of third degree of lower back

[4th] [5th] [6th] [7th] Additional Character Required   ✓ 3-character code

Unspecified laterality codes were excluded here.

● =New Code
▲ =Revised Code
▢ =Social determinants of health

Excludes1—Not coded here, do not use together

Excludes2—Not included here

T21.35X **Burn of third degree of buttock**
7th   Burn of third degree of anus

T21.36X **Burn of third degree of male genital region**
7th   Burn of third degree of penis or of scrotum or of testis

T21.37X **Burn of third degree of female genital region**
7th   Burn of third degree of labium (majus) (minus)
    Burn of third degree of perineum
    Burn of third degree of vulva
    Excludes2: burn of vagina (T28.3)

T21.39X **Burn of third degree of other site of trunk**
7th

T22   **BURN AND CORROSION OF SHOULDER AND UPPER**
4th   **LIMB, EXCEPT WRIST AND HAND**
    Excludes2: burn and corrosion of interscapular region (T21.-)
    burn and corrosion of wrist and hand (T23.-)

T22.0 **Burn of unspecified degree of shoulder and upper limb, except**
5th   **wrist and hand**
    Use additional external cause code to identify the source, place
    and intent of the burn (X00–X19, X75–X77, X96–X98, Y92)

T22.00X **Burn of unspecified degree of shoulder and upper**
7th   **limb, except wrist and hand, unspecified site**

T22.01 **Burn of unspecified**
6th   **degree of forearm**
    T22.011 **Burn of**
    7th   **unspecified**
       degree of
       right forearm

| 7th characters for categories |
| T20–T25 |
| A—initial encounter |
| D—subsequent encounter |
| S—sequela |

    T22.012 **Burn of unspecified degree of left forearm**
    7th

T22.02 **Burn of unspecified degree of elbow**
6th   **T22.021** **Burn of unspecified degree of right elbow**
    7th

    T22.022 **Burn of unspe-cified degree of left elbow**
    7th

T22.03 **Burn of unspecified degree of upper arm**
6th   **T22.031** **Burn of unspecified degree of right upper**
    7th   **arm**
    T22.032 **Burn of unspecified degree of left upper**
    7th   **arm**

T22.04 **Burn of unspecified degree of axilla**
6th   **T22.041** **Burn of unspecified degree of right axilla**
    7th

    T22.042 **Burn of unspecified degree of left axilla**
    7th

T22.05 **Burn of unspecified degree of shoulder**
6th   **T22.051** **Burn of unspecified degree of right**
    7th   **shoulder**
    T22.052 **Burn of unspecified degree of left shoulder**
    7th

T22.06 **Burn of unspecified degree of scapular region**
6th   **T22.061** **Burn of unspecified degree of right**
    7th   **scapular region**
    T22.062 **Burn of unspecified degree of left scapular**
    7th   **region**

T22.09 **Burn of unspecified degree of multiple sites of**
6th   **shoulder and upper limb, except wrist and hand**
    T22.091 **Burn of unspecified degree of multiple**
    7th   **sites of right shoulder and upper limb,**
       except wrist and hand
    T22.092 **Burn of unspecified degree of multiple**
    7th   **sites of left shoulder and upper limb,**
       except wrist and hand

T22.1 **Burn of first degree of shoulder and upper limb, except wrist**
5th   **and hand**
    Use additional external cause code to identify the source, place
    and intent of the burn (X00–X19, X75–X77, X96–X98, Y92)

T22.10X **Burn of first degree of shoulder and upper limb,**
7th   **except wrist and hand, unspecified site**

T22.11 **Burn of first degree of forearm**
6th   **T22.111** **Burn of first degree of right forearm**
    7th

    T22.112 **Burn of first degree of left forearm**
    7th

T22.12 **Burn of first degree of elbow**
6th   **T22.121** **Burn of first degree of right elbow**
    7th

    T22.122 **Burn of first degree of left elbow**
    7th

T22.13 **Burn of first degree of upper arm**
6th   **T22.131** **Burn of first degree of right upper arm**
    7th

    T22.132 **Burn of first degree of left upper arm**
    7th

T22.14 **Burn of first degree of axilla**
6th   **T22.141** **Burn of first degree of right axilla**
    7th

    T22.142 **Burn of first degree of left axilla**
    7th

T22.15 **Burn of first degree of shoulder**
6th   **T22.151** **Burn of first degree of right shoulder**
    7th

    T22.152 **Burn of first degree of left shoulder**
    7th

T22.16 **Burn of first degree of scapular region**
6th   **T22.161** **Burn of first degree of right scapular**
    7th   **region**
    T22.162 **Burn of first degree of left scapular region**
    7th

T22.19 **Burn of first degree of multiple sites of shoulder and**
6th   **upper limb, except wrist and hand**
    T22.191 **Burn of first degree of multiple sites of**
    7th   **right shoulder and upper limb, except**
       wrist and hand
    T22.192 **Burn of first degree of multiple sites of left**
    7th   **shoulder and upper limb, except wrist and**
       hand
    T22.199 **Burn of first degree of multiple sites of**
    7th   **unspecified shoulder and upper limb,**
       except wrist and hand

T22.2 **Burn of second degree of shoulder and upper limb, except**
5th   **wrist and hand**
    Use additional external cause code to identify the source, place
    and intent of the burn (X00–X19, X75–X77,X96–X98, Y92)

T22.20X **Burn of second degree of shoulder and upper limb,**
7th   **except wrist and hand, unspecified site**

T22.21 **Burn of second degree of forearm**
6th   **T22.211** **Burn of second degree of right forearm**
    7th

    T22.212 **Burn of second degree of left forearm**
    7th

    T22.219 **Burn of second degree of unspecified**
    7th   **forearm**

T22.22 **Burn of second degree of elbow**
6th   **T22.221** **Burn of second degree of right elbow**
    7th

    T22.222 **Burn of second degree of left elbow**
    7th

T22.23 **Burn of second degree of upper arm**
6th   **T22.231** **Burn of second degree of right upper arm**
    7th

    T22.232 **Burn of second degree of left upper arm**
    7th

T22.24 **Burn of second degree of axilla**
6th   **T22.241** **Burn of second degree of right axilla**
    7th

    T22.242 **Burn of second degree of left axilla**
    7th

T22.25 **Burn of second degree of shoulder**
6th   **T22.251** **Burn of second degree of right shoulder**
    7th

    T22.252 **Burn of second degree of left shoulder**
    7th

T22.26 **Burn of second degree of scapular region**
6th   **T22.261** **Burn of second degree of right scapular**
    7th   **region**

4th   5th   6th   7th   Additional Character Required   ✔   3-character code   Unspecified laterality codes were excluded here.   ● =New Code   ***Excludes1***—Not coded here, do not use together
                                                        ▲ =Revised Code   ***Excludes2***—Not included here
                                                        ⌑ =Social determinants of health

T22.262 **7th** Burn of second degree of left scapular region

T22.29 **6th** **Burn of second degree of multiple sites of shoulder and upper limb, except wrist and hand**

    T22.291 **7th** **Burn of second degree of multiple sites of right shoulder and upper limb, except wrist and hand**

    T22.292 **7th** **Burn of second degree of multiple sites of left shoulder and upper limb, except wrist and hand**

T22.3 **5th** **Burn of third degree of shoulder and upper limb, except wrist and hand**
Use additional external cause code to identify the source, place and intent of the burn (X00–X19, X75–X77, X96–X98, Y92)

  T22.31 **6th** **Burn of third degree of forearm**

    T22.311 **7th** **Burn of third degree of right forearm**

    T22.312 **7th** **Burn of third degree of left forearm**

    T22.319 **7th** **Burn of third degree of unspecified forearm**

  T22.32 **6th** **Burn of third degree of elbow**

    T22.321 **7th** **Burn of third degree of right elbow**

7th characters for categories T20–T25
A—initial encounter
D—subsequent encounter
S—sequela

    T22.322 **7th** **Burn of third degree of left elbow**

  T22.33 **6th** **Burn of third degree of upper arm**

    T22.331 **7th** **Burn of third degree of right upper arm**

    T22.332 **7th** **Burn of third degree of left upper arm**

  T22.34 **6th** **Burn of third degree of axilla**

    T22.341 **7th** **Burn of third degree of right axilla**

    T22.342 **7th** **Burn of third degree of left axilla**

  T22.35 **6th** **Burn of third degree of shoulder**

    T22.351 **7th** **Burn of third degree of right shoulder**

    T22.352 **7th** **Burn of third degree of left shoulder**

  T22.36 **6th** **Burn of third degree of scapular region**

    T22.361 **7th** **Burn of third degree of right scapular region**

    T22.362 **7th** **Burn of third degree of left scapular region**

  T22.39 **6th** **Burn of third degree of multiple sites of shoulder and upper limb, except wrist and hand**

    T22.391 **7th** **Burn of third degree of multiple sites of right shoulder and upper limb, except wrist and hand**

    T22.392 **7th** **Burn of third degree of multiple sites of left shoulder and upper limb, except wrist and hand**

T23 **4th** **BURN AND CORROSION OF WRIST AND HAND**

T23.0 **5th** **Burn of unspecified degree of wrist and hand**
Use additional external cause code to identify the source, place and intent of the burn (X00–X19, X75–X77, X96–X98, Y92)

  T23.00 **6th** **Burn of unspecified degree of hand, unspecified site**

    T23.001 **7th** **Burn of unspecified degree of right hand, unspecified site**

    T23.002 **7th** **Burn of unspecified degree of left hand, unspecified site**

    T23.009 **7th** **Burn of unspecified degree of unspecified hand, unspecified site**

  T23.01 **6th** **Burn of unspecified degree of thumb (nail)**

    T23.011 **7th** **Burn of unspecified degree of right thumb (nail)**

    T23.012 **7th** **Burn of unspecified degree of left thumb (nail)**

T23.02 **6th** **Burn of unspecified degree of single finger (nail) except thumb**

    T23.021 **7th** **Burn of unspecified degree of single right finger (nail) except thumb**

    T23.022 **7th** **Burn of unspecified degree of single left finger (nail) except thumb**

T23.03 **6th** **Burn of unspecified degree of multiple fingers (nail), not including thumb**

    T23.031 **7th** **Burn of unspecified degree of multiple right fingers (nail), not including thumb**

    T23.032 **7th** **Burn of unspecified degree of multiple left fingers (nail), not including thumb**

T23.04 **6th** **Burn of unspecified degree of multiple fingers (nail), including thumb**

    T23.041 **7th** **Burn of unspecified degree of multiple right fingers (nail), including thumb**

    T23.042 **7th** **Burn of unspecified degree of multiple left fingers (nail), including thumb**

T23.05 **6th** **Burn of unspecified degree of palm**

    T23.051 **7th** **Burn of unspecified degree of right palm**

    T23.052 **7th** **Burn of unspecified degree of left palm**

T23.06 **6th** **Burn of unspecified degree of back of hand**

    T23.061 **7th** **Burn of unspecified degree of back of right hand**

    T23.062 **7th** **Burn of unspecified degree of back of left hand**

T23.07 **6th** **Burn of unspecified degree of wrist**

    T23.071 **7th** **Burn of unspecified degree of right wrist**

    T23.072 **7th** **Burn of unspecified degree of left wrist**

T23.09 **6th** **Burn of unspecified degree of multiple sites of wrist and hand**

    T23.091 **7th** **Burn of unspecified degree of multiple sites of right wrist and hand**

    T23.092 **7th** **Burn of unspecified degree of multiple sites of left wrist and hand**

T23.1 **5th** **Burn of first degree of wrist and hand**
Use additional external cause code to identify the source, place and intent of the burn (X00–X19, X75–X77, X96–X98, Y92)

  T23.10 **6th** **Burn of first degree of hand, unspecified site**

    T23.101 **7th** **Burn of first degree of right hand, unspecified site**

    T23.102 **7th** **Burn of first degree of left hand, unspecified site**

  T23.11 **6th** **Burn of first degree of thumb (nail)**

    T23.111 **7th** **Burn of first degree of right thumb (nail)**

    T23.112 **7th** **Burn of first degree of left thumb (nail)**

  T23.12 **6th** **Burn of first degree of single finger (nail) except thumb**

    T23.121 **7th** **Burn of first degree of single right finger (nail) except thumb**

    T23.122 **7th** **Burn of first degree of single left finger (nail) except thumb**

  T23.13 **6th** **Burn of first degree of multiple fingers (nail), not including thumb**

    T23.131 **7th** **Burn of first degree of multiple right fingers (nail), not including thumb**

    T23.132 **7th** **Burn of first degree of multiple left fingers (nail), not including thumb**

  T23.14 **6th** **Burn of first degree of multiple fingers (nail), including thumb**

    T23.141 **7th** **Burn of first degree of multiple right fingers (nail), including thumb**

    T23.142 **7th** **Burn of first degree of multiple left fingers (nail), including thumb**

  T23.15 **6th** **Burn of first degree of palm**

    T23.151 **7th** **Burn of first degree of right palm**

CHAPTER 19. INJURY, POISONING AND CERTAIN OTHER CONSEQUENCES OF EXTERNAL CAUSES   (T22.262–T23.151)

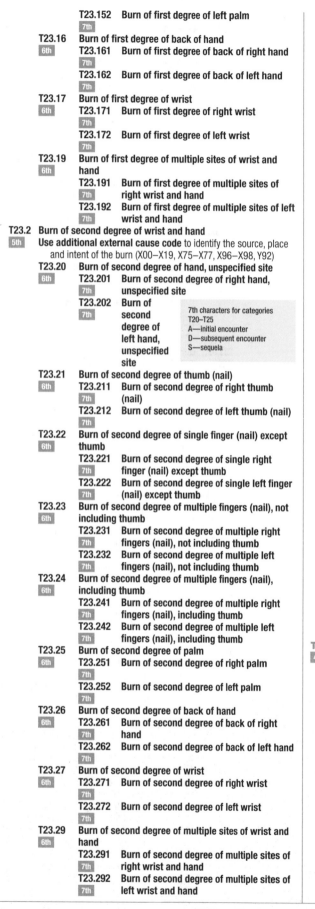

T23.152 Burn of first degree of left palm
7th

T23.16 Burn of first degree of back of hand
6th
T23.161 Burn of first degree of back of right hand
7th
T23.162 Burn of first degree of back of left hand
7th

T23.17 Burn of first degree of wrist
6th
T23.171 Burn of first degree of right wrist
7th
T23.172 Burn of first degree of left wrist
7th

T23.19 Burn of first degree of multiple sites of wrist and hand
6th
T23.191 Burn of first degree of multiple sites of right wrist and hand
7th
T23.192 Burn of first degree of multiple sites of left wrist and hand
7th

T23.2 Burn of second degree of wrist and hand
5th
Use additional external cause code to identify the source, place and intent of the burn (X00–X19, X75–X77, X96–X98, Y92)

T23.20 Burn of second degree of hand, unspecified site
6th
T23.201 Burn of second degree of right hand, unspecified site
7th
T23.202 Burn of second degree of left hand, unspecified site
7th

7th characters for categories T20–T25
A—initial encounter
D—subsequent encounter
S—sequela

T23.21 Burn of second degree of thumb (nail)
6th
T23.211 Burn of second degree of right thumb (nail)
7th
T23.212 Burn of second degree of left thumb (nail)
7th

T23.22 Burn of second degree of single finger (nail) except thumb
6th
T23.221 Burn of second degree of single right finger (nail) except thumb
7th
T23.222 Burn of second degree of single left finger (nail) except thumb
7th

T23.23 Burn of second degree of multiple fingers (nail), not including thumb
6th
T23.231 Burn of second degree of multiple right fingers (nail), not including thumb
7th
T23.232 Burn of second degree of multiple left fingers (nail), not including thumb
7th

T23.24 Burn of second degree of multiple fingers (nail), including thumb
6th
T23.241 Burn of second degree of multiple right fingers (nail), including thumb
7th
T23.242 Burn of second degree of multiple left fingers (nail), including thumb
7th

T23.25 Burn of second degree of palm
6th
T23.251 Burn of second degree of right palm
7th
T23.252 Burn of second degree of left palm
7th

T23.26 Burn of second degree of back of hand
6th
T23.261 Burn of second degree of back of right hand
7th
T23.262 Burn of second degree of back of left hand
7th

T23.27 Burn of second degree of wrist
6th
T23.271 Burn of second degree of right wrist
7th
T23.272 Burn of second degree of left wrist
7th

T23.29 Burn of second degree of multiple sites of wrist and hand
6th
T23.291 Burn of second degree of multiple sites of right wrist and hand
7th
T23.292 Burn of second degree of multiple sites of left wrist and hand
7th

T23.3 Burn of third degree of wrist and hand
5th
Use additional external cause code to identify the source, place and intent of the burn (X00–X19, X75–X77, X96–X98, Y92)

T23.30 Burn of third degree of hand, unspecified site
6th
T23.301 Burn of third degree of right hand, unspecified site
7th
T23.302 Burn of third degree of left hand, unspecified site
7th

T23.31 Burn of third degree of thumb (nail)
6th
T23.311 Burn of third degree of right thumb (nail)
7th
T23.312 Burn of third degree of left thumb (nail)
7th

T23.32 Burn of third degree of single finger (nail) except thumb
6th
T23.321 Burn of third degree of single right finger (nail) except thumb
7th
T23.322 Burn of third degree of single left finger (nail) except thumb
7th

T23.33 Burn of third degree of multiple fingers (nail), not including thumb
6th
T23.331 Burn of third degree of multiple right fingers (nail), not including thumb
7th
T23.332 Burn of third degree of multiple left fingers (nail), not including thumb
7th

T23.34 Burn of third degree of multiple fingers (nail), including thumb
6th
T23.341 Burn of third degree of multiple right fingers (nail), including thumb
7th
T23.342 Burn of third degree of multiple left fingers (nail), including thumb
7th

T23.35 Burn of third degree of palm
6th
T23.351 Burn of third degree of right palm
7th
T23.352 Burn of third degree of left palm
7th

T23.36 Burn of third degree of back of hand
6th
T23.361 Burn of third degree of back of right hand
7th
T23.362 Burn of third degree of back of left hand
7th

T23.37 Burn of third degree of wrist
6th
T23.371 Burn of third degree of right wrist
7th
T23.372 Burn of third degree of left wrist
7th

T23.39 Burn of third degree of multiple sites of wrist and hand
6th
T23.391 Burn of third degree of multiple sites of right wrist and hand
7th
T23.392 Burn of third degree of multiple sites of left wrist and hand
7th

T24 BURN AND CORROSION OF LOWER LIMB, EXCEPT
4th ANKLE AND FOOT
Excludes2: burn and corrosion of ankle and foot (T25.-)
burn and corrosion of hip region (T21.-)

T24.0 Burn of unspecified degree of lower limb, except ankle
5th and foot
Use additional external cause code to identify the source, place and intent of the burn (X00–X19, X75–X77, X96–X98, Y92)

T24.00 Burn of unspecified degree of unspecified site of
6th lower limb, except ankle and foot
T24.001 Burn of unspecified degree of unspecified site of right lower limb, except ankle and foot
7th
T24.002 Burn of unspecified degree of unspecified site of left lower limb, except ankle and foot
7th

T24.01 Burn of unspecified degree of thigh
6th
T24.011 Burn of unspecified degree of right thigh
7th
T24.012 Burn of unspecified degree of left thigh
7th

4th 5th 6th 7th Additional Character Required ✓ 3-character code

Unspecified laterality codes were excluded here.

• =New Code
▲ =Revised Code
▣ =Social determinants of health

Excludes1—Not coded here, do not use together
Excludes2—Not included here

390 PEDIATRIC ICD-10-CM 2021: A MANUAL FOR PROVIDER-BASED CODING

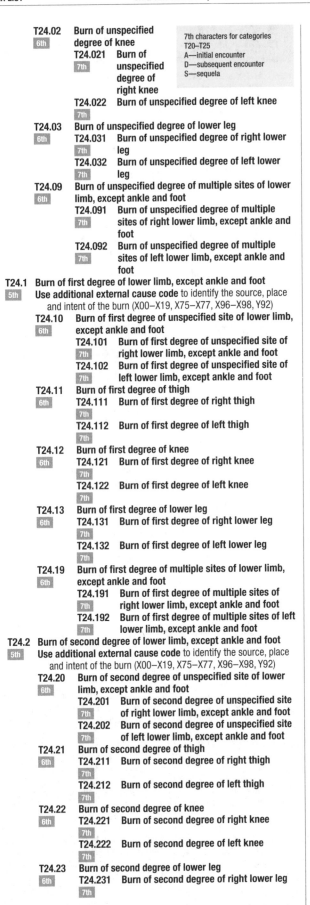

T24.02 **Burn of unspecified degree of knee** `6th`
 T24.021 **Burn of unspecified degree of right knee** `7th`
 T24.022 **Burn of unspecified degree of left knee** `7th`

7th characters for categories
T20–T25
A—initial encounter
D—subsequent encounter
S—sequela

T24.03 **Burn of unspecified degree of lower leg** `6th`
 T24.031 **Burn of unspecified degree of right lower leg** `7th`
 T24.032 **Burn of unspecified degree of left lower leg** `7th`

T24.09 **Burn of unspecified degree of multiple sites of lower limb, except ankle and foot** `6th`
 T24.091 **Burn of unspecified degree of multiple sites of right lower limb, except ankle and foot** `7th`
 T24.092 **Burn of unspecified degree of multiple sites of left lower limb, except ankle and foot** `7th`

T24.1 **Burn of first degree of lower limb, except ankle and foot** `5th`
 Use additional external cause code to identify the source, place and intent of the burn (X00–X19, X75–X77, X96–X98, Y92)

 T24.10 **Burn of first degree of unspecified site of lower limb, except ankle and foot** `6th`
 T24.101 **Burn of first degree of unspecified site of right lower limb, except ankle and foot** `7th`
 T24.102 **Burn of first degree of unspecified site of left lower limb, except ankle and foot** `7th`

 T24.11 **Burn of first degree of thigh** `6th`
 T24.111 **Burn of first degree of right thigh** `7th`
 T24.112 **Burn of first degree of left thigh** `7th`

 T24.12 **Burn of first degree of knee** `6th`
 T24.121 **Burn of first degree of right knee** `7th`
 T24.122 **Burn of first degree of left knee** `7th`

 T24.13 **Burn of first degree of lower leg** `6th`
 T24.131 **Burn of first degree of right lower leg** `7th`
 T24.132 **Burn of first degree of left lower leg** `7th`

 T24.19 **Burn of first degree of multiple sites of lower limb, except ankle and foot** `6th`
 T24.191 **Burn of first degree of multiple sites of right lower limb, except ankle and foot** `7th`
 T24.192 **Burn of first degree of multiple sites of left lower limb, except ankle and foot** `7th`

T24.2 **Burn of second degree of lower limb, except ankle and foot** `5th`
 Use additional external cause code to identify the source, place and intent of the burn (X00–X19, X75–X77, X96–X98, Y92)

 T24.20 **Burn of second degree of unspecified site of lower limb, except ankle and foot** `6th`
 T24.201 **Burn of second degree of unspecified site of right lower limb, except ankle and foot** `7th`
 T24.202 **Burn of second degree of unspecified site of left lower limb, except ankle and foot** `7th`

 T24.21 **Burn of second degree of thigh** `6th`
 T24.211 **Burn of second degree of right thigh** `7th`
 T24.212 **Burn of second degree of left thigh** `7th`

 T24.22 **Burn of second degree of knee** `6th`
 T24.221 **Burn of second degree of right knee** `7th`
 T24.222 **Burn of second degree of left knee** `7th`

 T24.23 **Burn of second degree of lower leg** `6th`
 T24.231 **Burn of second degree of right lower leg** `7th`
 T24.232 **Burn of second degree of left lower leg** `7th`

 T24.29 **Burn of second degree of multiple sites of lower limb, except ankle and foot** `6th`
 T24.291 **Burn of second degree of multiple sites of right lower limb, except ankle and foot** `7th`
 T24.292 **Burn of second degree of multiple sites of left lower limb, except ankle and foot** `7th`

T24.3 **Burn of third degree of lower limb, except ankle and foot** `5th`
 Use additional external cause code to identify the source, place and intent of the burn (X00–X19, X75–X77, X96–X98, Y92)

 T24.30 **Burn of third degree of unspecified site of lower limb, except ankle and foot** `6th`
 T24.301 **Burn of third degree of unspecified site of right lower limb, except ankle and foot** `7th`
 T24.302 **Burn of third degree of unspecified site of left lower limb, except ankle and foot** `7th`

 T24.31 **Burn of third degree of thigh** `6th`
 T24.311 **Burn of third degree of right thigh** `7th`
 T24.312 **Burn of third degree of left thigh** `7th`

 T24.32 **Burn of third degree of knee** `6th`
 T24.321 **Burn of third degree of right knee** `7th`
 T24.322 **Burn of third degree of left knee** `7th`

 T24.33 **Burn of third degree of lower leg** `6th`
 T24.331 **Burn of third degree of right lower leg** `7th`
 T24.332 **Burn of third degree of left lower leg** `7th`

 T24.39 **Burn of third degree of multiple sites of lower limb, except ankle and foot** `6th`
 T24.391 **Burn of third degree of multiple sites of right lower limb, except ankle and foot** `7th`
 T24.392 **Burn of third degree of multiple sites of left lower limb, except ankle and foot** `7th`

T25 **BURN AND CORROSION OF ANKLE AND FOOT** `4th`

 T25.0 **Burn of unspecified degree of ankle and foot** `5th`
 Use additional external cause code to identify the source, place and intent of the burn (X00–X19, X75–X77, X96–X98, Y92)

 T25.01 **Burn of unspecified degree of ankle** `6th`
 T25.011 **Burn of unspecified degree of right ankle** `7th`
 T25.012 **Burn of unspecified degree of left ankle** `7th`

 T25.02 **Burn of unspecified degree of foot** `6th`
 Excludes2: burn of unspecified degree of toe(s) (nail) (T25.03-)
 T25.021 **Burn of unspecified degree of right foot** `7th`
 T25.022 **Burn of unspecified degree of left foot** `7th`

 T25.03 **Burn of unspecified degree of toe(s) (nail)** `6th`
 T25.031 **Burn of unspecified degree of right toe(s) (nail)** `7th`
 T25.032 **Burn of unspecified degree of left toe(s) (nail)** `7th`

 T25.09 **Burn of unspecified degree of multiple sites of ankle and foot** `6th`
 T25.091 **Burn of unspecified degree of multiple sites of right ankle and foot** `7th`
 T25.092 **Burn of unspecified degree of multiple sites of left ankle and foot** `7th`

 T25.1 **Burn of first degree of ankle and foot** `5th`
 Use additional external cause code to identify the source, place and intent of the burn (X00–X19, X75–X77, X96–X98, Y92)

 T25.11 **Burn of first degree of ankle** `6th`
 T25.111 **Burn of first degree of right ankle** `7th`
 T25.112 **Burn of first degree of left ankle** `7th`

`4th` `5th` `6th` `7th` Additional Character Required   ✓ 3-character code

Unspecified laterality codes were excluded here.

• =New Code
▲ =Revised Code
▣ =Social determinants of health

Excludes1—Not coded here, do not use together
Excludes2—Not included here

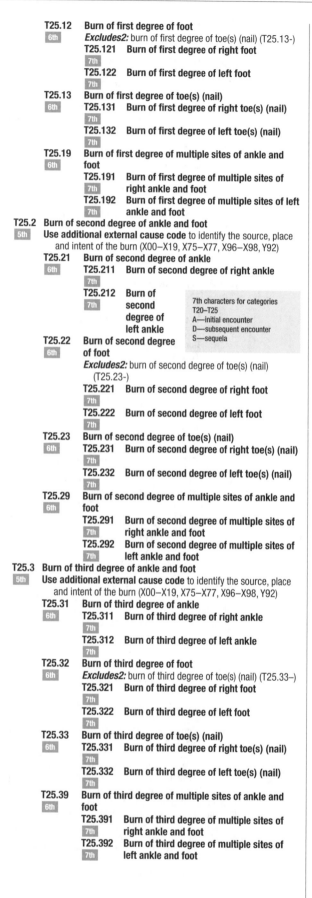

T25.12 Burn of first degree of foot
  6th   *Excludes2:* burn of first degree of toe(s) (nail) (T25.13-)

  T25.121 Burn of first degree of right foot
    7th

  T25.122 Burn of first degree of left foot
    7th

T25.13 Burn of first degree of toe(s) (nail)
  6th

  T25.131 Burn of first degree of right toe(s) (nail)
    7th

  T25.132 Burn of first degree of left toe(s) (nail)
    7th

T25.19 Burn of first degree of multiple sites of ankle and foot
  6th

  T25.191 Burn of first degree of multiple sites of right ankle and foot
    7th

  T25.192 Burn of first degree of multiple sites of left ankle and foot
    7th

T25.2 Burn of second degree of ankle and foot
  5th   Use additional external cause code to identify the source, place and intent of the burn (X00–X19, X75–X77, X96–X98, Y92)

  T25.21 Burn of second degree of ankle
    6th

    T25.211 Burn of second degree of right ankle
      7th

    T25.212 Burn of second degree of left ankle
      7th

  T25.22 Burn of second degree of foot
    6th   *Excludes2:* burn of second degree of toe(s) (nail) (T25.23-)

    T25.221 Burn of second degree of right foot
      7th

    T25.222 Burn of second degree of left foot
      7th

> 7th characters for categories
> T20–T25
> A—initial encounter
> D—subsequent encounter
> S—sequela

  T25.23 Burn of second degree of toe(s) (nail)
    6th

    T25.231 Burn of second degree of right toe(s) (nail)
      7th

    T25.232 Burn of second degree of left toe(s) (nail)
      7th

  T25.29 Burn of second degree of multiple sites of ankle and foot
    6th

    T25.291 Burn of second degree of multiple sites of right ankle and foot
      7th

    T25.292 Burn of second degree of multiple sites of left ankle and foot
      7th

T25.3 Burn of third degree of ankle and foot
  5th   Use additional external cause code to identify the source, place and intent of the burn (X00–X19, X75–X77, X96–X98, Y92)

  T25.31 Burn of third degree of ankle
    6th

    T25.311 Burn of third degree of right ankle
      7th

    T25.312 Burn of third degree of left ankle
      7th

  T25.32 Burn of third degree of foot
    6th   *Excludes2:* burn of third degree of toe(s) (nail) (T25.33–)

    T25.321 Burn of third degree of right foot
      7th

    T25.322 Burn of third degree of left foot
      7th

  T25.33 Burn of third degree of toe(s) (nail)
    6th

    T25.331 Burn of third degree of right toe(s) (nail)
      7th

    T25.332 Burn of third degree of left toe(s) (nail)
      7th

  T25.39 Burn of third degree of multiple sites of ankle and foot
    6th

    T25.391 Burn of third degree of multiple sites of right ankle and foot
      7th

    T25.392 Burn of third degree of multiple sites of left ankle and foot
      7th

(T26–T28) BURNS AND CORROSIONS CONFINED TO EYE AND INTERNAL ORGANS

T26 BURN AND CORROSION CONFINED TO EYE AND ADNEXA
  4th

  T26.0 Burn of eyelid and periocular area
    6th   Use additional external cause code to identify the source, place and intent of the burn (X00–X19, X75–X77, X96–X98, Y92)

> 7th characters for categories
> T26–T28
> A—initial encounter
> D—subsequent encounter
> S—sequela

    T26.01X Burn of right eyelid and periocular area
      7th

    T26.02X Burn of left eyelid and periocular area
      7th

T28 BURN AND CORROSION OF OTHER INTERNAL ORGANS
  4th   Use additional external cause code to identify the source and intent of the burn (X00–X19, X75–X77, X96–X98) and external cause code to identify place (Y92)

  T28.0XX Burn of mouth and pharynx
    7th

  T28.1XX Burn of esophagus
    7th

(T30–T32) BURNS AND CORROSIONS OF MULTIPLE AND UNSPECIFIED BODY REGIONS

T30 BURN AND CORROSION, BODY REGION UNSPECIFIED
  4th

  T30.0 Burn of unspecified body region, unspecified degree
    This code is not for inpatient use. Code to specified site and degree of burns
    Burn NOS
    Multiple burns NOS

> Note: No 7th characters are required for categories T30, T31, and T32.

  T30.4 Corrosion of unspecified body region, unspecified degree
    This code is not for inpatient use. Code to specified site and degree of corrosion
    Corrosion NOS
    Multiple corrosion NOS

T31 BURNS CLASSIFIED ACCORDING TO EXTENT OF BODY SURFACE INVOLVED
  4th

Note: This category is to be used as the primary code only when the site of the burn is unspecified. It should be used as a supplementary code with categories T20–T25 when the site is specified.

Please see full *ICD-10-CM* manual if reporting burns classified according to extent of body surface beyond 10% of body surface.

GUIDELINES

Assign codes from category T31, Burns classified according to extent of body surface involved, or T32, Corrosions classified according to extent of body surface involved, when the site of the burn is not specified or when there is a need for additional data. It is advisable to use category T31 as additional coding when needed to provide data for evaluating burn mortality, such as that needed by burn units. It is also advisable to use category T31 as an additional code for reporting purposes when there is mention of a third-degree burn involving 20 percent or more of the body surface.

Categories T31 and T32 are based on the classic "rule of nines" in estimating body surface involved: head and neck are assigned nine percent, each arm nine percent, each leg 18 percent, the anterior trunk 18 percent, posterior trunk 18 percent, and genitalia one percent. Providers may change these percentage assignments where necessary to accommodate infants and children who have proportionately larger heads than adults, and patients who have large buttocks, thighs, or abdomen that involve burns.

T31.0 Burns involving less than 10% of body surface
T31.1 Burns involving 10–19% of body surface
  5th   **T31.10** Burns involving 10–19% of body surface with 0% to 9% third degree burns
      Burns involving 10–19% of body surface NOS

T31.11   Burns involving 10–19% of body surface with 10–19% third degree burns

T32   **CORROSIONS CLASSIFIED ACCORDING TO EXTENT OF BODY SURFACE INVOLVED**
`4th`

> **Note:** This category is to be used as the primary code only when the site of the corrosion is unspecified. It may be used as a supplementary code with categories T20–T25 when the site is specified.
>
> **T32.0**   **Corrosions involving less than 10% of body surface**

(T36–T50) POISONING BY, ADVERSE EFFECTS OF AND UNDERDOSING OF DRUGS, MEDICAMENTS AND BIOLOGICAL SUBSTANCES

GUIDELINES

Codes in categories T36–T65 are combination codes that include the substance that was taken as well as the intent. No additional external cause code is required for poisonings, toxic effects, adverse effects and underdosing codes.

Do not code directly from the Table of Drugs

Do not code directly from the Table of Drugs and Chemicals. Always refer back to the Tabular List. *Refer to the ICD-10-CM manual for the Table of Drugs.*

Use as many codes as necessary to describe

Use as many codes as necessary to describe completely all drugs, medicinal or biological substances.

If the same code would describe the causative agent

If the same code would describe the causative agent for more than one adverse reaction, poisoning, toxic effect or underdosing, assign the code only once.

If two or more drugs, medicinal or biological substances

If two or more drugs, medicinal or biological substances are taken, code each individually unless a combination code is listed in the Table of Drugs and Chemicals. If multiple unspecified drugs, medicinal or biological substances were taken, assign the appropriate code from subcategory T50.91, Poisoning by, adverse effect of and underdosing of multiple unspecified drugs, medicaments and biological substances.

The occurrence of drug toxicity is classified in ICD-10-CM as follows:

ADVERSE EFFECT

When coding an adverse effect of a drug that has been correctly prescribed and properly administered, assign the appropriate code for the nature of the adverse effect followed by the appropriate code for the adverse effect of the drug (T36–T50). The code for the drug should have a 5th or 6th character "5" (for example T36.0X5-). Examples of the nature of an adverse effect are tachycardia, delirium, gastrointestinal hemorrhaging, vomiting, hypokalemia, hepatitis, renal failure, or respiratory failure.

POISONING

When coding a poisoning or reaction to the improper use of a medication (eg, overdose, wrong substance given or taken in error, wrong route of administration), first assign the appropriate code from categories T36–T50. The poisoning codes have an associated intent as their 5th or 6th character (accidental, intentional self-harm, assault and undetermined. **Use additional code(s)** for all manifestations of poisonings.

> If there is also a diagnosis of abuse or dependence of the substance, the abuse or dependence is assigned as an additional code.
>
> Examples of poisoning include:

Error was made in drug prescription

Errors made in drug prescription or in the administration of the drug by provider, nurse, patient, or other person.

Overdose of a drug intentionally taken

If an overdose of a drug was intentionally taken or administered and resulted in drug toxicity, it would be coded as a poisoning.

Nonprescribed drug taken with correctly prescribed and properly administered drug

If a nonprescribed drug or medicinal agent was taken in combination with a correctly prescribed and properly administered drug, any drug toxicity or other reaction resulting from the interaction of the two drugs would be classified as a poisoning.

Interaction of drug(s) and alcohol

When a reaction results from the interaction of a drug(s) and alcohol, this would be classified as poisoning.

> See Chapter 4 if poisoning is the result of insulin pump malfunctions.

UNDERDOSING

Underdosing refers to taking less of a medication than is prescribed by a provider or a manufacturer's instruction. Discontinuing the use of a prescribed medication on the patient's own initiative (not directed by the patient's provider) is also classified as an underdosing. For underdosing, assign the code from categories T36–T50 (fifth or sixth character "6").

> Codes for underdosing should never be assigned as principal or first-listed codes. If a patient has a relapse or exacerbation of the medical condition for which the drug is prescribed because of the reduction in dose, then the medical condition itself should be coded.
>
> Noncompliance (Z91.12-, Z91.13- and Z91.14-) or complication of care (Y63.6–Y63.9) codes are to be used with an underdosing code to indicate intent, if known.

Toxic Effects

When a harmful substance is ingested or comes in contact with a person, this is classified as a toxic effect. The toxic effect codes are in categories T51–T65.

> Toxic effect codes have an associated intent: accidental, intentional self-harm, assault and undetermined.

Includes: adverse effect of correct substance properly administered
     poisoning by overdose of substance
     poisoning by wrong substance given or taken in error
     underdosing by (inadvertently) (deliberately) taking less substance than prescribed or instructed

Code first, for adverse effects, the nature of the adverse effect, such as:
     adverse effect NOS (T88.7)
     aspirin gastritis (K29.-)
     blood disorders (D56–D76)
     contact dermatitis (L23–L25)
     dermatitis due to substances taken internally (L27.-)
     nephropathy (N14.0–N14.2)

Note: The drug giving rise to the adverse effect should be identified by use of codes from categories T36–T50 with fifth or sixth character 5.

Use additional code(s) to specify: manifestations of poisoning
     underdosing or failure in dosage during medical and surgical care (Y63.6, Y63.8–Y63.9)
     underdosing of medication regimen (Z91.12-, Z91.13-)

Excludes1: toxic reaction to local anesthesia in pregnancy (O29.3-)

Excludes2: abuse and dependence of psychoactive substances (F10–F19)
     abuse of non-dependence-producing substances (F55.-)
     drug reaction and poisoning affecting newborn (P00–P96)
     immunodeficiency due to drugs (D84.821)
     pathological drug intoxication (inebriation) (F10–F19)

T36   **POISONING BY, ADVERSE EFFECT OF AND UNDERDOSING OF SYSTEMIC ANTIBIOTICS**
`4th`

> ***Excludes1:*** antineoplastic antibiotics (T45.1-)
>   locally applied antibiotic NEC (T49.0)
>   topically used antibiotic for ear, nose and throat (T49.6)
>   topically used antibiotic for eye (T49.5)

7th characters for categories T36–T50
A—initial encounter
D—subsequent encounter
S—sequela

> **T36.0**   **Poisoning by, adverse effect of and underdosing of penicillins**
> `5th`
> > **T36.0X**   **Poisoning by, adverse effect of and underdosing of penicillins**
> > `6th`
> > > **T36.0X1**   **Poisoning by penicillins, accidental (unintentional)**
> > > `7th`   Poisoning by penicillins NOS
> > >
> > > **T36.0X5**   **Adverse effect of penicillins**
> > > `7th`
> > >
> > > **T36.0X6**   **Underdosing of penicillins**
> > > `7th`

    Additional Character Required   ✓   3-character code   Unspecified laterality codes were excluded here.

• =New Code
▲ =Revised Code
⌂ =Social determinants of health

Excludes1—Not coded here, do not use together
Excludes2—Not included here

T36.1 Poisoning by, adverse effect of and underdosing of
[5th] cephalosporins and other beta-lactam antibiotics

   T36.1X Poisoning by, adverse effect of and underdosing of
   [6th] cephalosporins and other beta-lactam antibiotics

      T36.1X1 Poisoning by cephalosporins and other
      [7th] beta-lactam antibiotics, accidental
      (unintentional)
         Poisoning by cephalosporins and other beta-
         lactam antibiotics NOS

      T36.1X5 Adverse effect of cephalosporins and
      [7th] other beta-lactam antibiotics

      T36.1X6 Underdosing of cephalosporins and other
      [7th] beta-lactam antibiotics

T36.3 Poisoning by, adverse effect of and underdosing of macrolides
[5th]

   T36.3X Poisoning by, adverse effect of and underdosing of
   [6th] macrolides

      T36.3X1 Poisoning by macrolides, accidental
      [7th] (unintentional)
         Poisoning by macrolides NOS

      T36.3X5 Adverse effect of macrolides
      [7th]

      T36.3X6 Underdosing of macrolides
      [7th]

T36.6 Poisoning by, adverse effect of and underdosing of rifampicins
[5th]

   T36.6X Poisoning by, adverse effect of and underdosing of
   [6th] rifampicins

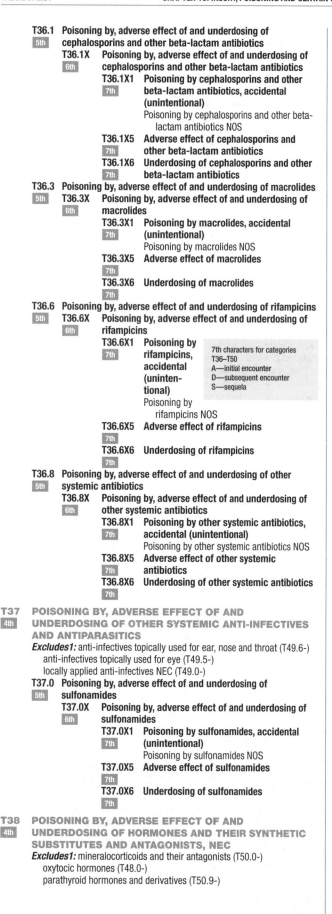

      T36.6X1 Poisoning by
      [7th] rifampicins,
      accidental
      (uninten-
      tional)
        Poisoning by
        rifampicins NOS

> 7th characters for categories
> T36–T50
> A—initial encounter
> D—subsequent encounter
> S—sequela

      T36.6X5 Adverse effect of rifampicins
      [7th]

      T36.6X6 Underdosing of rifampicins
      [7th]

T36.8 Poisoning by, adverse effect of and underdosing of other
[5th] systemic antibiotics

   T36.8X Poisoning by, adverse effect of and underdosing of
   [6th] other systemic antibiotics

      T36.8X1 Poisoning by other systemic antibiotics,
      [7th] accidental (unintentional)
         Poisoning by other systemic antibiotics NOS

      T36.8X5 Adverse effect of other systemic
      [7th] antibiotics

      T36.8X6 Underdosing of other systemic antibiotics
      [7th]

T37 POISONING BY, ADVERSE EFFECT OF AND
[4th] UNDERDOSING OF OTHER SYSTEMIC ANTI-INFECTIVES
AND ANTIPARASITICS

   Excludes1: anti-infectives topically used for ear, nose and throat (T49.6-)
      anti-infectives topically used for eye (T49.5-)
      locally applied anti-infectives NEC (T49.0-)

T37.0 Poisoning by, adverse effect of and underdosing of
[5th] sulfonamides

   T37.0X Poisoning by, adverse effect of and underdosing of
   [6th] sulfonamides

      T37.0X1 Poisoning by sulfonamides, accidental
      [7th] (unintentional)
         Poisoning by sulfonamides NOS

      T37.0X5 Adverse effect of sulfonamides
      [7th]

      T37.0X6 Underdosing of sulfonamides
      [7th]

T38 POISONING BY, ADVERSE EFFECT OF AND
[4th] UNDERDOSING OF HORMONES AND THEIR SYNTHETIC
SUBSTITUTES AND ANTAGONISTS, NEC

   Excludes1: mineralocorticoids and their antagonists (T50.0-)
      oxytocic hormones (T48.0-)
      parathyroid hormones and derivatives (T50.9-)

T38.2 Poisoning by, adverse effect of and underdosing of antithyroid
[5th] drugs

   T38.2X Poisoning by, adverse effect of and underdosing of
   [6th] antithyroid drugs

      T38.2X1 Poisoning by antithyroid drugs, accidental
      [7th] (unintentional)
         Poisoning by antithyroid drugs NOS

      T38.2X5 Adverse effect of antithyroid drugs
      [7th]

      T38.2X6 Underdosing of antithyroid drugs
      [7th]

T38.3 Poisoning by, adverse effect of and underdosing of insulin and
[5th] oral hypoglycemic [antidiabetic] drugs

   T38.3X Poisoning by, adverse effect of and underdosing of
   [6th] insulin and oral hypoglycemic [antidiabetic] drugs

      T38.3X1 Poisoning by insulin and oral
      [7th] hypoglycemic [antidiabetic] drugs,
      accidental (unintentional)
         Poisoning by insulin and oral hypoglycemic
         [antidiabetic] drugs NOS

      T38.3X5 Adverse effect of insulin and oral
      [7th] hypoglycemic [antidiabetic] drugs

      T38.3X6 Underdosing of insulin and oral
      [7th] hypoglycemic [antidiabetic] drugs

T39 POISONING BY, ADVERSE EFFECT OF AND
[4th] UNDERDOSING OF NONOPIOID ANALGESICS,
ANTIPYRETICS AND ANTIRHEUMATICS

T39.0 Poisoning by, adverse effect of and underdosing of salicylates
[5th]

   T39.01 Poisoning by, adverse effect of and underdosing of
   [6th] aspirin
      Poisoning by, adverse effect of and underdosing of
      acetylsalicylic acid

      T39.011 Poisoning by aspirin, accidental
      [7th] (unintentional)

      T39.012 Poisoning by aspirin, intentional self-harm
      [7th]

      T39.015 Adverse effect of aspirin
      [7th]

   T39.09 Poisoning by, adverse effect of and underdosing of
   [6th] other salicylates

      T39.091 Poisoning by salicylates, accidental
      [7th] (unintentional)
         Poisoning by salicylates NOS

      T39.092 Poisoning by salicylates, intentional self-
      [7th] harm

      T39.095 Adverse effect of salicylates
      [7th]

T39.1 Poisoning by, adverse effect of and underdosing of
[5th] 4-Aminophenol derivatives

   T39.1X Poisoning by, adverse effect of and underdosing of
   [6th] 4-Aminophenol derivatives

      T39.1X1 Poisoning by 4-Aminophenol derivatives,
      [7th] accidental (unintentional)
         Poisoning by 4-Aminophenol derivatives NOS

      T39.1X2 Poisoning by 4-Aminophenol derivatives,
      [7th] intentional self-harm

      T39.1X5 Adverse effect of 4-Aminophenol
      [7th] derivatives

T39.3 Poisoning by, adverse effect of and underdosing of other
[5th] nonsteroidal anti-inflammatory drugs [NSAID]

   T39.31 Poisoning by, adverse effect of and underdosing of
   [6th] propionic acid derivatives
      Poisoning by, adverse effect of and underdosing of
      fenoprofen/flurbiprofen/ibuprofen/ketoprofen/
      naproxen/oxaprozin

      T39.311 Poisoning by propionic acid derivatives,
      [7th] accidental (unintentional)

      T39.312 Poisoning by propionic acid derivatives,
      [7th] intentional self-harm

      T39.315 Adverse effect of propionic acid
      [7th] derivatives

   T39.39 Poisoning by, adverse effect of and under-dosing of
   [6th] other nonsteroidal anti-inflammatory drugs [NSAID]

[4th] [5th] [6th] [7th] Additional Character Required   ✓ 3-character code   Unspecified laterality codes were excluded here.

● =New Code
▲ =Revised Code
¤ =Social determinants of health

Excludes1—Not coded here, do not use together
Excludes2—Not included here

T39.391 Poisoning by other nonsteroidal anti-inflammatory drugs [NSAID], accidental (unintentional)
7th
Poisoning by other nonsteroidal anti-inflammatory drugs NOS

T39.392 Poisoning by other nonsteroidal anti-inflammatory drugs [NSAID], intentional self-harm
7th

T39.395 Adverse effect of other nonsteroidal anti-inflammatory drugs [NSAID]
7th

T40 POISONING BY, ADVERSE EFFECT OF AND UNDERDOSING OF NARCOTICS AND PSYCHODYSLEPTICS [HALLUCINOGENS]
4th
Excludes2: drug dependence and related mental and behavioral disorders due to psychoactive substance use (F10.–F19.-)

T40.2 Poisoning by, adverse effect of and underdosing of other opioids
5th

   T40.2X Poisoning by, adverse effect of and underdosing of other opioids
   6th

      T40.2X1 Poisoning by other opioids, accidental (unintentional)
      7th
      Poisoning by other opioids NOS

      T40.2X2 Poisoning by other opioids, intentional self-harm
      7th

      T40.2X5 Adverse effect of other opioids
      7th

T40.4 Poisoning by, adverse effect of and underdosing of other synthetic narcotics
5th

7th characters for categories T36–T50
A—initial encounter
D—subsequent encounter
S—sequela

   •**T40.41** Poisoning by fentanyl or fentanyl analogs
   6th

      •**T40.411** Poisoning by, adverse effect of and underdosing of fentanyl or fentanyl analogs, accidental (unintentional)
      7th

      •**T40.412** Poisoning by fentanyl or fentanyl analogs, intentional self-harm
      7th

      •**T40.413** Poisoning by fentanyl or fentanyl analogs, assault
      7th

      •**T40.414** Poisoning by fentanyl or fentanyl analogs, undetermined
      7th

      •**T40.415** Adverse effect of fentanyl or fentanyl analogs
      7th

      •**T40.416** Underdosing of fentanyl or fentanyl analogs
      7th

   •**T40.42** Poisoning by, adverse effect of and underdosing of tramadol
   6th

      •**T40.421** Poisoning by tramadol, accidental (unintentional)
      7th

      •**T40.422** Poisoning by tramadol, intentional self-harm
      7th

      •**T40.423** Poisoning by tramadol, assault
      7th

      •**T40.424** Poisoning by tramadol, undetermined
      7th

      •**T40.425** Adverse effect of tramadol
      7th

      •**T40.426** Underdosing of tramadol
      7th

   •**T40.49** Poisoning by, adverse effect of and underdosing of other synthetic narcotics
   6th

      •**T40.491** Poisoning by other synthetic narcotics, accidental (unintentional)
      7th

      •**T40.492** Poisoning by other synthetic narcotics, intentional self-harm
      7th

      •**T40.493** Poisoning by other synthetic narcotics, assault
      7th

      •**T40.494** Poisoning by other synthetic narcotics, undetermined
      7th

      •**T40.495** Adverse effect of other synthetic narcotics
      7th

      •**T40.496** Underdosing of other synthetic narcotics
      7th

T40.5 Poisoning by, adverse effect of and underdosing of cocaine
5th

   T40.5X Poisoning by, adverse effect of and underdosing of cocaine
   6th

      T40.5X1 Poisoning by cocaine, accidental (unintentional)
      7th
      Poisoning by cocaine NOS

      T40.5X2 Poisoning by cocaine, intentional self-harm
      7th

T42 POISONING BY, ADVERSE EFFECT OF AND UNDERDOSING OF ANTI-EPILEPTIC, SEDATIVE-HYPNOTIC AND ANTI-PARKINSONISM DRUGS
4th
Excludes2: drug dependence and related mental and behavioral disorders due to psychoactive substance use (F10.–F19.-)

T42.0 Poisoning by, adverse effect of and underdosing of hydantoin derivatives
5th

   T42.0X Poisoning by, adverse effect of and underdosing of hydantoin derivatives
   6th

      T42.0X1 Poisoning by hydantoin derivatives, accidental (unintentional)
      7th
      Poisoning by hydantoin derivatives NOS

      T42.0X2 Poisoning by hydantoin derivatives, intentional self-harm
      7th

      T42.0X5 Adverse effect of hydantoin derivatives
      7th

      T42.0X6 Underdosing of hydantoin derivatives
      7th

T42.3 Poisoning by, adverse effect of and underdosing of barbiturates
5th
Excludes1: poisoning by, adverse effect of and underdosing of thiobarbiturates (T41.1-)

   T42.3X Poisoning by, adverse effect of and underdosing of barbiturates
   6th

      T42.3X1 Poisoning by barbiturates, accidental (unintentional)
      7th
      Poisoning by barbiturates NOS

      T42.3X2 Poisoning by barbiturates, intentional self-harm
      7th

      T42.3X5 Adverse effect of barbiturates
      7th

      T42.3X6 Underdosing of barbiturates
      7th

T42.4 Poisoning by, adverse effect of and underdosing of benzodiazepines
5th

   T42.4X Poisoning by, adverse effect of and underdosing of benzodiazepines
   6th

      T42.4X1 Poisoning by benzodiazepines, accidental (unintentional)
      7th
      Poisoning by benzodiazepines NOS

      T42.4X2 Poisoning by benzodiazepines, intentional self-harm
      7th

      T42.4X5 Adverse effect of benzo-diazepines
      7th

      T42.4X6 Underdosing of benzodiazepines
      7th

T42.6 Poisoning by, adverse effect of and underdosing of other antiepileptic and sedative-hypnotic drugs
5th
Poisoning by, adverse effect of and underdosing of methaqualone
Poisoning by, adverse effect of and underdosing of valproic acid
Excludes1: poisoning by, adverse effect of and underdosing of carbamazepine (T42.1-)

   T42.6X Poisoning by, adverse effect of and underdosing of other antiepileptic and sedative-hypnotic drugs
   6th

      T42.6X5 Adverse effect of other antiepileptic and sedative-hypnotic drugs
      7th

T43 POISONING BY, ADVERSE EFFECT OF AND UNDERDOSING OF PSYCHOTROPIC DRUGS, NEC
4th
Excludes1: appetite depressants (T50.5-)
   barbiturates (T42.3-)
   benzodiazepines (T42.4-)
   methaqualone (T42.6-)
   psychodysleptics [hallucinogens] (T40.7–T40.9-)
Excludes2: drug dependence and related mental and behavioral disorders due to psychoactive substance use (F10.–F19.-)

4th	5th	6th	7th	Additional Character Required	✓	3-character code

Unspecified laterality codes were excluded here.

• =New Code
▲ =Revised Code
🔲 =Social determinants of health

Excludes1—Not coded here, do not use together
Excludes2—Not included here

T43.0 [5th] **Poisoning by, adverse effect of and underdosing of tricyclic and tetracyclic antidepressants**

    T43.01 [6th] **Poisoning by, adverse effect of and underdosing of tricyclic antidepressants**

        T43.011 [7th] **Poisoning by tricyclic antidepressants, accidental (unintentional)**
           Poisoning by tricyclic antidepressants NOS

        T43.012 [7th] **Poisoning by tricyclic antidepressants, intentional self-harm**

        T43.015 [7th] **Adverse effect of tricyclic antidepressants**

        T43.016 [7th] **Underdosing of tricyclic antidepressants**

    T43.02 [6th] **Poisoning by, adverse effect of and underdosing of tetracyclic antidepressants**

        T43.021 [7th] **Poisoning by tetracyclic antidepressants, accidental (unintentional)**
           Poisoning by tetracyclic antidepressants NOS

        T43.022 [7th] **Poisoning by tetracyclic antidepressants, intentional self-harm**

        T43.025 [7th] **Adverse effect of tetracyclic antidepressants**

        T43.026 [7th] **Underdosing of tetracyclic antidepressants**

T43.3 [5th] **Poisoning by, adverse effect of and underdosing of phenothiazine antipsychotics and neuroleptics**

    T43.3X [6th] **Poisoning by, adverse effect of and underdosing of phenothiazine antipsychotics and neuroleptics**

> 7th characters for categories T36–T50
> A—initial encounter
> D—subsequent encounter
> S—sequela

        T43.3X1 [7th] **Poisoning by phenothiazine antipsychotics and neuroleptics, accidental (unintentional)**
           Poisoning by phenothiazine antipsychotics and neuroleptics NOS

        T43.3X2 [7th] **Poisoning by phenothiazine antipsychotics and neuroleptics, intentional self-harm**

        T43.3X5 [7th] **Adverse effect of phenothiazine antipsychotics and neuroleptics**

        T43.3X6 [7th] **Underdosing of phenothiazine antipsychotics and neuroleptics**

T43.6 [5th] **Poisoning by, adverse effect of and underdosing of psychostimulants**

Excludes1: poisoning by, adverse effect of and underdosing of cocaine (T40.5-)

    T43.62 [6th] **Poisoning by, adverse effect of and underdosing of amphetamines**
    Poisoning by, adverse effect of and underdosing of methamphetamines

        T43.621 [7th] **Poisoning by amphetamines, accidental (unintentional)**
           Poisoning by amphetamines NOS

        T43.622 [7th] **Poisoning by amphetamines, intentional self-harm**

        T43.625 [7th] **Adverse effect of amphetamines**

    T43.63 [6th] **Poisoning by, adverse effect of and underdosing of methylphenidate**

        T43.631 [7th] **Poisoning by methyl-phenidate, accidental (unintentional)**
           Poisoning by methylphenidate NOS

        T43.632 [7th] **Poisoning by methylphenidate, intentional self-harm**

        T43.635 [7th] **Adverse effect of methylphenidate**

        T43.636 [7th] **Underdosing of methylphenidate**

    T43.64 [6th] **Poisoning by ecstacy**
    Poisoning by MDMA
    Poisoning by 3,4-methylenedioxymethamphetamine

        T43.641 [7th] **Poisoning by ecstasy, accidental (unintentional)**
           Poisoning by ecstasy NOS

        T43.642 [7th] **Poisoning by ecstasy, intentional self-harm**

        T43.643 [7th] **Poisoning by ecstasy, assault**

        T43.644 [7th] **Poisoning by ecstasy, undetermined**

T43.9 [5th] **Poisoning by, adverse effect of and underdosing of unspecified psychotropic drug**

    T43.91X [7th] **Poisoning by unspecified psychotropic drug, accidental (unintentional)**
    Poisoning by psychotropic drug NOS

    T43.92X [7th] **Poisoning by unspecified psychotropic drug, intentional self-harm**

    T43.95X [7th] **Adverse effect of unspecified psychotropic drug**

    T43.96X [7th] **Underdosing of unspecified psychotropic drug**

T44 [4th] **POISONING BY, ADVERSE EFFECT OF AND UNDERDOSING OF DRUGS PRIMARILY AFFECTING THE AUTONOMIC NERVOUS SYSTEM**

T44.5 [5th] **Poisoning by, adverse effect of and underdosing of predominantly beta-adrenoreceptor agonists**

Excludes1: poisoning by, adverse effect of and underdosing of beta-adrenoreceptor agonists used in asthma therapy (T48.6-)

    T44.5X [6th] **Poisoning by, adverse effect of and underdosing of predominantly beta-adrenoreceptor agonists**

        T44.5X1 [7th] **Poisoning by predominantly beta-adrenoreceptor agonists, accidental (unintentional)**
           Poisoning by predominantly beta-adrenoreceptor agonists NOS

        T44.5X2 [7th] **Poisoning by predominantly beta-adrenoreceptor agonists, intentional self-harm**

        T44.5X5 [7th] **Adverse effect of predominantly beta-adrenoreceptor agonists**

        T44.5X6 [7th] **Underdosing of predominantly beta-adrenoreceptor agonists**

T45 [4th] **POISONING BY, ADVERSE EFFECT OF AND UNDERDOSING OF PRIMARILY SYSTEMIC AND HEMATOLOGICAL AGENTS, NEC**

T45.0 [5th] **Poisoning by, adverse effect of and underdosing of antiallergic and antiemetic drugs**

Excludes1: poisoning by, adverse effect of and underdosing of phenothiazine-based neuroleptics (T43.3)

    T45.0X [6th] **Poisoning by, adverse effect of and underdosing of antiallergic and antiemetic drugs**

        T45.0X1 [7th] **Poisoning by antiallergic and antiemetic drugs, accidental (unintentional)**
           Poisoning by antiallergic and antiemetic drugs NOS

        T45.0X5 [7th] **Adverse effect of antiallergic and antiemetic drugs**

T45.4 [5th] **Poisoning by, adverse effect of and underdosing of iron and its compounds**

    T45.4X [6th] **Poisoning by, adverse effect of and underdosing of iron and its compounds**

        T45.4X1 [7th] **Poisoning by iron and its compounds, accidental (unintentional)**
           Poisoning by iron and its compounds NOS

        T45.4X2 [7th] **Poisoning by iron and its compounds, intentional self-harm**

        T45.4X5 [7th] **Adverse effect of iron and its compounds**

T46 [4th] **POISONING BY, ADVERSE EFFECT OF AND UNDERDOSING OF AGENTS PRIMARILY AFFECTING THE CARDIOVASCULAR SYSTEM**

Excludes1: poisoning by, adverse effect of and underdosing of metaraminol (T44.4)

[4th] [5th] [6th] [7th] Additional Character Required   ✔ 3-character code   Unspecified laterality codes were excluded here.   ● =New Code   ▲ =Revised Code   ☐ =Social determinants of health   *Excludes1*—Not coded here, do not use together   *Excludes2*—Not included here

T46.0 `5th` Poisoning by, adverse effect of and underdosing of cardiac-stimulant glycosides and drugs of similar action

    T46.0X `6th` Poisoning by, adverse effect of and underdosing of cardiac-stimulant glycosides and drugs of similar action

        T46.0X1 `7th` Poisoning by cardiac-stimulant glycosides and drugs of similar action, accidental (unintentional)
        Poisoning by cardiac-stimulant glycosides and drugs of similar action NOS

        T46.0X2 `7th` Poisoning by cardiac-stimulant glycosides and drugs of similar action, intentional self-harm

        T46.0X5 `7th` Adverse effect of cardiac-stimulant glycosides and drugs of similar action

T47 `4th` **POISONING BY, ADVERSE EFFECT OF AND UNDERDOSING OF AGENTS PRIMARILY AFFECTING THE GASTROINTESTINAL SYSTEM**

    T47.8 `5th` Poisoning by, adverse effect of and underdosing of other agents primarily affecting gastrointestinal system

        T47.8X `6th` Poisoning by, adverse effect of and underdosing of other agents primarily affecting gastro-intestinal system

        T47.8X5 `7th` Adverse effect of other agents primarily affecting gastrointestinal system

T48 `4th` **POISONING BY, ADVERSE EFFECT OF AND UNDERDOSING OF AGENTS PRIMARILY ACTING ON SMOOTH AND SKELETAL MUSCLES AND THE RESPIRATORY SYSTEM**

> 7th characters for categories
> T36–T50
> A—initial encounter
> D—subsequent encounter
> S—sequela

    T48.3 `5th` Poisoning by, adverse effect of and underdosing of antitussives

        T48.3X `6th` Poisoning by, adverse effect of and underdosing of antitussives

        T48.3X5 `7th` Adverse effect of antitussives

    T48.5 `5th` Poisoning by, adverse effect of and underdosing of other anti-common-cold drugs
    Poisoning by, adverse effect of and underdosing of decongestants
    Excludes2: poisoning by, adverse effect of and underdosing of antipyretics, NEC (T39.9-)
    poisoning by, adverse effect of and underdosing of non-steroidal antiinflammatory drugs (T39.3-)
    poisoning by, adverse effect of and underdosing of salicylates (T39.0-)

        T48.5X `6th` Poisoning by, adverse effect of and underdosing of other anti-common-cold drugs

        T48.5X5 `7th` Adverse effect of other anti-common-cold drugs

    T48.6 `5th` Poisoning by, adverse effect of and underdosing of antiasthmatics, NEC
    Poisoning by, adverse effect of and underdosing of beta-adrenoreceptor agonists used in asthma therapy
    Excludes1: poisoning by, adverse effect of and underdosing of beta-adrenoreceptor agonists not used in asthma therapy (T44.5)
    poisoning by, adverse effect of and underdosing of anterior pituitary [adenohypophyseal] hormones (T38.8)

        T48.6X `6th` Poisoning by, adverse effect of and underdosing of antiasthmatics

        T48.6X1 `7th` Poisoning by antiasthmatics, accidental (unintentional)
        Poisoning by antiasthmatics NOS

        T48.6X2 `7th` Poisoning by antiasthmatics, intentional self-harm

        T48.6X5 `7th` Adverse effect of anti-asthmatics

        T48.6X6 `7th` Underdosing of anti-asthmatics

T50 `4th` **POISONING BY, ADVERSE EFFECT OF AND UNDERDOSING OF DIURETICS AND OTHER AND UNSPECIFIED DRUGS, MEDICAMENTS AND BIOLOGICAL SUBSTANCES**

    T50.0 `5th` Poisoning by, adverse effect of and underdosing of mineralocorticoids and their antagonists

        T50.0X Poisoning by, adverse effect of and underdosing of mineralocorticoids and their antagonists

    T50.A `5th` Poisoning by, adverse effect of and underdosing of bacterial vaccines

        T50.A1 `6th` Poisoning by, adverse effect of and underdosing of pertussis vaccine, including combinations with a pertussis component

        T50.A15 `7th` Adverse effect of pertussis vaccine, including combinations with a pertussis component

        T50.A2 `6th` Poisoning by, adverse effect of and underdosing of mixed bacterial vaccines without a pertussis component

        T50.A25 `7th` Adverse effect of mixed bacterial vaccines without a pertussis component

        T50.A9 `6th` Poisoning by, adverse effect of and underdosing of other bacterial vaccines

        T50.A95 `7th` Adverse effect of other bacterial vaccines

        T50.A96 `7th` Underdosing of other bacterial vaccines

    T50.B `5th` Poisoning by, adverse effect of and underdosing of viral vaccines

        T50.B9 `6th` Poisoning by, adverse effect of and underdosing of other viral vaccines

        T50.B95 `7th` Adverse effect of other viral vaccines

    T50.9 `5th` Poisoning by, adverse effect of and underdosing of other and unspecified drugs, medicaments and biological substances

        T50.90 `6th` Poisoning by, adverse effect of and underdosing of unspecified drugs, medicaments and biological substances

        T50.901 `7th` Poisoning by unspecified drugs, medicaments and biological substances, accidental (unintentional)

        T50.902 `7th` Poisoning by unspecified drugs, medicaments and biological substances, intentional self-harm

        T50.905 `7th` Adverse effect of unspecified drugs, medicaments and biological substances

        T50.91 `6th` Poisoning by multiple unspecified drugs, medicaments and biological substances

        T50.911 `7th` Poisoning by multiple unspecified drugs, medicaments and biological substances, accidental (unintentional)

        T50.912 `7th` Poisoning by multiple unspecified drugs, medicaments and biological substances, intentional self-harm

        T50.914 `7th` Poisoning by multiple unspecified drugs, medicaments and biological substances, undetermined

        T50.915 `7th` Adverse effect of multiple unspecified drugs, medicaments and biological substances

        T50.916 `7th` Underdosing of multiple unspecified drugs, medicaments and biological substances

        T50.99 `6th` Poisoning by, adverse effect of and underdosing of other drugs, medicaments and biological substances

        T50.995 `7th` Adverse effect of other drugs, medicaments and biological substances

---

`4th` `5th` `6th` `7th` Additional Character Required   ✔   3-character code   Unspecified laterality codes were excluded here.

• =New Code
▲ =Revised Code
⌑ =Social determinants of health

Excludes1—Not coded here, do not use together
Excludes2—Not included here

CHAPTER 19. INJURY, POISONING AND CERTAIN OTHER CONSEQUENCES OF EXTERNAL CAUSES (T51–T60.0X4)

(T51–T65) TOXIC EFFECTS OF SUBSTANCES CHIEFLY NONMEDICINAL AS TO SOURCE

Note: When no intent is indicated code to accidental. Undetermined intent is only for use when there is specific documentation in the record that the intent of the toxic effect cannot be determined.

Note: Refer to the Table of Drugs first for a complete listing of chemicals and drugs. If the code is not listed in the tabular, please refer to the complete *ICD-10-CM* Manual.

Use additional code(s): for all associated manifestations of toxic effect, such as:
respiratory conditions due to external agents (J60–J70)
personal history of FB fully removed (Z87.821)
to identify any retained FB, if applicable (Z18.-)
Excludes1: contact with and (suspected) exposure to toxic substances (Z77.-)

T52 **TOXIC EFFECT OF ORGANIC SOLVENTS**
`4th`
    Excludes1: halogen derivatives of aliphatic and aromatic hydrocarbons (T53.-)

    T52.0 Toxic effects of petroleum products
`5th`
      Toxic effects of gasoline [petrol]
      Toxic effects of kerosene [paraffin oil]
      Toxic effects of paraffin wax
      Toxic effects of ether petroleum
      Toxic effects of naphtha petroleum
      Toxic effects of spirit petroleum

		7th characters for categories T52–T65 A—initial encounter D—subsequent encounter S—sequela

      T52.0X Toxic effects of petroleum products
`6th`
        T52.0X1 Toxic effect of petroleum products, accidental (unintentional)
`7th`
          Toxic effects of petroleum products NOS
        T52.0X2 Toxic effect of petroleum products, intentional self-harm
`7th`

		7th characters for categories T52–T65 A—initial encounter D—subsequent encounter S—sequela

    T52.8 Toxic effects of other organic solvents
`5th`
      T52.8X Toxic effects of other organic solvents
`6th`
        T52.8X1 Toxic effect of other organic solvents, accidental (unintentional)
`7th`
          Toxic effects of other organic solvents NOS
        T52.8X2 Toxic effect of other organic solvents, intentional self-harm
`7th`

T54 **TOXIC EFFECT OF CORROSIVE SUBSTANCES**
`4th`
    T54.3 Toxic effects of corrosive alkalis and alkali-like substances
`5th`
      Toxic effects of potassium hydroxide
      Toxic effects of sodium hydroxide
      T54.3X Toxic effects of corrosive alkalis and alkali-like substances
`6th`
        T54.3X1 Toxic effect of corrosive alkalis and alkali-like substances, accidental (unintentional)
`7th`
          Toxic effects of corrosive alkalis and alkali-like substances NOS
        T54.3X2 Toxic effect of corrosive alkalis and alkali-like substances, intentional self-harm
`7th`

T56 **TOXIC EFFECT OF METALS**
`4th`
    Includes: toxic effects of fumes and vapors of metals
      toxic effects of metals from all sources, except medicinal substances
    Use additional code to identify any retained metal FB, if applicable (Z18.0-, T18.1-)
    Excludes1: arsenic and its compounds (T57.0)
      manganese and its compounds (T57.2)
    T56.0 Toxic effects of lead and its compounds
`5th`
      T56.0X Toxic effects of lead and its compounds
`6th`
        T56.0X1 Toxic effect of lead and its compounds, accidental (unintentional)
`7th`
          Toxic effects of lead and its compounds NOS

T58 **TOXIC EFFECT OF CARBON MONOXIDE**
`4th`
    Includes: asphyxiation from carbon monoxide
      toxic effect of carbon monoxide from all sources
    T58.0 Toxic effect of carbon monoxide from motor vehicle exhaust
`5th`
      Toxic effect of exhaust gas from gas engine
      Toxic effect of exhaust gas from motor pump
      T58.01X Toxic effect of carbon monoxide from motor vehicle exhaust, accidental (unintentional)
`7th`
      T58.02X Toxic effect of carbon monoxide from motor vehicle exhaust, intentional self-harm
`7th`
      T58.03X Toxic effect of carbon monoxide from motor vehicle exhaust, assault
`7th`
      T58.04X Toxic effect of carbon monoxide from motor vehicle exhaust, undetermined
`7th`
    T58.1 Toxic effect of carbon monoxide from utility gas
`5th`
      Toxic effect of acetylene
      Toxic effect of gas NOS used for lighting, heating, cooking
      Toxic effect of water gas
      T58.11X Toxic effect of carbon monoxide from utility gas, accidental (unintentional)
`7th`
      T58.12X Toxic effect of carbon monoxide from utility gas, intentional self-harm
`7th`
      T58.13X Toxic effect of carbon monoxide from utility gas, assault
`7th`
      T58.14X Toxic effect of carbon monoxide from utility gas, undetermined
`7th`
    T58.9 Toxic effect of carbon monoxide from unspecified source
`5th`
      T58.91X Toxic effect of carbon monoxide from unspecified source, accidental (unintentional)
`7th`
      T58.92X Toxic effect of carbon monoxide from unspecified source, intentional self-harm
`7th`
      T58.93X Toxic effect of carbon monoxide from unspecified source, assault
`7th`
      T58.94X Toxic effect of carbon monoxide from unspecified source, undetermined
`7th`

T59 **TOXIC EFFECT OF OTHER GASES, FUMES AND VAPORS**
`4th`
    Includes: aerosol propellants
    Excludes1: chlorofluorocarbons (T53.5)
    T59.8 Toxic effect of other specified gases, fumes and vapors
`5th`
      T59.89 Toxic effect of other specified gases, fumes and vapors
`6th`
        T59.891 Toxic effect of other specified gases, fumes and vapors, accidental (unintentional)
`7th`
        T59.892 Toxic effect of other specified gases, fumes and vapors, intentional self-harm
`7th`
        T59.894 Toxic effect of other specified gases, fumes and vapors, undetermined
`7th`

T60 **TOXIC EFFECT OF PESTICIDES**
`4th`
    Includes: toxic effect of wood preservatives
    T60.0 Toxic effect of organophosphate and carbamate insecticides
`5th`
      T60.0X Toxic effect of organophosphate and carbamate insecticides
`6th`
        T60.0X1 Toxic effect of organophosphate and carbamate insecticides, accidental (unintentional)
`7th`
          Toxic effect of organophosphate and carbamate insecticides NOS
        T60.0X2 Toxic effect of organophosphate and carbamate insecticides, intentional self-harm
`7th`
        T60.0X3 Toxic effect of organophosphate and carbamate insecticides, assault
`7th`
        T60.0X4 Toxic effect of organophosphate and carbamate insecticides, undetermined
`7th`

`4th` `5th` `6th` `7th` Additional Character Required   ✓ 3-character code   Unspecified laterality codes were excluded here.   • =New Code   ▲ =Revised Code   ¤ =Social determinants of health   ***Excludes1***—Not coded here, do not use together   ***Excludes2***—Not included here

398   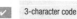   **PEDIATRIC ICD-10-CM 2021: A MANUAL FOR PROVIDER-BASED CODING**

T62 **TOXIC EFFECT OF OTHER NOXIOUS SUBSTANCES**
`4th` **EATEN AS FOOD**

Excludes1: allergic reaction to food, such as:
  anaphylactic shock (reaction) due to adverse food reaction (T78.0-)
  bacterial food borne intoxications (A05.-)
  dermatitis (L23.6, L25.4, L27.2)
  food protein-induced enterocolitis syndrome (K52.21)
  food protein-induced enteropathy (K52.22)
  gastroenteritis (noninfective) (K52.29)
  toxic effect of aflatoxin and other mycotoxins (T64)
  toxic effect of cyanides (T65.0-)
  toxic effect of hydrogen cyanide (T57.3-)
  toxic effect of mercury (T56.1-)

T62.0 **Toxic effect of ingested mushrooms**
  `5th` **T62.0X** **Toxic effect of ingested mushrooms**
    `6th` **T62.0X1** **Toxic effect of ingested mushrooms,**
      `7th` **accidental (unintentional)**
        Toxic effect of ingested mushrooms NOS
    T62.0X2 **Toxic effect of ingested mushrooms,**
      `7th` **intentional self-harm**

T63 **TOXIC EFFECT OF CONTACT WITH VENOMOUS ANIMALS**
`4th` **AND PLANTS**

Includes: bite or touch of venomous animal
  pricked or stuck by thorn or leaf

Excludes2: ingestion of toxic animal or plant (T61.-, T62.-)

T63.0 **Toxic effect of snake venom**
  `5th` **T63.00** **Toxic effect of unspecified snake venom**
    `6th` **T63.001** **Toxic effect of unspecified snake venom,**
      `7th` **accidental (unintentional)**
        Toxic effect of unspecified snake venom NOS

T63.3 **Toxic effect of venom of spider**
  `5th` **T63.30** **Toxic effect of unspecified spider venom**
    `6th` **T63.301** **Toxic effect of unspecified spider venom,**
      `7th` **accidental (unintentional)**
  T63.33 **Toxic effect of venom of brown recluse spider**
    `6th` **T63.331** **Toxic effect of venom of brown recluse**
      `7th` **spider, accidental (unintentional)**
    T63.332 **Toxic effect of venom of brown recluse**
      `7th` **spider, intentional self-harm**
    T63.333 **Toxic effect of venom of brown recluse**
      `7th` **spider, assault**
    T63.334 **Toxic effect**
      `7th` **of venom**
        of brown
        recluse
        spider,
        undeter-
        mined

7th characters for categories
T52–T65
A—initial encounter
D—subsequent encounter
S—sequela

T63.4 **Toxic effect of venom of other arthropods**
  `5th` **T63.42** **Toxic effect of venom of ants**
    `6th` **T63.421** **Toxic effect of venom of ants, accidental**
      `7th` **(unintentional)**
  T63.44 **Toxic effect of venom of bees**
    `6th` **T63.441** **Toxic effect of venom of bees, accidental**
      `7th` **(uninten-tional)**
  T63.45 **Toxic effect of venom of hornets**
    `6th` **T63.451** **Toxic effect of venom of hornets,**
      `7th` **accidental (unintentional)**
  T63.46 **Toxic effect of venom of wasps**
    Toxic effect of yellow jacket
    `6th` **T63.461** **Toxic effect of venom of wasps, accidental**
      `7th` **(unintentional)**
  T63.48 **Toxic effect of venom of other arthropod**
    `6th` **T63.481** **Toxic effect of venom of other arthropod,**
      `7th` **accidental (unintentional)**

T63.6 **Toxic effect of contact with other venomous marine animals**
  `5th` *Excludes1:* sea-snake venom (T63.09)
    Excludes2: poisoning by ingestion of shellfish (T61.78-)
  T63.62 **Toxic effect of contact with other jellyfish**
    `6th` **T63.621** **Toxic effect of contact with other jellyfish,**
      `7th` **accidental (unintentional)**

T63.9 Toxic effect of contact with unspecified venomous animal
  `5th` **T63.91X** Toxic effect of contact with unspecified venomous
    `7th` animal, accidental (unintentional)

T65 **TOXIC EFFECT OF OTHER AND UNSPECIFIED**
`4th` **SUBSTANCES**

T65.8 **Toxic effect of other specified substances**
  `5th` **T65.82** **Toxic effect of harmful algae and algae toxins**
    `6th` Toxic effect of (harmful) algae bloom NOS
      Toxic effect of blue-green algae bloom
      Toxic effect of brown tide
      Toxic effect of cyanobacteria bloom
      Toxic effect of Florida red tide
      Toxic effect of pfiesteria piscicida
      Toxic effect of red tide
    T65.821 **Toxic effect of harmful algae and algae**
      `7th` **toxins, accidental (unintentional)**
        Toxic effect of harmful algae and algae toxins
        NOS

T65.9 Toxic effect of unspecified substance
  `5th` **T65.91X** **Toxic effect of unspecified substance, accidental**
    `7th` **(unintentional)**
      Poisoning NOS
  T65.92X **Toxic effect of unspecified substance, intentional**
    `7th` **self-harm**

(T66–T78) OTHER AND UNSPECIFIED EFFECTS OF EXTERNAL CAUSES

T67 **EFFECTS OF HEAT AND LIGHT**
`4th` *Excludes1:* erythema [dermatitis] ab igne
  (L59.0)
  malignant hyperpyrexia due to
  anesthesia (T88.3)
  radiation-related disorders of the skin
  and subcutaneous tissue (L55–L59)

Excludes2: burns (T20–T31)
  sunburn (L55.-)
  sweat disorder due to heat (L74–L75)

7th characters for categories
T67–T78
A—initial encounter
D—subsequent encounter
S—sequela

T67.0 **Heatstroke and sunstroke**
  `5th` **Use additional code(s)** to identify any associated complications of
    heatstroke, such as:
    coma and stupor (R40.-)
    rhabdomyolysis (M62.82)
    SIRS (R65.1-)
  T67.01X **Heatstroke and sunstroke**
    `7th` Heat apoplexy
      Heat pyrexia
      Siriasis
      Thermoplegia
  T67.02X **Exertional heatstroke**
    `7th`
  T67.09X **Other heatstroke and sunstroke**
    `7th`

T67.1XX **Heat syncope**
  `7th` Heat collapse
T67.2XX **Heat cramp**
  `7th`
T67.3XX **Heat exhaustion, anhydrotic**
  `7th` Heat prostration due to water depletion
    Excludes1: heat exhaustion due to salt depletion (T67.4)
T67.4XX **Heat exhaustion due to salt depletion**
  `7th` Heat prostration due to salt (and water) depletion
T67.5XX **Heat exhaustion, unspecified**
  `7th` Heat prostration NOS
T67.6XX **Heat fatigue, transient**
  `7th`
T67.8XX **Other effects of heat and light**
  `7th`
T67.9XX **Effect of heat and light, unspecified**
  `7th`

T68 HYPOTHERMIA
[✓]
Accidental hypothermia
Hypothermia NOS
Use additional code to identify source of exposure:
Exposure to excessive cold of man-made origin (W93)
Exposure to excessive cold of natural origin (X31)
Excludes1: hypothermia following anesthesia (T88.51)
hypothermia not associated with low environmental temperature (R68.0)
hypothermia of newborn (P80.-)
Excludes2: frostbite (T33–T34)

T70 EFFECTS OF AIR PRESSURE AND WATER PRESSURE
[4th]
T70.0XX Otitic barotrauma
[7th]
Aero-otitis media
Effects of change in ambient atmospheric pressure
or water pressure on ears

T70.1XX Sinus barotrauma
[7th]
Aerosinusitis
Effects of change in ambient atmospheric pressure
on sinuses

T70.2 Other and unspecified effects of high altitude
[5th]
Excludes2: polycythemia due to high altitude (D75.1)

T70.20X Unspecified effects of high altitude
[7th]

T70.29X Other effects of high altitude
[7th]
Alpine sickness
Anoxia due to high altitude
Barotrauma NOS
Hypobaropathy
Mountain sickness

T71 ASPHYXIATION
[4th]
Mechanical suffocation
Traumatic suffocation
Excludes1: acute respiratory distress (syndrome) (J80)
anoxia due to high altitude (T70.2)
asphyxia NOS (R09.01)
asphyxia from carbon monoxide (T58.-)
asphyxia from inhalation of food or FB (T17.-)
asphyxia from other gases, fumes and vapors (T59.-)
respiratory distress (syndrome) in newborn (P22.-)

T71.1 Asphyxiation due to mechanical
[5th] **threat to breathing**
Suffocation due to mechanical
threat to breathing

7th characters for categories
T67–T78
A—initial encounter
D—subsequent encounter
S—sequela

T71.11 Asphyxiation due to
[6th] **smothering under pillow**
T71.111 Asphyxiation due to smothering under
[7th] **pillow, accidental**
Asphyxiation due to smothering under pillow NOS

T71.112 Asphyxiation due to smothering under
[7th] **pillow, intentional self-harm**

T71.113 Asphyxiation due to smothering under
[7th] **pillow, assault**

T71.114 Asphyxiation due to smothering under
[7th] **pillow, undetermined, initial encounter**

T71.12 Asphyxiation due to plastic bag
[6th]
T71.121 Asphyxiation due to plastic bag,
[7th] **accidental**
Asphyxiation due to plastic bag NOS

T71.122 Asphyxiation due to plastic bag,
[7th] **intentional self-harm**

T71.123 Asphyxiation due to plastic bag, assault
[7th]

T71.124 Asphyxiation due to plastic bag,
[7th] **undetermined**

T71.13 Asphyxiation due to being trapped in bed linens
[6th]
T71.131 Asphyxiation due to being trapped in bed
[7th] **linens, accidental**
Asphyxiation due to being trapped in bed linens NOS

T71.132 Asphyxiation due to being trapped in bed
[7th] **linens, intentional self-harm**

T71.133 Asphyxiation due to being trapped in bed
[7th] **linens, assault**

T71.134 Asphyxiation due to being trapped in bed
[7th] **linens, undetermined**

T71.14 Asphyxiation due to smothering under another
[6th] **person's body (in bed)**
T71.141 Asphyxiation due to smothering under
[7th] **another person's body (in bed), accidental**
Asphyxiation due to smothering under
another person's body (in bed) NOS

T71.143 Asphyxiation due to smothering under
[7th] **another person's body (in bed), assault**

T71.144 Asphyxiation due to smothering
[7th] **under another person's body (in bed), undetermined**

T71.15 Asphyxiation due to smothering in furniture
[6th]
T71.151 Asphyxiation due to smothering in
[7th] **furniture, accidental**
Asphyxiation due to smothering in furniture NOS

T71.152 Asphyxiation due to smothering in
[7th] **furniture, intentional self-harm**

T71.153 Asphyxiation due to smothering in
[7th] **furniture, assault**

T71.154 Asphyxiation due to smothering in
[7th] **furniture, undetermined**

T71.16 Asphyxiation due to hanging
[6th]
Hanging by window shade cord
Use additional code for any associated injuries, such as:
crushing injury of neck (S17.-)
fracture of cervical vertebrae (S12.0–S12.2-)
open wound of neck (S11.-)
T71.161 Asphyxiation due to hanging, accidental
[7th]
Asphyxiation due to hanging NOS
Hanging NOS

T71.162 Asphyxiation due to hanging, intentional
[7th] **self-harm**

T71.163 Asphyxiation due to hanging, assault
[7th]

T71.164 Asphyxiation due to hanging,
[7th] **undetermined**

T71.19 Asphyxiation due to mechanical threat to breathing
[6th] **due to other causes**
T71.191 Asphyxiation due to mechanical threat to
[7th] **breathing due to other causes, accidental**
Asphyxiation due to other causes NOS

T71.192 Asphyxiation due to mechanical threat to
[7th] **breathing due to other causes, intentional self-harm**

T71.193 Asphyxiation due to mechanical threat to
[7th] **breathing due to other causes, assault**

T71.194 Asphyxiation due to mechanical threat
[7th] **to breathing due to other causes, undetermined**

T71.2 Asphyxiation due to systemic oxygen deficiency due to low
[5th] **oxygen content in ambient air**
Suffocation due to systemic oxygen deficiency due to low oxygen
content in ambient air

T71.21X Asphyxiation due to cave-in or falling earth
[7th]
Use additional code for any associated cataclysm (X34–X38)

T71.22 Asphyxiation due to being trapped in a car trunk
[6th]
T71.221 Asphyxiation due to being trapped in a car
[7th] **trunk, accidental**

T71.222 Asphyxiation due to being trapped in a car
[7th] **trunk, intentional self-harm**

T71.223 Asphyxiation due to being trapped in a car
[7th] **trunk, assault**

T71.224 Asphyxiation due to being trapped in a car
[7th] **trunk, undetermined**

[4th] [5th] [6th] [7th] Additional Character Required [✓] 3-character code

Unspecified laterality codes were excluded here.

• =New Code
▲ =Revised Code
☐ =Social determinants of health

Excludes1—Not coded here, do not use together
Excludes2—Not included here

T71.23 [6th] Asphyxiation due to being trapped in a (discarded) refrigerator

  T71.231 [7th] Asphyxiation due to being trapped in a (discarded) refrigerator, accidental

  T71.232 [7th] Asphyxiation due to being trapped in a (discarded) refrigerator, intentional self-harm

  T71.233 [7th] Asphyxiation due to being trapped in a (discarded) refrigerator, assault

  T71.234 [7th] Asphyxiation due to being trapped in a (discarded) refrigerator, undetermined

  T71.29X [7th] Asphyxiation due to being trapped in other low oxygen environment

T71.9XX [7th] Asphyxiation due to unspecified cause

Suffocation (by strangulation) due to unspecified cause

Suffocation NOS

Systemic oxygen deficiency due to low oxygen content in ambient air or due to due to mechanical threat to breathing due to unspecified cause

Traumatic asphyxia NOS

T73 [4th] **EFFECTS OF OTHER DEPRIVATION**

T73.0XX [7th] **Starvation**

Deprivation of food

T73.1XX [7th] **Deprivation of water**

T73.2XX [7th] **Exhaustion due to exposure**

T73.3XX [7th] **Exhaustion due to excessive exertion**

Exhaustion due to overexertion

T73.8XX [7th] **Other effects of deprivation**

T74 [4th] **ADULT AND CHILD ABUSE, NEGLECT AND OTHER MALTREATMENT, CONFIRMED**

> **GUIDELINES**
>
> Sequence first the appropriate code from categories T74.- (Adult and child abuse, neglect and other maltreatment, confirmed) or T76.- (Adult and child abuse, neglect and other maltreatment, suspected) for abuse, neglect and other maltreatment, followed by any accompanying mental health or injury code(s).
>
> If the documentation in the medical record states abuse or neglect it is coded as confirmed (T74.-). It is coded as suspected if it is documented as suspected (T76.-).
>
> For cases of confirmed abuse or neglect an external cause code from the assault section (X92–Y08) should be added to identify the cause of any physical injuries. A perpetrator code (Y07) should be added when the perpetrator of the abuse is known. For suspected cases of abuse or neglect, do not report external cause or perpetrator code.
>
> If a suspected case of abuse, neglect or mistreatment is ruled out during an encounter code Z04.71, Encounter for examination and observation following alleged physical adult abuse, ruled out, or code Z04.72, Encounter for examination and observation following alleged child physical abuse, ruled out, should be used, not a code from T76.
>
> If a suspected case of alleged rape or sexual abuse is ruled out during an encounter code Z04.41, Encounter for examination and observation following alleged physical adult abuse, ruled out, or code Z04.42, Encounter for examination and observation following alleged rape or sexual abuse, ruled out, should be used, not a code from T76.
>
> | 7th characters for categories T67–T78 |
> | --- |
> | A—initial encounter |
> | D—subsequent encounter |
> | S—sequela |
>
> **For the victim of a patient suffering from Munchausen syndrome by proxy or Factitious disorder, assign the appropriate code from categories T74, Adult and child abuse, neglect and other maltreatment, confirmed, or T76, Adult and child abuse, neglect and other maltreatment, suspected.**
>
> **If a suspected case of forced sexual exploitation or forced labor exploitation is ruled out during an encounter, code Z04.81, Encounter for examination and observation of victim following forced sexual exploitation, or code Z04.82, Encounter for examination and observation of victim following forced labor exploitation, should be used, not a code from T76.**

Use additional code, if applicable, to identify any associated current injury external cause code to identify perpetrator, if known (Y07.-)

Excludes1: abuse and maltreatment in pregnancy (O9A.3-, O9A.4-, O9A.5-)

adult and child maltreatment, suspected (T76.-)

T74.0 [5th] **Neglect or abandonment, confirmed**

  ▢**T74.02X** [7th] **Child neglect or abandonment, confirmed**

T74.1 [5th] **Physical abuse, confirmed**

Excludes2: sexual abuse (T74.2-)

  ▢**T74.12X** [7th] **Child physical abuse, confirmed**

    Excludes2: shaken infant syndrome (T74.4)

T74.2 [5th] **Sexual abuse, confirmed**

Rape, confirmed

Sexual assault, confirmed

  ▢**T74.22X** [7th] **Child sexual abuse, confirmed**

T74.3 [5th] **Psychological abuse, confirmed**

  ▢**T74.32X** [7th] **Child psychological abuse, confirmed**

Bullying and intimidation, confirmed

Intimidation through social media, confirmed

T74.4XX [7th] **Shaken infant syndrome**

T74.5 [5th] **Forced sexual exploitation, confirmed**

  ▢**T74.51X** [7th] **Adult forced sexual exploitation, confirmed**

  ▢**T74.52X** [7th] **Child sexual exploitation, confirmed**

T74.6 [5th] **Forced labor exploitation, confirmed**

  ▢**T74.61X** [7th] **Adult forced labor exploitation, confirmed**

  ▢**T74.62X** [7th] **Child forced labor exploitation, confirmed**

▢**T74.9** [5th] **Unspecified maltreatment, confirmed**

  ▢**T74.92X** [7th] **Unspecified child maltreatment, confirmed**

T75 [4th] **OTHER AND UNSPECIFIED EFFECTS OF OTHER EXTERNAL CAUSES**

Excludes1: adverse effects NEC (T78.-)

Excludes2: burns (electric) (T20–T31)

T75.1XX [7th] **Unspecified effects of drowning and nonfatal submersion**

Immersion

Excludes1: specified effects of drowning —*code to* effects

T75.3XX [7th] **Motion sickness**

Airsickness

Seasickness

Travel sickness

Use additional external cause code to identify vehicle or type of motion (Y92.81-, Y93.5-)

T75.4XX [7th] **Electrocution**

Shock from electric current

Shock from electroshock gun (taser)

T75.8 [5th] **Other specified effects of external causes**

  T75.89X [7th] **Other specified effects of external causes**

T76 [4th] **ADULT AND CHILD ABUSE, NEGLECT AND OTHER MALTREATMENT, SUSPECTED**

> **GUIDELINES**
>
> See T74 for full guidelines.

Use additional code, if applicable, to identify any associated current injury

Excludes1: adult and child maltreatment, confirmed (T74.-)

suspected abuse and maltreatment in pregnancy (O9A.3-, O9A.4-, O9A.5-)

suspected adult physical abuse, ruled out (Z04.71)

suspected adult sexual abuse, ruled out (Z04.41)

suspected child physical abuse, ruled out (Z04.72)

suspected child sexual abuse, ruled out (Z04.42)

T76.0 [5th] **Neglect or abandonment, suspected**

  ▢**T76.02X** [7th] **Child neglect or abandonment, suspected**

T76.1 [5th] **Physical abuse, suspected**

| [4th] | [5th] | [6th] | [7th] | Additional Character Required | ✓ | 3-character code | Unspecified laterality codes were excluded here. | • =New Code ▲ =Revised Code ▢ =Social determinants of health | *Excludes1*—Not coded here, do not use together *Excludes2*—Not included here |

□**T76.12X Child physical abuse, suspected**
[7th]

T76.2 Sexual abuse, suspected
[5th] Rape, suspected
Excludes1: alleged abuse, ruled out (Z04.7)
□**T76.22X Child sexual abuse, suspected**
[7th]

T76.3 Psychological abuse, suspected
[5th] □**T76.32X Child psychological abuse, suspected**
[7th] Bullying and intimidation, suspected
Intimidation through social media, suspected

T76.5 Forced sexual exploitation, suspected
[5th] □**T76.52X Child sexual exploitation, suspected**
[7th]

T76.6 Forced labor exploitation, suspected
[5th] □**T76.62X Child forced labor exploitation, suspected**
[7th]

T76.9 Unspecified maltreatment, suspected
[5th] □**T76.92X Unspecified child maltreatment, suspected**
[7th]

T78 ADVERSE EFFECTS, NEC
[4th] *Excludes2:* complications of surgical and medical care NEC (T80–T88)
T78.0 Anaphylactic reaction due to food
[5th] Anaphylactic reaction due to adverse food reaction
Anaphylactic shock or reaction due to nonpoisonous foods
Anaphylactoid reaction due to food
T78.00X Anaphylactic reaction due to unspecified food
[7th]

T78.01X Anaphylactic reaction due to peanuts
[7th]

T78.02X Anaphylactic reaction due to shellfish (crustaceans)
[7th]

T78.03X Anaphylactic reaction due to other fish
[7th]

T78.04X Anaphylactic reaction due to fruits and vegetables
[7th]

T78.05X Anaphylactic reaction due to tree nuts and seeds
[7th] *Excludes2:* anaphylactic reaction due to peanuts (T78.01)

T78.06X Anaphylactic reaction due to food additives
[7th]

T78.07X Anaphylactic reaction due to milk and dairy products
[7th]

T78.08X Anaphylactic reaction due to eggs
[7th]

T78.09X Anaphylactic reaction due to other food products
[7th]

T78.1XX Other adverse food reactions, NEC
[7th] **Use additional code** to identify the type of reaction, if applicable

7th characters for categories T67–T78
A—initial encounter
D—subsequent encounter
S—sequela

Excludes1: anaphylactic reaction or shock due to adverse food reaction (T78.0-)
anaphylactic reaction due to food (T78.0-)
bacterial food borne intoxications (A05.-)
Excludes2: allergic and dietetic gastroenteritis and colitis (K52.29)
allergic rhinitis due to food (J30.5)
dermatitis due to food in contact with skin (L23.6, L24.6, L25.4)
dermatitis due to ingested food (L27.2)
food protein-induced enterocolitis syndrome (K52.21)
food protein-induced enteropathy (K52.22)

T78.2XX Anaphylactic shock, unspecified
[7th] Allergic shock
Anaphylactic reaction
Anaphylaxis
Excludes1: anaphylactic reaction or shock due to adverse effect of correct medicinal substance properly administered (T88.6)
anaphylactic reaction or shock due to adverse food reaction (T78.0-)
anaphylactic reaction or shock due to serum (T80.5-)

T78.3XX Angioneurotic edema
[7th] Allergic angioedema
Giant urticaria
Quincke's edema
Excludes1: serum urticaria (T80.6-)
urticaria (L50.-)

T78.4 Other and unspecified allergy
[5th] *Excludes1:* specified types of allergic reaction such as:
allergic diarrhea (K52.29)
allergic gastroenteritis and colitis (K52.29)
food protein-induced enterocolitis syndrome (K52.21)
food protein-induced enteropathy (K52.22)
dermatitis (L23–L25, L27.-)
hay fever (J30.1)
T78.40X Allergy, unspecified
[7th] Allergic reaction NOS
Hypersensitivity NOS
T78.49X Other allergy
[7th]

T78.8XX Other adverse effects, NEC
[7th]

(T79) CERTAIN EARLY COMPLICATIONS OF TRAUMA

T79 CERTAIN EARLY COMPLICATIONS OF TRAUMA, NEC
[4th] *Excludes2:* acute respiratory distress syndrome (J80)
complications occurring during or following medical procedures (T80–T88)
complications of surgical and medical care NEC (T80–T88)
newborn respiratory distress syndrome (P22.0)

7th characters for category T79
A—initial encounter
D—subsequent encounter
S—sequela

T79.4XX Traumatic shock
[7th] Shock (immediate) (delayed) following injury
Excludes1: anaphylactic shock due to adverse food reaction (T78.0-)
anaphylactic shock due to correct medicinal substance properly administered (T88.6)
anaphylactic shock due to serum (T80.5-)
anaphylactic shock NOS (T78.2)
anesthetic shock (T88.2)
electric shock (T75.4)
nontraumatic shock NEC (R57.-)
obstetric shock (O75.1)
postprocedural shock (T81.1-)
septic shock (R65.21)
shock complicating abortion or ectopic or molar pregnancy (O00–O07, O08.3)
shock due to lightning (T75.01)
shock NOS (R57.9)
T79.7XX Traumatic subcutaneous emphysema
[7th] *Excludes2:* emphysema NOS (J43)
emphysema (subcutaneous) resulting from a procedure (T81.82)

(T80–T88) COMPLICATIONS OF SURGICAL AND MEDICAL CARE, NEC

Use additional code for adverse effect, if applicable, to identify drug (T36–T50 with fifth or sixth character 5)
Use additional code(s) to identify the specified condition resulting from the complication
Use additional code to identify devices involved and details of circumstances (Y62–Y82)
Excludes2: any encounters with medical care for postprocedural conditions in which no complications are present, such as:
artificial opening status (Z93.-)
closure of external stoma (Z43.-)
fitting and adjustment of external prosthetic device (Z44.-)
burns and corrosions from local applications and irradiation (T20–T32)
complications of surgical procedures during pregnancy, childbirth and the puerperium (O00–O9A)

[4th] [5th] [6th] [7th] Additional Character Required   ✔ 3-character code   Unspecified laterality codes were excluded here.   ● =New Code   ▲ =Revised Code   □ =Social determinants of health   *Excludes1*—Not coded here, do not use together   *Excludes2*—Not included here

mechanical complication of respirator [ventilator] (J95.850)

poisoning and toxic effects of drugs and chemicals (T36–T65 with fifth or sixth character 1–4 or 6)

postprocedural fever (R50.82)

specified complications classified elsewhere, such as:

cerebrospinal fluid leak from spinal puncture (G97.0)

colostomy malfunction (K94.0-)

disorders of fluid and electrolyte imbalance (E86–E87)

functional disturbances following cardiac surgery (I97.0–I97.1)

intraoperative and postprocedural complications of specified body systems (D78.-, E36.-, E89.-, G97.3-, G97.4, H59.3-, H59.-, H95.2-, H95.3, I97.4-, I97.5, J95.6-, J95.7, K91.6-, L76.-, M96.-, N99.-)

ostomy complications (J95.0-, K94.-, N99.5-)

postgastric surgery syndromes (K91.1)

postlaminectomy syndrome NEC (M96.1)

postmastectomy lymphedema syndrome (I97.2)

postsurgical blind-loop syndrome (K91.2)

ventilator associated pneumonia (J95.851)

T80   **COMPLICATIONS FOLLOWING INFUSION, TRANSFUSION**
[4th]   **AND THERAPEUTIC INJECTION**

> *Includes:* complications following perfusion
>
> *Excludes2:* bone marrow transplant rejection (T86.01)
>
> febrile nonhemolytic transfusion reaction (R50.84)
>
> fluid overload due to transfusion (E87.71)
>
> posttransfusion purpura (D69.51)
>
> transfusion associated circulatory overload (TACO) (E87.71)
>
> transfusion (red blood cell) associated hemochromatosis (E83.111)
>
> transfusion related acute lung injury (TRALI) (J95.84)

> | 7th characters for category T80 |
> | --- |
> | A—initial encounter |
> | D—subsequent encounter |
> | S—sequela |

T80.0XX   **Air embolism following infusion, transfusion and**
[7th]   **therapeutic injection**

T80.2   **Infections following infusion, transfusion and therapeutic**
[5th]   **injection**

> *Use additional code* to identify the specific infection, such as: sepsis (A41.9)
>
> *Use additional code* (R65.2-) to identify severe sepsis, if applicable
>
> *Excludes2:* infections specified as due to prosthetic devices, implants and grafts (T82.6–T82.7, T83.5–T83.6, T84.5–T84.7, T85.7)
>
> postprocedural infections (T81.4-)

T80.21   **Infection due to central venous catheter**
[6th]   Infection due to pulmonary artery catheter (Swan-Ganz catheter)

    T80.211   **Bloodstream infection due to central**
    [7th]   **venous catheter**

      Catheter-related bloodstream infection (CRBSI) NOS

      Central line-associated blood-stream infection (CLABSI)

> | 7th characters for category T80 |
> | --- |
> | A—initial encounter |
> | D—subsequent encounter |
> | S—sequela |

      Bloodstream infection due to Hickman catheter/peripherally inserted central catheter (PICC)/portacath (port-a-cath)/pulmonary artery catheter/triple lumen catheter/umbilical venous catheter

    T80.212   **Local infection due to central venous**
    [7th]   **catheter**

      Exit or insertion site infection

      Local infection due to Hickman catheter/peripherally inserted central catheter (PICC)/portacath (port-a-cath)/pulmonary artery catheter/triple lumen catheter/umbilical venous catheter

      Port or reservoir infection

      Tunnel infection

T80.218   **Other infection due to central venous**
[7th]   **catheter**

> Other central line–associated infection/Hickman catheter/peripherally inserted central catheter (PICC)/portacath (port-a-cath)/pulmonary artery catheter/triple lumen catheter/umbilical venous catheter

T80.219   **Unspecified infection due to central**
[7th]   **venous catheter**

> Central line-associated infection NOS
>
> Unspecified infection due to Hickman catheter/peripherally inserted central catheter (PICC)/portacath (port-a-cath)/pulmonary artery catheter/triple lumen catheter/umbilical venous catheter

T80.22X   **Acute infection following transfusion, infusion, or**
[7th]   **injection of blood and blood products**

T80.29X   **Infection following other infusion, transfusion and**
[7th]   **therapeutic injection**

T80.3   **ABO incompatibility reaction due to transfusion of blood or**
[5th]   **blood products**

> *Excludes1:* minor blood group antigens reactions (Duffy) (E) (K(ell)) (Kidd) (Lewis) (M) (N) (P) (S) (T80.A-)

T80.30X   **ABO incompatibility**
[7th]   **reaction due to transfusion of blood or blood products, unspecified**

> ABO incompatibility blood transfusion NOS
>
> Reaction to ABO incompatibility from transfusion NOS

T80.5   **Anaphylactic reaction due to serum**
[5th]

> Allergic shock due to serum
>
> Anaphylactic shock due to serum
>
> Anaphylactoid reaction due to serum
>
> Anaphylaxis due to serum
>
> *Excludes1:* ABO incompatibility reaction due to transfusion of blood or blood products (T80.3-)
>
> allergic reaction or shock NOS (T78.2)
>
> anaphylactic reaction or shock NOS (T78.2)
>
> anaphylactic reaction or shock due to adverse effect of correct medicinal substance properly administered (T88.6)
>
> other serum reaction (T80.6-)

T80.51X   **Anaphylactic reaction due to administration of blood**
[7th]   **and blood products**

T80.52X   **Anaphylactic reaction due to vaccination**
[7th]

T80.59X   **Anaphylactic reaction due to other serum**
[7th]

T80.6   **Other serum reactions**
[5th]

> Intoxication by serum
>
> Protein sickness
>
> Serum rash
>
> Serum sickness
>
> Serum urticaria
>
> *Excludes2:* serum hepatitis (B16–B19)

T80.61X   **Other serum reaction due to administration of blood**
[7th]   **and blood products**

T80.62X   **Other serum reaction due to vaccination**
[7th]

T80.69X   **Other serum reaction due to other serum**
[7th]   **Code also,** if applicable, arthropathy in hypersensitivity reactions classified elsewhere (M36.4)

T80.8   **Other complications following infusion, transfusion and**
[5th]   **therapeutic injection**

T80.81   **Extravasation of vesicant agent**
[6th]   **Infiltration of vesicant agent**

    T80.810   **Extravasation of vesicant antineoplastic**
    [7th]   **chemotherapy**

      Infiltration of vesicant antineoplastic chemotherapy

    T80.818   **Extravasation of other vesicant agent**
    [7th]   Infiltration of other vesicant agent

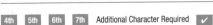 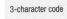 Additional Character Required   ✓ 3-character code   Unspecified laterality codes were excluded here.   ● =New Code   ▲ =Revised Code   ▫ =Social determinants of health   *Excludes1*—Not coded here, do not use together   *Excludes2*—Not included here

PEDIATRIC ICD-10-CM 2021: A MANUAL FOR PROVIDER-BASED CODING   **403**

T80.89X **Other complications following infusion, transfusion and therapeutic injection**
7th
Delayed serologic transfusion reaction (DSTR), unspecified incompatibility
Use additional code to identify graft-versus-host reaction, if applicable, (D89.81-)

T80.9 **Unspecified complication following infusion, transfusion and therapeutic injection**
5th

T80.90X **Unspecified complication following infusion and therapeutic injection**
7th

T80.91 **Hemolytic transfusion reaction, unspecified incompatibility**
6th
Excludes1: ABO incompatibility with hemolytic transfusion reaction (T80.31-)
Non-ABO incompatibility with hemolytic transfusion reaction (T80.A1-)
Rh incompatibility with hemolytic transfusion reaction (T80.41-)

T80.910 **Acute hemolytic transfusion reaction, unspecified incompatibility**
7th

T80.911 **Delayed hemolytic transfusion reaction, unspecified incompatibility**
7th

T80.919 **Hemolytic transfusion reaction, unspecified incompatibility, unspecified as acute or delayed**
7th
Hemolytic transfusion reaction NOS

T80.92X **Unspecified transfusion reaction**
7th
Transfusion reaction NOS

T81 **COMPLICATIONS OF PROCEDURES, NEC**
4th
Use additional code for adverse effect, if applicable, to identify drug (T36–T50 with fifth or sixth character 5)
Excludes2: complications following immunization (T88.0–T88.1)
complications following infusion, transfusion and therapeutic injection (T80.-)
complications of transplanted organs and tissue (T86.-)
specified complications classified elsewhere, such as:
complication of prosthetic devices, implants and grafts (T82–T85)
dermatitis due to drugs and medicaments (L23.3, L24.4, L25.1, L27.0–L27.1)
endosseous dental implant failure (M27.6-)
floppy iris syndrome (IFIS) (intraoperative) H21.81
intraoperative and postprocedural complications of specific body system (D78.-, E36.-, E89.-, G97.3-, G97.4, H59.3-, H59.-, H95.2-, H95.3, I97.4-, I97.5, J95, K91.-, L76.-, M96.-, N99.-)
ostomy complications (J95.0-, K94.-, N99.5-)
plateau iris syndrome (post-iridectomy) (postprocedural) H21.82
poisoning and toxic effects of drugs and chemicals (T36–T65 with fifth or sixth character 1–4 or 6)

T81.1 **Postprocedural shock**
5th
Shock during or resulting from a procedure, NEC
Excludes1: anaphylactic shock NOS (T78.2)
anaphylactic shock due to correct substance properly administered (T88.6)
anaphylactic shock due to serum (T80.5-)
anesthetic shock (T88.2)
electric shock (T75.4)
obstetric shock (O75.1)
septic shock (R65.21)
shock following abortion or ectopic or molar pregnancy (O00–O07, O08.3)
traumatic shock (T79.4)

> 7th characters for categories
> T81–T86
> A—initial encounter
> D—subsequent encounter
> S—sequela

T81.10X **Postprocedural shock unspecified**
7th
Collapse NOS during or resulting from a procedure, NEC
Postprocedural failure of peripheral circulation
Postprocedural shock NOS

T81.11X **Postprocedural cardiogenic shock**
7th

T81.12X **Postprocedural septic shock**
7th
Postprocedural endotoxic shock resulting from a procedure, NEC
Postprocedural gram-negative shock resulting from a procedure, NEC
Code first underlying infection
Use additional code, to identify any associated acute organ dysfunction, if applicable

T81.19X **Other postprocedural shock**
7th
Postprocedural hypovolemic shock

T81.3 **Disruption of wound, NEC**
5th
Disruption of any suture materials or other closure methods
Excludes1: breakdown (mechanical) of permanent sutures (T85.612)
displacement of permanent sutures (T85.622)
disruption of cesarean delivery wound (O90.0)
disruption of perineal obstetric wound (O90.1)
mechanical complication of permanent sutures NEC (T85.692)

T81.30X **Disruption of wound, unspecified**
7th
Disruption of wound NOS

T81.31X **Disruption of external operation (surgical) wound, NEC**
7th
Dehiscence of operation wound NOS
Disruption of operation wound NOS
Disruption or dehis-cence of closure of cornea
Disruption or dehiscence of closure of mucosa
Disruption or dehiscence of closure of skin and subcutaneous tissue
Full-thickness skin disruption or dehiscence
Superficial disruption or dehiscence of operation wound
Excludes1: dehiscence of amputation stump (T87.81)

T81.33X **Disruption of traumatic injury wound repair**
7th
Disruption or dehiscence of closure of traumatic laceration (external) (internal)

T81.4 **Infection following a procedure**
5th
Wound abscess following a procedure
Use additional code to identify infection
Use additional code (R65.2-) to identify severe sepsis, if applicable
Excludes2: bleb associated endophthalmitis (H59.4-)
infection due to infusion, transfusion and therapeutic injection (T80.2-)
infection due to prosthetic devices, implants and grafts (T82.6-T82.7, T83.5-T83.6, T84.5-T84.7, T85.7)
obstetric surgical wound infection (O86.0-)
postprocedural fever NOS (R50.82)
postprocedural retroperitoneal abscess (K68.11)

T81.40X **Infection following a procedure, unspecified**
7th

T81.41X **Infection following a procedure, superficial incisional surgical site**
7th
Subcutaneous abscess following a procedure
Stitch abscess following a procedure

T81.42X **Infection following a procedure, deep incisional surgical site**
7th
Intra-muscular abscess following a procedure

T81.43X **Infection following a procedure, organ and space surgical site**
7th
Intra-abdominal abscess following a procedure
Subphrenic abscess following a procedure

T81.44X **Sepsis following a procedure**
7th
Use additional code to identify the sepsis

T81.49X **Infection following a procedure, other surgical site**
7th

T81.8 **Other complications of procedures, NEC**
5th
Excludes2: hypothermia following anesthesia (T88.51)
malignant hyperpyrexia due to anesthesia (T88.3)

T81.89X **Other complications of procedures, NEC**
7th
Use additional code to specify complication, such as:
postprocedural delirium (F05)

T81.9XX **Unspecified complication of procedure**
7th

> 7th characters for categories
> T81–T86
> A—initial encounter
> D—subsequent encounter
> S—sequela

4th 5th 6th 7th Additional Character Required ✓ 3-character code

Unspecified laterality codes were excluded here.

● =New Code
▲ =Revised Code
☐ =Social determinants of health

Excludes1—Not coded here, do not use together
Excludes2—Not included here

T82 COMPLICATIONS OF CARDIAC AND VASCULAR
`4th` PROSTHETIC DEVICES, IMPLANTS AND GRAFTS

Excludes2: failure and rejection of transplanted organs and tissue (T86.-)

T82.7XX Infection and inflammatory reaction due to other cardiac
`7th` and vascular devices, implants and grafts

Use additional code to identify infection

T82.8 Other specified complications of cardiac and vascular
`5th` prosthetic devices, implants and grafts

    T82.84 Pain due to cardiac and vascular prosthetic devices,
    `6th` implants and grafts

        T82.847 Pain due to cardiac prosthetic devices,
        `7th` implants and grafts

        T82.848 Pain due to vascular prosthetic devices,
        `7th` implants and grafts

    T82.89 Other specified complication of cardiac and vascular
    `6th` prosthetic devices, implants and grafts

        T82.897 Other specified complication of cardiac
        `7th` prosthetic devices, implants and grafts

        T82.898 Other specified complication of vascular
        `7th` prosthetic devices, implants and grafts

T82.9XX Unspecified complication of cardiac and vascular prosthetic
`7th` device, implant and graft

T83 COMPLICATIONS OF GENITOURINARY PROSTHETIC
`4th` DEVICES, IMPLANTS AND GRAFTS

Excludes2: failure and rejection of transplanted organs and tissue (T86.-)

T83.0 Mechanical complication of urinary catheter
`5th`

    T83.09 Other mechanical complication of urinary catheter
    `6th`

      Obstruction (mechanical) of urinary catheter

      Perforation of urinary catheter

      Protrusion of urinary catheter

        T83.090 Other mechanical complication of
        `7th` cystostomy catheter

        T83.091 Other mechanical complication of
        `7th` indwelling urethral catheter

        T83.098 Other mechanical complication of other
        `7th` urinary catheter

          Other mechanical complication of Hopkins
            catheter

          Other mechanical complication of ileostomy
            catheter

          Other mechanical complication of urostomy
            catheter

T83.5 Infection and inflammatory reaction due to prosthetic device,
`5th` implant and graft in urinary system

Use additional code to identify infection

    T83.51 Infection and inflammatory reaction due to urinary
    `6th` catheter

      Excludes2: complications of stoma of urinary tract
      (N99.5-)

        T83.510 Infection and
        `7th` inflammatory
        reaction
        due to
        cystostomy
        catheter

> 7th characters for categories
> T81–T86
> A—initial encounter
> D—subsequent encounter
> S—sequela

        T83.511 Infection and inflammatory reaction due to
        `7th` indwelling urethral catheter

        T83.512 Infection and inflammatory reaction due to
        `7th` nephrostomy catheter

        T83.518 Infection and inflammatory reaction due to
        `7th` other urinary catheter

          Infection and inflammatory reaction due to
            Hopkins catheter or ileostomy catheter or
            urostomy catheter

    T83.59 Infection and inflammatory reaction due to
    `6th` prosthetic device, implant and graft in urinary
    system

        T83.591 Infection and inflammatory reaction due to
        `7th` implanted urinary sphincter

        T83.593 Infection and inflammatory reaction due to
        `7th` other urinary stents

          Infection and inflammatory reaction due to
            ileal conduit stents

          Infection and inflammatory reaction due to
            nephroureteral stent

        T83.598 Infection and inflammatory reaction due to
        `7th` other prosthetic device, implant and graft
        in urinary system

T83.9XX Unspecified complication of genitourinary prosthetic device,
`7th` implant and graft

T85 COMPLICATIONS OF OTHER INTERNAL PROSTHETIC
`4th` DEVICES, IMPLANTS AND GRAFTS

Excludes2: failure and rejection of transplanted organs and tissue (T86.-)

T85.0 Mechanical complication of ventricular intracranial
`5th` (communicating) shunt

    T85.01X Breakdown (mechanical) of ventricular intracranial
    `7th` (communicating) shunt

    T85.02X Displacement of ventricular intracranial
    `7th` (communicating) shunt

      Malposition of ventricular intracranial (communicating)
      shunt

    T85.03X Leakage of ventricular intracranial (communicating)
    `7th` shunt

    T85.09X Other mechanical complication of ventricular
    `7th` intracranial (communicating) shunt

      Obstruction (mechanical) of ventricular intracranial
      (communicating) shunt

      Perforation of ventricular intracranial (communicating)
      shunt

      Protrusion of ventricular intracranial (communicating)
      shunt

T85.6 Mechanical complication of other specified internal and
`5th` external prosthetic devices, implants and grafts

    T85.62 Displacement of other specified internal prosthetic
    `6th` devices, implants and grafts

      Malposition of other specified internal prosthetic devices,
      implants and grafts

        T85.624 Displacement of insulin pump

        T85.628 Displacement of other specified internal
        prosthetic devices, implants and grafts

    T85.69 Other mechanical complication of other specified
    `6th` internal prosthetic devices, implants and grafts

      Obstruction, mechanical of other specified internal
      prosthetic devices, implants and grafts

      Perforation of other specified internal prosthetic devices,
      implants and grafts

      Protrusion of other specified internal prosthetic devices,
      implants and grafts

        T85.694 Other mechanical complication of insulin
        `7th` pump

        T85.695 Other mechanical complication of other
        `7th` nervous system device, implant or graft

          Other mechanical complication of intrathecal
            infusion pump

        T85.698 Other mechanical complication of other
        `7th` specified internal prosthetic devices,
        implant and grafts

          Mechanical complication of nonabsorbable
            surgical material NOS

T85.7 Infection and inflammatory reaction due to other internal
`5th` prosthetic devices, implants and grafts

Use additional code to identify infection

    T85.79X Infection and inflammatory reaction due to other
    `7th` internal prosthetic devices, implants and grafts

T86 COMPLICATIONS OF TRANSPLANTED ORGANS
`4th` AND TISSUE

Codes under category T86, Complications of transplanted organs and
tissues, are for use for both complications and rejection of transplanted
organs. A transplant complication code is only assigned if the complication
affects the function of the transplanted organ. Two codes are required
to fully describe a transplant complication: the appropriate code from
category T86 and a secondary code that identifies the complication.

`4th` `5th` `6th` `7th` Additional Character Required   ✓   3-character code   Unspecified laterality codes were excluded here.   • =New Code   ▲ =Revised Code   ◘ =Social determinants of health   *Excludes1*—Not coded here, do not use together   *Excludes2*—Not included here

CHAPTER 19. INJURY, POISONING AND CERTAIN OTHER CONSEQUENCES OF EXTERNAL CAUSES   (T86.0–T88.9XX)

Pre-existing conditions or conditions that develop after the transplant are not coded as complications unless they affect the function of the transplanted organs.

See I.C.21 for transplant organ removal status

See I.C.2 for malignant neoplasm associated with transplanted organ.

Use additional code to identify other transplant complications, such as:
graft-versus-host disease (D89.81-)
malignancy associated with organ transplant (C80.2)
post-transplant lymphoproliferative disorders (PTLD) (D47.Z1)

T86.0 Complications of bone marrow transplant
> [5th] **T86.01X Bone marrow transplant rejection**
> [7th]
>
> **T86.02X Bone marrow transplant failure**
> [7th]

T86.1 Complications of kidney transplant
> [5th] Patients who have undergone kidney transplant may still have some form of CKD because the kidney transplant may not fully restore kidney function. Code T86.1- should be assigned for documented complications of a kidney transplant, such as transplant failure or rejection or other transplant complication. Code T86.1- should not be assigned for post kidney transplant patients who have CKD unless a transplant complication such as transplant failure or rejection is documented. If the documentation is unclear as to whether the patient has a complication of the transplant, query the provider.
>
> Conditions that affect the function of the transplanted kidney, other than CKD, should be assigned a code from subcategory T86.1, Complications of transplanted organ, kidney, and a secondary code that identifies the complication.
>
> For patients with CKD following a kidney transplant, but who do not have a complication such as failure or rejection, see section I.C.14 CKD and kidney transplant status.
>
> **T86.10X Unspecified complication of kidney transplant**
> [7th]
>
> **T86.11X Kidney transplant rejection**
> [7th]
>
> **T86.12X Kidney transplant failure**
> [7th]
>
> **T86.13X Kidney transplant infection**
> [7th] **Use additional code** to specify infection
>
> **T86.19X Other complication of kidney transplant**
> [7th]

T86.2 Complications of heart transplant
> [5th] *Excludes1:* complication of:
> artificial heart device (T82.5)
> heart-lung transplant (T86.3)
>
> **T86.21X Heart transplant rejection**
> [7th]
>
> **T86.22X Heart transplant failure**
> [7th]
>
> **T86.29 Other complications**
> [6th] **of heart transplant**
>> **T86.290 Cardiac**
>> [7th] **allograft**
>> **vasculopathy**
>> *Excludes1:*
>> atherosclerosis of coronary arteries (I25.75-, I25.76-, I25.81-)
>>
>> **T86.298 Other complications of heart transplant**
>> [7th]

7th characters for categories T81–T86
A—initial encounter
D—subsequent encounter
S—sequela

T86.3 Complications of heart-lung transplant
> [5th] **T86.30X Unspecified complication of heart-lung transplant**
> [7th]
>
> **T86.31X Heart-lung transplant rejection**
> [7th]
>
> **T86.32X Heart-lung transplant failure**
> [7th]
>
> **T86.33X Heart-lung transplant infection**
> [7th] **Use additional code** to specify infection
>
> **T86.39X Other complications of heart-lung transplant**
> [7th]

T86.4 Complications of liver transplant
> [5th] **T86.41X Liver transplant rejection**
> [7th]

T86.42X Liver transplant failure
[7th]

T86.5XX Complications of stem cell transplant
[7th] Complications from stem cells from peripheral blood
Complications from stem cells from umbilical cord

T86.8 Complications of other transplanted organs and tissues
> [5th] **T86.81 Complications of lung transplant**
> [6th] *Excludes1:* complication of heart-lung transplant (T86.3-)
>> **T86.810 Lung transplant rejection**
>> [7th]
>>
>> **T86.811 Lung transplant failure**
>> [7th]

T86.9 Complication of unspecified transplanted organ and tissue
> [5th] **T86.90X Unspecified complication of unspecified transplanted organ and tissue**
> [7th]

T88 OTHER COMPLICATIONS OF SURGICAL AND MEDICAL
[4th] **CARE, NEC**

Excludes2: complication following infusion, transfusion and therapeutic injection (T80.-)
complication following procedure NEC (T81.-)
complications of anesthesia in labor and delivery (O74.-)
complications of anesthesia in pregnancy (O29.-)
complications of anesthesia in puerperium (O89.-)
complications of devices, implants and grafts (T82–T85)
complications of obstetric surgery and procedure (O75.4)
dermatitis due to drugs and medicaments (L23.3, L24.4, L25.1, L27.0–L27.1)
poisoning and toxic effects of drugs and chemicals (T36–T65 with fifth or sixth character 1–4 or 6)
specified complications classified elsewhere

T88.0XX Infection following immunization
[7th] Sepsis following immunization

T88.1XX Other complications following immunization, NEC
[7th] Generalized vaccinia
Rash following immunization
Excludes1: vaccinia not from vaccine (B08.011)
Excludes2: anaphylactic shock due to serum (T80.5-)
other serum reactions (T80.6-)
postimmunization arthropathy (M02.2)
postimmunization encephalitis (G04.02)
postimmunization fever (R50.83)
Use additional code to identify the complication

T88.6XX Anaphylactic reaction due to adverse effect of correct drug
[7th] **or medicament properly administered**
Anaphylactic shock due to adverse effect of correct drug or medicament properly administered
Anaphylactoid reaction NOS
Use additional code for adverse effect, if applicable, to identify drug (T36–T50 with fifth or sixth character 5)
Excludes1: anaphylactic reaction due to serum (T80.5-)
anaphylactic shock or reaction due to adverse food reaction (T78.0-)

T88.7XX Unspecified adverse effect of drug or medicament
[7th] Drug hypersensitivity NOS
Drug reaction NOS
Use additional code for adverse effect, if applicable, to identify drug (T36–T50 with fifth or sixth character 5)
Excludes1: specified adverse effects of drugs and medicaments (A00–R94 and T80–T88.6, T88.8)

T88.8XX Other specified complications of surgical and medical care,
[7th] **NEC**

T88.9XX Complication of surgical and medical care, unspecified
[7th]

[4th] [5th] [6th] [7th] Additional Character Required   ✓ 3-character code   Unspecified laterality codes were excluded here.

• =New Code
▲ =Revised Code
⌂ =Social determinants of health

Excludes1—Not coded here, do not use together
Excludes2—Not included here

Chapter 20. External causes of morbidity (V00–Y99)

GUIDELINES

The external causes of morbidity codes should never be sequenced as the first-listed or principal diagnosis.

External cause codes are intended to provide data for injury research and evaluation of injury prevention strategies. These codes capture how the injury or health condition happened (cause), the intent (unintentional or accidental; or intentional, such as suicide or assault), the place where the event occurred, the activity of the patient at the time of the event, and the person's status (eg, civilian, military).

There is no national requirement for mandatory *ICD-10-CM* external cause code reporting. Unless a provider is subject to a state-based external cause code reporting mandate or these codes are required by a particular payer, reporting of *ICD-10-CM* codes in Chapter 20, External Causes of Morbidity, is not required. In the absence of a mandatory reporting requirement, providers are encouraged to voluntarily report external cause codes, as they provide valuable data for injury research and evaluation of injury prevention strategies.

General External Cause Coding Guidelines

USED WITH ANY CODE IN THE RANGE OF A00.0–T88.9, Z00–Z99
An external cause code may be used with any code in the range of A00.0–T88.9, Z00–Z99, classification that **represents** a health condition due to an external cause. Though they are most applicable to injuries, they are also valid for use with such things as infections or diseases due to an external source, and other health conditions, such as a heart attack that occurs during strenuous physical activity.

EXTERNAL CAUSE CODE USED FOR LENGTH OF TREATMENT
Assign the external cause code, with the appropriate 7th character (initial encounter, subsequent encounter or sequela) for each encounter for which the injury or condition is being treated.

Most categories in Chapter 20 have a 7th character requirement for each applicable code. Most categories in this chapter have three 7th character values: A, initial encounter, D, subsequent encounter and S, sequela. While the patient may be seen by a new or different provider over the course of treatment for an injury or condition, assignment of the 7th character for external cause should match the 7th character of the code assigned for the associated injury or condition for the encounter.

USE THE FULL RANGE OF EXTERNAL CAUSE CODES
Use the full range of external cause codes to completely describe the cause, the intent, the place of occurrence, and if applicable, the activity of the patient at the time of the event, and the patient's status, for all injuries, and other health conditions due to an external cause.

ASSIGN AS MANY EXTERNAL CAUSE CODES AS NECESSARY
Assign as many external cause codes as necessary to fully explain each cause. If only one external code can be recorded, assign the code most related to the principal diagnosis.

THE SELECTION OF THE APPROPRIATE EXTERNAL CAUSE CODE
The selection of the appropriate external cause code is guided by the Alphabetic Index of External Causes and by Inclusion and Exclusion notes in the Tabular List.

EXTERNAL CAUSE CODE CAN NEVER BE A PRINCIPAL DIAGNOSIS
An external cause code can never be a principal (first-listed) diagnosis.

COMBINATION EXTERNAL CAUSE CODES
Certain of the external cause codes are combination codes that identify sequential events that result in an injury, such as a fall which results in striking against an object. The injury may be due to either event or both. The combination external cause code used should correspond to the sequence of events regardless of which caused the most serious injury.

NO EXTERNAL CAUSE CODE NEEDED IN CERTAIN CIRCUMSTANCES
No external cause code from Chapter 20 is needed if the external cause and intent are included in a code from another chapter (eg, T36.0X1- Poisoning by penicillins, accidental (unintentional)).

Place of Occurrence Guideline
Refer to category Y92.

Activity Code
Refer to category Y93.

Place of Occurrence, Activity, and Status Codes Used with other External Cause Code

When applicable, place of occurrence, activity, and external cause status codes are sequenced after the main external cause code(s). Regardless of the number of external cause codes assigned, there should be only one place of occurrence code, one activity code, and one external cause status code assigned to an encounter.

If the Reporting Format Limits the Number of External Cause Codes

If the reporting format limits the number of external cause codes that can be used in reporting clinical data, report the code for the cause/intent most related to the principal diagnosis. If the format permits capture of additional external cause codes, the cause/intent, including medical misadventures, of the additional events should be reported rather than the codes for place, activity, or external status.

Multiple External Cause Coding Guidelines

More than one external cause code is required to fully describe the external cause of an illness or injury. The assignment of external cause codes should be sequenced in the following priority:

If two or more events cause separate injuries, an external cause code should be assigned for each cause. The first-listed external cause code will be selected in the following order:

External codes for child and adult abuse take priority over all other external cause codes.

See Chapter 19, Child and Adult abuse guidelines.

External cause codes for terrorism events take priority over all other external cause codes except child and adult abuse.

External cause codes for cataclysmic events take priority over all other external cause codes except child and adult abuse and terrorism.

External cause codes for transport accidents take priority over all other external cause codes except cataclysmic events, child and adult abuse and terrorism.

Activity and external cause status codes are assigned following all causal (intent) external cause codes.

The first-listed external cause code should correspond to the cause of the most serious diagnosis due to an assault, accident, or self-harm, following the order of hierarchy listed above.

Child and Adult Abuse Guideline
Refer to category Y07.

Unknown or Undetermined Intent Guideline

If the intent (accident, self-harm, assault) of the cause of an injury or other condition is unknown or unspecified, code the intent as accidental intent. All transport accident categories assume accidental intent.

USE OF UNDETERMINED INTENT
External cause codes for events of undetermined intent are only for use if the documentation in the record specifies that the intent cannot be determined.

Sequelae (Late Effects) of External Cause Guidelines

SEQUELAE EXTERNAL CAUSE CODES
Sequelae are reported using the external cause code with the 7th character "S" for sequela. These codes should be used with any report of a late effect or sequela resulting from a previous injury.

SEQUELA EXTERNAL CAUSE CODE WITH A RELATED CURRENT INJURY
A sequela external cause code should never be used with a related current nature of injury code.

USE OF SEQUELA EXTERNAL CAUSE CODES FOR SUBSEQUENT VISITS
Use a late effect external cause code for subsequent visits when a late effect of the initial injury is being treated. Do not use a late effect external cause code for subsequent visits for follow-up care (eg, to assess healing, to receive rehabilitative therapy) of the injury when no late effect of the injury has been documented.

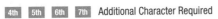 Additional Character Required ✓ 3-character code

•=New Code
▲=Revised Code

Excludes1—Not coded here, do not use together
Excludes2—Not included here

CHAPTER 20. EXTERNAL CAUSES OF MORBIDITY

CHAPTER 20. EXTERNAL CAUSES OF MORBIDITY (V00–V00.188)

Terrorism Guidelines (See *ICD-10-CM* manual for full guidelines.)

Cause of injury identified by the Federal Government (FBI) as terrorism
Cause of an injury is suspected to be the result of terrorism Code Y38.9, Terrorism, secondary effects

External cause status

Refer to category Y99.

Note: This chapter permits the classification of environmental events and circumstances as the cause of injury, and other adverse effects. Where a code from this section is applicable, it is intended that it shall be used secondary to a code from another chapter of the Classification indicating the nature of the condition. Most often, the condition will be classifiable to Chapter 19, Injury, poisoning and certain other consequences of external causes (S00–T88). Other conditions that may be stated to be due to external causes are classified in Chapters 1 to 18. For these conditions, codes from Chapter 20 should be used to provide additional information as to the cause of the condition.

ACCIDENTS (V00–X58)

(V00–V99) TRANSPORT ACCIDENTS

Note: This section is structured in 12 groups. Those relating to land transport accidents (V01–V89) reflect the victim's mode of transport and are subdivided to identify the victim's 'counterpart' or the type of event. The vehicle of which the injured person is an occupant is identified in the first two characters since it is seen as the most important factor to identify for prevention purposes. A transport accident is one in which the vehicle involved must be moving or running or in use for transport purposes at the time of the accident.

Use additional code to identify:
    Airbag injury (W22.1)
    Type of street or road (Y92.4-)
    Use of cellular telephone and other electronic equipment at the time of the
       transport accident (Y93.C-)

Excludes1: agricultural vehicles in stationary use or maintenance (W31.-)
    assault by crashing of motor vehicle (Y03.-)
    automobile or motor cycle in stationary use or maintenance- code to type of
       accident
    crashing of motor vehicle, undetermined intent (Y32)
    intentional self-harm by crashing of motor vehicle (X82)

Excludes2: transport accidents due to cataclysm (X34–X38)
    A traffic accident is any vehicle accident occurring on the public highway [ie, originating on, terminating on, or involving a vehicle partially on the highway]. A vehicle accident is assumed to have occurred on the public highway unless another place is specified, except in the case of accidents involving only off-road motor vehicles, which are classified as nontraffic accidents unless the contrary is stated.
    A nontraffic accident is any vehicle accident that occurs entirely in any place other than a public highway. Please see full *ICD-10-CM* manual for definitions of transport vehicles.

(V00–V09) PEDESTRIAN INJURED IN TRANSPORT ACCIDENT

Includes: person changing tire on transport vehicle
    person examining engine of vehicle broken down in (on side of) road
Excludes1: fall due to non-transport collision with other person (W03)
    pedestrian on foot falling (slipping) on ice and
      snow (W00.-)
    struck or bumped by another person (W51)

V00 [4th] **PEDESTRIAN CONVEYANCE ACCIDENT**
    Use additional place of occurrence and activity external cause codes, if known (Y92.-, Y93.-)
    Excludes1: collision with another person without fall (W51)
      fall due to person on foot colliding with another person on foot (W03)
      fall from non-moving wheelchair, nonmotorized scooter and motorized
        mobility scooter without collision (W05.-)
      pedestrian (conveyance) collision with other land transport vehicle
        (V01–V09)
      pedestrian on foot falling (slipping) on ice and snow (W00.-)

> **7th characters for category V00**
> A—initial encounter
> D—subsequent encounter
> S—sequela

V00.0 [5th] **Pedestrian on foot injured in collision with pedestrian conveyance**
    V00.01X [7th] Pedestrian on foot injured in collision with roller-skater
    V00.02X [7th] Pedestrian on foot injured in collision with skateboarder
    •**V00.031** [7th] Pedestrian on foot injured in collision with rider of standing electric scooter
    •**V00.038** [7th] Pedestrian on foot injured in collision with rider of other standing micro-mobility pedestrian conveyance
    V00.09X [7th] Pedestrian on foot injured in collision with other pedestrian conveyance

V00.1 [5th] **Rolling-type pedestrian conveyance accident**
    Excludes1: accident with baby stroller (V00.82-)
      accident with wheelchair (powered) (V00.81-)
      accident with motorized mobility scooter (V00.83-)
    V00.11 [6th] **In-line roller-skate accident**
      V00.111 [7th] Fall from in-line roller-skates
      V00.112 [7th] In-line roller-skater colliding with stationary object
      V00.118 [7th] Other in-line roller-skate accident
        Excludes1: roller-skater collision with other land transport vehicle (V01–V09 with 5th character 1)
    V00.12 [6th] **Non–in-line roller-skate accident**
      V00.121 [7th] Fall from non–in-line roller-skates
      V00.122 [7th] Non–in-line roller-skater colliding with stationary object
      V00.128 [7th] Other non–in-line roller-skating accident
        Excludes1: roller-skater collision with other land transport vehicle (V01–V09 with 5th character 1)
    V00.13 [6th] **Skateboard accident**
      V00.131 [7th] Fall from skateboard
      V00.132 [7th] Skateboarder colliding with stationary object
      V00.138 [7th] Other skateboard accident
        Excludes1: skateboarder collision with other land transport vehicle (V01–V09 with 5th character 2)
    V00.14 [6th] **Scooter (nonmotorized) accident**
      Excludes1: motorscooter accident (V20–V29)
      V00.141 [7th] Fall from scooter (nonmotorized)
      V00.142 [7th] Scooter (nonmotorized) colliding with stationary object
      V00.148 [7th] Other scooter (nonmotorized) accident
        Excludes1: scooter (nonmotorized) collision with other land transport vehicle (V01–V09 with fifth character 9)
    V00.15 [6th] **Heelies accident**
      Rolling shoe
      Wheeled shoe
      Wheelies accident
      V00.151 [7th] Fall from heelies
      V00.152 [7th] Heelies colliding with stationary object
      V00.158 [7th] Other heelies accident
    V00.18 [6th] **Accident on other rolling-type pedestrian conveyance**
      V00.181 [7th] Fall from other rolling-type pedestrian conveyance
      V00.182 [7th] Pedestrian on other rolling-type pedestrian conveyance colliding with stationary object
      V00.188 [7th] Other accident on other rolling-type pedestrian conveyance

---

[4th] [5th] [6th] [7th] Additional Character Required   3-character code

•=New Code   **Excludes1**—Not coded here, do not use together
▲=Revised Code   **Excludes2**—Not included here

V00.2 `5th` **Gliding-type pedestrian conveyance accident**

> 7th characters for categories V00 and V01
> A—initial encounter
> D—subsequent encounter
> S—sequela

    V00.21 `6th` **Ice-skates accident**
        V00.211 `7th` **Fall from ice-skates**
        V00.212 `7th` **Ice-skater colliding with stationary object**
        V00.218 `7th` **Other ice-skates accident**
          Excludes1: ice-skater collision with other land transport vehicle (V01–V09 with 5th character 9)

    V00.22 `6th` **Sled accident**
        V00.221 `7th` **Fall from sled**
        V00.222 `7th` **Sledder colliding with stationary object**
        V00.228 `7th` **Other sled accident**
          Excludes1: sled collision with other land transport vehicle (V01–V09 with 5th character 9)

V00.3 `5th` **Flat-bottomed pedestrian conveyance accident**

    V00.31 `6th` **Snowboard accident**
        V00.311 `7th` **Fall from snowboard**
        V00.312 `7th` **Snowboarder colliding with stationary object**
        V00.318 `7th` **Other snowboard accident**
          Excludes1: snowboarder collision with other land transport vehicle (V01–V09 with 5th character 9)

    V00.32 `6th` **Snow-ski accident**
        V00.321 `7th` **Fall from snow-skis**
        V00.322 `7th` **Snow-skier colliding with stationary object**
        V00.328 `7th` **Other snow-ski accident**
          Excludes1: snow-skier collision with other land transport vehicle (V01–V09 with 5th character 9)

    V00.38 `6th` **Other flat-bottomed pedestrian conveyance accident**
        V00.381 `7th` **Fall from other flat-bottomed pedestrian conveyance**
        V00.382 `7th` **Pedestrian on other flat-bottomed pedestrian conveyance colliding with stationary object**
        V00.388 `7th` **Other accident on other flat-bottomed pedestrian conveyance**

V00.8 `5th` **Accident on other pedestrian conveyance**

    V00.81 `6th` **Accident with wheelchair (powered)**
        V00.811 `7th` **Fall from moving wheelchair (powered)**
          Excludes1: fall from non-moving wheelchair (W05.0)
        V00.812 `7th` **Wheelchair (powered) colliding with stationary object**
        V00.818 `7th` **Other accident with wheelchair (powered)**

    V00.82 `6th` **Accident with baby stroller**
        V00.821 `7th` **Fall from baby stroller**
        V00.822 `7th` **Baby stroller colliding with stationary object**
        V00.828 `7th` **Other accident with baby stroller**

    • **V00.84** `6th` **Accident with standing micro-mobility pedestrian conveyance**
        • **V00.841** `7th` **Fall from standing electric scooter**
        • **V00.842** `7th` **Pedestrian on standing electric scooter colliding with stationary object**
        • **V00.848** `7th` **Other accident with standing micro-mobility pedestrian conveyance**
          Accident with hoverboard
          Accident with segway

V01 `4th` **PEDESTRIAN INJURED IN COLLISION WITH PEDAL CYCLE**

V01.0 `5th` **Pedestrian injured in collision with pedal cycle in nontraffic accident**
    V01.00X `7th` **Pedestrian on foot injured in collision with pedal cycle in nontraffic accident**
        Pedestrian NOS injured in collision with pedal cycle in nontraffic accident
    V01.01X `7th` **Pedestrian on roller-skates injured in collision with pedal cycle in nontraffic accident**
    V01.02X `7th` **Pedestrian on skateboard injured in collision with pedal cycle in nontraffic accident**
    • **V01.03** `6th` **Pedestrian on standing micro-mobility pedestrian conveyance injured in collision with pedal cycle in nontraffic accident**
        • **V01.031** `7th` **Pedestrian on standing electric scooter injured in collision with pedal cycle in nontraffic accident**
        • **V01.038** `7th` **Pedestrian on other standing micro-mobility pedestrian conveyance injured in collision with pedal cycle in nontraffic accident**
          Pedestrian on hoverboard injured in collision with pedal cycle in nontraffic accident
          Pedestrian on segway injured in collision with pedal cycle in nontraffic accident
    V01.09X `7th` **Pedestrian with other conveyance injured in collision with pedal cycle in nontraffic accident**
        Pedestrian with baby stroller injured in collision with pedal cycle in nontraffic accident
        Pedestrian on ice-skates or nonmotorized scooter or motorized mobility scooter or sled or snowboard or snow-skis or wheelchair (powered) injured in collision with pedal cycle in nontraffic accident

V01.1 `5th` **Pedestrian injured in collision with pedal cycle in traffic accident**
    V01.10X `7th` **Pedestrian on foot injured in collision with pedal cycle in traffic accident**
        Pedestrian NOS injured in collision with pedal cycle in traffic accident
    V01.11X `7th` **Pedestrian on roller-skates injured in collision with pedal cycle in traffic accident**
    V01.12X `7th` **Pedestrian on skateboard injured in collision with pedal cycle in traffic accident**
    • **V01.13** `6th` **Pedestrian on standing micro-mobility pedestrian conveyance injured in collision with pedal cycle in traffic accident**
        • **V01.131** `7th` **Pedestrian on standing electric scooter injured in collision with pedal cycle in traffic accident**
        • **V01.138** `7th` **Pedestrian on other standing micro-mobility pedestrian conveyance injured in collision with pedal cycle in traffic accident**
    V01.19X `7th` **Pedestrian with other conveyance injured in collision with pedal cycle in traffic accident**
        Pedestrian with baby stroller injured in collision with pedal cycle in traffic accident
        Pedestrian on ice-skates or nonmotorized scooter or motorized mobility scooter or sled or snowboard or snow-skis or wheelchair (powered) injured in collision with pedal cycle in traffic accident

V01.9 `5th` **Pedestrian injured in collision with pedal cycle, unspecified whether traffic or nontraffic accident**
    V01.90X `7th` **Pedestrian on foot injured in collision with pedal cycle, unspecified whether traffic or nontraffic accident**
        Pedestrian NOS injured in collision with pedal cycle, unspecified whether traffic or nontraffic accident
    V01.91X `7th` **Pedestrian on roller-skates injured in collision with pedal cycle, unspecified whether traffic or nontraffic accident**
    V01.92X `7th` **Pedestrian on skateboard injured in collision with pedal cycle, unspecified whether traffic or nontraffic accident**

`4th` `5th` `6th` `7th` Additional Character Required   ✔ 3-character code

•=New Code
▲=Revised Code

Excludes1—Not coded here, do not use together
Excludes2—Not included here

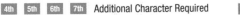 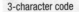

CHAPTER 20. EXTERNAL CAUSES OF MORBIDITY (V01.93–V04.031)

●**V01.93** **Pedestrian on standing micro-mobility pedestrian**
    6th **conveyance injured in collision with pedal cycle, unspecified whether traffic or nontraffic accident**

> 7th characters for categories
> V01–V04
> A—initial encounter
> D—subsequent encounter
> S—sequela

    ●**V01.931** **Pedestrian on standing electric scooter injured in collision with pedal cycle, unspecified whether traffic or nontraffic accident**
        7th

    ●**V01.938** **Pedestrian on other standing micro-mobility pedestrian conveyance injured in collision with pedal cycle, unspecified whether traffic or nontraffic accident**
        7th
        Pedestrian on hoverboard or segway injured in collision with pedal cycle, unspecified whether traffic or nontraffic accident

V01.99X **Pedestrian with other conveyance injured in collision with pedal cycle, unspecified whether traffic or nontraffic accident**
  7th
  Includes: Pedestrian with baby stroller, on ice-skates or nonmotorized scooter or motorized mobility scooter or sled or snowboard or snow-skis or wheelchair (powered) injured in collision with pedal cycle unspecified, whether traffic or nontraffic accident

V02 **PEDESTRIAN INJURED IN COLLISION WITH TWO- OR THREE-WHEELED MOTOR VEHICLE**
4th
Refer to the External Cause of Injuries Table

V03 **PEDESTRIAN INJURED IN COLLISION WITH CAR, PICK-UP TRUCK OR VAN**
4th

V03.0 **Pedestrian injured in collision with car, pick-up truck or van in nontraffic accident**
5th

  V03.00X **Pedestrian on foot injured in collision with car, pick-up truck or van in nontraffic accident**
    7th
    Pedestrian NOS injured in collision with car, pick-up truck or van in nontraffic accident

  V03.01X **Pedestrian on roller-skates injured in collision with car, pick-up truck or van in nontraffic accident**
    7th

  V03.02X **Pedestrian on skateboard injured in collision with car, pick-up truck or van in nontraffic accident**
    7th

  V03.03 **Pedestrian on standing micro-mobility pedestrian conveyance injured in collision with car, pick-up or van in nontraffic accident**

    ●**V03.031** **Pedestrian on standing electric scooter injured in collision with car, pick-up or van in nontraffic accident**
        7th

    ●**V03.038** **Pedestrian on other standing micro-mobility pedestrian conveyance injured in collision with car, pick-up or van in nontraffic accident**
        7th

  V03.09X **Pedestrian with other conveyance injured in collision with car, pick-up truck or van in nontraffic accident**
    7th
    Pedestrian with baby stroller or on ice-skates or nonmotorized scooter or motorized mobility scooter or sled or snowboard or snow-skis or wheelchair (powered) injured in collision with car, pick-up truck or van in nontraffic accident

V03.1 **Pedestrian injured in collision with car, pick-up truck or van in traffic accident**
5th

  V03.10X **Pedestrian on foot injured in collision with car, pick-up truck or van in traffic accident**
    7th
    Pedestrian NOS injured in collision with car, pick-up truck or van in traffic accident

  V03.11X **Pedestrian on roller-skates injured in collision with car, pick-up truck or van in traffic accident**
    7th

  V03.12X **Pedestrian on skateboard injured in collision with car, pick-up truck or van in traffic accident**
    7th

  ●**V03.13** **Pedestrian on standing micro-mobility pedestrian conveyance injured in collision with car, pick-up or van in traffic accident**
    6th

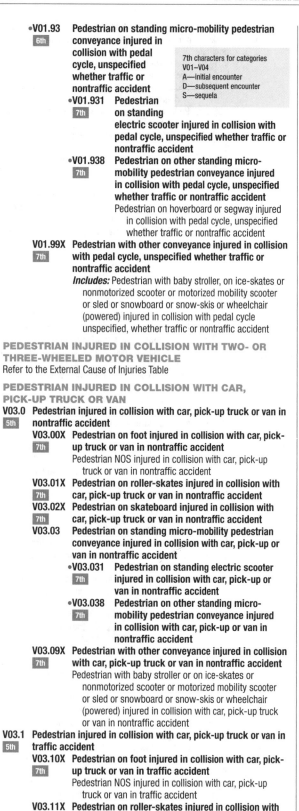

    ●**V03.131** **Pedestrian on standing electric scooter injured in collision with car, pick-up or van in traffic accident**
        7th

    ●**V03.138** **Pedestrian on other standing micro-mobility pedestrian conveyance injured in collision with car, pick-up or van in traffic accident**
        7th
        Pedestrian on hoverboard or segway injured in collision with car, pick-up or van in traffic accident

V03.19X **Pedestrian with other conveyance injured in collision with car, pick-up truck or van in traffic accident**
  7th
  Pedestrian with baby stroller or on ice-skates or nonmotorized scooter or motorized mobility scooter or sled or snowboard or snow-skis or wheelchair (powered) injured in collision with car, pick-up truck or van in traffic accident

V03.9 **Pedestrian injured in collision with car, pick-up truck or van, unspecified whether traffic or nontraffic accident**
5th

  V03.90X **Pedestrian on foot injured in collision with car, pick-up truck or van, unspecified whether traffic or nontraffic accident**
    7th
    Pedestrian NOS injured in collision with car, pick-up truck or van, unspecified whether traffic or nontraffic accident

  V03.91X **Pedestrian on roller-skates injured in collision with car, pick-up truck or van, unspecified whether traffic or nontraffic accident**
    7th

  V03.92X **Pedestrian on skateboard injured in collision with car, pick-up truck or van, unspecified whether traffic or nontraffic accident**
    7th

  ●**V03.93** **Pedestrian on standing micro-mobility pedestrian conveyance injured in collision with car, pick-up or van, unspecified whether traffic or nontraffic accident**
    7th

    ●**V03.931** **Pedestrian on standing electric scooter injured in collision with car, pick-up or van, unspecified whether traffic or nontraffic accident**
        7th

    ●**V03.938** **Pedestrian on other standing micro-mobility pedestrian conveyance injured in collision with car, pick-up or van, unspecified whether traffic or nontraffic accident**
        7th
        Pedestrian on hoverboard or segway injured in collision with car, pick-up or van, unspecified whether traffic or nontraffic accident

V03.99 **Pedestrian with other conveyance injured in collision with car, pick-up truck or van, unspecified whether traffic or nontraffic accident**

V04 **PEDESTRIAN INJURED IN COLLISION WITH HEAVY TRANSPORT VEHICLE OR BUS**
4th
Excludes1: pedestrian injured in collision with military vehicle (V09.01, V09.21)

V04.0 **Pedestrian injured in collision with heavy transport vehicle or bus in nontraffic accident**
5th

  V04.00X **Pedestrian on foot injured in collision with heavy transport vehicle or bus in nontraffic accident**
    7th
    Pedestrian NOS injured in collision with heavy transport vehicle or bus in nontraffic accident

  V04.01X **Pedestrian on roller-skates injured in collision with heavy transport vehicle or bus in nontraffic accident**
    7th

  V04.02X **Pedestrian on skateboard injured in collision with heavy transport vehicle or bus in nontraffic accident**
    7th

  ●**V04.03** **Pedestrian on standing micro-mobility pedestrian conveyance injured in collision with heavy transport vehicle or bus in nontraffic accident**
    6th

    ●**V04.031** **Pedestrian on standing electric scooter injured in collision with heavy transport vehicle or bus in nontraffic accident**
        7th

4th 5th 6th 7th Additional Character Required   ✓ 3-character code   ●=New Code   ***Excludes1***—Not coded here, do not use together
▲=Revised Code   ***Excludes2***—Not included here

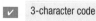

410   **PEDIATRIC ICD-10-CM 2021: A MANUAL FOR PROVIDER-BASED CODING**

• **V04.038 Pedestrian on other standing micro-mobility pedestrian conveyance injured in collision with heavy transport vehicle or bus in nontraffic accident**
[7th]

7th characters for categories V01–V04
A—initial encounter
D—subsequent encounter
S—sequela

Pedestrian on hoverboard or segway injured in collision with heavy transport vehicle or bus in nontraffic accident

V04.09X Pedestrian with other conveyance injured in collision with heavy transport vehicle or bus in nontraffic accident
[7th]

Pedestrian with baby stroller or on ice-skates or nonmotorized scooter or motorized mobility scooter or sled or snowboard or snow-skis or wheelchair (powered) injured in collision with heavy transport vehicle or bus in nontraffic accident

V04.1 Pedestrian injured in collision with heavy transport vehicle or bus in traffic accident
[5th]

V04.10X Pedestrian on foot injured in collision with heavy transport vehicle or bus in traffic accident
[7th]

Pedestrian NOS injured in collision with heavy transport vehicle or bus in traffic accident

V04.11X Pedestrian on roller-skates injured in collision with heavy transport vehicle or bus in traffic accident
[7th]

V04.12X Pedestrian on skateboard injured in collision with heavy transport vehicle or bus in traffic accident
[7th]

• **V04.13 Pedestrian on standing micro-mobility pedestrian conveyance injured in collision with heavy transport vehicle or bus in traffic accident**
[6th]

• **V04.131 Pedestrian on standing electric scooter injured in collision with heavy transport vehicle or bus in traffic accident**
[7th]

• **V04.138 Pedestrian on other standing micro-mobility pedestrian conveyance injured in collision with heavy transport vehicle or bus in traffic accident**
[7th]

Pedestrian on hoverboard or segway injured in collision with heavy transport vehicle or bus intraffic accident

V04.19X Pedestrian with other conveyance injured in collision with heavy transport vehicle or bus in traffic accident
[7th]

Pedestrian with baby stroller or on ice-skates or nonmotorized scooter or motorized mobility scooter or sled or snowboard or snow-skis or wheelchair (powered) injured in collision with heavy transport vehicle or bus in traffic accident

V05 PEDESTRIAN INJURED IN COLLISION WITH RAILWAY TRAIN OR RAILWAY VEHICLE
[7th]

Refer to the External Cause of Injuries Table

V06 PEDESTRIAN INJURED IN COLLISION WITH OTHER NONMOTOR VEHICLE
[7th]

Includes: collision with animal-drawn vehicle, animal being ridden, nonpowered streetcar

Excludes1: pedestrian injured in collision with pedestrian conveyance (V00.0-)

Refer to External Cause of Injuries Table

V09 PEDESTRIAN INJURED IN OTHER AND UNSPECIFIED TRANSPORT ACCIDENTS
[7th]

Refer to External Cause of Injuries Table

(V10–V19) PEDAL CYCLE RIDER INJURED IN TRANSPORT ACCIDENT

Includes: any non-motorized vehicle, excluding an animal-drawn vehicle, or a sidecar or trailer attached to the pedal cycle

Excludes2: rupture of pedal cycle tire (W37.0)

7th characters for categories V10–V18
A—initial encounter
D—subsequent encounter
S—sequela

V10 PEDAL CYCLE RIDER INJURED IN COLLISION WITH PEDESTRIAN OR ANIMAL
[4th]

Excludes1: pedal cycle rider collision with animal-drawn vehicle or animal being ridden (V16.-)

V10.0XX Pedal cycle driver injured in collision with pedestrian or animal in nontraffic accident
[7th]

V10.1XX Pedal cycle passenger injured in collision with pedestrian or animal in nontraffic accident
[7th]

V10.2XX Unspecified pedal cyclist injured in collision with pedestrian or animal in nontraffic accident
[7th]

V10.3XX Person boarding or alighting a pedal cycle injured in collision with pedestrian or animal
[7th]

V10.4XX Pedal cycle driver injured in collision with pedestrian or animal in traffic accident
[7th]

V10.5XX Pedal cycle passenger injured in collision with pedestrian or animal in traffic accident
[7th]

V10.9XX Unspecified pedal cyclist injured in collision with pedestrian or animal in traffic accident
[7th]

V11 PEDAL CYCLE RIDER INJURED IN COLLISION WITH OTHER PEDAL CYCLE
[4th]

V11.0XX Pedal cycle driver injured in collision with other pedal cycle in nontraffic accident
[7th]

V11.1XX Pedal cycle passenger injured in collision with other pedal cycle in nontraffic accident
[7th]

V11.2XX Unspecified pedal cyclist injured in collision with other pedal cycle in nontraffic accident
[7th]

V11.3XX Person boarding or alighting a pedal cycle injured in collision with other pedal cycle
[7th]

V11.4XX Pedal cycle driver injured in collision with other pedal cycle in traffic accident
[7th]

V11.5XX Pedal cycle passenger injured in collision with other pedal cycle in traffic accident
[7th]

V11.9XX Unspecified pedal cyclist injured in collision with other pedal cycle in traffic accident
[7th]

V15 PEDAL CYCLE RIDER INJURED IN COLLISION WITH RAILWAY TRAIN OR RAILWAY VEHICLE
[4th]

Refer to External Cause of Injuries Table

V16 PEDAL CYCLE RIDER INJURED IN COLLISION WITH OTHER NONMOTOR VEHICLE
[4th]

Includes: collision with animal-drawn vehicle, animal being ridden, streetcar

Refer to External Cause of Injuries Table

V13 PEDAL CYCLE RIDER INJURED IN COLLISION WITH CAR, PICK-UP TRUCK OR VAN
[4th]

V13.0XX Pedal cycle driver injured in collision with car, pick-up truck or van in nontraffic accident
[7th]

V13.1XX Pedal cycle passenger injured in collision with car, pick-up truck or van in nontraffic accident
[7th]

V13.2XX Unspecified pedal cyclist injured in collision with car, pick-up truck or van in nontraffic accident
[7th]

V13.3XX Person boarding or alighting a pedal cycle injured in collision with car, pick-up truck or van
[7th]

V13.4XX Pedal cycle driver injured in collision with car, pick-up truck or van in traffic accident
[7th]

V13.5XX Pedal cycle passenger injured in collision with car, pick-up truck or van in traffic accident
[7th]

V13.9XX Unspecified pedal cyclist injured in collision with car, pick-up truck or van in traffic accident
[7th]

V14 PEDAL CYCLE RIDER INJURED IN COLLISION WITH HEAVY TRANSPORT VEHICLE OR BUS
[4th]

Excludes1: pedal cycle rider injured in collision with military vehicle (V19.81)

CHAPTER 20. EXTERNAL CAUSES OF MORBIDITY (V04.038–V14)

[4th] [5th] [6th] [7th] Additional Character Required   ✔ 3-character code

•=New Code
▲=Revised Code

Excludes1—Not coded here, do not use together
Excludes2—Not included here

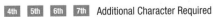

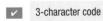

V14.0XX [7th] Pedal cycle driver injured in collision with heavy transport vehicle or bus in nontraffic accident

V14.1XX [7th] Pedal cycle passenger injured in collision with heavy transport vehicle or bus in nontraffic accident

7th characters for categories V10–V18
A—initial encounter
D—subsequent encounter
S—sequela

V14.2XX [7th] Unspecified pedal cyclist injured in collision with heavy transport vehicle or bus in nontraffic accident

V14.3XX [7th] Person boarding or alighting a pedal cycle injured in collision with heavy transport vehicle or bus

V14.4XX [7th] Pedal cycle driver injured in collision with heavy transport vehicle or bus in traffic accident

V14.5XX [7th] Pedal cycle passenger injured in collision with heavy transport vehicle or bus in traffic accident

V14.9XX [7th] Unspecified pedal cyclist injured in collision with heavy transport vehicle or bus in traffic accident

V12 [7th] **PEDAL CYCLE RIDER INJURED IN COLLISION WITH TWO- OR THREE-WHEELED MOTOR VEHICLE**
Refer to External Cause of Injuries Table

V17 [4th] **PEDAL CYCLE RIDER INJURED IN COLLISION WITH FIXED OR STATIONARY OBJECT**

V17.0XX [7th] Pedal cycle driver injured in collision with fixed or stationary object in nontraffic accident

V17.1XX [7th] Pedal cycle passenger injured in collision with fixed or stationary object in nontraffic accident

V17.2XX [7th] Unspecified pedal cyclist injured in collision with fixed or stationary object in nontraffic accident

V17.3XX [7th] Person boarding or alighting a pedal cycle injured in collision with fixed or stationary object

V17.4XX [7th] Pedal cycle driver injured in collision with fixed or stationary object in traffic accident

V17.5XX [7th] Pedal cycle passenger injured in collision with fixed or stationary object in traffic accident

V17.9XX [7th] Unspecified pedal cyclist injured in collision with fixed or stationary object in traffic accident

V18 [4th] **PEDAL CYCLE RIDER INJURED IN NONCOLLISION TRANSPORT ACCIDENT**
Includes: fall or thrown from pedal cycle (without antecedent collision)
    overturning pedal cycle NOS
    overturning pedal cycle without collision

V18.0XX [7th] Pedal cycle driver injured in noncollision transport accident in nontraffic accident

V18.1XX [7th] Pedal cycle passenger injured in noncollision transport accident in nontraffic accident

V18.2XX [7th] Unspecified pedal cyclist injured in noncollision transport accident in nontraffic accident

V18.3XX [7th] Person boarding or alighting a pedal cycle injured in noncollision transport accident

V18.4XX [7th] Pedal cycle driver injured in noncollision transport accident in traffic accident

V18.5XX [7th] Pedal cycle passenger injured in noncollision transport accident in traffic accident

V18.9XX [7th] Unspecified pedal cyclist injured in noncollision transport accident in traffic accident

V19 [4th] **PEDAL CYCLE RIDER INJURED IN OTHER AND UNSPECIFIED TRANSPORT ACCIDENTS**
Refer to External Cause of Injuries Table

(V20–V29) MOTORCYCLE RIDER INJURED IN TRANSPORT ACCIDENT

Includes: moped
    motorcycle with sidecar
    motorized bicycle
    motor scooter

Excludes1: three-wheeled motor vehicle (V30–V39)

7th characters for categories V20–V29
A—initial encounter
D—subsequent encounter
S—sequela

V20 [4th] **MOTORCYCLE RIDER INJURED IN COLLISION WITH PEDESTRIAN OR ANIMAL**
Excludes1: motorcycle rider collision with animal-drawn vehicle or animal being ridden (V26.-)

V20.0XX [7th] Motorcycle driver injured in collision with pedestrian or animal in nontraffic accident

V20.1XX [7th] Motorcycle passenger injured in collision with pedestrian or animal in nontraffic accident

V20.2XX [7th] Unspecified motorcycle rider injured in collision with pedestrian or animal in nontraffic accident

V20.3XX [7th] Person boarding or alighting a motorcycle injured in collision with pedestrian or animal

V20.4XX [7th] Motorcycle driver injured in collision with pedestrian or animal in traffic accident

V20.5XX [7th] Motorcycle passenger injured in collision with pedestrian or animal in traffic accident

V20.9XX [7th] Unspecified motorcycle rider injured in collision with pedestrian or animal in traffic accident

V21 [4th] **MOTORCYCLE RIDER INJURED IN COLLISION WITH PEDAL CYCLE**
Excludes1: motorcycle rider collision with animal-drawn vehicle or animal being ridden (V26.-)

V21.0XX [7th] Motorcycle driver injured in collision or with pedal cycle in nontraffic accident

V21.1XX [7th] Motorcycle passenger injured in collision with pedal cycle in nontraffic accident

V21.2XX [7th] Unspecified motorcycle rider injured in collision with pedal cycle in nontraffic accident

V21.3XX [7th] Person boarding or alighting a motorcycle injured in collision with pedal cycle

V21.4XX [7th] Motorcycle driver injured in collision with pedal cycle in traffic accident

V21.5XX [7th] Motorcycle passenger injured in collision with pedal cycle in traffic accident

V21.9XX [7th] Unspecified motorcycle rider injured in collision with pedal cycle in traffic accident

V22 [7th] **MOTORCYCLE RIDER INJURED IN COLLISION WITH TWO- OR THREE-WHEELED MOTOR VEHICLE**
Refer to External Cause of Injuries Table

V23 [4th] **MOTORCYCLE RIDER INJURED IN COLLISION WITH CAR, PICK-UP TRUCK OR VAN**

V23.0XX [7th] Motorcycle driver injured in collision with car, pick-up truck or van in nontraffic accident

V23.1XX [7th] Motorcycle passenger injured in collision with car, pick-up truck or van in nontraffic accident

V23.2XX [7th] Unspecified motorcycle rider injured in collision with car, pick-up truck or van in nontraffic accident

V23.3XX [7th] Person boarding or alighting a motorcycle injured in collision with car, pick-up truck or van

V23.4XX [7th] Motorcycle driver injured in collision with car, pick-up truck or van in traffic accident

V23.5XX [7th] Motorcycle passenger injured in collision with car, pick-up truck or van in traffic accident

V23.9XX [7th] Unspecified motorcycle rider injured in collision with car, pick-up truck or van in traffic accident

V24 [4th] **MOTORCYCLE RIDER INJURED IN COLLISION WITH HEAVY TRANSPORT VEHICLE OR BUS**
Excludes1: motorcycle rider injured in collision with military vehicle (V29.81)

V24.0XX [7th] Motorcycle driver injured in collision with heavy transport vehicle or bus in nontraffic accident

V24.1XX [7th] Motorcycle passenger injured in collision with heavy transport vehicle or bus in nontraffic accident

V24.2XX [7th] Unspecified motorcycle rider injured in collision with heavy transport vehicle or bus in nontraffic accident

V24.3XX [7th] Person boarding or alighting a motorcycle injured in collision with heavy transport vehicle or bus

V24.4XX [7th] Motorcycle driver injured in collision with heavy transport vehicle or bus in traffic accident

---

[4th] [5th] [6th] [7th] Additional Character Required   ✓ 3-character code

•=New Code
▲=Revised Code

Excludes1—Not coded here, do not use together
Excludes2—Not included here

V24.5XX Motorcycle passenger injured in collision with heavy
7th   transport vehicle or bus in
      traffic accident
V24.9XX Unspecified motorcycle rider
7th   injured in collision with heavy
      transport vehicle or bus in
      traffic accident

> 7th characters for categories
> V20–V29
> A—initial encounter
> D—subsequent encounter
> S—sequela

V25 MOTORCYCLE RIDER INJURED IN COLLISION WITH
4th RAILWAY TRAIN OR RAILWAY VEHICLE
Refer to External Cause of Injuries Table

V26 MOTORCYCLE RIDER INJURED IN COLLISION WITH
4th OTHER NONMOTOR VEHICLE
Includes: collision with animal-drawn vehicle, animal being ridden,
   streetcar
Refer to External Cause of Injuries Table

V27 MOTORCYCLE RIDER INJURED IN COLLISION WITH
4th FIXED OR STATIONARY OBJECT
V27.0XX Motorcycle driver injured in collision with fixed or
7th   stationary object in nontraffic accident
V27.1XX Motorcycle passenger injured in collision with fixed or
7th   stationary object in nontraffic accident
V27.2XX Unspecified motorcycle rider injured in collision with fixed
7th   or stationary object in nontraffic accident
V27.3XX Person boarding or alighting a motorcycle injured in
7th   collision with fixed or stationary object
V27.4XX Motorcycle driver injured in collision with fixed or
7th   stationary object in traffic accident
V27.5XX Motorcycle passenger injured in collision with fixed or
7th   stationary object in traffic accident
V27.9XX Unspecified motorcycle rider injured in collision with fixed
7th   or stationary object in traffic accident

V28 MOTORCYCLE RIDER INJURED IN NONCOLLISION
4th TRANSPORT ACCIDENT
Includes: fall or thrown from motorcycle (without antecedent collision)
   overturning motorcycle NOS
   overturning motorcycle without collision
V28.0XX Motorcycle driver injured in noncollision transport accident
7th   in nontraffic accident
V28.1XX Motorcycle passenger injured in noncollision transport
7th   accident in nontraffic accident
V28.2XX Unspecified motorcycle rider injured in noncollision
7th   transport accident in nontraffic accident
V28.3XX Person boarding or alighting a motorcycle injured in
7th   noncollision transport accident
V28.4XX Motorcycle driver injured in noncollision transport accident
7th   in traffic accident
V28.5XX Motorcycle passenger injured in noncollision transport
7th   accident in traffic accident
V28.9XX Unspecified motorcycle rider injured in noncollision
7th   transport accident in traffic accident

V29 MOTORCYCLE RIDER INJURED IN OTHER AND
4th UNSPECIFIED TRANSPORT ACCIDENTS
V29.0 Motorcycle driver injured in
5th   collision with other and
      unspecified motor vehicles
      in nontraffic accident

> 7th characters for category V29
> A—initial encounter
> D—subsequent encounter
> S—sequela

    V29.00X Motorcycle driver
    7th   injured in collision with
       unspecified motor vehicles in nontraffic accident
    V29.09X Motorcycle driver injured in collision with other
    7th   motor vehicles in nontraffic accident
V29.1 Motorcycle passenger injured in collision with other and
5th   unspecified motor vehicles in nontraffic accident
    V29.10X Motorcycle passenger injured in collision with
    7th   unspecified motor vehicles in nontraffic accident
    V29.19X Motorcycle passenger injured in collision with other
    7th   motor vehicles in nontraffic accident
V29.2 Unspecified motorcycle rider injured in collision with other and
5th   unspecified motor vehicles in nontraffic accident

V29.20X Unspecified motorcycle rider injured in collision with
7th   unspecified motor vehicles in nontraffic accident
      Motorcycle collision NOS, nontraffic
V29.29X Unspecified motorcycle rider injured in collision with
7th   other motor vehicles in nontraffic accident
V29.3XX Motorcycle rider (driver) (passenger) injured in unspecified
7th   nontraffic accident
      Motorcycle accident NOS, nontraffic
      Motorcycle rider injured in nontraffic accident NOS
V29.4 Motorcycle driver injured in collision with other and
5th   unspecified motor vehicles in traffic accident
    V29.40X Motorcycle driver injured in collision with
    7th   unspecified motor vehicles in traffic accident
    V29.49X Motorcycle driver injured in collision with other
    7th   motor vehicles in traffic accident
V29.5 Motorcycle passenger injured in collision with other and
5th   unspecified motor vehicles in traffic accident
    V29.50X Motorcycle passenger injured in collision with
    7th   unspecified motor vehicles in traffic accident
    V29.59X Motorcycle passenger injured in collision with other
    7th   motor vehicles in traffic accident
V29.6 Unspecified motorcycle rider injured in collision with other and
5th   unspecified motor vehicles in traffic accident
    V29.60X Unspecified motorcycle rider injured in collision with
    7th   unspecified motor vehicles in traffic accident
       Motorcycle collision NOS (traffic)
    V29.69X Unspecified motorcycle rider injured in collision with
    7th   other motor vehicles in traffic accident
V29.8 Motorcycle rider (driver) (passenger) injured in other specified
5th   transport accidents
    V29.81X Motorcycle rider (driver) (passenger) injured in
    7th   transport accident with military vehicle
    V29.88X Motorcycle rider (driver) (passenger) injured in other
    7th   specified transport accidents
V29.9XX Motorcycle rider (driver) (passenger) injured in unspecified
7th   traffic accident
      Motorcycle accident NOS

(V30–V39) OCCUPANT OF THREE-WHEELED MOTOR VEHICLE INJURED IN TRANSPORT ACCIDENT

Includes: motorized tricycle
   motorized rickshaw
   three-wheeled motor car

Excludes1: all-terrain vehicles (V86.-)
   motorcycle with sidecar (V20–V29)
   vehicle designed primarily for off-road use
   (V86.-)

> 7th characters for categories
> V30–V39
> A—initial encounter
> D—subsequent encounter
> S—sequela

V30 OCCUPANT OF THREE-WHEELED MOTOR VEHICLE
4th INJURED IN COLLISION WITH PEDESTRIAN OR ANIMAL
Excludes1: three-wheeled motor vehicle collision with animal-drawn
   vehicle or animal being ridden (V36.-)
V30.0XX Driver of three-wheeled motor vehicle injured in collision
7th   with pedestrian or animal in nontraffic accident
V30.1XX Passenger in three-wheeled motor vehicle injured in
7th   collision with pedestrian or animal in nontraffic accident
V30.2XX Person on outside of three-wheeled motor vehicle injured in
7th   collision with pedestrian or animal in nontraffic accident
V30.3XX Unspecified occupant of three-wheeled motor vehicle
7th   injured in collision with pedestrian or animal in nontraffic
      accident
V30.4XX Person boarding or alighting a three-wheeled motor vehicle
7th   injured in collision with pedestrian or animal
V30.5XX Driver of three-wheeled motor vehicle injured in collision
7th   with pedestrian or animal in traffic accident
V30.6XX Passenger in three-wheeled motor vehicle injured in
7th   collision with pedestrian or animal in traffic accident
V30.7XX Person on outside of three-wheeled motor vehicle injured in
7th   collision with pedestrian or animal in traffic accident
V30.9XX Unspecified occupant of three-wheeled motor vehicle
7th   injured in collision with pedestrian or animal in traffic
      accident

| 4th | 5th | 6th | 7th | Additional Character Required | ✓ | 3-character code |

•=New Code
▲=Revised Code

Excludes1—Not coded here, do not use together
Excludes2—Not included here

V31 `4th` **OCCUPANT OF THREE-WHEELED MOTOR VEHICLE INJURED IN COLLISION WITH PEDAL CYCLE**
Refer to the External Cause of Injuries Table

> 7th characters for categories
> V30–V39
> A—initial encounter
> D—subsequent encounter
> S—sequela

V32 `4th` **OCCUPANT OF THREE-WHEELED MOTOR VEHICLE INJURED IN COLLISION WITH TWO- OR THREE-WHEELED MOTOR VEHICLE**

V32.0XX `7th` Driver of three-wheeled motor vehicle injured in collision with two- or three-wheeled motor vehicle in nontraffic accident

V32.1XX `7th` Passenger in three-wheeled motor vehicle injured in collision with two- or three-wheeled motor vehicle in nontraffic accident

V32.2XX `7th` Person on outside of three-wheeled motor vehicle injured in collision with two- or three-wheeled motor vehicle in nontraffic accident

V32.3XX `7th` Unspecified occupant of three-wheeled motor vehicle injured in collision with two- or three-wheeled motor vehicle in nontraffic accident

V32.4XX `7th` Person boarding or alighting a three-wheeled motor vehicle injured in collision with two- or three-wheeled motor vehicle

V32.5XX `7th` Driver of three-wheeled motor vehicle injured in collision with two- or three-wheeled motor vehicle in traffic accident

V32.6XX `7th` Passenger in three-wheeled motor vehicle injured in collision with two- or three-wheeled motor vehicle in traffic accident

V32.7XX `7th` Person on outside of three-wheeled motor vehicle injured in collision with two- or three-wheeled motor vehicle in traffic accident

V32.9XX `7th` Unspecified occupant of three-wheeled motor vehicle injured in collision with two- or three-wheeled motor vehicle in traffic accident

V33 `4th` **OCCUPANT OF THREE-WHEELED MOTOR VEHICLE INJURED IN COLLISION WITH CAR, PICK-UP TRUCK OR VAN**

V33.0XX `7th` Driver of three-wheeled motor vehicle injured in collision with car, pick-up truck or van in nontraffic accident

V33.1XX `7th` Passenger in three-wheeled motor vehicle injured in collision with car, pick-up truck or van in nontraffic accident

V33.2XX `7th` Person on outside of three-wheeled motor vehicle injured in collision with car, pick-up truck or van in nontraffic accident

V33.3XX `7th` Unspecified occupant of three-wheeled motor vehicle injured in collision with car, pick-up truck or van in nontraffic accident

V33.4XX `7th` Person boarding or alighting a three-wheeled motor vehicle injured in collision with car, pick-up truck or van

V33.5XX `7th` Driver of three-wheeled motor vehicle injured in collision with car, pick-up truck or van in traffic accident

V33.6XX `7th` Passenger in three-wheeled motor vehicle injured in collision with car, pick-up truck or van in traffic accident

V33.7XX `7th` Person on outside of three-wheeled motor vehicle injured in collision with car, pick-up truck or van in traffic accident

V33.9XX `7th` Unspecified occupant of three-wheeled motor vehicle injured in collision with car, pick-up truck or van in traffic accident

V34 `4th` **OCCUPANT OF THREE-WHEELED MOTOR VEHICLE INJURED IN COLLISION WITH HEAVY TRANSPORT VEHICLE OR BUS**
Excludes1: occupant of three-wheeled motor vehicle injured in collision with military vehicle (V39.81)

V34.0XX `7th` Driver of three-wheeled motor vehicle injured in collision with heavy transport vehicle or bus in nontraffic accident

V34.1XX `7th` Passenger in three-wheeled motor vehicle injured in collision with heavy transport vehicle or bus in nontraffic accident

V34.2XX `7th` Person on outside of three-wheeled motor vehicle injured in collision with heavy transport vehicle or bus in nontraffic accident

V34.3XX `7th` Unspecified occupant of three-wheeled motor vehicle injured in collision with heavy transport vehicle or bus in nontraffic accident

V34.4XX `7th` Person boarding or alighting a three-wheeled motor vehicle injured in collision with heavy transport vehicle or bus

V34.5XX `7th` Driver of three-wheeled motor vehicle injured in collision with heavy transport vehicle or bus in traffic accident

V34.6XX `7th` Passenger in three-wheeled motor vehicle injured in collision with heavy transport vehicle or bus in traffic accident

V34.7XX `7th` Person on outside of three-wheeled motor vehicle injured in collision with heavy transport vehicle or bus in traffic accident

V34.9XX `7th` Unspecified occupant of three-wheeled motor vehicle injured in collision with heavy transport vehicle or bus in traffic accident

V35 `4th` **OCCUPANT OF THREE-WHEELED MOTOR VEHICLE INJURED IN COLLISION WITH RAILWAY TRAIN OR RAILWAY VEHICLE**
Refer to External Cause of Injuries Table

V36 `4th` **OCCUPANT OF THREE-WHEELED MOTOR VEHICLE INJURED IN COLLISION WITH OTHER NONMOTOR |VEHICLE**
Includes: collision with animal-drawn vehicle, animal being ridden, streetcar
Refer to External Cause of Injuries Table

V37 `4th` **OCCUPANT OF THREE-WHEELED MOTOR VEHICLE INJURED IN COLLISION WITH FIXED OR STATIONARY OBJECT**

V37.0XX `7th` Driver of three-wheeled motor vehicle injured in collision with fixed or stationary object in nontraffic accident

V37.1XX `7th` Passenger in three-wheeled motor vehicle injured in collision with fixed or stationary object in nontraffic accident

V37.2XX `7th` Person on outside of three-wheeled motor vehicle injured in collision with fixed or stationary object in nontraffic accident

V37.3XX `7th` Unspecified occupant of three-wheeled motor vehicle injured in collision with fixed or stationary object in nontraffic accident

V37.4XX `7th` Person boarding or alighting a three-wheeled motor vehicle injured in collision with fixed or stationary object

V37.5XX `7th` Driver of three-wheeled motor vehicle injured in collision with fixed or stationary object in traffic accident

V37.6XX `7th` Passenger in three-wheeled motor vehicle injured in collision with fixed or stationary object in traffic accident

V37.7XX `7th` Person on outside of three-wheeled motor vehicle injured in collision with fixed or stationary object in traffic accident

V37.9XX `7th` Unspecified occupant of three-wheeled motor vehicle injured in collision with fixed or stationary object in traffic accident

V38 `4th` **OCCUPANT OF THREE-WHEELED MOTOR VEHICLE INJURED IN NONCOLLISION TRANSPORT ACCIDENT**
Includes: fall or thrown from three-wheeled motor vehicle
overturning of three-wheeled motor vehicle NOS
overturning of three-wheeled motor vehicle without collision

V38.0XX `7th` Driver of three-wheeled motor vehicle injured in noncollision transport accident in nontraffic accident

V38.1XX `7th` Passenger in three-wheeled motor vehicle injured in noncollision transport accident in nontraffic accident

V38.2XX `7th` Person on outside of three-wheeled motor vehicle injured in noncollision transport accident in nontraffic accident

V38.3XX `7th` Unspecified occupant of three-wheeled motor vehicle injured in noncollision transport accident in nontraffic accident

V38.4XX `7th` Person boarding or alighting a three-wheeled motor vehicle injured in noncollision transport accident

V38.5XX `7th` Driver of three-wheeled motor vehicle injured in noncollision transport accident in traffic accident

V38.6XX `7th` Passenger in three-wheeled motor vehicle injured in noncollision transport accident in traffic accident

---

`4th` `5th` `6th` `7th` Additional Character Required   ✔ 3-character code   •=New Code   ▲=Revised Code   *Excludes1*—Not coded here, do not use together   *Excludes2*—Not included here

V38.7XX   Person on outside of three-wheeled motor vehicle injured in noncollision transport accident in traffic accident
7th

V38.9XX   Unspecified occupant of three-wheeled motor vehicle injured in noncollision transport accident in traffic accident
7th

7th characters for categories
V30–V39
A—initial encounter
D—subsequent encounter
S—sequela

V39   OCCUPANT OF THREE-WHEELED MOTOR VEHICLE INJURED IN OTHER AND UNSPECIFIED TRANSPORT ACCIDENTS
4th

V39.0   Driver of three-wheeled motor vehicle injured in collision with other and unspecified motor vehicles in nontraffic accident
5th

    V39.00X   Driver of three-wheeled motor vehicle injured in collision with unspecified motor vehicles in nontraffic accident
7th

    V39.09X   Driver of three-wheeled motor vehicle injured in collision with other motor vehicles in nontraffic accident
7th

V39.1   Passenger in three-wheeled motor vehicle injured in collision with other and unspecified motor vehicles in nontraffic accident
5th

    V39.10X   Passenger in three-wheeled motor vehicle injured in collision with unspecified motor vehicles in nontraffic accident
7th

    V39.19X   Passenger in three-wheeled motor vehicle injured in collision with other motor vehicles in nontraffic accident
7th

V39.2   Unspecified occupant of three-wheeled motor vehicle injured in accident
5th

    V39.20X   Unspecified occupant of three-wheeled motor vehicle injured in collision with unspecified motor vehicles in nontraffic accident
7th
       Collision NOS involving three-wheeled motor vehicle, nontraffic

    V39.29X   Unspecified occupant of three-wheeled
7th

V39.3XX   Occupant (driver) (passenger) of three-wheeled motor vehicle injured in unspecified nontraffic accident
7th
       Accident NOS involving three-wheeled motor vehicle, nontraffic
       Occupant of three-wheeled motor vehicle injured in nontraffic accident NOS

V39.4   Driver of three-wheeled motor vehicle injured in collision with other and unspecified motor vehicles in traffic accident
5th

    V39.40X   Driver of three-wheeled motor vehicle injured in collision with unspecified motor vehicles in traffic accident
7th

    V39.49X   Driver of three-wheeled motor vehicle injured in collision with other motor vehicles in traffic accident
7th

V39.5   Passenger in three-wheeled motor vehicle injured in collision with other and unspecified motor vehicles in traffic accident
5th

    V39.50X   Passenger in three-wheeled motor vehicle injured in collision with unspecified motor vehicles in traffic accident
7th

    V39.59X   Passenger in three-wheeled motor vehicle injured in collision with other motor vehicles in traffic accident
7th

V39.6   Unspecified occupant of three-wheeled motor vehicle injured in collision with other and unspecified motor vehicles in traffic accident
5th

    V39.60X   Unspecified occupant of three-wheeled motor vehicle injured in collision with unspecified motor vehicles in traffic accident
7th
       Collision NOS involving three-wheeled motor vehicle (traffic)

    V39.69X   Unspecified occupant of three-wheeled motor vehicle injured in collision with other motor vehicles in traffic accident
7th

V39.8   Occupant (driver) (passenger) of three-wheeled motor vehicle injured in other specified transport accidents
5th

    V39.81X   Occupant (driver) (passenger) of three-wheeled motor vehicle injured in transport accident with military vehicle
7th

V39.89X   Occupant (driver) (passenger) of three-wheeled motor vehicle injured in other specified transport accidents
7th

V39.9XX   Occupant (driver) (passenger) of three-wheeled motor vehicle injured in unspecified traffic accident
7th
       Accident NOS involving three-wheeled motor vehicle

(V40–V49) CAR OCCUPANT INJURED IN TRANSPORT ACCIDENT

Includes: a four-wheeled motor vehicle designed primarily for carrying passengers
   automobile (pulling a trailer or camper)
Excludes1: bus (V50–V59)
   minibus (V50–V59)
   minivan (V50–V59)
   motorcoach (V70–V79)
   pick-up truck (V50–V59)
   sport utility vehicle (SUV) (V50–V59)

7th characters for categories
V40–V49
A—initial encounter
D—subsequent encounter
S—sequela

V40   CAR OCCUPANT INJURED IN COLLISION WITH PEDESTRIAN OR ANIMAL
4th

   Excludes1: car collision with animal-drawn vehicle or animal being ridden (V46.-)

V40.0XX   Car driver injured in collision with pedestrian or animal in nontraffic accident
7th

V40.1XX   Car passenger injured in collision with pedestrian or animal in nontraffic accident
7th

V40.2XX   Person on outside of car injured in collision with pedestrian or animal in nontraffic accident
7th

V40.3XX   Unspecified car occupant injured in collision with pedestrian or animal in nontraffic accident
7th

V40.4XX   Person boarding or alighting a car injured in collision with pedestrian or animal
7th

V40.5XX   Car driver injured in collision with pedestrian or animal in traffic accident
7th

V40.6XX   Car passenger injured in collision with pedestrian or animal in traffic accident
7th

V40.7XX   Person on outside of car injured in collision with pedestrian or animal in traffic accident
7th

V40.9XX   Unspecified car occupant injured in collision with pedestrian or animal in traffic accident
7th

V41   CAR OCCUPANT INJURED IN COLLISION WITH PEDAL CYCLE
4th

   Refer to External Cause of Injuries Table

V42   CAR OCCUPANT INJURED IN COLLISION WITH TWO- OR THREE-WHEELED MOTOR VEHICLE
4th

V42.0XX   Car driver injured in collision with two- or three-wheeled motor vehicle in nontraffic accident
7th

V42.1XX   Car passenger injured in collision with two- or three-wheeled motor vehicle in nontraffic accident
7th

V42.2XX   Person on outside of car injured in collision with two- or three-wheeled motor vehicle in nontraffic accident
7th

V42.3XX   Unspecified car occupant injured in collision with two- or three-wheeled motor vehicle in nontraffic accident
7th

V42.4XX   Person boarding or alighting a car injured in collision with two- or three-wheeled motor vehicle
7th

V42.5XX   Car driver injured in collision with two- or three-wheeled motor vehicle in traffic accident
7th

V42.6XX   Car passenger injured in collision with two- or three-wheeled motor vehicle in traffic accident
7th

V42.7XX   Person on outside of car injured in collision with two- or three-wheeled motor vehicle in traffic accident
7th

V42.9XX   Unspecified car occupant injured in collision with two- or three-wheeled motor vehicle in traffic accident
7th

V43   CAR OCCUPANT INJURED IN COLLISION WITH CAR, PICK-UP TRUCK OR VAN
4th

V43.0   Car driver injured in collision with car, pick-up truck or van in nontraffic accident
5th

    V43.01X   Car driver injured in collision with sport utility vehicle in nontraffic accident
7th

    V43.02X   Car driver injured in collision with other type car in nontraffic accident
7th

4th   5th   6th   7th   Additional Character Required   ✔   3-character code

•=New Code   **Excludes1**—Not coded here, do not use together
▲=Revised Code   **Excludes2**—Not included here

V43.03X Car driver injured in collision with pick-up truck in
   7th   nontraffic accident

V43.04X Car driver injured in
   7th   collision with van in
        nontraffic accident

> 7th characters for categories
> V40–V49
> A—initial encounter
> D—subsequent encounter
> S—sequela

V43.1 Car passenger injured in collision
  5th   with car, pick-up truck or van in
       nontraffic accident

    V43.11X Car passenger injured in collision with sport utility
     7th   vehicle in nontraffic accident

    V43.12X Car passenger injured in collision with other type car
     7th   in nontraffic accident

    V43.13X Car passenger injured in collision with pick-up in
     7th   nontraffic accident

    V43.14X Car passenger injured in collision with van in
     7th   nontraffic accident

V43.2 Person on outside of car injured in collision with car, pick-up
  5th   truck or van in nontraffic accident

    V43.21X Person on outside of car injured in collision with
     7th   sport utility vehicle in nontraffic accident

    V43.22X Person on outside of car injured in collision with
     7th   other type car in nontraffic accident

    V43.23X Person on outside of car injured in collision with
     7th   pick-up truck in nontraffic accident

    V43.24X Person on outside of car injured in collision with van
     7th   in nontraffic accident

V43.3 Unspecified car occupant injured in collision with car, pick-up
  5th   truck or van in nontraffic accident

    V43.31X Unspecified car occupant injured in collision with
     7th   sport utility vehicle in nontraffic accident

    V43.32X Unspecified car occupant injured in collision with
     7th   other type car in nontraffic accident

    V43.33X Unspecified car occupant injured in collision with
     7th   pick-up truck in nontraffic accident

    V43.34X Unspecified car occupant injured in collision with
     7th   van in nontraffic accident

V43.4 Person boarding or alighting a car injured in collision with car,
  5th   pick-up truck or van

    V43.41X Person boarding or alighting a car injured in collision
     7th   with sport utility vehicle, initial encounter

    V43.42X Person boarding or alighting a car injured in collision
     7th   with other type car

    V43.43X Person boarding or alighting a car injured in collision
     7th   with pick-up truck

    V43.44X Person boarding or alighting a car injured in collision
     7th   with van

V43.5 Car driver injured in collision with car, pick-up truck or van in
  5th   traffic accident

    V43.51X Car driver injured in collision with sport utility
     7th   vehicle in traffic accident

    V43.52X Car driver injured in collision with other type car in
     7th   traffic accident

    V43.53X Car driver injured in collision with pick-up truck in
     7th   traffic accident

    V43.54X Car driver injured in collision with van in traffic
     7th   accident

V43.6 Car passenger injured in collision with car, pick-up truck or
  5th   van in traffic accident

    V43.61X Car passenger injured in collision with sport utility
     7th   vehicle in traffic accident

    V43.62X Car passenger injured in collision with other type car
     7th   in traffic accident

    V43.63X Car passenger injured in collision with pick-up truck
     7th   in traffic accident

    V43.64X Car passenger injured in collision with van in traffic
     7th   accident

V43.7 Person on outside of car injured in collision with car, pick-up
  5th   truck or van in traffic accident

    V43.71X Person on outside of car injured in collision with
     7th   sport utility vehicle in traffic accident

    V43.72X Person on outside of car injured in collision with
     7th   other type car in traffic accident

    V43.73X Person on outside of car injured in collision with
     7th   pick-up truck in traffic accident

    V43.74X Person on outside of car injured in collision with van
     7th   in traffic accident

V43.9 Unspecified car occupant injured in collision with car, pick-up
  5th   truck or van in traffic accident

    V43.91X Unspecified car occupant injured in collision with
     7th   sport utility vehicle in traffic accident

    V43.92X Unspecified car occupant injured in collision with
     7th   other type car in traffic accident

    V43.93X Unspecified car occupant injured in collision with
     7th   pick-up truck in traffic accident

    V43.94X Unspecified car occupant injured in collision with
     7th   van in traffic accident

V44 **CAR OCCUPANT INJURED IN COLLISION WITH HEAVY**
4th **TRANSPORT VEHICLE OR BUS**

Excludes1: car occupant injured in collision with military vehicle (V49.81)

V44.0XX Car driver injured in collision with heavy transport vehicle
 7th or bus in nontraffic accident

V44.1XX Car passenger injured in collision with heavy transport
 7th vehicle or bus in nontraffic accident

V44.2XX Person on outside of car injured in collision with heavy
 7th transport vehicle or bus in nontraffic accident

V44.3XX Unspecified car occupant injured in collision with heavy
 7th transport vehicle or bus in nontraffic accident

V44.4XX Person boarding or alighting a car injured in collision with
 7th heavy transport vehicle or bus

V44.5XX Car driver injured in collision with heavy transport vehicle
 7th or bus in traffic accident

V44.6XX Car passenger injured in collision with heavy transport
 7th vehicle or bus in traffic accident

V44.7XX Person on outside of car injured in collision with heavy
 7th transport vehicle or bus in traffic accident

V44.9XX Unspecified car occupant injured in collision with heavy
 7th transport vehicle or bus in traffic accident

V45 **CAR OCCUPANT INJURED IN COLLISION WITH RAILWAY**
4th **TRAIN OR RAILWAY VEHICLE**

V45.0XX Car driver injured in collision with railway train or railway
 7th vehicle in nontraffic accident

V45.1XX Car passenger injured in collision with railway train or
 7th railway vehicle in nontraffic accident

V45.2XX Person on outside of car injured in collision with railway
 7th train or railway vehicle in nontraffic accident

V45.3XX Unspecified car occupant injured in collision with railway
 7th train or railway vehicle in nontraffic accident

V45.4XX Person boarding or alighting a car injured in collision with
 7th railway train or railway vehicle

V45.5XX Car driver injured in collision with railway train or railway
 7th vehicle in traffic accident

V45.6XX Car passenger injured in collision with railway train or
 7th railway vehicle in traffic accident

V45.7XX Person on outside of car injured in collision with railway
 7th train or railway vehicle in traffic accident

V45.9XX Unspecified car occupant injured in collision with railway
 7th train or railway vehicle in traffic accident

V46 **CAR OCCUPANT INJURED IN COLLISION WITH OTHER**
6th **NONMOTOR VEHICLE**

Includes: collision with animal-drawn vehicle, animal being ridden,
streetcar

Refer to External Cause of Injuries Table

V47 **CAR OCCUPANT INJURED IN COLLISION WITH FIXED OR**
4th **STATIONARY OBJECT**

V47.0XX Car driver injured in collision with fixed or stationary object
 7th in nontraffic accident

V47.1XX Car passenger injured in collision with fixed or stationary
 7th object in nontraffic accident

V47.2XX Person on outside of car injured in collision with fixed or
 7th stationary object in nontraffic accident

V47.3XX Unspecified car occupant injured in collision with fixed or
 7th stationary object in nontraffic accident

V47.4XX Person boarding or alighting a car injured in collision with
 7th fixed or stationary object

V47.5XX Car driver injured in collision with fixed or stationary object
 7th in traffic accident

4th **5th** **6th** **7th** Additional Character Required   ✔ 3-character code

•=New Code   *Excludes1*—Not coded here, do not use together
▲=Revised Code   *Excludes2*—Not included here

V47.6XX Car passenger injured in collision with fixed or stationary
[7th] object in traffic accident

V47.7XX Person on outside of car
[7th] injured in collision with fixed
or stationary object in traffic
accident

V47.9XX Unspecified car occupant
[7th] injured in collision with fixed
or stationary object in traffic accident

7th characters for categories
V40–V49
A—initial encounter
D—subsequent encounter
S—sequela

V48 CAR OCCUPANT INJURED IN NONCOLLISION
[4th] TRANSPORT ACCIDENT
Includes: overturning car NOS
overturning car without collision

V48.0XX Car driver injured in noncollision transport accident in
[7th] nontraffic accident

V48.1XX Car passenger injured in noncollision transport accident in
[7th] nontraffic accident

V48.2XX Person on outside of car injured in noncollision transport
[7th] accident in nontraffic accident

V48.3XX Unspecified car occupant injured in noncollision transport
[7th] accident in nontraffic accident

V48.4XX Person boarding or alighting a car injured in noncollision
[7th] transport accident

V48.5XX Car driver injured in noncollision transport accident in
[7th] traffic accident

V48.6XX Car passenger injured in noncollision transport accident in
[7th] traffic accident

V48.7XX Person on outside of car injured in noncollision transport
[7th] accident in traffic accident

V48.9XX Unspecified car occupant injured in noncollision transport
[7th] accident in traffic accident

V49 CAR OCCUPANT INJURED IN OTHER AND UNSPECIFIED
[4th] TRANSPORT ACCIDENTS

V49.0 Driver injured in collision with other and unspecified motor
[5th] vehicles in nontraffic accident

   V49.00X Driver injured in collision with unspecified motor
   [7th] vehicles in nontraffic accident

   V49.09X Driver injured in collision with other motor vehicles
   [7th] in nontraffic accident

V49.1 Passenger injured in collision with other and unspecified
[5th] motor vehicles in nontraffic accident

   V49.10X Passenger injured in collision with unspecified motor
   [7th] vehicles in nontraffic accident

   V49.19X Passenger injured in collision with other motor
   [7th] vehicles in nontraffic accident

V49.2 Unspecified car occupant injured in collision with other and
[5th] unspecified motor vehicles in nontraffic accident

   V49.20X Unspecified car occupant injured in collision with
   [7th] unspecified motor vehicles in nontraffic accident
   Car collision NOS, nontraffic

   V49.29X Unspecified car occupant injured in collision with
   [7th] other motor vehicles in nontraffic accident

V49.3XX Car occupant (driver) (passenger) injured in unspecified
[7th] nontraffic accident
Car accident NOS, nontraffic
Car occupant injured in nontraffic accident NOS

V49.4 Driver injured in collision with other and unspecified motor
[5th] vehicles in traffic accident

   V49.40X Driver injured in collision with unspecified motor
   [7th] vehicles in traffic accident

   V49.49X Driver injured in collision with other motor vehicles
   [7th] in traffic accident

V49.5 Passenger injured in collision with other and unspecified
[5th] motor vehicles in traffic accident

   V49.50X Passenger injured in collision with unspecified motor
   [7th] vehicles in traffic accident

   V49.59X Passenger injured in collision with other motor
   [7th] vehicles in traffic accident

V49.6 Unspecified car occupant injured in collision with other and
[5th] unspecified motor vehicles in traffic accident

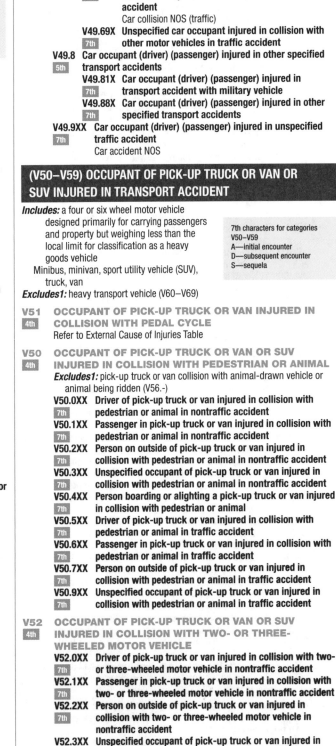

V49.60X Unspecified car occupant injured in collision with
[7th] other and unspecified motor vehicles in traffic
accident
Car collision NOS (traffic)

V49.69X Unspecified car occupant injured in collision with
[7th] other motor vehicles in traffic accident

V49.8 Car occupant (driver) (passenger) injured in other specified
[5th] transport accidents

   V49.81X Car occupant (driver) (passenger) injured in
   [7th] transport accident with military vehicle

   V49.88X Car occupant (driver) (passenger) injured in other
   [7th] specified transport accidents

V49.9XX Car occupant (driver) (passenger) injured in unspecified
[7th] traffic accident
Car accident NOS

(V50–V59) OCCUPANT OF PICK-UP TRUCK OR VAN OR SUV INJURED IN TRANSPORT ACCIDENT

Includes: a four or six wheel motor vehicle
designed primarily for carrying passengers
and property but weighing less than the
local limit for classification as a heavy
goods vehicle
Minibus, minivan, sport utility vehicle (SUV),
truck, van

7th characters for categories
V50–V59
A—initial encounter
D—subsequent encounter
S—sequela

Excludes1: heavy transport vehicle (V60–V69)

V51 OCCUPANT OF PICK-UP TRUCK OR VAN INJURED IN
[4th] COLLISION WITH PEDAL CYCLE
Refer to External Cause of Injuries Table

V50 OCCUPANT OF PICK-UP TRUCK OR VAN OR SUV
[4th] INJURED IN COLLISION WITH PEDESTRIAN OR ANIMAL
Excludes1: pick-up truck or van collision with animal-drawn vehicle or
animal being ridden (V56.-)

V50.0XX Driver of pick-up truck or van injured in collision with
[7th] pedestrian or animal in nontraffic accident

V50.1XX Passenger in pick-up truck or van injured in collision with
[7th] pedestrian or animal in nontraffic accident

V50.2XX Person on outside of pick-up truck or van injured in
[7th] collision with pedestrian or animal in nontraffic accident

V50.3XX Unspecified occupant of pick-up truck or van injured in
[7th] collision with pedestrian or animal in nontraffic accident

V50.4XX Person boarding or alighting a pick-up truck or van injured
[7th] in collision with pedestrian or animal

V50.5XX Driver of pick-up truck or van injured in collision with
[7th] pedestrian or animal in traffic accident

V50.6XX Passenger in pick-up truck or van injured in collision with
[7th] pedestrian or animal in traffic accident

V50.7XX Person on outside of pick-up truck or van injured in
[7th] collision with pedestrian or animal in traffic accident

V50.9XX Unspecified occupant of pick-up truck or van injured in
[7th] collision with pedestrian or animal in traffic accident

V52 OCCUPANT OF PICK-UP TRUCK OR VAN OR SUV
[4th] INJURED IN COLLISION WITH TWO- OR THREE-
WHEELED MOTOR VEHICLE

V52.0XX Driver of pick-up truck or van injured in collision with two-
[7th] or three-wheeled motor vehicle in nontraffic accident

V52.1XX Passenger in pick-up truck or van injured in collision with
[7th] two- or three-wheeled motor vehicle in nontraffic accident

V52.2XX Person on outside of pick-up truck or van injured in
[7th] collision with two- or three-wheeled motor vehicle in
nontraffic accident

V52.3XX Unspecified occupant of pick-up truck or van injured in
[7th] collision with two- or three-wheeled motor vehicle in
nontraffic accident

V52.4XX Person boarding or alighting a pick-up truck or van injured
[7th] in collision with two- or three-wheeled motor vehicle

V52.5XX Driver of pick-up truck or van injured in collision with two-
[7th] or three-wheeled motor vehicle in traffic accident

V52.6XX Passenger in pick-up truck or van injured in collision with
[7th] two- or three-wheeled motor vehicle in traffic accident

---

[4th] [5th] [6th] [7th] Additional Character Required   ✓ 3-character code

•=New Code
▲=Revised Code

Excludes1—Not coded here, do not use together
Excludes2—Not included here

CHAPTER 20. EXTERNAL CAUSES OF MORBIDITY   (V52.7XX–V59.09X)

V52.7XX Person on outside of pick-up truck or van injured in collision with two- or three-wheeled motor vehicle in traffic accident
7th

V52.9XX Unspecified occupant of pick-up truck or van injured in collision with two- or three-wheeled motor vehicle in traffic accident
7th

> 7th characters for categories
> V50–V59
> A—initial encounter
> D—subsequent encounter
> S—sequela

V53 OCCUPANT OF PICK-UP TRUCK OR VAN OR SUV
4th INJURED IN COLLISION WITH CAR, PICK-UP TRUCK OR VAN

V53.0XX Driver of pick-up truck or van injured in collision with car, pick-up truck or van in nontraffic accident
7th

V53.1XX Passenger in pick-up truck or van injured in collision with car, pick-up truck or van in nontraffic accident
7th

V53.2XX Person on outside of pick-up truck or van injured in collision with car, pick-up truck or van in nontraffic accident
7th

V53.3XX Unspecified occupant of pick-up truck or van injured in collision with car, pick-up truck or van in nontraffic accident
7th

V53.4XX Person boarding or alighting a pick-up truck or van injured in collision with car, pick-up truck or van
7th

V53.5XX Driver of pick-up truck or van injured in collision with car, pick-up truck or van in traffic accident
7th

V53.6XX Passenger in pick-up truck or van injured in collision with car, pick-up truck or van in traffic accident
7th

V53.7XX Person on outside of pick-up truck or van injured in collision with car, pick-up truck or van in traffic accident
7th

V53.9XX Unspecified occupant of pick-up truck or van injured in collision with car, pick-up truck or van in traffic accident
7th

V54 OCCUPANT OF PICK-UP TRUCK OR VAN OR SUV
4th INJURED IN COLLISION WITH HEAVY TRANSPORT VEHICLE OR BUS

Excludes1: occupant of pick-up truck or van injured in collision with military vehicle (V59.81)

V54.0XX Driver of pick-up truck or van injured in collision with heavy transport vehicle or bus in nontraffic accident
7th

V54.1XX Passenger in pick-up truck or van injured in collision with heavy transport vehicle or bus in nontraffic accident
7th

V54.2XX Person on outside of pick-up truck or van injured in collision with heavy transport vehicle or bus in nontraffic accident
7th

V54.3XX Unspecified occupant of pick-up truck or van injured in collision with heavy transport vehicle or bus in nontraffic accident
7th

V54.4XX Person boarding or alighting a pick-up truck or van injured in collision with heavy transport vehicle or bus
7th

V54.5XX Driver of pick-up truck or van injured in collision with heavy transport vehicle or bus in traffic accident
7th

V54.6XX Passenger in pick-up truck or van injured in collision with heavy transport vehicle or bus in traffic accident
7th

V54.7XX Person on outside of pick-up truck or van injured in collision with heavy transport vehicle or bus in traffic accident
7th

V54.9XX Unspecified occupant of pick-up truck or van injured in collision with heavy transport vehicle or bus in traffic accident
7th

V55 OCCUPANT OF PICK-UP TRUCK OR VAN OR SUV
4th INJURED IN COLLISION WITH RAILWAY TRAIN OR RAILWAY VEHICLE

V55.0XX Driver of pick-up truck or van injured in collision with railway train or railway vehicle in nontraffic accident
7th

V55.1XX Passenger in pick-up truck or van injured in collision with railway train or railway vehicle in nontraffic accident
7th

V55.2XX Person on outside of pick-up truck or van injured in collision with railway train or railway vehicle in nontraffic accident
7th

V55.3XX Unspecified occupant of pick-up truck or van injured in collision with railway train or railway vehicle in nontraffic accident
7th

V55.4XX Person boarding or alighting a pick-up truck or van injured in collision with railway train or railway vehicle
7th

V55.5XX Driver of pick-up truck or van injured in collision with railway train or railway vehicle in traffic accident
7th

V55.6XX Passenger in pick-up truck or van injured in collision with railway train or railway vehicle in traffic accident
7th

V55.7XX Person on outside of pick-up truck or van injured in collision with railway train or railway vehicle in traffic accident
7th

V55.9XX Unspecified occupant of pick-up truck or van injured in collision with railway train or railway vehicle in traffic accident
7th

V56 OCCUPANT OF PICK-UP TRUCK OR VAN INJURED IN
4th COLLISION WITH OTHER NONMOTOR VEHICLE

Includes: collision with animal-drawn vehicle, animal being ridden, streetcar
Refer to External Cause of Injuries Table

V57 OCCUPANT OF PICK-UP TRUCK
4th OR VAN OR SUV INJURED IN COLLISION WITH FIXED OR STATIONARY OBJECT

V57.0XX Driver of pick-up truck or van injured in collision with fixed or stationary object in nontraffic accident
7th

V57.1XX Passenger in pick-up truck or van injured in collision with fixed or stationary object in nontraffic accident
7th

V57.2XX Person on outside of pick-up truck or van injured in collision with fixed or stationary object in nontraffic accident
7th

V57.3XX Unspecified occupant of pick-up truck or van injured in collision with fixed or stationary object in nontraffic accident
7th

V57.4XX Person boarding or alighting a pick-up truck or van injured in collision with fixed or stationary object
7th

V57.5XX Driver of pick-up truck or van injured in collision with fixed or stationary object in traffic accident
7th

V57.6XX Passenger in pick-up truck or van injured in collision with fixed or stationary object in traffic accident
7th

V57.7XX Person on outside of pick-up truck or van injured in collision with fixed or stationary object in traffic accident
7th

V57.9XX Unspecified occupant of pick-up truck or van injured in collision with fixed or stationary object in traffic accident
7th

V58 OCCUPANT OF PICK-UP TRUCK OR VAN OR SUV
4th INJURED IN NONCOLLISION TRANSPORT ACCIDENT

Includes: overturning pick-up truck or van NOS
overturning pick-up truck or van without collision

V58.0XX Driver of pick-up truck or van injured in noncollision transport accident in nontraffic accident
7th

V58.1XX Passenger in pick-up truck or van injured in noncollision transport accident in nontraffic accident
7th

V58.2XX Person on outside of pick-up truck or van injured in noncollision transport accident in nontraffic accident
7th

V58.3XX Unspecified occupant of pick-up truck or van injured in noncollision transport accident in nontraffic accident
7th

V58.4XX Person boarding or alighting a pick-up truck or van injured in noncollision transport accident
7th

V58.5XX Driver of pick-up truck or van injured in noncollision transport accident in traffic accident
7th

V58.6XX Passenger in pick-up truck or van injured in noncollision transport accident in traffic accident
7th

V58.7XX Person on outside of pick-up truck or van injured in noncollision transport accident in traffic accident
7th

V58.9XX Unspecified occupant of pick-up truck or van injured in noncollision transport accident in traffic accident
7th

V59 OCCUPANT OF PICK-UP TRUCK OR VAN OR SUV
4th INJURED IN OTHER AND UNSPECIFIED TRANSPORT ACCIDENTS

V59.0 Driver of pick-up truck or van injured in collision with other and unspecified motor vehicles in nontraffic accident
5th

    V59.00X Driver of pick-up truck or van injured in collision with unspecified motor vehicles in nontraffic accident
    7th

    V59.09X Driver of pick-up truck or van injured in collision with other motor vehicles in nontraffic accident
    7th

4th 5th 6th 7th Additional Character Required   ✔ 3-character code

•=New Code   *Excludes1*—Not coded here, do not use together
▲=Revised Code   *Excludes2*—Not included here

 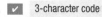

V59.1 Passenger in pick-up truck or van injured in collision with other and unspecified motor vehicles in nontraffic accident
> 5th

V59.10X Passenger in pick-up truck or van injured in collision with unspecified motor vehicles in nontraffic accident
> 7th

7th characters for categories V50–V59
A—initial encounter
D—subsequent encounter
S—sequela

V59.19X Passenger in pick-up truck or van injured in collision with other motor vehicles in nontraffic accident
> 7th

V59.2 Unspecified occupant of pick-up truck or van injured in collision with other and unspecified motor vehicles in nontraffic accident
> 5th

V59.20X Unspecified occupant of pick-up truck or van injured in collision with unspecified motor vehicles in nontraffic accident
> 7th
Collision NOS involving pick-up truck or van, nontraffic

V59.29X Unspecified occupant of pick-up truck or van injured in collision with other motor vehicles in nontraffic accident
> 7th

V59.3XX Occupant (driver) (passenger) of pick-up truck or van injured in unspecified nontraffic accident
> 7th
Accident NOS involving pick-up truck or van, nontraffic
Occupant of pick-up truck or van injured in nontraffic accident NOS

V59.4 Driver of pick-up truck or van injured in collision with other and unspecified motor vehicles in traffic accident
> 5th

V59.40X Driver of pick-up truck or van injured in collision with unspecified motor vehicles in traffic accident
> 7th

V59.49X Driver of pick-up truck or van injured in collision with other motor vehicles in traffic accident
> 7th

V59.5 Passenger in pick-up truck or van injured in collision with other and unspecified motor vehicles in traffic accident
> 5th

V59.50X Passenger in pick-up truck or van injured in collision with unspecified motor vehicles in traffic accident
> 7th

V59.59X Passenger in pick-up truck or van injured in collision with other motor vehicles in traffic accident
> 7th

V59.6 Unspecified occupant of pick-up truck or van injured in collision with other and unspecified motor vehicles in traffic accident
> 5th

V59.60X Unspecified occupant of pick-up truck or van injured in collision with unspecified motor vehicles in traffic accident
> 7th
Collision NOS involving pick-up truck or van (traffic)

V59.69X Unspecified occupant of pick-up truck or van injured in collision with other motor vehicles in traffic accident
> 7th

V59.8 Occupant (driver) (passenger) of pick-up truck or van injured in other specified transport accidents
> 5th

V59.81X Occupant (driver) (passenger) of pick-up truck or van injured in transport accident with military vehicle
> 7th

V59.88X Occupant (driver) (passenger) of pick-up truck or van injured in other specified transport accidents
> 7th

V59.9XX Occupant (driver) (passenger) of pick-up truck or van injured in unspecified traffic accident
> 7th
Accident NOS involving pick-up truck or van

(V60–V69) OCCUPANT OF HEAVY TRANSPORT VEHICLE INJURED IN TRANSPORT ACCIDENT

See complete *ICD-10-CM* manual for codes in categories V60–V69.

(V70–V79) BUS OCCUPANT INJURED IN TRANSPORT ACCIDENT

Includes: motorcoach
Excludes1: minibus (V50–V59)

V70 BUS OCCUPANT INJURED IN COLLISION WITH PEDESTRIAN OR ANIMAL
> 4th
Excludes1: bus collision with animal-drawn vehicle or animal being ridden (V76.-)

7th characters for categories V70–V79
A—initial encounter
D—subsequent encounter
S—sequela

V70.0XX Driver of bus injured in collision with pedestrian or animal in nontraffic accident
> 7th

V70.1XX Passenger on bus injured in collision with pedestrian or animal in nontraffic accident
> 7th

V70.2XX Person on outside of bus injured in collision with pedestrian or animal in nontraffic accident
> 7th

V70.3XX Unspecified occupant of bus injured in collision with pedestrian or animal in nontraffic accident
> 7th

V70.4XX Person boarding or alighting from bus injured in collision with pedestrian or animal
> 7th

V70.5XX Driver of bus injured in collision with pedestrian or animal in traffic accident
> 7th

V70.6XX Passenger on bus injured in collision with pedestrian or animal in traffic accident
> 7th

V70.7XX Person on outside of bus injured in collision with pedestrian or animal in traffic accident
> 7th

V70.9XX Unspecified occupant of bus injured in collision with pedestrian or animal in traffic accident
> 7th

V71 BUS OCCUPANT INJURED IN COLLISION WITH PEDAL CYCLE
Refer to External Cause of Injuries Table

V72 BUS OCCUPANT INJURED IN COLLISION WITH TWO- OR THREE-WHEELED MOTOR VEHICLE
> 4th

V72.0XX Driver of bus injured in collision with two- or three-wheeled motor vehicle in nontraffic accident
> 7th

V72.1XX Passenger on bus injured in collision with two- or three-wheeled motor vehicle in nontraffic accident
> 7th

V72.2XX Person on outside of bus injured in collision with two- or three-wheeled motor vehicle in nontraffic accident
> 7th

V72.3XX Unspecified occupant of bus injured in collision with two- or three-wheeled motor vehicle in nontraffic accident
> 7th

V72.4XX Person boarding or alighting from bus injured in collision with two- or three-wheeled motor vehicle
> 7th

V72.5XX Driver of bus injured in collision with two- or three-wheeled motor vehicle in traffic accident, sequela
> 7th

V72.6XX Passenger on bus injured in collision with two- or three-wheeled motor vehicle in traffic accident
> 7th

V72.7XX Person on outside of bus injured in collision with two- or three-wheeled motor vehicle in traffic accident
> 7th

V72.9XX Unspecified occupant of bus injured in collision with two- or three-wheeled motor vehicle in traffic accident
> 7th

V73 BUS OCCUPANT INJURED IN COLLISION WITH CAR, PICK-UP TRUCK OR VAN
> 4th

V73.0XX Driver of bus injured in collision with car, pick-up truck or van in nontraffic accident
> 7th

V73.1XX Passenger on bus injured in collision with car, pick-up truck or van in nontraffic accident
> 7th

V73.2XX Person on outside of bus injured in collision with car, pick-up truck or van in nontraffic accident
> 7th

V73.3XX Unspecified occupant of bus injured in collision with car, pick-up truck or van in nontraffic accident
> 7th

V73.4XX Person boarding or alighting from bus injured in collision with car, pick-up truck or van
> 7th

V73.5XX Driver of bus injured in collision with car, pick-up truck or van in traffic accident
> 7th

V73.6XX Passenger on bus injured in collision with car, pick-up truck or van in traffic accident
> 7th

V73.7XX Person on outside of bus injured in collision with car, pick-up truck or van in traffic accident
> 7th

V73.9XX Unspecified occupant of bus injured in collision with car, pick-up truck or van in traffic accident
> 7th

V74 BUS OCCUPANT INJURED IN COLLISION WITH HEAVY TRANSPORT VEHICLE OR BUS
> 4th
Excludes1: bus occupant injured in collision with military vehicle (V79.81)

V74.0XX Driver of bus injured in collision with heavy transport vehicle or bus in nontraffic accident
> 7th

V74.1XX Passenger on bus injured in collision with heavy transport vehicle or bus in nontraffic accident
> 7th

V74.2XX Person on outside of bus injured in collision with heavy transport vehicle or bus in nontraffic accident
> 7th

4th	5th	6th	7th	Additional Character Required	✓ 3-character code

•=New Code
▲=Revised Code

Excludes1—Not coded here, do not use together
Excludes2—Not included here

CHAPTER 20. EXTERNAL CAUSES OF MORBIDITY (V74.3XX–V79.9XX)

V74.3XX Unspecified occupant of bus injured in collision with heavy transport vehicle or bus in nontraffic accident
7th

V74.4XX Person boarding or alighting from bus injured in collision with heavy transport vehicle or bus
7th

V74.5XX Driver of bus injured in collision with heavy transport vehicle or bus in traffic accident
7th

V74.6XX Passenger on bus injured in collision with heavy transport vehicle or bus in traffic accident
7th

V74.7XX Person on outside of bus injured in collision with heavy transport vehicle or bus in traffic accident
7th

V74.9XX Unspecified occupant of bus injured in collision with heavy transport vehicle or bus in traffic accident
7th

> 7th characters for categories
> V70–V79
> A—initial encounter
> D—subsequent encounter
> S—sequela

V75 **BUS OCCUPANT INJURED IN COLLISION WITH RAILWAY**
4th **TRAIN OR RAILWAY VEHICLE**

V75.0XX Driver of bus injured in collision with railway train or railway vehicle in nontraffic accident
7th

V75.1XX Passenger on bus injured in collision with railway train or railway vehicle in nontraffic accident
7th

V75.2XX Person on outside of bus injured in collision with railway train or railway vehicle in nontraffic accident
7th

V75.3XX Unspecified occupant of bus injured in collision with railway train or railway vehicle in nontraffic accident
7th

V75.4XX Person boarding or alighting from bus injured in collision with railway train or railway vehicle
7th

V75.5XX Driver of bus injured in collision with railway train or railway vehicle in traffic accident
7th

V75.6XX Passenger on bus injured in collision with railway train or railway vehicle in traffic accident
7th

V75.7XX Person on outside of bus injured in collision with railway train or railway vehicle in traffic accident
7th

V75.9XX Unspecified occupant of bus injured in collision with railway train or railway vehicle in traffic accident
7th

V76 **BUS OCCUPANT INJURED IN COLLISION WITH OTHER**
7th **NONMOTOR VEHICLE**
Refer to External Cause of Injuries Table

V77 **BUS OCCUPANT INJURED IN COLLISION WITH FIXED OR**
4th **STATIONARY OBJECT**

V77.0XX Driver of bus injured in collision with fixed or stationary object in nontraffic accident
7th

V77.1XX Passenger on bus injured in collision with fixed or stationary object in nontraffic accident
7th

V77.2XX Person on outside of bus injured in collision with fixed or stationary object in nontraffic accident
7th

V77.3XX Unspecified occupant of bus injured in collision with fixed or stationary object in nontraffic accident
7th

V77.4XX Person boarding or alighting from bus injured in collision with fixed or stationary object
7th

V77.5XX Driver of bus injured in collision with fixed or stationary object in traffic accident
7th

V77.6XX Passenger on bus injured in collision with fixed or stationary object in traffic accident
7th

V77.7XX Person on outside of bus injured in collision with fixed or stationary object in traffic accident
7th

V77.9XX Unspecified occupant of bus injured in collision with fixed or stationary object in traffic accident
7th

V78 **BUS OCCUPANT INJURED IN NONCOLLISION**
4th **TRANSPORT ACCIDENT**
Includes: overturning bus NOS
overturning bus without collision

V78.0XX Driver of bus injured in noncollision transport accident in nontraffic accident
7th

V78.1XX Passenger on bus injured in noncollision transport accident in nontraffic accident
7th

V78.2XX Person on outside of bus injured in noncollision transport accident in nontraffic accident
7th

V78.3XX Unspecified occupant of bus injured in noncollision transport accident in nontraffic accident
7th

V78.4XX Person boarding or alighting from bus injured in noncollision transport accident
7th

V78.5XX Driver of bus injured in noncollision transport accident in traffic accident
7th

V78.6XX Passenger on bus injured in noncollision transport accident in traffic accident
7th

V78.7XX Person on outside of bus injured in noncollision transport accident in traffic accident
7th

V78.9XX Unspecified occupant of bus injured in noncollision transport accident in traffic accident
7th

V79 **BUS OCCUPANT INJURED IN OTHER AND UNSPECIFIED**
4th **TRANSPORT ACCIDENTS**

V79.0 Driver of bus injured in collision with other and unspecified
5th motor vehicles in nontraffic accident

> **V79.00X** Driver of bus injured in collision with unspecified
> 7th motor vehicles in nontraffic accident

> **V79.09X** Driver of bus injured in collision with other motor
> 7th vehicles in nontraffic accident

V79.1 Passenger on bus injured in collision with other and
5th unspecified motor vehicles in nontraffic accident

> **V79.10X** Passenger on bus injured in collision with
> 7th unspecified motor vehicles in nontraffic accident

> **V79.19X** Passenger on bus injured in collision with other
> 7th motor vehicles in nontraffic accident

V79.2 Unspecified bus occupant injured in collision with other and
5th unspecified motor vehicles in nontraffic accident

> **V79.20X** Unspecified bus occupant injured in collision with
> 7th unspecified motor vehicles in nontraffic accident
> Bus collision NOS, nontraffic

> **V79.29X** Unspecified bus occupant injured in collision with
> 7th other motor vehicles in nontraffic accident

V79.3XX Bus occupant (driver) (passenger) injured in unspecified
7th nontraffic accident
Bus accident NOS, nontraffic
Bus occupant injured in nontraffic accident NOS

V79.4 Driver of bus injured in collision with other and unspecified
5th motor vehicles in traffic accident

> **V79.40X** Driver of bus injured in collision with unspecified
> 7th motor vehicles in traffic accident

> **V79.49X** Driver of bus injured in collision with other motor
> 7th vehicles in traffic accident

V79.5 Passenger on bus injured in collision with other and
5th unspecified motor vehicles in traffic accident

> **V79.50X** Passenger on bus injured in collision with
> 7th unspecified motor vehicles in traffic accident

> **V79.59X** Passenger on bus injured in collision with other
> 7th motor vehicles in traffic accident

V79.6 Unspecified bus occupant injured in collision with other and
5th unspecified motor vehicles in traffic accident

> **V79.60X** Unspecified bus occupant injured in collision with
> 7th unspecified motor vehicles in traffic accident
> Bus collision NOS (traffic)

> **V79.69X** Unspecified bus occupant injured in collision with
> 7th other motor vehicles in traffic accident

V79.8 Bus occupant (driver) (passenger) injured in other specified
5th transport accidents

> **V79.81X** Bus occupant (driver) (passenger) injured in
> 7th transport accidents with military vehicle

> **V79.88X** Bus occupant (driver) (passenger) injured in other
> 7th specified transport accidents

V79.9XX Bus occupant (driver) (passenger) injured in unspecified
7th traffic accident
Bus accident NOS

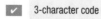

4th 5th 6th 7th Additional Character Required ✓ 3-character code

•=New Code *Excludes1*—Not coded here, do not use together
▲=Revised Code *Excludes2*—Not included here

(V80–V89) OTHER LAND TRANSPORT ACCIDENTS

V80 **ANIMAL-RIDER OR OCCUPANT OF ANIMAL-DRAWN VEHICLE INJURED IN TRANSPORT ACCIDENT**
`4th`

> 7th characters for categories
> V80–V89
> A—initial encounter
> D—subsequent encounter
> S—sequela

V80.0 Animal-rider or occupant of animal-drawn vehicle injured by fall from or being thrown from animal or animal-drawn vehicle in noncollision accident
`5th`

  V80.01 Animal-rider injured by fall from or being thrown from animal in noncollision accident
`6th`

    V80.010 Animal-rider injured by fall from or being thrown from horse in noncollision accident
`7th`

    V80.018 Animal-rider injured by fall from or being thrown from other animal in noncollision accident
`7th`

  V80.02X Occupant of animal-drawn vehicle injured by fall from or being thrown from animal-drawn vehicle in noncollision accident
`7th`
    Overturning animal-drawn vehicle NOS
    Overturning animal-drawn vehicle without collision

V80.1 Animal-rider or occupant of animal-drawn vehicle injured in collision with pedestrian or animal
`5th`
  Excludes1: animal-rider or animal-drawn vehicle collision with animal-drawn vehicle or animal being ridden (V80.7)

  V80.11X Animal-rider injured in collision with pedestrian or animal
`7th`

  V80.12X Occupant of animal-drawn vehicle injured in collision with pedestrian or animal
`7th`

V80.4 Animal-rider or occupant of animal-drawn vehicle injured in collision with car, pick-up truck, van, heavy transport vehicle or bus
`5th`
  Excludes1: animal-rider injured in collision with military vehicle (V80.910)
    occupant of animal-drawn vehicle injured in collision with military vehicle (V80.920)

  V80.41X Animal-rider injured in collision with car, pick-up truck, van, heavy transport vehicle or bus
`7th`

  V80.42X Occupant of animal-drawn vehicle injured in collision with car, pick-up truck, van, heavy transport vehicle or bus
`7th`

V80.8 Animal-rider or occupant of animal-drawn vehicle injured in collision with fixed or stationary object
`5th`

  V80.81X Animal-rider injured in collision with fixed or stationary object
`7th`

  V80.82X Occupant of animal-drawn vehicle injured in collision with fixed or stationary object
`7th`

V80.9 Animal-rider or occupant of animal-drawn vehicle injured in other and unspecified transport accidents
`5th`

  V80.91 Animal-rider injured in other and unspecified transport accidents
`6th`

    V80.919 Animal-rider injured in unspecified transport accident
`7th`
      Animal rider accident NOS

  V80.92 Occupant of animal-drawn vehicle injured in other and unspecified transport accidents
`6th`

    V80.929 Occupant of animal-drawn vehicle injured in unspecified transport accident
`7th`
      Animal-drawn vehicle accident NOS

V81 **OCCUPANT OF RAILWAY TRAIN OR RAILWAY VEHICLE INJURED IN TRANSPORT ACCIDENT**
`4th`
Includes: derailment of railway train or railway vehicle
  person on outside of train
Excludes1: streetcar (V82.-)
See complete *ICD-10-CM* manual for codes in category V81.

V82 **OCCUPANT OF POWERED STREETCAR INJURED IN TRANSPORT ACCIDENT**
`4th`
Includes: interurban electric car
  person on outside of streetcar
  tram (car)
  trolley (car)
Excludes1: bus (V70–V79)
  motorcoach (V70–V79)
  nonpowered streetcar (V76.-)
  train (V81.-)
See complete *ICD-10-CM* manual for codes in category V82.

V83 **OCCUPANT OF SPECIAL VEHICLE MAINLY USED ON INDUSTRIAL PREMISES INJURED IN TRANSPORT ACCIDENT**
`4th`
Includes: battery-powered airport passenger vehicle
  battery-powered truck (baggage) (mail)
  coal-car in mine
  forklift (truck)
  logging car
  self-propelled industrial truck
  station baggage truck (powered)
  tram, truck, or tub (powered) in mine or quarry
Excludes1: special construction vehicles (V85.-)
  special industrial vehicle in stationary use or maintenance (W31.-)
See complete *ICD-10-CM* manual for codes in category V83.

V84 **OCCUPANT OF SPECIAL VEHICLE MAINLY USED IN AGRICULTURE INJURED IN TRANSPORT ACCIDENT**
`4th`
Includes: self-propelled farm machinery
  tractor (and trailer)
Excludes1: animal-powered farm machinery accident (W30.8-)
  contact with combine harvester (W30.0)
  special agricultural vehicle in stationary use or maintenance (W30.-)

  V84.0XX Driver of special agricultural vehicle injured in traffic accident
`7th`

  V84.1XX Passenger of special agricultural vehicle injured in traffic accident
`7th`

  V84.2XX Person on outside of special agricultural vehicle injured in traffic accident
`7th`

  V84.3XX Unspecified occupant of special agricultural vehicle injured in traffic accident
`7th`

  V84.4XX Person injured while boarding or alighting from special agricultural vehicle
`7th`

  V84.5XX Driver of special agricultural vehicle injured in nontraffic accident
`7th`

  V84.6XX Passenger of special agricultural vehicle injured in nontraffic accident
`7th`

  V84.7XX Person on outside of special agricultural vehicle injured in nontraffic accident
`7th`

  V84.9XX Unspecified occupant of special agricultural vehicle injured in nontraffic accident
`7th`

V86 **OCCUPANT OF SPECIAL ALL-TERRAIN OR OTHER OFF-ROAD MOTOR VEHICLE, INJURED IN TRANSPORT ACCIDENT**
`4th`
Excludes1: special all-terrain vehicle in stationary use or maintenance (W31.-)
  sport-utility vehicle (V50–V59)
  three-wheeled motor vehicle designed for on-road use (V30–V39)

V86.0 Driver of special all-terrain or other off-road motor vehicle injured in traffic accident
`5th`

  V86.02X Driver of snowmobile injured in traffic accident
`7th`

  V86.03X Driver of dune buggy injured in traffic accident
`7th`

  V86.05X Driver of 3- or 4- wheeled all-terrain vehicle (ATV) injured in traffic accident
`7th`

  V86.06X Driver of dirt bike or motor/cross bike injured in traffic accident
`7th`

  V86.09X Driver of other special all-terrain or other off-road motor vehicle injured in traffic accident
`7th`
    Driver of go cart injured in traffic accident
    Driver of golf cart injured in traffic accident

CHAPTER 20. EXTERNAL CAUSES OF MORBIDITY (V80–V86.09X)

`4th` `5th` `6th` `7th` Additional Character Required   ✔ 3-character code

•=New Code
▲=Revised Code

Excludes1—Not coded here, do not use together
Excludes2—Not included here

V86.1 [5th] **Passenger of special all-terrain or other off-road motor vehicle injured in traffic accident**

    V86.12X [7th] **Passenger of snowmobile injured in traffic accident**

    V86.13X [7th] **Passenger of dune buggy injured in traffic accident**

7th characters for categories V80–V89
A—initial encounter
D—subsequent encounter
S—sequela

    V86.15X [7th] **Passenger of 3- or 4- wheeled ATV injured in traffic accident**

    V86.16X [7th] **Passenger of dirt bike or motor/cross bike injured in traffic accident**

    V86.19X [7th] **Passenger of other special all-terrain or other off-road motor vehicle injured in traffic accident**
        Passenger of go cart injured in traffic accident
        Passenger of golf cart injured in traffic accident

V86.3 [5th] **Unspecified occupant of special all-terrain or other off-road motor vehicle injured in traffic accident**

    V86.32X [7th] **Unspecific occupant of snowmobile injured in traffic accident**

    V86.33X [7th] **Unspecified occupant of dune buggy injured in traffic accident**

    V86.35X [7th] **Unspecified occupant of 3- or 4- wheeled ATV injured in traffic accident**

    V86.36X [7th] **Unspecified occupant of dirt bike or motor/cross bike injured in traffic accident**

    V86.39X [7th] **Unspecified occupant of other special all-terrain or other off-road motor vehicle injured in traffic accident**
        Passenger of go cart injured in traffic accident
        Passenger of golf cart injured in traffic accident

V86.5 [5th] **Driver of special all-terrain or other off-road motor vehicle injured in nontraffic accident**

    V86.52X [7th] **Driver of snowmobile injured in nontraffic accident**

    V86.53X [7th] **Driver of dune buggy injured in nontraffic accident**

    V86.55X [7th] **Driver of 3- or 4- wheeled ATV injured in nontraffic accident**

    V86.56X [7th] **Driver of dirt bike or motor/cross bike injured in nontraffic accident**

    V86.59X [7th] **Driver of other special all-terrain or other off-road motor vehicle injured in nontraffic accident**
        Driver of go cart injured in nontraffic accident
        Driver of golf cart injured in nontraffic accident

V86.6 [5th] **Passenger of special all-terrain or other off-road motor vehicle injured in nontraffic accident**

    V86.62X [7th] **Passenger of snowmobile injured in nontraffic accident**

    V86.63X [7th] **Passenger of dune buggy injured in nontraffic accident**

    V86.65X [7th] **Passenger of 3- or 4- wheeled ATV injured in nontraffic accident**

    V86.66X [7th] **Passenger of dirt bike or motor/cross bike injured in nontraffic accident**

    V86.69X [7th] **Passenger of other special all-terrain or other off-road motor vehicle injured in nontraffic accident**
        Passenger of go cart injured in nontraffic accident
        Passenger of golf cart injured in nontraffic accident

V86.9 [5th] **Unspecified occupant of special all-terrain or other off-road motor vehicle injured in nontraffic accident**

    V86.92X [7th] **Unspecific occupant of snowmobile injured in nontraffic accident**

    V86.93X [7th] **Unspecified occupant of dune buggy injured in nontraffic accident**

    V86.95X [7th] **Unspecified occupant of 3- or 4- wheeled ATV injured in nontraffic accident**

    V86.96X [7th] **Unspecified occupant of dirt bike or motor/cross bike injured in nontraffic accident**

V86.99X [7th] **Unspecified occupant of other special all-terrain or other off-road motor vehicle injured in nontraffic accident**
    Off-road motor-vehicle accident NOS
    Other motor-vehicle accident NOS
    Unspecified occupant of go cart injured in nontraffic accident
    Unspecified occupant of golf cart injured in nontraffic accident

V87 [4th] **TRAFFIC ACCIDENT OF SPECIFIED TYPE BUT VICTIM'S MODE OF TRANSPORT UNKNOWN**
    Excludes1: collision involving:
      pedal cycle (V10–V19)
      pedestrian (V01–V09)
    See complete *ICD-10-CM* manual for codes in category V87.

V88 [4th] **NONTRAFFIC ACCIDENT OF SPECIFIED TYPE BUT VICTIM'S MODE OF TRANSPORT UNKNOWN**
    Excludes1: collision involving:
      pedal cycle (V10–V19)
      pedestrian (V01–V09)
    See complete *ICD-10-CM* manual for codes in category V88.

V89 [4th] **MOTOR- OR NONMOTOR-VEHICLE ACCIDENT, TYPE OF VEHICLE UNSPECIFIED**

    V89.0XX [7th] **Person injured in unspecified motor-vehicle accident, nontraffic**
        Motor-vehicle accident NOS, nontraffic

    V89.1XX [7th] **Person injured in unspecified nonmotor-vehicle accident, nontraffic**
        Nonmotor-vehicle accident NOS (nontraffic)

    V89.2XX [7th] **Person injured in unspecified motor-vehicle accident, traffic**
        Motor-vehicle accident [MVA] NOS
        Road (traffic) accident NOS

    V89.3XX [7th] **Person injured in unspecified nonmotor-vehicle accident, traffic**
        Nonmotor-vehicle traffic accident NOS

    V89.9XX [7th] **Person injured in unspecified vehicle accident**
        Collision NOS

(V90–V94) WATER TRANSPORT ACCIDENTS

V90 [4th] **DROWNING AND SUBMERSION DUE TO ACCIDENT TO WATERCRAFT**
    Excludes1: fall into water not from watercraft (W16.-)
    water-transport-related drowning or submersion without accident to watercraft (V92.-)

7th characters for categories V90–V94
A—initial encounter
D—subsequent encounter
S—sequela

    V90.0 [5th] **Drowning and submersion due to watercraft overturning**

        V90.01X [7th] **Drowning and submersion due to passenger ship overturning**
            Drowning and submersion due to Ferry-boat overturning
            Drowning and submersion due to Liner overturning

        V90.02X [7th] **Drowning and submersion due to fishing boat overturning**

        V90.03X [7th] **Drowning and submersion due to other powered watercraft overturning**
            Drowning and submersion due to Hovercraft (on open water)/Jet ski overturning

        V90.04X [7th] **Drowning and submersion due to sailboat overturning**

        V90.05X [7th] **Drowning and submersion due to canoe or kayak overturning**

        V90.06X [7th] **Drowning and submersion due to (nonpowered) inflatable craft overturning**

        V90.08X [7th] **Drowning and submersion due to other unpowered watercraft overturning**
            Drowning and submersion due to windsurfer overturning

        V90.09X [7th] **Drowning and submersion due to unspecified watercraft overturning**
            Drowning and submersion due to boat/ship/watercraft NOS overturning

---

[4th] [5th] [6th] [7th]   Additional Character Required   3-character code

•=New Code
▲=Revised Code

Excludes1—Not coded here, do not use together
Excludes2—Not included here

V91 **OTHER INJURY DUE TO ACCIDENT TO WATERCRAFT**
4th *Includes:* any injury except drowning and
submersion as a result of an
accident to watercraft
Excludes1: civilian water transport
accident involving military watercraft
(V94.81-)
military watercraft accident in military or
war operations (Y36, Y37.-)
Excludes2: drowning and submersion due to accident to watercraft (V90.-)
See complete *ICD-10-CM* manual for codes in category V91.

> 7th characters for categories
> V90–V94
> A—initial encounter
> D—subsequent encounter
> S—sequela

V92 **DROWNING AND SUBMERSION DUE TO ACCIDENT**
4th **ON BOARD WATERCRAFT, WITHOUT ACCIDENT TO**
WATERCRAFT
Excludes1: civilian water transport accident involving military watercraft
(V94.81-)
drowning or submersion due to accident to watercraft (V90-V91)
drowning or submersion of diver who voluntarily jumps from boat not
involved in an accident (W16.711, W16.721)
fall into water without watercraft (W16.-)
military watercraft accident in military or war operations (Y36, Y37)
See complete *ICD-10-CM* manual for codes in category V92.

V93 **OTHER INJURY WHILE ON WATERCRAFT, WITHOUT**
4th **ACCIDENT TO WATERCRAFT**
V93.3 **Fall on board watercraft**
5th *Excludes1:* fall due to collision of watercraft (V91.2-)
V93.32X **Fall on board fishing boat**
7th
V93.33X **Fall on board other powered watercraft**
7th Fall on board Hovercraft/Jet ski (on open water)
V93.34X **Fall on board sailboat**
7th
V93.35X **Fall on board canoe or kayak**
7th
V93.36X **Fall on board (nonpowered) inflatable craft**
7th
V93.38X **Fall on board other unpowered watercraft**
7th
V93.39X **Fall on board unspecified watercraft**
7th Fall on board boat/ship/watercraft NOS
V93.8 **Other injury due to other accident on board watercraft**
5th Accidental poisoning by gases or fumes on watercraft
V93.82X **Other injury due to other accident on board fishing**
7th **boat**
V93.83X **Other injury due to other accident on board other**
7th **powered watercraft**
Other injury due to other accident on board Hovercraft
Other injury due to other accident on board Jet ski
V93.84X **Other injury due to other accident on board sailboat**
7th
V93.85X **Other injury due to other accident on board canoe or**
7th **kayak**
V93.86X **Other injury due to other accident on board**
7th **(nonpowered) inflatable craft**
V93.87X **Other injury due to other accident on board water-**
7th **skis**
Hit or struck by object while waterskiing
V93.88X **Other injury due to other accident on board other**
7th **unpowered watercraft**
Hit or struck by object while surfing
Hit or struck by object while on board windsurfer
V93.89X **Other injury due to other accident on board**
7th **unspecified watercraft**
Other injury due to other accident on board boat/ship/
watercraft NOS

V94 **OTHER AND UNSPECIFIED WATER TRANSPORT**
4th **ACCIDENTS**
Excludes1: military watercraft accidents in military or war operations
(Y36, Y37)
V94.3 **Injury to rider of (inflatable) watercraft being pulled behind**
5th **other watercraft**

V94.31X **Injury to rider of (inflatable) recreational watercraft**
7th **being pulled behind other watercraft**
Injury to rider of inner-tube pulled behind motor boat
V94.4XX **Injury to barefoot water-skier**
7th Injury to person being pulled behind boat or ship
V94.9XX **Unspecified water transport accident**
7th Water transport accident NOS
initial encounter accident
for definitions of transport

(V95–V97) AIR AND SPACE TRANSPORT ACCIDENTS

Excludes1: military aircraft accidents in military or war operations (Y36, Y37)
See complete *ICD-10-CM* manual for codes in categories V95–V97.

(V98–V99) OTHER AND UNSPECIFIED TRANSPORT ACCIDENTS

See complete *ICD-10-CM* manual for codes in categories V98–V99.

(W00–X58) OTHER EXTERNAL CAUSES OF ACCIDENTAL INJURY

(W00–W19) SLIPPING, TRIPPING, STUMBLING AND FALLS

Excludes1: assault involving a fall (Y01–Y02)
fall from animal (V80.-)
fall (in) (from) machinery (in operation)
(W28–W31)
fall (in) (from) transport vehicle (V01–V99)
intentional self-harm involving a fall (X80–X81)

> 7th characters for categories
> W00–W19
> A—initial encounter
> D—subsequent encounter
> S—sequela

Excludes2: at risk for fall (history of fall) Z91.81fall
(in) (from) burning building (X00.-)
fall into fire (X00–X04, X08)

W00 **FALL DUE TO ICE AND SNOW**
4th *Includes:* pedestrian on foot falling (slipping) on ice and snow
Excludes1: fall on (from) ice and snow involving pedestrian conveyance
(V00.-)
fall from stairs and steps not due to ice and snow (W10.-)
W00.0XX **Fall on same level due to ice and snow**
7th
W00.1XX **Fall from stairs and steps due to ice and snow**
7th
W00.2XX **Other fall from one level to another due to ice and snow**
7th
W00.9XX **Unspecified fall due to ice and snow**
7th

W01 **FALL ON SAME LEVEL FROM SLIPPING, TRIPPING AND**
4th **STUMBLING**
Includes: fall on moving sidewalk
Excludes1: fall due to bumping (striking) against object (W18.0-)
fall in shower or bathtub (W18.2-)
fall on same level NOS (W18.30)
fall on same level from slipping, tripping and stumbling due to ice or
snow (W00.0)
fall off or from toilet (W18.1-)
slipping, tripping and stumbling NOS (W18.40)
slipping, tripping and stumbling without falling (W18.4-)
W01.0XX **Fall on same level from slipping, tripping and stumbling**
7th **without subsequent striking against object**
Falling over animal
W01.1 **Fall on same level from slipping, tripping and stumbling with**
5th **subsequent striking against object**
W01.11 **Fall on same level from slipping, tripping and**
6th **stumbling with subsequent striking against sharp**
object
W01.110 **Fall on same level from slipping, tripping**
7th **and stumbling with subsequent striking**
against sharp glass
W01.118 **Fall on same level from slipping, tripping**
7th **and stumbling with subsequent striking**
against other sharp object

4th 5th 6th 7th Additional Character Required ✓ 3-character code

•=New Code
▲=Revised Code

Excludes1—Not coded here, do not use together
Excludes2—Not included here

CHAPTER 20. EXTERNAL CAUSES OF MORBIDITY (W01.119–W16.21)

W01.119 [7th] Fall on same level from slipping, tripping and stumbling with subsequent striking against unspecified sharp object

7th characters for categories W00–W19
A—initial encounter
D—subsequent encounter
S—sequela

W01.19 [6th] Fall on same level from slipping, tripping and stumbling with subsequent striking against other object

W01.190 [7th] Fall on same level from slipping, tripping and stumbling with subsequent striking against furniture

W01.198 [7th] Fall on same level from slipping, tripping and stumbling with subsequent striking against other object

W03 [7th] **OTHER FALL ON SAME LEVEL DUE TO COLLISION WITH ANOTHER PERSON**
Fall due to non-transport collision with other person
Excludes1: collision with another person without fall (W51)
crushed or pushed by a crowd or human stampede (W52)
fall involving pedestrian conveyance (V00-V09)
fall due to ice or snow (W00)
fall on same level NOS (W18.30)

W04 [7th] **FALL WHILE BEING CARRIED OR SUPPORTED BY OTHER PERSONS**
Accidentally dropped while being carried

W05 [7th] **FALL FROM NON-MOVING WHEELCHAIR, NONMOTORIZED SCOOTER AND MOTORIZED MOBILITY SCOOTER**
Excludes1: fall from moving wheelchair (powered) (V00.811)
fall from moving motorized mobility scooter (V00.831)
fall from nonmotorized scooter (V00.141)

W06 [7th] **FALL FROM BED**

W07 [7th] **FALL FROM CHAIR**

W08 [7th] **FALL FROM OTHER FURNITURE**

W09 [4th] **FALL ON AND FROM PLAYGROUND EQUIPMENT**
Excludes1: fall involving recreational machinery (W31)

W09.0XX [7th] Fall on or from playground slide

W09.1XX [7th] Fall from playground swing

W09.2XX [7th] Fall on or from jungle gym

W09.8XX [7th] Fall on or from other playground equipment

W10 [4th] **FALL ON AND FROM STAIRS AND STEPS**
Excludes1: Fall from stairs and steps due to ice and snow (W00.1)

W10.0XX [7th] Fall (on) (from) escalator

W10.1XX [7th] Fall (on) (from) sidewalk curb

W10.2XX [7th] Fall (on) (from) incline
Fall (on) (from) ramp

W10.8XX [7th] Fall (on) (from) other stairs and steps

W10.9XX [7th] Fall (on) (from) unspecified stairs and steps

W11 [7th] **FALL ON AND FROM LADDER**

W12 [7th] **FALL ON AND FROM SCAFFOLDING**

W13 [4th] **FALL FROM, OUT OF OR THROUGH BUILDING OR STRUCTURE**

W13.0XX [7th] Fall from, out of or through balcony
Fall from, out of or through railing

W13.1XX [7th] Fall from, out of or through bridge

W13.2XX [7th] Fall from, out of or through roof

W13.3XX [7th] Fall through floor

W13.4XX [7th] Fall from, out of or through window
Excludes2: fall with subsequent striking against sharp glass (W01.110)

W14 [7th] **FALL FROM TREE**

W15 [7th] **FALL FROM CLIFF**

W16 [4th] **FALL, JUMP OR DIVING INTO WATER**
Excludes1: accidental non-watercraft drowning and submersion not involving fall (W65–W74)
effects of air pressure from diving (W94.-)
fall into water from watercraft (V90–V94)
hitting an object or against bottom when falling from watercraft (V94.0)
Excludes2: striking or hitting diving board (W21.4)

W16.0 [5th] Fall into swimming pool
Excludes1: fall into empty swimming pool (W17.3)

W16.01 [6th] Fall into swimming pool striking water surface

W16.011 [7th] Fall into swimming pool striking water surface causing drowning and submersion
Excludes1: drowning and submersion while in swimming pool without fall (W67)

W16.012 [7th] Fall into swimming pool striking water surface causing other injury

W16.02 [6th] Fall into swimming pool striking bottom

W16.021 [7th] Fall into swimming pool striking bottom causing drowning and submersion
Excludes1: drowning and submersion while in swimming pool without fall (W67)

W16.022 [7th] Fall into swimming pool striking bottom causing other injury

W16.03 [6th] Fall into swimming pool striking wall

W16.031 [7th] Fall into swimming pool striking wall causing drowning and submersion
Excludes1: drowning and submersion while in swimming pool without fall (W67)

W16.032 [7th] Fall into swimming pool striking wall causing other injury

W16.1 [5th] Fall into natural body of water
Fall into lake
Fall into open sea
Fall into river
Fall into stream

W16.11 [6th] Fall into natural body of water striking water surface

W16.111 [7th] Fall into natural body of water striking water surface causing drowning and submersion
Excludes1: drowning and submersion while in natural body of water without fall (W69)

W16.112 [7th] Fall into natural body of water striking water surface causing other injury

W16.12 [6th] Fall into natural body of water striking bottom

W16.121 [7th] Fall into natural body of water striking bottom causing drowning and submersion
Excludes1: drowning and submersion while in natural body of water without fall (W69)

W16.122 [7th] Fall into natural body of water striking bottom causing other injury

W16.13 [6th] Fall into natural body of water striking side

W16.131 [7th] Fall into natural body of water striking side causing drowning and submersion
Excludes1: drowning and submersion while in natural body of water without fall (W69)

W16.132 [7th] Fall into natural body of water striking side causing other injury

W16.2 [5th] Fall in (into) filled bathtub or bucket of water

W16.21 [6th] Fall in (into) filled bathtub
Excludes1: fall into empty bathtub (W18.2)

[4th] [5th] [6th] [7th] Additional Character Required	3-character code	•=New Code	*Excludes1*—Not coded here, do not use together
		▲=Revised Code	*Excludes2*—Not included here

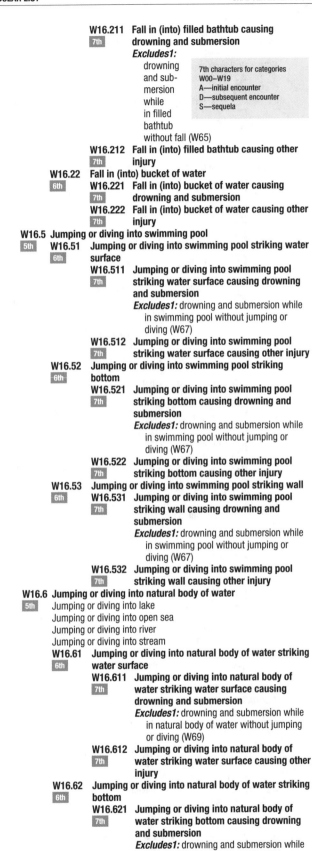

W16.211 Fall in (into) filled bathtub causing
7th **drowning and submersion**
Excludes1:
drowning and submersion while in filled bathtub without fall (W65)

7th characters for categories
W00–W19
A—initial encounter
D—subsequent encounter
S—sequela

W16.212 Fall in (into) filled bathtub causing other
7th **injury**

W16.22 Fall in (into) bucket of water
6th
    W16.221 Fall in (into) bucket of water causing
    7th **drowning and submersion**
    W16.222 Fall in (into) bucket of water causing other
    7th **injury**

W16.5 Jumping or diving into swimming pool
5th
    W16.51 Jumping or diving into swimming pool striking water
    6th **surface**
        W16.511 Jumping or diving into swimming pool
        7th **striking water surface causing drowning and submersion**
        Excludes1: drowning and submersion while in swimming pool without jumping or diving (W67)
        W16.512 Jumping or diving into swimming pool
        7th **striking water surface causing other injury**
    W16.52 Jumping or diving into swimming pool striking
    6th **bottom**
        W16.521 Jumping or diving into swimming pool
        7th **striking bottom causing drowning and submersion**
        Excludes1: drowning and submersion while in swimming pool without jumping or diving (W67)
        W16.522 Jumping or diving into swimming pool
        7th **striking bottom causing other injury**
    W16.53 Jumping or diving into swimming pool striking wall
    6th
        W16.531 Jumping or diving into swimming pool
        7th **striking wall causing drowning and submersion**
        Excludes1: drowning and submersion while in swimming pool without jumping or diving (W67)
        W16.532 Jumping or diving into swimming pool
        7th **striking wall causing other injury**

W16.6 Jumping or diving into natural body of water
5th
Jumping or diving into lake
Jumping or diving into open sea
Jumping or diving into river
Jumping or diving into stream
    W16.61 Jumping or diving into natural body of water striking
    6th **water surface**
        W16.611 Jumping or diving into natural body of
        7th **water striking water surface causing drowning and submersion**
        Excludes1: drowning and submersion while in natural body of water without jumping or diving (W69)
        W16.612 Jumping or diving into natural body of
        7th **water striking water surface causing other injury**
    W16.62 Jumping or diving into natural body of water striking
    6th **bottom**
        W16.621 Jumping or diving into natural body of
        7th **water striking bottom causing drowning and submersion**
        Excludes1: drowning and submersion while in natural body of water without jumping or diving (W69)
        W16.622 Jumping or diving into natural body of
        7th **water striking bottom causing other injury**

W17 OTHER FALL FROM ONE LEVEL TO ANOTHER
4th
W17.0XX Fall into well
7th
W17.1XX Fall into storm drain or manhole
7th
W17.2XX Fall into hole
7th
Fall into pit
W17.3XX Fall into empty swimming pool
7th
Excludes1: fall into filled swimming pool (W16.0-)
W17.4XX Fall from dock
7th
W17.8 Other fall from one level to another
5th
    W17.81X Fall down embankment (hill)*
    7th
    W17.82X Fall from (out of) grocery cart
    7th
    Fall due to grocery cart tipping over
    W17.89X Other fall from one level to another
    7th
    Fall from cherry picker/lifting device/sky lift

W18 OTHER SLIPPING, TRIPPING AND STUMBLING AND
4th **FALLS**
W18.0 Fall due to bumping against object
5th
Striking against object with subsequent fall
Excludes1: fall on same level due to slipping, tripping, or stumbling with subsequent striking against object (W01.1-)
    W18.00X Striking against unspecified object with subsequent
    7th **fall**
    W18.01X Striking against sports equipment with subsequent
    7th **fall**
    W18.02X Striking against glass with subsequent fall
    7th
    W18.09X Striking against other object with subsequent fall
    7th
W18.1 Fall from or off toilet
5th
    W18.11X Fall from or off toilet without subsequent striking
    7th **against object**
    Fall from (off) toilet NOS
    W18.12X Fall from or off toilet with subsequent striking
    7th **against object**
W18.2XX Fall in (into) shower or empty bathtub
7th
Excludes1: fall in full bathtub causing drowning or submersion (W16.21-)
W18.3 Other and unspecified fall on same level
5th
    W18.30X Fall on same level, unspecified
    7th
    W18.31X Fall on same level due to stepping on an object
    7th
    Fall on same level due to stepping on an animal
    Excludes1: slipping, tripping and stumbling without fall due to stepping on animal (W18.41)
    W18.39X Other fall on same level
    7th
W18.4 Slipping, tripping and stumbling without falling
5th
Excludes1: collision with another person without fall (W51)
    W18.40X Slipping, tripping and stumbling without falling,
    7th **unspecified**
    W18.41X Slipping, tripping and stumbling without falling due
    7th **to stepping on object**
    Slipping, tripping and stumbling without falling due to stepping on animal
    Excludes1: slipping, tripping and stumbling with fall due to stepping on animal (W18.31)
    W18.42X Slipping, tripping and stumbling without falling due
    7th **to stepping into hole or opening**
    W18.43X Slipping, tripping and stumbling without falling due
    7th **to stepping from one level to another**
    W18.49X Other slipping, tripping and stumbling without falling
    7th

W19 UNSPECIFIED FALL
Accidental fall NOS

4th 5th 6th 7th Additional Character Required   ✔ 3-character code

•=New Code   *Excludes1*—Not coded here, do not use together
▲=Revised Code   *Excludes2*—Not included here

CHAPTER 20. EXTERNAL CAUSES OF MORBIDITY   (W20–W49)

(W20–W49) EXPOSURE TO INANIMATE MECHANICAL FORCES

Excludes1: assault (X92–Y08)
  contact or collision with animals or persons
    (W50–W64)
  exposure to inanimate mechanical forces
    involving military or war operations
    (Y36.-, Y37.-)
  intentional self-harm (X71–X83)

> 7th characters for categories
> W20–W49
> A—initial encounter
> D—subsequent encounter
> S—sequela

W20 STRUCK BY THROWN, PROJECTED OR FALLING OBJECT
`7th`

Code first any associated:
  cataclysm (X34-X39)
  lightning strike (T75.00)
Excludes1: falling object in machinery accident (W24, W28-W31)
  falling object in transport accident (V01-V99)
  object set in motion by explosion (W35-W40)
  object set in motion by firearm (W32-W34)
  struck by thrown sports equipment (W21.-)

W21 STRIKING AGAINST OR STRUCK BY SPORTS EQUIPMENT
`4th`

Excludes1: assault with sports equipment (Y08.0-)
  striking against or struck by sports equipment with subsequent fall
    (W18.01)

W21.0 Struck by hit or thrown ball
`5th`

W21.00X Struck by hit or thrown ball, unspecified type
`7th`

W21.01X Struck by football
`7th`

W21.02X Struck by soccer ball
`7th`

W21.03X Struck by baseball
`7th`

W21.04X Struck by golf ball
`7th`

W21.05X Struck by basketball
`7th`

W21.06X Struck by volleyball
`7th`

W21.07X Struck by softball
`7th`

W21.09X Struck by other hit or thrown ball
`7th`

W21.1 Struck by bat, racquet or club
`5th`

W21.11X Struck by baseball bat
`7th`

W21.12X Struck by tennis racquet
`7th`

W21.13X Struck by golf club
`7th`

W21.19X Struck by other bat, racquet or club
`7th`

W21.2 Struck by hockey stick or puck
`5th`

W21.21 Struck by hockey stick
`6th`

W21.210 Struck by ice hockey stick
`7th`

W21.211 Struck by field hockey stick
`7th`

W21.22 Struck by hockey puck
`6th`

W21.220 Struck by ice hockey puck
`7th`

W21.221 Struck by field hockey puck
`7th`

W21.3 Struck by sports foot wear
`5th`

W21.31X Struck by shoe cleats
`7th`
  Stepped on by shoe cleats
W21.32X Struck by skate blades
`7th`
  Skated over by skate blades
W21.39X Struck by other sports foot wear
`7th`

W21.4XX Striking against diving board
`7th`
  Use additional code for subsequent falling into water, if
    applicable (W16.-)
W21.8 Striking against or struck by other sports equipment
`5th`
  W21.81X Striking against or struck by football helmet
  `7th`
  W21.89X Striking against or struck by other sports equipment
  `7th`
W21.9XX Striking against or struck by unspecified sports equipment
`7th`

W22 STRIKING AGAINST OR STRUCK BY OTHER OBJECTS
`4th`

Excludes1: striking against or struck by object with subsequent fall
  (W18.09)
W22.0 Striking against stationary object
`5th`
  Excludes1: striking against stationary sports equipment (W21.8)
  W22.01X Walked into wall
  `7th`
  W22.02X Walked into lamppost
  `7th`
  W22.03X Walked into furniture
  `7th`
  W22.04 Striking against wall of swimming pool
  `6th`
    W22.041 Striking against wall of swimming pool
    `7th`   **causing drowning and submersion**
      Excludes1: drowning and submersion while
        swimming without striking against wall
        (W67)
    W22.042 Striking against wall of swimming pool
    `7th`   **causing other injury**
  W22.09X Striking against other stationary object
  `7th`
W22.1 Striking against or struck by automobile airbag
`5th`
  W22.10X Striking against or struck by unspecified automobile
  `7th`   **airbag**
  W22.11X Striking against or struck by driver side automobile
  `7th`   **airbag**
  W22.12X Striking against or struck by front passenger side
  `7th`   **automobile airbag**
  W22.19X Striking against or struck by other automobile airbag
  `7th`
W22.8XX Striking against or struck by other objects
`7th`
  Striking against or struck by object NOS
    Excludes1: struck by thrown, projected or falling object (W20.-)

W23 CAUGHT, CRUSHED, JAMMED OR PINCHED IN OR BETWEEN OBJECTS
`4th`

Excludes1: injury caused by cutting or
    piercing instruments (W25–W27)
  injury caused by firearms malfunction
    (W32.1, W33.1-, W34.1-)
  injury caused by lifting and transmission devices (W24.-)
  injury caused by machinery (W28–W31)
  injury caused by nonpowered hand tools (W27.-)
  injury caused by transport vehicle being used as a means of
    transportation (V01–V99)
  injury caused by struck by thrown, projected or falling object (W20.-)
W23.0XX Caught, crushed, jammed, or pinched between moving
`7th`   **objects**
W23.1XX Caught, crushed, jammed, or pinched between stationary
`7th`   **objects**

W24 CONTACT WITH LIFTING AND TRANSMISSION DEVICES, NOT ELSEWHERE CLASSIFIED
`4th`

Excludes1: transport accidents (V01-V99)
W24.0XX Contact with lifting devices, not elsewhere classified
`7th`
  Contact with chain hoist
  Contact with drive belt
  Contact with pulley (block)
W24.1XX Contact with transmission devices, not elsewhere classified
`7th`
  Contact with transmission belt or cable

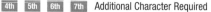

`4th` `5th` `6th` `7th` Additional Character Required   ✓ 3-character code

• =New Code   *Excludes1*—Not coded here, do not use together
▲ =Revised Code   *Excludes2*—Not included here

W25 **CONTACT WITH SHARP GLASS**
7th
Code first any associated:
injury due to flying glass from explosion
or firearm discharge (W32–W40)
transport accident (V00–V99)
Excludes1: fall on same level due to
slipping, tripping and stumbling with
subsequent striking against sharp glass (W01.110)
striking against sharp glass with subsequent fall (W18.02)
Excludes 2: glass embedded in skin (W45)

7th characters for categories
W20–W49
A—initial encounter
D—subsequent encounter
S—sequela

W26 **CONTACT WITH OTHER SHARP OBJECTS**
4th
Excludes 2: glass embedded in skin (W45)
W26.0XX **Contact with knife**
7th
W26.1XX **Contact with sword or dagger**
7th   **Excludes1:** contact with electric knife (W29.1)
W26.2XX **Contact with edge of stiff paper**
7th   Paper cut
W26.8XX **Contact with other sharp objects NEC**
7th   Contact with tin can lid
W26.9XX **Contact with unspecified sharp objects**
7th

W27 **CONTACT WITH NONPOWERED HAND TOOL**
4th
W27.0XX **Contact with workbench tool**
7th   Contact with auger
Contact with axe
Contact with chisel
Contact with handsaw
Contact with screwdriver
W27.1XX **Contact with garden tool**
7th   Contact with hoe
Contact with nonpowered lawn mower
Contact with pitchfork
Contact with rake
W27.2XX **Contact with scissors**
7th
W27.3XX **Contact with needle (sewing)**
7th   **Excludes1:** contact with hypodermic needle (W46.-)
W27.4XX **Contact with kitchen utensil**
7th   Contact with fork
Contact with ice-pick
Contact with can-opener NOS
W27.5XX **Contact with paper-cutter**
7th
W27.8XX **Contact with other nonpowered hand tool**
7th   Contact with nonpowered sewing machine
Contact with shovel

W28 **CONTACT WITH POWERED LAWN MOWER**
7th
Powered lawn mower (commercial) (residential)
Excludes1: contact with nonpowered lawn mower (W27.1)
Excludes2: exposure to electric current (W86.-)

(W29–W38)
See complete *ICD-10-CM* manual for codes in categories W29–W38.

W39 **DISCHARGE OF FIREWORK**
7th

(W40, W42)
See complete *ICD-10-CM* manual for codes in categories W40–W42.

W45 **FB OR OBJECT ENTERING THROUGH SKIN**
4th
Includes: foreign body or object embedded in skin
nail embedded in skin
Excludes2: contact with hand tools (nonpowered) (powered) (W27–W29)
contact with other sharp object(s) (W26.-)
contact with sharp glass (W25.-)
paper cut (W26.2-)
struck by objects (W20–W22)
W45.0XX **Nail entering through skin**
7th
W45.8XX **Other FB or object entering through skin**
7th   Splinter in skin NOS

W46 **CONTACT WITH HYPODERMIC NEEDLE**
4th
W46.0XX **Contact with hypodermic needle**
7th   Hypodermic needle stick NOS
W46.1XX **Contact with contaminated hypodermic needle**
7th

W49 **EXPOSURE TO OTHER INANIMATE MECHANICAL**
4th **FORCES**
Includes: exposure to abnormal gravitational [G] forces
exposure to inanimate mechanical forces NEC
Excludes1: exposure to inanimate mechanical forces involving military or
war operations (Y36.-, Y37.-)
W49.0 **Item causing external constriction**
5th   **W49.01X** **Hair causing external constriction**
7th
W49.02X **String or thread causing external constriction**
7th
W49.03X **Rubber band causing external constriction**
7th
W49.04X **Ring or other jewelry causing external constriction**
7th
W49.09X **Other specified item causing external constriction**
7th
W49.9XX **Exposure to other inanimate mechanical forces**
7th

(W50–W64) EXPOSURE TO ANIMATE MECHANICAL FORCES

Excludes1: Toxic effect of contact with venomous animals and plants (T63.-)

W50 **ACCIDENTAL HIT, STRIKE,**
4th **KICK, TWIST, OR SCRATCH BY**
ANOTHER PERSON
Includes: hit, strike, kick, twist, bite, or
scratch by another person NOS
Excludes1: assault by bodily force (Y04)
struck by objects (W20–W22)

7th characters for categories
W50–W64
A—initial encounter
D—subsequent encounter
S—sequela

W50.0XX **Accidental hit or strike by another person**
7th   Hit or strike by another person NOS
W50.1XX **Accidental kick by another person**
7th   Kick by another person NOS
W50.2XX **Accidental twist by another person**
7th   Twist by another person NOS
W50.3XX **Accidental bite by another person**
7th   Human bite
Bite by another person NOS
W50.4XX **Accidental scratch by another person**
7th   Scratch by another person NOS

W51 **ACCIDENTAL STRIKING AGAINST OR BUMPED INTO BY**
7th **ANOTHER PERSON**
Excludes1: assault by striking against or bumping into by another person
(Y04.2)
fall due to collision with another person (W03)

W52 **CRUSHED, PUSHED OR STEPPED ON BY CROWD OR**
7th **HUMAN STAMPEDE**
Crushed, pushed or stepped on by crowd or human stampede with or
without fall

W53 **CONTACT WITH RODENT**
4th
Includes: contact with saliva, feces or urine of rodent
W53.0 **Contact with mouse**
5th   **W53.01X** **Bitten by mouse**
7th
W53.09X **Other contact with mouse**
7th
W53.1 **Contact with rat**
5th   **W53.11X** **Bitten by rat**
7th
W53.19X **Other contact with rat**
7th
W53.2 **Contact with squirrel**
5th   **W53.21X** **Bitten by squirrel**
7th
W53.29X **Other contact with squirrel**
7th

 4th **5th** **6th** **7th** Additional Character Required   ✔ 3-character code

 •=New Code   **Excludes1**—Not coded here, do not use together
▲=Revised Code   **Excludes2**—Not included here

CHAPTER 20. EXTERNAL CAUSES OF MORBIDITY   (W53.8–W65)

W53.8 **Contact with other rodent**
- [5th] **W53.81X Bitten by other rodent**
  - [7th]
- **W53.89X Other contact with other rodent**
  - [7th]

> 7th characters for categories
> W50–W64
> A—initial encounter
> D—subsequent encounter
> S—sequela

W54 CONTACT WITH DOG
[4th] *Includes:* contact with saliva, feces or urine of dog

W54.0XX Bitten by dog
- [7th]

W54.1XX Struck by dog
- [7th] Knocked over by dog

> Report the injury code as primary

W54.8XX Other contact with dog
- [7th]

W55 CONTACT WITH OTHER MAMMALS
[4th] *Includes:* contact with saliva, feces or urine of mammal
Excludes1: animal being ridden—see transport accidents
     bitten or struck by dog (W54)
     bitten or struck by rodent (W53.-)
     contact with marine mammals (W56.-)

W55.0 Contact with cat
- [5th] **W55.01X Bitten by cat**
  - [7th]
- **W55.03X Scratched by cat**
  - [7th]
- **W55.09X Other contact with cat**
  - [7th]

W56 CONTACT WITH NONVENOMOUS MARINE ANIMAL
[4th] *Excludes1:* contact with venomous marine animal (T63.-)
See complete *ICD-10-CM* manual for codes in category W56.

W57 ACCIDENTAL BITTEN OR STUNG BY NONVENOMOUS INSECT AND OTHER NONVENOMOUS ARTHROPODS
[7th] *Excludes1:* contact with venomous insects and arthropods (T63.2-, T63.3-, T63.4-)

W58 CONTACT WITH CROCODILE OR ALLIGATOR
[4th] See complete *ICD-10-CM* manual for codes in category W58.

W59 CONTACT WITH OTHER NONVENOMOUS REPTILES
[4th] *Excludes1:* contact with venomous reptile (T63.0-, T63.1-)

W59.0 Contact with nonvenomous lizards
- [5th] **W59.01X Bitten by nonvenomous lizards**
  - [7th]
- **W59.02X Struck by nonvenomous lizards**
  - [7th]
- **W59.09X Other contact with nonvenomous lizards**
  - [7th] Exposure to nonvenomous lizards
  - Exposure to nonvenomous lizards

W59.1 Contact with nonvenomous snakes
- [5th] **W59.11X Bitten by nonvenomous snake**
  - [7th]
- **W59.12X Struck by nonvenomous snake**
  - [7th]
- **W59.13X Crushed by nonvenomous snake**
  - [7th]
- **W59.19X Other contact with nonvenomous snake**
  - [7th]

W59.2 Contact with turtles
- [5th] Excludes1: contact with tortoises (W59.8-)
- **W59.21X Bitten by turtle**
  - [7th]
- **W59.22X Struck by turtle**
  - [7th]
- **W59.29X Other contact with turtle**
  - [7th] Exposure to turtles

W59.8 Contact with other nonvenomous reptiles
- [5th] **W59.81X Bitten by other nonvenomous reptiles**
  - [7th]
- **W59.82X Struck by other nonvenomous reptiles**
  - [7th]
- **W59.83X Crushed by other nonvenomous reptiles**
  - [7th]
- **W59.89X Other contact with other nonvenomous reptiles**
  - [7th]

W60 CONTACT WITH NONVENOMOUS PLANT THORNS AND SPINES AND SHARP LEAVES
[7th] *Excludes1:* Contact with venomous plants (T63.7-)

W61 CONTACT WITH BIRDS (DOMESTIC) (WILD)
[4th] *Includes:* contact with excreta of birds

W61.0 Contact with parrot
- [5th] **W61.01X Bitten by parrot**
  - [7th]
- **W61.02X Struck by parrot**
  - [7th]
- **W61.09X Other contact with parrot**
  - [7th] Exposure to parrots

W61.1 Contact with macaw
- [5th] **W61.11X Bitten by macaw**
  - [7th]
- **W61.12X Struck by macaw**
  - [7th]
- **W61.19X Other contact with macaw**
  - [7th] Exposure to macaws

W61.3 Contact with chicken
- [5th] **W61.32X Struck by chicken**
  - [7th]
- **W61.33X Pecked by chicken**
  - [7th]
- **W61.39X Other contact with chicken**
  - [7th] Exposure to chickens

W61.4 Contact with turkey
- [5th] **W61.42X Struck by turkey**
  - [7th]
- **W61.43X Pecked by turkey**
  - [7th]
- **W61.49X Other contact with turkey**
  - [7th]

W61.5 Contact with goose
- [5th] **W61.51X Bitten by goose**
  - [7th]
- **W61.52X Struck by goose**
  - [7th]
- **W61.59X Other contact with goose**
  - [7th]

W61.6 Contact with duck
- [5th] **W61.61X Bitten by duck**
  - [7th]
- **W61.62X Struck by duck**
  - [7th]
- **W61.69X Other contact with duck**
  - [7th]

W61.9 Contact with other birds
- [5th] **W61.91X Bitten by other birds**
  - [7th]
- **W61.92X Struck by other birds**
  - [7th]
- **W61.99X Other contact with other birds**
  - [7th] Contact with bird NOS

W62 CONTACT WITH NONVENOMOUS AMPHIBIANS
[4th] *Excludes1:* contact with venomous amphibians (T63.81-R63.83)

W62.0XX Contact with nonvenomous frogs
- [7th]

W62.1XX Contact with nonvenomous toads
- [7th]

W62.9XX Contact with other nonvenomous amphibians
- [7th]

(W65–W74) ACCIDENTAL NON-TRANSPORT DROWNING AND SUBMERSION

Excludes1: accidental drowning and submersion due to fall into water (W16.-)
   accidental drowning and submersion due to water transport accident (V90.-, V92.-)
Excludes2: accidental drowning and submersion due to cataclysm (X34–X39)

> Report the injury code as primary
> A—initial encounter
> D—subsequent encounter
> S—sequela

[4th] [5th] [6th] [7th] Additional Character Required   ✔ 3-character code

•=New Code   *Excludes1*—Not coded here, do not use together
▲=Revised Code   *Excludes2*—Not included here

W65 [7th] **ACCIDENTAL DROWNING AND SUBMERSION WHILE IN BATHTUB**
Excludes1: accidental drowning and submersion due to fall in (into) bathtub (W16.211)

W67 [7th] **ACCIDENTAL DROWNING AND SUBMERSION WHILE IN SWIMMING-POOL**
Excludes1: accidental drowning and submersion due to fall into swimming pool (W16.011, W16.021, W16.031)
accidental drowning and submersion due to striking into wall of swimming pool (W22.041)

W69 [7th] **ACCIDENTAL DROWNING AND SUBMERSION WHILE IN NATURAL WATER**
Accidental drowning and submersion while in lake/open sea/river/stream
Excludes1: accidental drowning and submersion due to fall into natural body of water (W16.111, W16.121, W16.131)

W74 [7th] **UNSPECIFIED CAUSE OF ACCIDENTAL DROWNING AND SUBMERSION**
Drowning NOS

(W85–W99) EXPOSURE TO ELECTRIC CURRENT, RADIATION AND EXTREME AMBIENT AIR TEMPERATURE AND PRESSURE

Excludes1: exposure to: failure in dosage of radiation or temperature during surgical and medical care (Y63.2–Y63.5)
lightning (T75.0-)
natural cold (X31)
natural heat (X30)
natural radiation NOS (X39)
radiological procedure and radiotherapy (Y84.2)
sunlight (X32)

> 7th characters for categories
> W85–W99
> A—initial encounter
> D—subsequent encounter
> S—sequela

W86 [4th] **EXPOSURE TO OTHER SPECIFIED ELECTRIC CURRENT**
W86.0XX [7th] **Exposure to domestic wiring and appliances**

W86.1XX [7th] **Exposure to industrial wiring, appliances and electrical machinery**
Exposure to conductors
Exposure to control apparatus
Exposure to electrical equipment and machinery
Exposure to transformers

W86.8XX [7th] **Exposure to other electric current**
Exposure to wiring and appliances in or on farm (not farmhouse)
Exposure to wiring and appliances outdoors
Exposure to wiring and appliances in or on public building
Exposure to wiring and appliances in or on residential institutions
Exposure to wiring and appliances in or on schools

W89 [4th] **EXPOSURE TO MAN-MADE VISIBLE AND ULTRAVIOLET LIGHT**
Includes: exposure to welding light (arc)
Excludes2: exposure to sunlight (X32)
W89.1XX [7th] **Exposure to tanning bed**

W93 [4th] **EXPOSURE TO EXCESSIVE COLD OF MAN-MADE ORIGIN**
W93.0 [5th] **Contact with or inhalation of dry ice**
W93.01X [7th] **Contact with dry ice**

W93.02X [7th] **Inhalation of dry ice**

W93.1 [5th] **Contact with or inhalation of liquid air**
W93.11X [7th] **Contact with liquid air**
Contact with liquid hydrogen
Contact with liquid nitrogen

W93.12X [7th] **Inhalation of liquid air**
Inhalation of liquid hydrogen
Inhalation of liquid nitrogen

W93.2XX [7th] **Prolonged exposure in deep freeze unit or refrigerator**

W93.8XX [7th] **Exposure to other excessive cold of man-made origin**

W94 [4th] **EXPOSURE TO HIGH AND LOW AIR PRESSURE AND CHANGES IN AIR PRESSURE**
W94.0XX [7th] **Exposure to prolonged high air pressure**

W94.1 **Exposure to prolonged low air pressure**
[5th] **W94.11X** **Exposure to residence or prolonged visit at high altitude**
[7th]
W94.12X **Exposure to other prolonged low air pressure**
[7th]

W94.2 **Exposure to rapid changes in air pressure during ascent**
[5th] **W94.21X** **Exposure to reduction in atmospheric pressure while surfacing from deep-water diving**
[7th]
W94.22X **Exposure to reduction in atmospheric pressure while surfacing from underground**
[7th]
W94.23X **Exposure to sudden change in air pressure in aircraft during ascent**
[7th]
W94.29X **Exposure to other rapid changes in air pressure during ascent**
[7th]

W94.3 **Exposure to rapid changes in air pressure during descent**
[5th] **W94.31X** **Exposure to sudden change in air pressure in aircraft during descent**
[7th]
W94.32X **Exposure to high air pressure from rapid descent in water**
[7th]
W94.39X **Exposure to other rapid changes in air pressure during descent**
[7th]

(X00–X08) EXPOSURE TO SMOKE, FIRE AND FLAMES

Excludes1: arson (X97)
Excludes2: explosions (W35–W40)
lightning (T75.0-)
transport accident (V01–V99)

> 7th characters for categories
> X00–X08
> A—initial encounter
> D—subsequent encounter
> S—sequela

X00 [4th] **EXPOSURE TO UNCONTROLLED FIRE IN BUILDING OR STRUCTURE**
X00.1XX [7th] **Exposure to smoke in uncontrolled fire in building or structure**

X01 [4th] **EXPOSURE TO UNCONTROLLED FIRE, NOT IN BUILDING OR STRUCTURE**
Includes: exposure to forest fire
See complete *ICD-10-CM* manual for codes in category X01.

X02 [4th] **EXPOSURE TO CONTROLLED FIRE IN BUILDING OR STRUCTURE**
Includes: exposure to fire in fireplace
exposure to fire in stove
See complete *ICD-10-CM* manual for codes in category X02.

X03 [4th] **EXPOSURE TO CONTROLLED FIRE, NOT IN BUILDING OR STRUCTURE**
Includes: exposure to bon fire
exposure to camp-fire
exposure to trash fire
Includes: conflagration in building or structure
Code first any associated cataclysm
Excludes2: Exposure to ignition or melting of nightwear (X05)
Exposure to ignition or melting of other clothing and apparel (X06.-)
Exposure to other specified smoke, fire and flames (X08.-)
X03.1XX [7th] **Exposure to smoke in controlled fire, not in building or structure**

X04 [7th] **EXPOSURE TO IGNITION OF HIGHLY FLAMMABLE MATERIAL**
Exposure to ignition of gasoline
Exposure to ignition of kerosene
Exposure to ignition of petrol
Excludes2: exposure to ignition or melting of nightwear (X05)
exposure to ignition or melting of other clothing and apparel (X06)

[4th] [5th] [6th] [7th] Additional Character Required   ✔ 3-character code   •=New Code   ▲=Revised Code   *Excludes1*—Not coded here, do not use together   *Excludes2*—Not included here

PEDIATRIC ICD-10-CM 2021: A MANUAL FOR PROVIDER-BASED CODING   429

X05   **EXPOSURE TO IGNITION OR MELTING OF NIGHTWEAR**
`7th`

Excludes2: exposure to uncontrolled fire in
     building or structure (X00.-)
     exposure to uncontrolled fire, not in
     building or structure (X01.-)
     exposure to controlled fire in building or
     structure (X02.-)
     exposure to controlled fire, not in
     building or structure (X03.-)
     exposure to ignition of highly flammable materials (X04.-)

> 7th characters for categories
> X00–X08
> A—initial encounter
> D—subsequent encounter
> S—sequela

X06   **EXPOSURE TO IGNITION OR MELTING OF OTHER**
`4th`   **CLOTHING AND APPAREL**

     X06.0XX   **Exposure to ignition of plastic jewelry**
     `7th`

     X06.1XX   **Exposure to melting of plastic jewelry**
     `7th`

     X06.2XX   **Exposure to ignition of other clothing and apparel**
     `7th`

     X06.3XX   **Exposure to melting of other clothing and apparel**
     `7th`

X08   **EXPOSURE TO OTHER SPECIFIED SMOKE, FIRE**
`4th`   **AND FLAMES**
     See complete *ICD-10-CM* manual for codes in category X08.

(X10–X19) CONTACT WITH HEAT AND HOT SUBSTANCES

Excludes1:   exposure to excessive natural heat (X30)
     exposure to fire and flames (X00–X08)

X10   **CONTACT WITH HOT DRINKS,**
`4th`   **FOOD, FATS AND COOKING**
     OILS

> 7th characters for categories
> X10–X19
> A—initial encounter
> D—subsequent encounter
> S—sequela

     X10.0XX   **Contact with hot drinks**
     `7th`

     X10.1XX   **Contact with hot food**
     `7th`

     X10.2XX   **Contact with fats and cooking oils**
     `7th`

X11   **CONTACT WITH HOT TAP-WATER**
`4th`
     Includes: contact with boiling tap-water
         contact with boiling water NOS
     Excludes1: contact with water heated on stove (X12)
     X11.0XX   **Contact with hot water in bath or tub**
     `7th`   *Excludes1:* contact with running hot water in bath or tub
             (X11.1)
     X11.1XX   **Contact with running hot water**
     `7th`   Contact with hot water running out of hose
         Contact with hot water running out of tap
     X11.8XX   **Contact with other hot tap-water**
     `7th`   Contact with hot water in bucket
         Contact with hot tap-water NOS

X12   **CONTACT WITH OTHER HOT FLUIDS**
`7th`
     Contact with water heated on stove
     Excludes1: hot (liquid) metals (X18)

X13   **CONTACT WITH STEAM AND OTHER HOT VAPORS**
`4th`   **X13.0XX**   **Inhalation of steam and other hot vapors**
     `7th`

     X13.1XX   **Other contact with steam and other hot vapors**
     `7th`

X15   **CONTACT WITH HOT HOUSEHOLD APPLIANCES**
`4th`
     Excludes1: contact with heating appliances (X16)
         contact with powered household appliances (W29.-)
         exposure to controlled fire in building or structure due to household
         appliance (X02.8)
         exposure to household appliances electrical current (W86.0)
     X15.0XX   **Contact with hot stove (kitchen)**
     `7th`

     X15.1XX   **Contact with hot toaster**
     `7th`

     X15.2XX   **Contact with hotplate**
     `7th`

     X15.3XX   **Contact with hot saucepan**
     `7th`   **or skillet**
     X15.8XX   **Contact with other hot**
     `7th`   **household appliances**
         Contact with cooker/kettle/light
         bulbs

> 7th characters for categories
> X10–X19
> A—initial encounter
> D—subsequent encounter
> S—sequela

X16   **CONTACT WITH HOT HEATING APPLIANCES, RADIATORS**
`7th`   **AND PIPES**
     Excludes1: contact with powered appliances (W29.-)
         exposure to controlled fire in building or structure due to appliance
         (X02.8)
         exposure to industrial appliances electrical current (W86.1)

X17   **CONTACT WITH HOT ENGINES, MACHINERY AND TOOLS**
`7th`
     Excludes1: contact with hot heating appliances, radiators and pipes (X16)
         contact with hot household appliances (X15)

X18   **CONTACT WITH OTHER HOT METALS**
`7th`
     Contact with liquid metal

X19   **CONTACT WITH OTHER HEAT AND HOT SUBSTANCES**
`7th`
     Excludes1: objects that are not normally hot, e.g., an object made hot by a
         house fire (X00–X08)

(X30–X39) EXPOSURE TO FORCES OF NATURE

X30   **EXPOSURE TO EXCESSIVE NATURAL HEAT**
`7th`
     Exposure to excessive heat as the cause of sunstroke
         Exposure to heat NOS
     Excludes1: excessive heat of man-made
         origin (W92)
         exposure to man-made radiation (W89)
         exposure to sunlight (X32)
         exposure to tanning bed (W89)

> 7th characters for categories
> X30–X39
> A—initial encounter
> D—subsequent encounter
> S—sequela

X31   **EXPOSURE TO EXCESSIVE NATURAL COLD**
`7th`
     Excessive cold as the cause of chilblains NOS
     Excessive cold as the cause of immersion foot or hand
     Exposure to cold NOS
     Exposure to weather conditions

X32   **EXPOSURE TO SUNLIGHT**
`7th`
     Excludes1: man-made radiation (tanning bed) (W89)
     Excludes2: radiation-related disorders of the skin and subcutaneous tissue
         (L55–L59)

X34   **EARTHQUAKE**
`7th`
     Excludes2: tidal wave (tsunami) due to earthquake (X37.41)

X35   **VOLCANIC ERUPTION**
`7th`
     Excludes2: tidal wave (tsunami) due to volcanic eruption (X37.41)

X36   **AVALANCHE, LANDSLIDE AND OTHER EARTH**
`7th`   **MOVEMENTS**
     Includes: victim of mudslide of cataclysmic nature
     Excludes1: earthquake (X34)
     Excludes2: transport accident involving collision with avalanche or
         landslide not in motion (V01–V99)

X37   **CATACLYSMIC STORM**
`4th`   **X37.0XX**   **Hurricane**
     `7th`   Storm surge
     X37.1XX   **Tornado**
     `7th`   Cyclone
          Twister
     X37.2XX   **Blizzard (snow) (ice)**
     `7th`
     X37.3XX   **Dust storm**
     `7th`
     X37.4   **Tidal wave**
     `5th`   **X37.41X**   **Tidal wave due to earthquake or volcanic eruption**
         `7th`   Tidal wave NOS
               Tsunami
         X37.42X   **Tidal wave due to storm**
         `7th`
         X37.43X   **Tidal wave due to landslide**
         `7th`

`4th` `5th` `6th` `7th`   Additional Character Required   ✔   3-character code

•=New Code   *Excludes1*—Not coded here, do not use together
▲=Revised Code   *Excludes2*—Not included here

X37.8XX **Other cataclysmic storms**
7th   Cloudburst
Torrential rain
Excludes2: flood (X38)

X37.9XX **Unspecified cataclysmic storm**
7th   Storm NOS
Excludes1: collapse of dam or man-made structure causing earth movement (X36.0)

X38 **FLOOD**
7th   Flood arising from remote storm
Flood of cataclysmic nature arising from melting snow
Flood resulting directly from storm
Excludes1: collapse of dam or man-made structure causing earth movement (X36.0)
tidal wave NOS (X37.41)
tidal wave caused by storm (X37.42)

X39 **EXPOSURE TO OTHER FORCES OF NATURE**
4th   **X39.0** **Exposure to natural radiation**
5th   *Excludes1:* contact with and (suspected) exposure to radon and other naturally occurring radiation (Z77.123)
exposure to man-made radiation (W88–W90)
exposure to sunlight (X32)

X39.01X **Exposure to radon**
7th

X39.08X **Exposure to other natural radiation**
7th

X39.8XX **Other exposure to forces of nature**
7th

(X50–X58) ACCIDENTAL EXPOSURE TO OTHER SPECIFIED FACTORS

X50 **OVEREXERTION FROM MOVEMENT**
4th   **X50.0XX** **Overexertion from strenuous**
7th   **movement or load**
Lifting heavy objects
Lifting weights

X50.1XX **Overexertion from prolonged**
7th   **static or awkward postures**
Prolonged or static bending
Prolonged or static kneeling
Prolonged or static reaching
Prolonged or static sitting
Prolonged or static standing
Prolonged or static twisting

X50.3XX **Overexertion from repetitive movements**
7th   Use of hand as hammer

X50.9XX **Other and unspecified overexertion or strenuous**
7th   **movements or postures**
Contact pressure
Contact stress

X58 **EXPOSURE TO OTHER**
7th   **SPECIFIED FACTORS**
Accident NOS
Exposure NOS

> 7th characters for categories X30–X39
> A—initial encounter
> D—subsequent encounter
> S—sequela

> 7th characters for category X50
> A—initial encounter
> D—subsequent encounter
> S—sequela

> 7th characters for category X58
> A—initial encounter
> D—subsequent encounter
> S—sequela

(X71–X83) INTENTIONAL SELF-HARM

Purposely self-inflicted injury
Suicide (attempted)

X71 **INTENTIONAL SELF-HARM BY**
4th   **DROWNING AND SUBMERSION**
See complete *ICD-10-CM* manual for codes in category X71.

> 7th characters for category X71–X83
> A—initial encounter
> D—subsequent encounter
> S—sequela

X72 **INTENTIONAL SELF-HARM BY HANDGUN DISCHARGE**
7th   Intentional self-harm by gun/pistol/revolver for single hand use
Excludes1: Very pistol (X74.8)

X73 **INTENTIONAL SELF-HARM BY**
4th   **RIFLE, SHOTGUN AND LARGER**
   FIREARM DISCHARGE
Excludes1: airgun (X74.01)
See complete *ICD-10-CM* manual for codes in category X73.

> 7th characters for category X71–X83
> A—initial encounter
> D—subsequent encounter
> S—sequela

X74 **INTENTIONAL SELF-HARM BY OTHER AND UNSPECIFIED**
4th   **FIREARM AND GUN DISCHARGE**
See complete *ICD-10-CM* manual for codes in category X74.

X75 **INTENTIONAL SELF-HARM BY EXPLOSIVE MATERIAL**
7th

X76 **INTENTIONAL SELF-HARM BY SMOKE, FIRE AND**
7th   **FLAMES**

X77 **INTENTIONAL SELF-HARM BY STEAM, HOT VAPORS AND**
4th   **HOT OBJECTS**
See complete *ICD-10-CM* manual for codes in category X77.

X78 **INTENTIONAL SELF-HARM BY SHARP OBJECT**
4th   **X78.0XX** **Intentional self-harm by sharp glass**
7th

X78.1XX **Intentional self-harm by knife**
7th

X78.2XX **Intentional self-harm by sword or dagger**
7th

X78.8XX **Intentional self-harm by other sharp object**
7th

X78.9XX **Intentional self-harm by unspecified sharp object**
7th

X79 **INTENTIONAL SELF-HARM BY BLUNT OBJECT**
7th

X80 **INTENTIONAL SELF-HARM BY JUMPING FROM A HIGH**
7th   **PLACE**
Intentional fall from one level to another

X81 **INTENTIONAL SELF-HARM BY JUMPING OR LYING IN**
4th   **FRONT OF MOVING OBJECT**
See complete *ICD-10-CM* manual for codes in category X81.

X82 **INTENTIONAL SELF-HARM BY CRASHING OF MOTOR**
4th   **VEHICLE**
See complete *ICD-10-CM* manual for codes in category X82.

X83 **INTENTIONAL SELF-HARM BY OTHER SPECIFIED MEANS**
4th   *Excludes1:* intentional self-harm by poisoning or contact with toxic substance—See Table of Drugs and Chemicals
See complete *ICD-10-CM* manual for codes in category X83.

(X92–Y09) ASSAULT

Adult and child abuse, neglect and maltreatment are classified as assault. Any of the assault codes may be used to indicate the external cause of any injury resulting from the confirmed abuse.
    For confirmed cases of abuse, neglect and maltreatment, when the perpetrator is known, a code from Y07, Perpetrator of maltreatment and neglect, should accompany any other assault codes.

> 7th characters for categories X92–Y04
> A—initial encounter
> D—subsequent encounter
> S—sequela

Includes: homicide
injuries inflicted by another person with intent to injure or kill, by any means
Excludes1: injuries due to legal intervention (Y35.-)
injuries due to operations of war (Y36.-)
injuries due to terrorism (Y38.-)

X92 **ASSAULT BY DROWNING AND SUBMERSION**
4th   **X92.0XX** **Assault by drowning and submersion while in bathtub**
7th

X92.1XX **Assault by drowning and submersion while in swimming**
7th   **pool**

X92.2XX **Assault by drowning and submersion after push into**
7th   **swimming pool**

X92.3XX **Assault by drowning and submersion in natural water**
7th

X92.8XX **Other assault by drowning and submersion**
7th

4th   5th   6th   7th   Additional Character Required   ✔   3-character code

•=New Code
▲=Revised Code

Excludes1—Not coded here, do not use together
Excludes2—Not included here

CHAPTER 20. EXTERNAL CAUSES OF MORBIDITY (X37.8XX–X92.8XX)

X92.9XX **Assault by drowning and**
7th   **submission, unspecified**

> 7th characters for categories
> X92–Y04
> A—initial encounter
> D—subsequent encounter
> S—sequela

X93 **ASSAULT BY HANDGUN**
7th **DISCHARGE**
Assault by discharge of gun for single
    hand use
Assault by discharge of pistol
Assault by discharge of revolver
Excludes1: Very pistol (X95.8)

X94 **ASSAULT BY RIFLE, SHOTGUN AND LARGER FIREARM**
4th **DISCHARGE**
Excludes1: airgun (X95.01)
X94.1XX **Assault by hunting rifle**
7th

X95 **ASSAULT BY OTHER AND UNSPECIFIED FIREARM AND**
4th **GUN DISCHARGE**
X95.0 **Assault by gas, air or spring-operated guns**
5th   **X95.01X** **Assault by airgun discharge**
     7th   Assault by BB gun discharge
         Assault by pellet gun discharge
    X95.02X **Assault by paintball gun discharge**
     7th
    X95.09X **Assault by other gas, air or spring-operated gun**
     7th
X95.8XX **Assault by other firearm discharge**
7th   Assault by very pistol [flare] discharge
X95.9XX **Assault by unspecified firearm discharge**
7th

X96 **ASSAULT BY EXPLOSIVE MATERIAL**
4th *Excludes1:* incendiary device (X97)
     terrorism involving explosive material (Y38.2-)
See complete *ICD-10-CM* manual for codes in category X96.

X97 **ASSAULT BY SMOKE, FIRE AND FLAMES**
7th Assault by arson
Assault by cigarettes

X98 **ASSAULT BY STEAM, HOT VAPORS AND HOT OBJECTS**
4th **X98.0XX** **Assault by steam or hot vapors**
     7th
X98.1XX **Assault by hot tap water**
7th
X98.2XX **Assault by hot fluids**
7th
X98.3XX **Assault by hot household appliances**
7th
X98.8XX **Assault by other hot objects**
7th
X98.9XX **Assault by unspecified hot objects**
7th

X99 **ASSAULT BY SHARP OBJECT**
4th *Excludes1:* assault by strike by sports equipment (Y08.0-)
X99.0XX **Assault by sharp glass**
7th
X99.1XX **Assault by knife**
7th
X99.8XX **Assault by other sharp object**
7th
X99.9XX **Assault by unspecified sharp object**
7th   Assault by stabbing NOS

Y00 **ASSAULT BY BLUNT OBJECT**
7th *Excludes1:* assault by strike by sports equipment (Y08.0-)

Y01 **ASSAULT BY PUSHING FROM HIGH PLACE**
7th

Y02 **ASSAULT BY PUSHING OR PLACING VICTIM IN FRONT OF**
4th **MOVING OBJECT**
Y02.0XX **Assault by pushing or placing victim in front of motor**
7th   **vehicle**
Y02.1XX **Assault by pushing or placing victim in front of (subway)**
7th   **train**

Y02.8XX **Assault by pushing or placing victim in front of other**
7th   **moving object**

Y03 **ASSAULT BY CRASHING OF MOTOR VEHICLE**
4th **Y03.0XX** **Assault by being hit or run over by motor vehicle**
     7th
Y03.8XX **Other assault by crashing of motor vehicle**
7th

Y04 **ASSAULT BY BODILY FORCE**
4th *Excludes1:* assault by:
    submersion (X92.-)
    use of weapon (X93–X95, X99, Y00)
Y04.0XX **Assault by unarmed brawl or fight**
7th
Y04.1XX **Assault by human bite**
7th
Y04.2XX **Assault by strike against or bumped into by another person**
7th
Y04.8XX **Assault by other bodily force**
7th   Assault by bodily force NOS

Y07 **PERPETRATOR OF ASSAULT, MALTREATMENT AND**
4th **NEGLECT**
Adult and child abuse, neglect and maltreatment are classified as assault.
Any of the assault codes may be used to indicate the external cause of any
injury resulting from the confirmed abuse.
    For confirmed cases of abuse, neglect and maltreatment, when the
perpetrator is known, a code from Y07, Perpetrator of maltreatment and
neglect, should accompany any other assault codes.
    See Section I.C.19. Adult and child abuse, neglect and other
maltreatment
Note: Codes from this category are for use only in cases of **confirmed**
    abuse (T74.-)
Selection of the correct perpetrator code is based on the relationship
    between the perpetrator and the victim
Includes: perpetrator of abandonment
    perpetrator of emotional neglect
    perpetrator of mental cruelty
    perpetrator of physical abuse
    perpetrator of physical neglect
    perpetrator of sexual abuse
    perpetrator of torture
Y07.0 **Spouse or partner, perpetrator of maltreatment and neglect**
5th   Spouse or partner, perpetrator of maltreatment and neglect against
       spouse or partner
    Y07.01 **Husband, perpetrator of maltreatment and neglect**
    Y07.02 **Wife, perpetrator of maltreatment and neglect**
    Y07.03 **Male partner, perpetrator of maltreatment and**
        neglect
    Y07.04 **Female partner, perpetrator of maltreatment and**
        neglect
Y07.1 **Parent (adoptive) (biological), perpetrator of maltreatment**
5th **and neglect**
    Y07.11 **Biological father, perpetrator of maltreatment**
        and neglect
    Y07.12 **Biological mother, perpetrator of maltreatment**
        and neglect
    Y07.13 **Adoptive father, perpetrator of maltreatment**
        and neglect
    Y07.14 **Adoptive mother, perpetrator of maltreatment**
        and neglect
Y07.4 **Other family member, perpetrator of maltreatment and neglect**
5th **Y07.41** **Sibling, perpetrator of maltreatment and neglect**
     6th   *Excludes1:* stepsibling, perpetrator of maltreatment and
         neglect (Y07.435, Y07.436)
       Y07.410 **Brother, perpetrator of maltreatment and**
         neglect
       Y07.411 **Sister, perpetrator of maltreatment and**
         neglect
    Y07.42 **Foster parent, perpetrator of maltreatment and**
     6th   **neglect**
       Y07.420 **Foster father, perpetrator of maltreatment**
         and neglect

4th **5th** **6th** **7th**   Additional Character Required   ✔   3-character code   •=New Code   *Excludes1*—Not coded here, do not use together
                                                 ▲=Revised Code   *Excludes2*—Not included here

Y07.421   Foster mother, perpetrator of maltreatment and neglect

Y07.43 Stepparent or stepsibling, perpetrator of maltreatment and neglect
6th

Y07.430   Stepfather, perpetrator of maltreatment and neglect

Y07.432   Male friend of parent (co-residing in household), perpetrator of maltreatment and neglect

Y07.433   Stepmother, perpetrator of maltreatment and neglect

Y07.434   Female friend of parent (co-residing in household), perpetrator of maltreatment and neglect

Y07.435   Stepbrother, perpetrator or maltreatment and neglect

Y07.436   Stepsister, perpetrator of maltreatment and neglect

Y07.49 Other family member, perpetrator of maltreatment and neglect
6th

Y07.490   Male cousin, perpetrator of maltreatment and neglect

Y07.491   Female cousin, perpetrator of maltreatment and neglect

Y07.499   Other family member, perpetrator of maltreatment and neglect

Y07.5 Non-family member, perpetrator of maltreatment and neglect
5th   **Y07.50** Unspecified non-family member, perpetrator of maltreatment and neglect

Y07.51 Daycare provider, perpetrator of maltreatment and neglect
6th

Y07.510   At-home childcare provider, perpetrator of maltreatment and neglect

Y07.511   Daycare center childcare provider, perpetrator of maltreatment and neglect

Y07.519   Unspecified daycare provider, perpetrator of maltreatment and neglect

Y07.53 Teacher or instructor, perpetrator of maltreatment and neglect

Coach, perpetrator of maltreatment and neglect

Y07.59 Other non-family member, perpetrator of maltreatment and neglect

Y07.6 Multiple perpetrators of maltreatment and neglect

Y07.9 Unspecified perpetrator of maltreatment and neglect

Y08   ASSAULT BY OTHER SPECIFIED MEANS
4th

    Y08.0 Assault by strike by sport equipment
    5th   **Y08.01X Assault by strike by hockey stick**
      7th

      Y08.02X Assault by strike by baseball bat
      7th

      Y08.09X Assault by strike by other specified type of sport equipment
      7th

    Y08.8 Assault by other specified means
    5th   **Y08.81X Assault by crashing of aircraft**
      7th

      Y08.89X Assault by other specified means
      7th

Y09   ASSAULT BY UNSPECIFIED MEANS
7th

Assassination (attempted) NOS
Homicide (attempted) NOS
Manslaughter (attempted) NOS
Murder (attempted) NOS

(Y21–Y33) EVENT OF UNDETERMINED INTENT

Undetermined intent is only for use when there is specific documentation in the record that the intent of the injury cannot be determined. If no such documentation is present, code to accidental (unintentional).

See complete *ICD-10-CM* manual for codes in categories Y21–Y33.

(Y35–Y38) LEGAL INTERVENTION, OPERATIONS OF WAR, MILITARY OPERATIONS, AND TERRORISM

See complete *ICD-10-CM* manual for codes in categories Y35–Y38.

(Y62–Y69) MISADVENTURES TO PATIENTS DURING SURGICAL AND MEDICAL CARE

Excludes2: breakdown or malfunctioning of medical device (during procedure) (after implantation) (ongoing use) (Y70–Y82)
Excludes 1: surgical and medical procedures as the cause of abnormal reaction of the patient, without mention of misadventure at the time of the procedure (Y83–Y84)

See complete *ICD-10-CM* manual for codes in categories Y62–Y69.

(Y70–Y82) MEDICAL DEVICES ASSOCIATED WITH ADVERSE INCIDENTS IN DIAGNOSTIC AND THERAPEUTIC USE

Includes: breakdown or malfunction of medical devices (during use) (after implantation) (ongoing use)
Excludes2: misadventure to patients during surgical and medical care, classifiable to (Y62–Y69)

later complications following use of medical devices without breakdown or malfunctioning of device (Y83–Y84)

surgical and other medical procedures as the cause of abnormal reaction of the patient, or of later complication, without mention of misadventure at the time of the procedure (Y83–Y84)

See complete *ICD-10-CM* manual for codes in categories Y70 –Y82.

(Y83–Y84) SURGICAL AND OTHER MEDICAL PROCEDURES AS THE CAUSE OF ABNORMAL REACTION OF THE PATIENT, OR OF LATER COMPLICATION, WITHOUT MENTION OF MISADVENTURE AT THE TIME OF THE PROCEDURE

Excludes1: misadventures to patients during surgical and medical care, classifiable to (Y62–Y69)
Excludes2: breakdown or malfunctioning of medical device (after implantation) (during procedure) (ongoing use) (Y70–Y82)

See complete *ICD-10-CM* manual for codes in categories Y83–Y84.

(Y90–Y99) SUPPLEMENTARY FACTORS RELATED TO CAUSES OF MORBIDITY CLASSIFIED ELSEWHERE

Note: These categories may be used to provide supplementary information concerning causes of morbidity. They are not to be used for single-condition coding.

Y90   EVIDENCE OF ALCOHOL INVOLVEMENT DETERMINED
4th   **BY BLOOD ALCOHOL LEVEL**

Code first any associated alcohol related disorders (F10)
Y90.0 Blood alcohol level of less than 20 mg/100 ml
Y90.1 Blood alcohol level of 20–39 mg/100 ml
Y90.2 Blood alcohol level of 40–59 mg/100 ml
Y90.3 Blood alcohol level of 60–79 mg/100 ml
Y90.4 Blood alcohol level of 80–99 mg/100 ml
Y90.5 Blood alcohol level of 100–119 mg/100 ml
Y90.6 Blood alcohol level of 120–199 mg/100 ml
Y90.7 Blood alcohol level of 200–239 mg/100 ml
Y90.8 Blood alcohol level of 240 mg/100 ml or more
Y90.9 Presence of alcohol in blood, level not specified

Y92   PLACE OF OCCURRENCE OF THE EXTERNAL CAUSE
4th

GUIDELINE

When applicable, place of occurrence, activity, and external cause status codes are sequenced after the main external cause code(s). Regardless of the number of external cause codes assigned, there should be only one place of occurrence code, one activity code, and one external cause status code assigned to an encounter.

Codes from category Y92, Place of occurrence of the external cause, are secondary codes for use after other external cause codes to identify the location of the patient at the time of injury or other condition.

Generally, a place of occurrence code is assigned only once, at the initial encounter for treatment. However, in the rare instance that a new injury

---

4th **5th** **6th** **7th**   Additional Character Required   ✓   3-character code

•=New Code
▲=Revised Code

Excludes1—Not coded here, do not use together
Excludes2—Not included here

occurs during hospitalization, an additional place of occurrence code may be assigned. No 7th characters are used for Y92.

Do not use place of occurrence code Y92.9 if the place is not stated or is not applicable.

The following category is for use, when relevant, to identify the place of occurrence of the external cause. Use in conjunction with an activity code. Place of occurrence should be recorded only at the **initial encounter** for treatment.

Y92.0 **Non-institutional (private) residence as the place of**
[5th] **occurrence of the external cause**
> *Excludes1:* abandoned or derelict house (Y92.89)
> home under construction but not yet occupied (Y92.6-)
> institutional place of residence (Y92.1-)

  Y92.00 **Unspecified non-institutional (private) residence as**
  [6th] **the place of occurrence of the external cause**

    Y92.000 **Kitchen of unspecified non-institutional (private) residence as the place of occurrence of the external cause**

    Y92.001 **Dining room of unspecified non-institutional (private) residence as the place of occurrence of the external cause**

    Y92.002 **Bathroom of unspecified non-institutional (private) residence as the place of occurrence of the external cause**

    Y92.003 **Bedroom of unspecified non-institutional (private) residence as the place of occurrence of the external cause**

    Y92.007 **Garden or yard of unspecified non-institutional (private) residence as the place of occurrence of the external cause**

    Y92.008 **Other place in unspecified non-institutional (private) residence as the place of occurrence of the external cause**

    Y92.009 **Unspecified place in unspecified non-institutional (private) residence as the place of occurrence of the external cause**
      Home (NOS) as the place of occurrence of the external cause

Y92.1 **Institutional (nonprivate) residence as the place of occurrence**
[5th] **of the external cause**

  Y92.10 **Unspecified residential institution as the place of occurrence of the external cause**

  Y92.11 **Children's home and orphanage as the place of**
  [6th] **occurrence of the external cause**

    Y92.110 **Kitchen in children's home and orphanage as the place of occurrence of the external cause**

    Y92.111 **Bathroom in children's home and orphanage as the place of occurrence of the external cause**

    Y92.112 **Bedroom in children's home and orphanage as the place of occurrence of the external cause**

    Y92.113 **Driveway of children's home and orphanage as the place of occurrence of the external cause**

    Y92.114 **Garage of children's home and orphanage as the place of occurrence of the external cause**

    Y92.115 **Swimming-pool of children's home and orphanage as the place of occurrence of the external cause**

    Y92.116 **Garden or yard of children's home and orphanage as the place of occurrence of the external cause**

    Y92.118 **Other place in children's home and orphanage as the place of occurrence of the external cause**

    Y92.119 **Unspecified place in children's home and orphanage as the place of occurrence of the external cause**

  Y92.15 **Reform school as the place of occurrence of the**
  [6th] **external cause**

    Y92.150 **Kitchen in reform school as the place of occurrence of the external cause**

    Y92.151 **Dining room in reform school as the place of occurrence of the external cause**

    Y92.152 **Bathroom in reform school as the place of occurrence of the external cause**

    Y92.153 **Bedroom in reform school as the place of occurrence of the external cause**

    Y92.154 **Driveway of reform school as the place of occurrence of the external cause**

    Y92.155 **Garage of reform school as the place of occurrence of the external cause**

    Y92.156 **Swimming-pool of reform school as the place of occurrence of the external cause**

    Y92.157 **Garden or yard of reform school as the place of occurrence of the external cause**

    Y92.158 **Other place in reform school as the place of occurrence of the external cause**

    Y92.159 **Unspecified place in reform school as the place of occurrence of the external cause**

Y92.16 **School dormitory as the place of occurrence of the**
[6th] **external cause**
> *Excludes1:* reform school as the place of occurrence of
> the external cause (Y92.15-)
> school buildings and grounds as the place of
> occurrence of the external cause (Y92.2-)
> school sports and athletic areas as the place of
> occurrence of the external cause (Y92.3-)

    Y92.160 **Kitchen in school dormitory as the place of occurrence of the external cause**

    Y92.161 **Dining room in school dormitory as the place of occurrence of the external cause**

    Y92.162 **Bathroom in school dormitory as the place of occurrence of the external cause**

    Y92.163 **Bedroom in school dormitory as the place of occurrence of the external cause**

    Y92.168 **Other place in school dormitory as the place of occurrence of the external cause**

    Y92.169 **Unspecified place in school dormitory as the place of occurrence of the external cause**

Y92.2 **School, other institution and public administrative area as the**
[5th] **place of occurrence of the external cause**
> Building and adjacent grounds used by the general public or by a
> particular group of the public
> *Excludes1:* building under construction as the place of
> occurrence of the external cause (Y92.6)
> residential institution as the place of occurrence of the
> external cause (Y92.1)
> school dormitory as the place of occurrence of the
> external cause (Y92.16-)
> sports and athletics area of schools as the place of
> occurrence of the external cause (Y92.3-)

  Y92.21 **School (private) (public) (state) as the place of**
  [6th] **occurrence of the external cause**

    Y92.210 **Daycare center as the place of occurrence of the external cause**

    Y92.211 **Elementary school as the place of occurrence of the external cause**
      Kindergarten as the place of occurrence of the external cause

    Y92.212 **Middle school as the place of occurrence of the external cause**

    Y92.213 **High school as the place of occurrence of the external cause**

    Y92.214 **College as the place of occurrence of the external cause**
      University as the place of occurrence of the external cause

    Y92.215 **Trade school as the place of occurrence of the external cause**

    Y92.218 **Other school as the place of occurrence of the external cause**

 [4th] [5th] [6th] [7th] Additional Character Required   ✔ 3-character code   •=New Code   ▲=Revised Code   *Excludes1*—Not coded here, do not use together   *Excludes2*—Not included here

Y92.219 Unspecified school as the place of occurrence of the external cause

Y92.22 Religious institution as the place of occurrence of the external cause
Church as the place of occurrence of the external cause
Mosque as the place of occurrence of the external cause
Synagogue as the place of occurrence of the external cause

Y92.25 Cultural building as the place of occurrence of the external cause
Y92.250 Art Gallery as the place of occurrence of the external cause
Y92.251 Museum as the place of occurrence of the external cause
Y92.252 Music hall as the place of occurrence of the external cause
Y92.253 Opera house as the place of occurrence of the external cause
Y92.254 Theater (live) as the place of occurrence of the external cause
Y92.258 Other cultural public building as the place of occurrence of the external cause

Y92.26 Movie house or cinema as the place of occurrence of the external cause

Y92.29 Other specified public building as the place of occurrence of the external cause
Assembly hall as the place of occurrence of the external cause
Clubhouse as the place of occurrence of the external cause

Y92.3 Sports and athletics area as the place of occurrence of the external cause
Y92.31 Athletic court as the place of occurrence of the external cause
Excludes1: tennis court in private home or garden (Y92.09)
Y92.310 Basketball court as the place of occurrence of the external cause
Y92.311 Squash court as the place of occurrence of the external cause
Y92.312 Tennis court as the place of occurrence of the external cause
Y92.318 Other athletic court as the place of occurrence of the external cause

Y92.32 Athletic field as the place of occurrence of the external cause
Y92.320 Baseball field as the place of occurrence of the external cause
Y92.321 Football field as the place of occurrence of the external cause
Y92.322 Soccer field as the place of occurrence of the external cause
Y92.328 Other athletic field as the place of occurrence of the external cause
Cricket field as the place of occurrence of the external cause
Hockey field as the place of occurrence of the external cause

Y92.33 Skating rink as the place of occurrence of the external cause
Y92.330 Ice skating rink (indoor) (outdoor) as the place of occurrence of the external cause
Y92.331 Roller skating rink as the place of occurrence of the external cause

Y92.34 Swimming pool (public) as the place of occurrence of the external cause
Excludes1: swimming pool in private home or garden (Y92.016)

Y92.39 Other specified sports and athletic area as the place of occurrence of the external cause
Golf-course/gymnasium as the place of occurrence of the external cause

Y92.4 Street, highway and other paved roadways as the place of occurrence of the external cause
Excludes1: private driveway of residence (Y92.014, Y92.024, Y92.043, Y92.093, Y92.113, Y92.123, Y92.154, Y92.194)
Y92.41 Street and highway as the place of occurrence of the external cause
Y92.410 Unspecified street and highway as the place of occurrence of the external cause
Road NOS as the place of occurrence of the external cause
Y92.411 Interstate highway as the place of occurrence of the external cause
Freeway/Motorway as the place of occurrence of the external cause
Y92.412 Parkway as the place of occurrence of the external cause
Y92.413 State road as the place of occurrence of the external cause
Y92.414 Local residential or business street as the place of occurrence of the external cause
Y92.415 Exit ramp or entrance ramp of street or highway as the place of occurrence of the external cause

Y92.48 Other paved roadways as the place of occurrence of the external cause
Y92.480 Sidewalk as the place of occurrence of the external cause
Y92.481 Parking lot as the place of occurrence of the external cause
Y92.482 Bike path as the place of occurrence of the external cause
Y92.488 Other paved roadways as the place of occurrence of the external cause

Y92.7 Farm as the place of occurrence of the external cause
Ranch as the place of occurrence of the external cause
Excludes1: farmhouse and home premises of farm (Y92.01-)
Y92.71 Barn as the place of occurrence of the external cause
Y92.72 Chicken coop as the place of occurrence of the external cause
Hen house as the place of occurrence of the external cause
Y92.73 Farm field as the place of occurrence of the external cause
Y92.74 Orchard as the place of occurrence of the external cause
Y92.79 Other farm location as the place of occurrence of the external cause

Y92.83 Recreation area as the place of occurrence of the external cause
Y92.830 Public park as the place of occurrence of the external cause
Y92.831 Amusement park as the place of occurrence of the external cause
Y92.832 Beach/Seashore as the place of occurrence of the external cause
Y92.833 Campsite as the place of occurrence of the external cause
Y92.834 Zoological garden (Zoo) as the place of occurrence of the external cause
Y92.838 Other recreation area as the place of occurrence of the external cause

Y93 ACTIVITY CODES

GUIDELINE

Note: Category Y93 is provided for use to indicate the activity of the person seeking healthcare for an injury or health condition, such as a heart attack while shoveling snow, which resulted from, or was contributed to, by the activity. These codes are appropriate for use for both acute injuries, such as those from Chapter 19, and conditions that are due to the long-term, cumulative effects of an activity, such as those from Chapter 13. They are also appropriate for use with external cause codes for cause and intent if identifying the activity provides additional information on the event. These

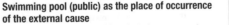

CHAPTER 20. EXTERNAL CAUSES OF MORBIDITY (Y92.219-Y93)

4th 5th 6th 7th Additional Character Required   ✔ 3-character code

• =New Code
▲ =Revised Code

Excludes1—Not coded here, do not use together
Excludes2—Not included here

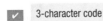

codes should be used in conjunction with codes for external cause status (Y99) and place of occurrence (Y92).

Assign a code from category Y93, Activity code, to describe the activity of the patient at the time the injury or other health condition occurred.

An activity code is used only once, at the initial encounter for treatment. Only one code from Y93 should be recorded on a medical record.

The activity codes are not applicable to poisonings, adverse effects, misadventures or sequela.

Do not assign Y93.9, Unspecified activity, if the activity is not stated.

A code from category Y93 is appropriate for use with external cause and intent codes if identifying the activity provides additional information about the event.

Y93.0 Activities involving walking and running
`5th`
    Excludes1: activity, walking an animal (Y93.K1)
        activity, walking or running on a treadmill (Y93.A1)

    Y93.01 Activity, walking, marching and hiking
        Activity, walking, marching and hiking on level or elevated terrain
        Excludes1: activity, mountain climbing (Y93.31)

    Y93.02 Activity, running

Y93.1 Activities involving water and water craft
`5th`
    Excludes1: activities involving ice (Y93.2-)

    Y93.11 Activity, swimming
    Y93.12 Activity, springboard and platform diving
    Y93.13 Activity, water polo
    Y93.14 Activity, water aerobics and water exercise
    Y93.15 Activity, underwater diving and snorkeling
        Activity, SCUBA diving
    Y93.16 Activity, rowing, canoeing, kayaking, rafting and tubing
    Y93.17 Activity, water skiing and wake boarding
    Y93.18 Activity, surfing, windsurfing and boogie boarding
        Activity, water sliding
    Y93.19 Activity, other involving water and watercraft
        Activity involving water NOS
        Activity, parasailing
        Activity, water survival training and testing

Y93.2 Activities involving ice and snow
`5th`
    Excludes1: activity, shoveling ice and snow (Y93.H1)

    Y93.21 Activity, ice skating
        Activity, figure skating (singles) (pairs)
        Activity, ice dancing
        Excludes1: activity, ice hockey (Y93.22)
    Y93.22 Activity, ice hockey
    Y93.23 Activity, snow (alpine) (downhill) skiing, snow-boarding, sledding, tobogganing and snow tubing
        Excludes1: activity, cross country skiing (Y93.24)
    Y93.24 Activity, cross country skiing
        Activity, nordic skiing
    Y93.29 Activity, other involving ice and snow
        Activity involving ice and snow NOS

Y93.3 Activities involving climbing, rappelling and jumping off
`5th`
    Excludes1: activity, hiking on level or elevated terrain (Y93.01)
        activity, jumping rope (Y93.56)
        activity, trampoline jumping (Y93.44)

    Y93.31 Activity, mountain climbing, rock climbing and wall climbing
    Y93.32 Activity, rappelling
    Y93.33 Activity, BASE jumping
        Activity, Building, Antenna, Span, Earth jumping
    Y93.34 Activity, bungee jumping
    Y93.35 Activity, hang gliding
    Y93.39 Activity, other involving climbing, rappelling and jumping off

Y93.4 Activities involving dancing and other rhythmic movement
`5th`
    Excludes1: activity, martial arts (Y93.75)

    Y93.41 Activity, dancing
    Y93.42 Activity, yoga
    Y93.43 Activity, gymnastics
        Activity, rhythmic gymnastics
        Excludes1: activity, trampolining (Y93.44)
    Y93.44 Activity, trampolining
    Y93.45 Activity, cheerleading

Y93.49 Activity, other involving dancing and other rhythmic movements

Y93.5 Activities involving other sports and athletics played individually
`5th`
    Excludes1: activity, dancing (Y93.41)
        activity, gymnastic (Y93.43)
        activity, trampolining (Y93.44)
        activity, yoga (Y93.42)

    Y93.51 Activity, roller skating (inline) and skateboarding
    Y93.52 Activity, horseback riding
    Y93.53 Activity, golf
    Y93.54 Activity, bowling
    Y93.55 Activity, bike riding
    Y93.56 Activity, jumping rope
    Y93.57 Activity, non-running track and field events
        Excludes1: activity, running (any form) (Y93.02)
    Y93.59 Activity, other involving other sports and athletics played individually
        Excludes1: activities involving climbing, rappelling, and jumping (Y93.3-)
        activities involving ice and snow (Y93.2-)
        activities involving walking and running (Y93.0-)
        activities involving water and watercraft (Y93.1-)

Y93.6 Activities involving other sports and athletics played as a team or group
`5th`
    Excludes1: activity, ice hockey (Y93.22)
        activity, water polo (Y93.13)

    Y93.61 Activity, American tackle football
        Activity, football NOS
    Y93.62 Activity, American flag or touch football
    Y93.63 Activity, rugby
    Y93.64 Activity, baseball
        Activity, softball
    Y93.65 Activity, lacrosse and field hockey
    Y93.66 Activity, soccer
    Y93.67 Activity, basketball
    Y93.68 Activity, volleyball (beach) (court)
    Y93.6A Activity, physical games generally associated with school recess, summer camp and children
        Including capture the flag/dodge ball/four square/kickball
    Y93.69 Activity, other involving other sports and athletics played as a team or group
        Activity, cricket

Y93.7 Activities involving other specified sports and athletics
`5th`
    Y93.71 Activity, boxing
    Y93.72 Activity, wrestling
    Y93.73 Activity, racquet and hand sports
        Activity, handball/racquetball/squash/tennis
    Y93.74 Activity, Frisbee
    Y93.75 Activity, martial arts
        Activity, combatives
    Y93.79 Activity, other specified sports and athletics
        Excludes1: sports and athletics activities specified in categories Y93.0–Y93.6

Y93.B Activities involving other muscle strengthening exercises
`5th`
    Y93.B1 Activity, exercise machines primarily for muscle strengthening
    Y93.B2 Activity, push-ups, pull-ups, sit-ups
    Y93.B3 Activity, free weights
        Activity, barbells/dumbbells
    Y93.B4 Activity, pilates
    Y93.B9 Activity, other involving muscle strengthening exercises
        Excludes1: activities involving muscle strengthening specified in categories Y93.0–Y93.A

Y93.C Activities involving computer technology and electronic devices
`5th`
    Excludes1: activity, electronic musical keyboard or instruments (Y93.J-)

    Y93.C1 Activity, computer keyboarding
        Activity, electronic game playing using keyboard or other stationary device

---

`4th` `5th` `6th` `7th`   Additional Character Required   ✔   3-character code

•=New Code   *Excludes1*—Not coded here, do not use together
▲=Revised Code   *Excludes2*—Not included here

 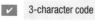

Y93.C2   **Activity, hand held interactive electronic device**
Activity, cellular telephone and communication device
Activity, electronic game playing using interactive device
Excludes1: activity, electronic game playing using
     keyboard or other stationary device (Y93.C1)

Y93.C9   **Activity, other involving computer technology and
electronic devices**

Y93.D   **Activities involving arts and handcrafts**
   `5th`
Excludes1: activities involving playing musical instrument (Y93.J-)

Y93.D1   **Activity, knitting and crocheting**

Y93.D2   **Activity, sewing**

Y93.D3   **Activity, furniture building and finishing**
Activity, furniture repair

Y93.D9   **Activity, other involving arts and handcrafts**

Y93.E   **Activities involving personal hygiene and interior property and
clothing maintenance**
   `5th`
Excludes1: activities involving cooking and grilling (Y93.G-)
     activities involving exterior property and land maintenance,
       building and construction (Y93.H-)
     activities involving caregiving (Y93.F-)
     activity, dishwashing (Y93.G1)
     activity, food preparation (Y93.G1)
     activity, gardening (Y93.H2)

Y93.E1   **Activity, personal bathing and showering**

Y93.E2   **Activity, laundry**

Y93.E3   **Activity, vacuuming**

Y93.E4   **Activity, ironing**

Y93.E5   **Activity, floor mopping and cleaning**

Y93.E6   **Activity, residential relocation**
Activity, packing up and unpacking involved in moving to
   a new residence

Y93.E8   **Activity, other personal hygiene**

Y93.E9   **Activity, other interior property and clothing
maintenance**

Y93.G   **Activities involving food preparation, cooking and grilling**
   `5th`
Y93.G1   **Activity, food preparation and clean up**
Activity, dishwashing

Y93.G2   **Activity, grilling and smoking food**

Y93.G3   **Activity, cooking and baking**
Activity, use of stove, oven and microwave oven

Y93.G9   **Activity, other involving cooking and grilling**

Y93.I   **Activities involving roller coasters and other types of external
motion**
   `5th`
Y93.I1   **Activity, roller coaster riding**

Y93.I9   **Activity, other involving external motion**

Y93.J   **Activities involving playing musical instrument**
   `5th`
Activity involving playing electric musical instrument

Y93.J1   **Activity, piano playing**
Activity, musical keyboard (electronic) playing

Y93.J2   **Activity, drum and other percussion instrument
playing**

Y93.J3   **Activity, string instrument playing**

Y93.J4   **Activity, winds and brass instrument playing**

Y93.K   **Activities involving animal care**
   `5th`
Excludes1: activity, horseback riding (Y93.52)

Y93.K1   **Activity, walking an animal**

Y93.K2   **Activity, milking an animal**

Y93.K3   **Activity, grooming and shearing an animal**

Y93.K9   **Activity, other involving animal care**

Y93.8   **Activities, other specified**
   `5th`
Y93.81   **Activity, refereeing a sports activity**

Y93.82   **Activity, spectator at an event**

Y93.83   **Activity, rough housing and horseplay**

Y93.84   **Activity, sleeping**

Y93.85   **Activity, choking game**
Activity, blackout or fainting or pass out game

Y93.89   **Activity, other specified**

Y95   **NOSOCOMIAL CONDITION**
   `✔`

Y99   **EXTERNAL CAUSE STATUS**
   `4th`

> **GUIDELINE**
>
> A code from category Y99, External cause status, should be assigned
> whenever any other external cause code is assigned for an encounter,
> including an Activity code, except for the events noted below. Assign a code
> from category Y99, External cause status, to indicate the work status of the
> person at the time the event occurred. The status code indicates whether
> the event occurred during military activity, whether a non-military person
> was at work, whether an individual including a student or volunteer was
> involved in a non-work activity at the time of the causal event.
>
> A code from Y99, External cause status, should be assigned, when
> applicable, with other external cause codes, such as transport accidents
> and falls. The external cause status codes are not applicable to poisonings,
> adverse effects, misadventures or late effects.
>
> Do not assign a code from category Y99 if no other external cause
> codes (cause, activity) are applicable for the encounter.
>
> An external cause status code is used only once, at the initial encounter
> for treatment. Only one code from Y99 should be recorded on a medical
> record.
>
> Do not assign code Y99.9, Unspecified external cause status, if the
> status is not stated.
>
> **Note:** A single code from category Y99 should be used in conjunction
> with the external cause code(s) assigned to a record to indicate the status
> of the person at the time the event occurred.

Y99.0   **Civilian activity done for income or pay**
Civilian activity done for financial or other compensation
Excludes1: military activity (Y99.1)
     volunteer activity (Y99.2)

Y99.2   **Volunteer activity**
Excludes1: activity of child or other family member assisting in
     compensated work of other family member (Y99.8)

Y99.8   **Other external cause status**
Activity NEC
Activity of child or other family member assisting in compensated
   work of other family member
Hobby not done for income
Leisure activity
Off-duty activity of military personnel
Recreation or sport not for income or while a student
Student activity
Excludes1: civilian activity done for income or compensation
   (Y99.0)
     military activity (Y99.1)

Y99.9   **Unspecified external cause status**

Chapter 21. Factors influencing health status and contact with health services (Z00–Z99)

GUIDELINES

Note: The chapter specific guidelines provide additional information about the use of Z codes for specified encounters.

Use of Z codes in any healthcare setting

Z codes are for use in any healthcare setting. Z codes may be used as either a first-listed (principal diagnosis code in the inpatient setting) or secondary code, depending on the circumstances of the encounter. Certain Z codes may only be used as first-listed or principal diagnosis.

Z codes indicate a reason for an encounter

Z codes are not procedure codes. A corresponding procedure code must accompany a Z code to describe any procedure performed.

Categories of Z codes

CONTACT/EXPOSURE
Refer to categories Z20 and Z77.

INOCULATIONS AND VACCINATIONS
Refer to category Z23.

STATUS
Status codes indicate that a patient is either a carrier of a disease or has the sequelae or residual of a past disease or condition. This includes such things as the presence of prosthetic or mechanical devices resulting from past treatment. A status code is informative, because the status may affect the course of treatment and its outcome. A status code is distinct from a history code. The history code indicates that the patient no longer has the condition.

A status code should not be used with a diagnosis code from one of the body system chapters, if the diagnosis code includes the information provided by the status code. For example, code Z94.1, Heart transplant status, should not be used with a code from subcategory T86.2, Complications of heart transplant. The status code does not provide additional information. The complication code indicates that the patient is a heart transplant patient.

For encounters for weaning from a mechanical ventilator, assign a code from subcategory J96.1, Chronic respiratory failure, followed by code Z99.11, Dependence on respirator [ventilator] status.

The status Z codes/categories are:
Z14, Z15, Z16, Z17, Z18, Z21, Z22, Z28.3, Z33.1, Z66, Z67, Z68, Z74.01, Z76.82, Z78, Z79, Z88 (Except: Z88.9), Z89, Z90, Z91.0-, Z93, Z94, Z95, Z96, Z97, Z98, Z99

HISTORY (OF)
There are two types of history Z codes, personal and family. *Refer to categories or codes Z80, Z81, Z82, Z83, Z84, Z85, Z86, Z87, Z91.4-, Z91.5, Z91.8- (Except: Z91.83), Z92 (Except: Z92.0 and Z92.82)*

SCREENING
Refer to categories Z11, Z12 and Z13 (except: Z13.9).

OBSERVATION
Refer to categories Z03 and Z04 for further details.

AFTERCARE
Aftercare visit codes cover situations when the initial treatment of a disease has been performed and the patient requires continued care during the healing or recovery phase, or for the long-term consequences of the disease. The aftercare Z code should not be used if treatment is directed at a current, acute disease. The diagnosis code is to be used in these cases. Exceptions to this rule are codes Z51.0, Encounter for antineoplastic radiation therapy, and codes from subcategory Z51.1, Encounter for antineoplastic chemotherapy and immunotherapy. These codes are to be first-listed, followed by the diagnosis code when a patient's encounter is solely to receive radiation therapy, chemotherapy, or immunotherapy for the treatment of a neoplasm. If the reason for the encounter is more than one type of antineoplastic therapy, code Z51.0 and a code from subcategory Z51.1 may be assigned together, in which case one of these codes would be reported as a secondary diagnosis.

The aftercare Z codes should also not be used for aftercare for injuries. For aftercare of an injury, assign the acute injury code with the appropriate 7th character (for subsequent encounter).

The aftercare codes are generally first-listed to explain the specific reason for the encounter. An aftercare code may be used as an additional code when some type of aftercare is provided in addition to the reason for admission and no diagnosis code is applicable. An example of this would be the closure of a colostomy during an encounter for treatment of another condition.

Aftercare codes should be used in conjunction with other aftercare codes or diagnosis codes to provide better detail on the specifics of an aftercare encounter visit, unless otherwise directed by the classification. Should a patient receive multiple types of antineoplastic therapy during the same encounter, code Z51.0, Encounter for antineoplastic radiation therapy, and codes from subcategory Z51.1, Encounter for antineoplastic chemotherapy and immunotherapy, may be used together on a record. The sequencing of multiple aftercare codes depends on the circumstances of the encounter.

Certain aftercare Z code categories need a secondary diagnosis code to describe the resolving condition or sequelae. For others, the condition is included in the code title.

Additional Z code aftercare category terms include fitting and adjustment, and attention to artificial openings.

Status Z codes may be used with aftercare Z codes to indicate the nature of the aftercare. For example code Z95.1, Presence of aortocoronary bypass graft, may be used with code Z48.812, Encounter for surgical aftercare following surgery on the circulatory system, to indicate the surgery for which the aftercare is being performed. A status code should not be used when the aftercare code indicates the type of status, such as using Z43.0, Encounter for attention to tracheostomy, with Z93.0, Tracheostomy status.

The aftercare Z category/codes: Z42, Z43, Z44, Z45, Z46, Z47, Z48, Z49 and Z51

FOLLOW-UP
The follow-up codes are used to explain continuing surveillance following completed treatment of a disease, condition, or injury. *Refer to categories Z08 and Z09.*

DONOR
Refer to the *ICD-10-CM* manual.

COUNSELING
Counseling Z codes are used when a patient or family member receives assistance in the aftermath of an illness or injury, or when support is required in coping with family or social problems. They are not used in conjunction with a diagnosis code when the counseling component of care is considered integral to standard treatment.

The counseling Z codes/categories: Z30.0-, Z31.5, Z31.6-, Z32.2, Z32.3, Z69, Z70, Z71 and Z76.81

NEWBORNS AND INFANTS
Newborn Z codes/categories: Z05, Z76.1, Z00.1- and Z38

ROUTINE AND ADMINISTRATIVE EXAMINATIONS
Pre-operative examination and pre-procedural laboratory examination Z codes are for use only in those situations when a patient is being cleared for a procedure or surgery and no treatment is given.

Refer to the Z codes/categories for routine and administrative examinations: Z00, Z01, Z02 (except: Z02.9) and Z32.0-

MISCELLANEOUS Z CODES
The miscellaneous Z codes capture a number of other health care encounters that do not fall into one of the other categories. Certain of these codes identify the reason for the encounter; others are for use as additional codes that provide useful information on circumstances that may affect a patient's care and treatment.

PROPHYLACTIC ORGAN REMOVAL
For encounters specifically for prophylactic removal of an organ refer to the full *ICD-10-CM* manual guidelines.

MISCELLANEOUS Z CODES/CATEGORIES:
Z28, (except: Z28.3), Z40, Z41 (except: Z41.9), Z53, Z55, Z56, Z57, Z58, Z59, Z60, Z62, Z63, Z64, Z65, Z72, Z73, Z74 (except: Z74.01), Z75, Z76.0, Z76.3, Z76.4, Z76.5, Z91.1-, Z91.84-, Z91.83 and Z91.89

NONSPECIFIC Z CODES
Certain Z codes are so non-specific, or potentially redundant with other codes in the classification, that there can be little justification for their use in the inpatient setting. Their use in the outpatient setting should be limited to those instances

---

   4th **5th** **6th** **7th** Additional Character Required   3-character code   Unspecified laterality codes were excluded here.   • =New Code ▲ =Revised Code ▫ =Social determinants of health   ***Excludes1***—Not coded here, do not use together ***Excludes2***—Not included here

when there is no further documentation to permit more precise coding. Otherwise, any sign or symptom or any other reason for visit that is captured in another code should be used.

NONSPECIFIC Z CODES:
Z02.9, Z04.9, Z13.9, Z41.9, Z52.9, Z86.59, Z88.9 and Z92.0

Z CODES THAT MAY ONLY BE PRINCIPAL/FIRST-LISTED DIAGNOSIS
The following Z codes/categories may only be reported as the principal/first-listed diagnosis, except when there are multiple encounters on the same day and the medical records for the encounters are combined: Z00, Z01, Z02, Z03, Z04, Z33.2, Z31.81, Z31.82, Z31.83, Z31.84, Z34, Z38, Z39, Z40, Z42, Z51.0, Z51.1-, Z52 (except: Z52.9), Z76.1, Z76.2 and Z99.12.

Note: Z codes represent reasons for encounters. A corresponding procedure code must accompany a Z code if a procedure is performed. Categories Z00–Z99 are provided for occasions when circumstances other than a disease, injury or external cause classifiable to categories A00–Y89 are recorded as 'diagnoses' or 'problems.' This can arise in two main ways:
a) When a person who may or may not be sick encounters the health services for some specific purpose, such as to receive limited care or service for a current condition, to donate an organ or tissue, to receive prophylactic vaccination (immunization), or to discuss a problem which is in itself not a disease or injury.
b) When some circumstance or problem is present which influences the person's health status but is not in itself a current illness or injury.

(Z00–Z13) PERSONS ENCOUNTERING HEALTH SERVICES FOR EXAMINATIONS

Note: Nonspecific abnormal findings disclosed at the time of these examinations are classified to categories R70–R94.
Excludes1: examinations related to pregnancy and reproduction (Z30–Z36, Z39.-)
Codes in categories Z00–Z04 "may only be reported as the principal/first-listed diagnosis, except when there are multiple encounters on the same day and the medical records for the encounters are combined."

Z00   ENCOUNTER FOR GENERAL EXAMINATION WITHOUT COMPLAINT, SUSPECTED OR REPORTED DIAGNOSIS
`4th`

GUIDELINES
The codes are not to be used if the examination is for diagnosis of a suspected condition or for treatment purposes. In such cases the diagnosis code is used. During a routine exam, should a diagnosis or condition be discovered, it should be coded as an additional code. Pre-existing and chronic conditions and history codes may also be included as additional codes as long as the examination is for administrative purposes and not focused on any particular condition.
　Some of the codes for routine health examinations distinguish between "with" and "without" abnormal findings. Code assignment depends on the information that is known at the time the encounter is being coded. For example, if no abnormal findings were found during the examination, but the encounter is being coded before test results are back, it is acceptable to assign the code for "without abnormal findings." When assigning a code for "with abnormal findings," additional code(s) should be assigned to identify the specific abnormal finding(s).
Excludes1: encounter for examination for administrative purposes (Z02.-)
Excludes2: encounter for pre-procedural examinations (Z01.81-)
　special screening examinations (Z11–Z13)

Z00.0   **Encounter for general adult medical examination**
`5th`   Encounter for adult periodic examination (annual) (physical) and any associated laboratory and radiologic examinations
Excludes1: encounter for examination of sign or symptom— code to sign or symptom
　general health check-up of infant or child (Z00.12.-)
　Z00.00   **Encounter for general adult medical examination without abnormal findings**
　　Encounter for adult health check-up NOS
　Z00.01   **Encounter for general adult medical examination with abnormal findings**
　　Use additional code to identify abnormal findings
Z00.1   **Encounter for newborn, infant and child health examinations**
`5th`

Z00.11   **Newborn health examination**
`6th`   *Refer to Chapter 16 for guidelines.*
　Health check for child under 29 days old
　Use additional code to identify any abnormal findings
　Excludes1: health check for child over 28 days old (Z00.12-)
　Z00.110   **Health examination for newborn; under 8 days old**
　　Health check for newborn under 8 days old
　Z00.111   **8 to 28 days old**
　　Health check for newborn 8 to 28 days old
　　Newborn weight check

Z00.12   **Encounter for routine child health examination;**
`6th`   Health check (routine) for child over 28 days old
　Immunizations appropriate for age
　Routine developmental screening of infant or child
　Routine vision and hearing testing

> Tip: An abnormal finding can be defined as an acute illness/injury/finding, unstable chronic illness, or abnormal screen

　Excludes1: health check for child under 29 days old (Z00.11-)
　health supervision of foundling or other healthy infant or child (Z76.1–Z76.2)
　newborn health examination (Z00.11-)
　Z00.121   **with abnormal findings**
　　Use additional code to identify abnormal findings
　Z00.129   **without abnormal findings**
　　Encounter for routine child health examination NOS

Z00.2   **Encounter for examination for period of rapid growth in childhood**
Z00.3   **Encounter for examination for adolescent development state**
　Encounter for puberty development state
Z00.7   **Encounter for examination for period of delayed growth in childhood**
`5th`
　Z00.70   **Encounter for examination for period of delayed growth in childhood without abnormal findings**
　Z00.71   **Encounter for examination for period of delayed growth in childhood with abnormal findings**
　　Use additional code to identify abnormal findings

Z01   ENCOUNTER FOR OTHER SPECIAL EXAMINATION WITHOUT COMPLAINT, SUSPECTED OR REPORTED DIAGNOSIS
`4th`

GUIDELINES
The codes are not to be used if the examination is for diagnosis of a suspected condition or for treatment purposes. In such cases the diagnosis code is used. During a routine exam, should a diagnosis or condition be discovered, it should be coded as an additional code. Pre-existing and chronic conditions and history codes may also be included as additional codes as long as the examination is for administrative purposes and not focused on any particular condition.
　Some of the codes for routine health examinations distinguish between "with" and "without" abnormal findings. Code assignment depends on the information that is known at the time the encounter is being coded. For example, if no abnormal findings were found during the examination, but the encounter is being coded before test results are back, it is acceptable to assign the code for "without abnormal findings." When assigning a code for "with abnormal findings," additional code(s) should be assigned to identify the specific abnormal finding(s).
Includes: routine examination of specific system
Note: Codes from category Z01 represent the reason for the encounter.
　A separate procedure code is required to identify any examinations or procedures performed
Excludes1: encounter for examination for administrative purposes (Z02.-)
　encounter for examination for suspected conditions, proven not to exist (Z03.-)
　encounter for laboratory and radiologic examinations as a component of general medical examinations (Z00.0-)
　encounter for laboratory, radiologic and imaging examinations for sign(s) and symptom(s)—**code to the sign(s) or symptom(s)**
Excludes2: screening examinations (Z11–Z13)

`4th` `5th` `6th` `7th` Additional Character Required   ✓   3-character code   Unspecified laterality codes were excluded here.   * =New Code   ▲ =Revised Code   ▫ =Social determinants of health   ***Excludes1***—Not coded here, do not use together   ***Excludes2***—Not included here

Z01.0 `5th` **Encounter for examination of eyes and vision;**
Excludes1: examination for driving license (Z02.4)

     Z01.00   **without abnormal findings**
     Encounter for examination of eyes and vision NOS

     Z01.01   **with abnormal findings**
     Use additional code to identify abnormal findings
     Excludes1: encounter for examination of eyes and
     vision with abnormal findings (Z01.01)
     encounter for examination of eyes and vision without
     abnormal findings (Z01.00)

     Z01.02 `6th` **Encounter for examination of eyes and vision following failed vision screening;**
       Z01.020   **without abnormal findings**
       Z01.021   **with abnormal findings**

Z01.1 `5th` **Encounter for examination of ears and hearing;**
     Z01.10   **Encounter for examination of ears and hearing without abnormal findings**
     Encounter for examination of ears and hearing NOS

     Z01.11 `6th` **Encounter for examination of ears and hearing with abnormal findings**
       Z01.110   **Encounter for hearing examination following failed hearing screening**
       Z01.118   **Encounter for examination of ears and hearing with other abnormal findings**
       Use additional code to identify abnormal findings

     Z01.12   **Encounter for hearing conservation and treatment**

Z01.3 `5th` **Encounter for examination of blood pressure**
     Z01.30   **Encounter for examination of blood pressure without abnormal findings**
     Encounter for examination of blood pressure NOS

     Z01.31   **Encounter for examination of blood pressure with abnormal findings**
     Use additional code to identify abnormal findings

Z01.4 `5th` **Encounter for gynecological examination**
Excludes2: pregnancy examination or test (Z32.0-)
     routine examination for contraceptive maintenance (Z30.4-)

     Z01.41 `6th` **Encounter for routine gynecological examination**
     Encounter for general gynecological examination with or without cervical smear
     Encounter for gynecological examination (general) (routine) NOS
     Encounter for pelvic examination (annual) (periodic)
     Use additional code: for screening for human papillomavirus, if applicable, (Z11.51)
     for screening vaginal pap smear, if applicable (Z12.72)
     to identify acquired absence of uterus, if applicable (Z90.71-)
     Excludes1: gynecologic examination status (Z08)
     screening cervical pap smear not a part of a routine gynecological examination (Z12.4)

       Z01.411   **Encounter for gynecological examination (general) (routine); with abnormal findings**
       Use additional code to identify abnormal findings
       Z01.419   **without abnormal findings**

     Z01.42   **Encounter for cervical smear to confirm findings of recent normal smear following initial abnormal smear**

Z01.8 `5th` **Encounter for other specified special examinations**
     Z01.81 `6th` **Encounter for preprocedural examinations**
     Pre-operative examination and pre-procedural laboratory examination Z codes are for use only in those situations when a patient is being cleared for a procedure or surgery and no treatment is given.
     Encounter for preoperative examinations
     Encounter for radiological and imaging examinations as part of preprocedural examination
       Z01.810   **Encounter for preprocedural; cardiovascular examination**
       Z01.811   **respiratory examination**

       Z01.812   **laboratory examination**
       Blood and urine tests prior to treatment or procedure

       Z01.818   **Encounter for other preprocedural examination**
       Encounter for preprocedural examination NOS
       Encounter for examinations prior to antineoplastic chemotherapy

     Z01.82   **Encounter for allergy testing**
     Excludes1: encounter for antibody response examination (Z01.84)

     Z01.84   **Encounter for antibody response examination**
     Encounter for immunity status testing
     Excludes1: encounter for allergy testing (Z01.82)

     Z01.89   **Encounter for other specified special examinations**

Z02 `4th` **ENCOUNTER FOR ADMINISTRATIVE EXAMINATION**

GUIDELINES

The codes are not to be used if the examination is for diagnosis of a suspected condition or for treatment purposes. In such cases the diagnosis code is used. During a routine exam, should a diagnosis or condition be discovered, it should be coded as an additional code. Pre-existing and chronic conditions and history codes may also be included as additional codes as long as the examination is for administrative purposes and not focused on any particular condition.

Some of the codes for routine health examinations distinguish between "with" and "without" abnormal findings. Code assignment depends on the information that is known at the time the encounter is being coded. For example, if no abnormal findings were found during the examination, but the encounter is being coded before test results are back, it is acceptable to assign the code for "without abnormal findings." When assigning a code for "with abnormal findings," additional code(s) should be assigned to identify the specific abnormal finding(s).

Z02.0 **Encounter for examination for admission to educational institution**
Encounter for examination for admission to preschool (education)
Encounter for examination for re-admission to school following illness or medical treatment

Z02.1 **Encounter for pre-employment examination**

Z02.2 **Encounter for examination for admission to residential institution**
Excludes1: examination for admission to prison (Z02.89)

Z02.3 **Encounter for examination for recruitment to armed forces**

Z02.4 **Encounter for examination for driving license**

Z02.5 **Encounter for examination for participation in sport**
Excludes1: blood-alcohol and blood-drug test (Z02.83)

Z02.6 **Encounter for examination for insurance purposes**

Z02.7 `5th` **Encounter for issue of medical certificate**
Excludes1: encounter for general medical examination (Z00–Z01, Z02.0–Z02.6, Z02.8–Z02.9)

     Z02.71   **Encounter for disability determination**
     Encounter for issue of medical certificate of incapacity or invalidity

     Z02.79   **Encounter for issue of other medical certificate**

Z02.8 `5th` **Encounter for other administrative examinations**
     Z02.82   **Encounter for adoption services**

     Z02.83   **Encounter for blood-alcohol and blood-drug test**
     Use additional code for findings of alcohol or drugs in blood (R78.-)

     Z02.89   **Encounter for other administrative examinations**
     Encounter for examination for admission to prison
     Encounter for examination for admission to summer camp
     Encounter for immigration or naturalization examination
     Encounter for premarital examination
     Excludes1: health supervision of foundling or other healthy infant or child (Z76.1–Z76.2)

Z02.9 **Encounter for administrative examinations, unspecified**

`4th` `5th` `6th` `7th` Additional Character Required   ✓ 3-character code   Unspecified laterality codes were excluded here.
   • =New Code   ▲ =Revised Code   ⊡ =Social determinants of health
   Excludes1—Not coded here, do not use together   *Excludes2*—Not included here

CHAPTER 21. FACTORS INFLUENCING HEALTH STATUS AND CONTACT WITH HEALTH SERVICES   (Z03–Z04.89)

Z03 ENCOUNTER FOR MEDICAL OBSERVATION FOR SUSPECTED DISEASES AND CONDITIONS RULED OUT
4th

GUIDELINES

This observation category is for use in very limited circumstances when a person is being observed for a suspected condition that is ruled out. The observation codes are not for use if an injury or illness or any signs or symptoms related to the suspected condition are present. In such cases the diagnosis/symptom code is used with the corresponding external cause code. The observation codes are primarily to be used as principal/first listed diagnosis. Additional codes may be used in addition to the observation code but only if they are unrelated to the suspected condition being observed.

This category is to be used when a person without a diagnosis is suspected of having an abnormal condition, without signs or symptoms, which requires study, but after examination and observation, is ruled out. This category is also for use for administrative and legal observation status.

An observation code may be assigned as a secondary diagnosis code when the patient is being observed for a condition that is ruled out and is unrelated to the principal/first-listed diagnosis (e.g., patient presents for treatment following injuries sustained in a motor vehicle accident and is also observed for suspected COVID-19 infection that is subsequently ruled out).

Excludes1: contact with and (suspected) exposures hazardous to health (Z77.-)

encounter for observation and evaluation of newborn for suspected diseases and conditions ruled out (Z05.-)

person with feared complaint in whom no diagnosis is made (Z71.1)

signs or symptoms under study—code to signs or symptoms

Z03.6 Encounter for observation for suspected toxic effect from ingested substance ruled out

Encounter for observation for suspected adverse effect from drug

Encounter for observation for suspected poisoning

Z03.7 Encounter for suspected maternal and fetal conditions ruled out
5th

GUIDELINES

Codes from subcategory Z03.7 may either be used as a first-listed or as an additional code assignment depending on the case. They are for use in very limited circumstances on a maternal record when an encounter is for a suspected maternal or fetal condition that is ruled out during that encounter (for example, a maternal or fetal condition may be suspected due to an abnormal test result). In addition, these codes are not for use if an illness or any signs or symptoms related to the suspected condition or problem are present. In such cases the diagnosis/symptom code is used.

Additional codes may be used in addition to the code from subcategory Z03.7, but only if they are unrelated to the suspected condition being evaluated.

Encounter for suspected maternal and fetal conditions not found

Excludes1: known or suspected fetal anomalies affecting management of mother, not ruled out (O26.-, O35.-, O36.-, O40.-, O41.-)

Z03.73 Encounter for suspected; fetal anomaly ruled out

Z03.74   problem with fetal growth ruled out

Z03.79   maternal and fetal conditions ruled out

Z03.8 Encounter for observation for other suspected diseases and conditions ruled out
5th

Z03.81 Encounter for observation for suspected exposure to; biological agents ruled out
6th

Z03.810   anthrax ruled out

Z03.818   other biological agents ruled out

•**Z03.82 Encounter for observation for suspected foreign body ruled out**
6th

Excludes1: retained foreign body (Z18.-)

retained foreign body in eyelid (H02.81)

residual foreign body in soft tissue (M79.5)

Excludes2: confirmed foreign body ingestion or aspiration including:

foreign body in alimentary tract (T18)

foreign body in ear (T16)

foreign body on external eye (T15)

foreign body in respiratory tract (T17)

•**Z03.821   Encounter for observation for suspected ingested foreign body ruled out**

•**Z03.822   Encounter for observation for suspected aspirated (inhaled) foreign body ruled out**

•**Z03.823   Encounter for observation for suspected inserted (injected) foreign body ruled out**

Encounter for observation for suspected inserted (injected) foreign body in eye, orifice or skin ruled out

Z03.89 Encounter for observation for other suspected diseases and conditions ruled out

Encounter for observation for suspected inserted (injected) foreign body in eye, orifice or skin ruled out

Z04 ENCOUNTER FOR EXAMINATION AND OBSERVATION FOR OTHER REASONS
4th

GUIDELINES

This observation category (excludes Z04.9) is for use in very limited circumstances when a person is being observed for a suspected condition that is ruled out. The observation codes are not for use if an injury or illness or any signs or symptoms related to the suspected condition are present. In such cases the diagnosis/symptom code is used with the corresponding external cause code. The observation codes are primarily to be used as principal diagnosis. Additional codes may be used in addition to the observation code but only if they are unrelated to the suspected condition being observed.

An observation code may be assigned as a secondary diagnosis code when the patient is being observed for a condition that is ruled out and is unrelated to the principal/first-listed diagnosis (e.g., patient presents for treatment following injuries sustained in a motor vehicle accident and is also observed for suspected COVID-19 infection that is subsequently ruled out).

Includes: encounter for examination for medicolegal reasons

This category is to be used when a person without a diagnosis is suspected of having an abnormal condition, without signs or symptoms, which requires study, but after examination and observation, is ruled out.

This category is also for use for administrative and legal observation status.

Z04.1 Encounter for examination and observation following; transport accident

Excludes1: encounter for examination and observation following work accident (Z04.2)

Do not report an external cause code with a Z04- code

Z04.2   work accident

Z04.3   other accident

Z04.4 Encounter for examination and observation following alleged rape
5th

Encounter for examination and observation of victim following alleged rape

Encounter for examination and observation of victim following alleged sexual abuse

Z04.42   Encounter for examination and observation following alleged child rape

Suspected child rape, ruled out

Suspected child sexual abuse, ruled out

Z04.7 Encounter for examination and observation following alleged; physical abuse
5th

Z04.72   child physical abuse

Suspected child physical abuse, ruled out

Excludes1: confirmed case of child physical abuse (T74.-)

encounter for examination and observation following alleged child sexual abuse (Z04.42)

suspected case of child physical abuse, not ruled out (T76.-)

Z04.8 Encounter for examination and observation for other specified reasons
5th

Encounter for examination and observation for request for expert evidence

Z04.81   Encounter for examination and observation of victim following forced sexual exploitation

Z04.82   Encounter for examination and observation of victim following forced labor exploitation

Z04.89   Encounter for examination and observation for other specified reasons

---

| **4th** | **5th** | **6th** | **7th** | Additional Character Required |  | 3-character code | Unspecified laterality codes were excluded here. | • =New Code
▲ =Revised Code
⌑ =Social determinants of health | **Excludes1**—Not coded here, do not use together
Excludes2—Not included here |

442   **PEDIATRIC ICD-10-CM 2021: A MANUAL FOR PROVIDER-BASED CODING**

Z04.9 Encounter for examination and observation for unspecified reason

Code is a nonspecific Z code, refer to Chapter 21 for guidelines.

Z05 [4th] ENCOUNTER FOR OBSERVATION AND EVALUATION OF NEWBORN FOR SUSPECTED DISEASES AND CONDITIONS RULED OUT

GUIDELINES

Use of Z05 codes

Assign a code from category Z05, Observation and evaluation of newborns and infants for suspected conditions ruled out, to identify those instances when a healthy newborn is evaluated for a suspected condition that is determined after study not to be present. Do not use a code from category Z05 when the patient has identified signs or symptoms of a suspected problem; in such cases code the sign or symptom.

Z05 on Other than the Birth Record

A code from category Z05 may also be assigned as a principal or first-listed code for readmissions or encounters when the code from category Z38 code no longer applies. Codes from category Z05 are for use only for healthy newborns and infants for which no condition after study is found to be present.

Z05 on a birth record

A code from category Z05 is to be used as a secondary code after the code from category Z38, Liveborn infants according to place of birth and type of delivery is listed first.

This category is to be used for newborns, within the neonatal period (the first 28 days of life), who are suspected of having an abnormal condition but without signs or symptoms, and which, after examination and observation, is ruled out.

An observation code may be assigned as a secondary diagnosis code when the patient is being observed for a condition that is ruled out and is unrelated to the principal/first-listed diagnosis (e.g., patient presents for treatment following injuries sustained in a motor vehicle accident and is also observed for suspected COVID-19 infection that is subsequently ruled out).

Z05.0 Observation and evaluation of newborn for suspected; cardiac condition ruled out

Z05.1 infectious condition ruled out

Z05.2 neurological condition ruled out

Z05.3 respiratory condition ruled out

Z05.4 genetic, metabolic or immunologic condition ruled out

    [5th] **Z05.41 genetic condition ruled out**

    Z05.42 metabolic condition ruled out

    Z05.43 immunologic condition ruled out

Z05.5 gastrointestinal condition ruled out

Z05.6 genitourinary condition ruled out

Z05.7 skin and subcutaneous tissue or musculoskeletal condition [5th] **ruled out**

    Z05.71 skin and subcutaneous tissue condition ruled out

    Z05.72 musculoskeletal condition ruled out

    Z05.73 connective tissue condition ruled out

Z05.8 Observation and evaluation of newborn for other specified suspected condition ruled out

Z05.9 Observation and evaluation of newborn for unspecified suspected condition ruled out

Z08 ✔ ENCOUNTER FOR FOLLOW-UP EXAMINATION AFTER COMPLETED TREATMENT FOR MALIGNANT NEOPLASM

GUIDELINES

The follow-up codes are used to explain continuing surveillance following completed treatment of a disease, condition, or injury. They imply that the condition has been fully treated and no longer exists. They should not be confused with aftercare codes, or injury codes with a 7th character for subsequent encounter, that explain ongoing care of a healing condition or its sequelae. Follow-up codes may be used in conjunction with history codes to provide the full picture of the healed condition and its treatment. The follow-up code is sequenced first, followed by the history code.

A follow-up code may be used to explain multiple visits. Should a condition be found to have recurred on the follow-up visit, then the diagnosis code for the condition should be assigned in place of the follow-up code.

Medical surveillance following completed treatment

Use additional code to identify any acquired absence of organs (Z90.-)

Use additional code to identify the personal history of malignant neoplasm (Z85.-)

Excludes1: aftercare following medical care (Z43–Z49, Z51)

Z09 ✔ ENCOUNTER FOR FOLLOW-UP EXAMINATION AFTER COMPLETED TREATMENT FOR CONDITIONS OTHER THAN MALIGNANT NEOPLASM

GUIDELINES

The follow-up codes are used to explain continuing surveillance following completed treatment of a disease, condition, or injury. They imply that the condition has been fully treated and no longer exists. They should not be confused with aftercare codes, or injury codes with a 7th character for subsequent encounter, that explain ongoing care of a healing condition or its sequelae. Follow-up codes may be used in conjunction with history codes to provide the full picture of the healed condition and its treatment. The follow-up code is sequenced first, followed by the history code.

A follow-up code may be used to explain multiple visits. Should a condition be found to have recurred on the follow-up visit, then the diagnosis code for the condition should be assigned in place of the follow-up code.

Medical surveillance following completed treatment

Use additional code to identify any applicable history of disease code (Z86.-. Z87.-)

Excludes1: aftercare following medical care (Z43–Z49, Z51)

    surveillance of contraception (Z30.4-)

    surveillance of prosthetic and other medical devices (Z44–Z46)

Z11 [4th] ENCOUNTER FOR SCREENING FOR INFECTIOUS AND PARASITIC DISEASES

GUIDELINES

Screening is the testing for disease or disease precursors in seemingly well individuals so that early detection and treatment can be provided for those who test positive for the disease (eg, screening mammogram).

The testing of a person to rule out or confirm a suspected diagnosis because the patient has some sign or symptom is a diagnostic examination, not a screening. In these cases, the sign or symptom is used to explain the reason for the test.

A screening code may be a first-listed code if the reason for the visit is specifically the screening exam. It may also be used as an additional code if the screening is done during an office visit for other health problems. A screening code is not necessary if the screening is inherent to a routine examination, such as a pap smear done during a routine pelvic examination. Should a condition be discovered during the screening then the code for the condition may be assigned as an additional diagnosis.

The Z code indicates that a screening exam is planned. A procedure code is required to confirm that the screening was performed.

Excludes1: encounter for diagnostic examination-code to sign or symptom

Z11.0 Encounter for screening for; intestinal infectious diseases

Z11.1 respiratory tuberculosis

    Encounter for screening for active tuberculosis disease

Z11.2 other bacterial diseases

Z11.3 infections with a predominantly sexual mode of transmission

    Excludes2: encounter for screening for HIV (Z11.4)

       encounter for screening for human papillomavirus (Z11.51)

Z11.4 HIV

Z11.5 Encounter for screening for; other viral diseases

[5th]   ***Excludes2:*** encounter for screening for viral intestinal disease (Z11.0)

    Z11.51 human papillomavirus (HPV)

    Z11.59 other viral diseases

Z11.6 Encounter for screening for other protozoal diseases and helminthiases

    Excludes2: encounter for screening for protozoal intestinal disease (Z11.0)

Z11.7 Encounter for testing for latent tuberculosis infection

Z11.8 Encounter for screening for other infectious and parasitic diseases

    Encounter for screening for chlamydia or rickettsial or spirochetal or mycoses

Z11.9 Encounter for screening for infectious and parasitic diseases, unspecified

CHAPTER 21. FACTORS INFLUENCING HEALTH STATUS AND CONTACT WITH HEALTH SERVICES (Z04.9–Z11.9)

    4th 5th 6th 7th Additional Character Required   3-character code

Unspecified laterality codes were excluded here.

• =New Code
▲ =Revised Code
▫ =Social determinants of health

Excludes1—Not coded here, do not use together
Excludes2—Not included here

PEDIATRIC ICD-10-CM 2021: A MANUAL FOR PROVIDER-BASED CODING   443

Z12 ENCOUNTER FOR SCREENING FOR MALIGNANT NEOPLASMS
`4th`

GUIDELINES

Screening is the testing for disease or disease precursors in seemingly well individuals so that early detection and treatment can be provided for those who test positive for the disease (eg, screening mammogram).

The testing of a person to rule out or confirm a suspected diagnosis because the patient has some sign or symptom is a diagnostic examination, not a screening. In these cases, the sign or symptom is used to explain the reason for the test.

A screening code may be a first-listed code if the reason for the visit is specifically the screening exam. It may also be used as an additional code if the screening is done during an office visit for other health problems. A screening code is not necessary if the screening is inherent to a routine examination, such as a pap smear done during a routine pelvic examination. Should a condition be discovered during the screening then the code for the condition may be assigned as an additional diagnosis.

The Z code indicates that a screening exam is planned. A procedure code is required to confirm that the screening was performed.

Use additional code to identify any family history of malignant neoplasm (Z80.-)

Excludes1: encounter for diagnostic examination-code to sign or symptom

Z12.3 Encounter for screening for malignant neoplasm of breast
- `5th` **Z12.31 Encounter for screening mammogram for malignant neoplasm of breast**
  - *Excludes1:* inconclusive mammogram (R92.2)
- **Z12.39 Encounter for other screening for malignant neoplasm of breast**

Z12.4 Encounter for screening for malignant neoplasm of cervix
Encounter for screening pap smear for malignant neoplasm of cervix
- *Excludes1:* when screening is part of general gynecological examination (Z01.4-)
- *Excludes2:* encounter for screening for human papillomavirus (Z11.51)

Z12.8 Encounter for screening for malignant neoplasm of; other sites
- `5th` **Z12.82 nervous system**
- **Z12.89 other sites**

Z12.9 Encounter for screening for malignant neoplasm, site unspecified

Z13 ENCOUNTER FOR SCREENING FOR OTHER DISEASES AND DISORDERS
`4th`

GUIDELINES

Screening is the testing for disease or disease precursors in seemingly well individuals so that early detection and treatment can be provided for those who test positive for the disease (eg, screening mammogram).

The testing of a person to rule out or confirm a suspected diagnosis because the patient has some sign or symptom is a diagnostic examination, not a screening. In these cases, the sign or symptom is used to explain the reason for the test.

A screening code may be a first-listed code if the reason for the visit is specifically the screening exam. It may also be used as an additional code if the screening is done during an office visit for other health problems. A screening code is not necessary if the screening is inherent to a routine examination, such as a pap smear done during a routine pelvic examination. Should a condition be discovered during the screening then the code for the condition may be assigned as an additional diagnosis.

The Z code indicates that a screening exam is planned. A procedure code is required to confirm that the screening was performed.
Excludes Z13.9.

Excludes1: encounter for diagnostic examination-code to sign or symptom

Z13.0 Encounter for screening for; diseases of the blood and blood-forming organs and certain disorders involving the immune mechanism

Z13.1 DM

Z13.2 nutritional, metabolic and other endocrine disorders
- `5th` **Z13.21 nutritional disorder**
- **Z13.22 metabolic disorder**
  - `6th` **Z13.220 lipoid disorders**
    Encounter for screening for cholesterol level or hypercholesterolemia or hyperlipidemia
  - **Z13.228 other metabolic disorders**

Z13.29 other suspected endocrine disorder
Excludes1: encounter for screening for DM (Z13.1)

Z13.3 Encounter for screening for mental health and behavioral disorders
`5th`
- **Z13.30 Encounter for screening examination for mental health and behavioral disorders, unspecified**
- **Z13.31 Encounter for screening for depression**
  Encounter for screening for depression, adult
  Encounter for screening for depression for child or adolescent
- **Z13.32 Encounter for screening for maternal depression**   Do not report **Z13.32** on the baby's record
  Encounter for screening for perinatal depression
- **Z13.39 Encounter for screening examination for other mental health and behavioral disorders**
  Encounter for screening for alcoholism
  Encounter for screening for intellectual disabilities

Z13.4 Encounter for screening for certain developmental disorders in childhood
`5th`
Encounter for screening for developmental handicaps in early childhood
Excludes2: encounter for routine child health examination (Z00.12-)
- **Z13.40 Encounter for screening for unspecified developmental delays**
- **Z13.41 Encounter for autism screening**
- **Z13.42 Encounter for screening for global developmental delays (milestones)**
  Encounter for screening for developmental handicaps in early childhood
- **Z13.49 Encounter for screening for other developmental delays**

Z13.5 eye and ear disorders
Excludes2: encounter for general hearing examination (Z01.1-)
encounter for general vision examination (Z01.0-)

Z13.6 cardiovascular disorders

Z13.7 genetic and chromosomal anomalies
`5th`
Excludes1: genetic testing for procreative management (Z31.4-)
- **Z13.71 Encounter for nonprocreative screening for genetic disease carrier status**
- **Z13.79 Encounter for other screening for genetic and chromosomal anomalies**

Z13.8 Encounter for screening for; other specified diseases and disorders
`5th`
Excludes2: screening for malignant neoplasms (Z12.-)
- **Z13.81 digestive system disorders**
  - `6th` **Z13.810 upper gastrointestinal disorder**
  - **Z13.811 lower gastrointestinal disorder**
    Excludes1: encounter for screening for intestinal infectious disease (Z11.0)
  - **Z13.818 other digestive system disorders**
- **Z13.82 Encounter for screening for musculoskeletal disorder**
  - `6th` **Z13.828 other musculoskeletal disorder**
- **Z13.83 respiratory disorder NEC**
  Excludes1: encounter for screening for respiratory tuberculosis (Z11.1)
- **Z13.84 dental disorders**
- **Z13.85 Encounter for screening for nervous system disorders**
  `6th`
  - **Z13.850 traumatic brain injury**
  - **Z13.858 other nervous system disorders**
- **Z13.88 disorder due to exposure to contaminants**
  Excludes1: those exposed to contaminants without suspected disorders (Z57.-, Z77.-)
- **Z13.89 other disorder**
  Encounter for screening for genitourinary disorders

Z13.9 Encounter for screening, unspecified
Code is a nonspecific Z code, refer to Chapter 21 for guidelines.

(Z14–Z15) GENETIC CARRIER AND GENETIC SUSCEPTIBILITY TO DISEASE

`4th` `5th` `6th` `7th` Additional Character Required   ☑ 3-character code   Unspecified laterality codes were excluded here.   • =New Code   ▲ =Revised Code   ¤ =Social determinants of health   *Excludes1*—Not coded here, do not use together   *Excludes2*—Not included here

Z14 **GENETIC CARRIER**
`4th` Genetic carrier status indicates that a person carries a gene, associated with a particular disease, which may be passed to offspring who may develop that disease. The person does not have the disease and is not at risk of developing the disease. Refer to Chapter 21 for status guidelines.
Z14.0 **Hemophilia A carrier**
　`5th` **Z14.01** **Asymptomatic hemophilia A carrier**
　　Z14.02 **Symptomatic hemophilia A carrier**
Z14.1 **Cystic fibrosis carrier**
Z14.8 **Genetic carrier of other disease**

(Z16) RESISTANCE TO ANTIMICROBIAL DRUGS

Z16 **RESISTANCE TO ANTIMICROBIAL DRUGS**
`4th` This code indicates that a patient has a condition that is resistant to antimicrobial drug treatment. Sequence the infection code first. This is a status category, refer to Chapter 21 for status guidelines.
Note: The codes in this category are provided for use as additional codes to identify the resistance and non-responsiveness of a condition to antimicrobial drugs.
Code first the infection
Excludes1: MRSA infection (A49.02)
　MRSA infection in diseases classified elsewhere (B95.62)
　MRSA pneumonia (J15.212)
　Sepsis due to MRSA (A41.02)
Z16.1 **Resistance to beta lactam antibiotics**
　`5th` **Z16.10** **Resistance to unspecified beta lactam antibiotics**
　　Z16.11 **Resistance to penicillins**
　　　Resistance to amoxicillin or ampicillin
　　Z16.12 **Extended spectrum beta lactamase (ESBL) resistance**
　　　Excludes 2: MRSA infection in diseases classified elsewhere (B95.62)
　　Z16.19 **other specified beta lactam antibiotics**
　　　Resistance to cephalosporins
Z16.2 **Resistance to; other antibiotics**
　`5th` **Z16.20** **unspecified antibiotic**
　　　Resistance to antibiotics NOS
　　Z16.21 **vancomycin**
　　Z16.22 **vancomycin related antibiotics**
　　Z16.23 **quinolones and fluoroquinolones**
　　Z16.24 **multiple antibiotics**
　　Z16.29 **other single specified antibiotic**
　　　Resistance to aminoglycosides or macrolides or sulfonamides or tetracyclines
Z16.3 **Resistance to; other antimicrobial drugs**
　`5th` ***Excludes1:*** resistance to antibiotics (Z16.1-, Z16.2-)
　　Z16.30 **unspecified antimicrobial drugs**
　　　Drug resistance NOS
　　Z16.32 **antifungal drug(s)**
　　Z16.33 **antiviral drug(s)**
　　　Z16.341 **single antimycobacterial drug**
　　　　Resistance to antimycobacterial drug NOS
　　　Z16.342 **multiple antimycobacterial drugs**
　　Z16.34 **Resistance to antimycobacterial drug(s)**
　　`6th` Resistance to tuberculostatics
　　Z16.35 **Resistance to multiple antimicrobial drugs**
　　　Excludes1: Resistance to multiple antibiotics only (Z16.24)
　　Z16.39 **other specified antimicrobial drug**

(Z18) RETAINED FB FRAGMENTS

Z18 **RETAINED FB FRAGMENTS**
`4th` *This is a status category, refer to Chapter 21 for status guidelines.*
Includes: embedded fragment (status)
　embedded splinter (status)
　retained FB status
Excludes1: artificial joint prosthesis status (Z96.6-)
　FB accidentally left during a procedure (T81.5-)
　FB entering through orifice (T15–T19)
　in situ cardiac device (Z95.-)
　organ or tissue replaced by means other than transplant (Z96.-, Z97.-)

organ or tissue replaced by transplant (Z94.-)
personal history of retained FB fully removed Z87.821
superficial FB (non-embedded splinter)—code to superficial FB, by site
Z18.1 **Retained metal fragments;**
　`5th` ***Excludes1:*** retained radioactive metal fragments (Z18.01–Z18.09)
　　Z18.10 **Retained metal fragments, unspecified**
　　　Retained metal fragment NOS
　　Z18.11 **Retained magnetic metal fragments**
　　Z18.12 **Retained nonmagnetic metal fragments**
Z18.2 **Retained plastic fragments**
　　Acrylics fragments
　　Diethylhexyl phthalates fragments
　　Isocyanate fragments
Z18.3 **Retained organic fragments**
　`5th` **Z18.31** **Retained animal quills or spines**
　　Z18.32 **Retained tooth**
　　Z18.33 **Retained wood fragments**
　　Z18.39 **Other retained organic fragments**
Z18.8 **Other specified retained FB**
　`5th` **Z18.81** **Retained glass fragments**
　　Z18.83 **Retained stone or crystalline fragments**
　　　Retained concrete or cement fragments
　　Z18.89 **Other specified retained FB fragments**
Z18.9 **Retained FB fragments, unspecified material**

(Z20–Z29) PERSONS WITH POTENTIAL HEALTH HAZARDS RELATED TO COMMUNICABLE DISEASES

GUIDELINES

Category Z20 indicates contact with, and suspected exposure to, communicable diseases. These codes are for patients who do not show any sign or symptom of a disease but are suspected to have been exposed to it by close personal contact with an infected individual or are in an area where a disease is epidemic.

Contact/exposure codes may be used as a first-listed code to explain an encounter for testing, or, more commonly, as a secondary code to identify a potential risk.

Z20 **CONTACT WITH AND (SUSPECTED) EXPOSURE TO**
`4th` **COMMUNICABLE DISEASES**
　Excludes1: carrier of infectious disease (Z22.-)
　　diagnosed current infectious or parasitic disease—see Alphabetic Index
　Excludes2: personal history of infectious and parasitic diseases (Z86.1-)
Z20.0 **Contact with and (suspected) exposure to intestinal infectious**
　`5th` **diseases;**
　　Z20.01 **due to E. coli**
　　Z20.09 **other intestinal infectious diseases**
Z20.1 **Contact with and (suspected) exposure to; tuberculosis**
Z20.2 **infections with a predominantly sexual mode of transmission**
Z20.3 **rabies**
Z20.4 **rubella**
Z20.5 **viral hepatitis**
Z20.6 **HIV**
　Excludes1: asymptomatic HIV
　　HIV infection status (Z21)
Z20.7 **pediculosis, acariasis and other infestations**
Z20.8 **Contact with and (suspected) exposure to; other**
　`5th` **communicable diseases**
　　Z20.81 **other bacterial communicable diseases**
　　`6th` **Z20.810** **anthrax**
　　　Z20.811 **meningococcus**
　　　Z20.818 **other bacterial communicable diseases**
　　　　Use Z20.818 for exposure to strep throat
　　Z20.82 **Contact with and (suspected) exposure to; other viral**
　　`6th` **communicable diseases**
　　　Z20.820 **varicella**
　　　Z20.821 **Zika virus**
　　　Z20.828 **other viral communicable diseases**
　　Z20.89 **other communicable diseases**
Z20.9 **unspecified communicable disease**

 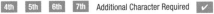 Additional Character Required ✓ 3-character code | Unspecified laterality codes were excluded here. | • =New Code ▲ =Revised Code ▣ =Social determinants of health | ***Excludes1***—Not coded here, do not use together ***Excludes2***—Not included here

PEDIATRIC ICD-10-CM 2021: A MANUAL FOR PROVIDER-BASED CODING   445

Z21   ASYMPTOMATIC HIV INFECTION STATUS

✔

This code indicates that a patient has tested positive for HIV but has manifested no signs or symptoms of the disease. This is a status code, refer to Chapter 21 for status guidelines.

HIV positive NOS

Code first HIV disease complicating pregnancy, childbirth and the puerperium, if applicable (O98.7-)

Excludes1: acquired immunodeficiency syndrome (B20)

contact with HIV (Z20.6)

exposure to HIV (Z20.6)

HIV disease (B20)

inconclusive laboratory evidence of HIV (R75)

Z22   CARRIER OF INFECTIOUS DISEASE

4th

Carrier status indicates that a person harbors the specific organisms of a disease without manifest symptoms and is capable of transmitting the infection. This is a status category, refer to Chapter 21 for status guidelines.

Includes: colonization status

suspected carrier

Excludes2: carrier of viral hepatitis (B18.-)

Z22.1   Carrier of other intestinal infectious diseases

Z22.2   Carrier of diphtheria

Z22.3   Carrier of other specified bacterial diseases

5th **Z22.31   Carrier of bacterial disease due to; meningococci**

Z22.32   Carrier of bacterial disease due to staphylococci

6th **Z22.321   Carrier or suspected carrier of MSSA**

MSSA colonization

Z22.322   Carrier or suspected carrier of MRSA

MRSA colonization

Z22.33   Carrier of bacterial disease due to streptococci

6th **Z22.330   Carrier of Group B streptococcus**

Excludes1: carrier of streptococcus group B (GBS) complicating pregnancy, childbirth and the puerperium (O99.82-)

Z22.338   Carrier of other streptococcus

Z22.39   Carrier of other specified bacterial diseases

Z22.4   Carrier of infections with a predominantly sexual mode of transmission

Z22.5   Carrier of viral hepatitis

Z22.6   Carrier of human T-lymphotropic virus type-1 [HTLV-1] infection

Z22.7   Latent tuberculosis

Latent tuberculosis infection (LTBI)

Excludes1: nonspecific reaction to cell mediated immunity measurement of gamma interferonantigen response without active tuberculosis (R76.12)

nonspecific reaction to tuberculin skin test without active tuberculosis (R76.11)

Z22.8   Carrier of other infectious diseases

Z22.9   Carrier of infectious disease, unspecified

Z23   ENCOUNTER FOR IMMUNIZATION

✔

GUIDELINES

Code Z23 is for encounters for inoculations and vaccinations. It indicates that a patient is being seen to receive a prophylactic inoculation against a disease. Procedure codes are required to identify the actual administration of the injection and the type(s) of immunizations given. Code Z23 may be used as a secondary code if the inoculation is given as a routine part of preventive health care, such as a well-baby visit.

Code first any routine childhood examination

Note: procedure codes are required to identify the types of immunizations given

> Tip: Z23 should be reported for every vaccine encounter

Z28   IMMUNIZATION NOT CARRIED OUT AND
4th **UNDERIMMUNIZATION STATUS**

Includes: vaccination not carried out

Z28.0   Immunization not carried out due to; contraindication

5th **Z28.01   acute illness of patient**

Z28.02   chronic illness or condition of patient

Z28.03   immune compromised state of patient

Z28.04   patient allergy to vaccine or component

Z28.09   other contraindication

Z28.1   Immunization not carried out due to patient decision for reasons of belief or group pressure

Immunization not carried out because of religious belief

Z28.2   Immunization not carried out due to; patient decision for other
5th **and unspecified reason**

Z28.20   patient decision for unspecified reason

Z28.21   patient refusal

Z28.29   patient decision for other reason

Z28.3   Underimmunization status

This is a status code, refer to Chapter 21 for status guidelines.

Delinquent immunization status

Lapsed immunization schedule status

Z28.8   Immunization not carried out; for other reason
5th **Z28.81   due to patient having had the disease**

Z28.82   because of caregiver refusal

Immunization not carried out because of parental or guardian refusal

Excludes1: immunization not carried out because of caregiver refusal because of religious belief (Z28.1)

Z28.83   due to unavailability of vaccine

Delay in delivery of vaccine

Lack of availability of vaccine

Manufacturer delay of vaccine

Z28.89   for other reason

Z28.9   Immunization not carried out for unspecified reason

Z29   ENCOUNTER FOR PROPHYLACTIC MEASURES
4th

Excludes 1: desensitization to allergens (Z51.6)

prophylactic surgery (Z40.-)

Z29.1   Encounter for prophylactic therapy
5th Encounter for administration of immunoglobulin

Z29.11   Encounter for prophylactic immunotherapy for RSV

Z29.12   Encounter for prophylactic antivenin

Z29.13   Encounter for prophylactic Rho(D) immune globulin

Z29.14   Encounter for prophylactic rabies immune globin

Z29.3   Encounter for prophylactic fluoride administration

Z29.8   Encounter for other specified prophylactic measures

Z29.9   Encounter for prophylactic measures, unspecified

(Z30–Z39) PERSONS ENCOUNTERING HEALTH SERVICES IN CIRCUMSTANCES RELATED TO REPRODUCTION

Z30   ENCOUNTER FOR CONTRACEPTIVE MANAGEMENT
4th **Z30.0   Encounter for general counseling and advice on contraception**
5th *Refer to Chapter 21 for guidelines on counseling.*

Z30.01   Encounter for initial prescription of; contraceptives
6th *Excludes1:* encounter for surveillance of contraceptives (Z30.4-)

Z30.011   contraceptive pills

Z30.012   emergency contraception

Encounter for postcoital contraception

Z30.013   injectable contraceptive

Z30.014   intrauterine contraceptive device

Excludes1: encounter for insertion of intrauterine contraceptive device (Z30.430, Z30.432)

Z30.015   vaginal ring hormonal contraceptive

Z30.016   transdermal patch hormonal contraceptive device

Z30.017   implantable subdermal contraceptive

Z30.018   other contraceptives

Encounter for initial prescription of barrier contraception or diaphragm

Z30.019   contraceptives, unspecified

Z30.02   Counseling and instruction in natural family planning to avoid pregnancy

Z30.09   Encounter for other general counseling and advice on contraception

Encounter for family planning advice NOS

Z30.4   Encounter for surveillance of contraceptives
5th **Z30.40   Encounter for surveillance of unspecified**

Z30.41   Encounter for surveillance of contraceptive pills

Encounter for repeat prescription for contraceptive pill

4th 5th 6th 7th Additional Character Required   ✔ 3-character code   Unspecified laterality codes were excluded here.   • =New Code   ▲ =Revised Code   ▯ =Social determinants of health   *Excludes1*—Not coded here, do not use together   *Excludes2*—Not included here

446   PEDIATRIC ICD-10-CM 2021: A MANUAL FOR PROVIDER-BASED CODING

Z30.42   Encounter for surveillance of injectable contraceptive

Z30.43   Encounter for surveillance of intrauterine contraceptive device
> **6th**

- **Z30.430**   Encounter for insertion of intrauterine contraceptive device
- **Z30.431**   Encounter for routine checking of intrauterine contraceptive device
- **Z30.432**   Encounter for removal of intrauterine contraceptive device
- **Z30.433**   Encounter for removal and reinsertion of intrauterine contraceptive device
  replacement of intrauterine contraceptive device

Z30.44   Encounter for surveillance of vaginal ring hormonal contraceptive device

Z30.45   Encounter for surveillance of transdermal patch hormonal contraceptive device

Z30.46   Encounter for surveillance of implantable subdermal contraceptive
Encounter for checking, reinsertion or removal of implantable subdermal contraceptive

Z30.49   Encounter for surveillance of other contraceptives
Encounter for surveillance of barrier contraception
Encounter for surveillance of diaphragm

Z30.8   Encounter for other contraceptive management
Encounter for postvasectomy sperm count
Encounter for routine examination for contraceptive maintenance
Excludes1: sperm count following sterilization reversal (Z31.42)
     sperm count for fertility testing (Z31.41)

Z30.9   Encounter for contraceptive management, unspecified

Z31   ENCOUNTER FOR PROCREATIVE MANAGEMENT
> **4th**

Excludes1: complications associated with artificial fertilization (N98.-)
     female infertility (N97.-)
     male infertility (N46.-)

Z31.5   Encounter for procreative genetic counseling
Refer to Chapter 21 for guidelines on counseling.

Z31.6   Encounter for general counseling and advice on procreation
> **5th**

Refer to Chapter 21 for guidelines on counseling.

- **Z31.69**   Encounter for other general counseling and advice on procreation

Z32   ENCOUNTER FOR PREGNANCY TEST AND CHILDBIRTH AND CHILDCARE INSTRUCTION
> **4th**

Z32.0   Encounter for pregnancy test
> **5th**

> **GUIDELINES**
>
> The codes are not to be used if the examination is for diagnosis of a suspected condition or for treatment purposes. In such cases the diagnosis code is used. During a routine exam, should a diagnosis or condition that is discovered, it should be coded as an additional code. Pre-existing and chronic conditions and history codes may also be included as additional codes as long as the examination is for administrative purposes and not focused on any particular condition.
>
> Some of the codes for routine health examinations distinguish between "with" and "without" abnormal findings. Code assignment depends on the information that is known at the time the encounter is being coded. For example, if no abnormal findings were found during the examination, but the encounter is being coded before test results are back, it is acceptable to assign the code for "without abnormal findings." When assigning a code for "with abnormal findings," additional code(s) should be assigned to identify the specific abnormal finding(s).

- **Z32.00**   Encounter for pregnancy test, result unknown
  Encounter for pregnancy test NOS
- **Z32.01**   Encounter for pregnancy test, result positive
- **Z32.02**   Encounter for pregnancy test, result negative

Z32.3   Encounter for childcare instruction
Encounter for prenatal or postpartum childcare instruction

Z33   PREGNANT STATE
> **4th**

Z33.1   Pregnant state, incidental
This is a status code, refer to Chapter 21 for status guidelines.
Pregnancy NOS
Pregnant state NOS
Excludes1: complications of pregnancy (O00–O9A)

Z38   LIVEBORN INFANTS ACCORDING TO PLACE OF BIRTH AND TYPE OF DELIVERY
> **4th**

> **GUIDELINES**
>
> When coding the birth episode in a newborn record, assign a code from category Z38, Liveborn infants according to place of birth and type of delivery, as the principal diagnosis. A code from category Z38 is assigned only once, to a newborn at the time of birth and throughout the initial stay at the birth hospital. If a newborn is transferred to another institution, a code from category Z38 should not be used at the receiving hospital.
>
> A code from category Z38 is used only on the newborn record, not on the mother's record. Codes in category Z38 "may only be reported as the principal/first-listed diagnosis, except when there are multiple encounters on the same day and the medical records for the encounters are combined." Refer to Chapter 16 for further guidelines.

Z38.0   Single liveborn infant, born in hospital
> **5th**

Single liveborn infant, born in birthing center or other health care facility

- **Z38.00**   Single liveborn infant, delivered vaginally
- **Z38.01**   Single liveborn infant, delivered by cesarean

Z38.1   Single liveborn infant, born outside hospital

Z38.2   Single liveborn infant, unspecified as to place of birth
Single liveborn infant NOS

Z38.3   Twin liveborn infant, born in hospital
> **5th**

- **Z38.30**   Twin liveborn infant, delivered vaginally
- **Z38.31**   Twin liveborn infant, delivered by cesarean

Z38.4   Twin liveborn infant, born outside hospital

Z38.5   Twin liveborn infant, unspecified as to place of birth

Z38.6   Other multiple liveborn infant, born in hospital
> **5th**

- **Z38.61**   Triplet liveborn infant, delivered vaginally
- **Z38.62**   Triplet liveborn infant, delivered by cesarean
- **Z38.63**   Quadruplet liveborn infant, delivered vaginally
- **Z38.64**   Quadruplet liveborn infant, delivered by cesarean
- **Z38.65**   Quintuplet liveborn infant, delivered vaginally
- **Z38.66**   Quintuplet liveborn infant, delivered by cesarean
- **Z38.68**   Other multiple liveborn infant, delivered vaginally
- **Z38.69**   Other multiple liveborn infant, delivered by cesarean

Z38.7   Other multiple liveborn infant, born outside hospital

Z38.8   Other multiple liveborn infant, unspecified as to place of birth

Z39   ENCOUNTER FOR MATERNAL POSTPARTUM CARE
> **4th**

Use only when billing under the mother

Z39.1   Encounter for care and examination of lactating mother
Encounter for supervision of lactation
Excludes1: disorders of lactation (O92.-)

(Z40–Z53) ENCOUNTERS FOR OTHER SPECIFIC HEALTH CARE

Categories Z40–Z53 are intended for use to indicate a reason for care. They may be used for patients who have already been treated for a disease or injury, but who are receiving aftercare or prophylactic care, or care to consolidate the treatment, or to deal with a residual state.

Z41   ENCOUNTER FOR PROCEDURES FOR PURPOSES OTHER THAN REMEDYING HEALTH STATE
> **4th**

Z41.2   Encounter for routine and ritual male circumcision

Z41.3   Encounter for ear piercing

Z41.8   Encounter for other procedures for purposes other than remedying health state

Z41.9   Encounter for procedure for purposes other than remedying health state, unspecified

Z43   ENCOUNTER FOR ATTENTION TO ARTIFICIAL OPENINGS
> **4th**

> **GUIDELINES**
>
> Aftercare visit codes cover situations when the initial treatment of a disease has been performed and the patient requires continued care during the healing or recovery phase, or for the long-term consequences of the disease. The aftercare Z code should not be used if treatment is directed at

---

   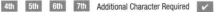 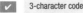

4th   **5th**   **6th**   **7th**   Additional Character Required   ✓   3-character code   Unspecified laterality codes were excluded here.   • =New Code   ▲ =Revised Code   ◘ =Social determinants of health   ***Excludes1***—Not coded here, do not use together   ***Excludes2***—Not included here

a current, acute disease. The diagnosis code is to be used in these cases.
Refer to Chapter 21 for aftercare guidelines.
Includes: closure of artificial openings
 passage of sounds or bougies through artificial openings
 reforming artificial openings
 removal of catheter from artificial openings
 toilet or cleansing of artificial openings
Excludes1: complications of external stoma (J95.0-, K94.-, N99.5-)
Excludes2: fitting and adjustment of prosthetic and other devices
 (Z44–Z46)
Z43.0 **Encounter for attention to tracheostomy**
Z43.1 **Encounter for attention to gastrostomy**
 Excludes 2: artificial opening status only, without need for care
 (Z93.-)
Z43.2 **Encounter for attention to ileostomy**
Z43.3 **Encounter for attention to colostomy**
Z43.4 **Encounter for attention to other artificial openings of digestive
 tract**
Z43.5 **Encounter for attention to cystostomy**
Z43.6 **Encounter for attention to other artificial openings of urinary
 tract**
 Encounter for attention to nephrostomy or ureterostomy or
 urethrostomy
Z43.7 **Encounter for attention to artificial vagina**
Z43.8 **Encounter for attention to other artificial openings**
Z43.9 **Encounter for attention to unspecified artificial opening**

Z45 **ENCOUNTER FOR ADJUSTMENT AND MANAGEMENT OF
 [4th] IMPLANTED DEVICE**
Includes: removal or replacement of implanted device
Excludes1: malfunction or other complications of device—see
 Alphabetical Index
Excludes2: encounter for fitting and adjustment of non-implanted device
 (Z46.-)
Z45.0 **Encounter for adjustment and management of cardiac device**
 [5th] Z45.01 **Encounter for adjustment and management of
 [6th] cardiac pacemaker**
 Encounter for adjustment and management of cardiac
 resynchronization therapy pacemaker (CRT-P)
 Excludes1: encounter for adjustment and management
 of automatic implantable cardiac defibrillator with
 synchronous cardiac pacemaker (Z45.02)
 Z45.010 **Encounter for checking and testing of
 cardiac pacemaker pulse generator
 [battery]**
 Encounter for replacing cardiac pacemaker
 pulse generator [battery]
 Z45.018 **Encounter for adjustment and
 management of other part of cardiac
 pacemaker**
 Excludes1: presence of other part of cardiac
 pacemaker (Z95.0)
 Excludes2: presence of prosthetic and other
 devices (Z95.1–Z95.5, Z95.811–Z97)
 Z45.02 **Encounter for adjustment and management of
 automatic implantable cardiac defibrillator**
 Encounter for adjustment and management of automatic
 implantable cardiac defibrillator with synchronous
 cardiac pacemaker
 Encounter for adjustment and management of cardiac
 resynchronization therapy defibrillator (CRT-D)
 Z45.09 **Encounter for adjustment and management of other
 cardiac device**

Z46 **ENCOUNTER FOR FITTING AND ADJUSTMENT OF OTHER
 [4th] DEVICES**
Includes: removal or replacement of other device
Excludes1: malfunction or other complications of device—see
 Alphabetical Index
Excludes2: encounter for fitting and management of implanted devices
 (Z45.-)
 issue of repeat prescription only (Z76.0)
 presence of prosthetic and other devices (Z95–Z97)

Z46.2 **Encounter for fitting and adjustment of other devices related
 to nervous system and special senses**
 Excludes2: encounter for adjustment and management of
 implanted nervous system device (Z45.4-)
 encounter for adjustment and management of implanted visual
 substitution device (Z45.31)
Z46.6 **Encounter for fitting and adjustment of urinary device**
 Excludes2: attention to artificial openings of urinary tract (Z43.5,
 Z43.6)
Z46.8 **Encounter for fitting and adjustment of other specified devices**
 [5th] Z46.81 **Encounter for fitting and adjustment of insulin pump**
 Encounter for insulin pump instruction and training
 Encounter for insulin pump titration
 Z46.82 **Encounter for fitting and adjustment of non-vascular
 catheter**
 Z46.89 **Encounter for fitting and adjustment of other
 specified devices**
 Encounter for fitting and adjustment of wheelchair
Z46.9 **Encounter for fitting and adjustment of unspecified device**

Z48 **ENCOUNTER FOR OTHER POSTPROCEDURAL
 [4th] AFTERCARE**

 GUIDELINES

Aftercare visit codes cover situations when the initial treatment of a
disease has been performed and the patient requires continued care during
the healing or recovery phase, or for the long-term consequences of the
disease. The aftercare Z code should not be used if treatment is directed at
a current, acute disease. The diagnosis code is to be used in these cases.
Refer to Chapter 21 for aftercare guidelines.
Excludes1: encounter for follow-up examination after completed treatment
 (Z08–Z09)
 encounter for aftercare following injury - code to Injury, by site, with
 appropriate 7th character for subsequent encounter
Excludes2: encounter for attention to artificial openings (Z43.-)
 encounter for fitting and adjustment of prosthetic and other devices
 (Z44–Z46)
Z48.0 **Encounter for; attention to dressings, sutures and drains**
 [5th] Excludes1: encounter for planned postprocedural wound closure
 (Z48.1)
 Do not report a Z48 code for an injury. Use the appropriate injury
 code.
 Z48.00 **change or removal of nonsurgical wound
 dressing**
 change or removal of wound dressing NOS
 Z48.01 **change or removal of surgical wound dressing**
 Z48.02 **removal of sutures**
 removal of staples
 Z48.03 **change or removal of drains**
Z48.1 **planned postprocedural wound closure**
 Excludes1: encounter for attention to dressings and sutures
 (Z48.0-)
Z48.2 **Encounter for aftercare following; organ transplant**
 [5th] Z48.21 **heart transplant**
 Z48.22 **kidney transplant**
 Z48.23 **liver transplant**
 Z48.24 **lung transplant**
 Z48.28 **multiple organ transplant**
 [6th] Z48.280 **heart-lung transplant**
 Z48.288 **multiple organ transplant**
 Z48.29 **other organ transplant**
 [6th] Z48.290 **bone marrow transplant**
 Z48.298 **other organ transplant**
Z48.3 **Aftercare following surgery for neoplasm**
 Use additional code to identify the neoplasm
Z48.8 **Encounter for other specified postprocedural aftercare**
 [5th] Z48.81 **Encounter for surgical aftercare following surgery
 [6th] on specified body systems**
 These codes identify the body system requiring
 aftercare. They are for use in conjunction with
 other aftercare codes to fully explain the aftercare
 encounter. The condition treated should also be coded
 if still present.

 [4th] [5th] [6th] [7th] Additional Character Required   3-character code   Unspecified laterality codes
were excluded here.   • =New Code
▲ =Revised Code
▯ =Social determinants of health   **Excludes1**—Not coded here, do not use together
Excludes2—Not included here

Excludes1: aftercare for injury—code the injury with 7th character D
aftercare following surgery for neoplasm (Z48.3)
Excludes2: aftercare following organ transplant (Z48.2-)
orthopedic aftercare (Z47.-)

- **Z48.810 Encounter for surgical aftercare following surgery on the sense organs**
- **Z48.811 Encounter for surgical aftercare following surgery on the nervous system**
  - **Excludes2:** encounter for surgical aftercare following surgery on the sense organs (Z48.810)
- **Z48.812 Encounter for surgical aftercare following surgery on the circulatory system**
- **Z48.813 Encounter for surgical aftercare following surgery on the respiratory system**
- **Z48.814 Encounter for surgical aftercare following surgery on the teeth or oral cavity**
- **Z48.815 Encounter for surgical aftercare following surgery on the digestive system**
- **Z48.816 Encounter for surgical aftercare following surgery on the genitourinary system**
  - **Excludes1:** encounter for aftercare following sterilization reversal (Z31.42)
- **Z48.817 Encounter for surgical aftercare following surgery on the skin and subcutaneous tissue**
- **Z48.89 Encounter for other specified surgical aftercare**

Z51 [4th] **ENCOUNTER FOR OTHER AFTERCARE AND MEDICAL CARE**

GUIDELINES

Aftercare visit codes cover situations when the initial treatment of a disease has been performed and the patient requires continued care during the healing or recovery phase, or for the long-term consequences of the disease. The aftercare Z code should not be used if treatment is directed at a current, acute disease. The diagnosis code is to be used in these cases. Refer to Chapter 21 for aftercare guidelines.
Code also condition requiring care
Excludes1: follow-up examination after treatment (Z08–Z09)
Excludes2: follow-up examination for medical surveillance after treatment (Z08–Z09)

- **Z51.0 Encounter for antineoplastic; radiation therapy**
  May only be reported as the principal/first-listed diagnosis, except when there are multiple encounters on the same day and the medical records for the encounters are combined.
- **Z51.1** [5th] **chemotherapy and immunotherapy**
  Codes Z51.1- may only be reported as the principal/first-listed diagnosis, except when there are multiple encounters on the same day and the medical records for the encounters are combined.
  Excludes2: encounter for chemotherapy and immunotherapy for non-neoplastic condition—code to condition
  - **Z51.11 chemotherapy**
  - **Z51.12 immunotherapy**
- **Z51.5 Encounter for palliative care**
- **Z51.6 Encounter for desensitization to allergens**
- **Z51.8 Encounter for other specified aftercare**
  [5th] **Excludes1:** holiday relief care (Z75.5)
  - **Z51.81 Encounter for therapeutic drug level monitoring**
    Code also any long-term (current) drug therapy (Z79.-)
    Excludes1: encounter for blood-drug test for administrative or medicolegal reasons (Z02.83)
  - **Z51.89 Encounter for other specified aftercare**

Z53 [4th] **PERSONS ENCOUNTERING HEALTH SERVICES FOR SPECIFIC PROCEDURES AND TREATMENT, NOT CARRIED OUT**

- **Z53.0 Procedure and treatment not carried out because of contraindication** [5th]
  - **Z53.01 Procedure and treatment not carried out due to patient smoking**
  - **Z53.09 Procedure and treatment not carried out because of other contraindication**

- **Z53.1 Procedure and treatment not carried out because of patient's decision for reasons of belief and group pressure**
- **Z53.2 Procedure and treatment not carried out because of patient's decision for other and unspecified reasons** [5th]
  - **Z53.20 Procedure and treatment not carried out because of patient's decision for unspecified reasons**
  - **Z53.21 Procedure and treatment not carried out due to patient leaving prior to being seen by healthcare provider**
  - **Z53.29 Procedure and treatment not carried out because of patient's decision for other reasons**
- **Z53.3 Procedure converted to open procedure** [5th]
  - **Z53.31 Laparoscopic surgical procedure converted to open procedure**
  - **Z53.32 Thoracoscopic surgical procedure converted to open procedure**
  - **Z53.33 Arthroscopic surgical procedure converted to open procedure**
  - **Z53.39 Other specified procedure converted to open procedure**
- **Z53.8 Procedure and treatment not carried out for other reasons**
- **Z53.9 Procedure and treatment not carried out, unspecified reason**

(Z55–Z65) PERSONS WITH POTENTIAL HEALTH HAZARDS RELATED TO SOCIOECONOMIC AND PSYCHOSOCIAL CIRCUMSTANCES

GUIDELINES (HEADER)

For social determinants of health, such as information found in categories Z55-Z65, Persons with potential health hazards related to socioeconomic and psychosocial circumstances, code assignment may be based on medical record documentation from clinicians involved in the care of the patient who are not the patient's provider since this information represents social information, rather than medical diagnoses. Report only as a secondary code.

Z55 [4th] **PROBLEMS RELATED TO EDUCATION AND LITERACY**
Excludes1: disorders of psychological development (F80–F89)
- □**Z55.0 Illiteracy and low-level literacy**
- □**Z55.1 Schooling unavailable and unattainable**
- □**Z55.2 Failed school examinations**
- □**Z55.3 Underachievement in school**
- □**Z55.4 Educational maladjustment and discord with teachers and classmates**
- □**Z55.8 Other problems related to education and literacy**
  Problems related to inadequate teaching
- □**Z55.9 Problems related to education and literacy, unspecified**
  Academic problems NOS

Z59 [4th] **PROBLEMS RELATED TO HOUSING AND ECONOMIC CIRCUMSTANCES**
Excludes2: problems related to upbringing (Z62.-)
- □**Z59.0 Homelessness**
- □**Z59.1 Inadequate housing**
  Lack of heating
  Restriction of space
  Technical defects in home preventing adequate care
  Unsatisfactory surroundings
  Excludes1: problems related to the natural and physical environment (Z77.1-)
- □**Z59.4 Lack of adequate food and safe drinking water**
  Inadequate drinking water supply
  Excludes1: effects of hunger (T73.0)
  inappropriate diet or eating habits (Z72.4)
  malnutrition (E40-E46)
- □**Z59.5 Extreme poverty**
- □**Z59.6 Low income**
- □**Z59.7 Insufficient social insurance and welfare support**
- □**Z59.8 Other problems related to housing and economic circumstances**
  Foreclosure on loan
  Isolated dwelling
  Problems with creditors
- □**Z59.9 Problem related to housing and economic circumstances, unspecified**

   | 4th | 5th | 6th | 7th | Additional Character Required | ✓ 3-character code | Unspecified laterality codes were excluded here. | • =New Code ▲ =Revised Code □ =Social determinants of health | **Excludes1**—Not coded here, do not use together **Excludes2**—Not included here

Z60 PROBLEMS RELATED TO SOCIAL ENVIRONMENT
4th

Z60.2 Problems related to living alone

□**Z60.3 Acculturation difficulty**
Problem with migration
Problem with social transplantation

□**Z60.4 Social exclusion and rejection**
Exclusion and rejection on the basis of personal characteristics, such as unusual physical appearance, illness or behavior
Excludes1: target of adverse discrimination such as for racial or religious reasons (Z60.5)

□**Z60.5 Target of (perceived) adverse discrimination and persecution**
Excludes1: social exclusion and rejection (Z60.4)

□**Z60.8 Other problems related to social environment**

□**Z60.9 Problem related to social environment, unspecified**

Z62 PROBLEMS RELATED TO UPBRINGING
4th

Includes: current and past negative life events in childhood
current and past problems of a child related to upbringing
Excludes2: maltreatment syndrome (T74.-)
problems related to housing and economic circumstances (Z59.-)

□**Z62.0 Inadequate parental supervision and control**

□**Z62.1 Parental overprotection**

□**Z62.2 Upbringing away from parents**
5th
Excludes1: problems with boarding school (Z59.3)

Z62.21 Child in welfare custody
Child in care of non-parental family member
Child in foster care
Excludes2: problem for parent due to child in welfare custody (Z63.5)

□**Z62.22 Institutional upbringing**
Child living in orphanage or group home

□**Z62.29 Other upbringing away from parents**

Z62.8 Other specified problems related to upbringing
5th

Z62.81 Personal history of abuse in childhood
6th

□**Z62.810 Personal history of; physical and sexual abuse in childhood**
Excludes1: current child physical abuse (T74.12, T76.12)
current child sexual abuse (T74.22, T76.22)

□**Z62.811 psychological abuse in childhood**
Excludes1: current child psychological abuse (T74.32, T76.32)

□**Z62.812 neglect in childhood**
Excludes1: current child neglect (T74.02, T76.02)

□**Z62.813 forced labor or sexual exploitation in childhood**
Excludes1: current exploitation or forced labor (T74.52-, T74.62-, T76.52-, T76.62-)

□**Z62.819 unspecified abuse in childhood**
Excludes1: current child abuse NOS (T74.92, T76.92)

Z62.82 Parent-child conflict
6th

□**Z62.820 Parent-biological child conflict**
Parent-child problem NOS

□**Z62.821 Parent-adopted child conflict**

□**Z62.822 Parent-foster child conflict**

Z62.89 Other specified problems related to upbringing
6th

□**Z62.890 Parent-child estrangement NEC**

□**Z62.891 Sibling rivalry**

□**Z62.898 Other specified problems related to upbringing**

□**Z62.9 Problem related to upbringing, unspecified**

Z63 OTHER PROBLEMS RELATED TO PRIMARY SUPPORT GROUP, INCLUDING FAMILY CIRCUMSTANCES
4th

Excludes2: maltreatment syndrome (T74.-, T76)
parent-child problems (Z62.-)
problems related to negative life events in childhood (Z62.-)
problems related to upbringing (Z62.-)

Z63.0 Problems in relationship with spouse or partner
Relationship distress with spouse or intimate partner
Excludes1: counseling for spousal or partner abuse problems (Z69.1)
counseling related to sexual attitude, behavior, and orientation (Z70.-)

Z63.3 Absence of family member
5th
Excludes1: absence of family member due to disappearance and death (Z63.4)
absence of family member due to separation and divorce (Z63.5)

□**Z63.31 Absence of family member due to military deployment**
Individual or family affected by other family member being on military deployment
Excludes1: family disruption due to return of family member from military deployment (Z63.71)

□**Z63.32 Other absence of family member**

□**Z63.4 Disappearance and death of family member**
Assumed death of family member
Bereavement

□**Z63.5 Disruption of family by separation and divorce**

Z63.6 Dependent relative needing care at home

Z63.7 Other stressful life events affecting family and household
5th

□**Z63.71 Stress on family due to return of family member from military deployment**
Individual or family affected by family member having returned from military deployment (current or past conflict)

□**Z63.72 Alcoholism and drug addiction in family**

□**Z63.79 Other stressful life events affecting family and household**
Anxiety (normal) about sick person in family
Health problems within family
Ill or disturbed family member
Isolated family

□**Z63.8 Other specified problems related to primary support group**
Family discord NOS
Family estrangement NOS
High expressed emotional level within family
Inadequate family support NOS
Inadequate or distorted communication within family

□**Z63.9 Problem related to primary support group, unspecified**
Relationship disorder NOS

Z64 PROBLEMS RELATED TO CERTAIN PSYCHOSOCIAL CIRCUMSTANCES
4th

Z64.0 Problems related to unwanted pregnancy

Z64.4 Discord with counselors
Discord with probation officer
Discord with social worker

Z65 PROBLEMS RELATED TO OTHER PSYCHOSOCIAL CIRCUMSTANCES
4th

Z65.3 Problems related to other legal circumstances
Arrest
Child custody or support proceedings
Litigation
Prosecution

Z65.4 Victim of crime and terrorism
Victim of torture

□**Z65.8 Other specified problems related to psychosocial circumstances**
Religious or spiritual problem

□**Z65.9 Problem related to unspecified psychosocial circumstances**

(Z66) DO NOT RESUSCITATE STATUS

Z66 DO NOT RESUSCITATE
☑ This code may be used when it is documented by the provider that a patient is on do not resuscitate status at any time during the stay. This is a status code, *refer to Chapter 21 for status guidelines.*
DNR status

  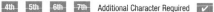 **4th** **5th** **6th** **7th** Additional Character Required ☑ 3-character code Unspecified laterality codes were excluded here. • =New Code ▲ =Revised Code ☒ =Social determinants of health *Excludes1*—Not coded here, do not use together *Excludes2*—Not included here

(Z67) BLOOD TYPE

Z67   BLOOD TYPE
`4th`
  Z67.1   Type A blood
  `5th` **Z67.10   Type A blood, Rh positive**
    Z67.11   Type A blood, Rh negative
  Z67.2   Type B blood
  `5th` **Z67.20   Type B blood, Rh positive**
    Z67.21   Type B blood, Rh negative
  Z67.3   Type AB blood
  `5th` **Z67.30   Type AB blood, Rh positive**
    Z67.31   Type AB blood, Rh negative
  Z67.4   Type O blood
  `5th` **Z67.40   Type O blood, Rh positive**
    Z67.41   Type O blood, Rh negative

(Z68) BODY MASS INDEX [BMI]

Z68   BODY MASS INDEX [BMI]
`4th`

> **GUIDELINES**
>
> This is a status category, refer to Chapter 21 for status guidelines. **BMI codes should only be assigned when the associated diagnosis (such as overweight or obesity) meets the definition of a reportable diagnosis (see Section III, Reporting Additional Diagnoses). Do not assign BMI codes during pregnancy. *See Section I.B.14 for BMI documentation by clinicians other than the patient's provider.***
> Kilograms per meters squared
> **Note:** BMI adult codes are for use for persons 20 years of age or older.
> BMI pediatric codes are for use for persons 2–19 years of age. These percentiles are based on the growth charts published by the Centers for Disease Control and Prevention (CDC)

  Z68.1   BMI 19.9 or less, adult
  Z68.2   BMI 20-29, adult
  `5th` **Z68.20   BMI 20.0-20.9, adult**
    Z68.21   BMI 21.0-21.9, adult
    Z68.22   BMI 22.0-22.9, adult
    Z68.23   BMI 23.0-23.9, adult
    Z68.24   BMI 24.0-24.9, adult
    Z68.25   BMI 25.0-25.9, adult
    Z68.26   BMI 26.0-26.9, adult
    Z68.27   BMI 27.0-27.9, adult
    Z68.28   BMI 28.0-28.9, adult
    Z68.29   BMI 29.0-29.9, adult
  Z68.3   BMI 30-39, adult
  `5th` **Z68.30   BMI 30.0-30.9, adult**
    Z68.31   BMI 31.0-31.9, adult
    Z68.32   BMI 32.0-32.9, adult
    Z68.33   BMI 33.0-33.9, adult
    Z68.34   BMI 34.0-34.9, adult
    Z68.35   BMI 35.0-35.9, adult
    Z68.36   BMI 36.0-36.9, adult
    Z68.37   BMI 37.0-37.9, adult
    Z68.38   BMI 38.0-38.9, adult
    Z68.39   BMI 39.0-39.9, adult
  Z68.4   Body mass index (BMI) 40 or greater, adult
  `5th` **Z68.41   Body mass index (BMI) 40.0-44.9, adult**
    Z68.42   Body mass index (BMI) 45.0-49.9, adult
    Z68.43   Body mass index (BMI) 50.0-59.9, adult
    Z68.44   Body mass index (BMI) 60.0-69.9, adult
    Z68.45   Body mass index (BMI) 70 or greater, adult
  Z68.5   BMI pediatric
  `5th` **Z68.51   BMI pediatric, less than 5th percentile for age**
    Z68.52   BMI pediatric, 5th percentile to less than 85th percentile for age
    Z68.53   BMI pediatric, 85th percentile to less than 95th percentile for age
    Z68.54   BMI pediatric, greater than or equal to 95th percentile for age

(Z69–Z76) PERSONS ENCOUNTERING HEALTH SERVICES IN OTHER CIRCUMSTANCES

Z69   ENCOUNTER FOR MENTAL HEALTH SERVICES FOR
`4th` **VICTIM AND PERPETRATOR OF ABUSE**

> **GUIDELINES**
>
> Counseling Z codes are used when a patient or family member receives assistance in the aftermath of an illness or injury, or when support is required in coping with family or social problems. They are not used in conjunction with a diagnosis code when the counseling component of care is considered integral to standard treatment.
> ***Includes:*** counseling for victims and perpetrators of abuse

  Z69.0   Encounter for mental health services for child abuse problems
  `5th` **Z69.01   Encounter for mental health services for; parental**
    `6th` **child abuse**
      ▫**Z69.010   victim of parental child abuse**
        Encounter for mental health services for victim of child abuse or neglect by parent
        Encounter for mental health services for victim of child psychological or sexual abuse by parent
      ▫**Z69.011   perpetrator of parental child abuse**
        Encounter for mental health services for perpetrator of parental child neglect
        Encounter for mental health services for perpetrator of parental child psychological or sexual abuse
        Excludes1: encounter for mental health services for non-parental child abuse (Z69.02-)
  `6th` **Z69.02   Encounter for mental health services for; non-parental child abuse**
      ▫**Z69.020   victim of non-parental child abuse**
        Encounter for mental health services for victim of non-parental child neglect
        Encounter for mental health services for victim of non-parental child psychological or sexual abuse
      ▫**Z69.021   perpetrator of non-parental child abuse**
        Encounter for mental health services for perpetrator of non-parental child neglect
        Encounter for mental health services for perpetrator of non-parental child psychological or sexual abuse
  Z69.1   Encounter for mental health services for; spousal or partner
  `5th` **abuse problems**
    Z69.11   victim of spousal or partner abuse
      Encounter for mental health services for victim of spouse or partner neglect
      Encounter for mental health services for victim of spouse or partner psychological abuse
      Encounter for mental health services for victim of spouse or partner violence, physical
    Z69.12   perpetrator of spousal or partner abuse
      Encounter for mental health services for perpetrator of spouse or partner neglect
      Encounter for mental health services for perpetrator of spouse or partner psychological abuse Encounter for mental health services for perpetrator of spouse or partner violence, physical Encounter for mental health services for perpetrator of spouse or partner violence, sexual
  Z69.8   Encounter for mental health services for victim or perpetrator
  `5th` **of other abuse**
    ▫**Z69.81   Encounter for mental health services for victim of other abuse**
      Encounter for mental health services for victim of non-spousal adult abuse
      Encounter for mental health services for victim of spouse or partner violence, sexual
      Encounter for rape victim counseling

CHAPTER 21. FACTORS INFLUENCING HEALTH STATUS AND CONTACT WITH HEALTH SERVICES   (Z67–Z69.81)

`4th` `5th` `6th` `7th`   Additional Character Required   ✓   3-character code   Unspecified laterality codes were excluded here.

• =New Code
▲ =Revised Code
▫ =Social determinants of health

Excludes1—Not coded here, do not use together
Excludes2—Not included here

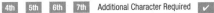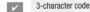

Z69.82   **Encounter for mental health services for perpetrator of other abuse**
Encounter for mental health services for perpetrator of non-spousal adult abuse

Z70   COUNSELING RELATED TO SEXUAL ATTITUDE, BEHAVIOR AND ORIENTATION
Includes: encounter for mental health services for sexual attitude, behavior and orientation
Excludes2: contraceptive or procreative counseling (Z30-Z31)

Z70.0   **Counseling related to sexual attitude**

Z70.1   **Counseling related to patient's sexual behavior and orientation**
Patient concerned regarding impotence
Patient concerned regarding non-responsiveness
Patient concerned regarding promiscuity
Patient concerned regarding sexual orientation

Z70.2   **Counseling related to sexual behavior and orientation of third party**
Advice sought regarding sexual behavior and orientation of child
Advice sought regarding sexual behavior and orientation of partner
Advice sought regarding sexual behavior and orientation of spouse

Z70.3   **Counseling related to combined concerns regarding sexual attitude, behavior and orientation**

Z70.8   **Other sex counseling**
Encounter for sex education

Z70.9   **Sex counseling, unspecified**

Z71   PERSONS ENCOUNTERING HEALTH SERVICES FOR OTHER COUNSELING AND MEDICAL ADVICE, NEC
Refer to category Z69 for guideline.
Excludes2: contraceptive or procreation counseling (Z30–Z31)
sex counseling (Z70.-)

Z71.0   **Person encountering health services to consult on behalf of another person**
Person encountering health services to seek advice or treatment for non-attending third party
Excludes2: anxiety (normal) about sick person in family (Z63.7)
expectant (adoptive) parent(s) pre-birth pediatrician visit (Z76.81)

Z71.2   **Person consulting for explanation of examination or test findings**

Z71.3   **Dietary counseling and surveillance**
Use additional code for any associated underlying medical condition
Use additional code to identify body mass index (BMI), if known (Z68.-)

Z71.4   **Alcohol abuse counseling and surveillance**
Use additional code for alcohol abuse or dependence (F10.-)
   Z71.41   **Alcohol abuse counseling and surveillance of alcoholic**
   ▫**Z71.42**   **Counseling for family member of alcoholic**
Counseling for significant other, partner, or friend of alcoholic

Z71.5   **Drug abuse counseling and surveillance**
Use additional code for drug abuse or dependence (F11–F16, F18–F19)
   Z71.51   **Drug abuse counseling and surveillance of drug abuser**
   ▫**Z71.52**   **Counseling for family member of drug abuser**
Counseling for significant other, partner, or friend of drug abuser

Z71.6   **Tobacco abuse counseling**
Use additional code for nicotine dependence (F17.-)

Z71.7   **HIV counseling**

Z71.8   **Other specified counseling**
Excludes2: counseling for contraception (Z30.0-)
   Z71.81   **Spiritual or religious counseling**
   Z71.82   **Exercise counseling**
   Z71.83   **Encounter for nonprocreative genetic counseling**
      Excludes1: counseling for genetics (Z31.5)
counseling for procreative management (Z31.6)
   Z71.84   **Encounter for health counseling related to travel**
Encounter for health risk and safety counseling for (international) travel

Code also, if applicable, encounter for immunization (Z23)
Excludes2: encounter for administrative examination (Z02.-)
encounter for other special examination without complaint, suspected or reported diagnosis (Z01.-)

Z71.89   **Other specified counseling**
Encounter for mental health services for victim of child abuse or neglect by parent
Encounter for mental health services for victim of child psychological or sexual abuse by parent

Z71.9   **Counseling, unspecified**
Encounter for medical advice NOS

Z72   PROBLEMS RELATED TO LIFESTYLE
Excludes2: problems related to life-management difficulty (Z73.-)
problems related to socioeconomic and psychosocial circumstances (Z55–Z65)

Z72.0   **Tobacco use**
Tobacco use NOS
Excludes1: history of tobacco dependence (Z87.891)
nicotine dependence (F17.2-)
tobacco dependence (F17.2-)
tobacco use during pregnancy (O99.33-)

Z72.3   **Lack of physical exercise**

Z72.4   **Inappropriate diet and eating habits**
Excludes1: behavioral eating disorders of infancy or childhood (F98.2.–F98.3)
eating disorders (F50.-)
lack of adequate food (Z59.4)
malnutrition and other nutritional deficiencies (E40–E64)

Z72.5   **High risk sexual behavior**
Promiscuity
Excludes1: paraphilias (F65)
   Z72.51   **High risk heterosexual behavior**
   Z72.52   **High risk homosexual behavior**
   Z72.53   **High risk bisexual behavior**

Z72.6   **Gambling and betting**
Excludes1: compulsive or pathological gambling (F63.0)

Z72.8   **Other problems related to lifestyle**
   Z72.81   **Antisocial behavior**
      Excludes1: conduct disorders (F91.-)
      Z72.810   **Child and adolescent antisocial behavior**
Antisocial behavior (child) (adolescent) without manifest psychiatric disorder
Delinquency NOS
Group delinquency
Offenses in the context of gang membership
Stealing in company with others
Truancy from school
   Z72.82   **Problems related to sleep**
      Z72.820   **Sleep deprivation**
Lack of adequate sleep
Excludes1: insomnia (G47.0-)
      Z72.821   **Inadequate sleep hygiene**
Bad sleep habits
Irregular sleep habits
Unhealthy sleep wake schedule
Excludes1: insomnia (F51.0-, G47.0-)
   Z72.89   **Other problems related to lifestyle**
Self-damaging behavior

Z72.9   **Problem related to lifestyle, unspecified**

Z73   PROBLEMS RELATED TO LIFE MANAGEMENT DIFFICULTY
Excludes2: problems related to socioeconomic and psychosocial circumstances (Z55–Z65)

Z73.4   **Inadequate social skills, NEC**

Z73.6   **Limitation of activities due to disability**
Excludes1: care-provider dependency (Z74.-)

Z73.8   **Other problems related to life management difficulty**
   Z73.81   **Behavioral insomnia of childhood**
      Z73.810   **Behavioral insomnia of childhood, sleep-onset association type**

 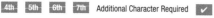 Additional Character Required   ✓   3-character code   Unspecified laterality codes were excluded here.   • =New Code   ▲ =Revised Code   ▫ =Social determinants of health   *Excludes1*—Not coded here, do not use together   *Excludes2*—Not included here

452   PEDIATRIC ICD-10-CM 2021: A MANUAL FOR PROVIDER-BASED CODING

	Z73.811	Behavioral insomnia of childhood, limit setting type
	Z73.812	Behavioral insomnia of childhood, combined type
	Z73.819	Behavioral insomnia of childhood, unspecified type
	Z73.82	Dual sensory impairment
	Z73.89	Other problems related to life management difficulty
Z73.9		Problem related to life management difficulty, unspecified

Z74 **[4th]** **PROBLEMS RELATED TO CARE PROVIDER DEPENDENCY**
Excludes2: dependence on enabling machines or devices NEC (Z99.-)

Z74.0 **Reduced mobility**
[5th] **Z74.09** **Other reduced mobility**
Chair ridden
Reduced mobility NOS
Excludes2: wheelchair dependence (Z99.3)

Z74.1 **Need for assistance with personal care**
Z74.2 **Need for assistance at home and no other household member able to render care**
Z74.3 **Need for continuous supervision**
Z74.8 **Other problems related to care provider dependency**
Z74.9 **Problem related to care provider dependency, unspecified**

Z75 **[4th]** **PROBLEMS RELATED TO MEDICAL FACILITIES AND OTHER HEALTH CARE**
Z75.0 **Medical services not available in home**
Excludes1: no other household member able to render care (Z74.2)
Z75.3 **Unavailability and inaccessibility of health-care facilities**
Excludes1: bed unavailable (Z75.1)

Z76 **[4th]** **PERSONS ENCOUNTERING HEALTH SERVICES IN OTHER CIRCUMSTANCES**
Z76.0 **Encounter for issue of repeat prescription**
Encounter for issue of repeat prescription for appliance or medicaments or spectacles
Excludes2: issue of medical certificate (Z02.7)
repeat prescription for contraceptive (Z30.4-)
Codes Z76.1 and Z76.2 may only be reported as the principal/first-listed diagnosis, except when there are multiple encounters on the same day and the medical records for the encounters are combined.
Z76.1 **Encounter for health supervision and care of foundling**
Refer to Chapter 16 for guidelines.
Z76.2 **Encounter for health supervision and care of other healthy infant and child**
Encounter for medical or nursing care or supervision of healthy infant under circumstances such as adverse socioeconomic conditions at home or such as awaiting foster or adoptive placement or such as maternal illness or such as number of children at home preventing or interfering with normal care
Z76.4 **Other boarder to healthcare facility**
Excludes1: homelessness (Z59.0)
Z76.5 **Malingerer [conscious simulation]**
Person feigning illness (with obvious motivation)
Excludes1: factitious disorder (F68.1-, F68.A)
peregrinating patient (F68.1-)
Z76.8 **Persons encountering health services in other specified**
[5th] **circumstances**
Z76.81 **Expectant parent(s) prebirth pediatrician visit**
Refer to Chapter 21 for guidelines on counseling.
Pre-adoption pediatrician visit for adoptive parent(s)
Z76.82 **Awaiting organ transplant status**
This is a status code, refer to Chapter 21 for status guidelines.
Patient waiting for organ availability
Z76.89 **Persons encountering health services in other specified circumstances**
Persons encountering health services NOS

(Z77–Z99) PERSONS WITH POTENTIAL HEALTH HAZARDS RELATED TO FAMILY AND PERSONAL HISTORY AND CERTAIN CONDITIONS INFLUENCING HEALTH STATUS

GUIDELINES
Contact/exposure codes may be used as a first-listed code to explain an encounter for testing, or, more commonly, as a secondary code to identify a potential risk.
Code also any follow-up examination (Z08–Z09)

Z77 **[4th]** **OTHER CONTACT WITH AND (SUSPECTED) EXPOSURES HAZARDOUS TO HEALTH**
Includes: contact with and (suspected) exposures to potential hazards to health
Excludes2: contact with and (suspected) exposure to communicable diseases (Z20.-)
exposure to (parental) (environmental) tobacco smoke in the perinatal period (P96.81)
newborn affected by noxious substances transmitted via placenta or breast milk (P04.-)
occupational exposure to risk factors (Z57.-)
retained FB (Z18.-)
retained FB fully removed (Z87.821)
toxic effects of substances chiefly nonmedicinal as to source (T51–T65)

Z77.0 **Contact with and (suspected) exposure to hazardous, chiefly**
[5th] **nonmedicinal, chemicals**
Z77.01 **Contact with and (suspected) exposure to;**
[6th] **hazardous metals**
Z77.010 **arsenic**
Z77.011 **lead**
Z77.012 **uranium**
Excludes1: retained depleted uranium fragments (Z18.01)
Z77.018 **other hazardous metals**
Contact with and (suspected) exposure to chromium compounds or nickel dust
Z77.02 **Contact with and (suspected) exposure to;**
[6th] **hazardous aromatic compounds**
Z77.020 **amines**
Z77.021 **benzene**
Z77.028 **other hazardous aromatic compounds**
Aromatic dyes NOS
Polycyclic aromatic hydrocarbons
Z77.09 **Contact with and (suspected) exposure to; other**
[6th] **hazardous, chiefly nonmedicinal, chemicals**
Z77.090 **asbestos**
Z77.098 **other hazardous, chiefly nonmedicinal, chemicals**
Dyes NOS
Z77.1 **Contact with and (suspected) exposure to; environmental**
[5th] **pollution and hazards in the physical environment**
Z77.12 **hazards in the physical environment**
[6th] **Z77.120** **mold (toxic)**
Z77.128 **other hazards in the physical environment**
Z77.2 **other hazardous substances**
[5th] **Z77.21** **potentially hazardous body fluids**
Z77.22 **environmental tobacco smoke (acute) (chronic)**
Exposure to second hand tobacco smoke (acute) (chronic)
Passive smoking (acute) (chronic)
Excludes1: nicotine dependence (F17.-)
tobacco use (Z72.0)
Excludes2: occupational exposure to environmental tobacco smoke (Z57.31)
Z77.29 **other hazardous substances**
Z77.9 **Other contact with and (suspected) exposures hazardous to health**

Z78 **[4th]** **OTHER SPECIFIED HEALTH STATUS**
This is a status category, refer to Chapter 21 for status guidelines.
Excludes2: asymptomatic HIV infection status (Z21)
postprocedural status (Z93–Z99)
sex reassignment status (Z87.890)

CHAPTER 21. FACTORS INFLUENCING HEALTH STATUS AND CONTACT WITH HEALTH SERVICES (Z73.811–Z78)

[4th] **[5th]** **[6th]** **[7th]** Additional Character Required	✔	3-character code	Unspecified laterality codes were excluded here.	• =New Code ▲ =Revised Code ▫ =Social determinants of health	*Excludes1*—Not coded here, do not use together *Excludes2*—Not included here

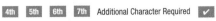

Z78.1   Physical restraint status
May be used when it is documented by the provider that a patient has been put in restraints during the current encounter. Please note that this code should not be reported when it is documented by the provider that a patient is temporarily restrained during a procedure.

Z78.9   Other specified health status

Z79   LONG TERM (CURRENT) DRUG THERAPY
`4th`

GUIDELINES

Codes from this category indicate a patient's continuous use of a prescribed drug (including such things as aspirin therapy) for the long-term treatment of a condition or for prophylactic use. It is not for use for patients who have addictions to drugs. This subcategory is not for use of medications for detoxification or maintenance programs to prevent withdrawal symptoms in patients with drug dependence (eg, methadone maintenance for opiate dependence). Assign the appropriate code for the drug dependence instead.

Assign a code from Z79 if the patient is receiving a medication for an extended period as a prophylactic measure (such as for the prevention of deep vein thrombosis) or as treatment of a chronic condition (such as arthritis) or a disease requiring a lengthy course of treatment (such as cancer). Do not assign a code from category Z79 for medication being administered for a brief period of time to treat an acute illness or injury (such as a course of antibiotics to treat acute bronchitis). This is a status category, refer to Chapter 21 for status guidelines.

Includes: long term (current) drug use for prophylactic purposes
Code also any therapeutic drug level monitoring (Z51.81)
Excludes2: drug abuse and dependence (F11–F19)
drug use complicating pregnancy, childbirth, and the puerperium (O99.32-)

Z79.1   Long term (current) use of; non-steroidal anti-inflammatories (NSAID)
Excludes2: long term (current) use of aspirin (Z79.82)

Z79.2   antibiotics

Z79.4   insulin
Excludes1: long term (current) use of oral antidiabetic drugs (Z79.84)
long term (current) use of oral hypoglycemic drugs (Z79.84)

Z79.5   steroids
`5th`
Z79.51   inhaled steroids
Z79.52   systemic steroids

Z79.8   Other long term (current) drug therapy
`5th`
Z79.82   Long term (current) use of aspirin
Z79.84   Long term (current) use of oral hypoglycemic drugs
Long term use of oral antidiabetic drugs
Excludes2: long term (current) use of insulin (Z79.4)
Z79.89   Other long term (current) drug therapy
`6th`   **Z79.899   Other long term (current) drug therapy**

Z80   FAMILY HISTORY OF PRIMARY MALIGNANT NEOPLASM
`4th`

GUIDELINES

Family history codes are for use when a patient has a family member(s) who has had a particular disease that causes the patient to be at higher risk of also contracting the disease. Family history codes may be used in conjunction with screening codes to explain the need for a test or procedure. History codes are also acceptable on any medical record regardless of the reason for visit. A history of an illness, even if no longer present, is important information that may alter the type of treatment ordered.

Z80.0   Family history of malignant neoplasm of digestive organs
Conditions classifiable to C15-C26

Z80.1   Family history of malignant neoplasm of trachea, bronchus and lung
Conditions classifiable to C33-C34

Z80.2   Family history of malignant neoplasm of other respiratory and intrathoracic organs
Conditions classifiable to C30-C32, C37-C39

Z80.3   Family history of malignant neoplasm of breast
Conditions classifiable to C50.-

Z80.4   Family history of malignant neoplasm of genital organs
`5th`   Conditions classifiable to C51-C63
Z80.41   Family history of malignant neoplasm of ovary
Z80.42   Family history of malignant neoplasm of prostate

Z80.43   Family history of malignant neoplasm of testis
Z80.49   Family history of malignant neoplasm of other genital organs

Z80.5   Family history of malignant neoplasm of urinary tract
`5th`   Conditions classifiable to C64–C68
Z80.51   Family history of malignant neoplasm of kidney
Z80.52   Family history of malignant neoplasm of bladder
Z80.59   Family history of malignant neoplasm of other urinary tract organ

Z80.6   Family history of leukemia
Conditions classifiable to C91–C95

Z80.7   Family history of other malignant neoplasms of lymphoid, hematopoietic and related tissues
Conditions classifiable to C81–C90, C96.-

Z80.8   Family history of malignant neoplasm of other organs or systems
Conditions classifiable to C00–C14, C40–C49, C69–C79

Z80.9   Family history of malignant neoplasm, unspecified
Conditions classifiable to C80.1

Z81   FAMILY HISTORY OF MENTAL AND BEHAVIORAL DISORDERS
`4th`

GUIDELINES

Family history codes are for use when a patient has a family member(s) who has had a particular disease that causes the patient to be at higher risk of also contracting the disease. family history codes may be used in conjunction with screening codes to explain the need for a test or procedure. History codes are also acceptable on any medical record regardless of the reason for visit. A history of an illness, even if no longer present, is important information that may alter the type of treatment ordered.

Z81.0   Family history of intellectual disabilities
Conditions classifiable to F70–F79

▫Z81.1   Family history of alcohol abuse and dependence
Conditions classifiable to F10.

Z81.2   Family history of tobacco abuse and dependence
Conditions classifiable to F17.-

Z81.3   Family history of other psychoactive substance abuse and dependence
Conditions classifiable to F11-F16, F18-F19

▫Z81.4   Family history of other substance abuse and dependence
Conditions classifiable to F55

Z81.8   Family history of other mental and behavioral disorders
Conditions classifiable elsewhere in F01–F99

Z82   FAMILY HISTORY OF CERTAIN DISABILITIES AND CHRONIC DISEASES (LEADING TO DISABLEMENT)
`4th`

GUIDELINES

Family history codes are for use when a patient has a family member(s) who has had a particular disease that causes the patient to be at higher risk of also contracting the disease. Family history codes may be used in conjunction with screening codes to explain the need for a test or procedure. History codes are also acceptable on any medical record regardless of the reason for visit. A history of an illness, even if no longer present, is important information that may alter the type of treatment ordered.

Z82.0   Family history of; epilepsy and other diseases of the nervous system
Conditions classifiable to G00–G99

Z82.1   blindness and visual loss
Conditions classifiable to H54.-

Z82.2   deafness and hearing loss
Conditions classifiable to H90–H91

Z82.3   Family history of stroke
Conditions classifiable to I60–I64

Z82.4   Family history of; ischemic heart disease and other diseases of the circulatory system
`5th`   Conditions classifiable to I00–I52, I65–I99
Z82.41   sudden cardiac death
Z82.49   ischemic heart disease and other diseases of the circulatory system

`4th` `5th` `6th` `7th`   Additional Character Required   ✔ 3-character code   Unspecified laterality codes were excluded here.   • =New Code   ▲ =Revised Code   ▫ =Social determinants of health   *Excludes1*—Not coded here, do not use together   *Excludes2*—Not included here

454   PEDIATRIC ICD-10-CM 2021: A MANUAL FOR PROVIDER-BASED CODING

Z82.5 **Family history of asthma and other chronic lower respiratory diseases**
Conditions classifiable to J40–J47
Excludes2: family history of other diseases of the respiratory system (Z83.6)

Z82.6 `5th` **Family history of; arthritis and other diseases of the musculoskeletal system and connective tissue**
Conditions classifiable to M00–M99

    Z82.61 **arthritis**
    Z82.62 **osteoporosis**
    Z82.69 **other diseases of the musculoskeletal system and connective tissue**

Z82.7 `5th` **Family history of; congenital malformations, deformations and chromosomal abnormalities**
Conditions classifiable to Q00–Q99

    Z82.71 **polycystic kidney**
    Z82.79 **other congenital malformations, deformations and chromosomal abnormalities**

Z82.8 **Family history of other disabilities and chronic diseases leading to disablement, NEC**

Z83 `4th` **FAMILY HISTORY OF OTHER SPECIFIC DISORDERS**

> **GUIDELINES**
>
> Family history codes are for use when a patient has a family member(s) who has had a particular disease that causes the patient to be at higher risk of also contracting the disease. family history codes may be used in conjunction with screening codes to explain the need for a test or procedure. History codes are also acceptable on any medical record regardless of the reason for visit. A history of an illness, even if no longer present, is important information that may alter the type of treatment ordered.
>
> *Excludes2:* contact with and (suspected) exposure to communicable disease in the family (Z20.-)

Z83.0 **Family history of human immunodeficiency virus [HIV] disease**
Conditions classifiable to B20

Z83.1 **Family history of other infectious and parasitic diseases**
Conditions classifiable to A00–B19, B25–B94, B99

Z83.2 **Family history of; diseases of the blood and blood-forming organs and certain disorders involving the immune mechanism**
Conditions classifiable to D50–D89

Z83.3 **DM**
Conditions classifiable to E08–E13

Z83.4 `5th` **other endocrine, nutritional and metabolic diseases**
Conditions classifiable to E00–E07, E15–E88

    Z83.41 **multiple endocrine neoplasia syndrome**
    Z83.42 **familial hypercholesterolemia**
    Z83.43 `6th` **disorders of lipoprotein metabolism and other lipidemia**

        Z83.430 **elevated lipoprotein(a)**
        Family history of elevated Lp(a)
        Z83.438 **other disorder of lipoprotein metabolism and other lipidemia**
        Family history of familial combined hyperlipidemia

    Z83.49 **other endocrine, nutritional and metabolic diseases**

Z83.5 `5th` **Family history of eye and ear disorders**

    Z83.51 `6th` **Family history of eye disorders**
    Conditions classifiable to H00–H53, H55–H59
    Excludes2: family history of blindness and visual loss (Z82.1)

        Z83.511 **Family history of glaucoma**
        Z83.518 **Family history of other specified eye disorder**

    Z83.52 **Family history of ear disorders**
    Conditions classifiable to H60–H83, H92–H95
    Excludes2: family history of deafness and hearing loss (Z82.2)

Z83.6 **other diseases of the respiratory system**
Conditions classifiable to J00–J39, J60–J99
Excludes2: family history of asthma and other chronic lower respiratory diseases (Z82.5)

Z83.7 `5th` **diseases of the digestive system**
Conditions classifiable to K00–K93

    Z83.71 **colonic polyps**
    Excludes2: family history of malignant neoplasm of digestive organs (Z80.0)
    Z83.79 **other diseases of the digestive system**

Z84 `4th` **FAMILY HISTORY OF OTHER CONDITIONS**

> **GUIDELINES**
>
> Family history codes are for use when a patient has a family member(s) who has had a particular disease that causes the patient to be at higher risk of also contracting the disease. Family history codes may be used in conjunction with screening codes to explain the need for a test or procedure. History codes are also acceptable on any medical record regardless of the reason for visit. A history of an illness, even if no longer present, is important information that may alter the type of treatment ordered.

Z84.0 **Family history of diseases of the skin and subcutaneous tissue**
Conditions classifiable to L00–L99

Z84.1 **Family history of disorders of kidney and ureter**
Conditions classifiable to N00–N29

Z84.2 **Family history of other diseases of the genitourinary system**
Conditions classifiable to N30–N99

Z84.3 **Family history of consanguinity**

Z84.8 **Family history of other specified conditions**
    `5th` **Z84.81** **Family history of carrier of genetic disease**
    Z84.82 **Family history of sudden infant death syndrome**
    Z84.89 **Family history of other specified conditions**

Z85 `4th` **PERSONAL HISTORY OF MALIGNANT NEOPLASM**

> **GUIDELINES**
>
> Personal history codes explain a patient's past medical condition that no longer exists and is not receiving any treatment, but that has the potential for recurrence, and therefore may require continued monitoring. These codes may be used in conjunction with follow-up codes to explain the need for a test or procedure. History codes are also acceptable on any medical record regardless of the reason for visit. A history of an illness, even if no longer present, is important information that may alter the type of treatment ordered.
>
> **Code first** any follow-up examination after treatment of malignant neoplasm (Z08)
> **Use additional code** to identify: alcohol use and dependence (F10.-)
> exposure to environmental tobacco smoke (Z77.22)
> history of tobacco dependence (Z87.891)
> occupational exposure to environmental tobacco smoke (Z57.31)
> tobacco dependence (F17.-)
> tobacco use (Z72.0)
> *Excludes2:* personal history of benign neoplasm (Z86.01-)
> personal history of carcinoma-in-situ (Z86.00-)

Z85.5 `5th` **Personal history of malignant neoplasm of urinary tract**
Conditions classifiable to C64–C68

    Z85.50 **Personal history of malignant neoplasm of; unspecified urinary tract organ**
    Z85.51 **bladder**
    Z85.52 `6th` **kidney**
    Excludes1: personal history of malignant neoplasm of renal pelvis (Z85.53)

        Z85.520 **Personal history of; malignant carcinoid tumor of kidney**
        Conditions classifiable to C7A.093
        Z85.528 **other malignant neoplasm of kidney**
        Conditions classifiable to C64

Z85.6 **Leukemia**
Conditions classifiable to C91–C95
Excludes1: leukemia in remission C91.0–C95.9 with 5th character 1

Z85.7 `5th` **Personal history of other malignant neoplasms of lymphoid, hematopoietic and related tissues**

    Z85.71 **Personal history of; Hodgkin lymphoma**
    Conditions classifiable to C81
    Z85.72 **non-Hodgkin lymphomas**
    Conditions classifiable to C82–C85

`4th` `5th` `6th` `7th` Additional Character Required ✓ 3-character code   Unspecified laterality codes were excluded here.

• =New Code
▲ =Revised Code
▫ =Social determinants of health

Excludes1—Not coded here, do not use together
Excludes2—Not included here

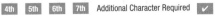

Z85.79 other malignant neoplasms of lymphoid, hematopoietic and related tissues
Conditions classifiable to C88–C90, C96
Excludes1: multiple myeloma in remission (C90.01)
plasma cell leukemia in remission (C90.11)
plasmacytoma in remission (C90.21)

Z85.8 **Malignant neoplasms of other organs and systems**
5th Conditions classifiable to C00–C14, C40–C49, C69–C79, C7A.098

Z85.82 **Personal history of malignant neoplasm of skin**
6th **Z85.820** **Personal history of malignant melanoma of skin**
Conditions classifiable to C43

Z85.83 **Personal history of malignant neoplasm of; bone and soft tissue**
6th Conditions classifiable to C40–C41; C45–C49
Z85.830 **bone**
Z85.831 **soft tissue**
Excludes2: personal history of malignant neoplasm of skin (Z85.82-)

Z85.84 **Personal history of; malignant neoplasm of eye and nervous tissue**
6th Conditions classifiable to C69–C72
Z85.840 **eye**
Z85.841 **brain**
Z85.848 **other parts of nervous tissue**

Z85.85 **Personal history of; malignant neoplasm of endocrine glands**
6th Conditions classifiable to C73–C75
Z85.850 **thyroid**
Z85.858 **other endocrine glands**

Z85.89 **other organs and systems**
Conditions classifiable to C7A.098, C76, C77–C79

Z85.9 **Personal history of malignant neoplasm, unspecified**
Conditions classifiable to C7A.00, C80.1

Z86 **PERSONAL HISTORY OF CERTAIN OTHER DISEASES**
4th

GUIDELINES

Personal history codes explain a patient's past medical condition that no longer exists and is not receiving any treatment, but that has the potential for recurrence, and therefore may require continued monitoring. These codes may be used in conjunction with follow-up codes to explain the need for a test or procedure. History codes are also acceptable on any medical record regardless of the reason for visit. A history of an illness, even if no longer present, is important information that may alter the type of treatment ordered.
Code first any follow-up examination after treatment (Z09)

Z86.0 **Personal history of in-situ and benign neoplasms and neoplasms of uncertain behavior**
5th *Excludes2:* personal history of malignant neoplasms (Z85.-)

Z86.00 **Personal history of in-situ neoplasm**
6th Conditions classifiable to D00–D09
Z86.000 **Personal history of in-situ neoplasm of breast**
Conditions classifiable to D05
Z86.001 **Personal history of in-situ neoplasm of cervix uteri**
Conditions classifiable to D06
Personal history of cervical intraepithelial neoplasia III [CIN III]
Z86.002 **Personal history of in-situ neoplasm of other and unspecified genital organs**
Conditions classifiable to D07
Personal history of high-grade prostatic intraepithelial neoplasia III [HGPIN III]
Personal history of vaginal intraepithelial neoplasia III [VAIN III]
Personal history of vulvar intraepithelial neoplasia III [VIN III]
Z86.003 **Personal history of in-situ neoplasm of oral cavity, esophagus and stomach**
Conditions classifiable to D00

Z86.004 **Personal history of in-situ neoplasm of other and unspecified digestive organs**
Conditions classifiable to D01
Personal history of anal intraepithelial neoplasia (AIN III)
Z86.005 **Personal history of in-situ neoplasm of middle ear and respiratory system**
Conditions classifiable to D02
Z86.006 **Personal history of melanoma in-situ**
Conditions classifiable to D03
Excludes2: sites other than skin—code to personal history of in-situ neoplasm of the site
Z86.007 **Personal history of in-situ neoplasm of skin**
Conditions classifiable to D04
Personal history of carcinoma in situ of skin
Z86.008 **Personal history of in-situ neoplasm of other site**
Conditions classifiable to D09

Z86.03 **Personal history of neoplasm of uncertain behavior**

Z86.1 **Personal history of infectious and parasitic diseases**
5th Conditions classifiable to A00–B89, B99
Excludes1: personal history of infectious diseases specific to a body system
sequelae of infectious and parasitic diseases (B90–B94)
Z86.11 **Personal history of; tuberculosis**
Z86.13 **malaria**
Z86.14 **MRSA infection**
Personal history of MRSA infection
Z86.15 **latent tuberculosis infection**
Z86.19 **other infectious and parasitic diseases**

Z86.2 **Personal history of diseases of the blood and blood-forming organs and certain disorders involving the immune mechanism**
Conditions classifiable to D50–D89

Z86.3 **Personal history of endocrine, nutritional and metabolic diseases**
5th Conditions classifiable to E00–E88
Z86.39 **other endocrine, nutritional and metabolic disease**

Z86.5 **Personal history of; mental and behavioral disorders**
5th Conditions classifiable to F40–F59
Z86.59 **other mental and behavioral disorders**
Code is a nonspecific Z code, refer to Chapter 21 for guidelines.

Z86.6 **Personal history of; diseases of the nervous system and sense organs**
5th Conditions classifiable to G00–G99, H00–H95
Z86.61 **infections of the central nervous system**
Personal history of encephalitis
Personal history of meningitis
Z86.69 **other diseases of the nervous system and sense organs**

Z86.7 **Personal history of; diseases of the circulatory system**
5th Conditions classifiable to I00–I99
Z86.73 **TIA and cerebral infarction without residual deficits**
Personal history of prolonged reversible ischemic neurological deficit (PRIND)
Personal history of stroke NOS without residual deficits
Excludes1: personal history of traumatic brain injury (Z87.820)
sequelae of cerebrovascular disease (I69.-)
Z86.74 **sudden cardiac arrest**
Personal history of sudden cardiac death successfully resuscitated
Z86.79 **other diseases of the circulatory system**

Z87 **PERSONAL HISTORY OF OTHER DISEASES AND CONDITIONS**
4th

GUIDELINES

Personal history codes explain a patient's past medical condition that no longer exists and is not receiving any treatment, but that has the potential

Unspecified laterality codes were excluded here.

• =New Code
▲ =Revised Code
▫ =Social determinants of health

Excludes1—Not coded here, do not use together
Excludes2—Not included here

for recurrence, and therefore may require continued monitoring. These codes may be used in conjunction with follow-up codes to explain the need for a test or procedure. History codes are also acceptable on any medical record regardless of the reason for visit. A history of an illness, even if no longer present, is important information that may alter the type of treatment ordered.

Code first any follow-up examination after treatment (Z09)

Z87.0 **Personal history of; diseases of the respiratory system**
> 5th   Conditions classifiable to J00–J99
>> **Z87.01**   **pneumonia (recurrent)**
>> **Z87.09**   **other diseases of the respiratory system**

Z87.3 **Personal history of diseases of the musculoskeletal system and connective tissue**
> 5th   Conditions classifiable to M00–M99
> *Excludes2:* personal history of (healed) traumatic fracture (Z87.81)
>> **Z87.39**   **other diseases of the musculoskeletal system and connective tissue**

Z87.4 **Personal history of; diseases of genitourinary system**
> 5th   Conditions classifiable to N00–N99
>> **Z87.44**   **diseases of urinary system**
>>> 6th   *Excludes1:* personal history of malignant neoplasm of cervix uteri (Z85.41)
>>> **Z87.440**   **urinary (tract) infections**
>>> **Z87.441**   **nephrotic syndrome**
>>> **Z87.442**   **urinary calculi**
>>>> Personal history of kidney stones
>>> **Z87.448**   **other diseases of urinary system**

Z87.7 **Personal history of (corrected) congenital malformations**
> 5th   Conditions classifiable to Q00–Q89 that have been repaired or corrected
> *Excludes1:* congenital malformations that have been partially corrected or repair but which still require medical treatment—**code to condition**
> *Excludes2:* other postprocedural states (Z98.-)
>> personal history of medical treatment (Z92.-)
>> presence of cardiac and vascular implants and grafts (Z95.-)
>> presence of other devices (Z97.-)
>> presence of other functional implants (Z96.-)
>> transplanted organ and tissue status (Z94.-)
>> **Z87.71**   **Personal history of; (corrected) congenital malformations of genitourinary system**
>>> 6th
>>> **Z87.710**   **(corrected) hypospadias**
>>> **Z87.718**   **other specified (corrected) congenital malformations of genitourinary system**
>> **Z87.72**   **Personal history of; (corrected) congenital malformations of nervous system and sense organs**
>>> 6th
>>> **Z87.720**   **(corrected) congenital malformations of eye**
>>> **Z87.721**   **(corrected) congenital malformations of ear**
>>> **Z87.728**   **other specified (corrected) congenital malformations of nervous system and sense organs**
>> **Z87.73**   **Personal history of; (corrected) congenital malformations of digestive system**
>>> 6th
>>> **Z87.730**   **(corrected) cleft lip and palate**
>>> **Z87.738**   **other specified (corrected) congenital malformations of digestive system**
>> **Z87.74**   **Personal history of; (corrected) congenital malformations of heart and circulatory system**
>> **Z87.75**   **(corrected) congenital malformations of respiratory system**
>> **Z87.76**   **(corrected) congenital malformations of integument, limbs and musculoskeletal system**
>> **Z87.79**   **other (corrected) congenital malformations**
>>> 6th   **Z87.790**   **(corrected) congenital malformations of face and neck**
>>> **Z87.798**   **other (corrected) congenital malformations**

Z87.8 **Personal history of; other specified conditions**
> 5th   **Z87.82**   **other (healed) physical injury and trauma**
>> 6th   Conditions classifiable to S00–T88, except traumatic fractures

>> **Z87.820**   **traumatic brain injury**
>>> *Excludes1:* personal history of TIA, and cerebral infarction without residual deficits (Z86.73)
>> **Z87.821**   **retained FB fully removed**
>> **Z87.828**   **other (healed) physical injury and trauma**
> **Z87.89**   **Personal history of; other specified conditions**
>> 6th   **Z87.891**   **nicotine dependence**
>>> *Excludes1:* current nicotine dependence (F17.2-)
>> **Z87.892**   **anaphylaxis**
>>> **Code also** allergy status such as:
>>> allergy status to drugs, medicaments and biological substances (Z88.-)
>>> allergy status, other than to drugs and biological substances (Z91.0-)
>> **Z87.898**   **other specified conditions**

Z88 **ALLERGY STATUS TO DRUGS, MEDICAMENTS AND BIOLOGICAL SUBSTANCES**
> 4th   This is a status category (excluding Z88.9), refer to Chapter 21 for status guidelines.
> *Excludes2:* Allergy status, other than to drugs and biological substances (Z91.0-)

Z88.0   **Allergy status to; penicillin**
Z88.1   **other antibiotic agents**
Z88.2   **sulfonamides status**
Z88.3   **other anti-infective agents**
Z88.4   **anesthetic agent**
Z88.5   **narcotic agent**
Z88.6   **analgesic agent**
Z88.7   **serum and vaccine**
Z88.8   **other drugs, medicaments and biological substances**
Z88.9   **unspecified drugs, medicaments and biological substances**
> Code is a nonspecific Z code, refer to Chapter 21 for guidelines.

Z90 **ACQUIRED ABSENCE OF ORGANS, NEC**
> 4th   This is a status category, refer to Chapter 21 for status guidelines.
> *Includes:* postprocedural or post-traumatic loss of body part NEC
> *Excludes1:* congenital absence—see Alphabetical Index
> *Excludes2:* postprocedural absence of endocrine glands (E89.-)
> **Note:** Use only if there are no complications or malfunctions of the organ or tissue replaced, the amputation site, or the equipment on which the patient is dependent.

Z90.4   **Acquired absence of; other specified parts of digestive tract**
> 5th   **Z90.49**   **other specified parts of digestive tract**
Z90.5   **Acquired absence of: kidney**
Z90.7   **genital organ(s)**
> 5th   *Excludes1:* personal history of sex reassignment (Z87.890)
> *Excludes2:* female genital mutilation status (N90.81-)
> **Z90.79**   **other genital organ(s)**
Z90.8   **Acquired absence of; other organs**
> 5th   **Z90.81**   **spleen**
> **Z90.89**   **other organs**

Z91 **PERSONAL RISK FACTORS, NEC**
> 4th   *Excludes2:* contact with and (suspected) exposures hazardous to health (Z77.-)
> exposure to pollution and other problems related to physical environment (Z77.1-)
> personal history of physical injury and trauma (Z87.81, Z87.82-)
> occupational exposure to risk factors (Z57.-)

Z91.0   **Allergy status, other than to drugs and biological substances**
> 5th   *This is a status sub-category, refer to Chapter 21 for status guidelines.*
> *Excludes2:* Allergy status to drugs, medicaments, and biological substances (Z88.-)
> **Z91.01**   **Food allergy status**
>> 6th   *Excludes2:* food additives allergy status (Z91.02)
>> **Z91.010**   **Allergy to; peanuts**
>> **Z91.011**   **milk products**
>>> *Excludes1:* lactose intolerance (E73.-)
>> **Z91.012**   **eggs**
>> **Z91.013**   **seafood**
>>> Allergy to shellfish or octopus or squid ink

4th   5th   6th   7th   Additional Character Required   ✓   3-character code   Unspecified laterality codes were excluded here.

• =New Code
▲ =Revised Code
¤ =Social determinants of health

Excludes1—Not coded here, do not use together
Excludes2—Not included here

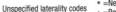

CHAPTER 21. FACTORS INFLUENCING HEALTH STATUS AND CONTACT WITH HEALTH SERVICES   (Z91.018–Z93.9)

         Z91.018   **other foods**
                    nuts other than peanuts
     Z91.02   **Food additives allergy status**
     Z91.03   **Insect allergy status**
       6th   **Z91.030**   **Bee allergy status**
              Z91.038   **Other insect allergy status**
     Z91.04   **Nonmedicinal substance allergy status**
       6th   **Z91.040**   **Latex allergy status**
                    Latex sensitivity status
              Z91.041   **Radiographic dye allergy status**
                    Allergy status to contrast media used for
                      diagnostic X-ray procedure
              Z91.048   **Other nonmedicinal substance allergy status**

Z91.1   **Patient's noncompliance with medical treatment and regimen**
   5th   **Z91.11**   **Patient's noncompliance with dietary regimen**
         Z91.12   **Patient's intentional underdosing of medication regimen**
       6th
           Code first underdosing of medication (T36–T50) with fifth or sixth character 6
           Excludes1: adverse effect of prescribed drug taken as directed–code to adverse effect poisoning (overdose)–code to poisoning
           Z91.120   **Patient's intentional underdosing of medication regimen due to financial hardship**
           Z91.128   **Patient's intentional underdosing of medication regimen for other reason**
         Z91.13   **Patient's unintentional underdosing of medication regimen**
       6th
           Code first underdosing of medication (T36–T50) with fifth or sixth character 6
           Excludes1: adverse effect of prescribed drug taken as directed—code to adverse effect poisoning (overdose)—code to poisoning
           Z91.138   **Patient's unintentional underdosing of medication regimen for other reason**
         Z91.14   **Patient's other noncompliance with medication regimen**
               Patient's underdosing of medication NOS
         Z91.15   **Patient's noncompliance with renal dialysis**
         Z91.19   **Patient's noncompliance with other medical treatment and regimen**
               Nonadherence to medical treatment

Z91.4   **Personal history of psychological trauma, NEC**

   5th

> **GUIDELINES**
>
> Personal history codes explain a patient's past medical condition that no longer exists and is not receiving any treatment, but that has the potential for recurrence, and therefore may require continued monitoring. These codes may be used in conjunction with follow-up codes to explain the need for a test or procedure. History codes are also acceptable on any medical record regardless of the reason for visit. A history of an illness, even if no longer present, is important information that may alter the type of treatment ordered.

         Z91.49   **Other personal history of psychological trauma, NEC**

Z91.5   **Personal history of self-harm**

> **GUIDELINES**
>
> Personal history codes explain a patient's past medical condition that no longer exists and is not receiving any treatment, but that has the potential for recurrence, and therefore may require continued monitoring. These codes may be used in conjunction with follow-up codes to explain the need for a test or procedure. History codes are also acceptable on any medical record regardless of the reason for visit. A history of an illness, even if no longer present, is important information that may alter the type of treatment ordered.

Personal history of parasuicide
Personal history of self-poisoning
Personal history of suicide attempt

Z91.8   **Other specified personal risk factors, NEC**

   5th

> **GUIDELINES**
>
> Personal history codes explain a patient's past medical condition that no longer exists and is not receiving any treatment, but that has the potential for recurrence, and therefore may require continued monitoring. These codes may be used in conjunction with follow-up codes to explain the need for a test or procedure. History codes are also acceptable on any medical record regardless of the reason for visit. A history of an illness, even if no longer present, is important information that may alter the type of treatment ordered. Excludes code Z91.83, Z91.84-.

         Z91.81   **History of falling**
              At risk for falling
         Z91.83   **Wandering in diseases classified elsewhere**
              Code first underlying disorder such as:
                Alzheimer's disease (G30.-)
                autism or pervasive developmental disorder (F84.-)
                intellectual disabilities (F70–F79)
                unspecified dementia with behavioral disturbance (F03.9-)
         Z91.84   **Oral health risk factors**
       6th   **Z91.841**   **Risk for dental caries, low**
              Z91.842   **Risk for dental caries, moderate**
              Z91.843   **Risk for dental caries, high**
              Z91.849   **Unspecified risk for dental caries**
         Z91.89   **Other specified personal risk factors, NEC**

Z92   **PERSONAL HISTORY OF MEDICAL TREATMENT**

   4th

> **GUIDELINES**
>
> Personal history codes explain a patient's past medical condition that no longer exists and is not receiving any treatment, but that has the potential for recurrence, and therefore may require continued monitoring. These codes may be used in conjunction with follow-up codes to explain the need for a test or procedure. History codes are also acceptable on any medical record regardless of the reason for visit. A history of an illness, even if no longer present, is important information that may alter the type of treatment ordered. Excludes codes Z92.0 and Z92.82.

Excludes2: postprocedural states (Z98.-)

Z92.2   **Personal history of; drug therapy**
   5th   ***Excludes2:*** long term (current) drug therapy (Z79.-)
         Z92.21   **antineoplastic chemotherapy**
         Z92.22   **monoclonal drug therapy**
         Z92.24   **steroid therapy**
       6th   **Z92.240**   **inhaled steroid therapy**
              Z92.241   **systemic steroid therapy**
                steroid therapy NOS
         Z92.25   **immunosuppression therapy**
              Excludes2: personal history of steroid therapy (Z92.24)
         Z92.29   **other drug therapy**
Z92.8   **Personal history of; other medical treatment**
   5th   **Z92.81**   **extracorporeal membrane oxygenation (ECMO)**

Z93   **ARTIFICIAL OPENING STATUS**

   4th   Note: Use only if there are no complications or malfunctions of the organ or tissue replaced, the amputation site, or the equipment on which the patient is dependent. This is a status category, refer to Chapter 21 for status guidelines.

Excludes1: artificial openings requiring attention or management (Z43.-)
              complications of external stoma (J95.0-, K94.-, N99.5-)

Z93.0   **Tracheostomy status**
Z93.1   **Gastrostomy status**
Z93.2   **Ileostomy status**
Z93.3   **Colostomy status**
Z93.4   **Other artificial openings of gastrointestinal tract status**
Z93.5   **Cystostomy status**
   5th   **Z93.50**   **Unspecified cystostomy status**
         Z93.51   **Cutaneous-vesicostomy status**
         Z93.52   **Appendico-vesicostomy status**
         Z93.59   **Other cystostomy status**
Z93.8   **Other artificial opening status**
Z93.9   **Artificial opening status, unspecified**

4th   **5th**   **6th**   **7th**   Additional Character Required   ✓ | 3-character code | Unspecified laterality codes were excluded here. | • =New Code   ▲ =Revised Code   ▫ =Social determinants of health | ***Excludes1***—Not coded here, do not use together   ***Excludes2***—Not included here

 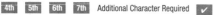

458   **PEDIATRIC ICD-10-CM 2021: A MANUAL FOR PROVIDER-BASED CODING**

Z94 **TRANSPLANTED ORGAN AND TISSUE STATUS**

`4th` Note: Use only if there are no complications or malfunctions of the organ or tissue replaced, the amputation site, or the equipment on which the patient is dependent. This is a status category, refer to Chapter 21 for status guidelines.

Includes: organ or tissue replaced by heterogenous or homogenous transplant

Excludes1: complications of transplanted organ or tissue—see Alphabetical Index

Excludes2: presence of vascular grafts (Z95.-)

Z94.0 **Kidney transplant status**

Z94.1 **Heart transplant status**

     Excludes1: artificial heart status (Z95.812)

         heart-valve replacement status (Z95.2–Z95.4)

Z94.2 **Lung transplant status**

Z94.3 **Heart and lungs transplant status**

Z94.4 **Liver transplant status**

Z94.5 **Skin transplant status**

     Autogenous skin transplant status

Z94.6 **Bone transplant status**

Z94.7 **Corneal transplant status**

Z94.8 **Other transplanted organ and tissue status**

     `5th` **Z94.81** **Bone marrow transplant status**

         Z94.82 **Intestine transplant status**

         Z94.83 **Pancreas transplant status**

         Z94.84 **Stem cells transplant status**

         Z94.89 **Other transplanted organ and tissue status**

Z94.9 **Transplanted organ and tissue status, unspecified**

Z95 **PRESENCE OF CARDIAC AND VASCULAR IMPLANTS AND GRAFTS**

`4th` This is a status category, refer to Chapter 21 for status guidelines.

Excludes2: complications of cardiac and vascular devices, implants and grafts (T82.-)

Z95.0 **Presence of cardiac pacemaker**

     Presence of cardiac resynchronization therapy (CRT-P) pacemaker

     Excludes1: adjustment or management of cardiac pacemaker (Z45.0-)

         presence of automatic (implantable) cardiac defibrillator with synchronous cardiac pacemaker (Z95.810)

Z95.2 **Presence of prosthetic heart valve**

     Presence of heart valve NOS

Z95.3 **Presence of xenogenic heart valve**

Z95.4 **Presence of other heart-valve replacement**

Z95.8 **Presence of other cardiac and vascular implants and grafts**

     `5th` **Z95.81** **Presence of other cardiac implants and grafts**

         `6th` **Z95.810** **Presence of automatic (implantable) cardiac defibrillator**

             Presence of automatic (implantable) cardiac defibrillator with synchronous cardiac pacemaker

             Presence of cardiac resynchronization therapy defibrillator (CRT-D)

             Presence of cardioverter-defibrillator (ICD)

         Z95.811 **Presence of heart assist device**

         Z95.812 **Presence of fully implantable artificial heart**

         Z95.818 **Presence of other cardiac implants and grafts**

Z96 **PRESENCE OF OTHER FUNCTIONAL IMPLANTS**

`4th` *Excludes2:* complications of internal prosthetic devices, implants and grafts (T82-T85)

     fitting and adjustment of prosthetic and other devices (Z44-Z46)

Z96.0 **Presence of urogenital implants**

Z96.1 **Presence of intraocular lens**

     Presence of pseudophakia

Z96.2 **Presence of otological and audiological implants**

     `5th` **Z96.21** **Cochlear implant status**

         Z96.22 **Myringotomy tube(s) status**

         Z96.29 **Presence of other otological and audiological implants**

             Presence of bone-conduction hearing device

             Presence of eustachian tube stent

             Stapes replacement

Z96.3 **Presence of artificial larynx**

Z96.4 **Presence of endocrine implants**

     `5th` **Z96.41** **Presence of insulin pump (external) (internal)**

         Z96.49 **Presence of other endocrine implants**

Z96.8 **Presence of other specified functional implants**

     `5th` **Z96.81** **Presence of artificial skin**

         Z96.82 **Presence of neurostimulator**

             Presence of brain neurostimulator

             Presence of gastric neurostimulator

             Presence of peripheral nerve neurostimulator

             Presence of sacral nerve neurostimulator

             Presence of spinal cord neurostimulator

             Presence of vagus nerve neurostimulator

         Z96.89 **Presence of other specified functional implants**

Z96.9 **Presence of functional implant, unspecified**

Z97 **PRESENCE OF OTHER DEVICES**

`4th` *Excludes1:* complications of internal prosthetic devices, implants and grafts (T82–T85)

Excludes 2: fitting and adjustment of prosthetic and other devices (Z44–Z46)

Z97.3 **Presence of spectacles and contact lenses**

Z97.4 **Presence of external hearing-aid**

Z97.5 **Presence of (intrauterine) contraceptive device**

     checking, reinsertion or removal of contraceptive device (Z30.43)

     Excludes1: checking, reinsertion or removal of implantable subdermal contraceptive (Z30.46)

         checking, reinsertion or removal of intrauterine contraceptive device (Z30.43-)

Z97.8 **Presence of other specified devices**

Z98 **OTHER POSTPROCEDURAL STATES**

`4th` This is a status category, refer to Chapter 21 for status guidelines.

Excludes2: aftercare (Z43–Z49, Z51)

     follow-up medical care (Z08–Z09)

     postprocedural complication—see Alphabetical Index

Z98.2 **Presence of cerebrospinal fluid drainage device**

     Presence of CSF shunt

Z98.8 **Other specified postprocedural states**

     `5th` **Z98.85** **Transplanted organ removal status**

         Assign code Z98.85, Transplanted organ removal status, to indicate that a transplanted organ has been previously removed. This code should not be assigned for the encounter in which the transplanted organ is removed. The complication necessitating removal of the transplant organ should be assigned for that encounter.

         See Chapter 19 for information on the coding of organ transplant complications.

         Transplanted organ previously removed due to complication, failure, rejection or infection

         Excludes1: encounter for removal of transplanted organ—code to complication of transplanted organ (T86.-)

     Z98.87 **Personal history of in utero procedure**

         `6th` **Z98.871** **Personal history of in utero procedure while a fetus**

     Z98.89 **Other specified postprocedural states**

         `6th` **Z98.890** **Other specified postprocedural states**

             Personal history of surgery, NEC

Z99 **DEPENDENCE ON ENABLING MACHINES AND DEVICES, NEC**

`4th` This is a status category, refer to Chapter 21 for status guidelines.

Z99.1 **Dependence on respirator**

     `5th` Dependence on ventilator

         Z99.11 **Dependence on respirator [ventilator] status**

             For encounters for weaning from a mechanical ventilator, assign a code from subcategory J96.1, Chronic respiratory failure, followed by code Z99.11, Dependence on respirator [ventilator] status.

CHAPTER 21. FACTORS INFLUENCING HEALTH STATUS AND CONTACT WITH HEALTH SERVICES   (Z94–Z99.11)

   `6th` `7th`   Additional Character Required   ✔  3-character code   Unspecified laterality codes were excluded here.

• =New Code
▲ =Revised Code
▯ =Social determinants of health

Excludes1—Not coded here, do not use together
Excludes2—Not included here

Z99.2 **Dependence on renal dialysis**
Hemodialysis status
Peritoneal dialysis status
Presence of arteriovenous shunt for dialysis
Renal dialysis status NOS
Excludes1: encounter for fitting and adjustment of dialysis catheter (Z49.0-)
Excludes2: noncompliance with renal dialysis (Z91.15)

Z99.3 **Dependence on wheelchair**
Wheelchair confinement status
Code first cause of dependence, such as:
    muscular dystrophy (G71.0-)
    obesity (E66.-)

Z99.8 **Dependence on other enabling machines and devices**

`5th` **Z99.81** **Dependence on supplemental oxygen**
Dependence on long-term oxygen

    Z99.89 **Dependence on other enabling machines and devices**
Dependence on machine or device NOS

(side text, left margin) CHAPTER 21. FACTORS INFLUENCING HEALTH STATUS AND CONTACT WITH HEALTH SERVICES   (Z99.2–Z99.89)

`4th` `5th` `6th` `7th` Additional Character Required   ✔ 3-character code   Unspecified laterality codes were excluded here.   • =New Code ▲ =Revised Code ◘ =Social determinants of health   ***Excludes1***—Not coded here, do not use together ***Excludes2***—Not included here

460   PEDIATRIC ICD-10-CM 2021: A MANUAL FOR PROVIDER-BASED CODING

Chapter 22. Codes for special purposes (U00–U85)

(U00–U49) PROVISIONAL ASSIGNMENT OF NEW DISEASES OF UNCERTAIN ETIOLOGY OR EMERGENCY USE

•U07 EMERGENCY USE OF U07

4th

GUIDELINES

For patients presenting with condition(s) related to vaping, assign code U07.0, Vaping-related disorder, as the principal diagnosis. For lung injury due to vaping, assign only code U07.0. Assign additional codes for other manifestations, such as acute respiratory failure (subcategory J96.0-) or pneumonitis (code J68.0). Associated respiratory signs and symptoms due to vaping, such as cough, shortness of breath, etc., are not coded separately, when a definitive diagnosis has been established. However, it would be appropriate to code separately any gastrointestinal symptoms, such as diarrhea and abdominal pain.

•U07.0 Vaping-related disorder
Dabbing related lung damage
Dabbing related lung injury
E-cigarette, or vaping, product use associated lung injury [EVALI]
Electronic cigarette related lung damage
Electronic cigarette related lung injury

Use additional code to identify manifestations, such as:
    abdominal pain (R10.84)
    acute respiratory distress syndrome (J80)
    diarrhea (R19.7)
    drug-induced interstitial lung disorder (J70.4)
    lipoid pneumonia (J69.1)
    weight loss (R63.4)

GUIDELINES

COVID-19 infection (infection due to SARS-CoV-2)

Code only confirmed cases

Code only a confirmed diagnosis of the 2019 novel coronavirus disease (COVID-19) as documented by the provider or documentation of a positive COVID-19 test result. For a confirmed diagnosis, assign code U07.1, COVID-19. This is an exception to the hospital inpatient guideline Section II, H. In this context, "confirmation" does not require documentation of a positive test result for COVID-19; the provider's documentation that the individual has COVID-19 is sufficient.

If the provider documents "suspected," "possible," "probable," or "inconclusive" COVID-19, do not assign code U07.1. Instead, code the signs and symptoms reported.

Sequencing of codes

When COVID-19 meets the definition of principal diagnosis, code U07.1, COVID-19, should be sequenced first, followed by the appropriate codes for associated manifestations, except when another guideline requires that certain codes be sequenced first, such as obstetrics, sepsis, or transplant complications.

For a COVID-19 infection that progresses to sepsis, see sepsis guidelines.

See Section I.C.16.h. for COVID-19 infection in newborn.
For a COVID-19 infection in a lung transplant patient, see Section I.C.19.g.3.a. Transplant complications other than kidney.

Acute respiratory manifestations of COVID-19

When the reason for the encounter/admission is a respiratory manifestation of COVID-19, assign code U07.1, COVID-19, as the principal/first-listed diagnosis and assign code(s) for the respiratory manifestation(s) as additional diagnoses.

The following conditions are examples of common respiratory manifestations of COVID-19.

PNEUMONIA
For a patient with pneumonia confirmed as due to COVID-19, assign codes U07.1, COVID-19, and J12.89, Other viral pneumonia.

ACUTE BRONCHITIS
For a patient with acute bronchitis confirmed as due to COVID-19, assign codes U07.1 and J20.8, Acute bronchitis due to other specified organisms. Bronchitis not otherwise specified (NOS) due to COVID-19 should be coded using code U07.1 and J40, Bronchitis, not specified as acute or chronic.

LOWER RESPIRATORY INFECTION
If the COVID-19 is documented as being associated with a lower respiratory infection, not otherwise specified (NOS), or an acute respiratory infection, NOS, codes U07.1 and J22, Unspecified acute lower respiratory infection, should be assigned. If the COVID-19 is documented as being associated with a respiratory infection, NOS, codes U07.1 and J98.8, Other specified respiratory disorders, should be assigned.

ACUTE RESPIRATORY DISTRESS SYNDROME
For acute respiratory distress syndrome (ARDS) due to COVID-19, assign codes U07.1, and J80, Acute respiratory distress syndrome.

ACUTE RESPIRATORY FAILURE
For acute respiratory failure due to COVID-19, assign code U07.1, and code J96.0-, Acute respiratory failure.

NON-RESPIRATORY MANIFESTATIONS OF COVID-19
When the reason for the encounter/admission is a non-respiratory manifestation (e.g., viral enteritis) of COVID-19, assign code U07.1, COVID-19, as the principal/first-listed diagnosis and assign code(s) for the manifestation(s) as additional diagnoses.

Exposure to COVID-19

For asymptomatic individuals with actual or suspected exposure to COVID-19, assign code Z20.828, Contact with and (suspected) exposure to other viral communicable diseases.

For symptomatic individuals with actual or suspected exposure to COVID-19 and the infection has been ruled out, or test results are inconclusive or unknown, assign code Z20.828, Contact with and (suspected) exposure to other viral communicable diseases. See Contact/Exposure guideline, for additional guidance regarding the use of category Z20 codes. If COVID-19 is confirmed see the COVID infection guideline.

Screening for COVID-19

During the COVID-19 pandemic, a screening code is generally not appropriate. For encounters for COVID-19 testing, including preoperative testing, code as exposure to COVID-19 (See Exposure guideline).

Coding guidance will be updated as new information concerning any changes in the pandemic status becomes available.

Signs and symptoms without definitive diagnosis of COVID-19

For patients presenting with any signs/symptoms associated with COVID-19 (such as fever, etc.) but a definitive diagnosis has not been established, assign the appropriate code(s) for each of the presenting signs and symptoms such as:
- R05 Cough
- R06.02 Shortness of breath
- R50.9 Fever, unspecified

If a patient with signs/symptoms associated with COVID-19 also has an actual or suspected contact with or exposure to COVID-19, assign Z20.828, Contact with and (suspected) exposure to other viral communicable diseases, as an additional code.

Asymptomatic individuals who test positive for COVID-19

For asymptomatic individuals who test positive for COVID-19, see code only confirmed cases guideline. Although the individual is

---

4th **5th** **6th** **7th** Additional Character Required   ✔ 3-character code

•=New Code
▲=Revised Code

Excludes1—Not coded here, do not use together
Excludes2—Not included here

asymptomatic, the individual has tested positive and is considered to have the COVID-19 infection.

Personal history of COVID-19

For patients with a history of COVID-19, assign code Z86.19, Personal history of other infectious and parasitic diseases.

Follow-up visits after COVID-19 infection has resolved

For individuals who previously had COVID-19 and are being seen for follow-up evaluation, and COVID-19 test results are negative, assign codes Z09, Encounter for follow-up examination after completed treatment for conditions other than malignant neoplasm, and Z86.19, Personal history of other infectious and parasitic diseases.

Encounter for antibody testing

For an encounter for antibody testing that is not being performed to confirm a current COVID-19 infection, nor is a follow-up test after resolution of COVID-19, assign Z01.84, Encounter for antibody response examination.

Follow the applicable guidelines above if the individual is being tested to confirm a current COVID-19 infection. For follow-up testing after a COVID-19 infection, see follow-up visits after COVID-19 infection has resolved guideline.

• **U07.1 COVID-19**
> **Use additional code** to identify pneumonia or other manifestations
> *Excludes1:* Coronavirus infection, unspecified (B34.2)
>> Coronavirus as the cause of diseases classified elsewhere (B97.2-)
>> Pneumonia due to SARS-associated coronavirus (J12.81)

CHAPTER 22. CODES FOR SPECIAL PURPOSES   (U07.1)

  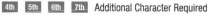 **4th** **5th** **6th** **7th** Additional Character Required   3-character code   •=New Code   *Excludes1*—Not coded here, do not use together
▲=Revised Code   *Excludes2*—Not included here

462   **PEDIATRIC ICD-10-CM 2021: A MANUAL FOR PROVIDER-BASED CODING**

ICD-10-CM EXTERNAL CAUSE
OF INJURIES TABLE

These tables are inserted for ease to locate an external cause code from a transport accident.
If not listed here, refer to the index. All codes require additional characters.
4th, 5th, 6th characters are "X" if not listed and all 7th characters (A, D, S) refer to encounter.

ICD-10-CM EXTERNAL CAUSE OF INJURIES TABLE

Collides with

	Pedestrian Conveyance	Car/Pick-up Truck/Van	Bike	Bus/HTV	Fixed Object	E-Scooter	Micro-Mobility	Train/Train Car	2 or 3 Motor Wheeler	Non-Motor Vehicle	Other (NOS)	Unspecified
Pedestrian on foot	V00.01 R V00.02 S V00.09 O	V03.00 N V03.10 T V03.90 U	V01.00 N V01.10 T V01.90 U	V04.00 N V04.10 T V04.90 U	Refer to W22	V00.031	V00.038	V05.00 N V05.10 T V05.90 U	V02.00 N V02.10 T V02.90 U	V06.00 N V06.10 T V06.90 U	V09.09 N V09.29 T	V09.00 N V09.20 T

Collides with

Activity of the Person Injured	Car/Pick-up Truck/Van	Bike	Bus/HTV	Fixed Object	Pedestrian or Animal	Train/Train Car	2 or 3 Motor Wheeler	Non-Motor Vehicle	Other (NOS)	Unspecified
In-line skater (I)/Roller skater (R)	V03.01 N V03.11 T V03.91 U	V01.01 N V01.11 T V01.91 U	V04.01 N V04.11 T V04.91 U	V00.112 I V00.122 R	V00.118 I V00.128 R	V05.01 N V05.11 T V05.91 U	V02.01 N V02.11 T V02.91 U	V06.01 N V06.11 T V06.91 U	V00.118 I V00.128 R	
Skateboarder	V03.02 N V03.12 T V03.92 U	V01.02 N V01.12 T V01.92 U	V04.02 N V04.12 T V04.92 U	V00.132	V00.138	V05.02 N V05.12 T V05.92 U	V02.02 N V02.12 T V02.92 U	V06.02 N V06.12 T V06.92 U	V00.138	
E-Scooter	V03.031 N V03.131 T V03.931 U	V01.031 N V01.131 T V01.931 U	V04.031 N V04.131 T V04.931 U	V00.842		V05.031 N V05.131 T V05.931 U	V02.031 N V02.131 T V02.931 U	V06.031 N V06.131 T V06.931 U		
Micro-mobility	V03.038 N V03.138 T V03.938 U	V01.038 N V01.138 T V01.938 U	V04.038 N V04.138 T V04.938 U			V05.038 N V05.138 T V05.938 U	V02.038 N V02.138 T V02.938 U	V06.038 N V06.138 T V06.938 U	V00.848	
Other (NOS)	V03.09 N V03.19 T V03.99 U	V01.09 N V01.19 T V01.99 U	V04.09 N V04.19 T V04.99 U			V05.09 N V05.19 T V05.99 U	V02.09 N V02.19 T V02.99 U	V06.09 N V06.19 T V06.99 U		
Scooter (Non-motorized)	V03.09 N V03.19 T V03.99 U	V01.09 N V01.19 T V01.99 U	V04.09 N V04.19 T V04.99 U	V00.142		V05.09 N V05.19 T V05.99 U	V02.09 N V02.19 T V02.99 U	V06.09 N V06.19 T V06.99 U		
Heelies	V03.09 N V03.19 T V03.99 U	V01.09 N V01.19 T V01.99 U	V04.09 N V04.19 T V04.99 U	V00.152		V05.09 N V05.19 T V05.99 U	V02.09 N V02.19 T V02.99 U	V06.09 N V06.19 T V06.99 U		
Ice-skater	V03.09 N V03.19 T V03.99 U	V01.09 N V01.19 T V01.99 U	V04.09 N V04.19 T V04.99 U	V00.212		V05.09 N V05.19 T V05.99 U	V02.09 N V02.19 T V02.99 U	V06.09 N V06.19 T V06.99 U		
Sledder	V03.09 N V03.19 T V03.99 U	V01.09 N V01.19 T V01.99 U	V04.09 N V04.19 T V04.99 U	V00.222		V05.09 N V05.19 T V05.99 U	V02.09 N V02.19 T V02.99 U	V06.09 N V06.19 T V06.99 U		
Snowboarder	V03.09 N V03.19 T V03.99 U	V01.09 N V01.19 T V01.99 U	V04.09 N V04.19 T V04.99 U	V00.312		V05.09 N V05.19 T V05.99 U	V02.09 N V02.19 T V02.99 U	V06.09 N V06.19 T V06.99 U		
Snowskier	V03.09 N V03.19 T V03.99 U	V01.09 N V01.19 T V01.99 U	V04.09 N V04.19 T V04.99 U	V00.322		V05.09 N V05.19 T V05.99 U	V02.09 N V02.19 T V02.99 U	V06.09 N V06.19 T V06.99 U		
Wheelchair	V03.09 N V03.19 T V03.99 U	V01.09 N V01.19 T V01.99 U	V04.09 N V04.19 T V04.99 U	V00.812		V05.09 N V05.19 T V05.99 U	V02.09 N V02.19 T V02.99 U	V06.09 N V06.19 T V06.99 U		

ªNon-motor vehicle includes streetcar, animal drawn vehicle, animal being ridden
I = In-line skates; R = roller skates; N = nontraffic accident; T = traffic accident; U = unspecified whether traffic or not
*Refer to the index

ICD-10-CM EXTERNAL CAUSE OF INJURIES TABLE

Collides with

Activity of the Person Injured	Car/Pick-up Truck/Van	Bike	Bus/HTV	Fixed Object	Pedestrian or Animal	Train/Train Car	2 or 3 Motor Wheeler	Non-Motor Vehicle	Other (NOS)	Unspecified
Bike										
Driver	V13.0 N / V13.4 T	V11.0 N / V11.4 T	V14.0 N / V14.4 T	V17.0 N / V17.4 T	V10.0 N / V10.4 T	V15.0 N / V15.4 T	V12.0 N / V12.4 T	V16.0 N / V16.4 T	V19.09 N / V19.49 T	V19.00 N / V19.40 T
Passenger	V13.1 N / V13.5 T	V11.1 N / V11.5 T	V14.1 N / V14.5 T	V17.1 N / V17.5 T	V10.1 N / V10.5 T	V15.1 N / V15.5 T	V12.1 N / V12.5 T	V16.1 N / V16.5 T	V19.19 N / V19.59 T	V19.10 N / V19.50 T
Boarding	V13.3	V11.3	V14.3	V17.3	V10.3	V15.3	V12.3	V16.3		
Unspecified	V13.2 N / V13.9 T	V11.2 N / V11.9 T	V14.2 N / V14.9 T	V17.2 N / V17.9 T	V10.2 N / V10.9 T	V15.2 N / V15.9 T	V12.2 N / V12.9 T	V16.2 N / V16.9 T	V19.29 N / V19.69 T	V19.20 N / V19.60 T
Motorcycle/Motor Scooter/ Moped										
Driver	V23.0 N / V23.4 T	V21.0 N / V21.4 T	V24.0 N / V24.4 T	V27.0 N / V27.4 T	V20.0 N / V20.4 T	V25.0 N / V25.4 T	V22.0 N / V22.4 T	V26.0 N / V26.4 T	V29.09 N / V29.49 T	V29.00 N / V29.40 T
Passenger	V23.1 N / V23.5 T	V21.1 N / V21.5 T	V24.1 N / V24.5 T	V27.1 N / V27.5 T	V20.1 N / V20.5 T	V25.1 N / V25.5 T	V22.1 N / V22.5 T	V26.1 N / V26.5 T	V29.19 N / V29.59 T	V29.10 N / V29.50 T
Boarding	V23.3	V21.3	V24.3	V27.3	V20.3	V25.3	V22.3	V26.3		
Unspecified	V23.2 N / V23.9 T	V21.2 N / V21.9 T	V24.2 N / V24.9 T	V27.2 N / V27.9 T	V20.2 N / V20.9 T	V25.2 N / V25.9 T	V22.2 N / V22.9 T	V26.2 N / V26.9 T	V29.29 N / V29.69 T	V29.20 N / V29.60 T
3-wheel vehicle										
Driver	V33.0 N / V33.5 T	V31.0 N / V31.5 T	V34.0 N / V34.5 T	V37.0 N / V37.5 T	V30.0 N / V30.5 T	V35.0 N / V35.5 T	V32.0 N / V32.5 T	V36.0 N / V36.5 T	V39.09 N / V39.49 T	V39.00 N / V39.40 T
Passenger	V33.1 N / V33.6 T	V31.1 N / V31.6 T	V34.1 N / V34.6 T	V37.1 N / V37.6 T	V30.1 N / V30.6 T	V35.1 N / V35.6 T	V32.1 N / V32.6 T	V36.1 N / V36.6 T	V39.19 N / V39.59 T	V39.10 N / V39.50 T
Rider on outside	V33.2 N / V33.7 T	V31.2 N / V31.7 T	V34.2 N / V34.7 T	V37.2 N / V37.7 T	V30.2 N / V30.7 T	V35.2 N / V35.7 T	V32.2 N / V32.7 T	V36.2 N / V36.7 T		
Boarding	V33.4	V31.4	V34.4	V37.4	V30.4	V35.4	V32.4	V36.4		
Unspecified	V33.3 N / V33.9 T	V31.3 N / V31.9 T	V34.3 N / V34.9 T	V37.3 N / V37.9 T	V30.3 N / V30.9 T	V35.3 N / V35.9 T	V32.3 N / V32.9 T	V36.3 N / V36.9 T	V39.29 N / V39.69 T	V39.20 N / V39.60 T
Car										
Driver	V43.0- N / V43.5- T	V41.0 N / V41.5 T	V44.0 N / V44.5 T	V47.0- N / V47.5- T	V40.0 N / V40.5 T	V45.0 N / V45.5 T	V42.0 N / V42.5 T		V49.09 N / V49.49 T	V49.00 N / V49.40 T
Passenger	V43.1- N / V43.6- T	V41.1 N / V41.6 T	V44.1 N / V44.6 T	V47.1- N / V47.6- T	V40.1 N / V40.6 T	V45.1 N / V45.6 T	V42.1 N / V42.6 T		V49.19 N / V49.59 T	V49.10 N / V49.50 T
Rider on outside	V43.2- N / V43.7- T	V41.2 N / V41.7 T	V44.2 N / V44.7 T	V47.2- N / V47.7- T	V40.2 N / V40.7 T	V45.2 N / V45.7 T	V42.2 N / V42.7 T		V59.3 N / V59.9 T	
Boarding	V43.4-	V41.4	V44.4	V47.4-	V40.4	V45.4	V42.4			
Unspecified	V43.3- N / V43.9- T	V41.3 N / V41.9 T	V44.3 N / V44.9 T	V47.3- N / V47.9- T	V40.3 N / V40.9 T	V45.3 N / V45.9 T	V42.3 N / V42.9 T		V49.29 N / V49.69 T	V49.20 N / V49.60 T
Pick-up Truck/Van/SUV										
Driver	V53.0 N / V53.5 T	V51.0 N / V51.5 T	V54.0 N / V54.5 T	V57.0 N / V57.5 T	V50.0 N / V50.5 T	V55.0 N / V55.5 T	V52.0 N / V52.5 T		V59.09 N / V59.49 T	V59.00 N / V59.40 T
Passenger	V53.1 N / V53.6 T	V51.1 N / V51.6 T	V54.1 N / V54.6 T	V57.1 N / V57.6 T	V50.1 N / V50.6 T	V55.1 N / V55.6 T	V52.1 N / V52.6 T		V59.19 N / V59.59 T	V59.10 N / V59.50 T

^aNon-motor vehicle includes streetcar, animal drawn vehicle, animal being ridden
I = In-line skates; R = roller skates; N = nontraffic accident; T = traffic accident; U = unspecified whether traffic or not
*Refer to the index

ICD-10-CM EXTERNAL CAUSE OF INJURIES TABLE

Activity of the Person Injured	Collides with									
	Car/Pick-up Truck/Van	Bike	Bus/HTV	Fixed Object	Pedestrian or Animal	Train/Train Car	2 or 3 Motor Wheeler	Non-Motor Vehicle	Other (NOS)	Unspecified
Rider on outside	V53.2 N / V53.7 T	V51.2 N / V51.7 T	V54.2 N / V54.7 T	V57.2 N / V57.7 T	V50.2 N / V50.7 T	V55.2 N / V55.7 T	V52.2 N / V52.7 T			
Boarding	V53.4	V51.4	V54.4	V57.4	V50.4	V55.4	V52.4			
Unspecified	V53.3 N / V53.9 T	V51.3 N / V51.9 T	V54.3 N / V54.9 T	V57.3 N / V57.9 T	V50.3 N / V50.9 T	V55.3 N / V55.9 T	V52.3 N / V52.9 T		V59.29 N / V59.69 T	V59.20 N / V59.60 T
Bus										
Driver	V73.0 N / V73.5 T	V71.0 N / V71.5 T	V74.0 N / V74.5 T	V77.0 N / V77.5 T	V70.0 N / V70.5 T	V75.0 N / V75.5 T	V72.0 N / V72.5 T	V76.0 N / V76.5 T	V79.09 N / V79.49 T	V79.00 N / V79.40 T
Passenger	V73.1 N / V73.6 T	V71.1 N / V71.6 T	V74.1 N / V74.6 T	V77.1 N / V77.6 T	V70.1 N / V70.6 T	V75.1 N / V75.6 T	V72.1 N / V72.6 T	V76.1 N / V76.6 T	V79.19 N / V79.59 T	V79.10 N / V79.50 T
Rider on outside	V73.2 N / V73.7 T	V71.2 N / V71.7 T	V74.2 N / V74.7 T	V77.2 N / V77.7 T	V70.2 N / V70.7 T	V75.2 N / V75.7 T	V72.2 N / V72.7 T	V76.2 N / V76.7 T		V79.3 N / V79.9 T
Boarding	V73.4	V71.4	V74.4	V77.4	V70.4	V75.4	V72.4	V76.4		
Unspecified	V73.3 N / V73.9 T	V71.3 N / V71.9 T	V74.3 N / V74.9 T	V77.3 N / V77.9 T	V70.3 N / V70.9 T	V75.3 N / V75.9 T	V72.3 N / V72.9 T	V76.3 N / V76.9 T	V79.29 N / V79.69 T	V79.20 N / V79.60 T
Animal Rider	V80.41	V80.21	V80.41	V80.81	*	V80.61	V80.31	V06.09	V80.918	V80.919
Animal-Drawn Vehicle	V80.42	V80.22	V80.42	V80.82	*	V80.62	V80.32	V06.09	V80.928	V80.929

Injured Person	Vehicle					
	Special Agriculture Vehicle	Snowmobile	Dune Buggy	3 or 4 Wheel ATV	Dirt Bike	Other ATV (eg, go-cart, golf cart)
Driver	V84.0 T / V84.5 N	V86.02 T / V86.52 N	V86.03 T / V86.53 N	V86.05 T / V86.55 N	V86.06 T / V86.56 N	V86.09 T / V86.59 N
Passenger	V84.1 T / V84.6 N	V86.12 T / V86.62 N	V86.13 T / V86.63 N	V86.15 T / V86.65 N	V86.16 T / V86.66 N	V86.19 T / V86.69 N
Outside rider	V84.2 T / V84.7 N	V86.22 T / V86.72 N	V86.23 T / V86.73 N	V86.25 T / V86.75 N	V86.26 T / V86.76 N	V86.29 T / V86.79 N
Unspecified	V84.3 T / V84.9 N	V86.32 T / V86.92 N	V86.33 T / V86.93 N	V86.35 T / V86.95 N	V86.36 T / V86.96 N	V86.39 T / V86.99 N
Boarding	V84.4	V86.42	V86.43	V86.45	V86.46	V86.49

ᵃNon-motor vehicle includes streetcar, animal drawn vehicle, animal being ridden
I = In-line skates; R = roller skates; N = nontraffic accident; T = traffic accident; U = unspecified whether traffic or not
*Refer to the index

ICD-10-CM EXTERNAL CAUSE
OF INJURIES INDEX

A

Refer to the External Cause of Injury Table first

Abandonment (causing exposure to weather conditions) (with intent to injure or kill) NEC X58

Abuse (adult) (child) (mental) (physical) (sexual) X58

Accident (to) X58

- aircraft (in transit) (powered)—*see also* Accident, transport, aircraft
  - due to, caused by cataclysm—*see* Forces of nature, by type
- animal-rider—*see* Accident, transport, animal-rider
- animal-drawn vehicle—*see* Accident, transport, animal-drawn vehicle occupant
- automobile—*see* Accident, transport, car occupant
- bare foot water skier V94.4
- boat, boating—*see also* Accident, watercraft
  - striking swimmer
    - powered V94.11
    - unpowered V94.12
- bus—*see* Accident, transport, bus occupant
- cable car, not on rails V98.0
  - on rails—*see* Accident, transport, streetcar occupant
- car—*see* Accident, transport, car occupant
- caused by, due to
  - animal NEC W64
  - chain hoist W24.0
  - cold (excessive)—*see* Exposure, cold
  - corrosive liquid, substance—*see* Table of Drugs and Chemicals
  - cutting or piercing instrument—*see* Contact, with, by type of instrument
  - drive belt W24.0
  - electric
    - current—*see* Exposure, electric current
    - motor (*see also* Contact, with, by type of machine) W31.3
      - current (of) W86.8
  - environmental factor NEC X58
  - explosive material—*see* Explosion
  - fire, flames—*see* Exposure, fire
  - firearm missile—*see* Discharge, firearm by type
  - heat (excessive)—*see* Heat
  - hot—*see* Contact, with, hot
  - ignition—*see* Ignition
  - lifting device W24.0
  - lightning—*see* subcategory T75.0
    - causing fire—*see* Exposure, fire
  - machine, machinery—*see* Contact, with, by type of machine
  - natural factor NEC X58
  - pulley (block) W24.0
  - radiation—*see* Radiation
  - steam X13.1
    - inhalation X13.0
    - pipe X16
  - thunderbolt—*see* subcategory T75.0
    - causing fire—*see* Exposure, fire
  - transmission device W24.1
- diving—*see also* Fall, into, water
  - with
    - drowning or submersion—*see* Drowning
- ice yacht V98.2
- in
  - medical, surgical procedure
    - as, or due to misadventure—*see* Misadventure
    - causing an abnormal reaction or later complication without mention of misadventure (*see also* Complication of or following, by type of procedure) Y84.9
- land yacht V98.1
- late effect of—*see* W00-X58 with 7th character S
- logging car—*see* Accident, transport, industrial vehicle occupant
- machine, machinery—*see also* Contact, with, by type of machine
  - on board watercraft V93.69
    - explosion—*see* Explosion, in, watercraft
    - fire—*see* Burn, on board watercraft
    - powered craft V93.63
      - ferry boat V93.61
      - fishing boat V93.62

Accident (to), *continued*
- ~ jet skis V93.63
- ~ liner V93.61
- ~ merchant ship V93.60
- ~ passenger ship V93.61
- ~ sailboat V93.64
- mobility scooter (motorized)—*see* Accident, transport, pedestrian, conveyance, specified type NEC
- motor scooter—*see* Accident, transport, motorcyclist
- motor vehicle NOS (traffic) (*see also* Accident, transport) V89.2
  - nontraffic V89.0
  - three-wheeled NOS—*see* Accident, transport, three-wheeled motor vehicle occupant
- motorcycle NOS—*see* Accident, transport, motorcyclist
- nonmotor vehicle NOS (nontraffic) (*see also* Accident, transport) V89.1
  - traffic NOS V89.3
- nontraffic (victim's mode of transport NOS) V88.9
  - collision (between) V88.7
    - bus and truck V88.5
    - car and:
      - ~ bus V88.3
      - ~ pickup V88.2
      - ~ three-wheeled motor vehicle V88.0
      - ~ train V88.6
      - ~ truck V88.4
      - ~ two-wheeled motor vehicle V88.0
      - ~ van V88.2
    - specified vehicle NEC and:
      - ~ three-wheeled motor vehicle V88.1
      - ~ two-wheeled motor vehicle V88.1
  - known mode of transport—*see* Accident, transport, by type of vehicle
  - noncollision V88.8
- on board watercraft V93.8-
  - inflatable V93.86
    - in tow
      - ~ recreational V94.31
      - ~ specified NEC V94.32
- parachutist V97.29
  - entangled in object V97.21
  - injured on landing V97.22
- pedal cycle—*see* Accident, transport, pedal cyclist
- pedestrian (on foot)
  - with
    - another pedestrian W51
      - ~ with fall W03
        - ◊ due to ice or snow W00.0
    - rider of
      - ~ electric scooter V00.031
      - ~ hoverboard V00.038
      - ~ micro-mobility pedestrian conveyance NEC V00.038
      - ~ Segway V00.038
    - transport vehicle—*see* Accident, transport
  - on pedestrian conveyance—*see* Accident, transport, pedestrian, conveyance
- quarry truck—*see* Accident, transport, industrial vehicle occupant
- railway vehicle (any) (in motion)—*see* Accident, transport, railway vehicle occupant
  - due to cataclysm—*see* Forces of nature, by type
- scooter (non-motorized)—*see* Accident, transport, pedestrian, conveyance, scooter
- skateboard—*see* Accident, transport, pedestrian, conveyance, skateboard
- ski(ing)—*see* Accident, transport, pedestrian, conveyance
  - lift V98.3
- specified cause NEC X58
- streetcar—*see* Accident, transport, streetcar occupant
- traffic (victim's mode of transport NOS) V87.9
  - collision (between) V87.7
    - bus and truck V87.5
    - car and:
      - ~ bus V87.3
      - ~ pickup V87.2
      - ~ three-wheeled motor vehicle V87.0
      - ~ train V87.6
      - ~ truck V87.4
      - ~ two-wheeled motor vehicle V87.0
      - ~ van V87.2

Accident (to), *continued*
- - specified vehicle NEC V86.39
    - ~ three-wheeled motor vehicle V87.1
    - ~ two-wheeled motor vehicle V87.1
  - known mode of transport—*see* Accident, transport, by type of vehicle
  - noncollision V87.8
- transport (involving injury to) V99
  - agricultural vehicle occupant (nontraffic) V84.-
  - aircraft V97.8-
    - occupant injured (in)
      - ~ nonpowered craft accident V96.9
        - ◊ balloon V96.0-
        - ◊ glider V96.2-
        - ◊ hang glider V96.1-
        - ◊ specified craft NEC V96.8
      - ~ powered craft accident V95.9
        - ◊ fixed wing NEC
          - » commercial V95.3-
          - » private V95.2-
        - ◊ glider (powered) V95.1-
        - ◊ helicopter V95.0-
        - ◊ specified craft NEC V95.8
        - ◊ ultralight V95.1-
      - ~ specified accident NEC V97.0
      - ~ while boarding or alighting V97.1
    - person (injured by)
      - ~ falling from, in or on aircraft V97.0
      - ~ machinery on aircraft V97.89
      - ~ on ground with aircraft involvement V97.39
      - ~ while boarding or alighting aircraft V97.1
  - airport (battery-powered) passenger vehicle—*see* Accident, transport, industrial vehicle occupant
  - all-terrain vehicle occupant (nontraffic) V86.99
    - driver V86.59
    - dune buggy—*see* Accident, transport, dune buggy occupant
    - hanger-on V86.79
    - passenger V86.69
  - animal-drawn vehicle occupant (in) V80.929
    - collision (with)
      - ~ animal V80.12
        - ◊ being ridden V80.711
      - ~ animal-drawn vehicle V80.721
      - ~ fixed or stationary object V80.82
      - ~ military vehicle V80.920
      - ~ nonmotor vehicle V80.791
      - ~ pedestrian V80.12
      - ~ specified motor vehicle NEC V80.52
      - ~ streetcar V80.731
    - noncollision V80.02
    - specified circumstance NEC V80.928
  - animal-rider V80.919
    - collision (with)
      - ~ animal V80.11
        - ◊ being ridden V80.710
      - ~ animal-drawn vehicle V80.720
      - ~ fixed or stationary object V80.81
      - ~ nonmotor vehicle V80.790
      - ~ pedestrian V80.11
      - ~ specified motor vehicle NEC V80.51
      - ~ streetcar V80.730
    - noncollision V80.018
      - ~ specified as horse rider V80.010
    - specified circumstance NEC V80.918
  - bus occupant V79.9
    - collision (with)
    - driver
      - ~ collision (with)
      - ~ noncollision accident (traffic) V78.5
        - ◊ nontraffic V78.0
    - noncollision accident (traffic) V78.9
      - ~ nontraffic V78.3
      - ~ while boarding or alighting V78.4
      - ~ noncollision accident (traffic) V78.7
        - ◊ nontraffic V78.2
    - passenger
      - ~ collision (with)
      - ~ noncollision accident (traffic) V78.6
        - ◊ nontraffic V78.1
    - specified type NEC V79.88
      - ~ military vehicle V79.81

Accident (to), *continued*
- cable car, not on rails V98.0
  - on rails—*see* Accident, transport, streetcar occupant
- car occupant V49.9
  - ambulance occupant—*see* Accident, transport, ambulance occupant
  - collision (with)
    - ◊ animal being ridden (traffic) V46.9
      - » nontraffic V46.3
      - » while boarding or alighting V46.4
    - ~ animal-drawn vehicle (traffic) V46.9
      - ◊ nontraffic V46.3
      - ◊ while boarding or alighting V46.4
    - ~ car (traffic) V43.92
      - ◊ nontraffic V43.32
      - ◊ while boarding or alighting V43.42
    - ~ motor vehicle NOS (traffic) V49.60
      - ◊ nontraffic V49.20
      - ◊ specified type NEC (traffic) V49.69
        - » nontraffic V49.29
    - ~ pickup truck (traffic) V43.93
      - ◊ nontraffic V43.33
      - ◊ while boarding or alighting V43.43
    - ~ specified vehicle NEC (traffic) V46.9
      - ◊ nontraffic V46.3
      - ◊ while boarding or alighting V46.4
    - ~ sport utility vehicle (traffic) V43.91
      - ◊ nontraffic V43.31
      - ◊ while boarding or alighting V43.41
    - ~ stationary object (traffic) V47.92
      - ◊ while boarding or alighting V47.4
    - ~ streetcar (traffic) V46.9
      - ◊ nontraffic V46.3
      - ◊ while boarding or alighting V46.4
    - ~ van (traffic) V43.94
      - ◊ nontraffic V43.34
      - ◊ while boarding or alighting V43.44
  - driver
    - ~ collision (with)
      - » animal being ridden (traffic) V46.5
        - ❖ nontraffic V46.0
      - ◊ animal-drawn vehicle (traffic) V46.5
        - » nontraffic V46.0
      - ◊ car (traffic) V43.52
        - » nontraffic V43.02
      - ◊ motor vehicle NOS (traffic) V49.40
        - » nontraffic V49.00
        - » specified type NEC (traffic) V49.49
          - ❖ nontraffic V49.09
      - ◊ pickup truck (traffic) V43.53
        - » nontraffic V43.03
      - ◊ specified vehicle NEC (traffic) V46.5
        - » nontraffic V46.0
      - ◊ sport utility vehicle (traffic) V43.51
        - » nontraffic V43.01
      - ◊ streetcar (traffic) V46.5
        - » nontraffic V46.0
      - ◊ van (traffic) V43.54
        - » nontraffic V43.04
    - ~ noncollision accident (traffic) V48.5
      - ◊ nontraffic V48.0
  - noncollision accident (traffic) V48.9
    - ~ nontraffic V48.3
    - ~ while boarding or alighting V48.4
  - nontraffic V49.3
  - hanger-on
    - ~ collision (with)
      - » animal being ridden (traffic) V46.7
        - ❖ nontraffic V46.2
      - ◊ animal-drawn vehicle (traffic) V46.7
        - » nontraffic V46.2
      - ◊ car (traffic) V43.72
        - » nontraffic V43.22
      - ◊ pickup truck (traffic) V43.73
        - » nontraffic V43.23
      - ◊ specified vehicle NEC (traffic) V46.7
        - » nontraffic V46.2
      - ◊ sport utility vehicle (traffic) V43.71
        - » nontraffic V43.21
      - ◊ stationary object (traffic) V47.7
        - » nontraffic V47.2

Accident (to), *continued*
- ◊ streetcar (traffic) V46.7
  - » nontraffic V46.2
- ◊ van (traffic) V43.74
  - » nontraffic V43.24
- ~ noncollision accident (traffic) V48.7
  - ◊ nontraffic V48.2
- passenger
  - ~ collision (with)
    - » animal being ridden (traffic) V46.6
      - ❖ nontraffic V46.1
    - ◊ animal-drawn vehicle (traffic) V46.6
      - » nontraffic V46.1
    - ◊ car (traffic) V43.62
      - » nontraffic V43.12
    - ◊ motor vehicle NOS (traffic) V49.50
      - » nontraffic V49.10
      - » specified type NEC (traffic) V49.59
        - ❖ nontraffic V49.19
    - ◊ pickup truck (traffic) V43.63
      - » nontraffic V43.13
    - ◊ specified vehicle NEC (traffic) V46.6
      - » nontraffic V46.1
    - ◊ sport utility vehicle (traffic) V43.61
      - » nontraffic V43.11
    - ◊ streetcar (traffic) V46.6
      - » nontraffic V46.1
    - ◊ van (traffic) V43.64
      - » nontraffic V43.14
  - ~ noncollision accident (traffic) V48.6
    - ◊ nontraffic V48.1
  - specified type NEC V49.88
- due to cataclysm—*see* Forces of nature, by type
- hoverboard V00.848
- ice yacht V98.2
- industrial vehicle occupant (nontraffic) V83.-
- land yacht V98.1
- logging car—*see* Accident, transport, industrial vehicle occupant
- motorcoach—*see* Accident, transport, bus occupant
- motorcyclist V29.9
  - collision (with)
    - ◊ animal being ridden (traffic) V26.9
      - » nontraffic V26.2
      - » while boarding or alighting V26.3
    - ~ animal-drawn vehicle (traffic) V26.9
      - ◊ nontraffic V26.2
      - ◊ while boarding or alighting V26.3
    - ~ motor vehicle NOS (traffic) V29.60
      - ◊ nontraffic V29.20
      - ◊ specified type NEC (traffic) V29.69
        - » nontraffic V29.29
    - ~ specified vehicle NEC (traffic) V26.9
      - ◊ nontraffic V26.2
      - ◊ while boarding or alighting V26.3
    - ~ streetcar (traffic) V26.9
      - ◊ nontraffic V26.2
      - ◊ while boarding or alighting V26.3
  - driver
    - ~ collision (with)
      - » animal being ridden (traffic) V26.4
        - ❖ nontraffic V26.0
      - ◊ animal-drawn vehicle (traffic) V26.4
        - » nontraffic V26.0
      - ◊ specified vehicle NEC (traffic) V26.4
        - » nontraffic V26.0
      - ◊ streetcar (traffic) V26.4
        - » nontraffic V26.0
    - ~ noncollision accident (traffic) V28.4
      - ◊ nontraffic V28.0
  - noncollision accident (traffic) V28.9
    - ~ nontraffic V28.2
    - ~ while boarding or alighting V28.3
  - nontraffic V29.3
  - passenger
    - ~ collision (with)
      - » animal being ridden (traffic) V26.5
        - ❖ nontraffic V26.1
      - ◊ animal-drawn vehicle (traffic) V26.5
        - » nontraffic V26.1
      - ◊ specified vehicle NEC (traffic) V26.5
      - ◊ streetcar (traffic) V26.5
        - » nontraffic V26.1

Accident (to), *continued*
- ~ noncollision accident (traffic) V28.5
  - ◊ nontraffic V28.1
- specified type NEC V29.88
  - ~ military vehicle V29.81
- motor vehicle NEC occupant (traffic) V86.39
- occupant (of)
  - aircraft (powered) V95.9
    - ~ nonpowered V96.9
    - ~ specified NEC V95.8
  - airport battery-powered vehicle—*see* Accident, transport, industrial vehicle occupant
  - all-terrain vehicle (ATV)—*see* Accident, transport, all-terrain vehicle occupant
  - animal-drawn vehicle—*see* Accident, transport, animal-drawn vehicle occupant
  - automobile—*see* Accident, transport, car occupant
  - balloon V96.00
  - battery-powered vehicle—*see* Accident, transport, industrial vehicle occupant
  - bicycle—*see* Accident, transport, pedal cyclist
    - ~ motorized—*see* Accident, transport, motorcycle rider
  - boat NEC—*see* Accident, watercraft
  - bus—*see* Accident, transport, bus occupant
  - cable car (on rails)—*see also* Accident, transport, streetcar occupant
    - ~ not on rails V98.0
  - car—*see also* Accident, transport, car occupant
    - ~ cable (on rails)—*see also* Accident, transport, streetcar occupant
      - ◊ not on rails V98.0
  - coach—*see* Accident, transport, bus occupant
  - farm machinery (self-propelled)—*see* Accident, transport, agricultural vehicle occupant
  - forklift—*see* Accident, transport, industrial vehicle occupant
  - glider (unpowered) V96.20
    - ~ hang V96.10
    - ~ powered (microlight) (ultralight)—*see* Accident, transport, aircraft, occupant, powered, glider
  - glider (unpowered) NEC V96.20
  - hang-glider V96.10
  - heavy (transport) vehicle—*see* Accident, transport, truck occupant
  - ice-yacht V98.2
  - kite (carrying person) V96.8
  - land-yacht V98.1
  - microlight—*see* Accident, transport, aircraft, occupant, powered, glider
  - motor scooter—*see* Accident, transport, motorcycle
  - motorcycle (with sidecar)—*see* Accident, transport, motorcycle
  - pedal cycle—*see also* Accident, transport, pedal cyclist
  - pick-up (truck)—*see* Accident, transport, pickup truck occupant
  - railway (train) (vehicle) (subterranean) (elevated)—*see* Accident, transport, railway vehicle occupant
    - ~ motorized—*see* Accident, transport, three-wheeled motor vehicle
    - ~ pedal driven—*see* Accident, transport, pedal cyclist
  - ship NOS V94.9
  - ski-lift (chair) (gondola) V98.3
  - sport utility vehicle—*see* Accident, transport, car occupant
  - streetcar (interurban) (operating on public street or highway)—*see* Accident, transport, streetcar occupant
  - three-wheeled vehicle (motorized)—*see also* Accident, transport, three-wheeled motor vehicle occupant
    - ~ nonmotorized—*see* Accident, transport, pedal cycle
  - tractor (farm) (and trailer)—*see* Accident, transport, agricultural vehicle occupant
  - train—*see* Accident, transport, railway vehicle occupant
  - tram—*see* Accident, transport, streetcar occupant

Accident (to), *continued*
- ■ tricycle—*see* Accident, transport, pedal cycle
  - ~ motorized—*see* Accident, transport, three-wheeled motor vehicle
- ■ trolley—*see* Accident, transport, streetcar occupant
- ■ ultralight—*see* Accident, transport, aircraft, occupant, powered, glider
- ■ van—*see* Accident, transport, van occupant
- ■ vehicle NEC V89.9
  - ~ heavy transport—*see* Accident, transport, truck occupant
  - ~ motor (traffic) NEC V89.2
    - ◊ nontraffic NEC V89.0
- ■ watercraft NOS V94.9
  - ~ causing drowning—*see* Drowning, resulting from accident to boat
- – parachutist V97.29
  - ■ after accident to aircraft—*see* Accident, transport, aircraft
  - ■ entangled in object V97.21
  - ■ injured on landing V97.22
- – pedal cyclist V19.9
  - ~ noncollision accident (traffic) V18.4
    - ◊ nontraffic V18.0
  - ■ noncollision accident (traffic) V18.9
    - ~ nontraffic V18.2
    - ~ while boarding or alighting V18.3
  - ■ nontraffic V19.3
  - ■ passenger
    - ~ noncollision accident (traffic) V18.5
      - ◊ nontraffic V18.1
  - ■ specified type NEC V19.88
    - ~ military vehicle V19.81
- – pedestrian
  - ■ conveyance (occupant) V09.9
    - ~ baby stroller V00.828
      - ◊ collision (with) V09.9
        - » stationary object V00.822
        - » vehicle V09.9
          - ★ nontraffic V09.00
          - ★ traffic V09.20
      - ◊ fall V00.821
      - ◊ nontraffic V09.1
        - » involving motor vehicle NEC V09.00
      - ◊ traffic V09.3
        - » involving motor vehicle NEC V09.20
    - ~ electric scooter (standing) (*see* External Cause of Injuries Table)
    - ~ flat-bottomed NEC V00.388
      - ◊ collision (with) V09.9
        - » stationary object V00.382
        - » vehicle V09.9
          - ★ nontraffic V09.00
          - ★ traffic V09.20
      - ◊ fall V00.381
      - ◊ nontraffic V09.1
        - » involving motor vehicle NEC V09.00
      - ◊ snow
        - » board—*see* Accident, transport, pedestrian, conveyance, snow board
        - » ski-—*see* Accident, transport, pedestrian, conveyance, skis (snow)
      - ◊ traffic V09.3
        - » involving motor vehicle NEC V09.20
    - ~ gliding type NEC V00.288
      - ◊ collision (with) V09.9
        - » stationary object V00.282
        - » vehicle V09.9
          - ★ nontraffic V09.00
          - ★ traffic V09.20
      - ◊ fall V00.281
      - ◊ heelies—*see* Accident, transport, pedestrian, conveyance, heelies
      - ◊ ice skate—*see* Accident, transport, pedestrian, conveyance, ice skate
      - ◊ nontraffic V09.1
        - » involving motor vehicle NEC V09.00
      - ◊ sled—*see* Accident, transport, pedestrian, conveyance, sled

Accident (to), *continued*
- ◊ traffic V09.3
  - » involving motor vehicle NEC V09.20
  - » wheelies—*see* Accident, transport, pedestrian, conveyance, heelies
- ~ heelies V00.158
  - ◊ fall V00.151
- ~ hoverboard—*see* External Cause of Injuries Table
- ~ ice skates V00.218
  - ◊ collision (with) V09.9
    - » vehicle V09.9
      - ★ nontraffic V09.00
      - ★ traffic V09.20
  - ◊ fall V00.211
  - ◊ nontraffic V09.1
    - » involving motor vehicle NEC V09.00
  - ◊ traffic V09.3
    - » involving motor vehicle NEC V09.20
- ~ micro-mobility pedestrian conveyance—*see* External Cause of Injuries Table
- ~ motorized mobility scooter V00.838
  - ◊ collision with stationary object V00.832
  - ◊ fall from V00.831
- ~ nontraffic V09.1
  - ◊ involving motor vehicle V09.00
    - » military V09.01
    - » specified type NEC V09.09
- ~ roller skates (non in-line) V00.128
  - ◊ collision (with) V09.9 stationary object V00.122
    - » vehicle V09.9
      - ★ nontraffic V09.00
      - ★ traffic V09.20
  - ◊ fall V00.121
  - ◊ in-line V00.118
    - » collision-—*see also* Accident, transport, pedestrian, conveyance occupant, roller skates, collision
      - ❖ with stationary object V00.112
    - » fall V00.111
  - ◊ nontraffic V09.1
    - » involving motor vehicle NEC V09.00
  - ◊ traffic V09.3
    - » involving motor vehicle NEC V09.20
- ~ rolling shoes V00.158
  - ◊ fall V00.151
- ~ rolling type NEC V00.188
  - ◊ collision (with) V09.9
    - » stationary object V00.182
    - » vehicle V09.9
      - ★ nontraffic V09.00
      - ★ traffic V09.20
  - ◊ fall V00.181
  - ◊ in-line roller skate—*see* Accident, transport, pedestrian, conveyance, roller skate, in-line
  - ◊ nontraffic V09.1
    - » involving motor vehicle NEC V09.00
  - ◊ roller skate—*see* Accident, transport, pedestrian, conveyance, roller skate
  - ◊ scooter (non-motorized)—*see* Accident, transport, pedestrian, conveyance, scooter
  - ◊ skateboard—*see* Accident, transport, pedestrian, conveyance, skateboard
  - ◊ traffic V09.3
    - » involving motor vehicle NEC V09.20
- ~ scooter (non-motorized) V00.148
  - ◊ collision (with) V09.9
    - » vehicle V09.9
      - ★ nontraffic V09.00
      - ★ traffic V09.20
  - ◊ fall V00.141
  - ◊ nontraffic V09.1
    - » involving motor vehicle NEC V09.00
  - ◊ traffic V09.3
    - » involving motor vehicle NEC V09.20
- ~ Segway—*see* External Cause of Injuries Table
- ~ skate board V00.138
  - ◊ collision (with) V09.9
    - » stationary object V00.132
    - » vehicle V09.9
      - ★ nontraffic V09.00
      - ★ traffic V09.20

Accident (to), *continued*
- ◊ fall V00.131
- ◊ nontraffic V09.1
  - » involving motor vehicle NEC V09.00
- ◊ traffic V09.3
  - » involving motor vehicle NEC V09.20
- ~ sled V00.228
  - ◊ collision (with) V09.9
    - » vehicle V09.9
      - ★ nontraffic V09.00
      - ★ traffic V09.20
  - ◊ fall V00.221
  - ◊ nontraffic V09.1
    - » involving motor vehicle NEC V09.00
  - ◊ traffic V09.3
    - » involving motor vehicle NEC V09.20
- ~ skis (snow) V00.328
  - ◊ collision (with) V09.9
    - » vehicle V09.9
      - ★ nontraffic V09.00
      - ★ traffic V09.20
  - ◊ fall V00.321
  - ◊ nontraffic V09.1
    - » involving motor vehicle NEC V09.00
  - ◊ traffic V09.3
    - » involving motor vehicle NEC V09.20
- ~ snow board V00.318
  - ◊ collision (with) V09.9
    - » vehicle V09.9
      - ★ nontraffic V09.00
      - ★ traffic V09.20
  - ◊ fall V00.311
  - ◊ nontraffic V09.1
    - » involving motor vehicle NEC V09.00
  - ◊ traffic V09.3
    - » involving motor vehicle NEC V09.20
- ~ specified type NEC V00.898
  - ◊ collision (with) V09.9
    - » stationary object V00.892
    - » vehicle V09.9
      - ★ nontraffic V09.00
      - ★ traffic V09.20
  - ◊ fall V00.891
  - ◊ nontraffic V09.1
    - » involving motor vehicle NEC V09.00
  - ◊ traffic V09.3
    - » involving motor vehicle NEC V09.20
- ~ traffic V09.3
  - ◊ involving motor vehicle V09.20
    - » military V09.21
    - » specified type NEC V09.29
- ~ wheelchair (powered) V00.818
  - ◊ collision (with) V09.9
    - » stationary object V00.812
    - » vehicle V09.9
      - ★ nontraffic V09.00
      - ★ traffic V09.20
  - ◊ fall V00.811
  - ◊ nontraffic V09.1
    - » involving motor vehicle NEC V09.00
  - ◊ traffic V09.3
    - » involving motor vehicle NEC V09.20
- ~ wheeled shoe V00.158
  - ◊ fall V00.151
- ■ on foot—*see also* Accident, pedestrian
  - ~ collision (with)
    - ◊ vehicle V09.9
      - ❖ nontraffic V09.00
      - ❖ traffic V09.20
  - ~ nontraffic V09.1
    - ◊ involving motor vehicle V09.00
      - » military V09.01
      - » specified type NEC V09.09
  - ~ traffic V09.3
    - ◊ involving motor vehicle V09.20
      - » military V09.21
      - » specified type NEC V09.29
- – person NEC (unknown way or transportation) V99
  - ■ collision (between)
    - ~ bus (with)
      - ◊ heavy transport vehicle (traffic) V87.5
        - » nontraffic V88.5

Accident (to), *continued*
  ~ car (with)
    ◊ nontraffic V88.5
    ◊ bus (traffic) V87.3
      » nontraffic V88.3
    ◊ heavy transport vehicle (traffic) V87.4
      » nontraffic V88.4
    ◊ pick-up truck or van (traffic) V87.2
      » nontraffic V88.2
    ◊ train or railway vehicle (traffic) V87.6
      » nontraffic V88.6
    ◊ two-or three-wheeled motor vehicle (traffic) V87.0
      » nontraffic V88.0
    ~ motor vehicle (traffic) NEC V87.7
      ◊ nontraffic V88.7
    ~ two-or three-wheeled vehicle (with) (traffic)
      ◊ motor vehicle NEC V87.1
        » nontraffic V88.1
    ■ nonmotor vehicle (collision) (noncollision) (traffic) V87.9
    ~ nontraffic V88.9
  – pickup truck occupant V59.9
    ■ collision (with)
      ~ animal (traffic) V50.9
        ◊ animal being ridden (traffic) V56.9
          » nontraffic V56.3
          » while boarding or alighting V56.4
      ~ animal-drawn vehicle (traffic) V56.9
        ◊ nontraffic V56.3
        ◊ while boarding or alighting V56.4
      ~ motor vehicle NOS (traffic) V59.60
        ◊ nontraffic V59.20
        ◊ specified type NEC (traffic) V59.69
          » nontraffic V59.29
      ~ specified vehicle NEC (traffic) V56.9
        ◊ nontraffic V56.3
        ◊ while boarding or alighting V56.4
      ~ streetcar (traffic) V56.9
        ◊ nontraffic V56.3
        ◊ while boarding or alighting V56.4
    ■ driver
      ~ collision (with)
        » animal being ridden (traffic) V56.5
          ❖ nontraffic V56.0
        ◊ animal-drawn vehicle (traffic) V56.5
          » nontraffic V56.0
        ◊ motor vehicle NOS (traffic) V59.40
          » nontraffic V59.00
          » specified type NEC (traffic) V59.49
            ❖ nontraffic V59.09
        ◊ specified vehicle NEC (traffic) V56.5
          » nontraffic V56.0
        ◊ streetcar (traffic) V56.5
          » nontraffic V56.0
      ~ noncollision accident (traffic) V58.5
        ◊ nontraffic V58.0
    ■ noncollision accident (traffic) V58.9
      ~ nontraffic V58.3
      ~ while boarding or alighting V58.4
    ■ nontraffic V59.3
    ■ hanger-on
      ~ collision (with)
        » animal being ridden (traffic) V56.7
          ❖ nontraffic V56.2
        ◊ animal-drawn vehicle (traffic) V56.7
          » nontraffic V56.2
        ◊ specified vehicle NEC (traffic) V56.7
          » nontraffic V56.2
        ◊ streetcar (traffic) V56.7
          » nontraffic V56.2
      ~ noncollision accident (traffic) V58.7
        ◊ nontraffic V58.2
    ■ passenger
      ~ collision (with)
        » animal being ridden (traffic) V56.6
          ❖ nontraffic V56.1
        ◊ animal-drawn vehicle (traffic) V56.6
          » nontraffic V56.1
        ◊ motor vehicle NOS (traffic) V59.50
          » nontraffic V59.10
          » specified type NEC (traffic) V59.59
            ❖ nontraffic V59.19

Accident (to), *continued*
        ◊ specified vehicle NEC (traffic) V56.6
          » nontraffic V56.1
        ◊ streetcar (traffic) V56.6
          » nontraffic V56.1
      ~ noncollision accident (traffic) V58.6
        ◊ nontraffic V58.1
    ■ specified type NEC V59.88
      ~ military vehicle V59.81
  – railway vehicle occupant V81.9
    ■ collision (with) V81.3
      ~ motor vehicle (non-military) (traffic) V81.1
        ◊ military V81.83
        ◊ nontraffic V81.0
      ~ rolling stock V81.2
      ~ specified object NEC V81.3
    ■ during derailment V81.7
    ■ explosion V81.81
    ■ fall (in railway vehicle) V81.5
      ~ during derailment V81.7
      ~ from railway vehicle V81.6
        ◊ during derailment V81.7
      ~ while boarding or alighting V81.4
    ■ fire V81.81
    ■ object falling onto train V81.82
    ■ specified type NEC V81.89
    ■ while boarding or alighting V81.4
  – ski lift V98.3
  – specified NEC V98.8
  – sport utility vehicle occupant
    ■ collision (with)
  – streetcar occupant V82.9
    ■ collision (with) V82.3
      ~ motor vehicle (traffic) V82.1
        ◊ nontraffic V82.0
      ~ rolling stock V82.2
    ■ during derailment V82.7
    ■ fall (in streetcar) V82.5
      ~ during derailment V82.7
      ~ from streetcar V82.6
        ◊ during derailment V82.7
        ◊ while boarding or alighting V82.4
      ~ while boarding or alighting V82.4
    ■ specified type NEC V82.8
    ■ while boarding or alighting V82.4
  – three-wheeled motor vehicle occupant V39.9
    ■ collision (with)
      ~ motor vehicle NOS (traffic) V39.60
        ◊ nontraffic V39.20
        ◊ specified type NEC (traffic) V39.69
          » nontraffic V39.29
    ■ driver
      ~ collision (with)
        ◊ motor vehicle NOS (traffic) V39.40
          » nontraffic V39.00
          » specified type NEC (traffic) V39.49
            ❖ nontraffic V39.09
      ~ noncollision accident (traffic) V38.5
        ◊ nontraffic V38.0
    ■ noncollision accident (traffic) V38.9
      ~ nontraffic V38.3
      ~ while boarding or alighting V38.4
    ■ nontraffic V39.3
    ■ hanger-on
      ~ noncollision accident (traffic) V38.7
        ◊ nontraffic V38.2
    ■ passenger
      ~ collision (with)
        ◊ motor vehicle NOS (traffic) V39.50
          » nontraffic V39.10
          » specified type NEC (traffic) V39.59
            ❖ nontraffic V39.19
      ~ noncollision accident (traffic) V38.6
        ◊ nontraffic V38.1
    ■ specified type NEC V39.89
      ~ military vehicle V39.81
  – tractor (farm) (and trailer)—*see* Accident, transport, agricultural vehicle occupant
  – tram—*see* Accident, transport, streetcar
  – trolley—*see* Accident, transport, streetcar
  – truck (heavy) occupant V69.9
    ■ collision (with)
      ~ animal (traffic) V60.9

Accident (to), *continued*
    ◊ being ridden (traffic) V66.9
      » nontraffic V66.3
      » while boarding or alighting V66.4
    ◊ nontraffic V60.3
    ◊ while boarding or alighting V60.4
    ~ animal-drawn vehicle (traffic) V66.9
      ◊ nontraffic V66.3
      ◊ while boarding or alighting V66.4
    ~ bus (traffic) V64.9
      ◊ nontraffic V64.3
      ◊ while boarding or alighting V64.4
    ~ car (traffic) V63.9
      ◊ nontraffic V63.3
      ◊ while boarding or alighting V63.4
    ~ motor vehicle NOS (traffic) V69.60
      ◊ nontraffic V69.20
      ◊ specified type NEC (traffic) V69.69
        » nontraffic V69.29
    ~ pedal cycle (traffic) V61.9
      ◊ nontraffic V61.3
      ◊ while boarding or alighting V61.4
    ~ pickup truck (traffic) V63.9
      ◊ nontraffic V63.3
      ◊ while boarding or alighting V63.4
    ~ railway vehicle (traffic) V65.9
      ◊ nontraffic V65.3
      ◊ while boarding or alighting V65.4
    ~ specified vehicle NEC (traffic) V66.9
      ◊ nontraffic V66.3
      ◊ while boarding or alighting V66.4
    ~ stationary object (traffic) V67.9
      ◊ nontraffic V67.3
      ◊ while boarding or alighting V67.4
    ~ streetcar (traffic) V66.9
      ◊ nontraffic V66.3
      ◊ while boarding or alighting V66.4
    ~ three wheeled motor vehicle (traffic) V62.9
      ◊ nontraffic V62.3
      ◊ while boarding or alighting V62.4
    ~ truck (traffic) V64.9
      ◊ nontraffic V64.3
      ◊ while boarding or alighting V64.4
    ~ two wheeled motor vehicle (traffic) V62.9
      ◊ nontraffic V62.3
      ◊ while boarding or alighting V62.4
    ~ van (traffic) V63.9
      ◊ nontraffic V63.3
      ◊ while boarding or alighting V63.4
  ■ driver
    ~ collision (with)
      ◊ animal (traffic) V60.5
        » being ridden (traffic) V66.5
          ❖ nontraffic V66.0
        » nontraffic V60.0
      ◊ animal-drawn vehicle (traffic) V66.5
        » nontraffic V66.0
      ◊ bus (traffic) V64.5
        » nontraffic V64.0
      ◊ car (traffic) V63.5
        » nontraffic V63.0
      ◊ motor vehicle NOS (traffic) V69.40
        » nontraffic V69.00
        » specified type NEC (traffic) V69.49
          ❖ nontraffic V69.09
      ◊ pedal cycle (traffic) V61.5
        » nontraffic V61.0
      ◊ pickup truck (traffic) V63.5
        » nontraffic V63.0
      ◊ railway vehicle (traffic) V65.5
        » nontraffic V65.0
      ◊ specified vehicle NEC (traffic) V66.5
        » nontraffic V66.0
      ◊ stationary object (traffic) V67.5
        » nontraffic V67.0
      ◊ streetcar (traffic) V66.5
        » nontraffic V66.0
      ◊ three wheeled motor vehicle (traffic) V62.5
        » nontraffic V62.0
      ◊ truck (traffic) V64.5
        » nontraffic V64.0
      ◊ two wheeled motor vehicle (traffic) V62.5
        » nontraffic V62.0

Accident (to), *continued*
◊ van (traffic) V63.5
» nontraffic V63.0
~ noncollision accident (traffic) V68.5
◊ nontraffic V68.0
■ hanger-on
~ collision (with)
◊ animal (traffic) V60.7
» being ridden (traffic) V66.7
❖ nontraffic V66.2
» nontraffic V60.2
◊ animal-drawn vehicle (traffic) V66.7
» nontraffic V66.2
◊ bus (traffic) V64.7
» nontraffic V64.2
◊ car (traffic) V63.7
» nontraffic V63.2
◊ pedal cycle (traffic) V61.7
» nontraffic V61.2
◊ pickup truck (traffic) V63.7
» nontraffic V63.2
◊ railway vehicle (traffic) V65.7
» nontraffic V65.2
◊ specified vehicle NEC (traffic) V66.7
» nontraffic V66.2
◊ stationary object (traffic) V67.7
» nontraffic V67.2
◊ streetcar (traffic) V66.7
» nontraffic V66.2
◊ three wheeled motor vehicle (traffic) V62.7
» nontraffic V62.2
◊ truck (traffic) V64.7
» nontraffic V64.2
◊ two wheeled motor vehicle (traffic) V62.7
» nontraffic V62.2
◊ van (traffic) V63.7
» nontraffic V63.2
~ noncollision accident (traffic) V68.7
◊ nontraffic V68.2
■ noncollision accident (traffic) V68.9
~ nontraffic V68.3
~ while boarding or alighting V68.4
■ nontraffic V69.3
■ passenger
~ collision (with)
◊ animal (traffic) V60.6
» being ridden (traffic) V66.6
❖ nontraffic V66.1
» nontraffic V60.1
◊ animal-drawn vehicle (traffic) V66.6
» nontraffic V66.1
◊ bus (traffic) V64.6
» nontraffic V64.1
◊ car (traffic) V63.6
» nontraffic V63.1
◊ motor vehicle NOS (traffic) V69.50
» nontraffic V69.10
» specified type NEC (traffic) V69.59
❖ nontraffic V69.19
◊ pedal cycle (traffic) V61.6
» nontraffic V61.1
◊ pickup truck (traffic) V63.6
» nontraffic V63.1
◊ railway vehicle (traffic) V65.6
» nontraffic V65.1
◊ specified vehicle NEC (traffic) V66.6
» nontraffic V66.1
◊ stationary object (traffic) V67.6
» nontraffic V67.1
◊ streetcar (traffic) V66.6
» nontraffic V66.1
◊ three wheeled motor vehicle (traffic) V62.6
» nontraffic V62.1
◊ truck (traffic) V64.6
» nontraffic V64.1
◊ two wheeled motor vehicle (traffic) V62.6
» nontraffic V62.1
◊ van (traffic) V63.6
» nontraffic V63.1
~ noncollision accident (traffic) V68.6
◊ nontraffic V68.1
■ pickup—*see* Accident, transport, pickup truck occupant

Accident (to), *continued*
■ specified type NEC V69.88
~ military vehicle V69.81
– van occupant V59.9
~ collision (with)
◊ animal (traffic) V50.9
◊ being ridden (traffic) V56.9
» nontraffic V56.3
» while boarding or alighting V56.4
~ animal-drawn vehicle (traffic) V56.9
◊ nontraffic V56.3
◊ while boarding or alighting V56.4
~ motor vehicle NOS (traffic) V59.60
◊ nontraffic V59.20
◊ specified type NEC (traffic) V59.69
» nontraffic V59.29
~ specified vehicle NEC (traffic) V56.9
◊ nontraffic V56.3
◊ while boarding or alighting V56.4
~ streetcar (traffic) V56.9
◊ nontraffic V56.3
◊ while boarding or alighting V56.4
■ driver
~ collision (with)
» animal being ridden (traffic) V56.5
❖ nontraffic V56.0
◊ animal-drawn vehicle (traffic) V56.5
» nontraffic V56.0
◊ motor vehicle NOS (traffic) V59.40
» nontraffic V59.00
» specified type NEC (traffic) V59.49
❖ nontraffic V59.09
◊ specified vehicle NEC (traffic) V56.5
◊ streetcar (traffic) V56.5
» nontraffic V56.0
~ noncollision accident (traffic) V58.5
◊ nontraffic V58.0
■ noncollision accident (traffic) V58.9
~ nontraffic V58.3
~ while boarding or alighting V58.4
■ nontraffic V59.3
■ hanger-on
~ collision (with)
» animal being ridden (traffic) V56.7
❖ nontraffic V56.2
◊ animal-drawn vehicle (traffic) V56.7
» nontraffic V56.2
◊ specified vehicle NEC (traffic) V56.7
» nontraffic V56.2
◊ streetcar (traffic) V56.7
» nontraffic V56.2
~ noncollision accident (traffic) V58.7
◊ nontraffic V58.2
■ passenger
~ collision (with)
» animal being ridden (traffic) V56.6
❖ nontraffic V56.1
◊ animal-drawn vehicle (traffic) V56.6
◊ motor vehicle NOS (traffic) V59.50
» nontraffic V59.10
» specified type NEC (traffic) V59.59
❖ nontraffic V59.19
◊ specified vehicle NEC (traffic) V56.6
» nontraffic V56.1
◊ streetcar (traffic) V56.6
» nontraffic V56.1
~ noncollision accident (traffic) V58.6
◊ nontraffic V58.1
■ specified type NEC V59.88
~ military vehicle V59.81
– watercraft occupant—*see* Accident, watercraft
• vehicle NEC V89.9
– animal-drawn NEC—*see* Accident, transport, animal-drawn vehicle occupant
– special
■ agricultural—*see* Accident, transport, agricultural vehicle occupant
– three-wheeled NEC (motorized)—*see* Accident, transport, three-wheeled motor vehicle occupant
• watercraft V94.9
– causing
■ drowning—*see* Drowning, due to, accident to, watercraft

Accident (to), *continued*
■ injury NEC V91.89
~ crushed between craft and object V91.19
◊ powered craft V91.1-
◊ unpowered craft V91.1-
~ fall on board V91.29
◊ powered craft V91.2-
◊ unpowered craft V91.2-
~ fire on board causing burn V91.09
◊ powered craft V91.0-
◊ unpowered craft V91.0-
~ hit by falling object V91.39
◊ powered craft V91.3-
◊ unpowered craft V91.3-
~ specified type NEC V91.89
◊ powered craft V91.8-
◊ unpowered craft V91.8-
– nonpowered, struck by
■ nonpowered vessel V94.22
■ powered vessel V94.21
– specified type NEC V94.89
– striking swimmer
■ powered V94.11
■ unpowered V94.12

Acid throwing (assault) Y08.89

Activity (involving) (of victim at time of event) Y93.9
• aerobic and step exercise (class) Y93.A3
• alpine skiing Y93.23
• animal care NEC Y93.K9
• arts and handcrafts NEC Y93.D9
• athletics NEC Y93.79
• athletics played as a team or group NEC Y93.69
• athletics played individually NEC Y93.59
• baking Y93.G3
• ballet Y93.41
• barbells Y93.B3
• BASE (Building, Antenna, Span, Earth) jumping Y93.33
• baseball Y93.64
• basketball Y93.67
• bathing (personal) Y93.E1
• beach volleyball Y93.68
• bike riding Y93.55
• blackout game Y93.85
• boogie boarding Y93.18
• bowling Y93.54
• boxing Y93.71
• brass instrument playing Y93.J4
• building construction Y93.H3
• bungee jumping Y93.34
• calisthenics Y93.A2
• canoeing (in calm and turbulent water) Y93.16
• capture the flag Y93.6A
• cardiorespiratory exercise NEC Y93.A9
• caregiving (providing) NEC Y93.F9
– bathing Y93.F1
– lifting Y93.F2
• cellular
– communication device Y93.C2
– telephone Y93.C2
• challenge course Y93.A5
• cheerleading Y93.45
• choking game Y93.85
• circuit training Y93.A4
• cleaning
– floor Y93.E5
• climbing NEC Y93.39
– mountain Y93.31
– rock Y93.31
– wall Y93.31
• clothing care and maintenance NEC Y93.E9
• combatives Y93.75
• computer
– keyboarding Y93.C1
– technology NEC Y93.C9
• confidence course Y93.A5
• construction (building) Y93.H3
• cooking and baking Y93.G3
• cool down exercises Y93.A2
• cricket Y93.69
• crocheting Y93.D1
• cross country skiing Y93.24
• dancing (all types) Y93.41

Activity (involving) (of victim at time of event), *continued*
- digging
  - dirt Y93.H1
- dirt digging Y93.H1
- dishwashing Y93.G1
- diving (platform) (springboard) Y93.12
  - underwater Y93.15
- dodge ball Y93.6A
- downhill skiing Y93.23
- drum playing Y93.J2
- dumbbells Y93.B3
- electronic
  - devices NEC Y93.C9
    - hand held interactive Y93.C2
  - game playing (using) (with)
    - interactive device Y93.C2
    - keyboard or other stationary device Y93.C1
- elliptical machine Y93.A1
- exercise(s)
  - machines ((primarily) for)
    - cardiorespiratory conditioning Y93.A1
    - muscle strengthening Y93.B1
  - muscle strengthening (non-machine) NEC Y93.B9
- external motion NEC Y93.I9
  - rollercoaster Y93.I1
- fainting game Y93.85
- field hockey Y93.65
- figure skating (pairs) (singles) Y93.21
- flag football Y93.62
- floor mopping and cleaning Y93.E5
- food preparation and clean up Y93.G1
- football (American) NOS Y93.61
  - flag Y93.62
  - tackle Y93.61
  - touch Y93.62
- four square Y93.6A
- free weights Y93.B3
- frisbee (ultimate) Y93.74
- furniture
  - building Y93.D3
  - finishing Y93.D3
  - repair Y93.D3
- game playing (electronic)
  - using keyboard or other stationary device Y93.C1
  - using interactive device Y93.C2
- gardening Y93.H2
- golf Y93.53
- grass drills Y93.A6
- grilling and smoking food Y93.G2
- grooming and shearing an animal Y93.K3
- guerilla drills Y93.A6
- gymnastics (rhythmic) Y93.43
- handball Y93.73
- handcrafts NEC Y93.D9
- hand held interactive electronic device Y93.C2
- hang gliding Y93.35
- hiking (on level or elevated terrain) Y93.01
- hockey (ice) Y93.22
  - field Y93.65
- horseback riding Y93.52
- household (interior) maintenance NEC Y93.E9
- ice NEC Y93.29
  - dancing or skating Y93.21
  - hockey Y93.22
- in-line roller skating Y93.51
- ironing Y93.E4
- judo Y93.75
- jumping (off) NEC Y93.39
  - BASE (Building, Antenna, Span, Earth) Y93.33
  - bungee Y93.34
  - jacks Y93.A2
  - rope Y93.56
- jumping jacks Y93.A2
- jumping rope Y93.56
- karate Y93.75
- kayaking (in calm and turbulent water) Y93.16
- keyboarding (computer) Y93.C1
- kickball Y93.6A
- knitting Y93.D1
- lacrosse Y93.65
- land maintenance NEC Y93.H9
- landscaping Y93.H2
- laundry Y93.E2

Activity (involving) (of victim at time of event), *continued*
- machines (exercise)
  - primarily for cardiorespiratory conditioning Y93.A1
  - primarily for muscle strengthening Y93.B1
- maintenance
  - exterior building NEC Y93.H9
  - household (interior) NEC Y93.E9
  - land Y93.H9
  - property Y93.H9
- marching (on level or elevated terrain) Y93.01
- martial arts Y93.75
- microwave oven Y93.G3
- milking an animal Y93.K2
- mopping (floor) Y93.E5
- mountain climbing Y93.31
- muscle strengthening
  - exercises (non-machine) NEC Y93.B9
  - machines Y93.B1
- musical keyboard (electronic) playing Y93.J1
- nordic skiing Y93.24
- obstacle course Y93.A5
- oven (microwave) Y93.G3
- packing up and unpacking in moving to a new residence Y93.E6
- parasailing Y93.19
- percussion instrument playing NEC Y93.J2
- personal
  - bathing and showering Y93.E1
  - hygiene NEC Y93.E8
  - showering Y93.E1
- physical games generally associated with school recess, summer camp and children Y93.6A
- physical training NEC Y93.A9
- piano playing Y93.J1
- pilates Y93.B4
- platform diving Y93.12
- playing musical instrument
  - brass instrument Y93.J4
  - drum Y93.J2
  - musical keyboard (electronic) Y93.J1
  - percussion instrument NEC Y93.J2
  - piano Y93.J1
  - string instrument Y93.J3
  - winds instrument Y93.J4
- property maintenance
  - exterior NEC Y93.H9
  - interior NEC Y93.E9
- pruning (garden and lawn) Y93.H2
- pull-ups Y93.B2
- push-ups Y93.B2
- racquetball Y93.73
- rafting (in calm and turbulent water) Y93.16
- raking (leaves) Y93.H1
- rappelling Y93.32
- refereeing a sports activity Y93.81
- residential relocation Y93.E6
- rhythmic gymnastics Y93.43
- rhythmic movement NEC Y93.49
- riding
  - horseback Y93.52
  - rollercoaster Y93.I1
- rock climbing Y93.31
- rollercoaster riding Y93.I1
- roller skating (in-line) Y93.51
- rough housing and horseplay Y93.83
- rowing (in calm and turbulent water) Y93.16
- rugby Y93.63
- running Y93.02
- SCUBA diving Y93.15
- sewing Y93.D2
- shoveling Y93.H1
  - dirt Y93.H1
  - snow Y93.H1
- showering (personal) Y93.E1
- sit-ups Y93.B2
- skateboarding Y93.51
- skating (ice) Y93.21
  - roller Y93.51
- skiing (alpine) (downhill) Y93.23
  - cross country Y93.24
  - nordic Y93.24
  - water Y93.17
- sledding (snow) Y93.23

Activity (involving) (of victim at time of event), *continued*
- sleeping (sleep) Y93.84
- smoking and grilling food Y93.G2
- snorkeling Y93.15
- snow NEC Y93.29
  - boarding Y93.23
  - shoveling Y93.H1
  - sledding Y93.23
  - tubing Y93.23
- soccer Y93.66
- softball Y93.64
- specified NEC Y93.89
- spectator at an event Y93.82
- sports NEC Y93.79
  - sports played as a team or group NEC Y93.69
  - sports played individually NEC Y93.59
- springboard diving Y93.12
- squash Y93.73
- stationary bike Y93.A1
- step (stepping) exercise (class) Y93.A3
- stepper machine Y93.A1
- stove Y93.G3
- string instrument playing Y93.J3
- surfing Y93.18
  - wind Y93.18
- swimming Y93.11
- tap dancing Y93.41
- tennis Y93.73
- tobogganing Y93.23
- touch football Y93.62
- track and field events (non-running) Y93.57
  - running Y93.02
- trampoline Y93.44
- treadmill Y93.A1
- trimming shrubs Y93.H2
- tubing (in calm and turbulent water) Y93.16
  - snow Y93.23
- ultimate frisbee Y93.74
- underwater diving Y93.15
- unpacking in moving to a new residence Y93.E6
- use of stove, oven and microwave oven Y93.G3
- vacuuming Y93.E3
- volleyball (beach) (court) Y93.68
- wake boarding Y93.17
- walking an animal Y93.K1
- walking (on level or elevated terrain) Y93.01
  - an animal Y93.K1
- wall climbing Y93.31
- warm up and cool down exercises Y93.A2
- water NEC Y93.19
  - aerobics Y93.14
  - craft NEC Y93.19
  - exercise Y93.14
  - polo Y93.13
  - skiing Y93.17
  - sliding Y93.18
  - survival training and testing Y93.19
- weeding (garden and lawn) Y93.H2
- wind instrument playing Y93.J4
- windsurfing Y93.18
- wrestling Y93.72
- yoga Y93.42

Adverse effect of drugs—*see* Table of Drugs and Chemicals

Air
- pressure
  - change, rapid
    - during
      - ascent W94.29
        - while (in) (surfacing from)
          - aircraft W94.23
          - deep water diving W94.21
          - underground W94.22
      - descent W94.39
        - in
          - aircraft W94.31
          - water W94.32
  - high, prolonged W94.0
  - low, prolonged W94.12
    - due to residence or long visit at high altitude W94.11

Alpine sickness W94.11

Altitude sickness W94.11

ACTIVITY (INVOLVING) (OF VICTIM AT TIME OF EVENT)–ALTITUDE SICKNESS

Anaphylactic shock, anaphylaxis—*see* Table of Drugs and Chemicals

Andes disease W94.11

Arachnidism, arachnoidism X58

Arson (with intent to injure or kill) X97

Asphyxia, asphyxiation
- by
  - food (bone) (seed) (*see* categories T17 and) T18
  - gas—*see also* Table of Drugs and Chemicals
- from
  - fire—*see also* Exposure, fire
  - ignition—*see* Ignition
  - vomitus T17.81

Aspiration
- food (any type) (into respiratory tract) (with asphyxia, obstruction respiratory tract, suffocation) (*see* categories T17 and) T18
- foreign body—*see* Foreign body, aspiration
- vomitus (with asphyxia, obstruction respiratory tract, suffocation) T17.81

Assassination (attempt)—*see* Assault

Assault (homicidal) (by) (in) Y09
- bite (of human being) Y04.1
- bodily force Y04.8
  - bite Y04.1
  - bumping into Y04.2
  - sexual (*see* subcategories T74.0,) T76.0
  - unarmed fight Y04.0
- brawl (hand) (fists) (foot) (unarmed) Y04.0
- burning, burns (by fire) NEC X97
  - acid Y08.89
  - caustic, corrosive substance Y08.89
  - chemical from swallowing caustic, corrosive substance—*see* Table of Drugs and Chemicals
  - cigarette(s) X97
  - hot object X98.9
    - fluid NEC X98.2
    - household appliance X98.3
    - specified NEC X98.8
    - steam X98.0
    - tap water X98.1
    - vapors X98.0
  - scalding X97
  - steam X98.0
  - vitriol Y08.89
- caustic, corrosive substance (gas) Y08.89
- crashing of
  - aircraft Y08.81
  - motor vehicle Y03.8
    - pushed in front of Y02.0
    - run over Y03.0
    - specified NEC Y03.8
- cutting or piercing instrument X99.9
  - dagger X99.2
  - glass X99.0
  - knife X99.1
  - specified NEC X99.8
  - sword X99.2
- dagger X99.2
- drowning (in) X92.9
  - bathtub X92.0
  - natural water X92.3
  - specified NEC X92.8
  - swimming pool X92.1
    - following fall X92.2
- dynamite X96.8
- explosive(s) (material) X96.9
- fight (hand) (fists) (foot) (unarmed) Y04.0
  - with weapon—*see* Assault, by type of weapon
- fire X97
- firearm X95.9
  - airgun X95.01
  - handgun X93
  - hunting rifle X94.1
  - larger X94.9
    - specified NEC X94.8
  - machine gun X94.2
  - shotgun X94.0
  - specified NEC X95.8
- gunshot (wound) NEC—*see* Assault, firearm, by type
- incendiary device X97

Assault (homicidal) (by) (in), *continued*
- injury Y09
  - to child due to criminal abortion attempt NEC Y08.89
- knife X99.1
- late effect of—*see* X92-Y08 with 7th character S
- placing before moving object NEC Y02.8
  - motor vehicle Y02.0
- poisoning—*see* categories T36-T65 with 7th character S
- puncture, any part of body—*see* Assault, cutting or piercing instrument
- pushing
  - before moving object NEC Y02.8
    - motor vehicle Y02.0
    - subway train Y02.1
    - train Y02.1
- from high place Y01
- rape T74.2-
- scalding —X97
- sexual (by bodily force) T74.2-
- shooting—*see* Assault, firearm
- specified means NEC Y08.89
- stab, any part of body—*see* Assault, cutting or piercing instrument
- steam X98.0
- striking against
  - other person Y04.2
  - sports equipment Y08.09
    - baseball bat Y08.02
    - hockey stick Y08.01
- struck by
  - sports equipment Y08.09
    - baseball bat Y08.02
    - hockey stick Y08.01
- submersion—*see* Assault, drowning
- violence Y09
- weapon Y09
  - blunt Y00
  - cutting or piercing—*see* Assault, cutting or piercing instrument
  - firearm—*see* Assault, firearm
- wound Y09
  - cutting—*see* Assault, cutting or piercing instrument
  - gunshot—*see* Assault, firearm
  - knife X99.1
  - piercing—*see* Assault, cutting or piercing instrument
  - puncture—*see* Assault, cutting or piercing instrument
  - stab—*see* Assault, cutting or piercing instrument

Attack by mammals NEC W55.89

Avalanche—*see* Landslide

B

Barotitis, barodontalgia, barosinusitis, barotrauma (otitic) (sinus)-—*see* Air, pressure

Battered (baby) (child) (person) (syndrome) X58

Bean in nose (*see* categories T17 and) T18

Bed set on fire NEC—*see* Exposure, fire, uncontrolled, building, bed

Bending, injury in—*see* category Y93

Bends-—*see* Air, pressure, change

Bite, bitten by
- alligator W58.01
- arthropod (nonvenomous) NEC W57
- bull W55.21
- cat W55.01
- cow W55.21
- crocodile W58.11
- dog W54.0
- goat W55.31
- hoof stock NEC W55.31
- horse W55.11
- human being (accidentally) W50.3
  - with intent to injure or kill Y04.1
  - as, or caused by, a crowd or human stampede (with fall) W52
  - assault Y04.1
  - in
    - fight Y04.1
- insect (nonvenomous) W57

Bite, bitten by, *continued*
- lizard (nonvenomous) W59.01
- mammal NEC W55.81
  - marine W56.31
- marine animal (nonvenomous) W56.81
- millipede W57
- moray eel W56.51
- mouse W53.01
- person(s) (accidentally) W50.3
  - with intent to injure or kill Y04.1
  - as, or caused by, a crowd or human stampede (with fall) W52
  - assault Y04.1
  - in
    - fight Y04.1
- pig W55.41
- raccoon W55.51
- rat W53.11
- reptile W59.81
  - lizard W59.01
  - snake W59.11
  - turtle W59.21
    - terrestrial W59.81
- rodent W53.81
  - mouse W53.01
  - rat W53.11
  - specified NEC W53.81
  - squirrel W53.21
- shark W56.41
- sheep W55.31
- snake (nonvenomous) W59.11
- spider (nonvenomous) W57
- squirrel W53.21

Blizzard X37.2

Blood alcohol level Y90.-

Blow X58

Blowing up—*see* Explosion

Brawl (hand) (fists) (foot) Y04.0

Breakage (accidental) (part of)
- ladder (causing fall) W11
- scaffolding (causing fall) W12

Broken
- glass, contact with—*see* Contact, with, glass

Bumping against, into (accidentally)
- object NEC W22.8
  - with fall—*see* Fall, due to, bumping against, object
  - caused by crowd or human stampede (with fall) W52
  - sports equipment W21.9
- person(s) W51
  - with fall W03
    - due to ice or snow W00.0
  - assault Y04.2
  - caused by, a crowd or human stampede (with fall) W52
- sports equipment W21.9

Burn, burned, burning (accidental) (by) (from) (on)
- acid NEC—*see* Table of Drugs and Chemicals
- bed linen—*see* Exposure, fire, uncontrolled, in building, bed
- blowtorch X08.8
  - with ignition of clothing NEC X06.2
    - nightwear X05
- bonfire, campfire (controlled)—*see also* Exposure, fire, controlled, not in building
  - uncontrolled—*see* Exposure, fire, uncontrolled, not in building
- candle X08.8
  - with ignition of clothing NEC X06.2
    - nightwear X05
- caustic liquid, substance (external) (internal) NEC—*see* Table of Drugs and Chemicals
- chemical (external) (internal)—*see also* Table of Drugs and Chemicals
- cigar(s) or cigarette(s) X08.8
  - with ignition of clothing NEC X06.2
    - nightwear X05
- clothes, clothing NEC (from controlled fire) X06.2
  - with conflagration—*see* Exposure, fire, uncontrolled, building

Burn, burned, burning (accidental) (by) (from) (on), *continued*

- not in building or structure—*see* Exposure, fire, uncontrolled, not in building
- cooker (hot) X15.8
  - stated as undetermined whether accidental or intentional Y27.3
- electric blanket X16
- engine (hot) X17
- fire, flames—*see* Exposure, fire
- flare, Very pistol—*see* Discharge, firearm NEC
- heat
  - from appliance (electrical) (household) (cooking object) X15.-
    - stated as undetermined whether accidental or intentional Y27.3
  - in local application or packing during medical or surgical procedure Y63.5
- heating
  - appliance, radiator or pipe X16
- hot
  - air X14.1
  - cooker X15.8
  - drink X10.0
  - engine X17
  - fat X10.2
  - fluid NEC X12
  - food X10.1
  - gases X14.1
  - heating appliance X16
  - household appliance NEC X15.8
  - kettle X15.8
  - liquid NEC X12
  - machinery X17
  - metal (molten) (liquid) NEC X18
  - object (not producing fire or flames) NEC X19
  - oil (cooking) X10.2
  - pipe(s) X16
  - radiator X16
  - saucepan (glass) (metal) X15.3
  - stove (kitchen) X15.0
  - substance NEC X19
    - caustic or corrosive NEC—*see* Table of Drugs and Chemicals
  - toaster X15.1
  - tool X17
  - vapor X13.1
  - water (tap)—*see* Contact, with, hot, tap water
- hotplate X15.2
- ignition—*see* Ignition
- inflicted by other person X97
  - by hot objects, hot vapor, and steam—*see* Assault, burning, hot object
- internal, from swallowed caustic, corrosive liquid, substance—*see* Table of Drugs and Chemicals
- iron (hot) X15.8
  - stated as undetermined whether accidental or intentional Y27.3
- kettle (hot) X15.8
  - stated as undetermined whether accidental or intentional Y27.3
- lamp (flame) X08.8
  - with ignition of clothing NEC X06.2
    - nightwear X05
- lighter (cigar) (cigarette) X08.8
  - with ignition of clothing NEC X06.2
    - nightwear X05
- lightning—*see* subcategory T75.0
  - causing fire—*see* Exposure, fire
- liquid (boiling) (hot) NEC X12
  - stated as undetermined whether accidental or intentional Y27.2
- on board watercraft
  - due to
    - accident to watercraft V91.09
      - ~ powered craft V91.0-
      - ~ unpowered craft V91.0-
    - fire on board V93.0-
    - specified heat source NEC on board V93.19
      - ~ ferry boat V93.11
      - ~ fishing boat V93.12
      - ~ jet skis V93.13
      - ~ liner V93.11

Burn, burned, burning (accidental) (by) (from) (on), *continued*

- ~ merchant ship V93.10
- ~ passenger ship V93.11
- ~ powered craft NEC V93.13
- ~ sailboat V93.14
- machinery (hot) X17
- matches X08.8
  - with ignition of clothing NEC X06.2
    - nightwear X05
- mattress—*see* Exposure, fire, uncontrolled, building, bed
- medicament, externally applied Y63.5
- metal (hot) (liquid) (molten) NEC X18
- nightwear (nightclothes, nightdress, gown, pajamas, robe) X05
- object (hot) NEC X19
- pipe (hot) X16
  - smoking X08.8
    - with ignition of clothing NEC X06.2
      - ~ nightwear X05
- powder—*see* Powder burn
- radiator (hot) X16
- saucepan (hot) (glass) (metal) X15.3
  - stated as undetermined whether accidental or intentional Y27.3
- self-inflicted X76
  - stated as undetermined whether accidental or intentional Y26
- steam X13.1
  - pipe X16
    - stated as undetermined whether accidental or intentional Y27.8
  - stated as undetermined whether accidental or intentional Y27.0
- stove (hot) (kitchen) X15.0
  - stated as undetermined whether accidental or intentional Y27.3
- substance (hot) NEC X19
  - boiling X12
    - stated as undetermined whether accidental or intentional Y27.2
  - molten (metal) X18
  - hot
    - household appliance X77.3
    - object X77.9
- stated as undetermined whether accidental or intentional Y27.0
- therapeutic misadventure
  - heat in local application or packing during medical or surgical procedure Y63.5
  - overdose of radiation Y63.2
- toaster (hot) X15.1
  - stated as undetermined whether accidental or intentional Y27.3
- tool (hot) X17
- torch, welding X08.8
  - with ignition of clothing NEC X06.2
    - nightwear X05
- trash fire (controlled)—*see* Exposure, fire, controlled, not in building
  - uncontrolled—*see* Exposure, fire, uncontrolled, not in building
- vapor (hot) X13.1
  - stated as undetermined whether accidental or intentional Y27.0
- Very pistol—*see* Discharge, firearm NEC

Butted by animal W55-

C

Caisson disease—*see* Air, pressure, change

Campfire (exposure to) (controlled)—*see also* Exposure, fire, controlled, not in building
- uncontrolled—*see* Exposure, fire, uncontrolled, not in building Car sickness T75.3

Cat
- bite W55.01
- scratch W55.03

Cataclysm, cataclysmic (any injury) NEC—*see* Forces of nature

Catching fire—*see* Exposure, fire

Caught
- between
  - folding object W23.0
  - objects (moving) (stationary and moving) W23.0
    - and machinery—*see* Contact, with, by type of machine
    - stationary W23.1
  - sliding door and door frame W23.0
- by, in
  - machinery (moving parts of)—*see* Contact, with, by type of machine
  - washing-machine wringer W23.0
- under packing crate (due to losing grip) W23.1

Cave-in caused by cataclysmic earth surface movement or eruption—*see* Landslide

Change(s) in air pressure—*see* Air, pressure, change

Choked, choking (on) (any object except food or vomitus)
- food (bone) (seed) (*see* categories T17 and) T18
- vomitus T17.81-

Cloudburst (any injury) X37.8

Cold, exposure to (accidental) (excessive) (extreme) (natural) (place) NEC—*see* Exposure, cold

Collapse
- building W20.1
  - burning (uncontrolled fire) X00.2
- dam or man-made structure (causing earth movement) X36.0
- machinery—*see* Contact, with, by type of machine
- structure W20.1
  - burning (uncontrolled fire) X00.2

Collision (accidental) NEC (*see also* Accident, transport) V89.9
- pedestrian W51
  - with fall W03
    - due to ice or snow W00.0
    - involving pedestrian conveyance—*see* Accident, transport, pedestrian, conveyance
  - and
    - crowd or human stampede (with fall) W52
    - object W22.8
      - ~ with fall—*see* Fall, due to, bumping against, object
- person(s)—*see* Collision, pedestrian
- transport vehicle NEC V89.9
  - and
    - avalanche, fallen or not moving—*see* Accident, transport
      - ~ falling or moving—*see* Landslide
    - landslide, fallen or not moving—*see* Accident, transport
      - ~ falling or moving—*see* Landslide
  - due to cataclysm—*see* Forces of nature, by type

Combustion, spontaneous—*see* Ignition

Complication (delayed) of or following (medical or surgical procedure) Y84.9
- with misadventure—*see* Misadventure
- amputation of limb(s) Y83.5
- anastomosis (arteriovenous) (blood vessel) (gastrojejunal) (tendon) (natural or artificial material) Y83.2
- aspiration (of fluid) Y84.4
  - tissue Y84.8
- biopsy Y84.8
- blood
  - sampling Y84.7
  - transfusion
    - procedure Y84.8
- bypass Y83.2
- catheterization (urinary) Y84.6
  - cardiac Y84.0
- colostomy Y83.3
- cystostomy Y83.3
- dialysis (kidney) Y84.1
- drug—*see* Table of Drugs and Chemicals
- due to misadventure—*see* Misadventure
- duodenostomy Y83.3
- electroshock therapy Y84.3
- external stoma, creation of Y83.3
- formation of external stoma Y83.3
- gastrostomy Y83.3
- graft Y83.2

Complication (delayed) of or following (medical or surgical procedure), *continued*

- hypothermia (medically-induced) Y84.8
- implant, implantation (of)
  - artificial
    - internal device (cardiac pacemaker) (electrodes in brain) (heart valve prosthesis) (orthopedic) Y83.1
    - material or tissue (for anastomosis or bypass) Y83.2
      - ~ with creation of external stoma Y83.3
  - natural tissues (for anastomosis or bypass) Y83.2
    - with creation of external stoma Y83.3
- infusion
  - procedure Y84.8
- injection—*see* Table of Drugs and Chemicals
  - procedure Y84.8
- insertion of gastric or duodenal sound Y84.5
- insulin-shock therapy Y84.3
- paracentesis (abdominal) (thoracic) (aspirative) Y84.4
- procedures other than surgical operation—*see* Complication of or following, by type of procedure
- radiological procedure or therapy Y84.2
- removal of organ (partial) (total) NEC Y83.6
- sampling
  - blood Y84.7
  - fluid NEC Y84.4
  - tissue Y84.8
- shock therapy Y84.3
- surgical operation NEC (*see also* Complication of or following, by type of operation) Y83.9
  - reconstructive NEC Y83.4
    - with
      - ~ anastomosis, bypass or graft Y83.2
      - ~ formation of external stoma Y83.3
  - specified NEC Y83.8
- transfusion—*see also* Table of Drugs and Chemicals
  - procedure Y84.8
- transplant, transplantation (heart) (kidney) (liver) (whole organ, any) Y83.0
  - partial organ Y83.4
- ureterostomy Y83.3
- vaccination—*see also* Table of Drugs and Chemicals
  - procedure Y84.8

Compression

- divers' squeeze—*see* Air, pressure, change
- trachea by
  - food (lodged in esophagus) (*see* categories T17 and T18
  - vomitus (lodged in esophagus) T17.81-
  Conflagration—*see* Exposure, fire, uncontrolled
  Constriction (external)
- hair W49.01
- jewelry W49.04
- ring W49.04
- rubber band W49.03
- specified item NEC W49.09
- string W49.02
- thread W49.02

Contact (accidental)

- with
  - abrasive wheel (metalworking) W31.1
  - alligator W58.0-
  - amphibian W62.9
    - frog W62.0
    - toad W62.1
  - animal (nonvenomous) NEC W64 (refer to specific animal by name in alphabetical order under "contact")
    - marine W56.8-
  - animate mechanical force NEC W64
  - arrow W21.89
    - not thrown, projected or falling W45.8
  - arthropods (nonvenomous) W57
  - axe W27.0
  - band-saw (industrial) W31.2
  - bayonet—*see* Bayonet wound
  - bee(s) X58
  - bench-saw (industrial) W31.2
  - bird W61.9-
  - blender W29.0

Contact (accidental), *continued*

- boiling water X12
  - stated as undetermined whether accidental or intentional Y27.2
- bore, earth-drilling or mining (land) (seabed) W31.0
- buffalo W55.39
- bull W55.2-
- bumper cars W31.81
- camel W55.39
- can
  - lid W26.8
  - opener W27.4
    - ~ powered W29.0
- cat W55.09
  - bite W55.01
  - scratch W55.03
- caterpillar (venomous) X58
- centipede (venomous) X58
- chain
  - hoist W24.0
    - ~ agricultural operations W30.89
  - saw W29.3
- chicken W61.3-
- chisel W27.0
- circular saw W31.2
- cobra X58
- combine (harvester) W30.0
- conveyer belt W24.1
- cooker (hot) X15.8
  - stated as undetermined whether accidental or intentional Y27.3
- coral X58
- cotton gin W31.82
- cow W55.2-
- crocodile W58.1-
- dagger W26.1
  - stated as undetermined whether accidental or intentional Y28.2
- dairy equipment W31.82
- dart W21.89
  - not thrown, projected or falling W26.8
- deer W55.39
- derrick W24.0
  - agricultural operations W30.89
    - ~ hay W30.2
- dog W54.-
- dolphin W56.0-
- donkey W55.39
- drill (powered) W29.8
  - earth (land) (seabed) W31.0
  - nonpowered W27.8
- drive belt W24.0
  - agricultural operations W30.89
- dry ice—*see* Exposure, cold, man-made
- dryer (clothes) (powered) (spin) W29.2
- duck W61.69
- earth(-)
  - drilling machine (industrial) W31.0
  - scraping machine in stationary use W31.83
- edge of stiff paper W26.2
- electric
  - beater W29.0
  - blanket X16
  - fan W29.2
    - ~ commercial W31.82
  - knife W29.1
  - mixer W29.0
- elevator (building) W24.0
  - agricultural operations W30.89
    - ~ grain W30.3
- engine(s), hot NEC X17
- excavating machine W31.0
- farm machine W30.9
- feces—*see* Contact, with, by type of animal
- fer de lance X58
- fish W56.5-
- flying horses W31.81
- forging (metalworking) machine W31.1
- fork W27.4
- forklift (truck) W24.0
  - agricultural operations W30.89
- frog W62.0

Contact (accidental), *continued*

- garden
  - cultivator (powered) W29.3
    - ~ riding W30.89
  - fork W27.1
- gas turbine W31.3
- Gila monster X58
- giraffe W55.39
- glass (sharp) (broken) W25
  - with subsequent fall W18.02
  - assault X99.0
  - due to fall—*see* Fall, by type
  - stated as undetermined whether accidental or intentional Y28.0
- goat W55.3-
- goose W61.5-
- hand
  - saw W27.0
  - tool (not powered) NEC W27.8
    - ~ powered W29.8
- harvester W30.0
- hay-derrick W30.2
- heat NEC X19
  - from appliance (electrical) (household)—*see* Contact, with, hot, household appliance
    - ~ heating appliance X16
- heating
  - appliance (hot) X16
  - pad (electric) X16
- hedge-trimmer (powered) W29.3
- hoe W27.1
- hoist (chain) (shaft) NEC W24.0
  - agricultural W30.89
- hoof stock NEC W55.3-
- hornet(s) X58
- horse W55.1-
- hot
  - air X14.1
    - ~ inhalation X14.0
  - cooker X15.8
  - drinks X10.0
  - engine X17
  - fats X10.2
  - fluids NEC X12
    - ~ assault X98.2
    - ~ undetermined whether accidental or intentional Y27.2
  - food X10.1
  - gases X14.1
    - ~ inhalation X14.0
  - heating appliance X16
  - household appliance X15.-
    - ~ assault X98.3
    - ~ object NEC X19
      - ◊ assault X98.8
      - ◊ stated as undetermined whether accidental or intentional Y27.9
    - ~ stated as undetermined whether accidental or intentional Y27.3
  - kettle X15.8
  - light bulb X15.8
  - liquid NEC (*see also* Burn) X12
    - ~ drinks X10.0
    - ~ stated as undetermined whether accidental or intentional Y27.2
    - ~ tap water X11.8
      - ◊ stated as undetermined whether accidental or intentional Y27.1
  - machinery X17
  - metal (molten) (liquid) NEC X18
  - object (not producing fire or flames) NEC X19
  - oil (cooking) X10.2
  - pipe X16
  - plate X15.2
  - radiator X16
  - saucepan (glass) (metal) X15.3
  - skillet X15.3
  - stove (kitchen) X15.0
  - substance NEC X19
  - tap-water X11.8
    - ~ assault X98.1

Contact (accidental), *continued*

- ~ heated on stove X12
  - ◊ stated as undetermined whether accidental or intentional Y27.2
- ~ in bathtub X11.0
- ~ running X11.1
- ~ stated as undetermined whether accidental or intentional Y27.1
  - ■ toaster X15.1
  - ■ tool X17
  - ■ vapors X13.1
    - ~ inhalation X13.0
  - ■ water (tap) X11.8
    - ~ boiling X12
      - ◊ stated as undetermined whether accidental or intentional Y27.2
    - ~ heated on stove X12
      - ◊ stated as undetermined whether accidental or intentional Y27.2
    - ~ in bathtub X11.0
    - ~ running X11.1
    - ~ stated as undetermined whether accidental or intentional Y27.1
- – hotplate X15.2
- – ice-pick W27.4
- – insect (nonvenomous) NEC W57
- – kettle (hot) X15.8
- – knife W26.0
  - ■ assault X99.1
  - ■ electric W29.1
  - ■ stated as undetermined whether accidental or intentional Y28.1
  - ■ suicide (attempt) X78.1
- – lathe (metalworking) W31.1
  - ■ turnings W45.8
  - ■ woodworking W31.2
- – lawnmower (powered) (ridden) W28
  - ■ causing electrocution W86.8
  - ■ unpowered W27.1
- – lift, lifting (devices) W24.0
  - ■ agricultural operations W30.89
  - ■ shaft W24.0
- – liquefied gas—*see* Exposure, cold, man-made
- – liquid air, hydrogen, nitrogen—*see* Exposure, cold, man-made
- – lizard (nonvenomous) W59.09
  - ■ bite W59.01
  - ■ strike W59.02
- – llama W55.39
- – macaw W61.1-
- – machine, machinery W31.9
  - ■ abrasive wheel W31.1
  - ■ agricultural including animal-powered W30.-
  - ■ band or bench or circular saw W31.2
  - ■ commercial NEC W31.82
  - ■ drilling, metal (industrial) W31.1
  - ■ earth-drilling W31.0
  - ■ earthmoving or scraping W31.89
  - ■ excavating W31.89
  - ■ forging machine W31.1
  - ■ gas turbine W31.3
  - ■ hot X17
  - ■ internal combustion engine W31.3
  - ■ land drill W31.0
  - ■ lathe W31.1
  - ■ lifting (devices) W24.0
  - ■ metal drill W31.1
  - ■ metalworking (industrial) W31.1
  - ■ milling, metal W31.1
  - ■ mining W31.0
  - ■ molding W31.2
  - ■ overhead plane W31.2
  - ■ power press, metal W31.1
  - ■ prime mover W31.3
  - ■ printing W31.89
  - ■ radial saw W31.2
  - ■ recreational W31.81
  - ■ roller-coaster W31.81
  - ■ rolling mill, metal W31.1
  - ■ sander W31.2
  - ■ seabed drill W31.0

Contact (accidental), *continued*

- ■ shaft
  - ~ hoist W31.0
  - ~ lift W31.0
- ■ specified NEC W31.89
- ■ spinning W31.89
- ■ steam engine W31.3
- ■ transmission W24.1
- ■ undercutter W31.0
- ■ water driven turbine W31.3
- ■ weaving W31.89
- ■ woodworking or forming (industrial) W31.2
- – mammal (feces) (urine) W55.89
  - ■ marine W56.39 (refer to specific animal by name)
    - ~ specified NEC W56.3-
  - ■ specified NEC W55.8-
- – marine
  - ■ animal W56.8- (refer to specific animal by name)
- – meat
  - ■ grinder (domestic) W29.0
    - ~ industrial W31.82
    - ~ nonpowered W27.4
  - ■ slicer (domestic) W29.0
    - ~ industrial W31.82
- – merry go round W31.81
- – metal, hot (liquid) (molten) NEC X18
- – millipede W57
- – nail W45.0
  - ■ gun W29.4
- – needle (sewing) W27.3
  - ■ hypodermic W46.0
    - ~ contaminated W46.1
- – object (blunt) NEC
  - ■ hot NEC X19
  - ■ sharp NEC W26.8
    - ~ inflicted by other person NEC W26.8
    - ~ self-inflicted X78.9
- – orca W56.2-
- – overhead plane W31.2
- – paper (as sharp object) W26.2
- – paper-cutter W27.5
- – parrot W61.0-
- – pig W55.4-
- – pipe, hot X16
- – pitchfork W27.1
- – plane (metal) (wood) W27.0
  - ■ overhead W31.2
- – plant thorns, spines, sharp leaves or other mechanisms W60
- – powered
  - ■ garden cultivator W29.3
  - ■ household appliance, implement, or machine W29.8
  - ■ saw (industrial) W31.2
    - ~ hand W29.8
- – printing machine W31.89
- – psittacine bird W61.2-
  - ■ strike W61.22
- – pulley (block) (transmission) W24.0
  - ■ agricultural operations W30.89
- – raccoon W55.5-
- – radial-saw (industrial) W31.2
- – radiator (hot) X16
- – rake W27.1
- – rattlesnake X58
- – reaper W30.0
- – reptile W59.8- (refer to specific reptile by name)
- – rivet gun (powered) W29.4
- – rodent (feces) (urine) W53.8-
  - ■ mouse W53.0-
  - ■ rat W53.1-
  - ■ specified NEC W53.8-
  - ■ squirrel W53.2-
- – roller coaster W31.81
- – rope NEC W24.0
  - ■ agricultural operations W30.89
- – saliva—*see* Contact, with, by type of animal
- – sander W29.8
  - ■ industrial W31.2
- – saucepan (hot) (glass) (metal) X15.3
- – saw W27.0
  - ■ band (industrial) W31.2
  - ■ bench (industrial) W31.2

Contact (accidental), *continued*

- ■ chain W29.3
- ■ hand W27.0
- – sawing machine, metal W31.1
- – scissors W27.2
- – scorpion X58
- – screwdriver W27.0
  - ■ powered W29.8
- – sea
  - ■ anemone, cucumber or urchin (spine) X58
  - ■ lion W56.1-
- – sewing-machine (electric) (powered) W29.2
  - ■ not powered W27.8
- – shaft (hoist) (lift) (transmission) NEC W24.0
  - ■ agricultural W30.89
- – shark W56.4-
- – shears (hand) W27.2
  - ■ powered (industrial) W31.1
    - ~ domestic W29.2
- – sheep W55.3-
- – shovel W27.8
- – snake (nonvenomous) W59.11
- – spade W27.1
- – spider (venomous) X58
- – spin-drier W29.2
- – spinning machine W31.89
- – splinter W45.8
- – sports equipment W21.9
- – staple gun (powered) W29.8
- – steam X13.1
  - ■ engine W31.3
  - ■ inhalation X13.0
  - ■ pipe X16
  - ■ shovel W31.89
- – stove (hot) (kitchen) X15.0
- – substance, hot NEC X19
  - ■ molten (metal) X18
- – sword W26.1
  - ■ assault X99.2
  - ■ stated as undetermined whether accidental or intentional Y28.2
- – tarantula X58
- – thresher W30.0
- – tin can lid W26.8
- – toad W62.1
- – toaster (hot) X15.1
- – tool W27.8
  - ■ hand (not powered) W27.8
    - ~ auger W27.0
    - ~ axe W27.0
    - ~ can opener W27.4
    - ~ chisel W27.0
    - ~ fork W27.4
    - ~ garden W27.1
    - ~ handsaw W27.0
    - ~ hoe W27.1
    - ~ ice-pick W27.4
    - ~ kitchen utensil W27.4
    - ~ manual
      - ◊ lawn mower W27.1
      - ◊ sewing machine W27.8
    - ~ meat grinder W27.4
    - ~ needle (sewing) W27.3
      - ◊ hypodermic W46.0
        - » contaminated W46.1
    - ~ paper cutter W27.5
    - ~ pitchfork W27.1
    - ~ rake W27.1
    - ~ scissors W27.2
    - ~ screwdriver W27.0
    - ~ specified NEC W27.8
    - ~ workbench W27.0
  - ■ hot X17
  - ■ powered W29.8
    - ~ blender W29.0
      - ◊ commercial W31.82
    - ~ can opener W29.0
      - ◊ commercial W31.82
    - ~ chainsaw W29.3
    - ~ clothes dryer W29.2
      - ◊ commercial W31.82
    - ~ dishwasher W29.2
      - ◊ commercial W31.82

CONTACT (ACCIDENTAL)–CONTACT (ACCIDENTAL)

Contact (accidental), *continued*
~ edger W29.3
~ electric fan W29.2
◊ commercial W31.82
~ electric knife W29.1
~ food processor W29.0
◊ commercial W31.82
~ garbage disposal W29.0
◊ commercial W31.82
~ garden tool W29.3
~ hedge trimmer W29.3
~ ice maker W29.0
◊ commercial W31.82
~ kitchen appliance W29.0
◊ commercial W31.82
~ lawn mower W28
~ meat grinder W29.0
◊ commercial W31.82
~ mixer W29.0
◊ commercial W31.82
~ rototiller W29.3
~ sewing machine W29.2
◊ commercial W31.82
~ washing machine W29.2
◊ commercial W31.82
– transmission device (belt, cable, chain, gear, pinion, shaft) W24.1
■ agricultural operations W30.89
– turbine (gas) (water-driven) W31.3
– turkey W61.4-
– turtle (nonvenomous) W59.2-
■ terrestrial W59.8-
– under-cutter W31.0
– vehicle
■ agricultural use (transport)—*see* Accident, transport, agricultural vehicle
~ not on public highway W30.81
■ industrial use (transport)—*see* Accident, transport, industrial vehicle
~ not on public highway W31.83
■ off-road use (transport)—*see* Accident, transport, all-terrain or off-road vehicle
~ not on public highway W31.83
– venomous animal/plant X58
– viper X58
– washing-machine (powered) W29.2
– wasp X58
– weaving-machine W31.89
– winch W24.0
■ agricultural operations W30.89
– wire NEC W24.0
■ agricultural operations W30.89
– wood slivers W45.8
– yellow jacket X58
– zebra W55.39

Coup de soleil X32

Crash
• aircraft (in transit) (powered) V95.9
– balloon V96.01
– fixed wing NEC (private) V95.21
■ commercial V95.31
– glider V96.21
■ hang V96.11
■ powered V95.11
– helicopter V95.01
– microlight V95.11
– nonpowered V96.9
■ specified NEC V96.8
– powered NEC V95.8
– stated as
■ homicide (attempt) Y08.81
■ suicide (attempt) X83.0
– ultralight V95.11
• transport vehicle NEC (*see also* Accident, transport) V89.9

Crushed (accidentally) X58
• between objects (moving) (stationary and moving) W23.0
– stationary W23.1
• by
– alligator W58.03
– avalanche NEC—*see* Landslide

Crushed (accidentally), *continued*
– cave-in W20.0
■ caused by cataclysmic earth surface movement—*see* Landslide
– crocodile W58.13
– crowd or human stampede W52
– falling
■ aircraft V97.39
■ earth, material W20.0
~ caused by cataclysmic earth surface movement—*see* Landslide
■ object NEC W20.8
– landslide NEC—*see* Landslide
– lizard (nonvenomous) W59.09
– machinery—*see* Contact, with, by type of machine
– reptile NEC W59.89
– snake (nonvenomous) W59.13
• in
– machinery—*see* Contact, with, by type of machine

Cut, cutting (any part of body) (accidental)—*see also* Contact, with, by object or machine
• during medical or surgical treatment as misadventure—*see* Index to Diseases and Injuries, Complications
• inflicted by other person—*see* Assault, cutting or piercing instrument
• machine NEC (*see also* Contact, with, by type of machine) W31.9
• self-inflicted—*see* Suicide, cutting or piercing instrument
• suicide (attempt)—*see* Suicide, cutting or piercing instrument

Cyclone (any injury) X37.1

D

Dehydration from lack of water X58

Deprivation X58

Derailment (accidental)
• railway (rolling stock) (train) (vehicle) (without antecedent collision) V81.7
– with antecedent collision—*see* Accident, transport, railway vehicle occupant
• streetcar (without antecedent collision) V82.7
– with antecedent collision—*see* Accident, transport, streetcar occupant

Descent
• parachute (voluntary) (without accident to aircraft) V97.29
– due to accident to aircraft—*see* Accident, transport, aircraft

Desertion X58

Destitution X58

Disability, late effect or sequela of injury—*see* Sequelae

Discharge (accidental)
• airgun W34.010
– assault X95.01
– stated as undetermined whether accidental or intentional Y24.0
• BB gun—*see* Discharge, airgun
• firearm (accidental) W34.00
– assault X95.9
– handgun (pistol) (revolver) W32.0
■ assault X93
■ stated as undetermined whether accidental or intentional Y22
– homicide (attempt) X95.9
– hunting rifle W33.02
■ assault X94.1
■ stated as undetermined whether accidental or intentional Y23.1
– larger W33.00
■ assault X94.9
■ hunting rifle—*see* Discharge, firearm, hunting rifle
■ shotgun—*see* Discharge, firearm, shotgun
■ specified NEC W33.09
~ assault X94.8
~ stated as undetermined whether accidental or intentional Y23.8
■ stated as undetermined whether accidental or intentional Y23.9

Discharge (accidental), *continued*
■ using rubber bullet
~ injuring
◊ bystander Y35.042
◊ law enforcement personnel Y35.041
◊ suspect Y35.043
– machine gun W33.03
■ assault X94.2
■ stated as undetermined whether accidental or intentional Y23.3
– pellet gun—*see* Discharge, airgun
– shotgun W33.01
■ assault X94.0
■ stated as undetermined whether accidental or intentional Y23.0
– specified NEC W34.09
■ assault X95.8
■ stated as undetermined whether accidental or intentional Y24.8
– stated as undetermined whether accidental or intentional Y24.9
– Very pistol W34.09
■ assault X95.8
■ stated as undetermined whether accidental or intentional Y24.8
• firework(s) W39
– stated as undetermined whether accidental or intentional Y25
• gas-operated gun NEC W34.018
– airgun—*see* Discharge, airgun
– assault X95.09
– paintball gun—*see* Discharge, paintball gun
– stated as undetermined whether accidental or intentional Y24.8
• gun NEC—*see also* Discharge, firearm NEC
– air—*see* Discharge, airgun
– BB—*see* Discharge, airgun
– for single hand use—*see* Discharge, firearm, handgun
– hand—*see* Discharge, firearm, handgun
– machine—*see* Discharge, firearm, machine gun
– other specified—*see* Discharge, firearm NEC
– paintball—*see* Discharge, paintball gun
– pellet—*see* Discharge, airgun
• handgun—*see* Discharge, firearm, handgun
• machine gun—*see* Discharge, firearm, machine gun
• paintball gun W34.011
– assault X95.02
– stated as undetermined whether accidental or intentional Y24.8
• rifle (hunting)—*see* Discharge, firearm, hunting rifle
• shotgun—*see* Discharge, firearm, shotgun
• spring-operated gun NEC W34.018
– assault / homicide (attempt) X95.09
– stated as undetermined whether accidental or intentional Y24.8

Diver's disease, palsy, paralysis, squeeze—*see* Air, pressure

Diving (into water)—*see* Accident, diving

Dog bite W54.0

Dragged by transport vehicle NEC (*see also* Accident, transport) V09.9

Drinking poison (accidental)—*see* Table of Drugs and Chemicals

Dropped (accidentally) while being carried or supported by other person W04

Drowning (accidental) W74
• assault X92.9
• due to
– accident (to)
■ machinery—*see* Contact, with, by type of machine
■ watercraft V90.89
~ burning V90.29
◊ powered V90.2-
◊ unpowered V90.2-
~ crushed V90.39
◊ powered V90.3-
◊ unpowered V90.3-
~ overturning V90.09
◊ powered V90.0-
◊ unpowered V90.0-

Drowning (accidental), *continued*
- ~ sinking V90.19
  - ◊ powered V90.1-
  - ◊ unpowered V90.1-
- ~ specified type NEC V90.89
  - ◊ powered V90.8-
  - ◊ unpowered V90.8-
- – avalanche—*see* Landslide
- – cataclysmic
  - ■ earth surface movement NEC—*see* Forces of nature, earth movement
  - ■ storm—*see* Forces of nature, cataclysmic storm
- – cloudburst X37.8
- – cyclone X37.1
- – fall overboard (from) V92.09
  - ■ powered craft V92.0-
  - ■ unpowered craft V92.0-
  - ■ resulting from
    - ~ accident to watercraft—*see* Drowning, due to, accident to, watercraft
    - ~ being washed overboard (from) V92.29
      - ◊ powered craft V92.2-
      - ◊ unpowered craft V92.2-
    - ~ motion of watercraft V92.19
      - ◊ powered craft V92.1-
      - ◊ unpowered craft V92.1-
- – hurricane X37.0
- – jumping into water from watercraft (involved in accident)—*see also* Drowning, due to, accident to, watercraft
  - ■ without accident to or on watercraft W16.711
- – torrential rain X37.8
- • following
  - – fall
    - ■ into
      - ~ bathtub W16.211
      - ~ bucket W16.221
      - ~ fountain—*see* Drowning, following, fall, into, water, specified NEC
      - ~ quarry—*see* Drowning, following, fall, into, water, specified NEC
      - ~ reservoir—*see* Drowning, following, fall, into, water, specified NEC
      - ~ swimming-pool W16.011
        - ◊ striking
          - » bottom W16.021
          - » wall W16.031
        - ◊ stated as undetermined whether accidental or intentional Y21.3
      - ~ water NOS W16.41
        - ◊ natural (lake) (open sea) (river) (stream) (pond) W16.111
          - » striking
            - ❖ bottom W16.121
            - ❖ side W16.131
        - ◊ specified NEC W16.311
          - » striking
            - ❖ bottom W16.321
            - ❖ wall W16.331
    - ■ overboard NEC—*see* Drowning, due to, fall overboard
  - – jump or dive
    - ■ from boat W16.711
      - ~ striking bottom W16.721
    - ■ into
      - ~ fountain—*see* Drowning, following, jump or dive, into, water, specified NEC
      - ~ quarry—*see* Drowning, following, jump or dive, into, water, specified NEC
      - ~ reservoir—*see* Drowning, following, jump or dive, into, water, specified NEC
      - ~ swimming-pool W16.511
        - ◊ striking
          - » bottom W16.521
          - » wall W16.531
      - ~ water NOS W16.91
        - ◊ natural (lake) (open sea) (river) (stream) (pond) W16.611
        - ◊ specified NEC W16.811
          - » striking
            - ❖ bottom W16.821
            - ❖ wall W16.831
        - ◊ striking bottom W16.621

Drowning (accidental), *continued*
- • in
  - – bathtub (accidental) W65
    - ■ assault X92.0
    - ■ following fall W16.211
      - ~ stated as undetermined whether accidental or intentional Y21.1
    - ■ stated as undetermined whether accidental or intentional Y21.0
  - – lake—*see* Drowning, in, natural water
  - – natural water (lake) (open sea) (river) (stream) (pond) W69
    - ■ assault X92.3
    - ■ following
      - ~ dive or jump W16.611
        - ◊ striking bottom W16.621
      - ~ fall W16.111
        - ◊ striking
          - » bottom W16.121
          - » side W16.131
    - ■ stated as undetermined whether accidental or intentional Y21.4
  - – quarry—*see* Drowning, in, specified place NEC
  - – quenching tank—*see* Drowning, in, specified place NEC
  - – reservoir—*see* Drowning, in, specified place NEC
  - – river—*see* Drowning, in, natural water
  - – sea—*see* Drowning, in, natural water
  - – specified place NEC W73
    - ■ assault X92.8
    - ■ following
      - ~ dive or jump W16.811
        - ◊ striking
          - » bottom W16.821
          - » wall W16.831
      - ~ fall W16.311
        - ◊ striking
          - » bottom W16.321
          - » wall W16.331
    - ■ stated as undetermined whether accidental or intentional Y21.8
  - – stream—*see* Drowning, in, natural water
  - – swimming-pool W67
    - ■ assault X92.1
      - ~ following fall X92.2
    - ■ following
      - ~ dive or jump W16.511
        - ◊ striking
          - » bottom W16.521
          - » wall W16.531
      - ~ fall W16.011
        - ◊ striking
          - » bottom W16.021
          - » wall W16.031
    - ■ stated as undetermined whether accidental or intentional Y21.2
      - ~ following fall Y21.3
      - ~ following fall X71.2
- • resulting from accident to watercraft *see* Drowning, due to, accident, watercraft
- • self-inflicted X71.9
- • stated as undetermined whether accidental or intentional Y21.9

E

Earth (surface) movement NEC—*see* Forces of nature, earth movement

Earth falling (on) W20.0
- • caused by cataclysmic earth surface movement or eruption—*see* Landslide

Earthquake (any injury) X34

Effect(s) (adverse) of
- • air pressure (any)-—*see* Air, pressure
- • cold, excessive (exposure to)—*see* Exposure, cold
- • heat (excessive)—*see* Heat
- • hot place (weather)—*see* Heat
- • insolation X30
- • late—*see* Sequelae
- • motion—*see* Motion
- • radiation—*see* Radiation
- • travel—*see* Travel

Electric shock (accidental) (by) (in)—*see* Exposure, electric current

Electrocution (accidental)—*see* Exposure, electric current

Endotracheal tube wrongly placed during anesthetic procedure

Entanglement
- • in
  - – bed linen, causing suffocation—*see* category T71
  - – wheel of pedal cycle V19.88

Entry of foreign body or material—*see* Foreign body

Environmental pollution related condition- *see* Z57

Exhaustion
- • cold—*see* Exposure, cold
- • due to excessive exertion—*see* category Y93
- • heat—*see* Heat

Explosion (accidental) (of) (with secondary fire) W40.9
- • acetylene W40.1
- • aerosol can W36.1
- • air tank (compressed) (in machinery) W36.2
- • aircraft (in transit) (powered) NEC V95.9
  - – balloon V96.05
  - – fixed wing NEC (private) V95.25
    - ■ commercial V95.35
  - – glider V96.25
    - ■ hang V96.15
    - ■ powered V95.15
  - – helicopter V95.05
  - – microlight V95.15
  - – nonpowered V96.9
    - ■ specified NEC V96.8
  - – powered NEC V95.8
  - – ultralight V95.15
- • anesthetic gas in operating room W40.1
- • bicycle tire W37.0
- • blasting (cap) (materials) W40.0
- • boiler (machinery), not on transport vehicle W35
  - – on watercraft—*see* Explosion, in, watercraft
- • butane W40.1
- • caused by other person X96.9
- • coal gas W40.1
- • detonator W40.0
- • dump (munitions) W40.8
- • dynamite W40.0
  - – in
    - ■ assault X96.8
- • explosive (material) W40.9
  - – gas W40.1
  - – specified NEC W40.8
    - ■ in
- • factory (munitions) W40.8
- • firearm (parts) NEC W34.19
  - – airgun W34.110
  - – BB gun W34.110
  - – gas, air or spring-operated gun NEC W34.118
  - – handgun W32.1
  - – hunting rifle W33.12
  - – larger firearm W33.10
    - ■ specified NEC W33.19
  - – machine gun W33.13
  - – paintball gun W34.111
  - – pellet gun W34.110
  - – shotgun W33.11
  - – Very pistol [flare] W34.19
- • fire-damp W40.1
- • fireworks W39
- • gas (coal) (explosive) W40.1
  - – cylinder W36.9
    - ■ aerosol can W36.1
    - ■ air tank W36.2
    - ■ pressurized W36.3
    - ■ specified NEC W36.8
- • gasoline (fumes) (tank) not in moving motor vehicle W40.1
  - – in motor vehicle—*see* Accident, transport, by type of vehicle
- • grain store W40.8
- • handgun (parts)—*see* Explosion, firearm, handgun (parts)
- • homicide (attempt) X96.9
  - – specified NEC X96.8
- • hose, pressurized W37.8

EXPLOSION (ACCIDENTAL) (OF) (WITH SECONDARY FIRE)–EXPOSURE (TO)

Explosion (accidental) (of) (with secondary fire), continued
- hot water heater, tank (in machinery) W35
  - on watercraft—see Explosion, in, watercraft
- in, on
  - dump W40.8
  - factory W40.8
  - watercraft V93.59
    - powered craft V93.53
      - ferry boat V93.51
      - fishing boat V93.52
      - jet skis V93.53
      - liner V93.51
      - merchant ship V93.50
      - passenger ship V93.51
      - sailboat V93.54
- machinery—see also Contact, with, by type of machine
  - on board watercraft—see Explosion, in, watercraft
  - pressure vessel—see Explosion, by type of vessel
- methane W40.1
- missile NEC W40.8
- munitions (dump) (factory) W40.8
- pipe, pressurized W37.8
- pressure, pressurized
  - cooker W38
  - gas tank (in machinery) W36.3
  - hose W37.8
  - pipe W37.8
  - specified device NEC W38
  - tire W37.8
    - bicycle W37.0
  - vessel (in machinery) W38
- propane W40.1
- self-inflicted X75
- steam or water lines (in machinery) W37.8
- stove W40.9
- stated as undetermined whether accidental or intentional Y25
- tire, pressurized W37.8
  - bicycle W37.0
- undetermined whether accidental or intentional Y25
- vehicle tire NEC W37.8
  - bicycle W37.0

Exposure (to) X58
- air pressure change—see Air, pressure
- cold (accidental) (excessive) (extreme) (natural) (place) X31
  - assault Y08.89
  - due to
    - man-made conditions W93.8
      - dry ice (contact) W93.01
        - inhalation W93.02
      - liquid air (contact) (hydrogen) (nitrogen) W93.11
        - inhalation W93.12
      - refrigeration unit (deep freeze) W93.2
    - weather (conditions) X31
  - self-inflicted X83.2
- due to abandonment or neglect X58
- electric current W86.8
  - appliance (faulty) W86.8
    - domestic W86.0
  - caused by other person Y08.89
  - conductor (faulty) W86.1
  - control apparatus (faulty) W86.1
  - electric power generating plant, distribution station W86.1
  - electroshock gun—see Exposure, electric current, taser
  - high-voltage cable W85
  - lightning—see subcategory T75.0
  - live rail W86.8
  - misadventure in medical or surgical procedure in electroshock therapy Y63.4
  - motor (electric) (faulty) W86.8
    - domestic W86.0
  - self-inflicted X83.1
  - specified NEC W86.8
    - domestic W86.0
  - stun gun—see Exposure, electric current, taser
  - taser W86.8
    - assault Y08.89
    - self-harm (intentional) X83.8
    - undetermined intent Y33

Exposure (to), continued
  - third rail W86.8
  - transformer (faulty) W86.1
  - transmission lines W85
- environmental tobacco smoke X58
- excessive
  - cold—see Exposure, cold
  - heat (natural) NEC X30
    - man-made W92
- factor(s) NOS X58
  - environmental NEC X58
    - man-made NEC W99
    - natural NEC—see Forces of nature
  - specified NEC X58
- fire, flames (accidental) X08.8
  - assault X97
  - campfire—see Exposure, fire, controlled, not in building
  - controlled (in)
    - with ignition (of) clothing (see also Ignition, clothes) X06.2
      - nightwear X05
    - bonfire—see Exposure, fire, controlled, not in building
    - brazier (in building or structure)—see also Exposure, fire, controlled, building
      - not in building or structure—see Exposure, fire, controlled, not in building
    - building or structure X02.0
      - with
        - fall from building X02.3
        - injury due to building collapse X02.2
        - from building X02.5
        - smoke inhalation X02.1
      - hit by object from building X02.4
      - specified mode of injury NEC X02.8
    - fireplace, furnace or stove—see Exposure, fire, controlled, building
    - not in building or structure X03.0
      - with
        - fall X03.3
        - smoke inhalation X03.1
      - hit by object X03.4
      - specified mode of injury NEC X03.8
    - trash—see Exposure, fire, controlled, not in building
  - fireplace—see Exposure, fire, controlled, building
  - fittings or furniture (in building or structure) (uncontrolled)—see Exposure, fire, uncontrolled, building
  - forest (uncontrolled)—see Exposure, fire, uncontrolled, not in building
  - grass (uncontrolled)—see Exposure, fire, uncontrolled, not in building
  - hay (uncontrolled)—see Exposure, fire, uncontrolled, not in building
  - ignition of highly flammable material X04
  - in, of, on, starting in
    - machinery—see Contact, with, by type of machine
    - motor vehicle (in motion) (see also Accident, transport, occupant by type of vehicle) V87.8
      - with collision—see Collision
    - railway rolling stock, train, vehicle V81.81
      - with collision—see Accident, transport, railway vehicle occupant
    - street car (in motion) V82.8
      - with collision—see Accident, transport, streetcar occupant
    - transport vehicle NEC—see also Accident, transport
      - with collision—see Collision
    - watercraft (in transit) (not in transit) V91.09
      - localized—see Burn, on board watercraft, due to, fire on board
      - powered craft V91.03
        - ferry boat V91.01
        - fishing boat V91.02
        - jet skis V91.03
        - liner V91.01
        - merchant ship V91.00
        - passenger ship V91.01

Exposure (to), continued
      - unpowered craft V91.08
        - canoe V91.05
        - inflatable V91.06
        - kayak V91.05
        - sailboat V91.04
        - surf-board V91.08
        - waterskis V91.07
        - windsurfer V91.08
  - lumber (uncontrolled)—see Exposure, fire, uncontrolled, not in building
  - prairie (uncontrolled)—see Exposure, fire, uncontrolled, not in building
  - resulting from
    - explosion—see Explosion
    - lightning X08.8
  - self-inflicted X76
  - specified NEC X08.8
  - started by other person X97
  - stove—see Exposure, fire, controlled, building
  - stated as undetermined whether accidental or intentional Y26
  - tunnel (uncontrolled)—see Exposure, fire, uncontrolled, not in building
  - uncontrolled
    - in building or structure X00.0
      - with
        - fall from building X00.3
        - injury due to building collapse X00.2
        - jump from building X00.5
        - smoke inhalation X00.1
      - bed X08.00
        - due to
          - cigarette X08.01
          - specified material NEC X08.09
      - furniture NEC X08.20
        - due to
          - cigarette X08.21
          - specified material NEC X08.29
      - hit by object from building X00.4
      - sofa X08.10
        - due to
          - cigarette X08.11
          - specified material NEC X08.19
      - specified mode of injury NEC X00.8
    - not in building or structure (any) X01.0
      - with
        - fall X01.3
        - smoke inhalation X01.1
      - hit by object X01.4
      - specified mode of injury NEC X01.8
  - undetermined whether accidental or intentional Y26
- forces of nature NEC—see Forces of nature
- G-forces (abnormal) W49.9
- gravitational forces (abnormal) W49.9
- heat (natural) NEC—see Heat
- high-pressure jet (hydraulic) (pneumatic) W49.9
- hydraulic jet W49.9
- inanimate mechanical force W49.9
- jet, high-pressure (hydraulic) (pneumatic) W49.9
- lightning—see subcategory T75.0
  - causing fire—see Exposure, fire
- mechanical forces NEC W49.9
  - animate NEC W64
  - inanimate NEC W49.9
- noise W42.9
  - supersonic W42.0
- noxious substance—see Table of Drugs and Chemicals
- pneumatic jet W49.9
- prolonged in deep-freeze unit or refrigerator W93.2
- radiation—see Radiation
- smoke—see also Exposure, fire
  - tobacco, second hand Z77.22
- specified factors NEC X58
- sunlight X32
  - man-made (sun lamp) W89.8
    - tanning bed W89.1
- supersonic waves W42.0
- transmission line(s), electric W85
- vibration W49.9

Exposure (to), *continued*
- waves
  - infrasound W49.9
  - sound W42.9
  - supersonic W42.0
- weather NEC—*see* Forces of nature

External cause status Y99.9
- child assisting in compensated work for family Y99.8
- civilian activity done for financial or other compensation Y99.0
- civilian activity done for income or pay Y99.0
- family member assisting in compensated work for other family member Y99.8
- hobby not done for income Y99.8
- leisure activity Y99.8
- military activity Y99.1
- off-duty activity of military personnel Y99.8
- recreation or sport not for income or while a student Y99.8
- specified NEC Y99.8
- student activity Y99.8
- volunteer activity Y99.2

F

Factors, supplemental
- alcohol
  - blood level Y90.-
- environmental-pollution-related condition- *see* Z57
- nosocomial condition Y95
- work-related condition Y99.0

Failure
- in suture or ligature during surgical procedure Y65.2
- mechanical, of instrument or apparatus (any) (during any medical or surgical procedure) Y65.8
- sterile precautions (during medical and surgical care)—*see* Misadventure, failure, sterile precautions, by type of procedure
- to
  - introduce tube or instrument Y65.4
    - endotracheal tube during anesthesia Y65.3
  - make curve (transport vehicle) NEC—*see* Accident, transport
  - remove tube or instrument Y65.4

Fall, falling (accidental) W19
- building W20.1
  - burning (uncontrolled fire) X00.3
- down
  - embankment W17.81
  - escalator W10.0
  - hill W17.81
  - ladder W11
  - ramp W10.2
  - stairs, steps W10.9
- due to
  - bumping against
    - object W18.00
      - ~ sharp glass W18.02
      - ~ specified NEC W18.09
      - ~ sports equipment W18.01
    - person W03
      - ~ due to ice or snow W00.0
      - ~ on pedestrian conveyance—*see* Accident, transport, pedestrian, conveyance
  - collision with another person W03
    - due to ice or snow W00.0
    - involving pedestrian conveyance—*see* Accident, transport, pedestrian, conveyance
  - grocery cart tipping over W17.82
  - ice or snow W00.9
    - from one level to another W00.2
      - ~ on stairs or steps W00.1
    - involving pedestrian conveyance—*see* Accident, transport, pedestrian, conveyance
    - on same level W00.0
  - slipping (on moving sidewalk) W01.0
    - with subsequent striking against object W01.10
      - ~ furniture W01.190
      - ~ sharp object W01.119
        - ◊ glass W01.110
        - ◊ power tool or machine W01.111

Fall, falling (accidental), *continued*
- ◊ specified NEC W01.118
- ~ specified NEC W01.198
- striking against
  - object W18.00
    - ~ sharp glass W18.02
    - ~ specified NEC W18.09
    - ~ sports equipment W18.01
  - person W03
    - ~ due to ice or snow W00.0
    - ~ on pedestrian conveyance—*see* Accident, transport, pedestrian, conveyance
- earth (with asphyxia or suffocation (by pressure))—*see* Earth, falling
- from, off, out of
  - aircraft NEC (with accident to aircraft NEC) V97.0
    - while boarding or alighting V97.1
  - balcony W13.0
  - bed W06
  - boat, ship, watercraft NEC (with drowning or submersion)—*see* Drowning, due to, fall overboard
    - with hitting bottom or object V94.0
  - bridge W13.1
  - building W13.9
    - burning (uncontrolled fire) X00.3
  - cavity W17.2
  - chair W07
  - cherry picker W17.89
  - cliff W15
  - dock W17.4
  - embankment W17.81
  - escalator W10.0
  - flagpole W13.8
  - furniture NEC W08
  - grocery cart W17.82
  - haystack W17.89
  - high place NEC W17.89
    - stated as undetermined whether accidental or intentional Y30
  - hole W17.2
  - incline W10.2
  - ladder W11
  - lifting device W17.89
  - machine, machinery—*see also* Contact, with, by type of machine
    - not in operation W17.89
  - manhole W17.1
  - mobile elevated work platform [MEWP] W17.89
  - motorized mobility scooter W05.2
  - one level to another NEC W17.89
    - intentional, purposeful, suicide (attempt) X80
    - stated as undetermined whether accidental or intentional Y30
  - pit W17.2
  - playground equipment W09.8
    - jungle gym W09.2
    - slide W09.0
    - swing W09.1
  - quarry W17.89
  - railing W13.9
  - ramp W10.2
  - roof W13.2
  - scaffolding W12
  - scooter (nonmotorized) W05.1
    - motorized mobility W05.2
  - sky lift W17.89
  - stairs, steps W10.9
    - curb W10.1
    - due to ice or snow W00.1
    - escalator W10.0
    - incline W10.2
    - ramp W10.2
    - sidewalk curb W10.1
    - specified NEC W10.8
    - standing
      - ~ electric scooter V00.841
      - ~ micro-mobility pedestrian conveyance V00.848
  - stepladder W11
  - storm drain W17.1
  - streetcar NEC V82.6
    - with antecedent collision—*see* Accident, transport, streetcar occupant
    - while boarding or alighting V82.4

Fall, falling (accidental), *continued*
- structure NEC W13.8
  - burning (uncontrolled fire) X00.3
- table W08
- toilet W18.11
  - with subsequent striking against object W18.12
- train NEC V81.6
  - during derailment (without antecedent collision) V81.7
    - ~ with antecedent collision—*see* Accident, transport, railway vehicle occupant
  - while boarding or alighting V81.4
- transport vehicle after collision—*see* Accident, transport, by type of vehicle, collision
- tree W14
- vehicle (in motion) NEC (*see also* Accident, transport) V89.9
  - motor NEC (*see also* Accident, transport, occupant, by type of vehicle) V87.8
  - stationary W17.89
    - ~ while boarding or alighting—*see* Accident, transport, by type of vehicle, while boarding or alighting
- viaduct W13.8
- wall W13.8
- watercraft—*see also* Drowning, due to, fall overboard
  - with hitting bottom or object V94.0
- well W17.0
- wheelchair, non-moving W05.0
  - powered—*see* Accident, transport, pedestrian, conveyance occupant, specified type NEC
- window W13.4
- in, on
  - aircraft NEC V97.0
    - with accident to aircraft V97.0
    - while boarding or alighting V97.1
  - bathtub (empty) W18.2
    - filled W16.212
      - ~ causing drowning W16.211
  - escalator W10.0
  - incline W10.2
  - ladder W11
  - machine, machinery—*see* Contact, with, by type of machine
  - object, edged, pointed or sharp (with cut)—*see* Fall, by type
  - playground equipment W09.8
    - jungle gym W09.2
    - slide W09.0
    - swing W09.1
  - ramp W10.2
  - scaffolding W12
  - shower W18.2
    - causing drowning W16.211
  - staircase, stairs, steps W10.9
    - curb W10.1
    - due to ice or snow W00.1
    - escalator W10.0
    - incline W10.2
    - specified NEC W10.8
  - streetcar (without antecedent collision) V82.5
    - with antecedent collision—*see* Accident, transport, streetcar occupant
    - while boarding or alighting V82.4
  - train (without antecedent collision) V81.5
    - with antecedent collision—*see* Accident, transport, railway vehicle occupant
    - during derailment (without antecedent collision) V81.7
      - ~ with antecedent collision—*see* Accident, transport, railway vehicle occupant
    - while boarding or alighting V81.4
  - transport vehicle after collision—*see* Accident, transport, by type of vehicle, collision
  - watercraft V93.39
    - due to
      - ~ accident to craft V91.29
        - ◊ powered craft V91.2-
        - ◊ unpowered craft V91.2-
    - powered craft V93.3-
    - unpowered craft V93.3-

Fall, falling (accidental), *continued*
- into
  - cavity W17.2
  - dock W17.4
  - fire—*see* Exposure, fire, by type
  - haystack W17.89
  - hole W17.2
  - lake—*see* Fall, into, water
  - manhole W17.1
  - moving part of machinery—*see* Contact, with, by type of machine
  - ocean—*see* Fall, into, water
  - opening in surface NEC W17.89
  - pit W17.2
  - pond—*see* Fall, into, water
  - quarry W17.89
  - river—*see* Fall, into, water
  - shaft W17.89
  - storm drain W17.1
  - stream—*see* Fall, into, water
  - swimming pool—*see also* Fall, into, water, in, swimming pool
    - empty W17.3
  - tank W17.89
  - water W16.42
    - causing drowning W16.41
    - from watercraft—*see* Drowning, due to, fall overboard
    - hitting diving board W21.4
    - in
      - ~ bathtub W16.212
        - ◊ causing drowning W16.211
      - ~ bucket W16.222
        - ◊ causing drowning W16.221
      - ~ natural body of water W16.112
        - ◊ causing drowning W16.111
        - ◊ striking
          - » bottom W16.122
            - ❖ causing drowning W16.121
          - » side W16.132
            - ❖ causing drowning W16.131
      - ~ specified water NEC W16.312
        - ◊ causing drowning W16.311
        - ◊ striking
          - » bottom W16.322
            - ❖ causing drowning W16.321
          - » wall W16.332
            - ❖ causing drowning W16.331
      - ~ swimming pool W16.012
        - ◊ causing drowning W16.011
        - ◊ striking
          - » bottom W16.022
            - ❖ causing drowning W16.021
          - » wall W16.032
            - » causing drowning W16.031
      - ~ utility bucket W16.222
        - ◊ causing drowning W16.221
  - well W17.0
- involving
  - bed W06
  - chair W07
  - furniture NEC W08
  - glass—*see* Fall, by type
  - playground equipment W09.8
    - jungle gym W09.2
    - slide W09.0
    - swing W09.1
  - roller blades—*see* Accident, transport, pedestrian, conveyance
  - skateboard(s)—*see* Accident, transport, pedestrian, conveyance
  - skates (ice) (in line) (roller)—*see* Accident, transport, pedestrian, conveyance
  - skis—*see* Accident, transport, pedestrian, conveyance
  - table W08
  - wheelchair, non-moving W05.0
    - powered—*see* Accident, transport, pedestrian, conveyance, specified type NEC
- object—*see* Struck by, object, falling
- off
  - toilet W18.11
    - with subsequent striking against object W18.12

Fall, falling (accidental), *continued*
- on same level W18.30
  - due to
    - specified NEC W18.39
    - stepping on an object W18.31
- out of
  - bed W06
  - building NEC W13.8
  - chair W07
  - furniture NEC W08
  - wheelchair, non-moving W05.0
    - powered—*see* Accident, transport, pedestrian, conveyance, specified type NEC
  - window W13.4
- over
  - animal W01.0
  - cliff W15
  - embankment W17.81
  - small object W01.0
- rock W20.8
- same level W18.30
  - from
    - being crushed, pushed, or stepped on by a crowd or human stampede W52
    - collision, pushing, shoving, by or with other person W03
    - slipping, stumbling, tripping W01.0
  - involving ice or snow W00.0
    - involving skates (ice) (roller), skateboard, skis—*see* Accident, transport, pedestrian, conveyance
- snowslide (avalanche)—*see* Landslide
- stone W20.8
- structure W20.1
  - burning (uncontrolled fire) X00.3
- through
  - bridge W13.1
  - floor W13.3
  - roof W13.2
  - wall W13.8
  - window W13.4
- timber W20.8
- tree (caused by lightning) W20.8
- while being carried or supported by other person(s) W04

Fallen on by
- animal (not being ridden) NEC W55.89

Felo-de-se—*see* Suicide

Fight (hand) (fists) (foot)—*see* Assault, fight

Fire (accidental)—*see* Exposure, fire

Firearm discharge—*see* Discharge, firearm

Fireworks (explosion) W39

Flash burns from explosion—*see* Explosion

Flood (any injury) (caused by) X38
- collapse of man-made structure causing earth movement X36.0
- tidal wave—*see* Forces of nature, tidal wave

Food (any type) in
- air passages (with asphyxia, obstruction, or suffocation) (*see* categories T17 and) T18
- alimentary tract causing asphyxia (due to compression of trachea) (*see* categories T17 and) T18

Forces of nature X39.8
- avalanche X36.1
  - causing transport accident—*see* Accident, transport, by type of vehicle
- blizzard X37.2
- cataclysmic storm X37.9
  - with flood X38
  - blizzard X37.2
  - cloudburst X37.8
  - cyclone X37.1
  - dust storm X37.3
  - hurricane X37.0
  - specified storm NEC X37.8
  - storm surge X37.0
  - tornado X37.1
  - twister X37.1
  - typhoon X37.0
- cloudburst X37.8
- cold (natural) X31

Fall, falling (accidental), *continued*
- cyclone X37.1
- dam collapse causing earth movement X36.0
- dust storm X37.3
- earth movement X36.1
  - earthquake X34
  - caused by dam or structure collapse X36.0
- earthquake X34
- flood (caused by) X38
  - dam collapse X36.0
  - tidal wave—*see* Forces of nature, tidal wave
- heat (natural) X30
- hurricane X37.0
- landslide X36.1
  - causing transport accident—*see* Accident, transport, by type of vehicle
- lightning—*see* subcategory T75.0
  - causing fire—*see* Exposure, fire
- mudslide X36.1
  - causing transport accident—*see* Accident, transport, by type of vehicle
- specified force NEC X39.8
- storm surge X37.0
- structure collapse causing earth movement X36.0
- sunlight X32
- tidal wave X37.41
  - due to
    - earthquake X37.41
    - landslide X37.43
    - storm X37.42
    - volcanic eruption X37.41
- tornado X37.1
- tsunami X37.41
- twister X37.1
- typhoon X37.0
- volcanic eruption X35

Foreign body
- aspiration—*see* Index to Diseases and Injuries, Foreign body, respiratory tract
- entering through skin W45.8
  - can lid W26.8
  - nail W45.0
  - paper W26.2
  - specified NEC W45.8
  - splinter W45.8

Forest fire (exposure to)—*see* Exposure, fire, uncontrolled, not in building

Found injured X58
- from exposure (to)—*see* Exposure
- on
  - highway, road (way), street V89.9
  - railway right of way V81.9

Fracture (circumstances unknown or unspecified) X58
- due to specified cause NEC X58

Frostbite X31
- due to man-made conditions—*see* Exposure, cold, man-made

Frozen—*see* Exposure, cold

G

Gunshot wound W34.00

H

Hailstones, injured by X39.8

Hanged herself or himself—*see* Hanging, self-inflicted

Hanging (accidental) (*see also* category) T71

Heat (effects of) (excessive) X30
- due to
  - man-made conditions W92
    - on board watercraft V93.29
      - ~ fishing boat V93.22
      - ~ merchant ship V93.20
      - ~ passenger ship V93.21
      - ~ sailboat V93.24
      - ~ specified powered craft NEC V93.23
  - weather (conditions) X30
- from
  - electric heating apparatus causing burning X16

Heat (effects of) (excessive), *continued*
- inappropriate in local application or packing in medical or surgical procedure Y63.5

Hemorrhage
- delayed following medical or surgical treatment without mention of misadventure—*see* Index to Diseases and Injuries, Complication(s)
- during medical or surgical treatment as misadventure—*see* Index to Diseases and Injuries, Complication(s)

High
- altitude (effects)—*see* Air, pressure, low
- level of radioactivity, effects—*see* Radiation
- pressure (effects)-—*see* Air, pressure, high
- temperature, effects—*see* Heat
- **Hit, hitting (accidental) by**—*see* Struck by
- **Hitting against**—*see* Striking against
- **Hot**
- place, effects—*see also* Heat
- weather, effects X30

House fire (uncontrolled)—*see* Exposure, fire, uncontrolled, building

Humidity, causing problem X39.8

Hunger X58

Hurricane (any injury) X37.0

Hypobarism, hypobaropathy—*see* Air, pressure, low

I

Ictus
- caloris—*see also* Heat
- solaris X30

Ignition (accidental) (*see also* Exposure, fire) X08.8
- anesthetic gas in operating room W40.1
- apparel X06.2
  - from highly flammable material X04
  - nightwear X05
- bed linen (sheets) (spreads) (pillows) (mattress)—*see* Exposure, fire, uncontrolled, building, bed
- benzine X04
- clothes, clothing NEC (from controlled fire) X06.2
  - from
    - highly flammable material X04
- ether X04
  - in operating room W40.1
- explosive material—*see* Explosion
- gasoline X04
- jewelry (plastic) (any) X06.0
- kerosene X04
- material
  - explosive—*see* Explosion
  - highly flammable with secondary explosion X04
- nightwear X05
- paraffin X04
- petrol X04

Immersion (accidental)—*see also* Drowning
- hand or foot due to cold (excessive) X31

Implantation of quills of porcupine W55.89

Inanition (from) (hunger) X58
- thirst X58

Inappropriate operation performed
- correct operation on wrong side or body part (wrong side) (wrong site) Y65.53
- operation intended for another patient done on wrong patient Y65.52
- wrong operation performed on correct patient Y65.51

Incident, adverse
- device
  - anesthesiology Y70.-
  - cardiovascular Y71.-
  - gastroenterology Y73.-
  - general
    - hospital Y74.-
    - surgical Y81.-
  - gynecological Y76.-
  - medical Y82.9
    - specified type NEC Y82.8
  - neurological Y75.-
  - obstetrical Y76.-
  - ophthalmic Y77.-

Incident, adverse, *continued*
  - orthopedic Y79.-
  - otorhinolaryngological Y72.-
  - personal use Y74.-
  - physical medicine Y80.-
  - plastic surgical Y81.-
  - radiological Y78.-
  - urology Y73.-

Incineration (accidental)—*see* Exposure, fire

Infanticide—*see* Assault

Infrasound waves (causing injury) W49.9

Ingestion
- foreign body (causing injury) (with obstruction) T17 or T18
- poisonous
  - plant(s) X58
  - substance NEC—*see* Table of Drugs and Chemicals

Inhalation
- excessively cold substance, man-made—*see* Exposure, cold, man-made
- food (any type) (into respiratory tract) (with asphyxia, obstruction respiratory tract, suffocation) (*see* categories T17 and) T18
- foreign body—*see* Foreign body, aspiration
- gastric contents (with asphyxia, obstruction respiratory passage, suffocation) T17.81-
- hot air or gases X14.0
- liquid air, hydrogen, nitrogen W93.12
- steam X13.0
  - assault X98.0
  - stated as undetermined whether accidental or intentional Y27.0
- toxic gas—*see* Table of Drugs and Chemicals
- vomitus (with asphyxia, obstruction respiratory passage, suffocation) T17.81-

Injury, injured (accidental(ly)) NOS X58
- by, caused by, from
  - assault—*see* Assault
- homicide (*see also* Assault) Y09
- inflicted (by)
  - other person
    - stated as
      - accidental X58
      - undetermined whether accidental or intentional Y33
- purposely (inflicted) by other person(s)—*see* Assault
- self-inflicted X83.8
  - stated as accidental X58
- specified cause NEC X58
- undetermined whether accidental or intentional Y33

Insolation, effects X30

Insufficient nourishment X58

Interruption of respiration (by)
- food (lodged in esophagus) (*see* categories T17 and) T18
- vomitus (lodged in esophagus) T17.81- Intoxication
- drug—*see* Table of Drugs and Chemicals
- poison—*see* Table of Drugs and Chemicals

J

Jammed (accidentally)
- between objects (moving) (stationary and moving) W23.0
  - stationary W23.1

Jumped, jumping
- before moving object NEC X81.8
  - motor vehicle X81.0
  - subway train X81.1
  - train X81.1
  - undetermined whether accidental or intentional Y31
- from
  - boat (into water) voluntarily, without accident (to or on boat) W16.712
    - with
      - accident to or on boat—*see* Accident, watercraft
      - drowning or submersion W16.711
    - striking bottom W16.722
      - causing drowning W16.721
  - building (*see also* Jumped, from, high place) W13.9
    - burning (uncontrolled fire) X00.5

Jumped, jumping, *continued*
  - high place NEC W17.89
    - suicide (attempt) X80
    - undetermined whether accidental or intentional Y30
  - structure (*see also* Jumped, from, high place) W13.9
    - burning (uncontrolled fire) X00.5
- into water W16.92
  - causing drowning W16.91
  - from, off watercraft—*see* Jumped, from, boat
  - in
    - natural body W16.612
      - causing drowning W16.611
      - striking bottom W16.622
        - causing drowning W16.621
    - specified place NEC W16.812
      - causing drowning W16.811
      - striking
        - bottom W16.822
          - causing drowning W16.821
        - wall W16.832
          - causing drowning W16.831
    - swimming pool W16.512
      - causing drowning W16.511
      - striking
        - bottom W16.522
          - causing drowning W16.521
        - wall W16.532
          - causing drowning W16.531

K

Kicked by
- animal NEC W55.82
- person(s) (accidentally) W50.1
  - with intent to injure or kill Y04.0
  - as, or caused by, a crowd or human stampede (with fall) W52
  - assault Y04.0
  - in
    - fight Y04.0

Kicking against
- object W22.8
  - sports equipment W21.9
  - stationary W22.09
    - sports equipment W21.89
- person—*see* Striking against, person
- sports equipment W21.9

Knocked down (accidentally) (by) NOS X58
- animal (not being ridden) NEC—*see also* Struck by, by type of animal
- crowd or human stampede W52
- person W51
  - in brawl, fight Y04.0
- transport vehicle NEC (*see also* Accident, transport) V09.9

L

Laceration NEC—*see* Injury

Lack of
- care (helpless person) (infant) (newborn) X58
- food except as result of abandonment or neglect X58
  - due to abandonment or neglect X58
- water except as result of transport accident X58
  - due to transport accident—*see* Accident, transport, by type
  - helpless person, infant, newborn X58

Landslide (falling on transport vehicle) X36.1
- caused by collapse of man-made structure X36.0

Late effect—*see* Sequelae

Lightning (shock) (stroke) (struck by)—*see* subcategory T75.0
- causing fire—*see* Exposure, fire

Loss of control (transport vehicle) NEC—*see* Accident, transport

Lying before train, vehicle or other moving object X81.8
- subway train X81.1
- train X81.1
- undetermined whether accidental or intentional Y31

MALFUNCTION (MECHANISM OR COMPONENT) (OF)—PLACE OF OCCURRENCE

M

Malfunction (mechanism or component) (of)
- firearm W34.10
  - airgun W34.110
  - BB gun W34.110
  - gas, air or spring-operated gun NEC W34.118
  - handgun W32.1
  - hunting rifle W33.12 larger firearm W33.10
    - specified NEC W33.19
  - machine gun W33.13
  - paintball gun W34.111
  - pellet gun W34.110
  - shotgun W33.11
  - specified NEC W34.19
  - Very pistol [flare] W34.19
- handgun—*see* Malfunction, firearm, handgun

Maltreatment—*see* Perpetrator

Mangled (accidentally) NOS X58

Manhandling (in brawl, fight) Y04.0

Manslaughter (nonaccidental)—*see* Assault

Mauled by animal NEC W55.89

Medical procedure, complication of (delayed or as an abnormal reaction without mention of misadventure)—*see* Complication of or following, by specified type of procedure
- due to or as a result of misadventure—*see* Misadventure

Melting (due to fire)—*see also* Exposure, fire
- apparel NEC X06.3
- clothes, clothing NEC X06.3
  - nightwear X05
- fittings or furniture (burning building) (uncontrolled fire) X00.8
- nightwear X05
- plastic jewelry X06.1

Mental cruelty X58

Military operations (injuries to military and civilians occurring during peacetime on military property and during routine military exercises and operations) (by) (from) (involving)—*Refer to ICD-10-CM Manual*

Misadventure(s) to patient(s) during surgical or medical care Y69
- contaminated medical or biological substance (blood, drug, fluid) Y64.9
  - administered (by) NEC Y64.9
    - immunization Y64.1
    - infusion Y64.0
    - injection Y64.1
    - specified means NEC Y64.8
    - transfusion Y64.0
    - vaccination Y64.1
- excessive amount of blood or other fluid during transfusion or infusion Y63.0
- failure
  - in dosage Y63.9
    - electroshock therapy Y63.4
    - inappropriate temperature (too hot or too cold) in local application and packing Y63.5
    - infusion
      - ~ excessive amount of fluid Y63.0
      - ~ incorrect dilution of fluid Y63.1
    - insulin-shock therapy Y63.4
    - nonadministration of necessary drug or biological substance Y63.6
    - overdose—*see* Table of Drugs and Chemicals
      - ~ radiation, in therapy Y63.2
    - radiation
      - ~ overdose Y63.2
    - specified procedure NEC Y63.8
    - transfusion
      - ~ excessive amount of blood Y63.0
  - mechanical, of instrument or apparatus (any) (during any procedure) Y65.8
  - sterile precautions (during procedure) Y62.9
    - aspiration of fluid or tissue (by puncture or catheterization, except heart) Y62.6
    - biopsy (except needle aspiration) Y62.8
      - ~ needle (aspirating) Y62.6
    - blood sampling Y62.6

Misadventure(s) to patient(s) during surgical or medical care, *continued*
- catheterization Y62.6
  - ~ heart Y62.5
- dialysis (kidney) Y62.2
- endoscopic examination Y62.4
- enema Y62.8
- immunization Y62.3
- infusion Y62.1
- injection Y62.3
- needle biopsy Y62.6
- paracentesis (abdominal) (thoracic) Y62.6
- perfusion Y62.2
- puncture (lumbar) Y62.6
- removal of catheter or packing Y62.8
- specified procedure NEC Y62.8
- surgical operation Y62.0
- transfusion Y62.1
- vaccination Y62.3
- suture or ligature during surgical procedure Y65.2
- to introduce or to remove tube or instrument—*see* Failure, to
- hemorrhage—*see* Index to Diseases and Injuries, Complication(s)
- inadvertent exposure of patient to radiation Y63.3
- inappropriate
  - operation performed—*see* Inappropriate operation performed
  - temperature (too hot or too cold) in local application or packing Y63.5
- infusion (*see also* Misadventure, by type, infusion) Y69
  - excessive amount of fluid Y63.0
  - incorrect dilution of fluid Y63.1
  - wrong fluid Y65.1
- nonadministration of necessary drug or biological substance Y63.6
- overdose—*see* Table of Drugs and Chemicals
  - radiation (in therapy) Y63.2
- perforation—*see* Index to Diseases and Injuries, Complication(s)
- performance of inappropriate operation—*see* Inappropriate operation performed
- puncture—*see* Index to Diseases and Injuries, Complication(s)
- specified type NEC Y65.8
  - failure
    - suture or ligature during surgical operation Y65.2
    - to introduce or to remove tube or instrument—*see* Failure, to
  - infusion of wrong fluid Y65.1
  - performance of inappropriate operation—*see* Inappropriate operation performed
  - transfusion of mismatched blood Y65.0
  - wrong
    - fluid in infusion Y65.1
    - placement of endotracheal tube during anesthetic procedure Y65.3
- transfusion—*see* Misadventure, by type, transfusion
  - excessive amount of blood Y63.0
  - mismatched blood Y65.0
- wrong
  - drug given in error—*see* Table of Drugs and Chemicals
  - fluid in infusion Y65.1
  - placement of endotracheal tube during anesthetic procedure Y65.3

Mismatched blood in transfusion Y65.0

Motion sickness T75.3

Mountain sickness W94.11

Mudslide (of cataclysmic nature)—*see* Landslide

N

Nail, contact with W45.0
- gun W29.4

Noise (causing injury) (pollution) W42.9
- supersonic W42.0

Nonadministration (of)
- drug or biological substance (necessary) Y63.6
- surgical and medical care Y66

Nosocomial condition Y95

O

Object
- falling
  - from, in, on, hitting
    - machinery—*see* Contact, with, by type of machine
- set in motion by
  - accidental explosion or rupture of pressure vessel W38
  - firearm—*see* Discharge, firearm, by type
  - machine(ry)—*see* Contact, with, by type of machine

Overdose (drug)—*see* Table of Drugs and Chemicals
- radiation Y63.2

Overexertion
- due to
  - other or unspecified movement X50.9
  - prolonged static or awkward postures X50.1
  - repetitive movements X50.3
  - strenuous movement X50.0

Overexposure (accidental) (to)
- cold (*see also* Exposure, cold) X31
  - due to man-made conditions—*see* Exposure, cold, man-made
- heat (*see also* Heat) X30
- radiation—*see* Radiation
- radioactivity W88.0
- sun (sunburn) X32
- weather NEC—*see* Forces of nature
- wind NEC—*see* Forces of nature

Overheated—*see* Heat

Overturning (accidental)
- machinery—*see* Contact, with, by type of machine
- transport vehicle NEC (*see also* Accident, transport) V89.9
- watercraft (causing drowning, submersion)—*see also* Drowning, due to, accident to, watercraft, overturning
  - causing injury except drowning or submersion—*see* Accident, watercraft, causing, injury NEC

P

Parachute descent (voluntary) (without accident to aircraft) V97.29
- due to accident to aircraft—*see* Accident, transport, aircraft

Pecked by bird W61.99

Perforation during medical or surgical treatment as misadventure—*see* Index to Diseases and Injuries, Complication(s)

Perpetrator, perpetration, of assault, maltreatment and neglect (by) Y07.-

Piercing—*see* Contact, with, by type of object or machine

Pinched
- between objects (moving) (stationary and moving) W23.0
  - stationary W23.1

Pinned under machine(ry)—*see* Contact, with, by type of machine

Place of occurrence Y92.9
- abandoned house Y92.89
- airplane Y92.813
- airport Y92.520
- ambulatory health services establishment NEC Y92.538
- ambulatory surgery center Y92.530
- amusement park Y92.831
- apartment (co-op) Y92.039
  - bathroom Y92.031
  - bedroom Y92.032
  - kitchen Y92.030
  - specified NEC Y92.038
- assembly hall Y92.29
- bank Y92.510
- barn Y92.71
- baseball field Y92.320
- basketball court Y92.310
- beach Y92.832
- boat Y92.814
- bowling alley Y92.39
- bridge Y92.89
- building under construction Y92.61

Place of occurrence, *continued*

- bus Y92.811
  - station Y92.521
- cafe Y92.511
- campsite Y92.833
- campus—*see* Place of occurrence, school
- canal Y92.89
- car Y92.810
- casino Y92.59
- church Y92.22
- cinema Y92.26
- clubhouse Y92.29
- coal pit Y92.64
- college (community) Y92.214
- condominium—*see* apartment
- construction area—Y92.6-
- convalescent home—Y92.129-
- court-house Y92.240
- cricket ground Y92.328
- cultural building Y92.25-
- dancehall Y92.252
- day nursery Y92.210
- dentist office Y92.531
- derelict house Y92.89
- desert Y92.820
- dock NOS Y92.89
- dockyard Y92.62
- doctor's office Y92.531
- dormitory—*see* institutional, school dormitory
- dry dock Y92.62
- factory (building) (premises) Y92.63
- farm (land under cultivation) (outbuildings) Y92.7-
- football field Y92.321
- forest Y92.821
- freeway Y92.411
- gallery Y92.250
- garage (commercial) Y92.59 (refer to specific residence)
- gas station Y92.524
- gasworks Y92.69
- golf course Y92.39
- gravel pit Y92.64
- grocery Y92.512
- gymnasium Y92.39
- handball court Y92.318
- harbor Y92.89
- harness racing course Y92.39
- healthcare provider office Y92.531
- highway (interstate) Y92.411
- hill Y92.828
- hockey rink Y92.330
- home—*see* residence
- hospice—Y92.129-
- hospital Y92.23-
  - patient room Y92.23-
- hotel Y92.59
- house—*see also* residence
  - abandoned Y92.89
  - under construction Y92.61
- industrial and construction area (yard) Y92.6-
- kindergarten Y92.211
- lacrosse field Y92.328
- lake Y92.828
- library Y92.241
- mall Y92.59
- market Y92.512
- marsh Y92.828
- military base—Y92.13-
- mosque Y92.22
- motel Y92.59
- motorway (interstate) Y92.411
- mountain Y92.828
- movie-house Y92.26
- museum Y92.251
- music-hall Y92.252
- not applicable Y92.9
- nuclear power station Y92.69
- nursing home—Y92.129-
- office building Y92.59
- offshore installation Y92.65
- opera-house Y92.253
- orphanage—Y92.11-
- outpatient surgery center Y92.530

Place of occurrence, *continued*

- park (public) Y92.830
  - amusement Y92.831
- parking garage Y92.89
  - lot Y92.481
- pavement Y92.480
- physician office Y92.531
- polo field Y92.328
- pond Y92.828
- post office Y92.242
- power station Y92.69
- prairie Y92.828
- prison—Y92.14-
- public
  - administration building Y92.24-
  - building NEC Y92.29
  - hall Y92.29
  - place NOS Y92.89
- race course Y92.39
- railway line (bridge) Y92.85
- ranch (outbuildings) Y92.7-
- recreation area Y92.838 (refer to specific sites)
- religious institution Y92.22
- reform school—*see* institutional, reform school
- residence (non-institutional) (private) Y92.009
  - apartment Y92.039
    - bathroom Y92.031
    - bedroom Y92.032
    - kitchen Y92.030
    - specified NEC Y92.038
  - boarding house Y92.04-
  - home, unspecified Y92.009
    - bathroom Y92.002
    - bedroom Y92.003
    - dining room Y92.001
    - garden Y92.007
    - kitchen Y92.000
  - house, single family Y92.019
    - bathroom Y92.012
    - bedroom Y92.013
    - dining room Y92.011
    - driveway Y92.014
    - garage Y92.015
    - garden Y92.017
    - kitchen Y92.010
    - specified NEC Y92.018
    - swimming pool Y92.016
    - yard Y92.017
  - institutional Y92.10
    - hospice Y92.12-
    - military base Y92.13-
    - nursing home Y92.12-
    - orphanage Y92.119
      - ~ bathroom Y92.111
      - ~ bedroom Y92.112
      - ~ driveway Y92.113
      - ~ garage Y92.114
      - ~ garden Y92.116
      - ~ kitchen Y92.110
      - ~ specified NEC Y92.118
      - ~ swimming pool Y92.115
      - ~ yard Y92.116
    - reform school Y92.15-
    - school dormitory Y92.169
      - ~ bathroom Y92.162
      - ~ bedroom Y92.163
      - ~ dining room Y92.161
      - ~ kitchen Y92.160
      - ~ specified NEC Y92.168
    - specified NEC Y92.199
      - ~ bathroom Y92.192
      - ~ bedroom Y92.193
      - ~ dining room Y92.191
      - ~ driveway Y92.194
      - ~ garage Y92.195
      - ~ garden Y92.197
      - ~ kitchen Y92.190
      - ~ specified NEC Y92.198
      - ~ swimming pool Y92.196
      - ~ yard Y92.197
  - mobile home Y92.029
    - bathroom Y92.022
    - bedroom Y92.023

Place of occurrence, *continued*

- dining room Y92.021
- driveway Y92.024
- garage Y92.025
- garden Y92.027
- kitchen Y92.020
- specified NEC Y92.028
- swimming pool Y92.026
- yard Y92.027
  - specified place in residence NEC Y92.008
  - specified residence type NEC Y92.09-
- restaurant Y92.511
- riding school Y92.39
- river Y92.828
- road Y92.410
- rodeo ring Y92.39
- rugby field Y92.328
- same day surgery center Y92.530
- sand pit Y92.64
- school (private) (public) (state) Y92.219
  - college Y92.214
  - daycare center Y92.210
  - elementary school Y92.211
  - high school Y92.213
  - kindergarten Y92.211
  - middle school Y92.212
  - specified NEC Y92.218
  - trace school Y92.215
  - university Y92.214
  - vocational school Y92.215
- sea (shore) Y92.832
- senior citizen center Y92.29
- service area (refer to specific site)
- shipyard Y92.62
- shop (commercial) Y92.513
- sidewalk Y92.480
- skating rink (roller) Y92.331
  - ice Y92.330
- soccer field Y92.322
- specified place NEC Y92.89
- sports area Y92.39 (also refer to specific sites)
  - athletic
    - court Y92.31-
    - field Y92.32-
  - golf course Y92.39
  - gymnasium Y92.39
  - riding school Y92.39
  - stadium Y92.39
  - swimming pool Y92.34
- squash court Y92.311
- stadium Y92.39
- steeple chasing course Y92.39
- store Y92.512
- stream Y92.828
- street and highway Y92.410
  - bike path Y92.482
  - freeway Y92.411
  - highway ramp Y92.415
  - interstate highway Y92.411
  - local residential or business street Y92.414
  - motorway Y92.411
  - parkway Y92.412
  - parking lot Y92.481
  - sidewalk Y92.480
  - specified NEC Y92.488
  - state road Y92.413
- subway car Y92.816
- supermarket Y92.512
- swamp Y92.828
- swimming pool (public) Y92.34
  - private (at) Y92.095 (refer to specific residence)
- synagogue Y92.22
- tennis court Y92.312
- theater Y92.254
- trade area Y92.59 (refer to specific site)
- trailer park, residential—*see* mobile home
- trailer site NOS Y92.89
- train Y92.815
  - station Y92.522
- truck Y92.812
- tunnel under construction Y92.69
- urgent (health) care center Y92.532
- university Y92.214

Place of occurrence, *continued*

- vehicle (transport) Y92.818
  - airplane Y92.813
  - boat Y92.814
  - bus Y92.811
  - car Y92.810
  - specified NEC Y92.818
  - subway car Y92.816
  - train Y92.815
  - truck Y92.812
- warehouse Y92.59
- water reservoir Y92.89
- wilderness area Y92.82-
- workshop Y92.69
- yard, private Y92.096 (refer to specific residence)
- youth center Y92.29
- zoo (zoological garden) Y92.834

Poisoning (accidental) (by)—*see also* Table of Drugs and Chemicals

- by plant, thorns, spines, sharp leaves or other mechanisms NEC X58
- carbon monoxide
  - generated by
    - motor vehicle—*see* Accident, transport
    - watercraft (in transit) (not in transit) V93.8-
- caused by injection of poisons into skin by plant thorns, spines, sharp leaves X58
  - marine or sea plants (venomous) X58
- exhaust gas
  - generated by
    - motor vehicle—*see* Accident, transport
    - watercraft (in transit) (not in transit) V93.89
      - ~ ferry boat V93.81
      - ~ fishing boat V93.82
      - ~ jet skis V93.83
      - ~ liner V93.81
      - ~ merchant ship V93.80
      - ~ passenger ship V93.81
      - ~ powered craft NEC V93.83
- fumes or smoke due to
  - explosion (*see also* Explosion) W40.9
  - fire—*see* Exposure, fire
  - ignition—*see* Ignition

Powder burn (by) (from)

- airgun W34.110
- BB gun W34.110
- firearm NEC W34.19
- gas, air or spring-operated gun NEC W34.118
- handgun W32.1
- hunting rifle W33.12
- larger firearm W33.10
  - specified NEC W33.19
- machine gun W33.13
- paintball gun W34.111
- pellet gun W34.110
- shotgun W33.11
- Very pistol [flare] W34.19

Premature cessation (of) surgical and medical care Y66

Privation (food) (water) X58

Procedure (operation)

- correct, on wrong side or body part (wrong side) (wrong site) Y65.53
- intended for another patient done on wrong patient Y65.52
- performed on patient not scheduled for surgery Y65.52
- performed on wrong patient Y65.52
- wrong, performed on correct patient Y65.51

Prolonged

- sitting in transport vehicle—*see* Travel, by type of vehicle
- stay in
  - high altitude as cause of anoxia, barodontalgia, barotitis or hypoxia W94.11
  - weightless environment X52

Pulling, excessive—*see* category Y93

Puncture, puncturing—*see also* Contact, with, by type of object or machine

- by
  - plant thorns, spines, sharp leaves or other mechanisms NEC W60

Place of occurrence, *continued*

- during medical or surgical treatment as misadventure—*see* Index to Diseases and Injuries, Complication(s)

Pushed, pushing (accidental) (injury in) (overexertion)—*see* category Y93

- by other person(s) (accidental) W51
  - with fall W03
    - due to ice or snow W00.0
  - as, or caused by, a crowd or human stampede (with fall) W52
  - before moving object NEC Y02.8
    - motor vehicle Y02.0
    - subway train Y02.1
    - train Y02.1
  - from
    - high place NEC
      - ~ in accidental circumstances W17.89
      - ~ stated as
        - ◊ intentional, homicide (attempt) Y01
        - ◊ undetermined whether accidental or intentional Y30
    - transport vehicle NEC (*see also* Accident, transport) V89.9

R

Radiation (exposure to) (refer to *ICD-10-CM* manual for more)

- infrared (heaters and lamps) W90.1
  - excessive heat from W92
- ionized, ionizing (particles, artificially accelerated)
  - radioisotopes W88.1
  - specified NEC W88.8
  - x-rays W88.0
- light sources (man-made visible and ultraviolet) W89.9
  - natural X32
  - specified NEC W89.8
  - tanning bed W89.1
  - welding light W89.0
- man-made visible light W89.9
  - specified NEC W89.8
  - tanning bed W89.1
  - welding light W89.0
- microwave W90.8
- misadventure in medical or surgical procedure Y63.2
- natural NEC X39.08
- overdose (in medical or surgical procedure) Y63.2
- sun X32
- ultraviolet (light) (man-made) W89.9
  - natural X32
  - specified NEC W89.8
  - tanning bed W89.1
  - welding light W89.0
- x-rays (hard) (soft) W88.0

Range disease W94.11

Rape (attempted) T74.2-

Rat bite W53.11

Reaction, abnormal to medical procedure (*see also* Complication of or following, by type of procedure) Y84.9

- with misadventure—*see* Misadventure
- biologicals or drugs or vaccine—*see* Table of Drugs and Chemicals

Recoil

- airgun W34.110
- BB gun W34.110
- firearm NEC W34.19
- gas, air or spring-operated gun NEC W34.118
- handgun W32.1
- hunting rifle W33.12
- larger firearm W33.10
  - specified NEC W33.19
- machine gun W33.13
- paintball gun W34.111
- pellet W34.110
- shotgun W33.11
- Very pistol [flare] W34.19

Reduction in

- atmospheric pressure—*see* Air, pressure, change

Rock falling on or hitting (accidentally) (person) W20.8

- in cave-in W20.0

Run over (accidentally) (by)

- animal (not being ridden) NEC W55.89
- machinery—*see* Contact, with, by specified type of machine
- transport vehicle NEC (*see also* Accident, transport) V09.9
  - motor NEC V09.20

Running

- before moving object X81.8
  - motor vehicle X81.0

Running off, away

- animal (being ridden) (*see also* Accident, transport) V80.918
  - not being ridden W55.89
- animal-drawn vehicle NEC (*see also* Accident, transport) V80.928
- highway, road (way), street
  - transport vehicle NEC (*see also* Accident, transport) V89.9

Rupture pressurized devices—*see* Explosion, by type of device

S

Saturnism—*see* Table of Drugs and Chemicals, lead

Scald, scalding (accidental) (by) (from) (in) X19

- air (hot) X14.1
- gases (hot) X14.1
- liquid (boiling) (hot) NEC X12
  - stated as undetermined whether accidental or intentional Y27.2
- local application of externally applied substance in medical or surgical care Y63.5
- metal (molten) (liquid) (hot) NEC X18
- self-inflicted X77.9
- stated as undetermined whether accidental or intentional Y27.8
- steam X13.1
  - assault X98.0
  - stated as undetermined whether accidental or intentional Y27.0
- vapor (hot) X13.1
  - assault X98.0
  - stated as undetermined whether accidental or intentional Y27.0

Scratched by

- cat W55.03
- person(s) (accidentally) W50.4
  - with intent to injure or kill Y04.0
  - as, or caused by, a crowd or human stampede (with fall) W52
  - assault Y04.0
  - in
    - fight Y04.0

Seasickness T75.3

Self-harm NEC—*see also* **External cause by type, undetermined whether accidental or intentional**

- intentional—*see* Suicide
- poisoning NEC—*see* Table of Drugs and Chemicals

Self-inflicted (injury) NEC—*see also* External cause by type, undetermined whether accidental or intentional

- intentional—*see* Suicide
- poisoning NEC—*see* Table of Drugs and Chemicals

Sequelae (of)

Use original code to define how the injury occurred with 7th character S

Shock

- electric—*see* Exposure, electric current
- from electric appliance (any) (faulty) W86.8
  - domestic W86.0

Shooting, shot (accidental(ly))—*see also* Discharge, firearm, by type

- herself or himself—*see* Discharge, firearm by type, self-inflicted
- inflicted by other person—*see* Discharge, firearm by type, homicide
  - accidental—*see* Discharge, firearm, by type of firearm

Shooting, shot (accidental(ly)), *continued*
- self-inflicted—*see* Discharge, firearm by type, suicide
  – accidental—*see* Discharge, firearm, by type of firearm
- suicide (attempt)—*see* Discharge, firearm by type, suicide

Shoving (accidentally) by other person—*see* Pushed, by other person

Sickness
- alpine W94.11
- motion—*see* Motion
- mountain W94.11

Sinking (accidental)
- watercraft (causing drowning, submersion)—*see also* Drowning, due to, accident to, watercraft, sinking
  – causing injury except drowning or submersion—*see* Accident, watercraft, causing, injury NEC

Siriasis X32

Slashed wrists—*see* Cut, self-inflicted

Slipping (accidental) (on same level) (with fall) W01.0
- on
  – ice W00.0
    ▪ with skates—*see* Accident, transport, pedestrian, conveyance
  – mud W01.0
  – oil W01.0
  – snow W00.0
    ▪ with skis—*see* Accident, transport, pedestrian, conveyance
  – surface (slippery) (wet) NEC W01.0
- without fall W18.40
  – due to
    ▪ specified NEC W18.49
    ▪ stepping from one level to another W18.43
    ▪ stepping into hole or opening W18.42
    ▪ stepping on object W18.41

Sliver, wood, contact with W45.8

Smoldering (due to fire)—*see* Exposure, fire

Sodomy (attempted) by force T74.2-

Sound waves (causing injury) W42.9
- supersonic W42.0

Splinter, contact with W45.8

Stab, stabbing—*see* Cut

Starvation X58

Status of external cause Y99.-

Stepped on
- by
  – animal (not being ridden) NEC W55.89
  – crowd or human stampede W52
  – person W50.0

Stepping on
- object W22.8
  – with fall W18.31
  – sports equipment W21.9
  – stationary W22.09
    ▪ sports equipment W21.89
- person W51
  – by crowd or human stampede W52
- sports equipment W21.9

Sting
- arthropod, nonvenomous W57
- insect, nonvenomous W57

Storm (cataclysmic)—*see* Forces of nature, cataclysmic storm

Straining, excessive—*see* category Y93

Strangling—*see* Strangulation

Strangulation (accidental)—*see* category T71

Strenuous movements—*see* category Y93

Striking against
- airbag (automobile) W22.10
  – driver side W22.11
  – front passenger side W22.12
  – specified NEC W22.19
- bottom when
  – diving or jumping into water (in) W16.822
    ▪ causing drowning W16.821

Striking against, *continued*
    ▪ from boat W16.722
      ~ causing drowning W16.721
    ▪ natural body W16.622
      ~ causing drowning W16.821
    ▪ swimming pool W16.522
      ~ causing drowning W16.521
  – falling into water (in) W16.322
    ▪ causing drowning W16.321
    ▪ fountain—*see* Striking against, bottom when, falling into water, specified NEC
    ▪ natural body W16.122
      ~ causing drowning W16.121
    ▪ reservoir—*see* Striking against, bottom when, falling into water, specified NEC
    ▪ specified NEC W16.322
      ~ causing drowning W16.321
    ▪ swimming pool W16.022
      ~ causing drowning W16.021
- diving board (swimming-pool) W21.4
- object W22.8
  – with
    ▪ drowning or submersion—*see* Drowning
    ▪ fall—*see* Fall, due to, bumping against, object
  – caused by crowd or human stampede (with fall) W52
  – furniture W22.03
  – lamppost W22.02
  – sports equipment W21.9
  – stationary W22.09
    ▪ sports equipment W21.89
  – wall W22.01
- person(s) W51
  – with fall W03
    ▪ due to ice or snow W00.0
  – as, or caused by, a crowd or human stampede (with fall) W52
  – assault Y04.2
- sports equipment W21.9
- wall (when) W22.01
  – diving or jumping into water (in) W16.832
    ▪ causing drowning W16.831
    ▪ swimming pool W16.532
      ~ causing drowning W16.531
  – falling into water (in) W16.332
    ▪ causing drowning W16.331
    ▪ fountain—*see* Striking against, wall when, falling into water, specified NEC
    ▪ natural body W16.132
      ~ causing drowning W16.131
    ▪ reservoir—*see* Striking against, wall when, falling into water, specified NEC
    ▪ specified NEC W16.332
      ~ causing drowning W16.331
    ▪ swimming pool W16.032
      ~ causing drowning W16.031
  – swimming pool (when) W22.042
    ▪ causing drowning W22.041
    ▪ diving or jumping into water W16.532
      ~ causing drowning W16.531
    ▪ falling into water W16.032
      ~ causing drowning W16.031

Struck (accidentally) by
- airbag (automobile) W22.10
  – driver side W22.11
  – front passenger side W22.12
  – specified NEC W22.19
- alligator W58.02
- animal (not being ridden) NEC W55.89
- avalanche—*see* Landslide
- ball (hit) (thrown) W21.00
  – assault Y08.09
  – baseball W21.03
  – basketball W21.05
  – golf ball W21.04
  – football W21.01
  – soccer W21.02
  – softball W21.07
  – specified NEC W21.09
  – volleyball W21.06
- bat or racquet
  – baseball bat W21.11
    ▪ assault Y08.02

Struck (accidentally) by, *continued*
  – golf club W21.13
    ▪ assault Y08.09
  – specified NEC W21.19
    ▪ assault Y08.09
  – tennis racquet W21.12
    ▪ assault Y08.09
- bullet—*see also* Discharge, firearm by type
- crocodile W58.12
- dog W54.1
- flare, Very pistol—*see* Discharge, firearm NEC
- hailstones X39.8
- hockey (ice)
  – field
    ▪ puck W21.221
    ▪ stick W21.211
  – puck W21.220
  – stick W21.210
    ▪ assault Y08.01
- landslide—*see* Landslide
- lightning—*see* subcategory T75.0
  – causing fire—*see* Exposure, fire
- machine—*see* Contact, with, by type of machine
- mammal NEC W55.89
  – marine W56.32
- marine animal W56.82
- object W22.8
  – blunt W22.8
    ▪ assault Y00
    ▪ undetermined whether accidental or intentional Y29
  – falling W20.8
    ▪ from, in, on
      ~ building W20.1
        ◊ burning (uncontrolled fire) X00.4
      ~ cataclysmic
        ◊ earth surface movement NEC—*see* Landslide
        ◊ storm—*see* Forces of nature, cataclysmic storm
      ~ cave-in W20.0
      ~ earthquake X34
      ~ machine (in operation)—*see* Contact, with, by type of machine
      ~ structure W20.1
        ◊ burning X00.4
      ~ transport vehicle (in motion)—*see* Accident, transport, by type of vehicle
      ~ watercraft V93.49
        ◊ due to
          » accident to craft V91.39
            ❖ powered craft V91.3-
            ❖ unpowered craft V91.3-
          ◊ powered craft V93.4-
          ◊ unpowered craft V93.4-
  – moving NEC W20.8
  – projected W20.8
    ▪ assault Y00
    ▪ in sports W21.9
      ~ assault Y08.09
      ~ ball W21.00
        ◊ baseball W21.03
        ◊ basketball W21.05
        ◊ football W21.01
        ◊ golf ball W21.04
        ◊ soccer W21.02
        ◊ softball W21.07
        ◊ specified NEC W21.09
        ◊ volleyball W21.06
      ~ bat or racquet
        ◊ baseball bat W21.11
          » assault Y08.02
        ◊ golf club W21.13
          » assault Y08.09
        ◊ specified NEC W21.19
          » assault Y08.09
        ◊ tennis racquet W21.12
          » assault Y08.09
      ~ hockey (ice)
        ◊ field
          » puck W21.221
          » stick W21.211
        ◊ puck W21.220

Struck (accidentally) by, *continued*
◊ stick W21.210
» assault Y08.01
~ specified NEC W21.89
– set in motion by explosion—*see* Explosion
– thrown W20.8
■ assault Y00
■ in sports W21.9
~ assault Y08.09
~ ball W21.00
◊ baseball W21.03
◊ basketball W21.05
◊ football W21.01
◊ golf ball W21.04
◊ soccer W21.02
◊ soft ball W21.07
◊ specified NEC W21.09
◊ volleyball W21.06
~ bat or racquet
◊ baseball bat W21.11
» assault Y08.02
◊ golf club W21.13
» assault Y08.09
◊ specified NEC W21.19
» assault Y08.09
◊ tennis racquet W21.12
» assault Y08.09
~ hockey (ice)
◊ field
» puck W21.221
» stick W21.211
◊ puck W21.220
◊ stick W21.210
» assault Y08.01
~ specified NEC W21.89
• other person(s) W50.0
– with
■ blunt object W22.8
~ intentional, homicide (attempt) Y00
~ sports equipment W21.9
~ undetermined whether accidental or intentional Y29
■ fall W03
~ due to ice or snow W00.0
– as, or caused by, a crowd or human stampede (with fall) W52
– assault Y04.2
– sports equipment W21.9
• sports equipment W21.9
– assault Y08.09
– ball W21.00
■ baseball W21.03
■ basketball W21.05
■ football W21.01
■ golf ball W21.04
■ soccer W21.02
■ soft ball W21.07
■ specified NEC W21.09
■ volleyball W21.06
– bat or racquet
■ baseball bat W21.11
~ assault Y08.02
■ golf club W21.13
~ assault Y08.09
■ specified NEC W21.19
■ tennis racquet W21.12
~ assault Y08.09
– cleats (shoe) W21.31
– foot wear NEC W21.39
– football helmet W21.81
– hockey (ice)
■ field
~ puck W21.221
~ stick W21.211
■ puck W21.220
■ stick W21.210
~ assault Y08.01
– skate blades W21.32
– specified NEC W21.89
■ assault Y08.09
• thunderbolt—*see* subcategory T75.0
– causing fire—*see* Exposure, fire

Struck (accidentally) by, *continued*
• transport vehicle NEC (*see also* Accident, transport) V09.9
– intentional, homicide (attempt) Y03.0
– motor NEC (*see also* Accident, transport) V09.20
• vehicle (transport) NEC—*see* Accident, transport, by type of vehicle
– stationary (falling from jack, hydraulic lift, ramp) W20.8

Stumbling
• over
– animal NEC W01.0
■ with fall W18.09
– carpet, rug or (small) object W22.8
■ with fall W18.09
– person W51
■ with fall W03
~ due to ice or snow W00.0
• without fall W18.40
– due to
■ specified NEC W18.49
■ stepping from one level to another W18.43
■ stepping into hole or opening W18.42
■ stepping on object W18.41

Submersion (accidental)—*see* Drowning
Suffocation (accidental) (by external means) (by pressure) (mechanical) (*see also* category) T71
• due to, by
– avalanche—*see* Landslide
– explosion—*see* Explosion
– fire—*see* Exposure, fire
– food, any type (aspiration) (ingestion) (inhalation) (*see* categories T17 and) T18
– ignition—*see* Ignition
– landslide—*see* Landslide
– machine(ry)—*see* Contact, with, by type of machine
– vomitus (aspiration) (inhalation) T17.81-
• in
– burning building X00.8

Suicide, suicidal (attempted) (by) X83.8
• blunt object X79
• burning, burns X76
– hot object X77.9
■ fluid NEC X77.2
■ household appliance X77.3
■ specified NEC X77.8
■ steam X77.0
■ tap water X77.1
■ vapors X77.0
• caustic substance—*see* Table of Drugs and Chemicals
• cold, extreme X83.2
• collision of motor vehicle with
– motor vehicle X82.0
– specified NEC X82.8
– train X82.1
– tree X82.2
• cut (any part of body) X78.9
• cutting or piercing instrument X78.9
– dagger X78.2
– glass X78.0
– knife X78.1
– specified NEC X78.8
– sword X78.2
• drowning (in) X71.9
– bathtub X71.0
– natural water X71.3
– specified NEC X71.8
– swimming pool X71.1
■ following fall X71.2
• electrocution X83.1
• explosive(s) (material) X75
• fire, flames X76
• firearm X74.9
– airgun X74.01
– handgun X72
– hunting rifle X73.1
– larger X73.9
■ specified NEC X73.8
– machine gun X73.2
– – paintball gun X74.02
– shotgun X73.0
– specified NEC X74.8

Suicide, suicidal (attempted) (by), *continued*
• hanging X83.8
• hot object—*see* Suicide, burning, hot object
• jumping
– before moving object X81.8
■ motor vehicle X81.0
■ subway train X81.1
■ train X81.1
– from high place X80
• lying before moving object, train, vehicle X81.8
• poisoning—*see* Table of Drugs and Chemicals
• puncture (any part of body)—*see* Suicide, cutting or piercing instrument
• scald—*see* Suicide, burning, hot object
• sharp object (any)—*see* Suicide, cutting or piercing instrument
• shooting—*see* Suicide, firearm
• specified means NEC X83.8
• stab (any part of body)—*see* Suicide, cutting or piercing instrument
• steam, hot vapors X77.0
• strangulation X83.8
• submersion—*see* Suicide, drowning
• suffocation X83.8
• wound NEC X83.8

Sunstroke X32
Supersonic waves (causing injury) W42.0
Surgical procedure, complication of (delayed or as an abnormal reaction without mention of misadventure)—*see also* Complication of or following, by type of procedure
• due to or as a result of misadventure—*see* Misadventure

Swallowed, swallowing
• foreign body T18
• poison—*see* Table of Drugs and Chemicals
• substance
– caustic or corrosive—*see* Table of Drugs and Chemicals
– poisonous—*see* Table of Drugs and Chemicals

T

Tackle in sport W03
Terrorism (involving) Y38.8-
Thirst X58
Thrown (accidentally)
• against part (any) of or object in transport vehicle (in motion) NEC—*see also* Accident, transport
• from
– high place, homicide (attempt) Y01
– machinery—*see* Contact, with, by type of machine
– transport vehicle NEC (*see also* Accident, transport) V89.9
– off—*see* Thrown, from
Thunderbolt—*see* subcategory T75.0
• causing fire—*see* Exposure, fire
Tidal wave (any injury) NEC—*see* Forces of nature, tidal wave
Took
• overdose (drug)—*see* Table of Drugs and Chemicals
• poison—*see* Table of Drugs and Chemicals
Tornado (any injury) X37.1
Torrential rain (any injury) X37.8
Torture X58
Trampled by animal NEC W55.89
Trapped (accidentally)
• between objects (moving) (stationary and moving)—*see* Caught
• by part (any) of
– motorcycle V29.88
– pedal cycle V19.88
– transport vehicle NEC (*see also* Accident, transport) V89.9
Travel (effects) (sickness) T75.3
Tree falling on or hitting (accidentally) (person) W20.8
Tripping
• over
– animal W01.0

Tripping, *continued*
- – carpet, rug or (small) object W22.8
  - ■ with fall W18.09
- – person W51
  - ■ with fall W03
    - ~ due to ice or snow W00.0
- • without fall W18.40
  - – due to
    - ■ specified NEC W18.49
    - ■ stepping from one level to another W18.43
    - ■ stepping into hole or opening W18.42
    - ■ stepping on object W18.41

Twisted by person(s) (accidentally) W50.2
- • with intent to injure or kill Y04.0
- • as, or caused by, a crowd or human stampede (with fall) W52
- • assault Y04.0
- • in fight Y04.0

Twisting, excessive—see category Y93

U

Underdosing of necessary drugs, medicaments or biological substances Y63.6

V

Vibration (causing injury) W49.9

Volcanic eruption (any injury) X35

Vomitus, gastric contents in air passages (with asphyxia, obstruction or suffocation) T17.81-

W

Walked into stationary object (any) W22.09
- • furniture W22.03
- • lamppost W22.02
- • wall W22.01

War operations (injuries to military personnel and civilians during war, civil insurrection and peacekeeping missions) (by) (from) (involving)—*Refer to ICD-10-CM Manual*

Washed
- • away by flood—*see* Flood
- • off road by storm (transport vehicle)—*see* Forces of nature, cataclysmic storm

Weather exposure NEC—*see* Forces of nature

Weightlessness (causing injury) (effects of) (in spacecraft, real or simulated) X52

Work related condition Y99.0

Wound (accidental) NEC (*see also* Injury) X58
- • battle (*see also* War operations) Y36.90
- • gunshot—*see* Discharge, firearm by type

Wrong
- • device implanted into correct surgical site Y65.51
- • fluid in infusion Y65.1
- • procedure (operation) on correct patient Y65.51
- • patient, procedure performed on Y65.52

TRIPPING–WRONG

Table of Drugs and Chemicals

The following table is a quick reference for all poisonings (accidental/unintentional, intentional/self-harm, assault), adverse effects, and underdosing as a result of a specific drug or chemical. The drugs/chemicals are listed alphabetically with their respective subcategory code. Every code is listed with a dash (-) to indicate that the next character is missing and should be reported with the fifth or sixth character as follows:

1	Poisoning, accidental, unintentional
2	Poisoning, intentional, self-harm
3	Poisoning, assault
4	Poisoning, undetermined
5	Adverse effect
6	Underdosing

DO NOT CODE FROM THE TABLE—ALWAYS REFER TO THE TABULAR. If the code requires an "encounter type," please refer to the tabular for more details.

EXAMPLE

Accidental Poisoning From Lysol—Initial Encounter
Lysol is listed as T54.1X-.
Lysol accidental poisoning would be T54.1X1-.
Lysol accidental poisoning, initial encounter, would be T54.1X1A.

Underdosing of Barbiturate—Follow-up Encounter
Barbiturate is listed as T42.3X-.
Underdosing of barbiturate would be T42.3X6-.
Underdosing of barbiturate, subsequent encounter, would be T42.3X6D.

Drug/Chemical	Code
1-propanol	T51.3X-
2-propanol	T51.2X-
2,4-D (dichlorophen-oxyacetic acid)	T60.3X-
2,4-toluene diisocyanate	T65.0X-
2,4,5-T (trichloro-phenoxyacetic acid)	T60.1X-
14-hydroxydihydro-morphinone	T40.2X-
ABOB	T37.5X-
Abrine	T62.2X-
Abrus (seed)	T62.2X-
Absinthe (beverage)	T51.0X-
Acaricide	T60.8X-
Acebutolol	T44.7X-
Acecarbromal	T42.6X-
Aceclidine	T44.1X-
Acedapsone	T37.0X-
Acefylline piperazine	T48.6X-
Acemorphan	T40.2X-
Acenocoumarin / Acenocoumarol	T45.51-
Acepifylline	T48.6X-
Acepromazine	T43.3X-
Acesulfamethoxypyridazine	T37.0X-
Acetal	T52.8X-
Acetaldehyde (vapor)	T52.8X-
liquid	T65.89-
P-Acetamidophenol	T39.1X-
Acetaminophen	T39.1X-
Acetaminosalol	T39.1X-
Acetanilide	T39.1X-
Acetarsol	T37.3X-
Acetazolamide	T50.2X-
Acetiamine	T45.2X-
Acetic	
acid	T54.2X-
w/sodium acetate (ointment)	T49.3X-
ester (solvent) (vapor)	T52.8X-
irrigating solution	T50.3X-
medicinal (lotion)	T49.2X-
anhydride	T65.89-
ether (vapor)	T52.8X-
Acetohexamide	T38.3X-
Acetohydroxamic acid	T50.99-
Acetomenaphthone	T45.7X-

Drug/Chemical	Code
Acetomorphine	T40.1X-
Acetone (oils)	T52.4X-
Acetonitrile	T52.8X-
Acetophenazine	T43.3X-
Acetophenetedin	T39.1X-
Acetophenone	T52.4X-
Acetorphine	T40.2X-
Acetosulfone (sodium)	T37.1X-
Acetrizoate (sodium)	T50.8X-
Acetrizoic acid	T50.8X-
Acetyl (bromide) (chloride)	T53.6X-
Acetylcarbromal	T42.6X-
Acetylcholine (chloride)	T44.1X-
derivative	T44.1X-
Acetylcysteine	T48.4X-
Acetyldigitoxin	T46.0X-
Acetyldigoxin	T46.0X-
Acetyldihydrocodeine	T40.2X-
Acetyldihydrocodeinone	T40.2X-
Acetylene (gas)	T59.89-
dichloride	T53.6X-
incomplete combustion of	T58.1-
industrial	T59.89-
tetrachloride	T53.6X-
vapor	T53.6X-
Acetylpheneturide	T42.6X-
Acetylphenylhydrazine	T39.8X-
Acetylsalicylic acid (salts)	T39.01-
enteric coated	T39.01-
Acetylsulfamethoxypyridazine	T37.0X-
Achromycin	T36.4X-
ophthalmic preparation	T49.5X-
topical NEC	T49.0X-
Aciclovir	T37.5X-
Acid (corrosive) NEC	T54.2X-
Acidifying agent NEC	T50.90-
Acipimox	T46.6X-
Acitretin	T50.99-
Aclarubicin	T45.1X-
Aclatonium napadisilate	T48.1X-
Aconite (wild)	T46.99-
Aconitine	T46.99-

1-PROPANOL–ACONITINE

ACONITUM FEROX–ALGLUCERASE

Drug/Chemical	Code
Aconitum ferox	T46.99-
Acridine	T65.6X-
vapor	T59.89-
Acriflavine	T37.9-
Acriflavinium chloride	T49.0X-
Acrinol	T49.0X-
Acrisorcin	T49.0X-
Acrivastine	T45.0X-
Acrolein (gas)	T59.89-
liquid	T54.1X-
Acrylamide	T65.89-
Acrylic resin	T49.3X-
Acrylonitrile	T65.89-
Actaea spicata	T62.2X-
berry	T62.1X-
Acterol	T37.3X-
ACTH	T38.81-
Actinomycin C	T45.1X-
Actinomycin D	T45.1X-
Activated charcoal—*see also Charcoal, medicinal*	T47.6X-
Acyclovir	T37.5X-
Adenine	T45.2X-
arabinoside	T37.5X-
Adenosine (phosphate)	T46.2X-
ADH	T38.89-
Adhesive NEC	T65.89-
Adicillin	T36.0X-
Adiphenine	T44.3X-
Adipiodone	T50.8X-
Adjunct, pharmaceutical	T50.90-
Adrenal (extract, cortex or medulla) (gluco or mineral corticoids) (hormones)	T38.0X-
ENT agent	T49.6X-
ophthalmic preparation	T49.5X-
topical NEC	T49.0X-
Adrenaline / Adrenalin	T44.5X-
Adrenergic NEC	T44.90-
blocking agent NEC	T44.8X-
beta, heart	T44.7X-
specified NEC	T44.99-
Adrenochrome	
(mono)semicarbazone	T46.99-
derivative	T46.99-
Adrenocorticotrophic hormone	T38.81-
Adrenocorticotrophin	T38.81-
Adriamycin	T45.1X-
Aerosol spray NEC	T65.9-
Aerosporin	T36.8X-
ENT agent	T49.6X-
ophthalmic preparation	T49.5X-
topical NEC	T49.0X-
Aethusa cynapium	T62.2X-
Afghanistan black	T40.7X-
Aflatoxin	T64.0-
Afloqualone	T42.8X-

Drug/Chemical	Code
African boxwood	T62.2X-
Agar	T47.4X-
Agonist (predominantly)	
alpha-adrenoreceptor	T44.4X-
beta-adrenoreceptor	T44.5X-
Agricultural agent NEC	T65.9-
Agrypnal	T42.3X-
AHLG	T50.Z1-
Air contaminant(s) type NOS	T65.9-
Ajmaline	T46.2X-
Akee	T62.1X-
Akrinol	T49.0X-
Akritoin	T37.8X-
Alacepril	T46.4X-
Alantolactone	T37.4X-
Albamycin	T36.8X-
Albendazole	T37.4X-
Albumin	T45.8X-
Albuterol	T48.6X-
Albutoin	T42.0X-
Alclometasone	T49.0X-
Alcohol	T51.9-
allyl	T51.8X-
amyl / butyl / propyl	T51.3X-
antifreeze / methyl	T51.1X-
beverage (grain, ethyl)	T51.0X-
dehydrated / denatured	T51.0X-
deterrent NEC	T50.6X-
diagnostic (gastric function)	T50.8X-
industrial	T51.0X-
isopropyl	T51.2X-
preparation for consumption	T51.0X-
radiator	T51.1X-
rubbing	T51.2X-
specified type NEC	T51.8X-
surgical	T51.0X-
vapor (any type of Alcohol)	T59.89-
wood	T51.1X-
Alcuronium (chloride)	T48.1X-
Aldactone	T50.0X-
Aldesulfone sodium	T37.1X-
Aldicarb	T60.0X-
Aldomet	T46.5X-
Aldosterone	T50.0X-
Aldrin (dust)	T60.1X-
Alexitol sodium	T47.1X-
Alfacalcidol	T45.2X-
Alfadolone	T41.1X-
Alfaxalone	T41.1X-
Alfentanil	T40.4X-
Alfuzosin (hydrochloride)	T44.8X-
Algae (harmful) (toxin)	T65.821
Algeldrate	T47.1X-
Algin	T47.8X-
Alglucerase	T45.3X-

Drug/Chemical	Code
Alidase	T45.3X-
Alimemazine	T43.3X-
Aliphatic thiocyanates	T65.0X-
Alizapride	T45.0X-
Alkali (caustic)	T54.3X-
Alkaline antiseptic solution (aromatic)	T49.6X-
Alkalinizing agents (medicinal)	T50.90-
Alkalizing agent NEC	T50.90-
Alka-seltzer	T39.01-
Alkavervir	T46.5X-
Alkonium (bromide)	T49.0X-
Alkylating drug NEC	T45.1X-
antimyeloproliferative or lymphatic	T45.1X-
Alkylisocyanate	T65.0X-
Allantoin	T49.4X-
Allegron	T43.01-
Allethrin	T49.0X-
Allobarbital	T42.3X-
Allopurinol	T50.4X-
Allyl	
Alcohol	T51.8X-
disulfide	T46.6X-
Allylestrenol	T38.5X-
Allylisopropylacetylurea	T42.6X-
Allylisopropylmalonylurea	T42.3X-
Allylthiourea	T49.3X-
Allyltribromide	T42.6X-
Allypropymal	T42.3X-
Almagate	T47.1X-
Almasilate	T47.1X-
Almitrine	T50.7X-
Aloes	T47.2X-
Aloglutamol	T47.1X-
Aloin	T47.2X-
Aloxidone	T42.2X-
Alpha	
acetyldigoxin	T46.0X-
adrenergic blocking drug	T44.6X-
amylase	T45.3X-
tocoferol (acetate) toco	T45.2X-
tocopherol	T45.2X-
Alphadolone	T41.1X-
Alphaprodine	T40.4X-
Alphaxalone	T41.1X-
Alprazolam	T42.4X-
Alprenolol	T44.7X-
Alprostadil	T46.7X-
Alsactide	T38.81-
Alseroxylon	T46.5X-
Alteplase	T45.61-
Altizide	T50.2X-
Altretamine	T45.1X-
Alum (medicinal)	T49.4X-
nonmedicinal (ammonium) (potassium)	T56.89-

Drug/Chemical	Code
Aluminium, aluminum	
acetate / chloride	T49.2X-
solution	T49.0X-
aspirin / bis (acetylsalicylate)	T39.01-
carbonate (gel, basic)	T47.1X-
chlorhydroxide-complex	T47.1X-
clofibrate	T46.6X-
diacetate	T49.2X-
glycinate	T47.1X-
hydroxide (gel)	T47.1X-
hydroxide-magn. carb. gel	T47.1X-
magnesium silicate	T47.1X-
nicotinate	T46.7X-
ointment (surgical) (topical)	T49.3X-
phosphate / silicate (sodium)	T47.1X-
salicylate	T39.09-
subacetate	T49.2X-
sulfate	T49.0X-
tannate	T47.6X-
Alurate	T42.3X-
Alverine	T44.3X-
Alvodine	T40.2X-
Amanita phalloides	T62.0X-
Amanitine	T62.0X-
Amantadine	T42.8X-
Ambazone	T49.6X-
Ambenonium (chloride)	T44.0X-
Ambroxol	T48.4X-
Ambuphylline	T48.6X-
Ambutonium bromide	T44.3X-
Amcinonide	T49.0X-
Amdinocilline	T36.0X-
Ametazole	T50.8X-
Amethocaine (regional, spinal)	T41.3X-
Amethopterin	T45.1X-
Amezinium metilsulfate	T44.99-
Amfebutamone	T43.29-
Amfepramone	T50.5X-
Amfetamine	T43.62-
Amfetaminil	T43.62-
Amfomycin	T36.8X-
Amidefrine mesilate	T48.5X-
Amidone	T40.3X-
Amidopyrine	T39.2X-
Amidotrizoate	T50.8X-
Amiflamine	T43.1X-
Amikacin	T36.5X-
Amikhelline	T46.3X-
Amiloride	T50.2X-
Aminacrine	T49.0X-
Amineptine	T43.01-
Aminitrozole	T37.3X-
Amino acids	T50.3X-
Aminoacetic acid (derivatives)	T50.3X-
Aminoacridine	T49.0X-

Drug/Chemical	Code
Aminobenzoic acid (-p)	T49.3X-
4-Aminobutyric acid	T43.8X-
Aminocaproic acid	T45.62-
Aminoethylisothiourium	T45.8X-
Aminofenazone	T39.2X-
Aminoglutethimide	T45.1X-
Aminohippuric acid	T50.8X-
Aminomethylbenzoic acid	T45.69-
Aminometradine	T50.2X-
Aminopentamide	T44.3X-
Aminophenazone	T39.2X-
Aminophenol	T54.0X-
4-Aminophenol derivatives	T39.1X-
Aminophenylpyridone	T43.59-
Aminophylline	T48.6X-
Aminopterin sodium	T45.1X-
Aminopyrine	T39.2X-
8-Aminoquinoline drugs	T37.2X-
Aminorex	T50.5X-
Aminosalicylic acid	T37.1X-
Aminosalylum	T37.1X-
Amiodarone	T46.2X-
Amiphenazole	T50.7X-
Amiquinsin	T46.5X-
Amisometradine	T50.2X-
Amisulpride	T43.59-
Amitriptyline	T43.01-
Amitriptylinoxide	T43.01-
Amlexanox	T48.6X-
Ammonia (fumes/vapor) (gas)	T59.89-
aromatic spirit	T48.99-
liquid (household)	T54.3X-
Ammoniated mercury	T49.0X-
Ammonium	
acid tartrate	T49.5X-
bromide	T42.6X-
carbonate	T54.3X-
chloride	T50.99-
expectorant	T48.4X-
compounds (household)NEC	T54.3X-
fumes (any usage)	T59.89-
industrial	T54.3X-
ichthyosulronate	T49.4X-
mandelate	T37.9-
sulfamate	T60.3X-
sulfonate resin	T47.8X-
Amobarbital (sodium)	T42.3X-
Amodiaquine	T37.2X-
Amopyroquin (e)	T37.2X-
Amoxapine	T43.01-
Amoxicillin	T36.0X-
Amperozide	T43.59-
Amphenidone	T43.59-
Amphetamine NEC	T43.62-

Drug/Chemical	Code
Amphomycin	T36.8X-
Amphotalide	T37.4X-
Amphotericin B	T36.7X-
topical	T49.0X-
Ampicillin	T36.0X-
Amprotropine	T44.3X-
Amsacrine	T45.1X-
Amygdaline	T62.2X-
Amyl	
acetate	T52.8X-
vapor	T59.89-
alcohol	T51.3X-
chloride	T53.6X-
formate	T52.8X-
nitrite	T46.3X-
propionate	T65.89-
Amylase	T47.5X-
Amyleine, regional	T41.3X-
Amylene	
dichloride	T53.6X-
hydrate	T51.3X-
Amylmetacresol	T49.6X-
Amylobarbitone	T42.3X-
Amylocaine, regional (infiltration) (subcutaneous) (nerve block) (spinal) (topical)	T41.3X-
Amylopectin	T47.6X-
Amytal (sodium)	T42.3X-
Anabolic steroid	T38.7X-
Analeptic NEC	T50.7X-
Analgesic	T39.9-
anti-inflammatory NEC	T39.9-
propionic acid derivative	T39.31-
antirheumatic NEC	T39.4X-
aromatic NEC	T39.1X-
narcotic NEC	T40.60-
non-narcotic NEC	T39.9-
pyrazole	T39.2X-
specified NEC	T39.8X-
Analgin	T39.2X-
Anamirta cocculus	T62.1X-
Ancillin	T36.0X-
Ancrod	T45.69-
Androgen	T38.7X-
Androgen-estrogen mixture	T38.7X-
Androstalone	T38.7X-
Androstanolone	T38.7X-
Androsterone	T38.7X-
Anemone pulsatilla	T62.2X-
Anesthesia	
caudal	T41.3X-
endotracheal	T41.0X-
epidural	T41.3X-
inhalation	T41.0X-
local (nerve or plexus blocking)	T41.3X-
mucosal	T41.3X-

Drug/Chemical	Code
Anesthesia, continued	
muscle relaxation	T48.1X-
potentiated	T41.20-
rectal (general)	T41.20-
local	T41.3X-
regional	T41.3X-
surface	T41.3X-
Anesthetic NEC	T41.41
with muscle relaxant	T41.20-
general	T41.20-
local	T41.3X-
gaseous NEC	T41.0X-
general NEC	T41.20-
halogenated hydrocarbon derivatives NEC	T41.0X-
infiltration NEC	T41.3X-
intravenous NEC	T41.1X-
local NEC	T41.3X-
rectal (general)	T41.20-
local	T41.3X-
regional NEC / spinal NEC	T41.3X-
thiobarbiturate	T41.1X-
topical	T41.3X-
Aneurine	T45.2X-
Angio-Conray	T50.8X-
Angiotensin	T44.5X-
Angiotensinamide	T44.99-
Anhydrohydroxy-progesterone	T38.5X-
Anhydron	T50.2X-
Anileridine	T40.4X-
Aniline (dye) (liquid)	T65.3X-
analgesic	T39.1X-
derivatives, therapeutic NEC	T39.1X-
vapor	T65.3X-
Aniscoropine	T44.3X-
Anise oil	T47.5X-
Anisidine	T65.3X-
Anisindione	T45.51-
Anisotropine methyl-bromide	T44.3X-
Anistreplase	T45.61-
Anorexiant (central)	T50.5X-
Anorexic agents	T50.5X-
Ansamycin	T36.6X-
Ant (bite) (sting)	T63.421
Antabuse	T50.6X-
Antacid NEC	T47.1X-
Antagonist	
Aldosterone	T50.0X-
alpha-adrenoreceptor	T44.6X-
anticoagulant	T45.7X-
beta-adrenoreceptor	T44.7X-
extrapyramidal NEC	T44.3X-
folic acid	T45.1X-
H2 receptor	T47.0X-
heavy metal	T45.8X-
narcotic analgesic	T50.7X-

Drug/Chemical	Code
Antagonist, continued	
opiate	T50.7X-
pyrimidine	T45.1X-
serotonin	T46.5X-
Antazolin (e)	T45.0X-
Anterior pituitary hormone NEC	T38.81-
Anthelmintic NEC	T37.4X-
Anthiolimine	T37.4X-
Anthralin	T49.4X-
Anthramycin	T45.1X-
Antiadrenergic NEC	T44.8X-
Antiallergic NEC	T45.0X-
Anti-anemic (drug) (preparation)	T45.8X-
Antiandrogen NEC	T38.6X-
Antianxiety drug NEC	T43.50-
Antiaris toxicaria	T65.89-
Antiarteriosclerotic drug	T46.6X-
Antiasthmatic drug NEC	T48.6X-
Antibiotic NEC	T36.9-
aminoglycoside	T36.5X-
anticancer	T45.1X-
antifungal	T36.7X-
antimycobacterial	T36.5X-
antineoplastic	T45.1X-
cephalosporin (group)	T36.1X-
chloramphenicol (group)	T36.2X-
ENT	T49.6X-
eye	T49.5X-
fungicidal (local)	T49.0X-
intestinal	T36.8X-
b-lactam NEC	T36.1X-
local	T49.0X-
macrolides	T36.3X-
polypeptide	T36.8X-
specified NEC	T36.8X-
tetracycline (group)	T36.4X-
throat	T49.6X-
Anticancer agents NEC	T45.1X-
Anticholesterolemic drug NEC	T46.6X-
Anticholinergic NEC	T44.3X-
Anticholinesterase	T44.0X-
organophosphorus	T44.0X-
insecticide	T60.0X-
nerve gas	T59.89-
reversible	T44.0X-
ophthalmological	T49.5X-
Anticoagulant NEC	T45.51-
Antagonist	T45.7X-
Anti-common-cold drug NEC	T48.5X-
Anticonvulsant	T42.71
barbiturate	T42.3X-
combination (with barbiturate)	T42.3X-
hydantoin	T42.0X-
hypnotic NEC	T42.6X-
oxazolidinedione	T42.2X-

ANTICONVULSANT–ANTINEOPLASTIC NEC

Drug/Chemical	Code
Anticonvulsant, continued	T42.71
pyrimidinedione	T42.6X-
specified NEC	T42.6X-
succinimide	T42.2X-
Anti-D immunoglobulin (human)	T50.Z1-
Antidepressant	T43.20-
monoamine oxidase inhibitor	T43.1X-
SSNRI	T43.21-
SSRI	T43.22-
specified NEC	T43.29-
tetracyclic	T43.02-
triazolopyridine	T43.21-
tricyclic	T43.01-
Antidiabetic NEC	T38.3X-
biguanide	T38.3X-
and sulfonyl combined	T38.3X-
combined	T38.3X-
sulfonylurea	T38.3X-
Antidiarrheal drug NEC	T47.6X-
absorbent	T47.6X-
Antidiphtheria serum	T50.Z1-
Antidiuretic hormone	T38.89-
Antidote NEC	T50.6X-
heavy metal	T45.8X-
Antidysrhythmic NEC	T46.2X-
Antiemetic drug	T45.0X-
Antiepilepsy agent	T42.71
combination or mixed	T42.5X-
specified, NEC	T42.6X-
Antiestrogen NEC	T38.6X-
Antifertility pill	T38.4X-
Antifibrinolytic drug	T45.62-
Antifilarial drug	T37.4X-
Antiflatulent	T47.5X-
Antifreeze	T65.9-
alcohol	T51.1X-
ethylene glycol	T51.8X-
Antifungal	
antibiotic (systemic)	T36.7X-
anti-infective NEC	T37.9-
disinfectant, local	T49.0X-
nonmedicinal (spray)	T60.3X-
topical	T49.0X-
Anti-gastric-secretion drug NEC	T47.1X-
Antigonadotrophin NEC	T38.6X-
Antihallucinogen	T43.50-
Antihelmintics	T37.4X-
Antihemophilic	
factor	T45.8X-
fraction	T45.8X-
globulin concentrate	T45.7X-
human plasma	T45.8X-
plasma, dried	T45.7X-
Antihemorrhoidal preparation	T49.2X-
Antiheparin drug	T45.7X-

Drug/Chemical	Code
Antihistamine	T45.0X-
Antihookworm drug	T37.4X-
Anti-human lymphocytic globulin	T50.Z1-
Antihyperlipidemic drug	T46.6X-
Antihypertensive drug NEC	T46.5X-
Anti-infective NEC	T37.9-
anthelmintic	T37.4X-
antibiotics	T36.9-
specified NEC	T36.8X-
antimalarial	T37.2X-
antimycobacterial NEC	T37.1X-
antibiotics	T36.5X-
antiprotozoal NEC	T37.3X-
blood	T37.2X-
antiviral	T37.5X-
arsenical	T37.8X-
bismuth, local	T49.0X-
ENT	T49.6X-
eye NEC	T49.5X-
heavy metals NEC	T37.8X-
local NEC	T49.0X-
specified NEC	T49.0X-
mixed	T37.9-
ophthalmic preparation	T49.5X-
topical NEC	T49.0X-
Anti-inflammatory drug NEC	T39.39-
local	T49.0X-
nonsteroidal NEC	T39.39-
propionic acid derivative	T39.31-
specified NEC	T39.39-
Antikaluretic	T50.3X-
Antiknock (tetraethyl lead)	T56.0X-
Antilipemic drug NEC	T46.6X-
Antimalarial	T37.2X-
prophylactic NEC	T37.2X-
pyrimidine derivative	T37.2X-
Antimetabolite	T45.1X-
Antimitotic agent	T45.1X-
Antimony (compounds) (vapor) NEC	T56.89-
anti-infectives	T37.8X-
dimercaptosuccinate	T37.3X-
hydride	T56.89-
pesticide (vapor)	T60.8X-
potassium (sodium)tartrate	T37.8X-
sodium dimercaptosuccinate	T37.3X-
tartrated	T37.8X-
Antimuscarinic NEC	T44.3X-
Antimycobacterial drug NEC	T37.1X-
antibiotics	T36.5X-
combination	T37.1X-
Antinausea drug	T45.0X-
Antinematode drug	T37.4X-
Antineoplastic NEC	T45.1X-
alkaloidal	T45.1X-
antibiotics	T45.1X-

Drug/Chemical	Code
Antineoplastic NEC, continued	T45.1X-
combination	T45.1X-
estrogen	T38.5X-
steroid	T38.7X-
Antiparasitic drug (systemic)	T37.9-
local	T49.0X-
specified NEC	T37.8X-
Antiparkinsonism drug NEC	T42.8X-
Antiperspirant NEC	T49.2X-
Antiphlogistic NEC	T39.4X-
Antiplatyhelmintic drug	T37.4X-
Antiprotozoal drug NEC	T37.3X-
blood	T37.2X-
local	T49.0X-
Antipruritic drug NEC	T49.1X-
Antipsychotic drug	T43.50-
specified NEC	T43.59-
Antipyretic	T39.9-
specified NEC	T39.8X-
Antipyrine	T39.2X-
Antirabies hyperimmune serum	T50.Z1-
Antirheumatic NEC	T39.4X-
Antirigidity drug NEC	T42.8X-
Antischistosomal drug	T37.4X-
Antiscorpion sera	T50.Z1-
Antiseborrheics	T49.4X-
Antiseptics (external) (medicinal)	T49.0X-
Antistine	T45.0X-
Antitapeworm drug	T37.4X-
Antitetanus immunoglobulin	T50.Z1-
Antithrombotic	T45.52-
Antithyroid drug NEC	T38.2X-
Antitoxin	T50.Z1-
Antitrichomonal drug	T37.3X-
Antituberculars	T37.1X-
antibiotics	T36.5X-
Antitussive NEC	T48.3X-
codeine mixture	T40.2X-
opiate	T40.2X-
Antivaricose drug	T46.8X-
Antivenin, antivenom (sera)	T50.Z1-
crotaline	T50.Z1-
spider bite	T50.Z1-
Antivertigo drug	T45.0X-
Antiviral drug NEC	T37.5X-
eye	T49.5X-
Antiwhipworm drug	T37.4X-
Antrol— *see also specific chemical*	T60.9-
fungicide	T60.9-
ANTU (alpha naphthylthiourea)	T60.4X-
Apalcillin	T36.0X-
APC	T48.5X-
Aplonidine	T44.4X-
Apomorphine	T47.7X-

Drug/Chemical	Code
Appetite depressants, central	T50.5X-
Apraclonidine (hydrochloride)	T44.4X-
Apresoline	T46.5X-
Aprindine	T46.2X-
Aprobarbital	T42.3X-
Apronalide	T42.6X-
Aprotinin	T45.62-
Aptocaine	T41.3X-
Aqua fortis	T54.2X-
Ara-A	T37.5X-
Ara-C	T45.1X-
Arachis oil	T49.3X-
cathartic	T47.4X-
Aralen	T37.2X-
Arecoline	T44.1X-
Arginine	T50.99-
glutamate	T50.99-
Argyrol	T49.0X-
ENT agent	T49.6X-
ophthalmic preparation	T49.5X-
Aristocort	T38.0X-
ENT agent	T49.6X-
ophthalmic preparation	T49.5X-
topical NEC	T49.0X-
Aromatics, corrosive	T54.1X-
disinfectants	T54.1X-
Arsenate of lead	T57.0X-
herbicide	T57.0X-
Arsenic, arsenicals (compounds) (dust) (vapor)NEC	T57.0X-
anti-infectives	T37.8X-
pesticide (dust) (fumes)	T57.0X-
Arsine (gas)	T57.0X-
Arsphenamine (silver)	T37.8X-
Arsthinol	T37.3X-
Artane	T44.3X-
Arthropod (venomous) NEC	T63.481
Articaine	T41.3X-
Asbestos	T57.8X-
Ascaridole	T37.4X-
Ascorbic acid	T45.2X-
Asiaticoside	T49.0X-
Asparaginase	T45.1X-
Aspidium (oleoresin)	T37.4X-
Aspirin (aluminum) (soluble)	T39.01-
Aspoxicillin	T36.0X-
Astemizole	T45.0X-
Astringent (local)	T49.2X-
specified NEC	T49.2X-
Astromicin	T36.5X-
Ataractic drug NEC	T43.50-
Atenolol	T44.7X-
Atonia drug, intestinal	T47.4X-
Atophan	T50.4X-
Atracurium besilate	T48.1X-

Drug/Chemical	Code
Atropine	T44.3X-
derivative	T44.3X-
methonitrate	T44.3X-
Attapulgite	T47.6X-
Auramine	T65.89-
dye	T65.6X-
fungicide	T60.3X-
Auranofin	T39.4X-
Aurantiin	T46.99-
Aureomycin	T36.4X-
ophthalmic preparation	T49.5X-
topical NEC	T49.0X-
Aurothioglucose	T39.4X-
Aurothioglycanide	T39.4X-
Aurothiomalate sodium	T39.4X-
Aurotioprol	T39.4X-
Automobile fuel	T52.0X-
Autonomic nervous system agent NEC	T44.90-
Avlosulfon	T37.1X-
Avomine	T42.6X-
Axerophthol	T45.2X-
Azacitidine	T45.1X-
Azacyclonol	T43.59-
Azadirachta	T60.2X-
Azanidazole	T37.3X-
Azapetine	T46.7X-
Azapropazone	T39.2X-
Azaribine	T45.1X-
Azaserine	T45.1X-
Azatadine	T45.0X-
Azatepa	T45.1X-
Azathioprine	T45.1X-
Azelaic acid	T49.0X-
Azelastine	T45.0X-
Azidocillin	T36.0X-
Azidothymidine	T37.5X-
Azinphos (ethyl) (methyl)	T60.0X-
Aziridine (chelating)	T54.1X-
Azithromycin	T36.3X-
Azlocillin	T36.0X-
Azobenzene smoke	T65.3X-
acaricide	T60.8X-
Azosulfamide	T37.0X-
AZT	T37.5X-
Aztreonam	T36.1X-
Azulfidine	T37.0X-
Azuresin	T50.8X-
Bacampicillin	T36.0X-
Bacillus	
lactobacillus	T47.8X-
subtilis	T47.6X-
Bacimycin	T49.0X-
ophthalmic preparation	T49.5X-

Drug/Chemical	Code
Bacitracin zinc	T49.0X-
with neomycin	T49.0X-
ENT agent	T49.6X-
ophthalmic preparation	T49.5X-
topical NEC	T49.0X-
Baclofen	T42.8X-
Baking soda	T50.99-
BAL	T45.8X-
Bambuterol	T48.6X-
Bamethan (sulfate)	T46.7X-
Bamifylline	T48.6X-
Bamipine	T45.0X-
Baneberry— *see Actaea spicata*	
Banewort— *see Belladonna*	
Barbenyl	T42.3X-
Barbexaclone	T42.6X-
Barbital (sodium)	T42.3X-
Barbitone	T42.3X-
Barbiturate NEC	T42.3X-
with tranquilizer	T42.3X-
anesthetic (intravenous)	T41.1X-
Barium (carbonate) (chloride) (sulfite)	T57.8X-
diagnostic agent	T50.8X-
pesticide / rodenticide	T60.4X-
sulfate (medicinal)	T50.8X-
Barrier cream	T49.3X-
Basic fuchsin	T49.0X-
Battery acid or fluid	T54.2X-
Bay rum	T51.8X-
BCG (vaccine)	T50.A9-
BCNU	T45.1X-
Bearsfoot	T62.2X-
Beclamide	T42.6X-
Beclomethasone	T44.5X-
Bee (sting) (venom)	T63.441
Befunolol	T49.5X-
Bekanamycin	T36.5X-
Belladonna— *see Nightshade*	T44.3X-
Bemegride	T50.7X-
Benactyzine	T44.3X-
Benadryl	T45.0X-
Benaprizine	T44.3X-
Benazepril	T46.4X-
Bencyclane	T46.7X-
Bendazol	T46.3X-
Bendrofluazide	T50.2X-
Bendroflumethiazide	T50.2X-
Benemid	T50.4X-
Benethamine penicillin	T36.0X-
Benexate	T47.1X-
Benfluorex	T46.6X-
Benfotiamine	T45.2X-
Benisone	T49.0X-
Benomyl	T60.0X-
Benoquin	T49.8X-

Drug/Chemical	Code
Benoxinate	T41.3X-
Benperidol	T43.4X-
Benproperine	T48.3X-
Benserazide	T42.8X-
Bentazepam	T42.4X-
Bentiromide	T50.8X-
Bentonite	T49.3X-
Benzalbutyramide	T46.6X-
Benzalkonium (chloride)	T49.0X-
ophthalmic preparation	T49.5X-
Benzamidosalicylate (calcium)	T37.1X-
Benzamine	T41.3X-
lactate	T49.1X-
Benzamphetamine	T50.5X-
Benzapril hydrochloride	T46.5X-
Benzathine benzylpenicillin	T36.0X-
Benzathine penicillin	T36.0X-
Benzatropine	T42.8X-
Benzbromarone	T50.4X-
Benzcarbimine	T45.1X-
Benzedrex	T44.99-
Benzedrine (amphetamine)	T43.62-
Benzenamine	T65.3X-
Benzene	T52.1X-
homologues (acetyl) (dimethyl) (methyl) (solvent)	T52.2X-
Benzethonium (chloride)	T49.0X-
Benzfetamine	T50.5X-
Benzhexol	T44.3X-
Benzhydramine (chloride)	T45.0X-
Benzidine	T65.89-
Benzilonium bromide	T44.3X-
Benzimidazole	T60.3X-
Benziodarone	T46.3X-
Benznidazole	T37.3X-
Benzocaine	T41.3X-
Benzodiapin	T42.4X-
Benzodiazepine NEC	T42.4X-
Benzoic acid	T49.0X-
with salicylic acid	T49.0X-
Benzoin (tincture)	T48.5X-
Benzol (benzene)	T52.1X-
vapor	T52.0X-
Benzomorphan	T40.2X-
Benzonatate	T48.3X-
Benzophenones	T49.3X-
Benzopyrone	T46.99-
Benzothiadiazides	T50.2X-
Benzoxonium chloride	T49.0X-
Benzoyl peroxide	T49.0X-
Benzoylpas calcium	T37.1X-
Benzperidin	T43.59-
Benzperidol	T43.59-
Benzphetamine	T50.5X-
Benzpyrinium bromide	T44.1X-
Benzquinamide	T45.0X-

Drug/Chemical	Code
Benzthiazide	T50.2X-
Benztropine	
anticholinergic	T44.3X-
antiparkinson	T42.8X-
Benzydamine	T49.0X-
Benzyl	
acetate	T52.8X-
alcohol	T49.0X-
benzoate	T49.0X-
Benzoic acid	T49.0X-
morphine	T40.2X-
nicotinate	T46.6X-
penicillin	T36.0X-
Benzylhydrochlorthiazide	T50.2X-
Benzylpenicillin	T36.0X-
Benzylthiouracil	T38.2X-
Bephenium hydroxy-naphthoate	T37.4X-
Bepridil	T46.1X-
Bergamot oil	T65.89-
Bergapten	T50.99-
Berries, poisonous	T62.1X-
Beryllium (compounds)	T56.7X-
b-acetyldigoxin	T46.0X-
beta adrenergic blocking agent, heart	T44.7X-
b-benzalbutyramide	T46.6X-
Betacarotene	T45.2X-
b-eucaine	T49.1X-
Beta-Chlor	T42.6X-
b-galactosidase	T47.5X-
Betahistine	T46.7X-
Betaine	T47.5X-
Betamethasone	T49.0X-
topical	T49.0X-
Betamicin	T36.8X-
Betanidine	T46.5X-
b-Sitosterol(s)	T46.6X-
Betaxolol	T44.7X-
Betazole	T50.8X-
Bethanechol	T44.1X-
chloride	T44.1X-
Bethanidine	T46.5X-
Betoxycaine	T41.3X-
Betula oil	T49.3X-
Bevantolol	T44.7X-
Bevonium metilsulfate	T44.3X-
Bezafibrate	T46.6X-
Bezitramide	T40.4X-
BHA	T50.99-
Bhang	T40.7X-
BHC (medicinal)	T49.0X-
nonmedicinal (vapor)	T53.6X-
Bialamicol	T37.3X-
Bibenzonium bromide	T48.3X-
Bibrocathol	T49.5X-
Bichloride of mercury— *see Mercury, chloride*	

Drug/Chemical	Code
Bichromates (calcium) (potassium) (sodium) (crystals)	T57.8X-
fumes	T56.2X-
Biclotymol	T49.6X-
Bicucculine	T50.7X-
Bifemelane	T43.29-
Biguanide derivatives, oral	T38.3X-
Bile salts	T47.5X-
Biligrafin	T50.8X-
Bilopaque	T50.8X-
Binifibrate	T46.6X-
Binitrobenzol	T65.3X-
Bioflavonoid(s)	T46.99-
Biological substance NEC	T50.90-
Biotin	T45.2X-
Biperiden	T44.3X-
Bisacodyl	T47.2X-
Bisbentiamine	T45.2X-
Bisbutiamine	T45.2X-
Bisdequalinium (salts) (diacetate)	T49.6X-
Bishydroxycoumarin	T45.51-
Bismarsen	T37.8X-
Bismuth salts	T47.6X-
aluminate	T47.1X-
anti-infectives	T37.8X-
formic iodide	T49.0X-
glycolylarsenate	T49.0X-
nonmedicinal (compounds)NEC	T65.9-
subcarbonate	T47.6X-
subsalicylate	T37.8X-
sulfarsphenamine	T37.8X-
Bisoprolol	T44.7X-
Bisoxatin	T47.2X-
Bisulepin (hydrochloride)	T45.0X-
Bithionol	T37.8X-
anthelminthic	T37.4X-
Bitolterol	T48.6X-
Bitoscanate	T37.4X-
Bitter almond oil	T62.8X-
Bittersweet	T62.2X-
Black	
flag	T60.9-
henbane	T62.2X-
leaf (40)	T60.9-
widow spider (bite)	T63.31-
antivenin	T50.Z1-
Blast furnace gas (carbon monoxide)	T58.8X-
Bleach	T54.9-
Bleaching agent (medicinal)	T49.4X-
Bleomycin	T45.1X-
Blockain (infiltration) (topical) (subcutaneous) (nerve block)	T41.3X-
Blockers, calcium channel	T46.1X-
Blood (derivatives) (natural) (plasma) (whole) (substitute)	T45.8X-
dried	T45.8X-
drug affecting NEC	T45.9-

Drug/Chemical	Code
Blood (derivatives) (natural) (plasma) (whole) (substitute), continued	T45.8X-
expander NEC	T45.8X-
fraction NEC	T45.8X-
Blue velvet	T40.2X-
Bone meal	T62.8X-
Bonine	T45.0X-
Bopindolol	T44.7X-
Boracic acid	T49.0X-
ENT agent	T49.6X-
ophthalmic preparation	T49.5X-
Borane complex	T57.8X-
Borate(s)	T57.8X-
buffer	T50.99-
cleanser	T54.9-
sodium	T57.8X-
Borax (cleanser)	T54.9-
Bordeaux mixture	T60.3X-
Boric acid	T49.0X-
ENT agent	T49.6X-
ophthalmic preparation	T49.5X-
Bornaprine	T44.3X-
Boron	T57.8X-
hydride NEC	T57.8X-
fumes or gas	T57.8X-
trifluoride	T59.89-
Botox	T48.29-
Botulinus anti-toxin (type A, B)	T50.Z1-
Brake fluid vapor	T59.89-
Brallobarbital	T42.3X-
Bran (wheat)	T47.4X-
Brass (fumes)	T56.89-
Brasso	T52.0X-
Bretylium tosilate	T46.2X-
Brevital (sodium)	T41.1X-
Brinase	T45.3X-
British antilewisite	T45.8X-
Brodifacoum	T60.4X-
Bromal (hydrate)	T42.6X-
Bromazepam	T42.4X-
Bromazine	T45.0X-
Brombenzylcyanide	T59.3X-
Bromelains	T45.3X-
Bromethalin	T60.4X-
Bromhexine	T48.4X-
Bromide salts	T42.6X-
Bromindione	T45.51-
Bromine	
compounds (medicinal)	T42.6X-
sedative	T42.6X-
vapor	T59.89-
Bromisoval	T42.6X-
Bromisovalum	T42.6X-
Bromobenzylcyanide	T59.3X-
Bromochlorosalicylani-lide	T49.0X-

Drug/Chemical	Code
Bromocriptine	T42.8X-
Bromodiphenhydramine	T45.0X-
Bromoform	T42.6X-
Bromophenol blue reagent	T50.99-
Bromopride	T47.8X-
Bromosalicylchloranitide	T49.0X-
Bromosalicylhydroxamic acid	T37.1X-
Bromo-seltzer	T39.1X-
Bromoxynil	T60.3X-
Bromperidol	T43.4X-
Brompheniramine	T45.0X-
Bromsulphthalein	T50.8X-
Bromural	T42.6X-
Bromvaletone	T42.6X-
Bronchodilator NEC	T48.6X-
Brotizolam	T42.4X-
Brovincamine	T46.7X-
Brown recluse spider (bite) (venom)	T63.33-
Brown spider (bite) (venom)	T63.39-
Broxaterol	T48.6X-
Broxuridine	T45.1X-
Broxyquinoline	T37.8X-
Bruceine	T48.29-
Brucia	T62.2X-
Brucine	T65.1X-
Bryonia	T47.2X-
Buclizine	T45.0X-
Buclosamide	T49.0X-
Budesonide	T44.5X-
Budralazine	T46.5X-
Bufferin	T39.01-
Buflomedil	T46.7X-
Buformin	T38.3X-
Bufotenine	T40.99-
Bufrolin	T48.6X-
Bufylline	T48.6X-
Bulk filler	T50.5X-
cathartic	T47.4X-
Bumetanide	T50.1X-
Bunaftine	T46.2X-
Bunamiodyl	T50.8X-
Bunazosin	T44.6X-
Bunitrolol	T44.7X-
Buphenine	T46.7X-
Bupivacaine (infiltration) (Nerve block) (spinal)	T41.3X-
Bupranolol	T44.7X-
Buprenorphine	T40.4X-
Bupropion	T43.29-
Burimamide	T47.1X-
Buserelin	T38.89-
Buspirone	T43.59-
Busulfan, busulphan	T45.1X-
Butabarbital (sodium)	T42.3X-
Butabarbitone	T42.3X-
Butabarpal	T42.3X-

Drug/Chemical	Code
Butacaine	T41.3X-
Butalamine	T46.7X-
Butalbital	T42.3X-
Butallylonal	T42.3X-
Butamben	T41.3X-
Butamirate	T48.3X-
Butane (distributed in mobile container or through pipes)	T59.89-
incomplete combustion	T58.1-
Butanilicaine	T41.3X-
Butanol	T51.3X-
Butanone, 2-butanone	T52.4X-
Butantrone	T49.4X-
Butaperazine	T43.3X-
Butazolidin	T39.2X-
Butetamate	T48.6X-
Butethal	T42.3X-
Butethamate	T44.3X-
Buthalitone (sodium)	T41.1X-
Butisol (sodium)	T42.3X-
Butizide	T50.2X-
Butobarbital (sodium)	T42.3X-
Butobarbitone	T42.3X-
Butoconazole (nitrate)	T49.0X-
Butorphanol	T40.4X-
Butriptyline	T43.01-
Butropium bromide	T44.3X-
Buttercups	T62.2X-
Butyl	
acetate (secondary)	T52.8X-
alcohol	T51.3X-
aminobenzoate	T41.3X-
butyrate	T52.8X-
carbinol or carbitol	T51.3X-
cellosolve	T52.3X-
chloral (hydrate)	T42.6X-
formate or lactate or propionate	T52.8X-
scopolamine bromide	T44.3X-
thiobarbital sodium	T41.1X-
Butylated hydroxy-anisole	T50.99-
Butylchloral hydrate	T42.6X-
Butyltoluene	T52.2X-
Butyn	T41.3X-
Butyrophenone (-based tranquilizers)	T43.4X-
Cabergoline	T42.8X-
Cacodyl, cacodylic acid	T57.0X-
Cactinomycin	T45.1X-
Cade oil	T49.4X-
Cadexomer iodine	T49.0X-
Cadmium (chloride) (fumes) (oxide)	T56.3X-
sulfide (medicinal) NEC	T49.4X-
Cadralazine	T46.5X-
Caffeine	T43.61-
Calabar bean	T62.2X-
Caladium seguinum	T62.2X-

Drug/Chemical	Code
Calamine (lotion)	T49.3X-
Calcifediol	T45.2X-
Calciferol	T45.2X-
Calcitonin	T50.99-
Calcitriol	T45.2X-
Calcium	T50.3X-
actylsalicylate	T39.01-
benzamidosalicylate	T37.1X-
bromide or bromolactobionate	T42.6X-
carbaspirin	T39.01-
carbimide	T50.6X-
carbonate	T47.1X-
chloride (anhydrous)	T50.99-
cyanide	T57.8X-
dioctyl sulfosuccinate	T47.4X-
disodium edathamil	T45.8X-
disodium edetate	T45.8X-
dobesilate	T46.99-
EDTA	T45.8X-
ferrous citrate	T45.4X-
folinate	T45.8X-
glubionate	T50.3X-
gluconate or – gluconogalactogluconate	T50.3X-
hydrate, hydroxide	T54.3X-
hypochlorite	T54.3X-
iodide	T48.4X-
ipodate	T50.8X-
lactate	T50.3X-
leucovorin	T45.8X-
mandelate	T37.9-
oxide	T54.3X-
pantothenate	T45.2X-
phosphate	T50.3X-
salicylate	T39.09-
salts	T50.3X-
Calculus-dissolving drug	T50.99-
Calomel	T49.0X-
Caloric agent	T50.3X-
Calusterone	T38.7X-
Camazepam	T42.4X-
Camomile	T49.0X-
Camoquin	T37.2X-
Camphor	
insecticide	T60.2X-
medicinal	T49.8X-
Camylofin	T44.3X-
Cancer chemo drug regimen	T45.1X-
Candeptin	T49.0X-
Candicidin	T49.0X-
Cannabinol	T40.7X-
Cannabis (derivatives)	T40.7X-
Canned heat	T51.1X-
Canrenoic acid	T50.0X-
Canrenone	T50.0X-
Cantharides, cantharidin, cantharis	T49.8X-

Drug/Chemical	Code
Canthaxanthin	T50.99-
Capillary-active drug NEC	T46.90-
Capreomycin	T36.8X-
Capsicum	T49.4X-
Captafol	T60.3X-
Captan	T60.3X-
Captodiame, captodiamine	T43.59-
Captopril	T46.4X-
Caramiphen	T44.3X-
Carazolol	T44.7X-
Carbachol	T44.1X-
Carbacrylamine (resin)	T50.3X-
Carbamate (insecticide)	T60.0X-
Carbamate (sedative)	T42.6X-
herbicide or insecticide	T60.0X-
Carbamazepine	T42.1X-
Carbamide	T47.3X-
peroxide	T49.0X-
topical	T49.8X-
Carbamylcholine chloride	T44.1X-
Carbaril	T60.0X-
Carbarsone	T37.3X-
Carbaryl	T60.0X-
Carbaspirin	T39.01-
Carbazochrome (salicylate) (sodium sulfonate)	T49.4X-
Carbenicillin	T36.0X-
Carbenoxolone	T47.1X-
Carbetapentane	T48.3X-
Carbethyl salicylate	T39.09-
Carbidopa (with levodopa)	T42.8X-
Carbimazole	T38.2X-
Carbinol	T51.1X-
Carbinoxamine	T45.0X-
Carbiphene	T39.8X-
Carbitol	T52.3X-
Carbo medicinalis	T47.6X-
Carbocaine (infiltration) (topical) (subcutaneous) (nerve block)	T41.3X-
Carbocisteine	T48.4X-
Carbocromen	T46.3X-
Carbol fuchsin	T49.0X-
Carbolic acid— *see also* Phenol	T54.0X-
Carbolonium (bromide)	T48.1X-
Carbomycin	T36.8X-
Carbon	
bisulfide (liquid) or vapor	T65.4X-
dioxide (gas)	T59.7X-
medicinal	T41.5X-
nonmedicinal	T59.7X-
snow	T49.4X-
disulfide (liquid) or vapor	T65.4X-
monoxide (from incomplete combustion)	T58.9-
blast furnace gas	T58.8X-
butane (distributed in mobile container or through pipes)	T58.1-
charcoal fumes or coal	T58.2X-

Drug/Chemical	Code
Carbon, continued	
coke (in domestic stoves, fireplaces)	T58.2X-
gas (piped)	T58.1-
solid (in domestic stoves, fireplaces)	T58.2X-
exhaust gas (motor)not in transit	T58.0-
combustion engine, any not in watercraft	T58.0-
farm tractor, not in transit	T58.0-
gas engine / motor pump	T58.01
motor vehicle, not in transit	T58.0-
fuel (in domestic use)	T58.2X-
gas (piped) (natural) or in mobile container	T58.1-
utility	T58.1-
in mobile container	T58.1-
illuminating gas	T58.1-
industrial fuels or gases, any	T58.8X-
kerosene (in domestic stoves, fireplaces)	T58.2X-
kiln gas or vapor	T58.8X-
motor exhaust gas, not in transit	T58.0-
piped gas (manufactured) (natural)	T58.1-
producer gas	T58.8X-
propane (distributed in mobile container)	T58.1-
distributed through pipes	T58.1-
specified source NEC	T58.8X-
stove gas (piped) / utility gas (piped) / water gas	T58.1-
wood (in domestic stoves, fireplaces)	T58.2X-
tetrachloride (vapor) NEC	T53.0X-
Carbonic acid gas	T59.7X-
anhydrase inhibitor NEC	T50.2X-
Carbophenothion	T60.0X-
Carboplatin	T45.1X-
Carboprost	T48.0X-
Carboquone	T45.1X-
Carbowax	T49.3X-
Carboxymethyl-cellulose	T47.4X-
S-Carboxymethyl-cysteine	T48.4X-
Carbrital	T42.3X-
Carbromal	T42.6X-
Carbutamide	T38.3X-
Carbuterol	T48.6X-
Cardiac medications (depressants) (rhythm regulater) NEC	T46.2X-
Cardiografin	T50.8X-
Cardio-green	T50.8X-
Cardiotonic (glycoside)NEC	T46.0X-
Cardiovascular drug NEC	T46.90-
Cardrase	T50.2X-
Carfecillin	T36.0X-
Carfenazine	T43.3X-
Carfusin	T49.0X-
Carindacillin	T36.0X-
Carisoprodol	T42.8X-
Carmellose	T47.4X-
Carminative	T47.5X-
Carmofur	T45.1X-
Carmustine	T45.1X-
Carotene	T45.2X-

Drug/Chemical	Code
Carphenazine	T43.3X-
Carpipramine	T42.4X-
Carprofen	T39.31-
Carpronium chloride	T44.3X-
Carrageenan	T47.8X-
Carteolol	T44.7X-
Carter's Little Pills	T47.2X-
Cascara (sagrada)	T47.2X-
Cassava	T62.2X-
Castellani's paint	T49.0X-
Castor (bean) (oil)	T62.2X-
Catalase	T45.3X-
Caterpillar (sting)	T63.431
Catha (edulis) (tea)	T43.69-
Cathartic NEC	T47.4X-
anthacene derivative	T47.2X-
bulk	T47.4X-
contact	T47.2X-
emollient NEC	T47.4X-
irritant NEC	T47.2X-
mucilage	T47.4X-
saline	T47.3X-
vegetable	T47.2X-
Cathine	T50.5X-
Cathomycin	T36.8X-
Cation exchange resin	T50.3X-
Caustic(s) NEC	T54.9-
alkali	T54.3X-
hydroxide	T54.3X-
potash	T54.3X-
soda	T54.3X-
specified NEC	T54.9-
Ceepryn	T49.0X-
ENT agent	T49.6X-
lozenges	T49.6X-
Cefacetrile	T36.1X-
Cefaclor	T36.1X-
Cefadroxil	T36.1X-
Cefalexin	T36.1X-
Cefaloglycin	T36.1X-
Cefaloridine	T36.1X-
Cefalosporins	T36.1X-
Cefalotin	T36.1X-
Cefamandole	T36.1X-
Cefamycin antibiotic	T36.1X-
Cefapirin	T36.1X-
Cefatrizine	T36.1X-
Cefazedone	T36.1X-
Cefazolin	T36.1X-
Cefbuperazone	T36.1X-
Cefetamet	T36.1X-
Cefixime	T36.1X-
Cefmenoxime	T36.1X-
Cefmetazole	T36.1X-
Cefminox	T36.1X-

Drug/Chemical	Code
Cefonicid	T36.1X-
Cefoperazone	T36.1X-
Ceforanide	T36.1X-
Cefotaxime	T36.1X-
Cefotetan	T36.1X-
Cefotiam	T36.1X-
Cefoxitin	T36.1X-
Cefpimizole	T36.1X-
Cefpiramide	T36.1X-
Cefradine	T36.1X-
Cefroxadine	T36.1X-
Cefsulodin	T36.1X-
Ceftazidime	T36.1X-
Cefteram	T36.1X-
Ceftezole	T36.1X-
Ceftizoxime	T36.1X-
Ceftriaxone	T36.1X-
Cefuroxime	T36.1X-
Cefuzonam	T36.1X-
Celestone	T38.0X-
topical	T49.0X-
Celiprolol	T44.7X-
Cell stimulants and proliferants	T49.8X-
Cellosolve	T52.9-
Cellulose	
cathartic	T47.4X-
hydroxyethyl	T47.4X-
nitrates (topical)	T49.3X-
oxidized	T49.4X-
Centipede (bite)	T63.41-
Central nervous system	
depressants	T42.71
anesthetic (general)NEC	T41.20-
gases NEC	T41.0X-
intravenous	T41.1X-
barbiturates	T42.3X-
benzodiazepines	T42.4X-
bromides	T42.6X-
cannabis sativa	T40.7X-
chloral hydrate	T42.6X-
ethanol	T51.0X-
hallucinogenics	T40.90-
hypnotics	T42.71
specified NEC	T42.6X-
muscle relaxants	T42.8X-
paraldehyde	T42.6X-
sedatives; sedative-hypnotics	T42.71
mixed NEC	T42.6X-
specified NEC	T42.6X-
muscle-tone depressants	T42.8X-
stimulants	T43.60-
amphetamines	T43.62-
analeptics	T50.7X-
antidepressants	T43.20-

Drug/Chemical	Code
Central nervous system, continued	
opiate antagonists	T50.7X-
specified NEC	T43.69-
Cephalexin	T36.1X-
Cephaloglycin	T36.1X-
Cephaloridine	T36.1X-
Cephalosporins	T36.1X-
N (adicillin)	T36.0X-
Cephalothin	T36.1X-
Cephalotin	T36.1X-
Cephradine	T36.1X-
Cerbera (odallam)	T62.2X-
Cerberin	T46.0X-
Cerebral stimulants	T43.60-
psychotherapeutic	T43.60-
specified NEC	T43.69-
Cerium oxalate	T45.0X-
Cerous oxalate	T45.0X-
Ceruletide	T50.8X-
Cetalkonium (chloride)	T49.0X-
Cethexonium chloride	T49.0X-
Cetiedil	T46.7X-
Cetirizine	T45.0X-
Cetomacrogol	T50.99-
Cetotiamine	T45.2X-
Cetoxime	T45.0X-
Cetraxate	T47.1X-
Cetrimide	T49.0X-
Cetrimonium (bromide)	T49.0X-
Cetylpyridinium chloride	T49.0X-
ENT agent or lozenges	T49.6X-
Cevitamic acid	T45.2X-
Chalk, precipitated	T47.1X-
Chamomile	T49.0X-
Ch'an su	T46.0X-
Charcoal	T47.6X-
activated— *see also Charcoal, medicinal*	T47.6X-
fumes (Carbon monoxide)	T58.2X-
industrial	T58.8X-
medicinal (activated)	T47.6X-
antidiarrheal	T47.6X-
poison control	T47.8X-
specified use other than for diarrhea	T47.8X-
topical	T49.8X-
Chaulmosulfone	T37.1X-
Chelating agent NEC	T50.6X-
Chelidonium majus	T62.2X-
Chemical substance NEC	T65.9-
Chenodeoxycholic acid	T47.5X-
Chenodiol	T47.5X-
Chenopodium	T37.4X-
Cherry laurel	T62.2X-
Chinidin (e)	T46.2X-
Chiniofon	T37.8X-
Chlophedianol	T48.3X-

Drug/Chemical	Code
Chloral	T42.6X-
derivative	T42.6X-
hydrate	T42.6X-
Chloralamide	T42.6X-
Chloralodol	T42.6X-
Chloralose	T60.4X-
Chlorambucil	T45.1X-
Chloramine	T57.8X-
topical	T49.0X-
Chloramphenicol	T36.2X-
ENT agent	T49.6X-
ophthalmic preparation	T49.5X-
topical NEC	T49.0X-
Chlorate (potassium) (sodium)NEC	T60.3X-
herbicide	T60.3X-
Chlorazanil	T50.2X-
Chlorbenzene, chlorbenzol	T53.7X-
Chlorbenzoxamine	T44.3X-
Chlorbutol	T42.6X-
Chlorcyclizine	T45.0X-
Chlordan (e) (dust)	T60.1X-
Chlordantoin	T49.0X-
Chlordiazepoxide	T42.4X-
Chlordiethyl benzamide	T49.3X-
Chloresium	T49.8X-
Chlorethiazol	T42.6X-
Chlorethyl— see Ethyl chloride	
Chloretone	T42.6X-
Chlorex	T53.6X-
insecticide	T60.1X-
Chlorfenvinphos	T60.0X-
Chlorhexadol	T42.6X-
Chlorhexamide	T45.1X-
Chlorhexidine	T49.0X-
Chlorhydroxyquinolin	T49.0X-
Chloride of lime (bleach)	T54.3X-
Chlorimipramine	T43.01-
Chlorinated	
camphene	T53.6X-
diphenyl	T53.7X-
hydrocarbons NEC (solvents)	T53.9-
lime (bleach)	T54.3X-
and boric acid solution	T49.0X-
naphthalene (insecticide)	T60.1X-
industrial (non-pesticide)	T53.7X-
pesticide NEC	T60.8X-
solution	T49.0X-
Chlorine (fumes) (gas)	T59.4X-
bleach	T54.3X-
compound gas NEC	T59.4X-
disinfectant	T59.4X-
releasing agents NEC	T59.4X-
Chlorisondamine chloride	T46.99-
Chlormadinone	T38.5X-

Drug/Chemical	Code
Chlormephos	T60.0X-
Chlormerodrin	T50.2X-
Chlormethiazole	T42.6X-
Chlormethine	T45.1X-
Chlormethylenecycline	T36.4X-
Chlormezanone	T42.6X-
Chloroacetic acid	T60.3X-
Chloroacetone	T59.3X-
Chloroacetophenone	T59.3X-
Chloroaniline	T53.7X-
Chlorobenzene, chlorobenzol	T53.7X-
Chlorobromomethane (fire extinguisher)	T53.6X-
Chlorobutanol	T49.0X-
Chlorocresol	T49.0X-
Chlorodehydro-methyltestosterone	T38.7X-
Chlorodinitrobenzene	T53.7X-
Chlorodiphenyl	T53.7X-
Chloroethane— see Ethyl chloride	
Chloroethylene	T53.6X-
Chlorofluorocarbons	T53.5X-
Chloroform (fumes) (vapor)	T53.1X-
anesthetic	T41.0X-
solvent	T53.1X-
water, concentrated	T41.0X-
Chloroguanide	T37.2X-
Chloromycetin	T36.2X-
ENT agent or otic solution	T49.6X-
ophthalmic preparation	T49.5X-
topical NEC	T49.0X-
Chloronitrobenzene	T53.7X-
Chlorophacinone	T60.4X-
Chlorophenol	T53.7X-
Chlorophenothane	T60.1X-
Chlorophyll	T50.99-
Chloropicrin (fumes)	T53.6X-
fumigant / pesticide	T60.8X-
fungicide	T60.3X-
Chloroprocaine (infiltration) (topical) (subcutaneous) (nerve block) (spinal)	T41.3X-
Chloroptic	T49.5X-
Chloropurine	T45.1X-
Chloropyramine	T45.0X-
Chloropyrifos	T60.0X-
Chloropyrilene	T45.0X-
Chloroquine	T37.2X-
Chlorothalonil	T60.3X-
Chlorothen	T45.0X-
Chlorothiazide	T50.2X-
Chlorothymol	T49.4X-
Chlorotrianisene	T38.5X-
Chlorovinyldichloro-arsine	T57.0X-
Chloroxine	T49.4X-
Chloroxylenol	T49.0X-
Chlorphenamine	T45.0X-

Drug/Chemical	Code
Chlorphenesin	T42.8X-
topical (antifungal)	T49.0X-
Chlorpheniramine	T45.0X-
Chlorphenoxamine	T45.0X-
Chlorphentermine	T50.5X-
Chlorproguanil	T37.2X-
Chlorpromazine	T43.3X-
Chlorpropamide	T38.3X-
Chlorprothixene	T43.4X-
Chlorquinaldol	T49.0X-
Chlorquinol	T49.0X-
Chlortalidone	T50.2X-
Chlortetracycline	T36.4X-
Chlorthalidone	T50.2X-
Chlorthion	T60.0X-
Chlorthiophos	T60.0X-
Chlortrianisene	T38.5X-
Chlor-Trimeton	T45.0X-
Chlorzoxazone	T42.8X-
Choke damp	T59.7X-
Cholagogues	T47.5X-
Cholebrine	T50.8X-
Cholecalciferol	T45.2X-
Cholecystokinin	T50.8X-
Cholera vaccine	T50.A9-
Choleretic	T47.5X-
Cholesterol-lowering agents	T46.6X-
Cholestyramine (resin)	T46.6X-
Cholic acid	T47.5X-
Choline	T48.6X-
chloride	T50.99-
dihydrogen citrate	T50.99-
salicylate	T39.09-
theophyllinate	T48.6X-
Cholinergic (drug)NEC	T44.1X-
muscle tone enhancer	T44.1X-
organophosphorus	T44.0X-
insecticide	T60.0X-
nerve gas	T59.89-
trimethyl ammonium propanediol	T44.1X-
Cholinesterase reactivator	T50.6X-
Cholografin	T50.8X-
Chorionic gonadotropin	T38.89-
Chromate	T56.2X-
dust or mist	T56.2X-
lead— see also lead	T56.0X-
paint	T56.0X-
Chromic	
acid	T56.2X-
dust or mist	T56.2X-
phosphate 32P	T45.1X-
Chromium	T56.2X-
compounds— see Chromate	
sesquioxide	T50.8X-
Chromomycin A3	T45.1X-

Drug/Chemical	Code
Chromonar	T46.3X-
Chromyl chloride	T56.2X-
Chrysarobin	T49.4X-
Chrysazin	T47.2X-
Chymar	T45.3X-
ophthalmic preparation	T49.5X-
Chymopapain	T45.3X-
Chymotrypsin	T45.3X-
ophthalmic preparation	T49.5X-
Cianidanol	T50.99-
Cianopramine	T43.01-
Cibenzoline	T46.2X-
Ciclacillin	T36.0X-
Ciclobarbital— see Hexobarbital	
Ciclonicate	T46.7X-
Ciclopirox (olamine)	T49.0X-
Ciclosporin	T45.1X-
Cicuta maculata or virosa	T62.2X-
Cicutoxin	T62.2X-
Cigarette lighter fluid	T52.0X-
Cigarettes (tobacco)	T65.22-
Ciguatoxin	T61.0-
Cilazapril	T46.4X-
Cimetidine	T47.0X-
Cimetropium bromide	T44.3X-
Cinchocaine	T41.3X-
Cinchona	T37.2X-
Cinchonine alkaloids	T37.2X-
Cinchophen	T50.4X-
Cinepazide	T46.7X-
Cinnamedrine	T48.5X-
Cinnarizine	T45.0X-
Cinoxacin	T37.8X-
Ciprofibrate	T46.6X-
Ciprofloxacin	T36.8X-
Cisapride	T47.8X-
Cisplatin	T45.1X-
Citalopram	T43.22-
Citanest (infiltration) (topical) (subcutaneous) (nerve block)	T41.3X-
Citric acid	T47.5X-
Citrovorum (factor)	T45.8X-
Claviceps purpurea	T62.2X-
Clavulanic acid	T36.1X-
Cleaner, cleansing agent, type not specified	T65.89-
of paint or varnish	T52.9-
specified type NEC	T65.89-
Clebopride	T47.8X-
Clefamide	T37.3X-
Clemastine	T45.0X-
Clematis vitalba	T62.2X-
Clemizole (penicillin)	T45.0X-
Clenbuterol	T48.6X-
Clidinium bromide	T44.3X-
Clindamycin	T36.8X-
Clinofibrate	T46.6X-

Drug/Chemical	Code
Clioquinol	T37.8X-
Cliradon	T40.2X-
Clobazam	T42.4X-
Clobenzorex	T50.5X-
Clobetasol	T49.0X-
Clobetasone	T49.0X-
Clobutinol	T48.3X-
Clocortolone	T38.0X-
Clodantoin	T49.0X-
Clodronic acid	T50.99-
Clofazimine	T37.1X-
Clofedanol	T48.3X-
Clofenamide	T50.2X-
Clofenotane	T49.0X-
Clofezone	T39.2X-
Clofibrate	T46.6X-
Clofibride	T46.6X-
Cloforex	T50.5X-
Clomethiazole	T42.6X-
Clometocillin	T36.0X-
Clomifene	T38.5X-
Clomiphene	T38.5X-
Clomipramine	T43.01-
Clomocycline	T36.4X-
Clonazepam	T42.4X-
Clonidine	T46.5X-
Clonixin	T39.8X-
Clopamide	T50.2X-
Clopenthixol	T43.4X-
Cloperastine	T48.3X-
Clophedianol	T48.3X-
Cloponone	T36.2X-
Cloprednol	T38.0X-
Cloral betaine	T42.6X-
Cloramfenicol	T36.2X-
Clorazepate (dipotassium)	T42.4X-
Clorexolone	T50.2X-
Clorfenamine	T45.0X-
Clorgiline	T43.1X-
Clorotepine	T44.3X-
Clorox (bleach)	T54.9-
Clorprenaline	T48.6X-
Clortermine	T50.5X-
Clotiapine	T43.59-
Clotiazepam	T42.4X-
Clotibric acid	T46.6X-
Clotrimazole	T49.0X-
Cloxacillin	T36.0X-
Cloxazolam	T42.4X-
Cloxiquine	T49.0X-
Clozapine	T42.4X-
Coagulant NEC	T45.7X-

Drug/Chemical	Code
Coal (carbon monoxide from)— *see also Carbon, monoxide, coal*	T58.2X-
oil— *see Kerosene*	
tar	T49.1X-
fumes	T59.89-
medicinal (ointment)	T49.4X-
analgesics NEC	T39.2X-
naphtha (solvent)	T52.0X-
Cobalamine	T45.2X-
Cobalt (nonmedicinal) (fumes) (industrial)	T56.89-
medicinal (trace) (chloride)	T45.8X-
Cobra (venom)	T63.041
Coca (leaf)	T40.5X-
Cocaine	T40.5X-
topical anesthetic	T41.3X-
Cocarboxylase	T45.3X-
Coccidioidin	T50.8X-
Cocculus indicus	T62.1X-
Cochineal	T65.6X-
medicinal products	T50.99-
Codeine	T40.2X-
Cod-liver oil	T45.2X-
Coenzyme A	T50.99-
Coffee	T62.8X-
Cogalactoiso-merase	T50.99-
Cogentin	T44.3X-
Coke fumes or gas (carbon monoxide)	T58.2X-
industrial use	T58.8X-
Colace	T47.4X-
Colaspase	T45.1X-
Colchicine	T50.4X-
Colchicum	T62.2X-
Cold cream	T49.3X-
Colecalciferol	T45.2X-
Colestipol	T46.6X-
Colestyramine	T46.6X-
Colimycin	T36.8X-
Colistimethate	T36.8X-
Colistin	T36.8X-
sulfate (eye preparation)	T49.5X-
Collagen	T50.99-
Collagenase	T49.4X-
Collodion	T49.3X-
Colocynth	T47.2X-
Colophony adhesive	T49.3X-
Colorant— *see also Dye*	T50.99-
Combustion gas (after combustion) — *see Carbon, monoxide*	
prior to combustion	T59.89-
Compazine	T43.3X-
Compound	
42 (warfarin)	T60.4X-
269 (endrin)	T60.1X-
497 (dieldrin)	T60.1X-
1080 (sodium fluoroacetate)	T60.4X-

CLIOQUINOL–COMPOUND

Drug/Chemical	Code
Compound, continued	
3422 (parathion)	T60.0X-
3911 (phorate)	T60.0X-
3956 (toxaphene)	T60.1X-
4049 (malathion)	T60.0X-
4069 (malathion)	T60.0X-
4124 (dicapthon)	T60.0X-
E (cortisone)	T38.0X-
F (hydrocortisone)	T38.0X-
Congener, anabolic	T38.7X-
Congo red	T50.8X-
Coniine, conine	T62.2X-
Conium (maculatum)	T62.2X-
Conjugated estrogenic substances	T38.5X-
Contac	T48.5X-
Contact lens solution	T49.5X-
Contraceptive (oral)	T38.4X-
vaginal	T49.8X-
Contrast medium, radiography	T50.8X-
Convallaria glycosides	T46.0X-
Convallaria majalis	T62.2X-
berry	T62.1X-
Copper (dust) (fumes) (nonmedicinal) NEC	T56.4X-
arsenate, arsenite	T57.0X-
insecticide	T60.2X-
emetic	T47.7X-
fungicide	T60.3X-
gluconate	T49.0X-
insecticide	T60.2X-
medicinal (trace)	T45.8X-
oleate	T49.0X-
sulfate	T56.4X-
cupric	T56.4X-
fungicide	T60.3X-
medicinal	
ear	T49.6X-
emetic	T47.7X-
eye	T49.5X-
cuprous	T56.4X-
fungicide	T60.3X-
medicinal	
ear	T49.6X-
emetic	T47.7X-
eye	T49.5X-
Copperhead snake (bite) (venom)	T63.06-
Coral (sting)	T63.69-
snake (bite) (venom)	T63.02-
Corbadrine	T49.6X-
Cordite	T65.89-
vapor	T59.89-
Cordran	T49.0X-
Corn cures	T49.4X-
Corn starch	T49.3X-
Cornhusker's lotion	T49.3X-
Coronary vasodilator NEC	T46.3X-

Drug/Chemical	Code
Corrosive NEC	T54.9-
acid NEC	T54.2X-
aromatics	T54.1X-
disinfectant	T54.1X-
fumes NEC	T54.9-
specified NEC	T54.9-
sublimate	T56.1X-
Cortate	T38.0X-
Cort-Dome	T38.0X-
ENT agent	T49.6X-
ophthalmic preparation	T49.5X-
topical NEC	T49.0X-
Cortef	T38.0X-
ENT agent	T49.6X-
ophthalmic preparation	T49.5X-
topical NEC	T49.0X-
Corticosteroid	T38.0X-
ENT agent	T49.6X-
mineral	T50.0X-
ophthalmic	T49.5X-
topical NEC	T49.0X-
Corticotropin	T38.81-
Cortisol	T49.0X-
ENT agent	T49.6X-
ophthalmic preparation	T49.5X-
topical NEC	T49.0X-
Cortisone (acetate)	T38.0X-
ENT agent	T49.6X-
ophthalmic preparation	T49.5X-
topical NEC	T49.0X-
Cortivazol	T38.0X-
Cortogen	T38.0X-
ENT agent	T49.6X-
ophthalmic preparation	T49.5X-
Cortone	T38.0X-
ENT agent	T49.6X-
ophthalmic preparation	T49.5X-
Cortril	T38.0X-
ENT agent	T49.6X-
ophthalmic preparation	T49.5X-
topical NEC	T49.0X-
Corynebacterium parvum	T45.1X-
Cosmetic preparation	T49.8X-
Cosmetics	T49.8X-
Cosyntropin	T38.81-
Cotarnine	T45.7X-
Co-trimoxazole	T36.8X-
Cottonseed oil	T49.3X-
Cough mixture (syrup)	T48.4X-
containing opiates	T40.2X-
expectorants	T48.4X-
Coumadin	T45.51-
rodenticide	T60.4X-
Coumaphos	T60.0X-
Coumarin	T45.51-

Drug/Chemical	Code
Coumetarol	T45.51-
Cowbane	T62.2X-
Cozyme	T45.2X-
Crack	T40.5X-
Crataegus extract	T46.0X-
Creolin	T54.1X-
disinfectant	T54.1X-
Creosol (compound)	T49.0X-
Creosote (coal tar) (beechwood)	T49.0X-
medicinal (expectorant) (syrup)	T48.4X-
Cresol(s)	T49.0X-
and soap solution	T49.0X-
Cresyl acetate	T49.0X-
Cresylic acid	T49.0X-
Crimidine	T60.4X-
Croconazole	T37.8X-
Cromoglicic acid	T48.6X-
Cromolyn	T48.6X-
Cromonar	T46.3X-
Cropropamide	T39.8X-
with crotethamide	T50.7X-
Crotamiton	T49.0X-
Crotethamide	T39.8X-
with cropropamide	T50.7X-
Croton (oil)	T47.2X-
chloral	T42.6X-
Crude oil	T52.0X-
Cryogenine	T39.8X-
Cryolite (vapor)	T60.1X-
insecticide	T60.1X-
Cryptenamine (tannates)	T46.5X-
Crystal violet	T49.0X-
Cuckoopint	T62.2X-
Cumetharol	T45.51-
Cupric	
acetate	T60.3X-
acetoarsenite	T57.0X-
arsenate	T57.0X-
gluconate	T49.0X-
oleate	T49.0X-
sulfate	T56.4X-
Cuprous sulfate— *see also Copper sulfate*	T56.4X-
Curare, curarine	T48.1X-
Cyamemazine	T43.3X-
Cyamopsis tetragono-loba	T46.6X-
Cyanacetyl hydrazide	T37.1X-
Cyanic acid (gas)	T59.89-
Cyanide(s) (compounds) (potassium) (sodium)NEC	T65.0X-
dust or gas (inhalation)NEC	T57.3X-
fumigant	T65.0X-
hydrogen	T57.3X-
mercuric— *see Mercury*	
pesticide (dust) (fumes)	T65.0X-
Cyanoacrylate adhesive	T49.3X-
Cyanocobalamin	T45.8X-

Drug/Chemical	Code
Cyanogen (chloride) (gas)NEC	T59.89-
Cyclacillin	T36.0X-
Cyclaine	T41.3X-
Cyclamate	T50.99-
Cyclamen europaeum	T62.2X-
Cyclandelate	T46.7X-
Cyclazocine	T50.7X-
Cyclizine	T45.0X-
Cyclobarbital	T42.3X-
Cyclobarbitone	T42.3X-
Cyclobenzaprine	T48.1X-
Cyclodrine	T44.3X-
Cycloguanil embonate	T37.2X-
Cyclohexane	T52.8X-
Cyclohexanol	T51.8X-
Cyclohexanone	T52.4X-
Cycloheximide	T60.3X-
Cyclohexyl acetate	T52.8X-
Cycloleucin	T45.1X-
Cyclomethycaine	T41.3X-
Cyclopentamine	T44.4X-
Cyclopenthiazide	T50.2X-
Cyclopentolate	T44.3X-
Cyclophosphamide	T45.1X-
Cycloplegic drug	T49.5X-
Cyclopropane	T41.29-
Cyclopyrabital	T39.8X-
Cycloserine	T37.1X-
Cyclosporin	T45.1X-
Cyclothiazide	T50.2X-
Cycrimine	T44.3X-
Cyhalothrin	T60.1X-
Cymarin	T46.0X-
Cypermethrin	T60.1X-
Cyphenothrin	T60.2X-
Cyproheptadine	T45.0X-
Cyproterone	T38.6X-
Cysteamine	T50.6X-
Cytarabine	T45.1X-
Cytisus	T62.2X-
Cytochrome C	T47.5X-
Cytomel	T38.1X-
Cytosine arabinoside	T45.1X-
Cytoxan	T45.1X-
Cytozyme	T45.7X-
2,4-D	T60.3X-
Dacarbazine	T45.1X-
Dactinomycin	T45.1X-
DADPS	T37.1X-
Dakin's solution	T49.0X-
Dalapon (sodium)	T60.3X-
Dalmane	T42.4X-
Danazol	T38.6X-
Danilone	T45.51-
Danthron	T47.2X-

Drug/Chemical	Code
Dantrolene	T42.8X-
Dantron	T47.2X-
Daphne (gnidium) (mezereum)	T62.2X-
berry	T62.1X-
Dapsone	T37.1X-
Daraprim	T37.2X-
Darnel	T62.2X-
Darvon	T39.8X-
Daunomycin	T45.1X-
Daunorubicin	T45.1X-
DBI	T38.3X-
D-Con	T60.9-
insecticide	T60.2X-
rodenticide	T60.4X-
DDAVP	T38.89-
DDE (bis [chlorophenyl]-dichloroethylene)	T60.2X-
DDS	T37.1X-
DDT (dust)	T60.1X-
Deadly nightshade	T62.2X-
berry	T62.1X-
Deamino-D-arginine vasopressin	T38.89-
Deanol (aceglumate)	T50.99-
Debrisoquine	T46.5X-
Decaborane	T57.8X-
fumes	T59.89-
Decadron	T38.0X-
topical NEC	T49.0X-
Decahydronaphthalene	T52.8X-
Decalin	T52.8X-
Decamethonium (bromide)	T48.1X-
Decholin	T47.5X-
Declomycin	T36.4X-
Decongestant, nasal (mucosa)	T48.5X-
Deet	T60.8X-
Deferoxamine	T45.8X-
Deflazacort	T38.0X-
Deglycyrrhizinized extract of licorice	T48.4X-
Dehydrocholic acid	T47.5X-
Dehydroemetine	T37.3X-
Dekalin	T52.8X-
Delalutin	T38.5X-
Delorazepam	T42.4X-
Delphinium	T62.2X-
Deltamethrin	T60.1X-
Deltasone	T38.0X-
Deltra	T38.0X-
Delvinal	T42.3X-
Demecarium (bromide)	T49.5X-
Demeclocycline	T36.4X-
Demecolcine	T45.1X-
Demegestone	T38.5X-
Demelanizing agents	T49.8X-
Demephion -O and -S	T60.0X-
Demerol	T40.2X-
Demethylchlortetracycline	T36.4X-

Drug/Chemical	Code
Demethyltetracycline	T36.4X-
Demeton -O and -S	T60.0X-
Demulcent (external)	T49.3X-
Demulen	T38.4X-
Denatured alcohol	T51.0X-
Dendrid	T49.5X-
Dental drug, topical application NEC	T49.7X-
Dentifrice	T49.7X-
Deodorant spray (feminine hygiene)	T49.8X-
Deoxycortone	T50.0X-
2-Deoxy-5-fluorouridine	T45.1X-
5-Deoxy-5-fluorouridine	T45.1X-
Deoxyribonuclease (pancreatic)	T45.3X-
Depilatory	T49.4X-
Deprenalin	T42.8X-
Deprenyl	T42.8X-
Depressant, appetite	T50.5X-
Depressant	
appetite (central)	T50.5X-
cardiac	T46.2X-
central nervous system (anesthetic)— *see also Central nervous system, depressants*	T42.7-
general anesthetic	T41.20-
muscle tone	T42.8X-
muscle tone, central	T42.8X-
psychotherapeutic	T43.50-
Deptropine	T45.0X-
Dequalinium (chloride)	T49.0X-
Derris root	T60.2X-
Deserpidine	T46.5X-
Desferrioxamine	T45.8X-
Desipramine	T43.01-
Deslanoside	T46.0X-
Desloughing agent	T49.4X-
Desmethylimipramine	T43.01-
Desmopressin	T38.89-
Desocodeine	T40.2X-
Desogestrel	T38.5X-
Desomorphine	T40.2X-
Desonide	T49.0X-
Desoximetasone	T49.0X-
Desoxycorticosteroid	T50.0X-
Desoxycortone	T50.0X-
Desoxyephedrine	T43.62-
Detaxtran	T46.6X-
Detergent	T49.2X-
external medication	T49.2X-
local	T49.2X-
medicinal	T49.2X-
nonmedicinal	T55.1X-
specified NEC	T55.1X-
Deterrent, alcohol	T50.6X-
Detoxifying agent	T50.6X-
Detrothyronine	T38.1X-
Dettol (external medication)	T49.0X-

Drug/Chemical	Code	Drug/Chemical	Code
Dexamethasone	T38.0X-	Dibekacin	T36.5X-
ENT agent	T49.6X-	Dibenamine	T44.6X-
ophthalmic preparation	T49.5X-	Dibenzepin	T43.01-
topical NEC	T49.0X-	Dibenzheptropine	T45.0X-
Dexamfetamine	T43.62-	Dibenzyline	T44.6X-
Dexamphetamine	T43.62-	Diborane (gas)	T59.89-
Dexbrompheniramine	T45.0X-	Dibromochloropropane	T60.8X-
Dexchlorpheniramine	T45.0X-	Dibromodulcitol	T45.1X-
Dexedrine	T43.62-	Dibromoethane	T53.6X-
Dexetimide	T44.3X-	Dibromomannitol	T45.1X-
Dexfenfluramine	T50.5X-	Dibromopropamidine isethionate	T49.0X-
Dexpanthenol	T45.2X-	Dibrompropamidine	T49.0X-
Dextran (40) (70) (150)	T45.8X-	Dibucaine	T41.3X-
Dextriferron	T45.4X-	Dibunate sodium	T48.3X-
Dextro calcium pantothenate	T45.2X-	Dibutoline sulfate	T44.3X-
Dextro pantothenyl alcohol	T45.2X-	Dicamba	T60.3X-
Dextroamphetamine	T43.62-	Dicapthon	T60.0X-
Dextromethorphan	T48.3X-	Dichlobenil	T60.3X-
Dextromoramide	T40.4X-	Dichlone	T60.3X-
topical	T49.8X-	Dichloralphenozone	T42.6X-
Dextropropoxyphene	T40.4X-	Dichlorbenzidine	T65.3X-
Dextrorphan	T40.2X-	Dichlorhydrin	T52.8X-
Dextrose	T50.3X-	Dichlorhydroxyquinoline	T37.8X-
concentrated solution, intravenous	T46.8X-	Dichlorobenzene	T53.7X-
Dextrothyroxin	T38.1X-	Dichlorobenzyl alcohol	T49.6X-
Dextrothyroxine sodium	T38.1X-	Dichlorodifluoromethane	T53.5X-
DFP	T44.0X-	Dichloroethane	T52.8X-
DHE	T37.3X-	Sym-Dichloroethyl ether	T53.6X-
45	T46.5X-	Dichloroethyl sulfide, not in war	T59.89-
Diabinese	T38.3X-	Dichloroethylene	T53.6X-
Diacetone alcohol	T52.4X-	Dichloroformoxine, not in war	T59.89-
Diacetyl monoxime	T50.99-	Dichlorohydrin, alpha-dichlorohydrin	T52.8X-
Diacetylmorphine	T40.1X-	Dichloromethane (solvent) (vapor)	T53.4X-
Diachylon plaster	T49.4X-	Dichloronaphthoquinone	T60.3X-
Diaethylstilboestrolum	T38.5X-	Dichlorophen	T37.4X-
Diagnostic agent NEC	T50.8X-	2,4-Dichlorophenoxyacetic acid	T60.3X-
Dial (soap)	T49.2X-	Dichloropropene	T60.3X-
sedative	T42.3X-	Dichloropropionic acid	T60.3X-
Dialkyl carbonate	T52.9-	Dichlorphenamide	T50.2X-
Diallylbarbituric acid	T42.3X-	Dichlorvos	T60.0X-
Diallymal	T42.3X-	Diclofenac	T39.39-
Dialysis solution (intraperitoneal)	T50.3X-	Diclofenamide	T50.2X-
Diaminodiphenylsulfone	T37.1X-	Diclofensine	T43.29-
Diamorphine	T40.1X-	Diclonixine	T39.8X-
Diamox	T50.2X-	Dicloxacillin	T36.0X-
Diamthazole	T49.0X-	Dicophane	T49.0X-
Dianthone	T47.2X-	Dicoumarol, dicoumarin, dicumarol	T45.51-
Diaphenylsulfone	T37.0X-	Dicrotophos	T60.0X-
Diasone (sodium)	T37.1X-	Dicyanogen (gas)	T65.0X-
Diastase	T47.5X-	Dicyclomine	T44.3X-
Diatrizoate	T50.8X-	Dicycloverine	T44.3X-
Diazepam	T42.4X-	Dideoxycytidine	T37.5X-
Diazinon	T60.0X-	Dideoxyinosine	T37.5X-
Diazomethane (gas)	T59.89-	Dieldrin (vapor)	T60.1X-
Diazoxide	T46.5X-	Diemal	T42.3X-

Drug/Chemical	Code
Dienestrol	T38.5X-
Dienoestrol	T38.5X-
Dietetic drug NEC	T50.90-
Diethazine	T42.8X-
Diethyl	
barbituric acid / carbinol	T42.3X-
carbamazine	T37.4X-
carbonate / oxide	T52.8X-
ether (vapor)— *see also ether*	T41.0X-
propion	T50.5X-
stilbestrol	T38.5X-
toluamide (nonmedicinal)	T60.8X-
medicinal	T49.3X-
Diethylcarbamazine	T37.4X-
Diethylene	
dioxide	T52.8X-
glycol (monoacetate) (monobutyl ether) (monoethyl ether)	T52.3X-
Diethylhexylphthalate	T65.89-
Diethylpropion	T50.5X-
Diethylstilbestrol	T38.5X-
Diethylstilboestrol	T38.5X-
Diethylsulfone-diethylmethane	T42.6X-
Diethyltoluamide	T49.0X-
Diethyltryptamine (DET)	T40.99-
Difebarbamate	T42.3X-
Difencloxazine	T40.2X-
Difenidol	T45.0X-
Difenoxin	T47.6X-
Difetarsone	T37.3X-
Diffusin	T45.3X-
Diflorasone	T49.0X-
Diflos	T44.0X-
Diflubenzuron	T60.1X-
Diflucortolone	T49.0X-
Diflunisal	T39.09-
Difluoromethyldopa	T42.8X-
Difluorophate	T44.0X-
Digestant NEC	T47.5X-
Digitalin (e)	T46.0X-
Digitalis (leaf) (glycoside)	T46.0X-
Digitoxin	T46.0X-
Digitoxose	T46.0X-
Digoxin	T46.0X-
Digoxine	T46.0X-
Dihydralazine	T46.5X-
Dihydrazine	T46.5X-
Dihydrocodeine	T40.2X-
Dihydrocodeinone	T40.2X-
Dihydroergocornine	T46.7X-
Dihydroergocristine (mesilate)	T46.7X-
Dihydroergokryptine	T46.7X-
Dihydroergotamine	T46.5X-
Dihydroergotoxine (mesilate)	T46.7X-
Dihydrohydroxycodeinone	T40.2X-
Dihydrohydroxymorphinone	T40.2X-

Drug/Chemical	Code
Dihydroisocodeine	T40.2X-
Dihydromorphine	T40.2X-
Dihydromorphinone	T40.2X-
Dihydrostreptomycin	T36.5X-
Dihydrotachysterol	T45.2X-
Dihydroxyaluminum aminoacetate	T47.1X-
Dihydroxyaluminum sodium carbonate	T47.1X-
Dihydroxyanthraquinone	T47.2X-
Dihydroxycodeinone	T40.2X-
Dihydroxypropyl theophylline	T50.2X-
Diiodohydroxyquin	T37.8X-
topical	T49.0X-
Diiodohydroxyquinoline	T37.8X-
Diiodotyrosine	T38.2X-
Diisopromine	T44.3X-
Diisopropylamine	T46.3X-
Diisopropylfluorophos-phonate	T44.0X-
Dilantin	T42.0X-
Dilaudid	T40.2X-
Dilazep	T46.3X-
Dill	T47.5X-
Diloxanide	T37.3X-
Diltiazem	T46.1X-
Dimazole	T49.0X-
Dimefline	T50.7X-
Dimefox	T60.0X-
Dimemorfan	T48.3X-
Dimenhydrinate	T45.0X-
Dimercaprol (British anti-lewisite)	T45.8X-
Dimercaptopropanol	T45.8X-
Dimestrol	T38.5X-
Dimetane	T45.0X-
Dimethicone	T47.1X-
Dimethindene	T45.0X-
Dimethisoquin	T49.1X-
Dimethisterone	T38.5X-
Dimethoate	T60.0X-
Dimethocaine	T41.3X-
Dimethoxanate	T48.3X-
Dimethyl	
arsine, arsinic acid	T57.0X-
carbinol	T51.2X-
carbonate	T52.8X-
diguanide	T38.3X-
ketone (vapor)	T52.4X-
meperidine	T40.2X-
parathion	T60.0X-
phthlate	T49.3X-
polysiloxane	T47.8X-
sulfate (fumes)	T59.89-
liquid	T65.89-
sulfoxide (nonmedicinal)	T52.8X-
medicinal	T49.4X-
tryptamine	T40.99-
tubocurarine	T48.1X-

Drug/Chemical	Code
Dimethylamine sulfate	T49.4X-
Dimethylformamide	T52.8X-
Dimethyltubocurarinium chloride	T48.1X-
Dimeticone	T47.1X-
Dimetilan	T60.0X-
Dimetindene	T45.0X-
Dimetotiazine	T43.3X-
Dimorpholamine	T50.7X-
Dimoxyline	T46.3X-
Dinitrobenzene	T65.3X-
vapor	T59.89-
Dinitrobenzol	T65.3X-
vapor	T59.89-
Dinitrobutylphenol	T65.3X-
Dinitro (-ortho-) cresol (pesticide) (spray)	T65.3X-
Dinitrocyclohexylphenol	T65.3X-
Dinitrophenol	T65.3X-
Dinoprost	T48.0X-
Dinoprostone	T48.0X-
Dinoseb	T60.3X-
Dioctyl sulfosuccinate (calcium) (sodium)	T47.4X-
Diodone	T50.8X-
Diodoquin	T37.8X-
Dionin	T40.2X-
Diosmin	T46.99-
Dioxane	T52.8X-
Dioxathion	T60.0X-
Dioxin	T53.7X-
Dioxopromethazine	T43.3X-
Dioxyline	T46.3X-
Dipentene	T52.8X-
Diperodon	T41.3X-
Diphacinone	T60.4X-
Diphemanil	T44.3X-
metilsulfate	T44.3X-
Diphenadione	T45.51-
rodenticide	T60.4X-
Diphenhydramine	T45.0X-
Diphenidol	T45.0X-
Diphenoxylate	T47.6X-
Diphenylamine	T65.3X-
Diphenylbutazone	T39.2X-
Diphenylchloroarsine, not in war	T57.0X-
Diphenylhydantoin	T42.0X-
Diphenylmethane dye	T52.1X-
Diphenylpyraline	T45.0X-
Diphtheria	
antitoxin	T50.Z1-
vaccine — See also Vaccines	T50.A9-
Diphylline	T50.2X-
Dipipanone	T40.4X-
Dipivefrine	T49.5X-
Diplovax	T50.B9-
Diprophylline	T50.2X-
Dipropyline	T48.29-

Drug/Chemical	Code
Dipyridamole	T46.3X-
Dipyrone	T39.2X-
Diquat (dibromide)	T60.3X-
Disinfectant	T65.89-
alkaline	T54.3X-
aromatic	T54.1X-
intestinal	T37.8X-
Disipal	T42.8X-
Disodium edetate	T50.6X-
Disoprofol	T41.29-
Disopyramide	T46.2X-
Distigmine (bromide)	T44.0X-
Disulfamide	T50.2X-
Disulfanilamide	T37.0X-
Disulfiram	T50.6X-
Disulfoton	T60.0X-
Dithiazanine iodide	T37.4X-
Dithiocarbamate	T60.0X-
Dithranol	T49.4X-
Diucardin	T50.2X-
Diupres	T50.2X-
Diuretic NEC	T50.2X-
benzothiadiazine	T50.2X-
carbonic acid anhydrase inhibitors	T50.2X-
furfuryl NEC	T50.2X-
loop (high-ceiling)	T50.1X-
mercurial NEC or osmotic	T50.2X-
purine or saluretic NEC	T50.2X-
sulfonamide	T50.2X-
thiazide NEC or xanthine	T50.2X-
Diurgin	T50.2X-
Diuril	T50.2X-
Diuron	T60.3X-
Divalproex	T42.6X-
Divinyl ether	T41.0X-
Dixanthogen	T49.0X-
Dixyrazine	T43.3X-
D-lysergic acid diethylamide	T40.8X-
DMCT	T36.4X-
DMSO— see Dimethyl sulfoxide	
DNBP	T60.3X-
DNOC	T65.3X-
Dobutamine	T44.5X-
DOCA	T38.0X-
Docusate sodium	T47.4X-
Dodicin	T49.0X-
Dofamium chloride	T49.0X-
Dolophine	T40.3X-
Doloxene	T39.8X-
Domestic gas (after combustion)— see Gas, utility	
prior to combustion	T59.89-
Domiodol	T48.4X-
Domiphen (bromide)	T49.0X-
Domperidone	T45.0X-
Dopa	T42.8X-

DOPAMINE–EPAB

Drug/Chemical	Code
Dopamine	T44.99-
Doriden	T42.6X-
Dormiral	T42.3X-
Dormison	T42.6X-
Dornase	T48.4X-
Dorsacaine	T41.3X-
Dosulepin	T43.01-
Dothiepin	T43.01-
Doxantrazole	T48.6X-
Doxapram	T50.7X-
Doxazosin	T44.6X-
Doxepin	T43.01-
Doxifluridine	T45.1X-
Doxorubicin	T45.1X-
Doxycycline	T36.4X-
Doxylamine	T45.0X-
Dramamine	T45.0X-
Drano (drain cleaner)	T54.3X-
Dressing, live pulp	T49.7X-
Drocode	T40.2X-
Dromoran	T40.2X-
Dromostanolone	T38.7X-
Dronabinol	T40.7X-
Droperidol	T43.59-
Dropropizine	T48.3X-
Drostanolone	T38.7X-
Drotaverine	T44.3X-
Drotrecogin alfa	T45.51-
Drug NEC	T50.90-
specified NEC	T50.99-
DTaP	T50.A1
DTIC	T45.1X-
Duboisine	T44.3X-
Dulcolax	T47.2X-
Duponol (C) (EP)	T49.2X-
Durabolin	T38.7X-
Dyclone	T41.3X-
Dyclonine	T41.3X-
Dydrogesterone	T38.5X-
Dye NEC	T65.6X-
antiseptic	T49.0X-
diagnostic agents	T50.8X-
pharmaceutical NEC	T50.90-
Dyflos	T44.0X-
Dymelor	T38.3X-
Dynamite	T65.3X-
fumes	T59.89-
Dyphylline	T44.3X-
Ear drug NEC	T49.6X-
Ear preparations	T49.6X-
Echothiophate, echothiopate, ecothiopate	T49.5X-
Econazole	T49.0X-
Ecothiopate iodide	T49.5X-
Ecstasy	T43.64-
Ectylurea	T42.6X-

Drug/Chemical	Code
Edathamil disodium	T45.8X-
Edecrin	T50.1X-
Edetate, disodium (calcium)	T45.8X-
Edoxudine	T49.5X-
Edrophonium	T44.0X-
chloride	T44.0X-
EDTA	T50.6X-
Eflornithine	T37.2X-
Efloxate	T46.3X-
Elase	T49.8X-
Elastase	T47.5X-
Elaterium	T47.2X-
Elcatonin	T50.99-
Elder	T62.2X-
berry, (unripe)	T62.1X-
Electrolyte balance drug	T50.3X-
Electrolytes NEC	T50.3X-
Electrolytic agent NEC	T50.3X-
Elemental diet	T50.90-
Elliptinium acetate	T45.1X-
Embramine	T45.0X-
Emepronium (salts) (bromide)	T44.3X-
Emetic NEC	T47.7X-
Emetine	T37.3X-
Emollient NEC	T49.3X-
Emorfazone	T39.8X-
Emylcamate	T43.59-
Enalapril	T46.4X-
Enalaprilat	T46.4X-
Encainide	T46.2X-
Endocaine	T41.3X-
Endosulfan	T60.2X-
Endothall	T60.3X-
Endralazine	T46.5X-
Endrin	T60.1X-
Enflurane	T41.0X-
Enhexymal	T42.3X-
Enocitabine	T45.1X-
Enovid	T38.4X-
Enoxacin	T36.8X-
Enoxaparin (sodium)	T45.51-
Enpiprazole	T43.59-
Enprofylline	T48.6X-
Enprostil	T47.1X-
ENT preparations (anti-infectives)	T49.6X-
Enterogastrone	T38.89-
Enviomycin	T36.8X-
Enzodase	T45.3X-
Enzyme NEC	T45.3X-
depolymerizing	T49.8X-
fibrolytic	T45.3X-
gastric / intestinal	T47.5X-
local action / proteolytic	T49.4X-
thrombolytic	T45.3X-
EPAB	T41.3X-

Drug/Chemical	Code
Epanutin	T42.0X-
Ephedra	T44.99-
Ephedrine	T44.99-
Epichlorhydrin, epichlorohydrin	T52.8X-
Epicillin	T36.0X-
Epiestriol	T38.5X-
Epimestrol	T38.5X-
Epinephrine	T44.5X-
Epirubicin	T45.1X-
Epitiostanol	T38.7X-
Epitizide	T50.2X-
EPN	T60.0X-
EPO	T45.8X-
Epoetin alpha	T45.8X-
Epomediol	T50.99-
Epoprostenol	T45.521
Epoxy resin	T65.89-
Eprazinone	T48.4X-
Epsilon amino-caproic acid	T45.62-
Epsom salt	T47.3X-
Eptazocine	T40.4X-
Equanil	T43.59-
Equisetum	T62.2X-
diuretic	T50.2X-
Ergobasine	T48.0X-
Ergocalciferol	T45.2X-
Ergoloid mesylates	T46.7X-
Ergometrine	T48.0X-
Ergonovine	T48.0X-
Ergot NEC	T64.81
derivative or medicinal (alkaloids) or prepared	T48.0X-
Ergotamine	T46.5X-
Ergotocine	T48.0X-
Ergotrate	T48.0X-
Eritrityl tetranitrate	T46.3X-
Erythrityl tetranitrate	T46.3X-
Erythrol tetranitrate	T46.3X-
Erythromycin (salts)	T36.3X-
ophthalmic preparation	T49.5X-
topical NEC	T49.0X-
Erythropoietin	T45.8X-
human	T45.8X-
Escin	T46.99-
Esculin	T45.2X-
Esculoside	T45.2X-
ESDT (ether-soluble tar distillate)	T49.1X-
Eserine	T49.5X-
Esflurbiprofen	T39.31-
Eskabarb	T42.3X-
Eskalith	T43.8X-
Esmolol	T44.7X-
Estanozolol	T38.7X-
Estazolam	T42.4X-

Drug/Chemical	Code
Estradiol	T38.5X-
with testosterone	T38.7X-
benzoate	T38.5X-
Estramustine	T45.1X-
Estriol	T38.5X-
Estrogen	T38.5X-
Estrone	T38.5X-
Estropipate	T38.5X-
Etacrynate sodium	T50.1X-
Etacrynic acid	T50.1X-
Etafedrine	T48.6X-
Etafenone	T46.3X-
Etambutol	T37.1X-
Etamiphyllin	T48.6X-
Etamivan	T50.7X-
Etamsylate	T45.7X-
Etebenecid	T50.4X-
Ethacridine	T49.0X-
Ethacrynic acid	T50.1X-
Ethadione	T42.2X-
Ethambutol	T37.1X-
Ethamide	T50.2X-
Ethamivan	T50.7X-
Ethamsylate	T45.7X-
Ethanol (beverage)	T51.0X-
Ethanolamine oleate	T46.8X-
Ethaverine	T44.3X-
Ethchlorvynol	T42.6X-
Ethebenecid	T50.4X-
Ether (vapor)	T41.0X-
anesthetic	T41.0X-
divinyl	T41.0X-
ethyl (medicinal)	T41.0X-
nonmedicinal	T52.8X-
solvent	T52.8X-
Ethiazide	T50.2X-
Ethidium chloride (vapor)	T59.89-
Ethinamate	T42.6X-
Ethinylestradiol, ethinyloestradiol	T38.5X-
with	
levonorgestrel or norethisterone	T38.4X-
Ethiodized oil (131 I)	T50.8X-
Ethion	T60.0X-
Ethionamide	T37.1X-
Ethioniamide	T37.1X-
Ethisterone	T38.5X-
Ethobral	T42.3X-
Ethocaine (infiltration) (topical) (nervel block) (spinal)	T41.3X-
Ethoheptazine	T40.4X-
Ethopropazine	T44.3X-
Ethosuximide	T42.2X-
Ethotoin	T42.0X-
Ethoxazene	T37.9-
Ethoxazorutoside	T46.99-
2-Ethoxyethanol	T52.3X-

ETHOXZOLAMIDE–EX-LAX (PHENOLPHTHALEIN)

Drug/Chemical	Code
Ethoxzolamide	T50.2X-
Ethyl	
acetate	T52.8X-
alcohol (beverage)	T51.0X-
aldehyde (vapor)	T59.89-
liquid	T52.8X-
aminobenzoate	T41.3X-
aminophenothiazine	T43.3X-
benzoate	T52.8X-
biscoumacetate	T45.51-
bromide (anesthetic)	T41.0X-
carbamate	T45.1X-
carbinol	T51.3X-
carbonate	T52.8X-
chaulmoograte	T37.1X-
chloride (anesthetic)	T41.0X-
anesthetic (local)	T41.3X-
inhaled	T41.0X-
local	T49.4X-
solvent	T53.6X-
dibunate	T48.3X-
dichloroarsine (vapor)	T57.0X-
estranol	T38.7X-
ether— *see also ether*	T52.8X-
formate NEC (solvent)	T52.0X-
fumarate	T49.4X-
hydroxyisobutyrate NEC (solvent)	T52.8X-
iodoacetate	T59.3X-
lactate NEC (solvent)	T52.8X-
loflazepate	T42.4X-
mercuric chloride	T56.1X-
methylcarbinol	T51.8X-
morphine	T40.2X-
noradrenaline	T48.6X-
oxybutyrate NEC (solvent)	T52.8X-
Ethylene (gas)	T59.89-
anesthetic (general)	T41.0X-
chlorohydrin	T52.8X-
vapor	T53.6X-
dichloride	T52.8X-
vapor	T53.6X-
dinitrate	T52.3X-
glycol(s)	T52.8X-
dinitrate	T52.3X-
monobutyl ether	T52.3X-
imine	T54.1X-
oxide (fumigant) (nonmedicinal)	T59.89-
medicinal	T49.0X-
Ethylenediamine theophylline	T48.6X-
Ethylenediaminetetra-acetic acid	T50.6X-
Ethylenedinitrilotetra-acetate	T50.6X-
Ethylestrenol	T38.7X-
Ethylhydroxycellulose	T47.4X-

Drug/Chemical	Code
Ethylidene	
chloride NEC	T53.6X-
diacetate	T60.3X-
dicoumarin / dicoumarol	T45.51-
diethyl ether	T52.0X-
Ethylmorphine	T40.2X-
Ethylnorepinephrine	T48.6X-
Ethylparachlorophen-oxyisobutyrate	T46.6X-
Ethynodiol	T38.4X-
with mestranol diacetate	T38.4X-
Etidocaine (infiltration) (subcutaneous) (nerve block)	T41.3X-
Etidronate	T50.99-
Etidronic acid (disodium salt)	T50.99-
Etifoxine	T42.6X-
Etilefrine	T44.4X-
Etilfen	T42.3X-
Etinodiol	T38.4X-
Etiroxate	T46.6X-
Etizolam	T42.4X-
Etodolac	T39.39-
Etofamide	T37.3X-
Etofibrate	T46.6X-
Etofylline	T46.7X-
clofibrate	T46.6X-
Etoglucid	T45.1X-
Etomidate	T41.1X-
Etomide	T39.8X-
Etomidoline	T44.3X-
Etoposide	T45.1X-
Etorphine	T40.2X-
Etoval	T42.3X-
Etozolin	T50.1X-
Etretinate	T50.99-
Etryptamine	T43.69-
Etybenzatropine	T44.3X-
Etynodiol	T38.4X-
Eucaine	T41.3X-
Eucalyptus oil	T49.7X-
Eucatropine	T49.5X-
Eucodal	T40.2X-
Euneryl	T42.3X-
Euphthalmine	T44.3X-
Eurax	T49.0X-
Euresol	T49.4X-
Euthroid	T38.1X-
Evans blue	T50.8X-
Evipal	T42.3X-
sodium	T41.1X-
Evipan	T42.3X-
sodium	T41.1X-
Exalamide	T49.0X-
Exalgin	T39.1X-
Excipients, pharmaceutical	T50.90-
Exhaust gas (engine) (motor vehicle)	T58.0-
Ex-Lax (phenolphthalein)	T47.2X-

Drug/Chemical	Code
Expectorant NEC	T48.4X-
Extended insulin zinc suspension	T38.3X-
External medications (skin) (mucous membrane)	T49.9-
dental agent	T49.7X-
ENT agent	T49.6X-
ophthalmic preparation	T49.5X-
specified NEC	T49.8X-
Extrapyramidal antagonist NEC	T44.3X-
Eye agents (anti-infective)	T49.5X-
Eye drug NEC	T49.5X-
FAC (fluorouracil + doxorubicin + cyclophosphamide)	T45.1X-
Factor	
I (fibrinogen)	T45.8X-
III (thromboplastin)	T45.8X-
VIII (antihemophilic Factor) (concentrate)	T45.8X-
IX complex	T45.7X-
human	T45.8X-
Famotidine	T47.0X-
Fat suspension, intravenous	T50.99-
Fazadinium bromide	T48.1X-
Febarbamate	T42.3X-
Fecal softener	T47.4X-
Fedrilate	T48.3X-
Felodipine	T46.1X-
Felypressin	T38.89-
Femoxetine	T43.22-
Fenalcomine	T46.3X-
Fenamisal	T37.1X-
Fenazone	T39.2X-
Fenbendazole	T37.4X-
Fenbutrazate	T50.5X-
Fencamfamine	T43.69-
Fendiline	T46.1X-
Fenetylline	T43.69-
Fenflumizole	T39.39-
Fenfluramine	T50.5X-
Fenobarbital	T42.3X-
Fenofibrate	T46.6X-
Fenoprofen	T39.31-
Fenoterol	T48.6X-
Fenoverine	T44.3X-
Fenoxazoline	T48.5X-
Fenproporex	T50.5X-
Fenquizone	T50.2X-
Fentanyl	T40.4X-
Fentanyl/fentanyl analogs	T40.41-
Fentazin	T43.3X-
Fenthion	T60.0X-
Fenticlor	T49.0X-
Fenylbutazone	T39.2X-
Feprazone	T39.2X-
Fer de lance (bite) (venom)	T63.06-

Drug/Chemical	Code
Ferric— *see also Iron*	
chloride	T45.4X-
citrate	T45.4X-
hydroxide	T45.4X-
pyrophosphate	T45.4X-
Ferritin	T45.4X-
Ferrocholinate	T45.4X-
Ferrodextrane	T45.4X-
Ferropolimaler	T45.4X-
Ferrous— *see also Iron*	T45.4X-
Ferrous fumerate, gluconate, lactate, salt NEC, sulfate (medicinal)	T45.4X-
Ferrovanadium (fumes)	T59.89-
Ferrum— *see Iron*	
Fertilizers NEC	T65.89-
with herbicide mixture	T60.3X-
Fetoxilate	T47.6X-
Fiber, dietary	T47.4X-
Fiberglass	T65.831
Fibrinogen (human)	T45.8X-
Fibrinolysin (human)	T45.69-
Fibrinolysis	
affecting drug	T45.60-
inhibitor NEC	T45.62-
Fibrinolytic drug	T45.61-
Filix mas	T37.4X-
Filtering cream	T49.3X-
Fiorinal	T39.01-
Firedamp	T59.89-
Fish, noxious, nonbacterial	T61.9-
ciguatera	T61.0-
scombroid	T61.1-
shell	T61.781-
specified NEC	T61.771-
Flagyl	T37.3X-
Flavine adenine dinucleotide	T45.2X-
Flavodic acid	T46.99-
Flavoxate	T44.3X-
Flaxedil	T48.1X-
Flaxseed (medicinal)	T49.3X-
Flecainide	T46.2X-
Fleroxacin	T36.8X-
Floctafenine	T39.8X-
Flomax	T44.6X-
Flomoxef	T36.1X-
Flopropione	T44.3X-
Florantyrone	T47.5X-
Floraquin	T37.8X-
Florinef	T38.0X-
ENT agent	T49.6X-
ophthalmic preparation	T49.5X-
topical NEC	T49.0X-
Flowers of sulfur	T49.4X-
Floxuridine	T45.1X-
Fluanisone	T43.4X-

FLUBENDAZOLE–FOXGLOVE

Drug/Chemical	Code
Flubendazole	T37.4X-
Fluclorolone acetonide	T49.0X-
Flucloxacillin	T36.0X-
Fluconazole	T37.8X-
Flucytosine	T37.8X-
Fludeoxyglucose (18F)	T50.8X-
Fludiazepam	T42.4X-
Fludrocortisone	T50.0X-
ENT agent	T49.6X-
ophthalmic preparation	T49.5X-
topical NEC	T49.0X-
Fludroxycortide	T49.0X-
Flufenamic acid	T39.39-
Fluindione	T45.51-
Flumequine	T37.8X-
Flumethasone	T49.0X-
Flumethiazide	T50.2X-
Flumidin	T37.5X-
Flunarizine	T46.7X-
Flunidazole	T37.8X-
Flunisolide	T48.6X-
Flunitrazepam	T42.4X-
Fluocinolone (acetonide)	T49.0X-
Fluocinonide	T49.0X-
Fluocortin (butyl)	T49.0X-
Fluocortolone	T49.0X-
Fluohydrocortisone	T38.0X-
ENT agent	T49.6X-
ophthalmic preparation	T49.5X-
topical NEC	T49.0X-
Fluonid	T49.0X-
Fluopromazine	T43.3X-
Fluoracetate	T60.8X-
Fluorescein	T50.8X-
Fluorhydrocortisone	T50.0X-
Fluoride (nonmedicinal) (pesticide) (sodium) NEC	T60.8X-
medicinal NEC	T50.99-
dental use	T49.7X-
not pesticide NEC	T54.9-
stannous	T49.7X-
Fluorinated corticosteroids	T38.0X-
Fluorine (gas)	T59.5X-
Fluoristan	T49.7X-
Fluormetholone	T49.0X-
Fluoroacetate	T60.8X-
Fluorocarbon monomer	T53.6X-
Fluorocytosine	T37.8X-
Fluorodeoxyuridine	T45.1X-
Fluorometholone	T49.0X-
ophthalmic preparation	T49.5X-
Fluorophosphate insecticide	T60.0X-
Fluorosol	T46.3X-
Fluorouracil	T45.1X-
Fluorphenylalanine	T49.5X-
Fluothane	T41.0X-

Drug/Chemical	Code
Fluoxetine	T43.22-
Fluoxymesterone	T38.7X-
Flupenthixol	T43.4X-
Flupentixol	T43.4X-
Fluphenazine	T43.3X-
Fluprednidene	T49.0X-
Fluprednisolone	T38.0X-
Fluradoline	T39.8X-
Flurandrenolide	T49.0X-
Flurandrenolone	T49.0X-
Flurazepam	T42.4X-
Flurbiprofen	T39.31-
Flurobate	T49.0X-
Fluroxene	T41.0X-
Fluspirilene	T43.59-
Flutamide	T38.6X-
Flutazolam	T42.4X-
Fluticasone propionate	T38.0X-
Flutoprazepam	T42.4X-
Flutropium bromide	T48.6X-
Fluvoxamine	T43.22-
Folacin	T45.8X-
Folic acid	T45.8X-
with ferrous salt	T45.2X-
antagonist	T45.1X-
Folinic acid	T45.8X-
Folium stramoniae	T48.6X-
Follicle-stimulating hormone, human	T38.81-
Folpet	T60.3X-
Fominoben	T48.3X-
Food, foodstuffs, noxious, nonbacterial, NEC	T62.9-
berries	T62.1X-
mushrooms	T62.0X-
plants	T62.2X-
seafood	T61.9-
specified NEC	T61.8X-
seeds	T62.2X-
shellfish	T61.781
specified NEC	T62.8X-
Fool's parsley	T62.2X-
Formaldehyde (solution), gas or vapor	T59.2X-
fungicide	T60.3X-
Formalin	T59.2X-
fungicide	T60.3X-
vapor	T59.2X-
Formic acid	T54.2X-
vapor	T59.89-
Foscarnet sodium	T37.5X-
Fosfestrol	T38.5X-
Fosfomycin	T36.8X-
Fosfonet sodium	T37.5X-
Fosinopril	T46.4X-
sodium	T46.4X-
Fowler's solution	T57.0X-
Foxglove	T62.2X-

Drug/Chemical	Code
Framycetin	T36.5X-
Frangula	T47.2X-
extract	T47.2X-
Frei antigen	T50.8X-
Freon	T53.5X-
Fructose	T50.3X-
Frusemide	T50.1X-
FSH	T38.81-
Ftorafur	T45.1X-
Fuel	
automobile	T52.0X-
exhaust gas, not in transit	T58.0-
vapor NEC	T52.0X-
gas (domestic use) / utility / in mobile container / piped	T59.89-
industrial, incomplete combustion	T58.8X-
Fugillin	T36.8X-
Fulminate of mercury	T56.1X-
Fulvicin	T36.7X-
Fumadil	T36.8X-
Fumagillin	T36.8X-
Fumaric acid	T49.4X-
Fumes (from)	T59.9-
corrosive NEC	T54.9-
freons	T53.5X-
hydrocarbons (all types)	T59.89-
nitrogen dioxide	T59.0X-
petroleum (liquefied) (distributed)	T59.89-
polyester	T59.89-
specified source NEC	T59.89-
sulfur dioxide	T59.1X-
Fumigant NEC	T60.9-
Fungi, noxious, used as food	T62.0X-
Fungicide NEC (nonmedicinal)	T60.3X-
Fungizone	T36.7X-
topical	T49.0X-
Furacin	T49.0X-
Furadantin	T37.9-
Furazolidone	T37.8X-
Furazolium chloride	T49.0X-
Furfural	T52.8X-
Furnace (coal burning) (domestic), gas from	T58.2X-
industrial	T58.8X-
Furniture polish	T65.89-
Furosemide	T50.1X-
Furoxone	T37.9-
Fursultiamine	T45.2X-
Fusafungine	T36.8X-
Fusel oil (any) (amyl) (butyl) (propyl), vapor	T51.3X-
Fusidate (ethanolamine) (sodium)	T36.8X-
Fusidic acid	T36.8X-
Fytic acid, nonasodium	T50.6X-
GABA	T43.8X-
Gadopentetic acid	T50.8X-
Galactose	T50.3X-
b-Galactosidase	T47.5X-

Drug/Chemical	Code
Galantamine	T44.0X-
Gallamine (triethiodide)	T48.1X-
Gallium citrate	T50.99-
Gallopamil	T46.1X-
Gamboge	T47.2X-
Gamimune	T50.Z1-
Gamma globulin	T50.Z1-
Gamma-aminobutyric acid	T43.8X-
Gamma-benzene hexachloride (medicinal)	T49.0X-
nonmedicinal, vapor	T53.6X-
Gamma-BHC (medicinal)	T49.0X-
Gamulin	T50.Z1-
Ganciclovir (sodium)	T37.5X-
Ganglionic blocking drug NEC	T44.2X-
specified NEC	T44.2X-
Ganja	T40.7X-
Garamycin	T36.5X-
ophthalmic preparation	T49.5X-
topical NEC	T49.0X-
Gardenal	T42.3X-
Gardepanyl	T42.3X-
Gas NEC	T59.9-
acetylene	T59.89-
incomplete combustion of	T58.1-
air contaminants, source or type not specified	T59.9-
anesthetic	T41.0X-
blast furnace	T58.8X-
chlorine	T59.4X-
coal	T58.2X-
cyanide	T57.3X-
dicyanogen	T65.0X-
exhaust	T58.0-
prior to combustion	T59.89-
from wood- or coal-burning stove or fireplace	T58.2X-
industrial use	T58.8X-
prior to combustion	T59.89-
utility (in mobile container or piped)	T59.89-
garage	T58.0-
hydrocarbon NEC (piped)	T59.89-
hydrocyanic acid	T65.0X-
illuminating (after combustion)	T58.1-
prior to combustion	T59.89-
kiln	T58.8X-
lacrimogenic	T59.3X-
marsh	T59.89-
motor exhaust, not in transit	T58.0-
natural	T59.89-
oil	T52.0X-
petroleum (liquefied) (distributed in mobile containers) (piped)	T59.89-
producer	T58.8X-
refrigerant (chlorofluoro-carbon)	T53.5X-
not chlorofluoro-carbon	T59.89-
sewer	T59.9-
specified source NEC	T59.9-

Drug/Chemical	Code
Gas NEC, continued	T59.9-
stove (after combustion)	T58.1-
prior to combustion	T59.89-
tear	T59.3X-
therapeutic	T41.5X-
utility (for cooking, heating, or lighting) (piped) (mobile container) NEC	T59.89-
water	T58.1-
Gasoline	T52.0X-
vapor	T52.0X-
Gastric enzymes	T47.5X-
Gastrografin	T50.8X-
Gastrointestinal drug	T47.9-
biological	T47.8X-
specified NEC	T47.8X-
Gaultheria procumbens	T62.2X-
Gefarnate	T44.3X-
Gelatin (intravenous)	T45.8X-
absorbable (sponge)	T45.7X-
Gelfilm	T49.8X-
Gelfoam	T45.7X-
Gelsemine	T50.99-
Gelsemium (sempervirens)	T62.2X-
Gemeprost	T48.0X-
Gemfibrozil	T46.6X-
Gemonil	T42.3X-
Gentamicin	T36.5X-
ophthalmic preparation	T49.5X-
topical NEC	T49.0X-
Gentian	T47.5X-
violet	T49.0X-
Gepefrine	T44.4X-
Gestonorone caproate	T38.5X-
Gexane	T49.0X-
Gila monster (venom)	T63.11-
Ginger	T47.5X-
Gitalin	T46.0X-
Gitaloxin	T46.0X-
Gitoxin	T46.0X-
Glafenine	T39.8X-
Glandular extract (medicinal)NEC	T50.Z9-
Glaucarubin	T37.3X-
Glibenclamide	T38.3X-
Glibornuride	T38.3X-
Gliclazide	T38.3X-
Glimidine	T38.3X-
Glipizide	T38.3X-
Gliquidone	T38.3X-
Glisolamide	T38.3X-
Glisoxepide	T38.3X-
Globin zinc insulin	T38.3X-
Globulin (antilymphocytic) (antirhesus) (antivenin) (antiviral)	T50.Z1-
Glucagon	T38.3X-
Glucocorticoids	T38.0X-

Drug/Chemical	Code
Glucocorticosteroid	T38.0X-
Gluconic acid	T50.99-
Glucosamine sulfate	T39.4X-
Glucose	T50.3X-
with sodium chloride	T50.3X-
Glucosulfone sodium	T37.1X-
Glucurolactone	T47.8X-
Glue NEC	T52.8X-
Glutamic acid	T47.5X-
Glutaral (medicinal)	T49.0X-
nonmedicinal	T65.89-
Glutaraldehyde (nonmedicinal)	T65.89-
medicinal	T49.0X-
Glutathione	T50.6X-
Glutethimide	T42.6X-
Glyburide	T38.3X-
Glycerin	T47.4X-
Glycerol	T47.4X-
borax	T49.6X-
intravenous	T50.3X-
iodinated	T48.4X-
Glycerophosphate	T50.99-
Glyceryl	
gualacolate	T48.4X-
nitrate	T46.3X-
triacetate (topical)	T49.0X-
trinitrate	T46.3X-
Glycine	T50.3X-
Glyclopyramide	T38.3X-
Glycobiarsol	T37.3X-
Glycols (ether)	T52.3X-
Glyconiazide	T37.1X-
Glycopyrrolate	T44.3X-
Glycopyrronium (bromide)	T44.3X-
Glycoside, cardiac (stimulant)	T46.0X-
Glycyclamide	T38.3X-
Glycyrrhiza extract	T48.4X-
Glycyrrhizic acid	T48.4X-
Glycyrrhizinate potassium	T48.4X-
Glymidine sodium	T38.3X-
Glyphosate	T60.3X-
Glyphylline	T48.6X-
Gold	
colloidal (l98Au)	T45.1X-
salts	T39.4X-
Golden sulfide of antimony	T56.89-
Goldylocks	T62.2X-
Gonadal tissue extract	T38.90-
female	T38.5X-
male	T38.7X-
Gonadorelin	T38.89-
Gonadotropin	T38.89-
chorionic	T38.89-
pituitary	T38.81-
Goserelin	T45.1X-

Drug/Chemical	Code
Grain alcohol	T51.0X-
Gramicidin	T49.0X-
Granisetron	T45.0X-
Gratiola officinalis	T62.2X-
Grease	T65.89-
Green hellebore	T62.2X-
Green soap	T49.2X-
Grifulvin	T36.7X-
Griseofulvin	T36.7X-
Growth hormone	T38.81-
Guaiac reagent	T50.99-
Guaiacol derivatives	T48.4X-
Guaifenesin	T48.4X-
Guaimesal	T48.4X-
Guaiphenesin	T48.4X-
Guamecycline	T36.4X-
Guanabenz	T46.5X-
Guanacline	T46.5X-
Guanadrel	T46.5X-
Guanatol	T37.2X-
Guanethidine	T46.5X-
Guanfacine	T46.5X-
Guano	T65.89-
Guanochlor	T46.5X-
Guanoclor	T46.5X-
Guanoctine	T46.5X-
Guanoxabenz	T46.5X-
Guanoxan	T46.5X-
Guar gum (medicinal)	T46.6X-
Hachimycin	T36.7X-
Hair	
dye	T49.4X-
preparation NEC	T49.4X-
Halazepam	T42.4X-
Halcinolone	T49.0X-
Halcinonide	T49.0X-
Halethazole	T49.0X-
Hallucinogen NOS	T40.90-
specified NEC	T40.99-
Halofantrine	T37.2X-
Halofenate	T46.6X-
Halometasone	T49.0X-
Haloperidol	T43.4X-
Haloprogin	T49.0X-
Halotex	T49.0X-
Halothane	T41.0X-
Haloxazolam	T42.4X-
Halquinols	T49.0X-
Hamamelis	T49.2X-
Haptendextran	T45.8X-
Harmonyl	T46.5X-
Hartmann's solution	T50.3X-
Hashish	T40.7X-
Hawaiian Woodrose seeds	T40.99-
HCB	T60.3X-

Drug/Chemical	Code
HCH	T53.6X-
medicinal	T49.0X-
HCN	T57.3X-
Headache cures, drugs, powders NEC	T50.90-
Heavenly Blue (morning glory)	T40.99-
Heavy metal antidote	T45.8X-
Hedaquinium	T49.0X-
Hedge hyssop	T62.2X-
Heet	T49.8X-
Helenin	T37.4X-
Helium (nonmedicinal)NEC	T59.89-
medicinal	T48.99-
Hellebore (black) (green) (white)	T62.2X-
Hematin	T45.8X-
Hematinic preparation	T45.8X-
Hematological agent	T45.9-
specified NEC	T45.8X-
Hemlock	T62.2X-
Hemostatic	T45.62-
drug, systemic	T45.62-
Hemostyptic	T49.4X-
Henbane	T62.2X-
Heparin (sodium)	T45.51-
action reverser	T45.7X-
Heparin-fraction	T45.51-
Heparinoid (systemic)	T45.51-
Hepatic secretion stimulant	T47.8X-
Hepatitis B	
immune globulin	T50.Z1-
vaccine	T50.B9-
Hepronicate	T46.7X-
Heptabarb	T42.3X-
Heptabarbital	T42.3X-
Heptabarbitone	T42.3X-
Heptachlor	T60.1X-
Heptalgin	T40.2X-
Heptaminol	T46.3X-
Herbicide NEC	T60.3X-
Heroin	T40.1X-
Herplex	T49.5X-
HES	T45.8X-
Hesperidin	T46.99-
Hetacillin	T36.0X-
Hetastarch	T45.8X-
HETP	T60.0X-
Hexachlorobenzene (vapor)	T60.3X-
Hexachlorocyclohexane	T53.6X-
Hexachlorophene	T49.0X-
Hexadiline	T46.3X-
Hexadimethrine (bromide)	T45.7X-
Hexadylamine	T46.3X-
Hexaethyl tetraphos-phate	T60.0X-
Hexafluorenium bromide	T48.1X-
Hexafluronium (bromide)	T48.1X-
Hexa-germ	T49.2X-

HEXAHYDROBENZOL–HYDROCYANIC ACID (LIQUID)

Drug/Chemical	Code
Hexahydrobenzol	T52.8X-
Hexahydrocresol(s)	T51.8X-
arsenide	T57.0X-
arseniurated	T57.0X-
cyanide	T57.3X-
gas	T59.89-
Fluoride (liquid)	T57.8X-
vapor	T59.89-
phophorated	T60.0X-
sulfate	T57.8X-
sulfide (gas)	T59.6X-
arseniurated	T57.0X-
sulfurated	T57.8X-
Hexahydrophenol	T51.8X-
Hexalen	T51.8X-
Hexamethonium bromide	T44.2X-
Hexamethylene	T52.8X-
Hexamethylmelamine	T45.1X-
Hexamidine	T49.0X-
Hexamine (mandelate)	T37.8X-
Hexanone, 2-hexanone	T52.4X-
Hexanuorenium	T48.1X-
Hexapropymate	T42.6X-
Hexasonium iodide	T44.3X-
Hexcarbacholine bromide	T48.1X-
Hexemal	T42.3X-
Hexestrol	T38.5X-
Hexethal (sodium)	T42.3X-
Hexetidine	T37.8X-
Hexobarbital	T42.3X-
rectal	T41.29-
sodium	T41.1X-
Hexobendine	T46.3X-
Hexocyclium (metilsulfate)	T44.3X-
Hexoestrol	T38.5X-
Hexone	T52.4X-
Hexoprenaline	T48.6X-
Hexylcaine	T41.3X-
Hexylresorcinol	T52.2X-
HGH (human growth hormone)	T38.81-
Hinkle's pills	T47.2X-
Histalog	T50.8X-
Histamine (phosphate)	T50.8X-
Histoplasmin	T50.8X-
Holly berries	T62.2X-
Homatropine	T44.3X-
methylbromide	T44.3X-
Homochlorcyclizine	T45.0X-
Homosalate	T49.3X-
Homo-tet	T50.Z1-
Hormone	T38.80-
adrenal cortical steroids	T38.0X-
androgenic	T38.7X-
anterior pituitary NEC	T38.81-
antidiabetic agents	T38.3X-

Drug/Chemical	Code
Hormone, continued	T38.80-
antidiuretic	T38.89-
cancer therapy	T45.1X-
follicle stimulating	T38.81-
gonadotropic	T38.89-
pituitary	T38.81-
growth	T38.81-
luteinizing	T38.81-
ovarian	T38.5X-
oxytocic	T48.0X-
parathyroid (derivatives)	T50.99-
pituitary (posterior)NEC	T38.89-
anterior	T38.81-
specified, NEC	T38.89-
thyroid	T38.1X-
Hornet (sting)	T63.451
Horse anti-human lymphocytic serum	T50.Z1-
Horticulture agent NEC	T65.9-
with pesticide	T60.9-
Human	
albumin	T45.8X-
growth hormone (HGH)	T38.81-
immune serum	T50.Z1-
Hyaluronidase	T45.3X-
Hyazyme	T45.3X-
Hycodan	T40.2X-
Hydantoin derivative NEC	T42.0X-
Hydeltra	T38.0X-
Hydergine	T44.6X-
Hydrabamine penicillin	T36.0X-
Hydralazine	T46.5X-
Hydrargaphen	T49.0X-
Hydrargyri amino-chloridum	T49.0X-
Hydrastine	T48.29-
Hydrazine	T54.1X-
monoamine oxidase inhibitors	T43.1X-
Hydrazoic acid, azides	T54.2X-
Hydriodic acid	T48.4X-
Hydrocarbon gas	T59.89-
Hydrochloric acid (liquid)	T54.2X-
medicinal (digestant)	T47.5X-
vapor	T59.89-
Hydrochlorothiazide	T50.2X-
Hydrocodone	T40.2X-
Hydrocortisone (derivatives)	T49.0X-
aceponate	T49.0X-
ENT agent	T49.6X-
ophthalmic preparation	T49.5X-
topical NEC	T49.0X-
Hydrocortone	T38.0X-
ENT agent	T49.6X-
ophthalmic preparation	T49.5X-
topical NEC	T49.0X-
Hydrocyanic acid (liquid)	T57.3X-
gas	T65.0X-

Drug/Chemical	Code
Hydroflumethiazide	T50.2X-
Hydrofluoric acid (liquid)	T54.2X-
vapor	T59.89-
Hydrogen	T59.89-
arsenide	T57.0X-
arseniureted	T57.0X-
chloride	T57.8X-
cyanide (salts) (gas)	T57.3X-
Fluoride (vapor)	T59.5X-
peroxide	T49.0X-
phosphureted	T57.1X-
sulfide (sulfureted)	T59.6X-
arseniureted	T57.0X-
Hydromethylpyridine	T46.7X-
Hydromorphinol	T40.2X-
Hydromorphinone	T40.2X-
Hydromorphone	T40.2X-
Hydromox	T50.2X-
Hydrophilic lotion	T49.3X-
Hydroquinidine	T46.2X-
Hydroquinone	T52.2X-
vapor	T59.89-
Hydrosulfuric acid (gas)	T59.6X-
Hydrotalcite	T47.1X-
Hydrous wool fat	T49.3X-
Hydroxide, caustic	T54.3X-
Hydroxocobalamin	T45.8X-
Hydroxyamphetamine	T49.5X-
Hydroxycarbamide	T45.1X-
Hydroxychloroquine	T37.8X-
Hydroxydihydrocodeinone	T40.2X-
Hydroxyestrone	T38.5X-
Hydroxyethyl starch	T45.8X-
Hydroxymethylpenta-none	T52.4X-
Hydroxyphenamate	T43.59-
Hydroxyphenylbutazone	T39.2X-
Hydroxyprogesterone	T38.5X-
caproate	T38.5X-
Hydroxyquinoline (derivatives) NEC	T37.8X-
Hydroxystilbamidine	T37.3X-
Hydroxytoluene (nonmedicinal)	T54.0X-
medicinal	T49.0X-
Hydroxyurea	T45.1X-
Hydroxyzine	T43.59-
Hyoscine	T44.3X-
Hyoscyamine	T44.3X-
Hyoscyamus	T44.3X-
dry extract	T44.3X-
Hypaque	T50.8X-
Hypertussis	T50.Z1-
Hypnotic	T42.71
anticonvulsant	T42.71
specified NEC	T42.6X-
Hypochlorite	T49.0X-
Hypophysis, posterior	T38.89-

Drug/Chemical	Code
Hypotensive NEC	T46.5X-
Hypromellose	T49.5X-
Ibacitabine	T37.5X-
Ibopamine	T44.99-
Ibufenac	T39.31-
Ibuprofen	T39.31-
Ibuproxam	T39.31-
Ibuterol	T48.6X-
Ichthammol	T49.0X-
Ichthyol	T49.4X-
Idarubicin	T45.1X-
Idrocilamide	T42.8X-
Ifenprodil	T46.7X-
Ifosfamide	T45.1X-
Iletin	T38.3X-
Ilex	T62.2X-
Illuminating gas (after combustion)	T58.1-
prior to combustion	T59.89-
Ilopan	T45.2X-
Iloprost	T46.7X-
Ilotycin	T36.3X-
ophthalmic preparation	T49.5X-
topical NEC	T49.0X-
Imidazole-4-carboxamide	T45.1X-
Iminostilbene	T42.1X-
Imipenem	T36.0X-
Imipramine	T43.01-
Immu-G	T50.Z1-
Immuglobin	T50.Z1-
Immune (globulin) (serum)	T50.Z1-
Immunoglobin human (intravenous) (normal)	T50.Z1-
Immunosuppressive drug	T45.1X-
Immu-tetanus	T50.Z1-
Indalpine	T43.22-
Indanazoline	T48.5X-
Indandione (derivatives)	T45.51-
Indapamide	T46.5X-
Indendione (derivatives)	T45.51-
Indenolol	T44.7X-
Inderal	T44.7X-
Indian	
hemp	T40.7X-
tobacco	T62.2X-
Indigo carmine	T50.8X-
Indobufen	T45.521
Indocin	T39.2X-
Indocyanine green	T50.8X-
Indometacin	T39.39-
Indomethacin	T39.39-
farnesil	T39.4X-
Indoramin	T44.6X-
Industrial	
alcohol	T51.0X-
fumes	T59.89-
solvents (fumes) (vapors)	T52.9-

Drug/Chemical	Code
Influenza vaccine	T50.B9-
Ingested substance NEC	T65.9-
INH	T37.1X-
Inhibitor	
angiotensin-converting enzyme	T46.4X-
carbonic anhydrase	T50.2X-
fibrinolysis	T45.62-
monoamine oxidase NEC	T43.1X-
hydrazine	T43.1X-
postsynaptic	T43.8X-
prothrombin synthesis	T45.51-
Ink	T65.89-
Inorganic substance NEC	T57.9-
Inosine pranobex	T37.5X-
Inositol	T50.99-
nicotinate	T46.7X-
Inproquone	T45.1X-
Insect (sting), venomous	T63.481
ant	T63.421
bee	T63.441
caterpillar	T63.431
hornet	T63.451
wasp	T63.461
Insecticide NEC	T60.9-
carbamate	T60.0X-
chlorinated	T60.1X-
mixed	T60.9-
organochlorine	T60.1X-
organophosphorus	T60.0X-
Insular tissue extract	T38.3X-
Insulin (amorphous) (globin) (isophane) (Lente) (NPH) (Semilente) (Ultralente)	T38.3X-
defalan	T38.3X-
human	T38.3X-
injection, soluble (biphasic)	T38.3X-
intermediate acting	T38.3X-
protamine zinc	T38.3X-
slow acting	T38.3X-
zinc protamine injection/suspension (amorphous) (crystalline)	T38.3X-
Interferon (alpha) (beta) (gamma)	T37.5X-
Intestinal motility control drug	T47.6X-
biological	T47.8X-
Intranarcon	T41.1X-
Intravenous	
amino acids or fat suspensions	T50.99-
Inulin	T50.8X-
Invert sugar	T50.3X-
Iobenzamic acid	T50.8X-
Iocarmic acid	T50.8X-
Iocetamic acid	T50.8X-
Iodamide	T50.8X-

Drug/Chemical	Code
Iodide NEC— *see also Iodine*	T49.0X-
mercury (ointment)	T49.0X-
methylate	T49.0X-
potassium (expectorant)NEC	T48.4X-
Iodinated	
contrast medium	T50.8X-
glycerol	T48.4X-
human serum albumin (131I)	T50.8X-
Iodine (antiseptic, external) (tincture) NEC	T49.0X-
125— *see also Radiation sickness, and Exposure to radioactivce isotopes*	T50.8X-
therapeutic	T50.99-
131— *see also Radiation sickness, and Exposure to radioactivce isotopes*	T50.8X-
therapeutic	T38.2X-
diagnostic	T50.8X-
for thyroid conditions (antithyroid)	T38.2X-
solution	T49.0X-
vapor	T59.89-
Iodipamide	T50.8X-
Iodized (poppy seed) oil	T50.8X-
Iodobismitol	T37.8X-
Iodochlorhydroxyquin	T37.8X-
topical	T49.0X-
Iodochlorhydroxyquinoline	T37.8X-
Iodocholesterol (131I)	T50.8X-
Iodoform	T49.0X-
Iodohippuric acid	T50.8X-
Iodopanoic acid	T50.8X-
Iodophthalein (sodium)	T50.8X-
Iodopyracet	T50.8X-
Iodoquinol	T37.8X-
Iodoxamic acid	T50.8X-
Iofendylate	T50.8X-
Ioglycamic acid	T50.8X-
Iohexol	T50.8X-
Ion exchange resin	
anion	T47.8X-
cation	T50.3X-
cholestyramine	T46.6X-
intestinal	T47.8X-
Iopamidol	T50.8X-
Iopanoic acid	T50.8X-
Iophenoic acid	T50.8X-
Iopodate, sodium	T50.8X-
Iopodic acid	T50.8X-
Iopromide	T50.8X-
Iopydol	T50.8X-
Iotalamic acid	T50.8X-
Iothalamate	T50.8X-
Iothiouracil	T38.2X-
Iotrol	T50.8X-
Iotrolan	T50.8X-
Iotroxate	T50.8X-
Iotroxic acid	T50.8X-

Drug/Chemical	Code
Ioversol	T50.8X-
Ioxaglate	T50.8X-
Ioxaglic acid	T50.8X-
Ioxitalamic acid	T50.8X-
Ipecac	T47.7X-
Ipecacuanha	T48.4X-
Ipodate, calcium	T50.8X-
Ipral	T42.3X-
Ipratropium (bromide)	T48.6X-
Ipriflavone	T46.3X-
Iprindole	T43.01-
Iproclozide	T43.1X-
Iprofenin	T50.8X-
Iproheptine	T49.2X-
Iproniazid	T43.1X-
Iproplatin	T45.1X-
Iproveratril	T46.1X-
Iron (compounds) (medicinal) NEC	T45.4X-
ammonium/dextran injection/salts/sorbitex/sorbitol citric acid complex	T45.4X-
nonmedicinal	T56.89-
Irrigating fluid (vaginal)	T49.8X-
eye	T49.5X-
Isepamicin	T36.5X-
Isoaminile (citrate)	T48.3X-
Isoamyl nitrite	T46.3X-
Isobenzan	T60.1X-
Isobutyl acetate	T52.8X-
Isocarboxazid	T43.1X-
Isoconazole	T49.0X-
Isocyanate	T65.0X-
Isoephedrine	T44.99-
Isoetarine	T48.6X-
Isoethadione	T42.2X-
Isoetharine	T44.5X-
Isoflurane	T41.0X-
Isoflurophate	T44.0X-
Isomaltose, ferric complex	T45.4X-
Isometheptene	T44.3X-
Isoniazid	T37.1X-
with	
rifampicin	T36.6X-
thioacetazone	T37.1X-
Isonicotinic acid hydrazide	T37.1X-
Isonipecaine	T40.4X-
Isopentaquine	T37.2X-
Isophane insulin	T38.3X-
Isophorone	T65.89-
Isophosphamide	T45.1X-
Isopregnenone	T38.5X-
Isoprenaline	T48.6X-
Isopromethazine	T43.3X-
Isopropamide	T44.3X-
iodide	T44.3X-
Isopropanol	T51.2X-

Drug/Chemical	Code
Isopropyl	
acetate	T52.8X-
alcohol	T51.2X-
medicinal	T49.4X-
ether	T52.8X-
Isopropylaminophenazone	T39.2X-
Isoproterenol	T48.6X-
Isosorbide dinitrate	T46.3X-
Isothipendyl	T45.0X-
Isotretinoin	T50.99-
Isoxazolyl penicillin	T36.0X-
Isoxicam	T39.39-
Isoxsuprine	T46.7X-
Ispagula	T47.4X-
husk	T47.4X-
Isradipine	T46.1X-
I-thyroxine sodium	T38.1X-
Itraconazole	T37.8X-
Itramin tosilate	T46.3X-
Ivermectin	T37.4X-
Izoniazid	T37.1X-
with thioacetazone	T37.1X-
Jalap	T47.2X-
Jamaica	
dogwood (bark)	T39.8X-
ginger	T65.89-
root	T62.2X-
Jatropha	T62.2X-
curcas	T62.2X-
Jectofer	T45.4X-
Jellyfish (sting)	T63.62-
Jequirity (bean)	T62.2X-
Jimson weed (stramonium)	T62.2X-
Josamycin	T36.3X-
Juniper tar	T49.1X-
Kallidinogenase	T46.7X-
Kallikrein	T46.7X-
Kanamycin	T36.5X-
Kantrex	T36.5X-
Kaolin	T47.6X-
light	T47.6X-
Karaya (gum)	T47.4X-
Kebuzone	T39.2X-
Kelevan	T60.1X-
Kemithal	T41.1X-
Kenacort	T38.0X-
Keratolytic drug NEC	T49.4X-
anthracene	T49.4X-
Keratoplastic NEC	T49.4X-
Kerosene, kerosine (fuel) (solvent)NEC	T52.0X-
insecticide	T52.0X-
vapor	T52.0X-
Ketamine	T41.29-
Ketazolam	T42.4X-
Ketazon	T39.2X-

KETOBEMIDONE–LEVOPROXYPHYLLINE

Drug/Chemical	Code
Ketobemidone	T40.4X-
Ketoconazole	T49.0X-
Ketols	T52.4X-
Ketone oils	T52.4X-
Ketoprofen	T39.31-
Ketorolac	T39.8X-
Ketotifen	T45.0X-
Khat	T43.69-
Khellin	T46.3X-
Khelloside	T46.3X-
Kiln gas or vapor (carbon monoxide)	T58.8X-
Kitasamycin	T36.3X-
Konsyl	T47.4X-
Kosam seed	T62.2X-
Krait (venom)	T63.09-
Kwell (insecticide)	T60.1X-
anti-infective (topical)	T49.0X-
Labetalol	T44.8X-
Laburnum (seeds)	T62.2X-
leaves	T62.2X-
Lachesine	T49.5X-
Lacidipine	T46.5X-
Lacquer	T65.6X-
Lacrimogenic gas	T59.3X-
Lactated potassic saline	T50.3X-
Lactic acid	T49.8X-
Lactobacillus (all forms or compounds)	T47.6X-
Lactoflavin	T45.2X-
Lactose (as excipient)	T50.90-
Lactuca (virosa) (extract)	T42.6X-
Lactucarium	T42.6X-
Lactulose	T47.3X-
Laevo— see Levo-	
Lanatosides	T46.0X-
Lanolin	T49.3X-
Largactil	T43.3X-
Larkspur	T62.2X-
Laroxyl	T43.01-
Lasix	T50.1X-
Lassar's paste	T49.4X-
Latamoxef	T36.1X-
Latex	T65.81-
Lathyrus (seed)	T62.2X-
Laudanum	T40.0X-
Laudexium	T48.1X-
Laughing gas	T41.0X-
Laurel, black or cherry	T62.2X-
Laurolinium	T49.0X-
Lauryl sulfoacetate	T49.2X-
Laxative NEC	T47.4X-
osmotic	T47.3X-
saline	T47.3X-
stimulant	T47.2X-
L-dopa	T42.8X-

Drug/Chemical	Code
Lead (dust) (fumes) (vapor) NEC	T56.0X-
acetate	T49.2X-
alkyl (fuel additive)	T56.0X-
anti-infectives	T37.8X-
antiknock compound (tetraethyl)	T56.0X-
arsenate, arsenite (dust) (herbicide) (insecticide) (vapor)	T57.0X-
carbonate (paint)	T56.0X-
chromate (paint)	T56.0X-
dioxide	T56.0X-
inorganic	T56.0X-
iodide (pigment) (paint)	T56.0X-
monoxide (dust) (paint)	T56.0X-
organic	T56.0X-
oxide (paint)	T56.0X-
salts	T56.0X-
specified compound NEC	T56.0X-
tetra-ethyl	T56.0X-
Lebanese red	T40.7X-
Lefetamine	T39.8X-
Lenperone	T43.4X-
Lente lietin (insulin)	T38.3X-
Leptazol	T50.7X-
Leptophos	T60.0X-
Leritine	T40.2X-
Letosteine	T48.4X-
Letter	T38.1X-
Lettuce opium	T42.6X-
Leucinocaine	T41.3X-
Leucocianidol	T46.99-
Leucovorin (factor)	T45.8X-
Leukeran	T45.1X-
Leuprolide	T38.89-
Levalbuterol	T48.6X-
Levallorphan	T50.7X-
Levamisole	T37.4X-
Levanil	T42.6X-
Levarterenol	T44.4X-
Levdropropizine	T48.3X-
Levobunolol	T49.5X-
Levocabastine (hydrochloride)	T45.0X-
Levocarnitine	T50.99-
Levodopa (w carbidopa)	T42.8X-
Levo-dromoran	T40.2X-
Levoglutamide	T50.99-
Levoid	T38.1X-
Levo-iso-methadone	T40.3X-
Levomepromazine	T43.3X-
Levonordefrin	T49.6X-
Levonorgestrel	T38.4X-
with ethinylestradiol	T38.5X-
Levopromazine	T43.3X-
Levoprome	T42.6X-
Levopropoxyphene	T40.4X-
Levopropylhexedrine	T50.5X-
Levoproxyphylline	T48.6X-

Drug/Chemical	Code
Levorphanol	T40.4X-
Levothyroxine	T38.1X-
sodium	T38.1X-
Levsin	T44.3X-
Levulose	T50.3X-
Lewisite (gas), not in war	T57.0X-
Librium	T42.4X-
Lidex	T49.0X-
Lidocaine	T41.3X-
regional	T41.3X-
spinal	T41.3X-
Lidofenin	T50.8X-
Lidoflazine	T46.1X-
Lighter fluid	T52.0X-
Lignin hemicellulose	T47.6X-
Lignocaine	T41.3X-
regional	T41.3X-
spinal	T41.3X-
Ligroin (e) (solvent)	T52.0X-
vapor	T59.89-
Ligustrum vulgare	T62.2X-
Lily of the valley	T62.2X-
Lime (chloride)	T54.3X-
Limonene	T52.8X-
Lincomycin	T36.8X-
Lindane (insecticide) (nonmedicinal) (vapor)	T53.6X-
medicinal	T49.0X-
Liniments NEC	T49.9-
Linoleic acid	T46.6X-
Linolenic acid	T46.6X-
Linseed	T47.4X-
Liothyronine	T38.1X-
Liotrix	T38.1X-
Lipancreatin	T47.5X-
Lipo-alprostadil	T46.7X-
Lipo-Lutin	T38.5X-
Lipotropic drug NEC	T50.90-
Liquefied petroleum gases	T59.89-
piped (pure or mixed with air)	T59.89-
Liquid	
paraffin	T47.4X-
petrolatum	T47.4X-
topical	T49.3X-
specified NEC	T65.89-
substance	T65.9-
Liquor creosolis compositus	T65.89-
Liquorice	T48.4X-
extract	T47.8X-
Lisinopril	T46.4X-
Lisuride	T42.8X-
Lithane	T43.8X-
Lithium	T56.89-
gluconate	T43.59-
salts (carbonate)	T43.59-
Lithonate	T43.8X-

Drug/Chemical	Code
Liver	
extract	T45.8X-
for parenteral use	T45.8X-
fraction 1	T45.8X-
hydrolysate	T45.8X-
Lizard (bite) (venom)	T63.121
LMD	T45.8X-
Lobelia	T62.2X-
Lobeline	T50.7X-
Local action drug NEC	T49.8X-
Locorten	T49.0X-
Lofepramine	T43.01-
Lolium temulentum	T62.2X-
Lomotil	T47.6X-
Lomustine	T45.1X-
Lonidamine	T45.1X-
Loperamide	T47.6X-
Loprazolam	T42.4X-
Lorajmine	T46.2X-
Loratidine	T45.0X-
Lorazepam	T42.4X-
Lorcainide	T46.2X-
Lormetazepam	T42.4X-
Lotions NEC	T49.9-
Lotusate	T42.3X-
Lovastatin	T46.6X-
Lowila	T49.2X-
Loxapine	T43.59-
Lozenges (throat)	T49.6X-
LSD	T40.8X-
L-Tryptophan— see amino acid	
Lubricant, eye	T49.5X-
Lubricating oil NEC	T52.0X-
Lucanthone	T37.4X-
Luminal	T42.3X-
Lung irritant (gas)NEC	T59.9-
Luteinizing hormone	T38.81-
Lutocylol	T38.5X-
Lutromone	T38.5X-
Lututrin	T48.29-
Lye (concentrated)	T54.3X-
Lygranum (skin test)	T50.8X-
Lymecycline	T36.4X-
Lymphogranuloma venereum antigen	T50.8X-
Lynestrenol	T38.4X-
Lyovac Sodium Edecrin	T50.1X-
Lypressin	T38.89-
Lysergic acid diethylamide	T40.8X-
Lysergide	T40.8X-
Lysine vasopressin	T38.89-
Lysol	T54.1X-
Lysozyme	T49.0X-
Lytta (vitatta)	T49.8X-
Mace	T59.3X-
Macrogol	T50.99-

LEVORPHANOL–MACROGOL

527

Drug/Chemical	Code
Macrolide	
anabolic drug	T38.7X-
antibiotic	T36.3X-
Mafenide	T49.0X-
Magaldrate	T47.1X-
Magic mushroom	T40.99-
Magnamycin	T36.8X-
Magnesia magma	T47.1X-
Magnesium NEC	T56.89-
carbonate	T47.1X-
citrate	T47.4X-
hydroxide (oxide)	T47.1X-
peroxide	T49.0X-
salicylate	T39.09-
silicofluoride	T50.3X-
sulfate	T47.4X-
thiosulfate	T45.0X-
trisilicate	T47.1X-
Malathion (medicinal) (insecticide)	T49.0X-
insecticide	T60.0X-
Male fern extract	T37.4X-
M-AMSA	T45.1X-
Mandelic acid	T37.8X-
Manganese (dioxide) (salts)	T57.2X-
medicinal	T50.99-
Mannitol	T47.3X-
hexanitrate	T46.3X-
Mannomustine	T45.1X-
MAO inhibitors	T43.1X-
Mapharsen	T37.8X-
Maphenide	T49.0X-
Maprotiline	T43.02-
Marcaine (infiltration) (subcutaneous) (nerve block)	T41.3X-
Marezine	T45.0X-
Marihuana	T40.7X-
Marijuana	T40.7X-
Marine (sting)	T63.69-
animals (sting)	T63.69-
plants (sting)	T63.71-
Marplan	T43.1X-
Marsh gas	T59.89-
Marsilid	T43.1X-
Matulane	T45.1X-
Mazindol	T50.5X-
MCPA	T60.3X-
MDMA	T43.64-
Meadow saffron	T62.2X-
Measles virus vaccine (attenuated)	T50.B9-
Meat, noxious	T62.8X-
Meballymal	T42.3X-
Mebanazine	T43.1X-
Mebaral	T42.3X-
Mebendazole	T37.4X-
Mebeverine	T44.3X-
Mebhydrolin	T45.0X-

Drug/Chemical	Code
Mebumal	T42.3X-
Mebutamate	T43.59-
Mecamylamine	T44.2X-
Mechlorethamine	T45.1X-
Mecillinam	T36.0X-
Meclizine (hydrochloride)	T45.0X-
Meclocycline	T36.4X-
Meclofenamate	T39.39-
Meclofenamic acid	T39.39-
Meclofenoxate	T43.69-
Meclozine	T45.0X-
Mecobalamin	T45.8X-
Mecoprop	T60.3X-
Mecrilate	T49.3X-
Mecysteine	T48.4X-
Medazepam	T42.4X-
Medicament NEC	T50.90-
Medinal	T42.3X-
Medomin	T42.3X-
Medrogestone	T38.5X-
Medroxalol	T44.8X-
Medroxyprogesterone acetate (depot)	T38.5X-
Medrysone	T49.0X-
Mefenamic acid	T39.39-
Mefenorex	T50.5X-
Mefloquine	T37.2X-
Mefruside	T50.2X-
Megahallucinogen	T40.90-
Megestrol	T38.5X-
Meglumine	
antimoniate	T37.8X-
diatrizoate	T50.8X-
iodipamide	T50.8X-
iotroxate	T50.8X-
MEK (methyl ethyl ketone)	T52.4X-
Meladinin	T49.3X-
Meladrazine	T44.3X-
Melaleuca alternifolia oil	T49.0X-
Melanizing agents	T49.3X-
Melanocyte-stimulating hormone	T38.89-
Melarsonyl potassium	T37.3X-
Melarsoprol	T37.3X-
Melia azedarach	T62.2X-
Melitracen	T43.01-
Mellaril	T43.3X-
Meloxine	T49.3X-
Melperone	T43.4X-
Melphalan	T45.1X-
Memantine	T43.8X-
Menadiol (sodium sulfate)	T45.7X-
Menadione	T45.7X-
sodium bisulfite	T45.7X-
Menaphthone	T45.7X-
Menaquinone	T45.7X-
Menatetrenone	T45.7X-

Drug/Chemical	Code
Meningococcal vaccine	T50.A9-
Menningovax (-AC) (-C)	T50.A9-
Menotropins	T38.81-
Menthol	T48.5X-
Mepacrine	T37.2X-
Meparfynol	T42.6X-
Mepartricin	T36.7X-
Mepazine	T43.3X-
Mepenzolate	T44.3X-
bromide	T44.3X-
Meperidine	T40.4X-
Mephebarbital	T42.3X-
Mephenamin (e)	T42.8X-
Mephenesin	T42.8X-
Mephenhydramine	T45.0X-
Mephenoxalone	T42.8X-
Mephentermine	T44.99-
Mephenytoin	T42.0X-
with phenobarbital	T42.3X-
Mephobarbital	T42.3X-
Mephosfolan	T60.0X-
Mepindolol	T44.7X-
Mepiperphenidol	T44.3X-
Mepitiostane	T38.7X-
Mepivacaine (epidural)	T41.3X-
Meprednisone	T38.0X-
Meprobam	T43.59-
Meprobamate	T43.59-
Meproscillarin	T46.0X-
Meprylcaine	T41.3X-
Meptazinol	T39.8X-
Mepyramine	T45.0X-
Mequitazine	T43.3X-
Meralluride	T50.2X-
Merbaphen	T50.2X-
Merbromin	T49.0X-
Mercaptobenzothiazole salts	T49.0X-
Mercaptomerin	T50.2X-
Mercaptopurine	T45.1X-
Mercumatilin	T50.2X-
Mercuramide	T50.2X-
Mercurochrome	T49.0X-
Mercurophylline	T50.2X-
Mercury, mercurial, mercuric, mercurous (compounds) (cyanide) (fumes) (nonmedicinal) (vapor) NEC	T56.1X-
ammoniated	T49.0X-
anti-infective	
local	T49.0X-
systemic	T37.8X-
topical	T49.0X-
chloride (ammoniated)	T49.0X-
diuretic NEC	T50.2X-
fungicide (organic)	T56.1X-
oxide, yellow	T49.0X-
Mersalyl	T50.2X-

Drug/Chemical	Code
Merthiolate	T49.0X-
ophthalmic preparation	T49.5X-
Meruvax	T50.B9-
Mesalazine	T47.8X-
Mescal buttons	T40.99-
Mescaline	T40.99-
Mesna	T48.4X-
Mesoglycan	T46.6X-
Mesoridazine	T43.3X-
Mestanolone	T38.7X-
Mesterolone	T38.7X-
Mestranol	T38.5X-
Mesulergine	T42.8X-
Mesulfen	T49.0X-
Mesuximide	T42.2X-
Metabutethamine	T41.3X-
Metactesylacetate	T49.0X-
Metacycline	T36.4X-
Metaldehyde (snail killer) NEC	T60.8X-
Metals (heavy) (nonmedicinal)	T56.9-
dust, fumes, or vapor NEC	T56.9-
light NEC	T56.9-
dust, fumes, or vapor NEC	T56.9-
specified NEC	T56.89-
thallium	T56.81-
Metamfetamine	T43.62-
Metamizole sodium	T39.2X-
Metampicillin	T36.0X-
Metamucil	T47.4X-
Metandienone	T38.7X-
Metandrostenolone	T38.7X-
Metaphen	T49.0X-
Metaphos	T60.0X-
Metapramine	T43.01-
Metaproterenol	T48.29-
Metaraminol	T44.4X-
Metaxalone	T42.8X-
Metenolone	T38.7X-
Metergoline	T42.8X-
Metescufylline	T46.99-
Metetoin	T42.0X-
Metformin	T38.3X-
Methacholine	T44.1X-
Methacycline	T36.4X-
Methadone	T40.3X-
Methallenestril	T38.5X-
Methallenoestril	T38.5X-
Methamphetamine	T43.62-
Methampyrone	T39.2X-
Methandienone	T38.7X-
Methandriol	T38.7X-
Methandrostenolone	T38.7X-
Methane	T59.89-
Methanethiol	T59.89-
Methaniazide	T37.1X-

Drug/Chemical	Code
Methanol (vapor)	T51.1X-
Methantheline	T44.3X-
Methanthelinium bromide	T44.3X-
Methaphenilene	T45.0X-
Methapyrilene	T45.0X-
Methaqualone (compound)	T42.6X-
Metharbital	T42.3X-
Methazolamide	T50.2X-
Methdilazine	T43.3X-
Methedrine	T43.62-
Methenamine (mandelate)	T37.8X-
Methenolone	T38.7X-
Methergine	T48.0X-
Methetoin	T42.0X-
Methiacil	T38.2X-
Methicillin	T36.0X-
Methimazole	T38.2X-
Methiodal sodium	T50.8X-
Methionine	T50.99-
Methisazone	T37.5X-
Methisoprinol	T37.5X-
Methitural	T42.3X-
Methixene	T44.3X-
Methobarbital, methobarbitone	T42.3X-
Methocarbamol	T42.8X-
skeletal muscle relaxant	T48.1X-
Methohexital	T41.1X-
Methohexitone	T41.1X-
Methoin	T42.0X-
Methopholine	T39.8X-
Methopromazine	T43.3X-
Methorate	T48.3X-
Methoserpidine	T46.5X-
Methotrexate	T45.1X-
Methotrimeprazine	T43.3X-
Methoxa-Dome	T49.3X-
Methoxamine	T44.4X-
Methoxsalen	T50.99-
Methoxyaniline	T65.3X-
Methoxybenzyl penicillin	T36.0X-
Methoxychlor	T53.7X-
Methoxy-DDT	T53.7X-
2-Methoxyethanol	T52.3X-
Methoxyflurane	T41.0X-
Methoxyphenamine	T48.6X-
Methoxypromazine	T43.3X-
5-Methoxypsoralen (5-MOP)	T50.99-
8-Methoxypsoralen (8-MOP)	T50.99-
Methscopolamine bromide	T44.3X-
Methsuximide	T42.2X-
Methyclothiazide	T50.2X-
Methyl	
acetate	T52.4X-
acetone	T52.4X-
acrylate	T65.89-

Drug/Chemical	Code
Methyl, continued	
alcohol	T51.1X-
aminophenol	T65.3X-
amphetamine	T43.62-
androstanolone	T38.7X-
atropine	T44.3X-
benzene	T52.2X-
benzoate	T52.8X-
benzol	T52.2X-
bromide (gas)	T59.89-
fumigant	T60.8X-
butanol	T51.3X-
carbinol	T51.1X-
carbonate	T52.8X-
CCNU	T45.1X-
cellosolve	T52.9-
cellulose	T47.4X-
chloride (gas)	T59.89-
chloroformate	T59.3X-
cyclohexane	T52.8X-
cyclohexanol	T51.8X-
cyclohexanone	T52.8X-
cyclohexyl acetate	T52.8X-
demeton	T60.0X-
dihydromorphinone	T40.2X-
ergometrine	T48.0X-
ergonovine	T48.0X-
ethyl ketone	T52.4X-
glucamine antimonate	T37.8X-
hydrazine	T65.89-
iodide	T65.89-
isobutyl ketone	T52.4X-
isothiocyanate	T60.3X-
mercaptan	T59.89-
morphine NEC	T40.2X-
nicotinate	T49.4X-
paraben	T49.0X-
parafynol	T42.6X-
parathion	T60.0X-
peridol	T43.4X-
phenidate	T43.631
ENT agent	T49.6X
ophthalmic preparation	T49.5X-
topical NEC	T49.0X-
propylcarbinol	T51.3X-
rosaniline NEC	T49.0X-
salicylate	T49.2X-
sulfate (fumes)	T59.89-
liquid	T52.8X-
sulfonal	T42.6X-
testosterone	T38.7X-
thiouracil	T38.2X-
Methylamphetamine	T43.62-
Methylated spirit	T51.1X-
Methylatropine nitrate	T44.3X-

Drug/Chemical	Code
Methylbenactyzium bromide	T44.3X-
Methylbenzethonium chloride	T49.0X-
Methylcellulose	T47.4X-
laxative	T47.4X-
Methylchlorophenoxy-acetic acid	T60.3X-
Methyldopa	T46.5X-
Methyldopate	T46.5X-
Methylene	
blue	T50.6X-
chloride or dichloride (solvent)NEC	T53.4X-
Methylenedioxyamphetamine	T43.62-
Methylenedioxymethamphetamine	T43.64-
Methylergometrine	T48.0X-
Methylergonovine	T48.0X-
Methylestrenolone	T38.5X-
Methylethyl cellulose	T50.99-
Methylhexabital	T42.3X-
Methylmorphine	T40.2X-
Methylparaben (ophthalmic)	T49.5X-
Methylparafynol	T42.6X-
Methylpentynol, methylpenthynol	T42.6X-
Methylphenidate	T43.631
Methylphenobarbital	T42.3X-
Methylpolysiloxane	T47.1X-
Methylprednisolone	T38.0X-
Methylrosaniline	T49.0X-
Methylrosanilinium chloride	T49.0X-
Methyltestosterone	T38.7X-
Methylthionine chloride	T50.6X-
Methylthioninium chloride	T50.6X-
Methylthiouracil	T38.2X-
Methyprylon	T42.6X-
Methysergide	T46.5X-
Metiamide	T47.1X-
Meticillin	T36.0X-
Meticrane	T50.2X-
Metildigoxin	T46.0X-
Metipranolol	T49.5X-
Metirosine	T46.5X-
Metisazone	T37.5X-
Metixene	T44.3X-
Metizoline	T48.5X-
Metoclopramide	T45.0X-
Metofenazate	T43.3X-
Metofoline	T39.8X-
Metolazone	T50.2X-
Metopon	T40.2X-
Metoprine	T45.1X-
Metoprolol	T44.7X-
Metrifonate	T60.0X-
Metrizamide	T50.8X-
Metrizoic acid	T50.8X-
Metronidazole	T37.8X-
Metycaine (infiltration) (topical) (subcutaneous) (nerve block)	T41.3X-

Drug/Chemical	Code
Metyrapone	T50.8X-
Mevinphos	T60.0X-
Mexazolam	T42.4X-
Mexenone	T49.3X-
Mexiletine	T46.2X-
Mezereon	T62.2X-
berries	T62.1X-
Mezlocillin	T36.0X-
Mianserin	T43.02-
Micatin	T49.0X-
Miconazole	T49.0X-
Micronomicin	T36.5X-
Midazolam	T42.4X-
Midecamycin	T36.3X-
Mifepristone	T38.6X-
Milk of magnesia	T47.1X-
Millipede (tropical) (venomous)	T63.41-
Miltown	T43.59-
Milverine	T44.3X-
Minaprine	T43.29-
Minaxolone	T41.29-
Mineral	
acids	T54.2X-
oil (laxative) (medicinal)	T47.4X-
emulsion	T47.2X-
nonmedicinal	T52.0X-
topical	T49.3X-
salt NEC	T50.3X-
spirits	T52.0X-
Mineralocorticosteroid	T50.0X-
Minocycline	T36.4X-
Minoxidil	T46.7X-
Miokamycin	T36.3X-
Miotic drug	T49.5X-
Mipafox	T60.0X-
Mirex	T60.1X-
Mirtazapine	T43.02-
Misonidazole	T37.3X-
Misoprostol	T47.1X-
Mithramycin	T45.1X-
Mitobronitol	T45.1X-
Mitoguazone	T45.1X-
Mitolactol	T45.1X-
Mitomycin	T45.1X-
Mitopodozide	T45.1X-
Mitotane	T45.1X-
Mitoxantrone	T45.1X-
Mivacurium chloride	T48.1X-
Miyari bacteria	T47.6X-
MMR vaccine	T50.B9-
Moclobemide	T43.1X-
Moderil	T46.5X-
Mofebutazone	T39.2X-
Molindone	T43.59-
Molsidomine	T46.3X-

Drug/Chemical	Code
Mometasone	T49.0X-
Monistat	T49.0X-
Monkshood	T62.2X-
Monoamine oxidase inhibitor NEC	T43.1X-
hydrazine	T43.1X-
Monobenzone	T49.4X-
Monochloroacetic acid	T60.3X-
Monochlorobenzene	T53.7X-
Monoethanolamine (oleate)	T46.8X-
Monooctanoin	T50.99-
Monophenylbutazone	T39.2X-
Monosodium glutamate	T65.89-
Monosulfiram	T49.0X-
Monoxidine hydrochloride	T46.1X-
Monuron	T60.3X-
Moperone	T43.4X-
Mopidamol	T45.1X-
MOPP (mechloreth-amine + vincristine + prednisone + procarbazine)	T45.1X-
Morfin	T40.2X-
Morinamide	T37.1X-
Morning glory seeds	T40.99-
Moroxydine	T37.5X-
Morphazinamide	T37.1X-
Morphine	T40.2X-
antagonist	T50.7X-
Morpholinylethylmorphine	T40.2X-
Morsuximide	T42.2X-
Mosapramine	T43.59-
Moth balls (naphthalene)	T60.2X-
paradichlorobenzene	T60.1X-
Motor exhaust gas	T58.0-
Mouthwash (antiseptic)	T49.6X-
Moxastine	T45.0X-
Moxaverine	T44.3X-
Moxisylyte	T46.7X-
Mucilage, plant	T47.4X-
Mucolytic drug	T48.4X-
Mucomyst	T48.4X-
Mucous membrane agents (external)	T49.9-
specified NEC	T49.8X-
Multiple unspec drugs	T50.91-
Mumps	
immune globulin (human)	T50.Z1-
skin test antigen	T50.8X-
Mupirocin	T49.0X-
Muromonab-CD3	T45.1X-
Muscle-action drug NEC	T48.20-
Muscle affecting agents NEC	T48.20-
oxytocic	T48.0X-
relaxants	T48.20-
central nervous system	T42.8X-
skeletal	T48.1X-
smooth	T44.3X-
Mushroom, noxious	T62.0X-

Drug/Chemical	Code
Mussel, noxious	T61.781
Mustard (emetic) (black)	T47.7X-
gas, not in war	T59.9-
nitrogen	T45.1X-
Mustine	T45.1X-
M-vac	T45.1X-
Mycifradin	T36.5X-
topical	T49.0X-
Mycitracin	T36.8X-
ophthalmic preparation	T49.5X-
Mycostatin	T36.7X-
topical	T49.0X-
Mycotoxins (NEC)	T64.81
aflatoxin	T64.0-
Mydriacyl	T44.3X-
Mydriatic drug	T49.5X-
Myelobromal	T45.1X-
Myleran	T45.1X-
Myochrysin (e)	T39.2X-
Myoneural blocking agents	T48.1X-
Myralact	T49.0X-
Myristica fragrans	T62.2X-
Myristicin	T65.89-
Mysoline	T42.3X-
Nabilone	T40.7X-
Nabumetone	T39.39-
Nadolol	T44.7X-
Nafcillin	T36.0X-
Nafoxidine	T38.6X-
Naftazone	T46.99-
Naftidrofuryl (oxalate)	T46.7X-
Naftifine	T49.0X-
Nail polish remover	T52.9-
Nalbuphine	T40.4X-
Naled	T60.0X-
Nalidixic acid	T37.8X-
Nalorphine	T50.7X-
Naloxone	T50.7X-
Naltrexone	T50.7X-
Namenda	T43.8X-
Nandrolone	T38.7X-
Naphazoline	T48.5X-
Naphtha (painters') (petroleum)	T52.0X-
solvent	T52.0X-
vapor	T52.0X-
Naphthalene (non-chlorinated)	T60.2X-
chlorinated	T60.1X-
vapor	T60.1X-
insecticide or moth repellent	T60.2X-
chlorinated	T60.1X-
vapor	T60.2X-
chlorinated	T60.1X-
Naphthol	T65.89-
Naphthylamine	T65.89-
Naphthylthiourea (ANTU)	T60.4X-

Drug/Chemical	Code
Naproxen (Naprosyn)	T39.31-
Narcotic (drug)	T40.60-
analgesic NEC	T40.60-
antagonist	T50.7X-
specified NEC	T40.69-
synthetic (other)	T40.49-
Narcotine	T48.3X-
Nardil	T43.1X-
Nasal drug NEC	T49.6X-
Natamycin	T49.0X-
Natural	
blood (product)	T45.8X-
gas (piped)	T59.89-
incomplete combustion	T58.1-
Nealbarbital	T42.3X-
Nectadon	T48.3X-
Nedocromil	T48.6X-
Nefopam	T39.8X-
Nematocyst (sting)	T63.69-
Nembutal	T42.3X-
Nemonapride	T43.59-
Neoarsphenamine	T37.8X-
Neocinchophen	T50.4X-
Neomycin (derivatives)	T36.5X-
with bacitracin	T49.0X-
with neostigmine	T44.0X-
ENT agent	T49.6X-
ophthalmic preparation	T49.5X-
topical NEC	T49.0X-
Neonal	T42.3X-
Neoprontosil	T37.0X-
Neosalvarsan	T37.8X-
Neosilversalvarsan	T37.8X-
Neosporin	T36.8X-
ENT agent	T49.6X-
opthalmic preparation	T49.5X-
topical NEC	T49.0X-
Neostigmine bromide	T44.0X-
Neraval	T42.3X-
Neravan	T42.3X-
Nerium oleander	T62.2X-
Nerve gas, not in war	T59.9-
Nesacaine (infiltration) (subcutaneous) (nerve block)	T41.3X-
Netilmicin	T36.5X-
Neurobarb	T42.3X-
Neuroleptic drug NEC	T43.50-
Neuromuscular blocking drug	T48.1X-
Neutral insulin injection	T38.3X-
Neutral spirits (beverage)	T51.0X-
Niacin	T46.7X-
Niacinamide	T45.2X-
Nialamide	T43.1X-
Niaprazine	T42.6X-
Nicametate	T46.7X-
Nicardipine	T46.1X-

Drug/Chemical	Code
Nicergoline	T46.7X-
Nickel (carbonyl) (tetra-carbonyl) (fumes) (vapor)	T56.89-
Nickelocene	T56.89-
Niclosamide	T37.4X-
Nicofuranose	T46.7X-
Nicomorphine	T40.2X-
Nicorandil	T46.3X-
Nicotiana (plant)	T62.2X-
Nicotinamide	T45.2X-
Nicotine (insecticide) (spray) (sulfate) NEC	T60.2X-
from tobacco	T65.29-
cigarettes	T65.22-
not insecticide	T65.29-
Nicotinic acid	T46.7X-
Nicotinyl alcohol	T46.7X-
Nicoumalone	T45.51-
Nifedipine	T46.1X-
Nifenazone	T39.2X-
Nifuraldezone	T37.9-
Nifuratel	T37.8X-
Nifurtimox	T37.3X-
Nifurtoinol	T37.8X-
Nightshade, deadly (solanum)	T62.2X-
berry	T62.1X-
Nikethamide	T50.7X-
Nilstat	T36.7X-
topical	T49.0X-
Nilutamide	T38.6X-
Nimesulide	T39.39-
Nimetazepam	T42.4X-
Nimodipine	T46.1X-
Nimorazole	T37.3X-
Nimustine	T45.1X-
Niridazole	T37.4X-
Nisentil	T40.2X-
Nisoldipine	T46.1X-
Nitramine	T65.3X-
Nitrate, organic	T46.3X-
Nitrazepam	T42.4X-
Nitrefazole	T50.6X-
Nitrendipine	T46.1X-
Nitric	
acid (liquid)	T54.2X-
vapor	T59.89-
oxide (gas)	T59.0X-
Nitrimidazine	T37.3X-
Nitrite, amyl (medicinal) (vapor)	T46.3X-
Nitroaniline	T65.3X-
vapor	T59.89-
Nitrobenzene, nitrobenzol (vapor)	T65.3X-
Nitrocellulose	T65.89-
lacquer	T65.89-
Nitrodiphenyl	T65.3X-
Nitrofural	T49.0X-
Nitrofurantoin	T37.8X-

Drug/Chemical	Code
Nitrofurazone	T49.0X-
Nitrogen	T59.0X-
mustard	T45.1X-
Nitroglycerin, nitro-glycerol (medicinal)	T46.3X-
nonmedicinal	T65.5X-
fumes	T65.5X-
Nitroglycol	T52.3X-
Nitrohydrochloric acid	T54.2X-
Nitromersol	T49.0X-
Nitronaphthalene	T65.89-
Nitrophenol	T54.0X-
Nitropropane	T52.8X-
Nitroprusside	T46.5X-
Nitrosodimethylamine	T65.3X-
Nitrothiazol	T37.4X-
Nitrotoluene, nitrotoluol	T65.3X-
vapor	T65.3X-
Nitrous	
acid (liquid)	T54.2X-
fumes	T59.89-
ether spirit	T46.3X-
oxide	T41.0X-
Nitroxoline	T37.8X-
Nitrozone	T49.0X-
Nizatidine	T47.0X-
Nizofenone	T43.8X-
Noctec	T42.6X-
Noludar	T42.6X-
Nomegestrol	T38.5X-
Nomifensine	T43.29-
Nonoxinol	T49.8X-
Nonylphenoxy (polyethoxy-ethanol)	T49.8X-
Noptil	T42.3X-
Noradrenaline	T44.4X-
Noramidopyrine	T39.2X-
methanesulfonate sodium	T39.2X-
Norbormide	T60.4X-
Nordazepam	T42.4X-
Norepinephrine	T44.4X-
Norethandrolone	T38.7X-
Norethindrone	T38.4X-
Norethisterone (acetate) (enantate)	T38.4X-
with ethinylestradiol	T38.5X-
Noretynodrel	T38.5X-
Norfenefrine	T44.4X-
Norfloxacin	T36.8X-
Norgestrel	T38.4X-
Norgestrienone	T38.4X-
Norlestrin	T38.4X-
Norlutin	T38.4X-
Normal serum albumin (human), salt-poor	T45.8X-
Normethandrone	T38.5X-
Normorphine	T40.2X-

Drug/Chemical	Code
Norpseudoephedrine	T50.5X-
Nortestosterone (furanpropionate)	T38.7X-
Nortriptyline	T43.01-
Noscapine	T48.3X-
Nose preparations	T49.6X-
Novobiocin	T36.5X-
Novocain (infiltration) (topical) (spinal)	T41.3X-
Noxious foodstuff	T62.9-
specified NEC	T62.8X-
Noxiptiline	T43.01-
Noxytiolin	T49.0X-
NPH Iletin (insulin)	T38.3X-
Numorphan	T40.2X-
Nunol	T42.3X-
Nupercaine (spinal anesthetic)	T41.3X-
topical (surface)	T41.3X-
Nutmeg oil (liniment)	T49.3X-
Nutritional supplement	T50.90-
Nux vomica	T65.1X-
Nydrazid	T37.1X-
Nylidrin	T46.7X-
Nystatin	T36.7X-
topical	T49.0X-
Nytol	T45.0X-
Obidoxime chloride	T50.6X-
Octafonium (chloride)	T49.3X-
Octamethyl pyrophos-phoramide	T60.0X-
Octanoin	T50.99-
Octatropine methyl-bromide	T44.3X-
Octotiamine	T45.2X-
Octoxinol (9)	T49.8X-
Octreotide	T38.99-
Octyl nitrite	T46.3X-
Oestradiol	T38.5X-
Oestriol	T38.5X-
Oestrogen	T38.5X-
Oestrone	T38.5X-
Ofloxacin	T36.8X-
Oil (of)	T65.89-
bitter almond	T62.8X-
cloves	T49.7X-
colors	T65.6X-
fumes	T59.89-
lubricating	T52.0X-
Niobe	T52.8X-
vitriol (liquid)	T54.2X-
fumes	T54.2X-
wintergreen (bitter) NEC	T49.3X-
Oily preparation (for skin)	T49.3X-
Ointment NEC	T49.3X-
Olanzapine	T43.59-
Oleander	T62.2X-
Oleandomycin	T36.3X-
Oleandrin	T46.0X-
Oleic acid	T46.6X-

Drug/Chemical	Code
Oleovitamin A	T45.2X-
Oleum ricini	T47.2X-
Olive oil (medicinal)NEC	T47.4X-
Olivomycin	T45.1X-
Olsalazine	T47.8X-
Omeprazole	T47.1X-
OMPA	T60.0X-
Oncovin	T45.1X-
Ondansetron	T45.0X-
Ophthaine	T41.3X-
Ophthetic	T41.3X-
Opiate NEC	T40.60-
antagonists	T50.7X-
Opioid NEC	T40.2X-
Opipramol	T43.01-
Opium alkaloids (total)	T40.0X-
Oracon	T38.4X-
Oragrafin	T50.8X-
Oral contraceptives	T38.4X-
Oral rehydration salts	T50.3X-
Orazamide	T50.99-
Orciprenaline	T48.29-
Organidin	T48.4X-
Organonitrate NEC	T46.3X-
Organophosphates	T60.0X-
Orimune	T50.B9-
Orinase	T38.3X-
Ormeloxifene	T38.6X-
Ornidazole	T37.3X-
Ornithine aspartate	T50.99-
Ornoprostil	T47.1X-
Orphenadrine (hydrochloride)	T42.8X-
Ortal (sodium)	T42.3X-
Orthoboric acid	T49.0X-
ENT agent	T49.6X-
ophthalmic preparation	T49.5X-
Orthocaine	T41.3X-
Orthodichlorobenzene	T53.7X-
Ortho-Novum	T38.4X-
Orthotolidine (reagent)	T54.2X-
Osmic acid (liquid) (fumes)	T54.2X-
Osmotic diuretics	T50.2X-
Otilonium bromide	T44.3X-
Otorhinolaryngological drug NEC	T49.6X-
Ouabain (e)	T46.0X-
Ovarian (hormone) (stimulant)	T38.5X-
Ovral	T38.4X-
Ovulen	T38.4X-
Oxacillin	T36.0X-
Oxalic acid	T54.2X-
ammonium salt	T50.99-
Oxamniquine	T37.4X-
Oxanamide	T43.59-
Oxandrolone	T38.7X-
Oxantel	T37.4X-

Drug/Chemical	Code
Oxapium iodide	T44.3X-
Oxaprotiline	T43.02-
Oxaprozin	T39.31-
Oxatomide	T45.0X-
Oxazepam	T42.4X-
Oxazimedrine	T50.5X-
Oxazolam	T42.4X-
Oxazolidine derivatives	T42.2X-
Oxazolidinedione (derivative)	T42.2X-
Oxcarbazepine	T42.1X-
Oxedrine	T44.4X-
Oxeladin (citrate)	T48.3X-
Oxendolone	T38.5X-
Oxetacaine	T41.3X-
Oxethazine	T41.3X-
Oxetorone	T39.8X-
Oxiconazole	T49.0X-
Oxidizing agent NEC	T54.9-
Oxipurinol	T50.4X-
Oxitriptan	T43.29-
Oxitropium bromide	T48.6X-
Oxodipine	T46.1X-
Oxolamine	T48.3X-
Oxolinic acid	T37.8X-
Oxomemazine	T43.3X-
Oxophenarsine	T37.3X-
Oxprenolol	T44.7X-
Oxsoralen	T49.3X-
Oxtriphylline	T48.6X-
Oxybate sodium	T41.29-
Oxybuprocaine	T41.3X-
Oxybutynin	T44.3X-
Oxychlorosene	T49.0X-
Oxycodone	T40.2X-
Oxyfedrine	T46.3X-
Oxygen	T41.5X-
Oxylone	T49.0X-
ophthalmic preparation	T49.5X-
Oxymesterone	T38.7X-
Oxymetazoline	T48.5X-
Oxymetholone	T38.7X-
Oxymorphone	T40.2X-
Oxypertine	T43.59-
Oxyphenbutazone	T39.2X-
Oxyphencyclimine	T44.3X-
Oxyphenisatine	T47.2X-
Oxyphenonium bromide	T44.3X-
Oxypolygelatin	T45.8X-
Oxyquinoline (derivatives)	T37.8X-
Oxytetracycline	T36.4X-
Oxytocic drug NEC	T48.0X-
Oxytocin (synthetic)	T48.0X-
Ozone	T59.89-
PABA	T49.3X-
Packed red cells	T45.8X-

Drug/Chemical	Code
Padimate	T49.3X-
Paint NEC	T65.6X-
cleaner	T52.9-
fumes NEC	T59.89-
lead (fumes)	T56.0X-
solvent NEC	T52.8X-
stripper	T52.8X-
Palfium	T40.2X-
Palm kernel oil	T50.99-
Paludrine	T37.2X-
PAM (pralidoxime)	T50.6X-
Pamaquine (naphthoute)	T37.2X-
Panadol	T39.1X-
Pancreatic	
digestive secretion stimulant	T47.8X-
dornase	T45.3X-
Pancreatin	T47.5X-
Pancrelipase	T47.5X-
Pancuronium (bromide)	T48.1X-
Pangamic acid	T45.2X-
Panthenol	T45.2X-
topical	T49.8X-
Pantopon	T40.0X-
Pantothenic acid	T45.2X-
Panwarfin	T45.51-
Papain (digestant)	T47.5X-
Papaveretum	T40.0X-
Papaverine	T44.3X-
Para-acetamidophenol	T39.1X-
Para-aminobenzoic acid	T49.3X-
Para-aminophenol derivatives	T39.1X-
Para-aminosalicylic acid	T37.1X-
Paracetaldehyde	T42.6X-
Paracetamol	T39.1X-
Parachlorophenol (camphorated)	T49.0X-
Paracodin	T40.2X-
Paradione	T42.2X-
Paraffin(s) (wax)	T52.0X-
liquid (medicinal)	T47.4X-
nonmedicinal	T52.0X-
Paraformaldehyde	T60.3X-
Paraldehyde	T42.6X-
Paramethadione	T42.2X-
Paramethasone	T38.0X-
acetate	T49.0X-
Paraoxon	T60.0X-
Paraquat	T60.3X-
Parasympatholytic NEC	T44.3X-
Parasympathomimetic drug NEC	T44.1X-
Parathion	T60.0X-
Parathormone	T50.99-
Parathyroid extract	T50.99-
Paratyphoid vaccine	T50.A9-
Paredrine	T44.4X-
Paregoric	T40.0X-

Drug/Chemical	Code
Pargyline	T46.5X-
Paris green (insecticide)	T57.0X-
Parnate	T43.1X-
Paromomycin	T36.5X-
Paroxypropione	T45.1X-
Parzone	T40.2X-
PAS	T37.1X-
Pasiniazid	T37.1X-
PBB (polybrominated biphenyls)	T65.89-
PCB	T65.89-
PCP	
meaning pentachlorophenol	T60.1X-
fungicide / herbicide	T60.3X-
insecticide	T60.1X-
meaning phencyclidine	T40.99-
Peach kernel oil (emulsion)	T47.4X-
Peanut oil (emulsion)NEC	T47.4X-
topical	T49.3X-
Pearly Gates (morning glory seeds)	T40.99-
Pecazine	T43.3X-
Pectin	T47.6X-
Pefloxacin	T37.8X-
Pegademase, bovine	T50.Z9-
Pelletierine tannate	T37.4X-
Pemirolast (potassium)	T48.6X-
Pemoline	T50.7X-
Pempidine	T44.2X-
Penamecillin	T36.0X-
Penbutolol	T44.7X-
Penethamate	T36.0X-
Penfluridol	T43.59-
Penflutizide	T50.2X-
Pengitoxin	T46.0X-
Penicillamine	T50.6X-
Penicillin (any)	T36.0X-
Penicillinase	T45.3X-
Penicilloyl polylysine	T50.8X-
Penimepicycline	T36.4X-
Pentachloroethane	T53.6X-
Pentachloronaphthalene	T53.7X-
Pentachlorophenol (pesticide)	T60.1X-
fungicide / herbicide	T60.3X-
insecticide	T60.1X-
Pentaerythritol	T46.3X-
chloral	T42.6X-
tetranitrate NEC	T46.3X-
Pentaerythrityl tetranitrate	T46.3X-
Pentagastrin	T50.8X-
Pentalin	T53.6X-
Pentamethonium bromide	T44.2X-
Pentamidine	T37.3X-
Pentanol	T51.3X-
Pentapyrrolinium (bitartrate)	T44.2X-
Pentaquine	T37.2X-
Pentazocine	T40.4X-

Drug/Chemical	Code
Pentetrazole	T50.7X-
Penthienate bromide	T44.3X-
Pentifylline	T46.7X-
Pentobarbital (sodium)	T42.3X-
Pentobarbitone	T42.3X-
Pentolonium tartrate	T44.2X-
Pentosan polysulfate (sodium)	T39.8X-
Pentostatin	T45.1X-
Pentothal	T41.1X-
Pentoxifylline	T46.7X-
Pentoxyverine	T48.3X-
Pentrinat	T46.3X-
Pentylenetetrazole	T50.7X-
Pentylsalicylamide	T37.1X-
Pentymal	T42.3X-
Peplomycin	T45.1X-
Peppermint (oil)	T47.5X-
Pepsin (digestant)	T47.5X-
Pepstatin	T47.1X-
Peptavlon	T50.8X-
Perazine	T43.3X-
Percaine (spinal)	T41.3X-
topical (surface)	T41.3X-
Perchloroethylene	T53.3X-
medicinal	T37.4X-
vapor	T53.3X-
Percodan	T40.2X-
Percogesic	T45.0X-
Percorten	T38.0X-
Pergolide	T42.8X-
Pergonal	T38.81-
Perhexilene	T46.3X-
Perhexiline (maleate)	T46.3X-
Periactin	T45.0X-
Periciazine	T43.3X-
Periclor	T42.6X-
Perindopril	T46.4X-
Perisoxal	T39.8X-
Peritoneal dialysis solution	T50.3X-
Peritrate	T46.3X-
Perlapine	T42.4X-
Permanganate	T65.89-
Permethrin	T60.1X-
Pernocton	T42.3X-
Pernoston	T42.3X-
Peronine	T40.2X-
Perphenazine	T43.3X-
Pertofrane	T43.01-
Pertussis immune serum (human)	T50.Z1-
Peruvian balsam	T49.0X-
Peruvoside	T46.0X-
Pesticide (dust) (fumes) (vapor) NEC	T60.9-
arsenic	T57.0X-
chlorinated	T60.1X-
cyanide / kerosene	T65.0X-

Drug/Chemical	Code
Pesticide (dust) (fumes) (vapor) NEC, continued	T60.9-
mixture (of compounds)	T60.9-
naphthalene	T60.2X-
organochlorine (compounds)	T60.1X-
petroleum (distillate) (products)NEC	T60.8X-
specified ingredient NEC	T60.8X-
strychnine	T65.1X-
thallium	T60.4X-
Pethidine	T40.4X-
Petrichloral	T42.6X-
Petrol	T52.0X-
vapor	T52.0X-
Petrolatum	T49.3X-
hydrophilic	T49.3X-
liquid	T47.4X-
topical	T49.3X-
nonmedicinal	T52.0X-
red veterinary	T49.3X-
white	T49.3X-
Petroleum (products) NEC	T52.0X-
jelly	T49.3X-
pesticide	T60.8X-
solids	T52.0X-
solvents	T52.0X-
vapor	T52.0X-
Peyote	T40.99-
Phanodorm, phanodorn	T42.3X-
Phanquinone	T37.3X-
Phanquone	T37.3X-
Pharmaceutical (adjunct) (excipient) (sweetner) NEC	T50.90-
Phemitone	T42.3X-
Phenacaine	T41.3X-
Phenacemide	T42.6X-
Phenacetin	T39.1X-
Phenadoxone	T40.2X-
Phenaglycodol	T43.59-
Phenantoin	T42.0X-
Phenaphthazine reagent	T50.99-
Phenazocine	T40.4X-
Phenazone	T39.2X-
Phenazopyridine	T39.8X-
Phenbenicillin	T36.0X-
Phenbutrazate	T50.5X-
Phencyclidine	T40.99-
Phendimetrazine	T50.5X-
Phenelzine	T43.1X-
Phenemal	T42.3X-
Phenergan	T42.6X-
Pheneticillin	T36.0X-
Pheneturide	T42.6X-
Phenformin	T38.3X-
Phenglutarimide	T44.3X-
Phenicarbazide	T39.8X-
Phenindamine	T45.0X-
Phenindione	T45.51-

Drug/Chemical	Code
Pheniprazine	T43.1X-
Pheniramine	T45.0X-
Phenisatin	T47.2X-
Phenmetrazine	T50.5X-
Phenobal	T42.3X-
Phenobarbital	T42.3X-
with mephenytoin	T42.3X-
with phenytoin	T42.3X-
sodium	T42.3X-
Phenobarbitone	T42.3X-
Phenobutiodil	T50.8X-
Phenoctide	T49.0X-
Phenol	T49.0X-
disinfectant	T54.0X-
in oil injection	T46.8X-
medicinal	T49.1X-
nonmedicinal NEC	T54.0X-
pesticide	T60.8X-
red	T50.8X-
Phenolic preparation	T49.1X-
Phenolphthalein	T47.2X-
Phenolsulfonphthalein	T50.8X-
Phenomorphan	T40.2X-
Phenonyl	T42.3X-
Phenoperidine	T40.4X-
Phenopyrazone	T46.99-
Phenoquin	T50.4X-
Phenothiazine (psychotropic)NEC	T43.3X-
insecticide	T60.2X-
Phenothrin	T49.0X-
Phenoxybenzamine	T46.7X-
Phenoxyethanol	T49.0X-
Phenoxymethyl penicillin	T36.0X-
Phenprobamate	T42.8X-
Phenprocoumon	T45.51-
Phensuximide	T42.2X-
Phentermine	T50.5X-
Phenthicillin	T36.0X-
Phentolamine	T46.7X-
Phenyl	
butazone	T39.2X-
enediamine	T65.3X-
hydrazine	T65.3X-
antineoplastic	T45.1X-
salicylate	T49.3X-
Phenylalanine mustard	T45.1X-
Phenylbutazone	T39.2X-
Phenylenediamine	T65.3X-
Phenylephrine	T44.4X-
Phenylethylbiguanide	T38.3X-
Phenylmercuric (acetate) (borate) (nitrate)	T49.0X-
Phenylmethylbarbitone	T42.3X-
Phenylpropanol	T47.5X-
Phenylpropanolamine	T44.99-
Phenylsulfthion	T60.0X-

Drug/Chemical	Code
Phenyltoloxamine	T45.0X-
Phenyramidol, phenyramidon	T39.8X-
Phenytoin	T42.0X-
with Phenobarbital	T42.3X-
pHisoHex	T49.2X-
Pholcodine	T48.3X-
Pholedrine	T46.99-
Phorate	T60.0X-
Phosdrin	T60.0X-
Phosfolan	T60.0X-
Phosgene (gas)	T59.89-
Phosphamidon	T60.0X-
Phosphate	T65.89-
laxative	T47.4X-
organic	T60.0X-
solvent	T52.9-
tricresyl	T65.89-
Phosphine (fumigate)	T57.1X-
Phospholine	T49.5X-
Phosphoric acid	T54.2X-
Phosphorus (compound)NEC	T57.1X-
pesticide	T60.0X-
Phthalates	T65.89-
Phthalic anhydride	T65.89-
Phthalimidoglutarimide	T42.6X-
Phthalylsulfathiazole	T37.0X-
Phylloquinone	T45.7X-
Physeptone	T40.3X-
Physostigma venenosum	T62.2X-
Physostigmine	T49.5X-
Phytolacca decandra	T62.2X-
berries	T62.1X-
Phytomenadione	T45.7X-
Phytonadione	T45.7X-
Picoperine	T48.3X-
Picosulfate (sodium)	T47.2X-
Picric (acid)	T54.2X-
Picrotoxin	T50.7X-
Piketoprofen	T49.0X-
Pilocarpine	T44.1X-
Pilocarpus (jaborandi)extract	T44.1X-
Pilsicainide (hydrochloride)	T46.2X-
Pimaricin	T36.7X-
Pimeclone	T50.7X-
Pimelic ketone	T52.8X-
Pimethixene	T45.0X-
Piminodine	T40.2X-
Pimozide	T43.59-
Pinacidil	T46.5X-
Pinaverium bromide	T44.3X-
Pinazepam	T42.4X-
Pindolol	T44.7X-
Pindone	T60.4X-
Pine oil (disinfectant)	T65.89-
Pinkroot	T37.4X-

Drug/Chemical	Code
Pipadone	T40.2X-
Pipamazine	T45.0X-
Pipamperone	T43.4X-
Pipazetate	T48.3X-
Pipemidic acid	T37.8X-
Pipenzolate bromide	T44.3X-
Piperacetazine	T43.3X-
Piperacillin	T36.0X-
Piperazine	T37.4X-
estrone sulfate	T38.5X-
Piper cubeba	T62.2X-
Piperidione	T48.3X-
Piperidolate	T44.3X-
Piperocaine (all types)	T41.3X-
Piperonyl butoxide	T60.8X-
Pipethanate	T44.3X-
Pipobroman	T45.1X-
Pipotiazine	T43.3X-
Pipoxizine	T45.0X-
Pipradrol	T43.69-
Piprinhydrinate	T45.0X-
Pirarubicin	T45.1X-
Pirazinamide	T37.1X-
Pirbuterol	T48.6X-
Pirenzepine	T47.1X-
Piretanide	T50.1X-
Piribedil	T42.8X-
Piridoxilate	T46.3X-
Piritramide	T40.4X-
Piromidic acid	T37.8X-
Piroxicam	T39.39-
beta-cyclodextrin complex	T39.8X-
Pirozadil	T46.6X-
Piscidia (bark) (erythrina)	T39.8X-
Pitch	T65.89-
Pitkin's solution	T41.3X-
Pitocin	T48.0X-
Pitressin (tannate)	T38.89-
Pituitary extracts (posterior)	T38.89-
anterior	T38.81-
Pituitrin	T38.89-
Pivampicillin	T36.0X-
Pivmecillinam	T36.0X-
Placental hormone	T38.89-
Placidyl	T42.6X-
Plague vaccine	T50.A9-
Plant	
food or fertilizer NEC	T65.89-
containing herbicide	T60.3X-
noxious, used as food	T62.2X-
berries	T62.1X-
seeds	T62.2X-
specified type NEC	T62.2X-
Plasma	T45.8X-
Plasmanate	T45.8X-

Drug/Chemical	Code
Plasminogen (tissue) activator	T45.61-
Plaster dressing	T49.3X-
Plastic dressing	T49.3X-
Plegicil	T43.3X-
Plicamycin	T45.1X-
Podophyllotoxin	T49.8X-
Podophyllum (resin)	T49.4X-
Poison NEC	T65.9-
Poisonous berries	T62.1X-
Pokeweed (any part)	T62.2X-
Poldine metilsulfate	T44.3X-
Polidexide (sulfate)	T46.6X-
Polidocanol	T46.8X-
Poliomyelitis vaccine	T50.B9-
Polish (car) (floor) (furniture) (metal) (porcelain) (silver)	T65.89-
Poloxalkol	T47.4X-
Poloxamer	T47.4X-
Polyaminostyrene resins	T50.3X-
Polycarbophil	T47.4X-
Polychlorinated biphenyl	T65.89-
Polycycline	T36.4X-
Polyester fumes	T59.89-
Polyester resin hardener	T52.9-
fumes	T59.89-
Polyestradiol phosphate	T38.5X-
Polyethanolamine alkyl sulfate	T49.2X-
Polyethylene adhesive	T49.3X-
Polyferose	T45.4X-
Polygeline	T45.8X-
Polymyxin	T36.8X-
B	T36.8X-
ENT agent	T49.6X-
ophthalmic preparation	T49.5X-
topical NEC	T49.0X-
E sulfate (eye preparation)	T49.5X-
Polynoxylin	T49.0X-
Polyoestradiol phosphate	T38.5X-
Polyoxymethyleneurea	T49.0X-
Polysilane	T47.8X-
Polytetrafluoroethylene (inhaled)	T59.89-
Polythiazide	T50.2X-
Polyvidone	T45.8X-
Polyvinylpyrrolidone	T45.8X-
Pontocaine (hydrochloride) (infiltration) (topical)	T41.3X-
Porfiromycin	T45.1X-
Posterior pituitary hormone NEC	T38.89-
Pot	T40.7X-
Potash (caustic)	T54.3X-
Potassic saline injection (lactated)	T50.3X-
Potassium (salts) NEC	T50.3X-
aminobenzoate	T45.8X-
aminosalicylate	T37.1X-
antimony ' tartrate'	T37.8X-
arsenite (solution)	T57.0X-
bichromate	T56.2X-

Drug/Chemical	Code
Potassium (salts) NEC, continued	T50.3X-
bisulfate	T47.3X-
bromide	T42.6X-
canrenoate	T50.0X-
carbonate	T54.3X-
chlorate NEC	T65.89-
chloride	T50.3X-
citrate	T50.99-
cyanide	T65.0X-
ferric hexacyanoferrate (medicinal)	T50.6X-
nonmedicinal	T65.89-
Fluoride	T57.8X-
glucaldrate	T47.1X-
hydroxide	T54.3X-
iodate	T49.0X-
iodide	T48.4X-
nitrate	T57.8X-
oxalate	T65.89-
perchlorate (nonmedicinal)NEC	T65.89-
antithyroid	T38.2X-
medicinal	T38.2X-
Permanganate (nonmedicinal)	T65.89-
medicinal	T49.0X-
sulfate	T47.2X-
Potassium-removing resin	T50.3X-
Potassium-retaining drug	T50.3X-
Povidone	T45.8X-
iodine	T49.0X-
Practolol	T44.7X-
Prajmalium bitartrate	T46.2X-
Pralidoxime (iodide) (chloride)	T50.6X-
Pramiverine	T44.3X-
Pramocaine	T49.1X-
Pramoxine	T49.1X-
Prasterone	T38.7X-
Pravastatin	T46.6X-
Prazepam	T42.4X-
Praziquantel	T37.4X-
Prazitone	T43.29-
Prazosin	T44.6X-
Prednicarbate	T49.0X-
Prednimustine	T45.1X-
Prednisolone	T38.0X-
ENT agent	T49.6X-
ophthalmic preparation	T49.5X-
steaglate	T49.0X-
topical NEC	T49.0X-
Prednisone	T38.0X-
Prednylidene	T38.0X-
Pregnandiol	T38.5X-
Pregneninolone	T38.5X-
Preludin	T43.69-
Premarin	T38.5X-
Premedication anesthetic	T41.20-
Prenalterol	T44.5X-

Drug/Chemical	Code
Prenoxdiazine	T48.3X-
Prenylamine	T46.3X-
Preparation H	T49.8X-
Preparation, local	T49.4X-
Preservative (nonmedicinal)	T65.89-
medicinal	T50.90-
wood	T60.9-
Prethcamide	T50.7X-
Pride of China	T62.2X-
Pridinol	T44.3X-
Prifinium bromide	T44.3X-
Prilocaine	T41.3X-
Primaquine	T37.2X-
Primidone	T42.6X-
Primula (veris)	T62.2X-
Prinadol	T40.2X-
Priscol, Priscoline	T44.6X-
Pristinamycin	T36.3X-
Privet	T62.2X-
berries	T62.1X-
Privine	T44.4X-
Pro-Banthine	T44.3X-
Probarbital	T42.3X-
Probenecid	T50.4X-
Probucol	T46.6X-
Procainamide	T46.2X-
Procaine	T41.3X-
benzylpenicillin	T36.0X-
nerve block (periphreal) (plexus)	T41.3X-
penicillin G	T36.0X-
regional / spinal	T41.3X-
Procalmidol	T43.59-
Procarbazine	T45.1X-
Procaterol	T44.5X-
Prochlorperazine	T43.3X-
Procyclidine	T44.3X-
Producer gas	T58.8X-
Profadol	T40.4X-
Profenamine	T44.3X-
Profenil	T44.3X-
Proflavine	T49.0X-
Progabide	T42.6X-
Progesterone	T38.5X-
Progestin	T38.5X-
oral contraceptive	T38.4X-
Progestogen NEC	T38.5X-
Progestone	T38.5X-
Proglumide	T47.1X-
Proguanil	T37.2X-
Prolactin	T38.81-
Prolintane	T43.69-
Proloid	T38.1X-
Proluton	T38.5X-
Promacetin	T37.1X-
Promazine	T43.3X-

POTASSIUM (SALTS) NEC–PROMAZINE

Drug/Chemical	Code
Promedol	T40.2X-
Promegestone	T38.5X-
Promethazine (teoclate)	T43.3X-
Promin	T37.1X-
Pronase	T45.3X-
Pronestyl (hydrochloride)	T46.2X-
Pronetalol	T44.7X-
Prontosil	T37.0X-
Propachlor	T60.3X-
Propafenone	T46.2X-
Propallylonal	T42.3X-
Propamidine	T49.0X-
Propane (in mobile container)	T59.89-
distributed through pipes	T59.89-
incomplete combustion	T58.1-
Propanidid	T41.29-
Propanil	T60.3X-
1-Propanol	T51.3X-
2-Propanol	T51.2X-
Propantheline (bromide)	T44.3X-
Proparacaine	T41.3X-
Propatylnitrate	T46.3X-
Propicillin	T36.0X-
Propiolactone	T49.0X-
Propiomazine	T45.0X-
Propionaidehyde (medicinal)	T42.6X-
Propionate (calcium) (sodium)	T49.0X-
Propion gel	T49.0X-
Propitocaine	T41.3X-
Propofol	T41.29-
Propoxur	T60.0X-
Propoxycaine (infiltration) (spinal) (subcutaneous) (nerve block) (topical)	T41.3X-
Propoxyphene	T40.4X-
Propranolol	T44.7X-
Propyl	
alcohol	T51.3X-
carbinol	T51.3X-
hexadrine	T44.4X-
iodone	T50.8X-
thiouracil	T38.2X-
Propylaminopheno-thiazine	T43.3X-
Propylene	T59.89-
Propylhexedrine	T48.5X-
Propyliodone	T50.8X-
Propylparaben (ophthalmic)	T49.5X-
Propylthiouracil	T38.2X-
Propyphenazone	T39.2X-
Proquazone	T39.39-
Proscillaridin	T46.0X-
Prostacyclin	T45.521
Prostaglandin (I2)	T45.521
E1	T46.7X-
E2	T48.0X-
F2 alpha	T48.0X-

Drug/Chemical	Code
Prostigmin	T44.0X-
Prosultiamine	T45.2X-
Protamine sulfate	T45.7X-
zinc insulin	T38.3X-
Protease	T47.5X-
Protectant, skin NEC	T49.3X-
Protein hydrolysate	T50.99-
Prothiaden— *see Dothiepin hydrochloride*	
Prothionamide	T37.1X-
Prothipendyl	T43.59-
Prothoate	T60.0X-
Prothrombin	
activator	T45.7X-
synthesis inhibitor	T45.51-
Protionamide	T37.1X-
Protirelin	T38.89-
Protokylol	T48.6X-
Protopam	T50.6X-
Protoveratrine(s) (A) (B)	T46.5X-
Protriptyline	T43.01-
Provera	T38.5X-
Provitamin A	T45.2X-
Proxibarbal	T42.3X-
Proxymetacaine	T41.3X-
Proxyphylline	T48.6X-
Prozac— *see Fluoxetine hydrochloride*	
Prunus	
laurocerasus	T62.2X-
virginiana	T62.2X-
Prussian blue	
commercial	T65.89-
therapeutic	T50.6X-
Prussic acid	T65.0X-
vapor	T57.3X-
Pseudoephedrine	T44.99-
Psilocin	T40.99-
Psilocybin	T40.99-
Psilocybine	T40.99-
Psoralene (nonmedicinal)	T65.89-
Psoralens (medicinal)	T50.99-
PSP (phenolsulfonphthalein)	T50.8X-
Psychodysleptic drug NOS	T40.90-
specified NEC	T40.99-
Psychostimulant	T43.60-
amphetamine	T43.62-
caffeine	T43.61-
methylphenidate	T43.631
specified NEC	T43.69-
Psychotherapeutic drug NEC	T43.9-
antidepressants	T43.20-
specified NEC	T43.8X-
tranquilizers NEC	T43.50-
Psychotomimetic agents	T40.90-
Psychotropic drug NEC	T43.9-
specified NEC	T43.8X-

Drug/Chemical	Code
Psyllium hydrophilic mucilloid	T47.4X-
Pteroylglutamic acid	T45.8X-
Pteroyltriglutamate	T45.1X-
PTFE— *see Polytetrafluoroethylene*	
Pulp	
devitalizing paste	T49.7X-
dressing	T49.7X-
Pulsatilla	T62.2X-
Pumpkin seed extract	T37.4X-
Purex (bleach)	T54.9-
Purgative NEC— *see also Cathartic*	T47.4X-
Purine analogue (antineoplastic)	T45.1X-
Purine diuretics	T50.2X-
Purinethol	T45.1X-
PVP	T45.8X-
Pyrabital	T39.8X-
Pyramidon	T39.2X-
Pyrantel	T37.4X-
Pyrathiazine	T45.0X-
Pyrazinamide	T37.1X-
Pyrazinoic acid (amide)	T37.1X-
Pyrazole (derivatives)	T39.2X-
Pyrazolone analgesic NEC	T39.2X-
Pyrethrin, pyrethrum (nonmedicinal)	T60.2X-
Pyrethrum extract	T49.0X-
Pyribenzamine	T45.0X-
Pyridine	T52.8X-
aldoxime methiodide	T50.6X-
aldoxime methyl chloride	T50.6X-
vapor	T59.89-
Pyridium	T39.8X-
Pyridostigmine bromide	T44.0X-
Pyridoxal phosphate	T45.2X-
Pyridoxine	T45.2X-
Pyrilamine	T45.0X-
Pyrimethamine (w/ sulfadoxine)	T37.2X-
Pyrimidine antagonist	T45.1X-
Pyriminil	T60.4X-
Pyrithione zinc	T49.4X-
Pyrithyldione	T42.6X-
Pyrogallic acid	T49.0X-
Pyrogallol	T49.0X-
Pyroxylin	T49.3X-
Pyrrobutamine	T45.0X-
Pyrrolizidine alkaloids	T62.8X-
Pyrvinium chloride	T37.4X-
PZI	T38.3X-
Quaalude	T42.6X-
Quarternary ammonium	
anti-infective	T49.0X-
ganglion blocking	T44.2X-
parasympatholytic	T44.3X-
Quazepam	T42.4X-
Quicklime	T54.3X-
Quillaja extract	T48.4X-

Drug/Chemical	Code
Quinacrine	T37.2X-
Quinaglute	T46.2X-
Quinalbarbital	T42.3X-
Quinalbarbitone sodium	T42.3X-
Quinalphos	T60.0X-
Quinapril	T46.4X-
Quinestradiol	T38.5X-
Quinestradol	T38.5X-
Quinestrol	T38.5X-
Quinethazone	T50.2X-
Quingestanol	T38.4X-
Quinidine	T46.2X-
Quinine	T37.2X-
Quiniobine	T37.8X-
Quinisocaine	T49.1X-
Quinocide	T37.2X-
Quinoline (derivatives)NEC	T37.8X-
Quinupramine	T43.01-
Quotane	T41.3X-
Rabies	
immune globulin (human)	T50.Z1-
vaccine	T50.B9-
Racemoramide	T40.2X-
Racemorphan	T40.2X-
Racepinefrin	T44.5X-
Raclopride	T43.59-
Radiator alcohol	T51.1X-
Radioactive drug NEC	T50.8X-
Radio-opaque (drugs) (materials)	T50.8X-
Ramifenazone	T39.2X-
Ramipril	T46.4X-
Ranitidine	T47.0X-
Ranunculus	T62.2X-
Rat poison NEC	T60.4X-
Rattlesnake (venom)	T63.01-
Raubasine	T46.7X-
Raudixin	T46.5X-
Rautensin	T46.5X-
Rautina	T46.5X-
Rautotal	T46.5X-
Rauwiloid	T46.5X-
Rauwoldin	T46.5X-
Rauwolfia (alkaloids)	T46.5X-
Razoxane	T45.1X-
Realgar	T57.0X-
Recombinant (R)— *see specific protein*	
Red blood cells, packed	T45.8X-
Red squill (scilliroside)	T60.4X-
Reducing agent, industrial NEC	T65.89-
Refrigerant gas (CFC)	T53.5X-
not chlorofluoro-carbon	T59.89-
Regroton	T50.2X-
Rehydration salts (oral)	T50.3X-
Rela	T42.8X-

Drug/Chemical	Code
Relaxant, muscle	
anesthetic	T48.1X-
central nervous system	T42.8X-
skeletal NEC	T48.1X-
smooth NEC	T44.3X-
Remoxipride	T43.59-
Renese	T50.2X-
Renografin	T50.8X-
Replacement solution	T50.3X-
Reproterol	T48.6X-
Rescinnamine	T46.5X-
Reserpin (e)	T46.5X-
Resorcin, resorcinol (nonmedicinal)	T65.89-
medicinal	T49.4X-
Respaire	T48.4X-
Respiratory drug NEC	T48.90-
antiasthmatic NEC	T48.6X-
anti-common-cold NEC	T48.5X-
expectorant NEC	T48.4X-
stimulant	T48.90-
Retinoic acid	T49.0X-
Retinol	T45.2X-
Rh (D) immune globulin (human)	T50.Z1-
Rhodine	T39.01-
RhoGAM	T50.Z1-
Rhubarb	
dry extract	T47.2X-
tincture, compound	T47.2X-
Ribavirin	T37.5X-
Riboflavin	T45.2X-
Ribostamycin	T36.5X-
Ricin	T62.2X-
Ricinus communis	T62.2X-
Rickettsial vaccine NEC	T50.A9-
Rifabutin	T36.6X-
Rifamide	T36.6X-
Rifampicin	T36.6X-
with isoniazid	T37.1X-
Rifampin	T36.6X-
Rifamycin	T36.6X-
Rifaximin	T36.6X-
Rimantadine	T37.5X-
Rimazolium metilsulfate	T39.8X-
Rimifon	T37.1X-
Rimiterol	T48.6X-
Ringer (lactate) solution	T50.3X-
Ristocetin	T36.8X-
Ritalin	T43.631
Ritodrine	T44.5X-
Rociverine	T44.3X-
Rocky Mtn spotted fever vaccine	T50.A9-
Rodenticide NEC	T60.4X-
Rohypnol	T42.4X-
Rokitamycin	T36.3X-

Drug/Chemical	Code
Rolaids	T47.1X-
Rolitetracycline	T36.4X-
Romilar	T48.3X-
Ronifibrate	T46.6X-
Rosaprostol	T47.1X-
Rose bengal sodium (131I)	T50.8X-
Rose water ointment	T49.3X-
Rosoxacin	T37.8X-
Rotenone	T60.2X-
Rotoxamine	T45.0X-
Rough-on-rats	T60.4X-
Roxatidine	T47.0X-
Roxithromycin	T36.3X-
Rt-PA	T45.61-
Rubbing alcohol	T51.2X-
Rubefacient	T49.4X-
Rubidium chloride Rb82	T50.8X-
Rubidomycin	T45.1X-
Rue	T62.2X-
Rufocromomycin	T45.1X-
Russel's viper venin	T45.7X-
Ruta (graveolens)	T62.2X-
Rutinum	T46.99-
Rutoside	T46.99-
Sabadilla (plant) (pesticide)	T62.2X-
Saccharated iron oxide	T45.8X-
Saccharin	T50.90-
Saccharomyces boulardii	T47.6X-
Safflower oil	T46.6X-
Safrazine	T43.1X-
Salazosulfapyridine	T37.0X-
Salbutamol	T48.6X-
Salicylamide	T39.09-
Salicylate NEC	T39.09-
methyl	T49.3X-
theobromine calcium	T50.2X-
Salicylazosulfapyridine	T37.0X-
Salicylhydroxamic acid	T49.0X-
Salicylic acid	T49.4X-
with benzoic acid	T49.4X-
congeners/derivatives/salts	T39.09-
Salinazid	T37.1X-
Salmeterol	T48.6X-
Salol	T49.3X-
Salsalate	T39.09-
Salt substitute	T50.90-
Salt-replacing drug	T50.90-
Salt-retaining mineralocorticoid	T50.0X-
Saluretic NEC	T50.2X-
Saluron	T50.2X-
Salvarsan 606 (neosilver) (silver)	T37.8X-
Sambucus canadensis	T62.2X-
berry	T62.1X-
Sandril	T46.5X-
Sanguinaria canadensis	T62.2X-

Drug/Chemical	Code
Saniflush (cleaner)	T54.2X-
Santonin	T37.4X-
Santyl	T49.8X-
Saralasin	T46.5X-
Sarcolysin	T45.1X-
Sarkomycin	T45.1X-
Saroten	T43.01-
Savin (oil)	T49.4X-
Scammony	T47.2X-
Scarlet red	T49.8X-
Scheele's green	T57.0X-
insecticide	T57.0X-
Schizontozide (blood) (tissue)	T37.2X-
Schradan	T60.0X-
Schweinfurth green	T57.0X-
insecticide	T57.0X-
Scilla, rat poison	T60.4X-
Scillaren	T60.4X-
Sclerosing agent	T46.8X-
Scombrotoxin	T61.1-
Scopolamine	T44.3X-
Scopolia extract	T44.3X-
Scouring powder	T65.89-
Sea	
anemone (sting)	T63.631
cucumber (sting)	T63.69-
snake (bite) (venom)	T63.09-
urchin spine (puncture)	T63.69-
Seafood	T61.9-
specified NEC	T61.8X-
Secbutabarbital	T42.3X-
Secbutabarbitone	T42.3X-
Secnidazole	T37.3X-
Secobarbital	T42.3X-
Seconal	T42.3X-
Secretin	T50.8X-
Sedative NEC	T42.71
mixed NEC	T42.6X-
Sedormid	T42.6X-
Seed disinfectant or dressing	T60.8X-
Seeds (poisonous)	T62.2X-
Selegiline	T42.8X-
Selenium NEC (fumes)	T56.89-
disulfide or sulfide	T49.4X-
Selenomethionine (75Se)	T50.8X-
Selsun	T49.4X-
Semustine	T45.1X-
Senega syrup	T48.4X-
Senna	T47.2X-
Sennoside A+B	T47.2X-
Septisol	T49.2X-
Seractide	T38.81-
Serax	T42.4X-
Serenesil	T42.6X-
Serenium (hydrochloride)	T37.9-

Drug/Chemical	Code
Serepax— see Oxazepam	
Sermorelin	T38.89-
Sernyl	T41.1X-
Serotonin	T50.99-
Serpasil	T46.5X-
Serrapeptase	T45.3X-
Serum	
antibotulinus	T50.Z1-
anticytotoxic	T50.Z1-
antidiphtheria	T50.Z1-
antimeningococcus	T50.Z1-
anti-Rh	T50.Z1-
anti-snake-bite	T50.Z1-
antitetanic	T50.Z1-
antitoxic	T50.Z1-
complement (inhibitor)	T45.8X-
convalescent	T50.Z1-
hemolytic complement	T45.8X-
immune (human)	T50.Z1-
protective NEC	T50.Z1-
Setastine	T45.0X-
Setoperone	T43.59-
Sewer gas	T59.9-
Shampoo	T55.0X-
Shellfish, noxious, nonbacterial	T61.781
Sildenafil	T46.7X-
Silibinin	T50.99-
Silicone NEC	T65.89-
medicinal	T49.3X-
Silvadene	T49.0X-
Silver	T49.0X-
anti-infectives	T49.0X-
arsphenamine	T37.8X-
colloidal	T49.0X-
nitrate	T49.0X-
ophthalmic preparation	T49.5X-
toughened (keratolytic)	T49.4X-
nonmedicinal (dust)	T56.89-
protein	T49.5X-
salvarsan	T37.8X-
sulfadiazine	T49.4X-
Silymarin	T50.99-
Simaldrate	T47.1X-
Simazine	T60.3X-
Simethicone	T47.1X-
Simfibrate	T46.6X-
Simvastatin	T46.6X-
Sincalide	T50.8X-
Sinequan	T43.01-
Singoserp	T46.5X-
Sintrom	T45.51-
Sisomicin	T36.5X-
Sitosterols	T46.6X-
Skeletal muscle relaxants	T48.1X-

Drug/Chemical	Code
Skin	
agents (external)	T49.9-
specified NEC	T49.8X-
test antigen	T50.8X-
Sleep-eze	T45.0X-
Sleeping draught, pill	T42.71
Smallpox vaccine	T50.B1-
Smelter fumes NEC	T56.9-
Smog	T59.1X-
Smoke NEC	T59.81-
Smooth muscle relaxant	T44.3X-
Snail killer NEC	T60.8X-
Snake venom or bite	T63.00-
hemocoagulase	T45.7X-
Snuff	T65.21-
Soap (powder) (product)	T55.0X-
enema	T47.4X-
medicinal, soft	T49.2X-
superfatted	T49.2X-
Sobrerol	T48.4X-
Soda (caustic)	T54.3X-
bicarb	T47.1X-
Sodium	
acetosulfone	T37.1X-
acetrizoate	T50.8X-
acid phosphate	T50.3X-
alginate	T47.8X-
amidotrizoate	T50.8X-
aminopterin	T45.1X-
amylosulfate	T47.8X-
amytal	T42.3X-
antimony gluconate	T37.3X-
arsenate	T57.0X-
aurothiomalate	T39.4X-
aurothiosulfate	T39.4X-
barbiturate	T42.3X-
basic phosphate	T47.4X-
bicarbonate	T47.1X-
bichromate	T57.8X-
biphosphate	T50.3X-
bisulfate	T65.89-
borate	
cleanser	T57.8X-
eye	T49.5X-
therapeutic	T49.8X-
bromide	T42.6X-
cacodylate (nonmedicinal)NEC	T50.8X-
anti-infective	T37.8X-
herbicide	T60.3X-
calcium edetate	T45.8X-
carbonate NEC	T54.3X-
chlorate NEC	T65.89-
herbicide	T54.9-

Drug/Chemical	Code
chloride	T50.3X-
with glucose	T50.3X-
chromate	T65.89-
citrate	T50.99-
cromoglicate	T48.6X-
cyanide	T65.0X-
cyclamate	T50.3X-
dehydrocholate	T45.8X-
diatrizoate	T50.8X-
dibunate	T48.4X-
dioctyl sulfosuccinate	T47.4X-
dipantoyl ferrate	T45.8X-
edetate	T45.8X-
ethacrynate	T50.1X-
feredetate	T45.8X-
fluoride— *see Fluoride*	
fluoroacetate (dust) (pesticide)	T60.4X-
free salt	T50.3X-
fusidate	T36.8X-
glucaldrate	T47.1X-
glucosulfone	T37.1X-
glutamate	T45.8X-
hydrogen carbonate	T50.3X-
hydroxide	T54.3X-
hypochlorite (bleach)NEC	T54.3X-
disinfectant	T54.3X-
medicinal (anti-infective) (external)	T49.0X-
vapor	T54.3X-
hyposulfite	T49.0X-
indigotin disulfonate	T50.8X-
iodide	T50.99-
I-131	T50.8X-
therapeutic	T38.2X-
iodohippurate (131I)	T50.8X-
iopodate	T50.8X-
iothalamate	T50.8X-
iron edetate	T45.4X-
lactate (compound solution)	T45.8X-
lauryl (sulfate)	T49.2X-
L-triiodothyronine	T38.1X-
magnesium citrate	T50.99-
mersalate	T50.2X-
metasilicate	T65.89-
metrizoate	T50.8X-
monofluoroacetate (pesticide)	T60.1X-
morrhuate	T46.8X-
nafcillin	T36.0X-
nitrate (oxidizing agent)	T65.89-
nitrite	T50.6X-
nitroferricyanide	T46.5X-
nitroprusside	T46.5X-
oxalate	T65.89-
oxide/peroxide	T65.89-
oxybate	T41.29-
para-aminohippurate	T50.8X-

SODIUM–STANOZOLOL

Drug/Chemical	Code
Sodium, continued	
perborate (nonmedicinal)NEC	T65.89-
medicinal	T49.0X-
soap	T55.0X-
percarbonate— *see Sodium, perborate*	
pertechnetate Tc99m	T50.8X-
phosphate	
cellulose	T45.8X-
dibasic	T47.2X-
monobasic	T47.2X-
phytate	T50.6X-
picosulfate	T47.2X-
polyhydroxyaluminium monocarbonate	T47.1X-
polystyrene sulfonate	T50.3X-
propionate	T49.0X-
propyl hydroxybenzoate	T50.99-
psylliate	T46.8X-
removing resins	T50.3X-
salicylate	T39.09-
salt NEC	T50.3X-
selenate	T60.2X-
stibogluconate	T37.3X-
sulfate	T47.4X-
sulfoxone	T37.1X-
tetradecyl sulfate	T46.8X-
thiopental	T41.1X-
thiosalicylate	T39.09-
thiosulfate	T50.6X-
tolbutamide	T38.3X-
(L)-triiodothyronine	T38.1X-
tyropanoate	T50.8X-
valproate	T42.6X-
versenate	T50.6X-
Sodium-free salt	T50.90-
Sodium-removing resin	T50.3X-
Soft soap	T55.0X-
Solanine	T62.2X-
berries	T62.1X-
Solanum dulcamara	T62.2X-
berries	T62.1X-
Solapsone	T37.1X-
Solar lotion	T49.3X-
Solasulfone	T37.1X-
Soldering fluid	T65.89-
Solid substance	T65.9-
specified NEC	T65.89-
Solvent, industrial NEC	T52.9-
naphtha	T52.0X-
petroleum	T52.0X-
specified NEC	T52.8X-
Soma	T42.8X-
Somatorelin	T38.89-
Somatostatin	T38.99-
Somatotropin	T38.81-
Somatrem	T38.81-

Drug/Chemical	Code
Somatropin	T38.81-
Sominex	T45.0X-
Somnos	T42.6X-
Somonal	T42.3X-
Soneryl	T42.3X-
Soothing syrup	T50.90-
Sopor	T42.6X-
Soporific	T42.71
Soporific drug	T42.71
specified type NEC	T42.6X-
Sorbide nitrate	T46.3X-
Sorbitol	T47.4X-
Sotalol	T44.7X-
Sotradecol	T46.8X-
Soysterol	T46.6X-
Spacoline	T44.3X-
Spanish fly	T49.8X-
Sparine	T43.3X-
Sparteine	T48.0X-
Spasmolytic	
anticholinergics	T44.3X-
autonomic	T44.3X-
bronchial NEC	T48.6X-
quaternary ammonium	T44.3X-
skeletal muscle NEC	T48.1X-
Spectinomycin	T36.5X-
Speed	T43.62-
Spermicide	T49.8X-
Spider (bite) (venom)	T63.39-
antivenin	T50.Z1-
Spigelia (root)	T37.4X-
Spindle inactivator	T50.4X-
Spiperone	T43.4X-
Spiramycin	T36.3X-
Spirapril	T46.4X-
Spirilene	T43.59-
Spirit(s) (neutral) NEC	T51.0X-
beverage / industrial/ mineral/surgical	T51.0X-
Spironolactone	T50.0X-
Spiroperidol	T43.4X-
Sponge, absorbable (gelatin)	T45.7X-
Sporostacin	T49.0X-
Spray (aerosol)	T65.9-
cosmetic	T65.89-
medicinal NEC	T50.90-
Spurge flax	T62.2X-
Spurges	T62.2X-
Sputum viscosity-lowering drug	T48.4X-
Squill	T46.0X-
rat poison	T60.4X-
Squirting cucumber (cathartic)	T47.2X-
Stains	T65.6X-
Stannous fluoride	T49.7X-
Stanolone	T38.7X-
Stanozolol	T38.7X-

Drug/Chemical	Code
Staphisagria or stavesacre (pediculicide)	T49.0X-
Starch	T50.90-
Stelazine	T43.3X-
Stemetil	T43.3X-
Stepronin	T48.4X-
Sterculia	T47.4X-
Sternutator gas	T59.89-
Steroid	T38.0X-
anabolic	T38.7X-
androgenic	T38.7X-
antineoplastic, hormone	T38.7X-
estrogen	T38.5X-
ENT agent	T49.6X-
ophthalmic preparation	T49.5X-
topical NEC	T49.0X-
Stibine	T56.89-
Stibogluconate	T37.3X-
Stibophen	T37.4X-
Stilbamidine (isetionate)	T37.3X-
Stilbestrol	T38.5X-
Stilboestrol	T38.5X-
Stimulant	
central nervous system	T43.60-
analeptics / opiate antagonist	T50.7X-
psychotherapeutic NEC	T43.60-
specified NEC	T43.69-
respiratory	T48.90-
Stone-dissolving drug	T50.90-
Storage battery (cells) (acid)	T54.2X-
Stovaine (infiltration) (topical) (subcutaneous) (nerve block) (spinal)	T41.3X-
Stovarsal	T37.8X-
Stoxil	T49.5X-
Stramonium	T48.6X-
natural state	T62.2X-
Streptodornase	T45.3X-
Streptoduocin	T36.5X-
Streptokinase	T45.61-
Streptomycin (derivative)	T36.5X-
Streptonivicin	T36.5X-
Streptovarycin	T36.5X-
Streptozocin	T45.1X-
Streptozotocin	T45.1X-
Stripper (paint) (solvent)	T52.8X-
Strobane	T60.1X-
Strofantina	T46.0X-
Strophanthin (g) (k)	T46.0X-
Strophanthus	T46.0X-
Strophantin	T46.0X-
Strophantin-g	T46.0X-
Strychnine (nonmedicinal) (pesticide) (salts)	T65.1X-
medicinal	T48.29-
Styramate	T42.8X-
Styrene	T65.89-
Succinimide, antiepileptic or anticonvulsant	T42.2X-

Drug/Chemical	Code
Succinylcholine	T48.1X-
Succinylsulfathiazole	T37.0X-
Sucralfate	T47.1X-
Sucrose	T50.3X-
Sufentanil	T40.4X-
Sulbactam	T36.0X-
Sulbenicillin	T36.0X-
Sulbentine	T49.0X-
Sulfacetamide	T49.0X-
ophthalmic preparation	T49.5X-
Sulfachlorpyridazine	T37.0X-
Sulfacitine	T37.0X-
Sulfadiasulfone sodium	T37.0X-
Sulfadiazine	T37.0X-
silver (topical)	T49.0X-
Sulfadimethoxine	T37.0X-
Sulfadimidine	T37.0X-
Sulfadoxine	T37.0X-
with pyrimethamine	T37.2X-
Sulfaethidole	T37.0X-
Sulfafurazole	T37.0X-
Sulfaguanidine	T37.0X-
Sulfalene	T37.0X-
Sulfaloxate	T37.0X-
Sulfaloxic acid	T37.0X-
Sulfamazone	T39.2X-
Sulfamerazine	T37.0X-
Sulfameter	T37.0X-
Sulfamethazine	T37.0X-
Sulfamethizole	T37.0X-
Sulfamethoxazole	T37.0X-
with trimethoprim	T36.8X-
Sulfamethoxydiazine	T37.0X-
Sulfamethoxypyridazine	T37.0X-
Sulfamethylthiazole	T37.0X-
Sulfametoxydiazine	T37.0X-
Sulfamidopyrine	T39.2X-
Sulfamonomethoxine	T37.0X-
Sulfamoxole	T37.0X-
Sulfamylon	T49.0X-
Sulfan blue (diagnostic dye)	T50.8X-
Sulfanilamide	T37.0X-
Sulfanilylguanidine	T37.0X-
Sulfaperin	T37.0X-
Sulfaphenazole	T37.0X-
Sulfaphenylthiazole	T37.0X-
Sulfaproxyline	T37.0X-
Sulfapyridine	T37.0X-
Sulfapyrimidine	T37.0X-
Sulfarsphenamine	T37.8X-
Sulfasalazine	T37.0X-
Sulfasuxidine	T37.0X-
Sulfasymazine	T37.0X-
Sulfated amylopectin	T47.8X-
Sulfathiazole	T37.0X-

Drug/Chemical	Code
Sulfatostearate	T49.2X-
Sulfinpyrazone	T50.4X-
Sulfiram	T49.0X-
Sulfisomidine	T37.0X-
Sulfisoxazole	T37.0X-
ophthalmic preparation	T49.5X-
Sulfobromophthalein (sodium)	T50.8X-
Sulfobromphthalein	T50.8X-
Sulfogaiacol	T48.4X-
Sulfomyxin	T36.8X-
Sulfonal	T42.6X-
Sulfonamide NEC	T37.0X-
eye	T49.5X-
Sulfonazide	T37.1X-
Sulfones	T37.1X-
Sulfonethylmethane	T42.6X-
Sulfonmethane	T42.6X-
Sulfonphthal, sulfonphthol	T50.8X-
Sulfonylurea derivatives, oral	T38.3X-
Sulforidazine	T43.3X-
Sulfoxone	T37.1X-
Sulfur, sulfurated, sulfuric, (compounds NEC) (medicinal)	T49.4X-
acid	T54.2X-
dioxide (gas)	T59.1X-
hydrogen	T59.6X-
ointment	T49.0X-
pesticide (vapor)	T60.9-
vapor NEC	T59.89-
Sulfuric acid	T54.2X-
Sulglicotide	T47.1X-
Sulindac	T39.39-
Sulisatin	T47.2X-
Sulisobenzone	T49.3X-
Sulkowitch's reagent	T50.8X-
Sulmetozine	T44.3X-
Suloctidil	T46.7X-
Sulphadiazine	T37.0X-
Sulphadimethoxine	T37.0X-
Sulphadimidine	T37.0X-
Sulphadione	T37.1X-
Sulphafurazole	T37.0X-
Sulphamethizole	T37.0X-
Sulphamethoxazole	T37.0X-
Sulphan blue	T50.8X-
Sulphaphenazole	T37.0X-
Sulphapyridine	T37.0X-
Sulphasalazine	T37.0X-
Sulphinpyrazone	T50.4X-
Sulpiride	T43.59-
Sulprostone	T48.0X-
Sulpyrine	T39.2X-
Sultamicillin	T36.0X-
Sulthiame	T42.6X-
Sultiame	T42.6X-

Drug/Chemical	Code
Sultopride	T43.59-
Sumatriptan	T39.8X-
Sunflower seed oil	T46.6X-
Superinone	T48.4X-
Suprofen	T39.31-
Suramin (sodium)	T37.4X-
Surfacaine	T41.3X-
Surital	T41.1X-
Sutilains	T45.3X-
Suxamethonium (chloride)	T48.1X-
Suxethonium (chloride)	T48.1X-
Suxibuzone	T39.2X-
Sweet niter spirit	T46.3X-
Sweet oil (birch)	T49.3X-
Sweetener	T50.90-
Sym-dichloroethyl ether	T53.6X-
Sympatholytic NEC	T44.8X-
haloalkylamine	T44.8X-
Sympathomimetic NEC	T44.90-
anti-common-cold	T48.5X-
bronchodilator	T48.6X-
specified NEC	T44.99-
Synagis	T50.B9-
Synalar	T49.0X-
Synthetic narcotics (other)	T40.49-
Synthroid	T38.1X-
Syntocinon	T48.0X-
Syrosingopine	T46.5X-
Systemic drug	T45.9-
specified NEC	T45.8X-
2,4,5-T	T60.3X-
Tablets— *see also specified substance*	T50.90-
Tace	T38.5X-
Tacrine	T44.0X-
Tadalafil	T46.7X-
Talampicillin	T36.0X-
Talbutal	T42.3X-
Talc powder	T49.3X-
Talcum	T49.3X-
Taleranol	T38.6X-
Tamoxifen	T38.6X-
Tamsulosin	T44.6X-
Tandearil, tanderil	T39.2X-
Tannic acid (Tannin)	T49.2X-
medicinal (astringent)	T49.2X-
Tansy	T62.2X-
TAO	T36.3X-
Tapazole	T38.2X-
Tar NEC	T52.0X-
camphor	T60.1X-
distillate	T49.1X-
fumes	T59.89-
medicinal (ointment)	T49.1X-
Taractan	T43.59-
Tarantula (venomous)	T63.321

Drug/Chemical	Code
Tartar emetic	T37.8X-
Tartaric acid	T65.89-
Tartrate, laxative	T47.4X-
Tartrated antimony (anti-infective)	T37.8X-
Tauromustine	T45.1X-
TCA— *see* Trichloroacetic acid	
TCDD	T53.7X-
TDI (vapor)	T65.0X-
Teclothiazide	T50.2X-
Teclozan	T37.3X-
Tegafur	T45.1X-
Tegretol	T42.1X-
Teicoplanin	T36.8X-
Telepaque	T50.8X-
Tellurium	T56.89-
TEM	T45.1X-
Temazepam	T42.4X-
Temocillin	T36.0X-
Tenamfetamine	T43.62-
Teniposide	T45.1X-
Tenitramine	T46.3X-
Tenoglicin	T48.4X-
Tenonitrozole	T37.3X-
Tenoxicam	T39.39-
TEPA	T45.1X-
TEPP	T60.0X-
Teprotide	T46.5X-
Terazosin	T44.6X-
Terbufos	T60.0X-
Terbutaline	T48.6X-
Terconazole	T49.0X-
Terfenadine	T45.0X-
Teriparatide (acetate)	T50.99-
Terizidone	T37.1X-
Terlipressin	T38.89-
Terodiline	T46.3X-
Teroxalene	T37.4X-
Terpin (cis)hydrate	T48.4X-
Terramycin	T36.4X-
Tertatolol	T44.7X-
Tessalon	T48.3X-
Testolactone	T38.7X-
Testosterone	T38.7X-
Tetanus toxoid or vaccine	T50.A9-
antitoxin	T50.Z1-
immune globulin (human)	T50.Z1-
toxoid	T50.A9-
with diphtheria toxoid	T50.A2-
with pertussis	T50.A1-
Tetrabenazine	T43.59-
Tetracaine	T41.3X-
Tetrachlorethylene— *see Tetrachloroethylene*	
Tetrachlormethiazide	T50.2X-
2,3,7,8-Tetrachlorodibenzo-p-dioxin	T53.7X-

Drug/Chemical	Code
Tetrachloroethane	T53.6X-
vapor	T53.6X-
paint or varnish	T53.6X-
Tetrachloroethylene (liquid)	T53.3X-
medicinal	T37.4X-
vapor	T53.3X-
Tetracosactide	T38.81-
Tetracosactrin	T38.81-
Tetracycline	T36.4X-
ophthalmic preparation	T49.5X-
topical NEC	T49.0X-
Tetradifon	T60.8X-
Tetradotoxin	T61.771
Tetraethyl	
lead	T56.0X-
pyrophosphate	T60.0X-
Tetraethylammonium chloride	T44.2X-
Tetraethylthiuram disulfide	T50.6X-
Tetrahydroaminoacridine	T44.0X-
Tetrahydrocannabinol	T40.7X-
Tetrahydrofuran	T52.8X-
Tetrahydronaphthalene	T52.8X-
Tetrahydrozoline	T49.5X-
Tetralin	T52.8X-
Tetramethrin	T60.2X-
Tetramethylthiuram (disulfide) NEC	T60.3X-
medicinal	T49.0X-
Tetramisole	T37.4X-
Tetranicotinoyl fructose	T46.7X-
Tetrazepam	T42.4X-
Tetronal	T42.6X-
Tetryl	T65.3X-
Tetrylammonium chloride	T44.2X-
Tetryzoline	T49.5X-
Thalidomide	T45.1X-
Thallium (compounds) (dust) NEC	T56.81-
pesticide	T60.4X-
THC	T40.7X-
Thebacon	T48.3X-
Thebaine	T40.2X-
Thenoic acid	T49.6X-
Thenyldiamine	T45.0X-
Theobromine (calcium salicylate)	T48.6X-
sodium salicylate	T48.6X-
Theophyllamine	T48.6X-
Theophylline	T48.6X-
Thiabendazole	T37.4X-
Thialbarbital	T41.1X-
Thiamazole	T38.2X-
Thiambutosine	T37.1X-
Thiamine	T45.2X-
Thiamphenicol	T36.2X-
Thiamylal (sodium)	T41.1X-
Thiazesim	T43.29-
Thiazides (diuretics)	T50.2X-

Drug/Chemical	Code
Thiazinamium metilsulfate	T43.3X-
Thiethylperazine	T43.3X-
Thimerosal	T49.0X-
ophthalmic preparation	T49.5X-
Thioacetazone	T37.1X-
Thiobarbital sodium	T41.1X-
Thiobarbiturate anesthetic	T41.1X-
Thiobismol	T37.8X-
Thiobutabarbital sodium	T41.1X-
Thiocarbamate (insecticide)	T60.0X-
Thiocarbamide	T38.2X-
Thiocarbarsone	T37.8X-
Thiocarlide	T37.1X-
Thioctamide	T50.99-
Thioctic acid	T50.99-
Thiofos	T60.0X-
Thioglycolate	T49.4X-
Thioglycolic acid	T65.89-
Thioguanine	T45.1X-
Thiomercaptomerin	T50.2X-
Thiomerin	T50.2X-
Thiomersal	T49.0X-
Thionazin	T60.0X-
Thiopental (sodium)	T41.1X-
Thiopentone (sodium)	T41.1X-
Thiopropazate	T43.3X-
Thioproperazine	T43.3X-
Thioridazine	T43.3X-
Thiosinamine	T49.3X-
Thiotepa	T45.1X-
Thiothixene	T43.4X-
Thiouracil (benzyl) (methyl) (propyl)	T38.2X-
Thiourea	T38.2X-
Thiphenamil	T44.3X-
Thiram	T60.3X-
medicinal	T49.2X-
Thonzylamine (systemic)	T45.0X-
mucosal decongestant	T48.5X-
Thorazine	T43.3X-
Thorium dioxide suspension	T50.8X-
Thornapple	T62.2X-
Throat drug NEC	T49.6X-
Thrombin	T45.7X-
Thrombolysin	T45.61-
Thromboplastin	T45.7X-
Thurfyl nicotinate	T46.7X-
Thymol	T49.0X-
Thymopentin	T37.5X-
Thymoxamine	T46.7X-
Thymus extract	T38.89-
Thyreotrophic hormone	T38.81-
Thyroglobulin	T38.1X-
Thyroid (hormone)	T38.1X-
Thyrolar	T38.1X-
Thyrotrophin	T38.81-

Drug/Chemical	Code
Thyrotropic hormone	T38.81-
Thyroxine	T38.1X-
Tiabendazole	T37.4X-
Tiamizide	T50.2X-
Tianeptine	T43.29-
Tiapamil	T46.1X-
Tiapride	T43.59-
Tiaprofenic acid	T39.31-
Tiaramide	T39.8X-
Ticarcillin	T36.0X-
Ticlatone	T49.0X-
Ticlopidine	T45.521
Ticrynafen	T50.1X-
Tidiacic	T50.99-
Tiemonium	T44.3X-
iodide	T44.3X-
Tienilic acid	T50.1X-
Tifenamil	T44.3X-
Tigan	T45.0X-
Tigloidine	T44.3X-
Tilactase	T47.5X-
Tiletamine	T41.29-
Tilidine	T40.4X-
Timepidium bromide	T44.3X-
Timiperone	T43.4X-
Timolol	T44.7X-
Tin (chloride) (dust) (oxide) NEC	T56.6X-
anti-infectives	T37.8X-
Tindal	T43.3X-
Tinidazole	T37.3X-
Tinoridine	T39.8X-
Tiocarlide	T37.1X-
Tioclomarol	T45.51-
Tioconazole	T49.0X-
Tioguanine	T45.1X-
Tiopronin	T50.99-
Tiotixene	T43.4X-
Tioxolone	T49.4X-
Tipepidine	T48.3X-
Tiquizium bromide	T44.3X-
Tiratricol	T38.1X-
Tisopurine	T50.4X-
Titanium (compounds) (vapor)	T56.89-
dioxide/ointment/oxide	T49.3X-
tetrachloride	T56.89-
Titanocene	T56.89-
Titroid	T38.1X-
Tizanidine	T42.8X-
TMTD	T60.3X-
TNT (fumes)	T65.3X-
Toadstool	T62.0X-
Tobacco NEC	T65.29-
cigarettes	T65.22-
Indian	T62.2X-
smoke, second-hand	T65.22-

Drug/Chemical	Code
Tobramycin	T36.5X-
Tocainide	T46.2X-
Tocoferol	T45.2X-
Tocopherol (acetate)	T45.2X-
Tocosamine	T48.0X-
Todralazine	T46.5X-
Tofisopam	T42.4X-
Tofranil	T43.01-
Toilet deodorizer	T65.89-
Tolamolol	T44.7X-
Tolazamide	T38.3X-
Tolazoline	T46.7X-
Tolbutamide (sodium)	T38.3X-
Tolciclate	T49.0X-
Tolmetin	T39.39-
Tolnaftate	T49.0X-
Tolonidine	T46.5X-
Toloxatone	T42.6X-
Tolperisone	T44.3X-
Tolserol	T42.8X-
Toluene (liquid)	T52.2X-
diisocyanate	T65.0X-
Toluidine (vapor)	T65.89-
Toluol (liquid)	T52.2X-
vapor	T52.2X-
Toluylenediamine	T65.3X-
Tolylene-2,4-diisocyanate	T65.0X-
Tonic NEC	T50.90-
Topical action drug NEC	T49.9-
ear, nose or throat	T49.6X-
eye	T49.5X-
skin	T49.9-
specified NEC	T49.8X-
Toquizine	T44.3X-
Toremifene	T38.6X-
Tosylchloramide sodium	T49.8X-
Toxaphene (dust) (spray)	T60.1X-
Toxin, diphtheria (Schick Test)	T50.8X-
Tractor fuel NEC	T52.0X-
Tragacanth	T50.99-
Tramadol	T40.42-
Tramazoline	T48.5X-
Tranexamic acid	T45.62-
Tranilast	T45.0X-
Tranquilizer NEC	T43.50-
with hypnotic or sedative	T42.6X-
benzodiazepine NEC	T42.4X-
butyrophenone NEC	T43.4X-
carbamate	T43.59-
dimethylamine / ethylamine	T43.3X-
hydroxyzine	T43.59-
major NEC	T43.50-
penothiazine NEC / piperazine NEC	T43.3X-
piperidine / propylamine	T43.3X-

Drug/Chemical	Code
Tranquilizer NEC, continued	T43.50-
specified NEC	T43.59-
thioxanthene NEC	T43.59-
Tranxene	T42.4X-
Tranylcypromine	T43.1X-
Trapidil	T46.3X-
Trasentine	T44.3X-
Travert	T50.3X-
Trazodone	T43.21-
Trecator	T37.1X-
Treosulfan	T45.1X-
Tretamine	T45.1X-
Tretinoin	T49.0X-
Tretoquinol	T48.6X-
Triacetin	T49.0X-
Triacetoxyanthracene	T49.4X-
Triacetyloleandomycin	T36.3X-
Triamcinolone	T38.0X-
ENT agent	T49.6X-
hexacetonide	T49.0X-
ophthalmic preparation	T49.5X-
topical NEC	T49.0X-
Triampyzine	T44.3X-
Triamterene	T50.2X-
Triazine (herbicide)	T60.3X-
Triaziquone	T45.1X-
Triazolam	T42.4X-
Triazole (herbicide)	T60.3X-
Tribenoside	T46.99-
Tribromacetaldehyde	T42.6X-
Tribromoethanol, rectal	T41.29-
Tribromomethane	T42.6X-
Trichlorethane	T53.2X-
Trichlorethylene	T53.2X-
Trichlorfon	T60.0X-
Trichlormethiazide	T50.2X-
Trichlormethine	T45.1X-
Trichloroacetic acid, Trichloracetic acid	T54.2X-
medicinal	T49.4X-
Trichloroethane	T53.2X-
Trichloroethanol	T42.6X-
Trichloroethyl phosphate	T42.6X-
Trichloroethylene (liquid) (vapor)	T53.2X-
anesthetic (gas)	T41.0X-
Trichlorofluoromethane NEC	T53.5X-
Trichloronate	T60.0X-
2,4,5-Trichlorophen-oxyacetic acid	T60.3X-
Trichloropropane	T53.6X-
Trichlorotriethylamine	T45.1X-
Trichomonacides NEC	T37.3X-
Trichomycin	T36.7X-
Triclobisonium chloride	T49.0X-
Triclocarban	T49.0X-
Triclofos	T42.6X-
Triclosan	T49.0X-

Drug/Chemical	Code
Tricresyl phosphate	T65.89-
solvent	T52.9-
Tricyclamol chloride	T44.3X-
Tridesilon	T49.0X-
Tridihexethyl iodide	T44.3X-
Tridione	T42.2X-
Trientine	T45.8X-
Triethanolamine NEC	T54.3X-
Triethanomelamine	T45.1X-
Triethylenemelamine	T45.1X-
Triethylenephosphoramide	T45.1X-
Triethylenethiophosphoramide	T45.1X-
Trifluoperazine	T43.3X-
Trifluoroethyl vinyl ether	T41.0X-
Trifluperidol	T43.4X-
Triflupromazine	T43.3X-
Trifluridine	T37.5X-
Triflusal	T45.521
Trihexyphenidyl	T44.3X-
Triiodothyronine	T38.1X-
Trilene	T41.0X-
Trilostane	T38.99-
Trimebutine	T44.3X-
Trimecaine	T41.3X-
Trimeprazine (tartrate)	T44.3X-
Trimetaphan camsilate	T44.2X-
Trimetazidine	T46.7X-
Trimethadione	T42.2X-
Trimethaphan	T44.2X-
Trimethidinium	T44.2X-
Trimethobenzamide	T45.0X-
Trimethoprim (w/ sulfamethoxazole)	T37.8X-
Trimethylcarbinol	T51.3X-
Trimethylpsoralen	T49.3X-
Trimeton	T45.0X-
Trimetrexate	T45.1X-
Trimipramine	T43.01-
Trimustine	T45.1X-
Trinitrine	T46.3X-
Trinitrobenzol	T65.3X-
Trinitrophenol	T65.3X-
Trinitrotoluene (fumes)	T65.3X-
Trional	T42.6X-
Triorthocresyl phosphate	T65.89-
Trioxide of arsenic	T57.0X-
Trioxysalen	T49.4X-
Tripamide	T50.2X-
Triparanol	T46.6X-
Tripelennamine	T45.0X-
Triperiden	T44.3X-
Triperidol	T43.4X-
Triphenylphosphate	T65.89-
Triple bromides	T42.6X-
Triple carbonate	T47.1X-
Triprolidine	T45.0X-

Drug/Chemical	Code
Trisodium hydrogen edetate	T50.6X-
Trisoralen	T49.3X-
Trisulfapyrimidines	T37.0X-
Trithiozine	T44.3X-
Tritiozine	T44.3X-
Tritoqualine	T45.0X-
Trofosfamide	T45.1X-
Troleandomycin	T36.3X-
Trolnitrate (phosphate)	T46.3X-
Tromantadine	T37.5X-
Trometamol	T50.2X-
Tromethamine	T50.2X-
Tronothane	T41.3X-
Tropacine	T44.3X-
Tropatepine	T44.3X-
Tropicamide	T44.3X-
Trospium chloride	T44.3X-
Troxerutin	T46.99-
Troxidone	T42.2X-
Tryparsamide	T37.3X-
Trypsin	T45.3X-
Tryptizol	T43.01-
TSH	T38.81-
Tuaminoheptane	T48.5X-
Tuberculin (PPD)	T50.8X-
Tubocurare	T48.1X-
Tubocurarine (chloride)	T48.1X-
Tulobuterol	T48.6X-
Turpentine (spirits of)	T52.8X-
vapor	T52.8X-
Tybamate	T43.59-
Tyloxapol	T48.4X-
Tymazoline	T48.5X-
Tyropanoate	T50.8X-
Tyrothricin	T49.6X-
ENT agent	T49.6X-
ophthalmic preparation	T49.5X-
Ufenamate	T39.39-
Ultraviolet light protectant	T49.3X-
Undecenoic acid	T49.0X-
Undecoylium	T49.0X-
Undecylenic acid (derivatives)	T49.0X-
Unna's boot	T49.3X-
Unsaturated fatty acid	T46.6X-
Unspecified drug or substance	T50.90-
Unspecified drug or substance, multiple	T50.91-
Uracil mustard	T45.1X-
Uramustine	T45.1X-
Urapidil	T46.5X-
Urari	T48.1X-
Urate oxidase	T50.4X-
Urea	T47.3X-
peroxide	T49.0X-
stibamine	T37.4X-
topical	T49.8X-

Drug/Chemical	Code
Urethane	T45.1X-
Uric acid metabolism drug NEC	T50.4X-
Uricosuric agent	T50.4X-
Urinary anti-infective	T37.8X-
Urofollitropin	T38.81-
Urokinase	T45.61-
Urokon	T50.8X-
Ursodeoxycholic acid	T50.99-
Ursodiol	T50.99-
Urtica	T62.2X-
Vaccine NEC	T50.Z9-
antineoplastic	T50.Z9-
bacterial NEC	T50.A9-
with	
other bacterial component	T50.A2-
pertussis component	T50.A1-
viral-rickettsial component	T50.A2-
mixed NEC	T50.A2-
BCG	T50.A9-
cholera	T50.A9-
diphtheria	T50.A9-
with tetanus	T50.A2-
and pertussis	T50.A1-
influenza	T50.B9-
measles, mumps and rubella (MMR)	T50.B9-
meningococcal	T50.A9-
paratyphoid	T50.A9-
plague	T50.A9-
poliomyelitis	T50.B9-
rabies	T50.B9-
respiratory syncytial virus	T50.B9-
rickettsial NEC	T50.A9-
with	
bacterial component	T50.A2-
Rocky Mountain spotted fever	T50.A9-
sabin oral	T50.B9-
smallpox	T50.B1-
TAB	T50.A9-
tetanus	T50.A9-
typhoid	T50.A9-
typhus	T50.A9-
viral NEC	T50.B9-
yellow fever	T50.B9-
Vaccinia immune globulin	T50.Z1-
Vaginal contraceptives	T49.8X-
Valerian (root) (tincture)	T42.6X-
tincture	T42.6X-
Valethamate bromide	T44.3X-
Valisone	T49.0X-
Valium	T42.4X-
Valmid	T42.6X-
Valnoctamide	T42.6X-
Valproate (sodium)	T42.6X-
Valproic acid	T42.6X-
Valpromide	T42.6X-

Drug/Chemical	Code
Vanadium	T56.89-
Vancomycin	T36.8X-
Vapor— see also Gas	T59.9-
kiln (carbon monoxide)	T58.8X-
specified source NEC	T59.89-
Vardenafil	T46.7X-
Varicose reduction drug	T46.8X-
Varnish	T65.4X-
cleaner	T52.9-
Vaseline	T49.3X-
Vasodilan	T46.7X-
Vasodilator	
coronary NEC	T46.3X-
peripheral NEC	T46.7X-
Vasopressin	T38.89-
Vasopressor drugs	T38.89-
Vecuronium bromide	T48.1X-
Vegetable extract, astringent	T49.2X-
Venlafaxine	T43.21-
Venom, venomous (bite) (sting)	T63.9-
amphibian NEC	T63.831
animal NEC	T63.89-
ant	T63.421
arthropod NEC	T63.481
bee	T63.441
centipede	T63.41-
fish	T63.59-
frog	T63.81-
hornet	T63.451
insect NEC	T63.481
lizard	T63.121
marine	
animals	T63.69-
bluebottle	T63.61-
jellyfish NEC	T63.62-
Portatese Man-o-war	T63.61-
sea anemone	T63.631
specified NEC	T63.69-
fish	T63.59-
plants	T63.71-
sting ray	T63.51-
millipede (tropical)	T63.41-
plant NEC	T63.79-
marine	T63.71-
reptile	T63.19-
gila monster	T63.11-
lizard NEC	T63.12-
scorpion	T63.2X-
snake	T63.00-
African NEC	T63.081
American (North) (South)NEC	T63.06-
Asian	T63.08-
Australian	T63.07-
cobra	T63.041
coral snake	T63.02-

VENOM, VENOMOUS (BITE) (STING)–XANTHINE DIURETICS

Drug/Chemical	Code
Venom, venomous (bite) (sting), continued	T63.9-
rattlesnake	T63.01-
specified NEC	T63.09-
taipan	T63.03-
specified NEC	T63.89-
spider	T63.30-
black widow	T63.31-
brown recluse	T63.33-
specified NEC	T63.39-
tarantula	T63.321
sting ray	T63.51-
toad	T63.821
wasp	T63.461
Venous sclerosing drug NEC	T46.8X-
Ventolin— *see* Albuterol	
Veramon	T42.3X-
Verapamil	T46.1X-
Veratrine	T46.5X-
Veratrum	
album	T62.2X-
alkaloids	T46.5X-
viride	T62.2X-
Verdigris	T60.3X-
Veronal	T42.3X-
Veroxil	T37.4X-
Versenate	T50.6X-
Versidyne	T39.8X-
Vetrabutine	T48.0X-
Vidarabine	T37.5X-
Vienna	
green	T57.0X-
insecticide	T60.2X-
red	T57.0X-
pharmaceutical dye	T50.99-
Vigabatrin	T42.6X-
Viloxazine	T43.29-
Viminol	T39.8X-
Vinbarbital, vinbarbitone	T42.3X-
Vinblastine	T45.1X-
Vinburnine	T46.7X-
Vincamine	T45.1X-
Vincristine	T45.1X-
Vindesine	T45.1X-
Vinesthene, vinethene	T41.0X-
Vinorelbine tartrate	T45.1X-
Vinpocetine	T46.7X-
Vinyl	
acetate	T65.89-
bital	T42.3X-
bromide	T65.89-
chloride	T59.89-
ether	T41.0X-
Vinylbital	T42.3X-
Vinylidene chloride	T65.89-

Drug/Chemical	Code
Vioform	T37.8X-
topical	T49.0X-
Viomycin	T36.8X-
Viosterol	T45.2X-
Viper (venom)	T63.09-
Viprynium	T37.4X-
Viquidil	T46.7X-
Viral vaccine NEC	T50.B9-
Virginiamycin	T36.8X-
Virugon	T37.5X-
Viscous agent	T50.90-
Visine	T49.5X-
Visnadine	T46.3X-
Vitamin NEC	T45.2X-
A, B, B1 or B2 or B6 or B12 or B15, C, D, D2, D3, E (acetate) NEC	T45.2X-
nicotinic acid	T46.7X-
hematopoietic	T45.8X-
K, K1, K2, NEC	T45.7X-
PP	T45.2X-
ulceroprotectant	T47.1X-
Vleminckx's solution	T49.4X-
Voltaren— *see* Diclofenac sodium	
Warfarin	T45.51-
rodenticide	T60.4X-
sodium	T45.51-
Wasp (sting)	T63.461
Water	
balance drug	T50.3X-
distilled	T50.3X-
hemlock	T62.2X-
moccasin (venom)	T63.06-
purified	T50.3X-
Wax (paraffin) (petroleum)	T52.0X-
automobile	T65.89-
Weed killers NEC	T60.3X-
Welldorm	T42.6X-
White	
arsenic	T57.0X-
hellebore	T62.2X-
lotion (keratolytic)	T49.4X-
spirit	T52.0X-
Whitewash	T65.89-
Whole blood (human)	T45.8X-
Wild (black cherry) (poisonous plants NEC)	T62.2X-
Window cleaning fluid	T65.89-
Wintergreen (oil)	T49.3X-
Wisterine	T62.2X-
Witch hazel	T49.2X-
Wood alcohol or spirit	T51.1X-
Wool fat (hydrous)	T49.3X-
Woorali	T48.1X-
Wormseed, American	T37.4X-
Xamoterol	T44.5X-
Xanthine diuretics	T50.2X-

Drug/Chemical	Code
Xanthinol nicotinate	T46.7X-
Xanthotoxin	T49.3X-
Xantinol nicotinate	T46.7X-
Xantocillin	T36.0X-
Xenon (127Xe) (133Xe)	T50.8X-
Xenysalate	T49.4X-
Xibornol	T37.8X-
Xigris	T45.51-
Xipamide	T50.2X-
Xylene (vapor)	T52.2X-
Xylocaine (infiltration) (topical)	T41.3X-
Xylol (vapor)	T52.2X-
Xylometazoline	T48.5X-
Yeast (dried)	T45.2X-
Yellow (jasmine)	T62.2X-
phenolphthalein	T47.2X-
Yew	T62.2X-
Yohimbic acid	T40.99-
Zactane	T39.8X-
Zalcitabine	T37.5X-
Zaroxolyn	T50.2X-
Zephiran (topical)	T49.0X-
ophthalmic preparation	T49.5X-
Zeranol	T38.7X-
Zerone	T51.1X-
Zidovudine	T37.5X-
Zimeldine	T43.22-

Drug/Chemical	Code
Zinc (compounds) (fumes) (vapor)NEC	T56.5X-
anti-infectives (bacitracin)	T49.0X-
antivaricose	T46.8X-
chloride (mouthwash)	T49.6X-
chromate	T56.5X-
gelatin or oxide (plaster)	T49.3X-
peroxide	T49.0X-
pesticides	T56.5X-
phosphide or pyrithionate	T60.4X-
stearate	T49.3X-
sulfate	T49.5X-
ENT agent	T49.6X-
ophthalmic solution	T49.5X-
topical NEC	T49.0X-
undecylenate	T49.0X-
Zineb	T60.0X-
Zinostatin	T45.1X-
Zipeprol	T48.3X-
Zofenopril	T46.4X-
Zolpidem	T42.6X-
Zomepirac	T39.39-
Zopiclone	T42.6X-
Zorubicin	T45.1X-
Zotepine	T43.59-
Zovant	T45.51-
Zoxazolamine	T42.8X-
Zuclopenthixol	T43.4X-
Zygadenus (venenosus)	T62.2X-
Zyprexa	T43.59-

XANTHINOL NICOTINATE-ZYPREXA

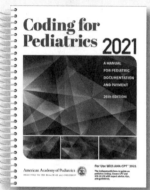
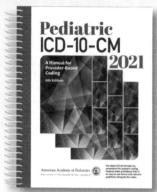
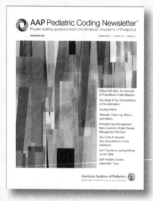
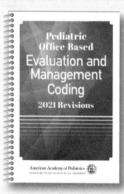
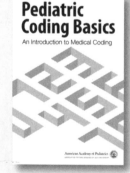
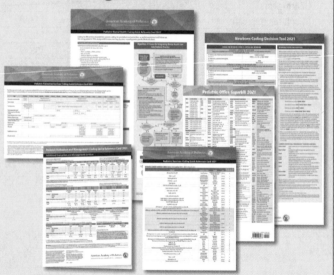
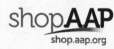